P9-EDI-851

Psychosocial Components of Occupational Therapy

Psychosocial Components of Occupational Therapy

Anne Cronin Mosey, OTR, Ph.D., FAOTA

Professor of Occupational Therapy
New York University
New York, New York

Raven Press New York

Raven Press, 1185 Avenue of the Americas, New York, New York 10036

Made in the United States of America

Library of Congress Cataloging-in-Publication Data

Mosey, Anne Cronin.
Psychosocial components of occupational therapy.

Includes bibliographies and index.
1. Occupational therapy—Psychological aspects.
2. Occupational therapy—Social aspects. I. Title.
RM735.M57 1986 615.8′5152 86-535
ISBN 0-89004-334-5

The material contained in this volume was submitted as previously unpublished material, except in the instances in which credit has been given to the source from which some of the illustrative material was derived.

Great care has been taken to maintain the accuracy of the information contained in the volume. However, Raven Press cannot be held responsible for errors or for any consequences arising from the use of the information contained herein.

0 9 8 7 6 5 4 3 2

To the people involved in writing this book:
Those who reconciled differences,
Those who grew,
Those who were hurt.

Acknowledgments

Above all I would like to acknowledge those students, colleagues, and friends who were often bored and sometimes neglected but who, nevertheless, offered me encouragement and reassurance that the task would be accomplished.

More specifically, I am grateful to: Deborah Labovitz, who creatively arranged my academic assignments; Beatriz Abreu, who urged me to refine the performance components; and Sharon Lefkofsky, Ruth Meyers, and Brena Manoly, who reviewed sections of the manuscript, providing assistance with structure and content.

Many thanks to all of you.

Preface

This text is concerned with the psychosocial components of occupational therapy as they relate to all areas of specialization. Its purpose is to provide an overview of the psychosocial components—both the body of knowledge and approaches to evaluation and intervention. As used here, *psychosocial components* refers to the performance components of (a) sensory integration, (b) cognitive function, (c) psychological function, and (d) social interaction; and to all of the occupational performances: (a) family interaction, (b) activities of daily living, (c) school/work, (d) play/leisure/recreation, and (e) temporal adaptation.

Research for this text involved a survey of occupational therapy literature and the literature of those disciplines and professions from which the profession has selected relevant theories. In the interest of space and consideration for the reader, difficult decisions had to be made in regards to what would be included in the text and the depth in which some aspects would be presented. It is hoped, therefore, that the reader will take the opportunity to explore the various references, and beyond.

My main goal in writing this text was to draw together the literature basic to the psychosocial components in some systematized fashion. In so doing, it was anticipated that: (a) basic professional students would be able to begin study in this area in an organized manner; (b) advanced professional students would have a point of departure for analysis, critical evaluation, and research; and (c) clinicians would have a readily available reference to assist them in dealing with the psychosocial problems of their clients. It is to these various groups, then, that this text is addressed.

The psychosocial components of occupational therapy are not only taken into consideration in all areas of specialization. They are also fundamental to the understanding of our clients, ourselves as therapists, and the tools that we use in practice. Thus, this book is not designed for any one academic course. It is designed to be used in a variety of courses, as a basic text or as supplementary reading.

Finally, in researching and writing this book, I gained a much deeper appreciation of how rich and complex is our body of knowledge and how varied our practice. It is an experience I hope that the reader will share.

Anne Cronin Mosey
January 1986

Contents

Introduction

The psychosocial components of occupational therapy are those areas of human function that enable the individual (a) to perceive the world as comprehensible, safe, responsive to personal action, and a source of need satisfaction; and (b) to engage in various required and desired social roles on the basis of these perceptions. Psychosocial components do not include an individual's physical capacity to act in relation to the environment. Although the latter is an important part of the occupational therapy process, it will not be addressed in this text. Rather, this text will explore the knowledge, skills, and attitudes that are fundamental to adaptation irrespective of the individual's current physical status.

As may be evident to the reader, the author is employing the mind–body dichotomy so traditional in Western thought. This dichotomy is, of course, ultimately not valid; however, to study a particular phenomenon it is sometimes necessary to separate the phenomenon from its substratum. This is a temporary measure that allows us to examine the phenomenon in depth and detail. Certainly the whole—the individual—is greater than the sum of his parts; separating the psychosocial components from all of the other aspects of the individual is somewhat artificial.

There is, however, another purpose in employing the mind–body dichotomy. In the course of its development, occupational therapy has organized its practice and thus, in part, its thinking around various areas of specialization. These areas are defined sometimes by age (e.g., pediatrics and geriatrics), sometimes by anatomical structures (e.g., the hand), and sometimes by a broad area of dysfunction (e.g., physical disabilities). Such a custom is not unusual in a profession, nor is it necessarily detrimental to the services offered. Nevertheless, at times, specialization can lead to a degree of fragmentation. This is particularly true in the case of psychosocial components.

Traditionally, in both education and practice, psychosocial components have been of primary concern in relation to psychiatric patients. This is not to say that occupational therapists who work with individuals other than psychiatric clients are unconcerned about the psychosocial adjustment of their clients. They are, but this concern is often secondary: evaluation and intervention in this area may not be as carefully planned as in others, and, in the rush and demands of the clinical setting, it is sometimes almost forgotten.

In addition, in the occupational therapy literature, the psychosocial adaptation of the nonpsychiatric client is addressed as if it were somehow separate or different than the psychosocial adaptation of the psychiatric client. Thus, for example, "psychological adjustment to physical disability" and "death and dying" are dealt with as entities existing somehow detached from the various frames of reference in occupational therapy that deal with psychosocial function and dysfunction.

Finally, the psychosocial adaptation of family members or of individuals significant to the client is often not given sufficient attention. Concern about families is indeed evident, but the degree to which such concern is acted on is probably not very high. There is recognition that families often need assistance to adapt. How the occupational therapist goes about giving such assistance, however, is not clearly defined. Even if described, it is, again, usually detached from the various frames of reference of occupational therapy.

For the reasons listed above, this text will focus on the psychosocial components of the occupational therapy process. The usefulness of the methods of evaluation and intervention proposed are, on the whole, not limited by medical diagnosis, age, or whether the individual was initially identified as a client or as a family member. Thus, the emphasis in this text is on people: on helping people to adapt, and to participate in the life of their community in a way that enables them to satisfy their own needs and the needs of others.

The individuals of concern in this text may be (a) those people who, in the the typical course of growth and development, did not develop the knowledge, skills, and attitudes fundamental to continued adaptation; (b) those people who, because of congenital or early childhood deficit, need considerable support and assistance to learn how to adapt; (c) those people who, because of physical change (e.g., disease, trauma, aging), must acquire new or additional means of adapting; and (d) those people whose life situation has been so seriously altered that the old or usual ways of adapting are no longer effective. Any given individual in need of assistance may, of course, fit easily into more than one of these categories. The categories are only delimited to give the reader some idea of the scope of the text. Furthermore, these categories do not in any way indicate that individuals in different categories would be assisted in dissimilar ways. This is not necessarily the case.

The term "adaptation" has been employed repeatedly without any definition. As used in this text, adaptation is the process of making adjustments either in behavior or in the environment that enhance personal survival and contribute to the realization of personal potential. Adaptation is thus described as having two interrelated parts: the individual modifies his own thoughts, feelings, and actions, and also attempts to manipulate the environment—human and nonhuman—to make it more comfortable. Adaptation is an important concept in occupational therapy. In fact, it has been suggested as a unifying concept underlying our various specialized areas of practice.

The approach of this text is pluralistic. Various orientations or frames of reference relative to the psychosocial components of occupational therapy are presented and reviewed. This is in contrast to a more monistic approach in which a single orientation would be presented as the basis for practice. The attempt to articulate a monistic approach is currently a common theme in the occupational therapy literature. This is the expression of a belief that we as a profession should have one agreed-on theoretical base and method of application for dealing with each, or all, aspects of our domain of concern.

I disagree with this approach for two reasons. First, we are far from agreement as to how to bring about change in many areas of our domain of concern. Second, and perhaps more important, a singular approach would ultimately be extremely detrimental to the profession's growth if not its existence. It would seem that diversity—a variety of orientations and points of view—is a far healthier state of affairs, and potentially far more adaptive for the profession.

In using a pluralistic approach, I sometimes offer critical comments. It is not my intention, however, to promote any particular frame of reference. Rather, I suggest some populations and settings in which a particular frame of reference may be appropriate. It is, nevertheless, up to the reader—the practitioner—to select the frame of reference most suited to the client's setting and most compatible with the practitioner's own theoretical and philosophical positions.

One final introductory comment. The term *psychosocial components* is somewhat of a misnomer; I use it because it is common in the occupational therapy literature. However, the area of psychosocial components comprises more than the performance components of psychological function and social interaction. It also includes sensory integration and cognitive function and all of the occupational performances—family interaction, activities of daily living, school/work, play/leisure/recreation, and temporal adaptation. In this text I exclude motor function and visual perception. All of the above terms are defined in Chapter 1; sufficient for now is a repetition of the definition presented initially: the psychosocial components of occupational therapy are those areas of human function that enable the individual (a) to perceive the world as comprehensible, safe, responsive to personal action, and a source of need satisfaction; and (b) to engage in various required and desired social roles on the basis of these perceptions.

Part 1

An Overview

Prior to discussing the psychosocial components of occupational therapy, it seems appropriate to place this aspect of the profession into some perspective. The first chapter briefly defines the various parts of the profession and describes the relationship between the parts. The second chapter is devoted to a discussion of the psychosocial components of occupational therapy from a historical point of view.

1 The Profession

For the purpose of describing occupational therapy, this chapter is divided into four sections: definition; configuration, a description of the dynamic relationship of the parts of the profession; an outline of the profession's model, the reservoir of its knowledge and beliefs; and frames of reference, the structures used by the profession to link theory to practice.

DEFINITION OF OCCUPATIONAL THERAPY

For the purpose of this text occupational therapy will be defined as the art and science of using selected theories as a guide for collaborating with a client to assess that individual's ability to engage in the performance of life tasks and, if necessary, to assist the individual in acquiring the knowledge, skills, and attitudes necessary for the performance of required life tasks. Of primary concern to the occupational therapist are individuals whose abilities to cope with tasks of living are threatened or impaired by biological, psychological, or sociological stress, trauma, or deficit. Fundamental to the practice of occupational therapy is concern for and use of the nonhuman environment. The nonhuman environment is viewed as an entity to be mastered, an aid to facilitate the performance of life tasks, and a vehicle for assisting in the development of sensory, perceptual, cognitive, and motor skills and need-fulfilling intrapersonal and interpersonal relationships. Concurrently, the practice of occupational therapy requires skillful execution of personal interactions on the part of the therapist (711).

The first concept of the definition that may need clarification is "art." Art is the composition of any artifact or interpersonal experience that diminishes the isolation of the individual; that reaffirms the power of the human mind, body, and spirit; and that assists the individual in discovering meaning in existence. That which is identified as art assists in fulfilling the universal need for kinship and relatedness to others and the need for a sense of individuality and selfness (174).

Occupational therapy has been defined as a science for three reasons. First, it is based on the end result of scientific inquiry. It is based on a number of theoretical systems. Second, it makes use of scientific procedures and rules to assist in the development, verification, refinement, or refutation of theories specific to the practice of occupational therapy. Thirdly, practitioners use scientific principles to analyze and synthesize data derived from client interaction to determine areas of function and dysfunction and to design appropriate strategies for intervention.

The term "client" will be used throughout this text to designate the individual who is involved in a collaborative relationship with an occupational therapist. The term has the connotation of an individual who freely and knowledgeably seeks assistance with an understanding of both his or her rights and responsibilities.

Occupational therapy is concerned with an individual's ability to engage in the performance of life tasks. Life task refers to all of those activities one must be able to perform to meet one's own needs and to be a contributing member of a community. Thus, occupational therapists are involved in helping clients to engage in appropriate familial roles; to care for their personal needs such as grooming, shopping, and cooking; to maintain satisfactory interpersonal relationships; to participate in the world of work; and to engage in satisfying recreational and avocational pursuits. Life tasks, as defined above, are frequently referred to as "occupational performance" in the literature. It is the latter term that will be used most frequently in this text.

The term "nonhuman environment" refers to all aspects of the environment that are not human. It includes natural objects such as plants, animals, the wind, fields, and mountains as well as man-made objects such as books, works of art, household furnishings, and computers. As an entity to be mastered, the occupational therapist is concerned with helping clients to manipulate the nonhuman environment. As an aid to facilitate the performance of life tasks, the occupational therapist may provide and teach the client how to use various devices that will permit the client to become more independent. Finally, the nonhuman environment is used as a vehicle for the development of skills. For example, to assist in the development of self-understanding, the therapist might involve a client in various self-expressive activities such as drawing or sculpting.

As the last part of the definition indicates, the practice of occupational therapy requires skillful execution of personal interactions on the part of the therapist. The occupational therapist is concerned with promoting growth, development, improved functioning, and a greater ability on the part of the client to cope with and gain satisfaction from life. This process is facilitated by establishing rapport and a comfortable, unconstrained relationship characterized by perception of the client as a unique, knowledgeable person worthy of respect and love. The occupational therapist is an intrinsic part of each activity, which is designed to enhance the functioning of a client. The occupational therapist acts in such a way so as to assist the client in acquiring more appreciation, more expression, and more functional use of latent inner resources.

THE CONFIGURATION

Occupational therapy may be thought of as having six parts: a philosophical foundation, a model, frames of reference, practice, data, and research (711). These parts are in a dynamic relationship with each other (Fig. 1-1). Similar to other professions, occupational therapy is founded on philosophy: the critical evaluation of the facts of experience (221,554,701,738,782,844,848). Although philosophy as a discipline is concerned with a broad spectrum of phenomena, only four areas are particularly important to occupational therapy: philosophical assumptions, ethics, art, and science. Philosophical assumptions regarding the nature of the individual and the individual's relationship to the human and nonhuman environments are fundamental to occupational therapy. These assumptions are drawn from various schools or systems of philosophy. Occupational therapy's ethical code is derived from the philosophical study of that which is moral and of value in human conduct. An understanding of the art of occupational therapy is derived from the philosophical study of aesthetics. The philosophy of science provides guidelines for the development of our body of knowledge.

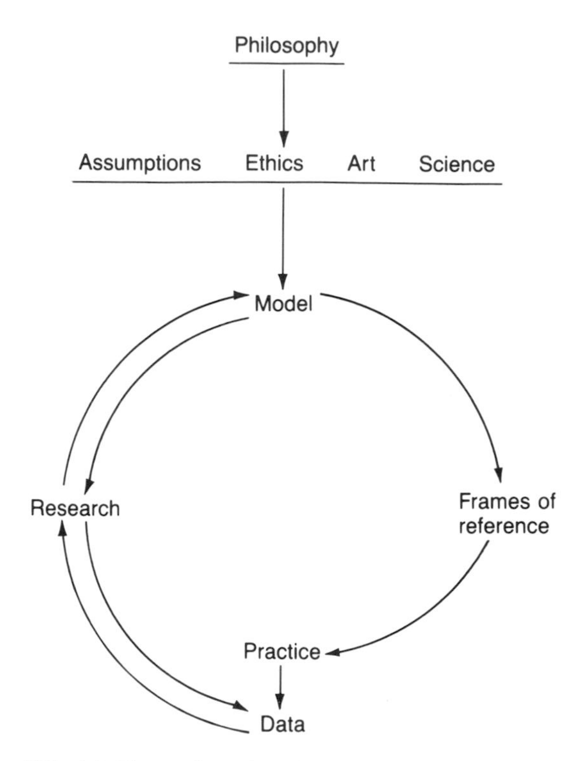

FIG. 1-1. The configuration of occupational theory: A loop.

All professions have a model. A model is the particular way in which a profession perceives itself, its relationship to other professions, and its association with the society to which it is responsible. A model is the reservoir of the collective knowledge and beliefs of a profession. It is characterized by a description of the profession's philosophical assumptions, ethical code, body of knowledge, domain of concern, the nature of and principles for sequencing the various aspects of practice, and the profession's legitimate tools. A more detailed description of the occupational therapy model is given later.

Although professions have only one model, they usually have a variety of frames of reference. Frames of reference, derived from a profession's model, provide guidance in day-to-day interaction with clients. A frame of reference is far more limited than a model. It is usually based on only a small part of the profession's body of knowledge and is addressed to a narrow range of a profession's domain of concern. Although the concept of frame of reference will be described more fully later, a formal definition may be useful at this point. A frame of reference is defined as a set of interrelated, internally consistent concepts, definitions, and postulates derived from or compatible with empirical data, providing a systematic description of or prescription for particular designs of the environment for the purpose of facilitating evaluation and effecting change.

A frame of reference is a link between theory and practice. It describes a particular area of the profession's domain of concern. It provides an outline of behaviors that indicate whether a client is in a state of function or dysfunction in the specified area.

Finally, a frame of reference delineates the types of interactions considered to eliminate or minimize dysfunction. The latter is derived from the theoretical base of the frame of reference. A frame of reference is not a formula for action; it is, rather, only a guide.

Practice is the application of one or more frames of reference in interaction between client and practitioner. Practice is the essence of any profession. The roles of consultant, administrator, scholar, or educator are important, but the major function of these roles is to support, enhance, and refine practice.

Data used in context of the occupational therapy configuration refers to information generated through practice. The majority of this information is concerned with the client's response to the evaluation and intervention process. This is essentially unsystematized data. If properly considered, however, it can lead to the formation of tentative hypotheses. The data generated from practice may, on the other hand, be derived from systematic observation. For this to occur, the practitioner follows a predetermined structured research plan designed to yield specific data. Depending on the hypothesis being tested, the data generated may be used to determine the effectiveness of a given frame of reference or they may be used to develop, refute, refine, or verify one or more theories that support the practice of occupational therapy.

The components of the occupational therapy configuration have been briefly discussed in isolation, not in their relationship one with the other. The term "loop" is used to identify this relationship for it has the connotation of that which unfolds or encircles in a continuous pattern. The arrows in Fig. 1-1 are a means of indicating directionality for this recurrent process.

Occupational therapy has its origin in philosophy. It is from philosophy that we derive and understand our assumptions, ethics, art, and science. Using this philosophical understructure, the profession has developed its own unique model over a period of time. The various frames of reference of the profession are formulated out of the content of the profession's model. If a particular frame of reference deviates too far from the parameters of the profession's model, its use may be questioned by the profession and others. Frames of reference provide guidance for practice. Practice, in turn, generates data that may be used to gain knowledge about the effectiveness of practice or to refine the theoretical foundation of the profession.

At this point in the loop, the flow of events ceases to be unidirectional. Unsystematized data, prior to being useful to a profession, must be subjected to rigorous study. This is indicated by the double arrows between data and research. Knowledge of research methodology enables the investigator to plan how data are to be collected and analyzed. There is, one will note, no direct relationship between research and practice and between research and frames of reference. Research findings influence, directly, only the body of knowledge of a profession: a component of a profession's model.

If research findings were directly applied to frames of reference, the body of knowledge of a profession would, over a period of time, become irrelevant, and suited only for study as historical trivia. Similarly, if research findings were directly applied to practice, the function of frames of reference as a guide for practice would become obsolete.

Research findings, then, are first used in relationship to modifying or supporting the theoretical foundation of a profession. If a particular theory is altered through research findings, this will lead to alteration in those frames of reference that make use of that particular theoretical system. In turn, this will lead to alterations in practice. Research, then, is relevant and important to practice but it influences practice only after findings are incorporated into the model of a profession and appropriate frames of reference. Finally, the arrows in Fig. 1-1 indicate that a profession's model may directly influence research. Essentially, this arrow denotes a profession's responsibility to study its own theoretical foundation continually.

In summary, the occupational therapy configuration is a schematic representation of the relationship between the profession's philosophical foundation, its model, the various frames of reference, practice, and the data generated by practice and research. The relationship is continuous, a process that enriches us as practitioners and our clients.

THE MODEL

As previously defined, a profession's model is the typical way in which the profession perceives itself, its relationship to other professions, and its association with the society to which it is responsible. The model of a profession is characterized by a description of six elements: the profession's philosophical assumptions, ethical code, body of knowledge, domain of concern, nature of and principles for sequencing the various aspects of practice, and the profession's legitimate tools. The model of a profession is, in general, accepted by the members of the profession and by society. However, the content of a profession's model is ever changing. For example, new theoretical systems may be added and other theoretical systems that cannot be verified may be deleted; the domain of concern of a profession may contract because another profession may be seen as having more expertise in a particular area; or a new legitimate tool may be added or further refined. A model is dynamic, with each part interrelated. Change in one part usually leads to change in several other parts. As the reservoir of a profession's knowledge and beliefs, a model provides a sense of unity and identity for a profession (75,341,457, 572,666,715,780,828,861,892,1036).

Philosophical Assumptions

Philosophical assumptions are basic beliefs about the nature of human life, the individual, society, and the universe, and the relationship between these various elements. The philosophical assumptions of a profession state how the members of the profession view the individual, his or her interrelatedness with the environment, and the profession's goals or purpose. The philosophical assumptions of a profession have a pervasive influence on the other components of a profession's model.

There are seven philosophical assumptions of occupational therapy.

1. Each individual has the right to a meaningful existence; to an existence that allows one to be productive; to experience pleasure and joy; to love and be loved; and to live in surroundings that are safe, supportive, and comfortable.
2. Each individual is influenced by stage-specific maturation of the species, the social nature of the species, and the cognitive structure of the species.
3. Each individual has inherent needs for work, play, and rest that must be satisfied in a relatively equal balance.
4. Each individual has the right to seek his or her potential through personal choice within the context of some social constraints.
5. Each individual is only able to reach his or her potential through purposeful interaction with the human and nonhuman environment.
6. Each individual is only able to be understood within the context of his or her environment of family, community, and cultural group.
7. Occupational therapy is concerned with promoting functional independence through intervention directed toward facilitating participation in major social roles (occupational performances) and the development of the physical, cognitive, psychological, and social skills (performance components) that are fundamental to these roles. The extent to which intervention is focused on occupational performances or performance components is dependent on the needs of a particular client at any given point in time (28,248,267,291,450,485,678,794, 796,798,825,885,1045).

Ethical Code

The ethical code of a profession serves as a guide for practitioners in determining what is moral behavior relative to clients and colleagues. In addition, it serves as a contract with the society to which the profession is responsible (147,369,844,1005). The ethical code of occupational therapy is quite lengthy and has been published elsewhere (30). However, to give the reader some idea of our code, an oath derived from the code is presented below (711). Similar to other health professions, our code of ethics has been derived, in part, from the Hippocratic Oath of medicine. The occupational therapy oath is rendered, hopefully, in the spirit of the Hippocratic Oath, with its reverence for the responsibilities and privileges of practice, teaching, and scholarly pursuits.

> As an occupational therapist I will: revere the quality of life as life itself; assist all who request my help according to my ability and judgment; provide sufficient information to enable my client or those responsible for my client to make informed decisions regarding intervention; respect my client's right to self-determination; protect the confidence of my client, sharing only with those others who are immediately involved with my client's care; be goal directed and objective in my evaluation and intervention but above all I will be with my

client in the stress of evaluation and the work of intervention; make only recommendations that I judge as being beneficial to my client; maintain my competence and represent that competence accurately; accept my own limitations and when indicated seek the assistance of those with different or greater knowledge and skill; ask only a reasonable fee for service; take responsibility for participating in formulating the policies and standards of my profession; build upon the knowledge and skills of those who have come before me, giving full recognition to their contributions; share my knowledge and skills with those who will follow through publication and teaching; respect my colleagues to the extent that they deserve my respect; sanction those colleagues who are incompetent or unethical in practice; be accountable for all my decisions and actions.

To the members of my profession and the society to which I am responsible and serve, I make this pledge with full understanding of the actions required by this oath.

Body of Knowledge

The body of knowledge (also referred to as theoretical foundation) of a profession is an ordered set of selected theoretical systems that serve as the scientific bases for practice. These theoretical systems are derived from a number of different disciplines and professions and from the scholarly pursuits of the profession itself. A profession's body of knowledge is considered to be unique in two ways. First, it is specifically selected and formulated to have relevance to the profession. Second, it is unique in its totality, not in its various elements. Some aspects of the body of knowledge of all professions are shared with other professions (776,892).

The body of knowledge of occupational therapy consists of selected theories from the biological sciences, psychology, sociology, the arts, medicine, and theories generated through the practice of occupational therapy. The following outline indicates broad areas or theories that form the substratum for practice. The theoretical systems relevant to the psychosocial components of occupational therapy will be presented in greater detail later in the text (25,445,960).

- *Biological Sciences* Anatomy; physiology; neuroanatomy; neurophysiology; biomechanics; development and maturation of the neuromuscular, skeletal, sensory, and endocrine systems; the various relationships between the biological systems; conservation of physical energy.
- *Psychology* Development and maintenance of cognitive processes, learning, personality development, measurement and testing, psychoanalytic theory, object relations, ego psychology, psychodynamics, symbolism, psychosocial development, the psychological impact of stress, the psychosocial aspects of various life stages, the psychological components of disability and chronic illness, psychological needs, the counseling process, industrial psychology, the significance of play and recreation in the life cycle.
- *Sociology* The dynamics of primary and secondary groups; the dynamics of the family; the process of child rearing; varieties of life styles; development of morality and a system of values; the structure and process of groups that can be directed toward facilitating growth, need satisfaction, and the maintenance of function; human relations; communication theory; the nature of work; occupational choice, career change, and various career patterns; the structure and dynamics of a community; community resources; the nature of various social systems; cultural differences in life styles, values, and norms; role theory; industrial sociology relative to management, supervision, and administration.
- *The Arts* Fine, applied, industrial, and manual arts; dance; music; literature.
- *Medicine* The sequelae of disease, trauma, genetic deficits, and stress; the positive and negative factors that influence intervention relative to sequelae; the course and prognosis of various diagnostic categories; general principles of rehabilitation.
- *Occupational Therapy* The nature of the nonhuman environment as it influences development and the alteration of dysfunction; the nature and use of purposeful activities to develop, maintain, and facilitate function; the dynamics and processes of activity groups; the design and fabrication of functional aids and adaptive equipment and the impact of these aids and equipment on the ability of the individual to function comfortably in his selected life style; the various means whereby the function and dysfunction of concern to the occupational therapist are identified; the means by which dysfunction is prevented, minimized, or eliminated; the use of functional capacities to minimize deficits in other areas of function.

As mentioned, the body of knowledge of occupational therapy, similar to all other parts of its model, changes over time. Thus, what is outlined above may soon be dated.

Domain of Concern

A profession's domain of concern involves those areas of human experience in which practitioners of the profession offer assistance to others. It is essentially a statement of what the profession believes to be its area of expertise. The domain of concern of occupational therapy is here described as being composed of performance components and occupational performances within the context of age and an individual's enviroment (29,189, 190,445,616,618,787,794,800,820,885,960). Figure 1-2, an attempt to illustrate the domain of concern of occupational therapy and the relationship between its component parts (711), will be defined only briefly here. More elaborate explanation will be provided later.

Performance Components

Performance components are the building blocks from which occupational performances are fashioned. They are integrated, elaborated, and refined in a variety of ways that enable the individual to engage in a number of occupational performances.

Motor function is the ability to use one's body to act effectively relative to the environment. Sensory integration is a subcortical process that involves receiving, selecting, combining, and coordinating vestibular, proprioceptive, and tactile information for functional use. Visual perception, a primarily cortical process, involves the recognition, discrimination, and interpretation of visual stimuli relative to the tangible concrete properties of objects and events. Cognitive function, a cortical process, involves the use of information for the purpose of thinking and problem solving.

Psychological function, strongly influenced by the emotional or feeling part of human experience, is the process of using information from past events and information currently available from the environment in such a way as to view oneself, others, and one's life situation realistically.

Social interaction is the process of interacting and engaging with others in casual and sustained relationships individually and in the context of a variety of small groups.

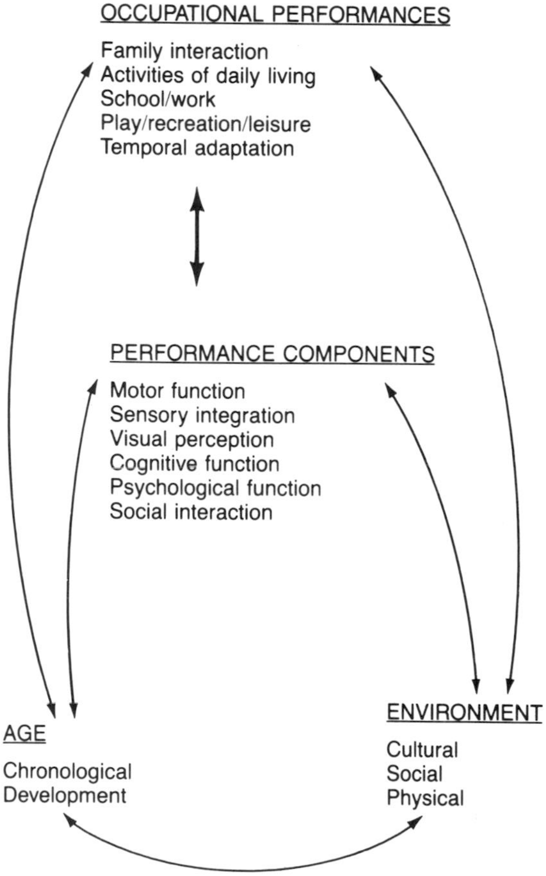

Occupational Performances

Occupational performances are fairly large organized patterns of behavior through which an individual engages in and meets the demands of the environment. The first four are frequently referred to as social roles.

Family interaction involves nuclear, extended, and expanded familial roles in addition to (a) those relationships dealing with the typical familial issues of intimacy, emotional support, sexuality, and child rearing, which are seen by the participants as being family-like in nature and (b) preparation for entering into new familial roles through such interactings as dating and courtship.

Activities of daily living are all those activities that one must engage in or accomplish in order to participate with comfort in other facets of life. These activities may be subdivided into self-care, communication, and travel. Activities of daily living also include the responsibilities of being a homemaker or home manager.

School/work concerns the various social roles involved in being a student and in being a participant in remunerative employment.

Play/leisure/recreation refers to solitary or shared experiences engaged in for the purpose of amusement, relaxation, or self-actualization. The formation and maintenance of various types of friend relationships are an important part of this aspect of human interactions.

Temporal adaptation is the organization of one's time in such a way as to fulfill the responsibilities adequately and to enjoy the pleasures of one's required and/or desired roles.

OCCUPATIONAL PERFORMANCES
Family interaction
Activities of daily living
School/work
Play/recreation/leisure
Temporal adaptation

PERFORMANCE COMPONENTS
Motor function
Sensory integration
Visual perception
Cognitive function
Psychological function
Social interaction

AGE
Chronological
Development

ENVIRONMENT
Cultural
Social
Physical

FIG. 1-2. Domain of concern: Occupational therapy. (Revised by Lisa Jones.)

Age

The idea of age or place in the life cycle can be conceived of as chronological age, the number of days, months, and years an individual has lived since the day of birth; and developmental age, the level of function in performance components and occupational performance in comparison to the approximate age-specific norms of the individual's cultural group. Developmental age is not necessarily related to chronological age.

Environment

Environment refers to the aggregate of surrounding things, conditions, or influences as they affect an individual's existence or development. Cultural environment involves an individual's past, present, and anticipated future involvement in a cultural system—the social structures, values, norms, and expectations that are accepted and shared by a group of people.

Social environment is the matrix of people with whom an individual presently relates and to whom she or he will need to relate to in the future. These people may be family, friends, co-workers, fellow residents, and individuals who are in control of or provide community services.

Physical environment is the material surroundings in which the individual lives now or is likely to live in the future. This includes such things as food, clothing and shelter, possible architectural barriers, the complexity of the environment, ambience, the degree of physical safety, and the opportunity to be surrounded by nonhuman objects that have personal meaning to the individual.

With this final definition of the elements of occupational therapy's domain of concern, the reader is referred again to Fig. 1-2. Performance components are placed in the center of the schematic representation, for they are considered to be the core of the occupational therapy process. This is where the evaluation and intervention processes usually begin. Occupational performances, age, and environment are considered to be the parameters. In general, the arrows connecting the parts of the domain of concern are meant to indicate the interrelationship of all parts of the domain of concern. Thus, evaluation and intervention relative to performance components always take into consideration the client's age, current and possible future involvement in the various areas of occupational performance, and the client's past, present, and anticipated future environment. In addition, age and culture group membership, for example, will help the therapist to determine whether the client's functioning in the areas of occupational performance is within the range of what is considered to be acceptable limits. Knowledge of age, a client's past engagement in occupational performances, and the client's past and anticipated future environment assist the therapist in designing plans for intervention that are most likely to provide a firm groundwork for the client's successful return to full participation in the life of the community.

The arrow connecting performance components and occupational performances is stylistically different to indicate the special relationship between these parts of the domain of concern. As mentioned, performance components form the building blocks for occupational performances. In turn, performance components are developed and refined throughout the life cycle primarily through engaging in occupational performances. In intervention, the occupational therapists frequently use the tasks or activities associated with occupational performances, e.g., preparing a meal, using a computer, games, to facilitate adequate development of performance components.

As may have been evident, there is considerable overlapping between and among the various parts of the occupational therapy domain of concern. Although this initially may be somewhat confusing, there are distinct differences. At times, it is necessary to divide to understand. One of the major assets of the occupational therapy domain of concern is the interrelatedness of its parts. Like a puzzle, we may admire each piece but it is the parts together that give us appreciation of the whole.

The Nature of and Principles for Sequencing the Various Aspects of Practice

The nature of practice is essentially a definition of the various aspects of practice. Principles for sequencing the various aspects of practice refer to the way in which a profession goes about the process of problem identification and proceeds through to problem solution relative to assisting a client (45,194,380,697). This part of the occupational therapy model is outlined in Fig. 1-3.

Evaluation is a collaborative process between client, therapist, and significant others to assess whether an individual requires assistance in meeting health needs in his or her current environment, is in need of intervention directed toward prevention, is able to benefit from involvement in the change process, or is in need of a program of maintenance or management. Screening is the process of ascertaining whether an individual has problems in functioning that may be ameliorated through the occupational therapy process. The purpose of formal evaluation is to verify the existence of the problems

Evaluation
  Screening
  Formal evaluation
Intervention
  Meeting health needs
  Prevention
  Management
  The change process
  Maintenance
Termination

Communication

FIG. 1-3. The aspects and sequence of occupational therapy practice. (Adapted from refs. 29,129,190,623, and 960.)

found in screening, to define the problems further, or to dismiss the results of screening as spurious.

Evaluation is concerned with identifying areas of function and dysfunction through the observation of specified behaviors. Function refers to the capacity to engage comfortably at an age-appropriate level in the various performance components and occupational performances within the context of one's cultural, social, and physical environment. In contrast, dysfunction refers to the inability to engage comfortably at an age-appropriate level in the various performance components and occupational performances within the context of one's cultural, social, and physical environment. Behavior indicative of function and dysfunction are those behaviors that provide evidence or indicate whether an individual is competent in the performance components and occupational performances.

Evaluation takes place prior to and periodically during intervention. It is concerned with identifying the current status of the individual. Intervention, on the other hand, involves some maintenance or modification of current status.

Intervention is a collaborative effort on the part of client and therapist directed toward goals that they have previously established. For the sake of clarity and specificity, intervention can be subdivided into five types: meeting health needs, prevention, the change process, maintenance, and management.

1. Meeting health needs is the process of satisfying or fulfilling inherent human needs so that an individual may experience a sense of physical, psychological, and social well-being. These needs are considered to be shared by all individuals regardless of their current state of health. Health needs may be differentiated from those needs that arise from the consequence of physical or psychological dysfunction. Thus, for example, the need for love and acceptance is considered to be a health need. Extreme psychological dependency of an adult is not considered to be a health need. The latter is evidence of dysfunction and would be dealt with in the change process.

2. Prevention is the process of facilitating the development of skills in potential areas of dysfunction and promoting skills in areas of function. As used in this text, prevention refers to intervention prior to any evidence of dysfunction. Prevention is often initiated with individuals who are considered to be "at risk" relative to the development of dysfunction.

3. The change process is concerned with the development or restoration of function to the highest possible level. The therapist and client anticipate and work toward significant change. The change process is directed toward enhancing the client's ability in the various areas of performance components and occupational performances. For example, the therapist may be concerned with increasing the client's physical coordination or in identifying and developing the skills necessary for participation in recreational activities enjoyable to the client.

4. Maintenance is the process of preserving and supporting an individual's current level of function. There are two somewhat different types of maintenance. One process involves maintaining function in one or more areas while attempting to alter dysfunction in other selected areas. The other type of maintenance is entirely separate from the change process in relationship to time. Subsequent to the termination of the change process, the therapist may continue to be concerned with maintenance of the degree of function that has been attained.

5. Management is the process of minimizing undesirable or disruptive behavior so that one can deal more directly and effectively with areas of dysfunction. It is not concerned with changing that behavior per se. If the change process is successful, it is assumed such behavior will gradually disappear as the individual acquires more functional skills in dealing with the self and the environment.

Intervention for the sake of clarification has been described above as having five distinct parts. As may be apparent, there is some overlapping or areas of commonality between the five aspects of intervention. They have been separated here to describe the distinct differences. In the actual intervention process, the various aspects of intervention may blend one with the other. A note of caution: in this possible blending, a wise therapist knows each ingredient included in any particular plan for intervention.

The length of intervention varies but in the majority of cases it is time limited. Termination is the process of bringing to an end a particular relationship or, at times, one aspect of a relationship. In the latter case, for example, the therapist and client may bring the change process to a point of closure but their relationship may continue relative to maintenance of function.

The last aspect of practice is communication. This includes the giving and receiving of information between: (a) the client and therapist; (b) family members or others significant to the client and the therapist; and (c) other team members and the therapist. This type of communication is primarily verbal in nature. Written communication is also very important and includes evaluation summaries, plans for intervention, termination reports, and other types of documentation.

The sequence of the various aspects of practice is typically as follows. Initial evaluation is directed toward determining the need for occupational therapy intervention and the type(s) of intervention required. Periodic evaluation takes place throughout the intervention process. After initial evaluation, if intervention is indicated, the therapist is first concerned with meeting health needs and prevention. Maintenance of current function is the next priority. If necessary, intervention is then directed toward management. This accomplished, the therapist focuses attention on the change process. In the change process, intervention is usually first directed toward dysfunction in performance components. As a client becomes more skilled in performance components, more concentrated effort is directed toward occupational performances. For example, as cognitive function increases, the therapist and client may spend an increasing amount of time in developing adequate work habits. When a sufficient level of function in one or more of the performance components cannot be attained by the client, the therapist assists the client in developing substitute skills. A substitute skill is a skill that serves as a means of compensating for lack of function in one or more of the performance components. For example, an individual who is unable to regain an adequate degree of motor function in one hand may be assisted in learning how to become competent in performing a number of activities with the use of only the noninvolved hand. Next, the therapist assists the client in identifying and planning the ways in which function will be maintained after termination of intervention. The final step of the occupational therapy process is termination.

The typical sequence of practice outlined above is general in nature. The sequence may be altered because of the special needs of a particular client or the environment in which evaluation and intervention take place. Communication takes place throughout the evaluation–intervention–termination sequence.

Legitimate Tools

Legitimate tools are the sixth and last component of a profession's model. As previously defined, legitimate tools are the permissible means by which the practitioners of a given profession fulfill their responsibility to society. It is through the use of its tools that a profession attempts to achieve its goals in meeting specific needs of society.

It appears from a review of the literature and from practice that occupational therapy has six legitimate tools. These are the nonhuman environment, conscious use of self, the teaching-learning process, purposeful activities, activity groups, and activity analysis and synthesis. A short definition of these tools follows; a more detailed description is provided in Part 3.

The nonhuman environment, as previously defined, refers to all aspects of the environment that are not human. Occupational therapists view the nonhuman environment as an entity to be mastered, an aid to facilitate the performance of life tasks, and a vehicle for assisting in the development of sensory, perceptual, cognitive, and motor skills and need-fulfilling intrapersonal and interpersonal relationships.

Conscious use of self involves a planned interaction with another person in order to alleviate fear or anxiety; provide reassurance; obtain necessary information; provide information; give advice; and to assist the other individual to gain more appreciation of, more expression of, and more functional use of his or her latent inner resources. Such a relationship is concerned with promoting growth and development, improving and maintaining function, and fostering a greater ability to cope with the stresses of life. Conscious use of self also includes the therapist's use of her body to provide physical support, maintain appropriate positioning, and other necessary physical manipulations.

The teaching-learning process is an interaction between client and therapist designed to help the client acquire new and more adaptive knowledge, skills, and attitudes. In its application, this tool may be based on one or more of the various theories of learning.

Purposeful activities are doing processes directed toward a planned or hypothesized end result. In contrast, random activities are undirected and without a predetermined goal. An activity is only purposeful if it is congruent with

> The individual's sensory, motor, cognitive, psychological and social maturation . . . developmental needs and skill readiness . . . and recognized by the individual's social and cultural groups as relevant to their values and needs (209, p. 308).

Purposeful activities are doing processes which involve

> Investigating, trying out and gaining evidence of one's capacities for experiencing, responding, managing, creating and controlling. (209, p. 308)

Activity groups are primary groups made up of and designed to assist individuals who share common concerns or problems related to the acquisition or maintenance of performance components or occupational performances. They are also used as a means of satisfying health needs. Activities are either an integral part of the groups' here-and-now interaction or a specific gestalt of activities, engaged in by group members outside of the context of the group, that become the focus for group discussion.

Purposeful activities and activity groups are selected and designed for evaluation and intervention through analysis and synthesis of activities. Activity analysis is the process of examining an activity to distinguish its component parts. Activity synthesis is the process of combining component parts of the human and nonhuman environment so as to design an activity suitable for evaluation of or intervention in various areas of human function.

Except for activity analysis and synthesis, there is, again, considerable overlap between the legitimate tools of occupational therapy. The first four tools may be used singly but more often they are used in combination.

In summary, this section has described the various components of the occupational therapy model—philosophical assumptions, ethical code, body of knowledge, domain of concern, the nature of and principles for sequencing the various aspects of practice, and legitimate tools. The final element of the configuration of occupational therapy to be discussed is frames of reference.

FRAMES OF REFERENCE

The model of the profession defines and delineates the broad outlines of the profession as it is understood by its members and by society. Frames of reference further delineate a particular area or aspect of the profession and, as such, are the link between the profession's model and practice. In a more narrow sense, frames of reference are the intermediary step between a profession's body of knowledge and clinical application. As previously defined, a frame of reference is a set of interrelated, internally consistent concepts, definitions, and postulates derived from or compatible with empirical data that provides a systematic description of or prescription for particular designs of the environment for the purpose of facilitating evaluation and effecting change relative to a specified part of the profession's domain of concern.

Frames of reference are a necessary part of the configuration of the profession because of the nature of theory. Theory or theoretical systems are descriptive: they state the relationship between various phenomena. Theory is not designed to deal with practical situations. It does not answer the questions of how, when, relative to whom, and so on. The essence of the problem, then, is how to structure scientific knowledge so it may be applied in day-to-day situations. This is the function of frames of reference. They are prescriptive and normative in nature and ideally answer the questions of how, when, and relative to whom. They provide a schema for the practitioner (75,119,140,174,307,346,427,627,646,720, 777,780,917).

In addition to being the link between a profession's body of knowledge and practice, frames of reference also reflect the other components of a profession's model. The philosophical assumptions and ethical code of a profession are embodied within its frames of reference. Frames of reference give life and meaning to the abstraction of assumptions and ethics. Frames of reference more specifically define and amplify one or more aspects of the profession's collective domain of concern. The sequence of practice of a profession is followed in its frames of reference. The tools suggested are an elaboration of one or more of the tools considered legitimate by the profession.

Although, ideally, a profession's frames of reference are addressed to all aspects of practice, this is not the case in occupational therapy. At the present time, our frames of reference are primarily concerned with the change process. Guidelines for prevention of dysfunction and maintenance of function can be deduced from our current frames of reference. The processes of meeting health needs and management present a somewhat different problem. Guidelines for these types of intervention cannot be deduced from our current frames of reference. In addition, and perhaps more important, there is no integrated theoretical system basic to these two areas of intervention. There are some theoretical postulates, but they do not combine easily into a unified whole. In Chapter 17, meeting health needs and management are further defined; evaluation relative to the need for intervention and suggested ways of intervening are described. The theoretical base provided is, at best, both pragmatic and eclectic. These are areas of intervention that have received little attention by the profession.

Structure

The content of various frames of reference related to the psychosocial components of occupational therapy will be explored in detail in Part 5. Just as one may speak of the structure of theory regardless of content, so also can one speak of the structure of a frame of reference without reference to content.

The structure of a frame of reference is made up of:

- A statement of the theoretical base.
- Delineation of function-dysfunction continuums.
- A listing of behaviors indicative of function and dysfunction.
- Postulates regarding change.

The theoretical base of a frame of reference delineates the theoretical systems that are necessary for an adequate description of one or more elements of the domain of concern and fundamental to modifying dysfunction in the specified areas. It is referred to as the base of a frame of reference because it identifies the parameters of the frame of reference and serves as the matrix from which all other parts are deduced. A theoretical base may be formulated from one theoretical system, or concepts, definitions, and postulates may be drawn from several different theoretical systems. The latter is more often the case.

Function-dysfunction continuums are a delineation of the component parts of the specified area addressed in the frame of reference. The term "continuum" was chosen to indicate that there is essentially no break or line of demarcation between that which is considered function and that which is considered dysfunction. Function is considered to be relative to age, cultural background, and the expected environment of the client.

A frame of reference may have one or several function-dysfunction continuums. Most have more than one continuum but there is no particular number that is appropriate. The criteria for judging numerical adequacy is whether the continuums identify all of the component parts of the human function(s) to which the frame of reference is addressed. If there is more than one continuum, these continuums should be relatively mutually exclusive and stated on the same conceptual level.

Behaviors indicative of function and dysfunction are those behaviors that serve to identify function or dysfunction relative to each of the continuums. These behaviors are stated in the most specific way possible. However, the degree of specificity often depends on the type of frame of reference. They tend to be more specific in acquisitional frames of reference, for example, than in analytical frames of reference.

Behavior indicative of function and dysfunction provides the foundation for devising evaluation strategies. Activities are analyzed relative to the probability of eliciting behaviors indicative of function and dysfunction as enumerated in a particular frame of reference. Activities are synthesized based on knowledge of the gestalt of behaviors the therapist wishes to observe. An illustration of synthesis is selecting an activity for evaluation that is likely to elicit a number of different behaviors indicative of function and dysfunction rather than an activity that is likely to elicit only one such behavior. (The evaluation process will be discussed in much greater detail in Parts 4 and 5.)

Postulates regarding change are descriptive or prescriptive statements, deduced from the theoretical base, which state the principles by which an individual is assisted in moving from a state of dysfunction to a state of function. Postulates regarding change state the nature, quality, quantity, and sequence of interaction with the human and nonhuman environment that is believed to facilitate change. They also state principles that guide the practitioner in selection of immediate and long-term goals, the step-by-step progression of intervention in each area of dysfunction, and the postulates that are applicable during each stage of intervention.

Postulates regarding change form the basis for activity analysis and synthesis relative to the change process. Activities are analyzed according to whether and to what degree they embody the environmental characteristics stated in a postulate as being instrumental in bringing about positive change. Activities are synthesized to be as consistent as possible with the entire postulate regarding change for a specific area of dysfunction.

In summary, the structure of a frame of reference consists of a theoretical base, function-dysfunction continuums, behavior indicative of function and dysfunction, and postulates regarding change. Frames of reference provide the theoretical rationale for the change process. They also provide the conceptual framework for activity analysis and synthesis relative to designing activities for evaluation and intervention.

Types

This section will briefly discuss the three major categories of frames of reference currently used in occupational therapy: analytical, developmental, and acquisitional. A more detailed discussion will be presented in Part 5.

Analytical frames of reference provide a structure for linking psychodynamic theories, the symbolic potential and reality aspects of purposeful activities, and the process of altering intrapsychic content.

There are three assumptions basic to analytical frames of reference (289,290,307,317,427,492,646,969).

1. Intrapsychic content is the major factor that influences behavior. Intrapsychic content here refers to needs, primitive impulses, drives, emotions, feelings, ideas, and so forth.
2. Intrapsychic content can best be altered by bringing it to a point where it can be examined and evaluated in the context of a shared reality. This process is often referred to as communication.
3. Repeated interactions in situations that elicit intrapsychic conflicts, with guidance, facilitate conflict resolution and the addition of new, more adaptive intrapsychic content. This process is often referred to as "working through." The last two assumptions are considered to be the sequence of events in the change process. One part of the sequence without the other is not believed to be conducive to permanent change.

In analytic frames of reference, purposeful activities are viewed in part as being concerned with action, the meaning of action, its use in communicating intrapsychic content, and the use of such nonverbal communication for the benefit of the client. The symbolic potential of activities—the actions, the objects used in the action process as well as those that result from the action, and the interpersonal relationships that influence the action and are in turn influenced by it—is emphasized. Activities are considered (a) to have inherent characteristics that elicit expression of specific intrapsychic content, (b) to serve as a basis for a shared reality, and (c) to provide an experiential laboratory for the introjection of new intrapsychic content.

Developmental frames of reference provide a structure for linking theories of human development, the age-specific nature of many activities, and the process of acquiring the basic skills necessary for successful interaction in the environment.

There are three assumptions basic to developmental frames of reference (58,64,67,74,339,616,618,703,801, 938,960).

1. Behavior is primarily influenced by the extent to which the individual has mastered previous aspects of development.

2. In the typical developmental process, the individual progresses through specific stages of development in various areas of human function. In each stage the individual's behavior or skill is qualitatively different than at a past or future stage in that particular area. Qualitative differences refers to the idea that something new is added at each stage. This is not addition of more refined skill. Rather something entirely new is added to the individual's repertoire of behavior. An example of qualitative difference can be seen in the child's development of group interaction skill. Initially the child plays alone or with an adult. This is followed by parallel play with other children, then the sharing of short-term activities, and so forth. Behavior from a previous stage is usually integrated with the new emerging stage.

3. Interacting in an environment that simulates the usual optimal enviroment for the acquisition of a particular stage of development in a given area of human function will allow the individual to acquire the necessary behavior in an integrated manner. This is sometimes referred to as the recapitulation of development. The individual must master all stages of development in a particular area to reach the appropriate age specific level in that area of function.

In developmental frames of reference, purposeful activities are sometimes considered relative to their symbolic potential for gratifying infantile needs. This orientation is somewhat different than in analytical frames of reference. The symbolic potential of activities in analytical frames of reference is considered in order to facilitate communication and working through. Gratification of infantile needs is definitely not a part of analytical frames of reference; it is, however, a part of some developmental frames of reference. In other developmental frames of reference the reality of the activity irrespective of possible latent or overt symbolic potential is given priority. Activities are primarily viewed as a vehicle for the learning of skills rather than an entity to be mastered in and of themselves. Finally, considerable emphasis is placed on the age-specific characteristics of activities.

Acquisitional frames of reference provide a structure for linking learning theories, the reality aspect of purposeful activities, and the process of acquiring specific skills needed for successful participation in the environment.

There are three assumptions basic to acquisitional frames of reference (307,427,646,705,960,969).

1. Behavior is primarily influenced by interaction with the external environment. Intrapsychic content, if addressed, is considered to be the by-product of one's repertoire of behavior. Thus, it is believed that overt behavior or the skills that an individual has is responsible for intrapsychic content. If there is a change in behavior, this will be reflected in intrapsychic content. The reverse is not believed to be possible.

2. Areas of function included in acquisitional frames of reference are quantitative and non-stage-specific. Non-stage-specific refers to the idea that there are no identifiable stages of development for a particular area

of function. The individual acquires increased or more refined skill in a particular area but this is a difference of quantity, not quality. An example of the increase in quantity is the individual's acquisition of knowledge.

3. Adaptive behavior is acquired by direct interaction in an environment designed for learning a particular skill. Recapitulation is not seen as necessary.

In acquisitional frames of reference, the symbolic potential of purposeful activities is rarely if ever considered. The reality of the activity is given primary emphasis. Activities are far more likely to be viewed as entities to be mastered in and of themselves rather than vehicles for the learning of "other skills." The age-specific characteristics of an activity may be taken into consideration but it is not emphasized to the same extent as in developmental frames of reference.

As will be discussed in Part 5, not all of the current frames of reference that deal with the psychosocial components of occupational therapy fall easily into one of the categories outlined above. There are variations within a number of frames of reference that make them difficult to place. In the absence of a more refined taxonomy, however, these categories will be used in this text.

SUMMARY

This chapter has presented an overview of the configuration of occupational therapy. It has identified and described the relationship between our philosophical foundation, model, frames or reference, practice, data, and research. The model of occupational therapy was considered in some detail with a description of our philosophical assumptions, code of ethics, body of knowledge, domain of concern, nature of and principles of sequencing the various aspects of practice, and legitimate tools. The concept of frame of reference was defined. The purpose or function of frames of reference and their structure was outlined. A taxonomy of frames of reference which are addressed to the psychosocial components of occupational therapy was described. The assumptions of the three types of frames of reference was presented as well as their different orientation to the analysis and synthesis of purposeful activities.

2 Historical Perspective

In the last chapter the psychosocial components of occupational therapy were placed within the much wider perspective of the totality of the profession: within the configuration of occupational therapy. In this chapter the psychosocial components of occupational therapy are discussed from a historical perspective (17,19,21,23, 82,101,115,116,237,439,443,707,794,802,920,956,1011, 1012,1040). The purpose of this chapter is to follow the threads of the various types of intervention, frames of reference, and tools of occupational therapy as they have evolved to the present. It should be noted that this is not, in any sense, a complete history. Little attention is given to changes in professional education, to the structure, function, and issues of the American Occupational Therapy Association, or to remediation relative to deficits in motor function and visual perception.

To provide some order to the chapter it is divided into four sections. In the first section, the Beginning, the formation of the National Society for the Promotion of Occupational Therapy (now the American Occupational Therapy Association) in March 1917 serves as the point of departure for this historical survey. The founders and their ideas about occupational therapy are introduced.

The second section is Physical Medicine. Occupational therapy has always been closely identified with medicine, although, as will be discussed later, this has not always been a comfortable alliance. Nevertheless, it has had considerable impact on the profession. In addition, selected social phenomena have influenced medicine and, in turn, have been influenced by medicine. This section will first focus on physical medicine and related social phenomena. With that as a background, the psychosocial components of occupational therapy will be explored relative to physical medicine.

The format of the third section, Psychiatry, is similar to that outlined for physical medicine. In the Introduction one of the purposes of this text was identified as an attempt to present the psychosocial component of occupational therapy regardless of diagnostic category. The reason for a definite distinction here between physical medicine and psychiatry is that historically these two branches of medicine and occupational therapy have been separated for some time. Thus, a more accurate picture can be provided by heeding this divergence.

The fourth section, In Search of Identity, traces the steps taken by occupational therapy to define itself. From initial reliance on medicine, it has struggled to identify its focus of intervention, formulate frames of reference, and articulate a comprehensive theory. In so doing, occupational therapy is in the process of coming of age and its relationship with medicine has been redefined.

THE BEGINNING

A small institution in Clifton Springs, New York called Consolation House would appear to be a fitting setting for the formal beginning of occupational therapy. This was an institution founded by George Edward Barton, an architect, where, through participation in various activities (occupations), people were assisted in recovering from the effects of illness.

The National Society for the Promotion of Occupational Therapy had five charter members. George Edward Barton formulated the term "occupational therapy." He defined this term as the

> science of instructing and encouraging the sick in such labors as will involve those energies and activities producing a beneficial therapeutic effect (82, p. 60).

He defined the purpose of occupational therapy

> to divert the patient's mind, to exercise some particular set of muscles or a limb or perhaps to merely relieve the tedium of convalescence (82, p. 60).

William Rush Dunton, Jr. was a staff psychiatrist at Sheppard and Enoch Pratt Asylum in Baltimore. He became aware of therapeutic effects of activities as he observed patients' participation in an arts and crafts program. He said that the purpose of occupational therapy was

> to divert the patient's attention from unpleasant subjects, to keep the patient's train of thought in more healthy channels, to control attention, to secure rest, to train in mental processes by educating hands, eyes, muscles... to serve as a safety valve, to provide a new vocation (251, p. 3).

Herbert J. Hall, a physician, prescribed occupations for his patients because he felt they were a "potent factor in the maintenance of physical, mental and moral health in the individual and the community" (382, p. 12). He was given a grant of one thousand dollars by Harvard University to study the effect of occupations in the treatment of neurasthenia (a psychological disorder characterized by feelings of weakness and a general lowering of bodily and mental tone). He used various arts and crafts and found that they had a "normalizing effect."

Eleanor Clark Slagle, as a social work student, became interested in arts and crafts for the mentally ill when she observed the detrimental effects of enforced idleness on hospitalized patients. Through her work with patients she developed a method of treatment that was to become known as "habit training." Her orientation will be described more fully later in this chapter. Briefly, Slagle believed that remedial occupation "serves to overcome some habits, to modify others and to construct new ones to the end that habit reactions will be favorable to the restoration and maintenance of health (904, p. 40)." She also felt that a balanced program of work, play and rest was beneficial for mentally ill patients (904).

Susan E. Tracy, a nurse, first became aware of the importance of some kind of occupation to make prolonged bedrest less anxiety provoking and more acceptable to patients. She also had experience in the care of psychiatric patients. For all patients, Tracy encouraged occupations in order to foster "the patient's physical improvement, his educational advancement, his financial betterment" (443, p. 132).

For all of the founders of the profession, "occupation" seems to have been derived from the verb to occupy; to be engaged in some activity, to fill up time and space. The importance of activity in distracting patients from pain, anxiety, and boredom, in organizing one's daily life, in maintaining or restoring physical strength and endurance, and in contributing to a healthy psychological state of being seems to have been recognized by each of the founders. Although specifically stated only by Tracy, all of the founders seemed to have distinguished occupation from "busy work" or whiling away time doing nothing of particular importance. Here then at its very beginning the first and primary tool of occupational therapy, purposeful activities, had its origin. Tracy, Dunton, and, particularly, Slagle emphasized the educational aspect of occupations. Educational both in the sense of how to present and teach activities to patients and also in the sense of the development of skills and attitudes necessary for productive living. Thus, the teaching-learning process also became a tool of occupational therapy from its inception.

The founders of occupational therapy seemed to have made little distinction between the benefits of occupation relative to diagnostic category. Therefore, it made little difference if one had physical or emotional problems; activities were beneficial for all, except perhaps the most acutely ill. For the founders, there was a recognized relationship between the mind and the body. Physical activity was seen as of the utmost importance in assisting those with psychological difficulties. The use of activities to maintain a positive psychological outlook for those recovering from physical disease or injury was often emphasized. It was only later in its development that occupational therapy began to make the distinction between individuals with physical problems and those with emotional or psychiatric problems.

The terms "to maintain" or "to restore" are frequent in the writings of the founders. It is evident that they recognized the difference between these two processes. Thus, two of the aspects of intervention—the maintenance of function and the change process—were identifiable at the beginning of the profession. It is also interesting to note, however, that restoration or the change process was viewed as a somewhat more prestigious undertaking. Maintenance of function was considered a respectable concern, but somehow not quite as worthy. This differential view of change versus maintenance has continued to this day. At times, in fact, maintenance has been seen as the responsibility of an undefined somebody else. This is not entirely true today but the change process remains more respected and valued. Social factors have influenced this point of view. The economics of the health delivery system are such that one is far more likely to receive remuneration for facilitating change than for assisting in the maintenance of function.

Finally, the purpose of the National Society for the Promotion of Occupational Therapy was outlined in its constitution—"the advancement of occupation as a therapeutic measure, the study of the effects of occupation upon the human being and the dissemination of scientific knowledge of this subject" (443, p. 10). This is a succinct statement of the tasks that are the responsibility of all occupational therapists.

The five individuals who were the founders of occupational therapy laid the groundwork for the profession. It has changed and evolved over time but their influence can still be felt almost 70 years later.

PHYSICAL MEDICINE

Changes in Medicine

The medical scene was far different in 1917 than it is today (123,292,300,304,414,599,828,892). Infectious disease was unrestrained, sanitation practices were often poor, immunology was in its infancy, and there were no antibiotics. Infant and early childhood mortality was high as was mortality due to childbirth and industrial and farm accidents. The population of the United States was relatively young, with few people over 60 years of age.

Medical practice was primarily concerned with the care of acute conditions. This occurred because of the predominance of acute conditions and relatively few people who lived long enough to develop chronic conditions. The major chronic disease was tuberculosis, which was primarily treated by rest and diet. People did not survive spinal cord injuries; the incidence of cerebral vascular accidents and cardiopulmonary disease was low because of the youthfulness of the population. There was essentially no treatment for cancer. Rehabilitation as we know it today did not exist. Hospitalization for medical and surgical conditions was very long and often included a lengthy period of convalescence. This was also true for those injured in World War I.

Between the two world wars there were many advances in medical and surgical techniques, immunology came of age, and there was a steady decrease in infant and childhood mortality. The economic depression of the 1930s led to a decrease in length of hospitalization and the beginning of third-party payment for hospitalization. Although there was some interest in the idea of rehabilitation, the depression impeded any real development.

World War II resulted in many changes in physical medicine, perhaps the most important being the introduction of antibiotics. This led to a marked decrease in mortality from infectious disease. A substantial number of those injured in the war survived. Many more people lived beyond 65 years of age.

With the survival of a massive number of war injured, the rehabilitation movement was born. Medicine was confronted with developing the means for dealing with the severely impaired individual. Society's support of this undertaking was motivated by both humanitarian and economic interests. Enabling the handicapped individual to be independent, particularly financially independent, was seen as ultimately less expensive than custodial care. The rehabilitation movement was essentially a revolutionary phase of medicine. Up to this time medicine had been primarily concerned with sustaining life. Once sustained, the quality of life was not considered within medicine's domain of concern. In addition, medicine's orientation had been acute care. Only in occasional medical crises were the techniques of acute care necessary or appropriate in the rehabilitation process.

The theoretical foundation of medicine did not provide the basis for the rehabilitation process and, in general, organized medicine did not support the rehabilitation movement. The lack of support was covert because any negative statement regarding rehabilitation would have been considered callous and unpatriotic. Within organized medicine the rehabilitation process was viewed as tangential to medicine and was accorded low status. This stance has continued with some minor modification to this day.

The lack of a theoretical foundation and support from organized medicine was a handicap for physicians concerned about rehabilitation. Nevertheless the movement was launched with a good deal of success. Reasons for this success were twofold. The war injured were young, basically healthy and motivated: ideal candidates for rehabilitation. Physicians sought the assistance of the emerging health professions: occupational therapy, physical therapy, and speech therapy to name a few. These professions were also young, basically healthy and motivated. They arrived on the scene with little tradition, experience with chronic patients, a pragmatic approach to problem solving, and a strong desire to prove their worth as members of the health team. In this exciting and provocative environment, techniques were developed, often by trial and error, and the beginning of a body of knowledge was formulated.

The end of World War II saw a marked increase in the birth rate. With advances in immunology and availability of antibiotics, infant and early childhood mortality further decreased. American society was inundated by and preoccupied with the care of its children. The poliomyelitis epidemics of the late 1940s and early 1950s primarily affected children and were no respecters of class. Many children were left severely disabled. Society demanded that something be done. Federal agencies were formed and a considerable amount of public monies allocated for both research and the care of the children handicapped by poliomyelitis. The orientation and, with some modification, the techniques of rehabilitation were applied to combat the disabling sequelae of poliomyelitis. Additional techniques were developed and the rehabilitative body of knowledge grew. Rehabilitative effects were highly successful, for the most part, for essentially the same reasons as outlined above relative to those disabled in World War II. The development of the Sabin and Salk vaccines brought an end to the epidemics.

With society's continued preoccupation with its children, Federal agencies in place, money available, and documented evidence of the effectiveness of rehabilitation, attention was turned to the congenitally impaired, often multiply handicapped child. The problems posed by such individuals with motor, sensory, and cognitive deficits were in many cases far more complex than those of earlier candidates for rehabilitation. The term "rehabilitation," to restore to former capacity, was no longer applicable. These individuals had never had the skills necessary for adaptation. Thus a new term, "habilitation," to develop the capacity to function, came into use. Although habilitation was somewhat less successful than rehabilitation had been up to this point, concern for handicapped children continued. Initially the habilitation process tended to be clinically based or take place within special schools. In 1976, Public Law 94-142, Education for All Handicapped Children Act was enacted. This law required, among other things, that handicapped children and adolescents be educated in the least restricted environment. This brought many previously sheltered children into the mainstream of public education. Members of the habilitation team followed these children into the public school system, providing intervention for the children and support for the educators unfamiliar with teaching handicapped individuals.

Concomitant with its concern for children, society was also confronted with an increase of chronic conditions in the adult population. More people survived disease and injury, and the population of the United States was aging. This was a relatively new phenomenon. Medicine's orientation to acute conditions was once more eroded. There was a steady increase in the incidence of arthritis, cardiopulmonary conditions, cerebral vascular accidents, cancer, and traumatic injury. Medical and surgical means to deal with these conditions advanced but the conditions per se defied eradication. Rehabilitation techniques were also used but with much less dramatic results. Many individuals had to cope with both the debilitating effects of chronic illness and a marked change in life style.

The population of the United States continues to age. With decrease in the birth rate, the median age is now over 30 years of age, with approximately 25 million people over the age of 65 years. These demographic trends will more than likely continue. This is a phenomenon that will have ramifications throughout the entire social system. For medicine, the need for orientation to chronic conditions has become a paramount necessity. The health problems of individuals over 65 are just beginning to be studied. Knowledge of the aging process is embryonic at best. What is apparent is that medicine must give considerably more attention not only to the physical problems of the aged, but to the psychological components of the aging process as well.

Occupational Therapy

Occupational therapy's beginning at the dawn of World War I gave it little time to move beyond the collective knowledge of its founders before being called on to provide assistance to the wounded. Occupational therapists were appointed by the Surgeon General as Reconstruction Aides "to furnish forms of occupation to convalescents in long illnesses and to give to patients the therapeutic benefit of activity (443, p. 11)." These aides served in hospitals in both the United States and Europe (443).

The other initial involvement of occupational therapists in physical medicine was in tuberculosis sanitariums. There were a considerable number of such institutions with large populations. Treatment consisted of prolonged and complete bedrest, a nutritious diet, and fresh air. Patients were gradually allowed out of bed for a few hours each day and were permitted to engage in some restricted activities. Convalescence in the sanitarium continued for a number of months, if not years. Occupational therapists were primarily involved with distracting patients from pain, anxiety, and boredom through the use of activities. Occupational therapists contributed to the physical aspects of convalescence by grading activities relative to time and effort required. The grading of activities relative to time and effort was the beginning of activity analysis and synthesis.

Aside from concern about increasing endurance, muscle strength, and vital capacity, intervention by occupational therapists was primarily oriented to the psychosocial components of occupational therapy. Meeting health needs, not change, was the primary focus. Meeting health needs, then, came to be a part of occupational therapy intervention very early in its history.

With the end of World War I and its aftermath, occupational therapists continued to work in tuberculosis sanitariums. However, for the first time in any great number, they moved into general hospitals to work on the medical and surgical units. Convalescence continued to be lengthy. Thus, meeting health needs was an important contribution to the overall well-being of patients. During the economic depression of the 1930s, however, meetings patients' health needs became a luxury that hospitals could ill afford. Many occupational therapists lost their jobs. Occupational therapists would return to medical and surgical wards after World War II but never in large numbers. The importance of meeting health needs in physical medicine entered a hiatus from which it is only just beginning to recover.

As mentioned, World War II provided the impetus for the rehabilitation movement. Occupational therapists became members of rehabilitation teams bringing with them their concern for and skill in meeting health needs. No one cared. Meeting health needs was not seen as a priority in the complex and largely uncharted course that lay ahead. Physical restoration was almost the singular focus. It was an exciting and productive time. Occupational therapists contributed to and learned much through participation in the rehabilitation movement.

But something was lost. The psychosocial components of occupational therapy—both relative to meeting health needs and the change process—were either ignored or given only covert attention. In relationship to meeting health needs, programs of diversional activities were developed. Occupational therapists found participation in such programs unprestigious. Responsibility for diversional activities was delegated or actually given to others. In relationship to the change process, occupational therapy's understanding of how to facilitate psychological and social adjustment to physical disabilities was not very advanced at this time. Because of the lack of knowledge, occupational therapists were more than willing to leave this area of practice to others. The fact that these mostly unspecified "others" were not particularly concerned and were also lacking in knowledge and skill seemed not to be of major interest to occupational therapists, or for that matter, to the rehabilitation team.

Occupational therapists now have considerably more knowledge and skill in facilitating psychosocial adaptation and use this in the process of physical rehabilitation. But the schism between the physical and psychosocial components of the practice of occupational therapy, which began with the rehabilitation movement, is only in the initial stages of healing.

Occupational therapists, being an integral part of the rehabilitation team, participated in the rehabilitation of individuals disabled by poliomyelitis. However, it was the problems presented by the multiply handicapped child that brought a new challenge and diversity to the profession. Habilitation required a broader perspective and for the first time a concentrated focus on child and adolescent development. Age as a significant factor in the occupational therapy process was recognized. Children were not little adults, they were indeed very different. The natural sequence of maturation and development had to be taken into consideration in evaluation and intervention.

One of the consequences of the rehabilitation movement with its team structure was an attempt by occupational therapists to define their uniqueness. This was particularly true in relationship to physical therapists. Although this differentiation process continues to this day, one major point of contrast was identified. Occupational therapists were oriented to the promotion of function. It is imperative to strengthen muscles, increase range of motion, and develop coordinated patterns of movement. However, all of this is irrelevant if the individual is unable to use these abilities in a functional manner. Thus, occupational therapists, at least in part, focused their attention on the practical tasks of activities of daily living, work, and play. Although these aspects of human experiences had been seen as important by the founders of the profession, they were reaffirmed through participation in the rehabilitation movement. This emphasis was of particular significance in working with the multiply handicapped child. It gave focus to the occupational therapist's role and to the occupational therapy process.

In working with the multiply handicapped, neurologically impaired child, it became evident that many of them had difficulty in academic learning that was unrelated to intellectual capacity. In the late 1950s A. Jean Ayres began to study this phenomenon and identified an essential process necessary for competence in these areas. This is now referred to as sensory integration, one of the performance components of occupational therapy. Originally studied in relationship to the multiply handicapped child, evidence of deficit in sensory integrative capacities has been found in individuals described as learning disabled who are not handicapped in any other way.

With the passage of PL 94-142, occupational therapists, similar to other members of the habilitation team, moved into the public school system. In such a context occupational therapists with their understanding of sensory integration have been able to identify and provide assistance to children with learning problems. In working with such children, it became evident that although sensory integrative deficits were present, many of these children have secondary emotional difficulties. The lack of academic skills in an environment that places a high premium on such skills is often devastating to a child's sense of self-worth. A cycle of self-defeating and maladapative behavior and additional difficulty in learning develops. To break into this cycle, occupational therapists found it necessary to deal with cognitive, psychological, and social components as well as sensory integration. Here was a point of the coming together of what is referred to in this text as the psychosocial components of occupational therapy. This amalgamation of the sensory integrative component with the traditional psychosocial components (cognition, psychological function, and social interaction) occurred at about the same time in the area of psychiatry. However, as will be discussed in the final section of this chapter, the marriage of these components is not entirely characterized by conjugal bliss.

Similar to medicine, by the late 1950s occupational therapists were involved in helping adults with chronic conditions. A rehabilitative approach was often effective in increasing function but such an approach only dealt with part of the problem. What was needed was a long-term orientation that emphasized the maintenance of function. Although there had been some concern previously with this aspect of intervention, it now became a prominent feature of the occupational therapy process. This concern was also a significant factor in motivating occupational therapists to move out into the community. Many adults with chronic conditions were not in need of long-term hospitalization but rather lived and often worked in the community. Outpatient and eventually home care became fairly common settings for the practice of occupational therapy.

With the aging of the population, occupational therapists became increasingly interested in the elderly. Because of the problems presented by the aged and the increased sophistication of occupational therapy, there was a tendency toward a more integrative approach. Physical as well as psychosocial components were addressed simultaneously within the context of age and environment. The occupational performances of family interaction, activities of daily living, recreation, and, to some extent, temporal adaptation were taken into consideration. In addition, all aspects of intervention were given fairly equal attention. The "parts" of the occupational domain of concern and aspects of practice were brought together in a much closer proximity than had occurred previously.

Working with the elderly contributed to the theoretical foundation and ultimately to the practice of occupational therapy in two ways. Occupational therapists were confronted repeatedly with death and dying. Thus, it was necessary for the profession to develop techniques for helping others to deal with this aspect of the human experience. Attention was given both to the dying individual and to those who suffered loss through death. In considering the phenomenon of loss, occupational therapists realized that the idea of loss, mourning, and readjustment was a phenomenon applicable in many situations. Thus, attention was given to loss as a consequence of deprivation of physical capacity, life style, social roles, and cultural grounding. This added a needed dimension to the occupational therapy process.

The other contribution to occupational therapy made through working with the elderly had to do with human growth and development. Occupational therapy originally was concerned with the adult population. This was seen as a homogeneous population without any discernible developmental stages. After World War II, the profession in part turned to problems of children and adolescents. Theories regarding development in these stages of the life cycle became part of the theoretical foundation of occupational therapy. With increasing concern for the elderly population, theories regarding the final stages of the life cycle were added. It is only just recently that occupational therapy has begun to add theories regarding human development between 18 and 65 years of age to their body of knowledge. This somewhat disjointed sequence of events is not really the fault of occupational therapy. As will be discussed in Chapter 5, this is also a reflection of the study of human growth and development as a discipline. With the addition of the middle parts of the life cycle to the theoretical foundation of occupational therapy, age, as one parameter of the occupational therapy domain of concern, was given adequate substance.

PSYCHIATRY

Changes in Medicine

As a backdrop to looking at occupational therapy in psychiatry, it is necessary to review some of the major movements in the treatment of mental illness (5,10,54, 315,562,563,649,864,1051). Prior to the Civil War, individuals identified as insane were both cruelly neglected and badly mistreated. Somewhat after the Civil War, medicine, previously not particularly concerned, began to take a humanistic approach to the care of the insane. (Humanism is a system or mode of thought and action in which human interest, values, and dignity predominate; an orientation that was common in many parts of American society at this time.) It was felt that the insane should be treated with tenderness, compassion, and sympathy. Large state hospitals were built. People considered too peculiar or incompetent to participate in the life of the community were sent to these hospitals, far distant from populous areas. (There were a few private sanitariums but these accounted for only a very small number of hospitalized patients.) Individuals who went to state hospitals were for the most part expected to remain there for the rest of their lives. Return to home and community was not anticipated. Drugs and other types of therapy as we know them today did not exist.

Out of the humanistic orientation a type of treatment did, however, evolve. Formulated by Samuel Tuke, and other Europeans and Americans, this approach came to be referred to as "moral treatment" (115,962,1033). Emphasis was placed on the need for work and diversions to combat the effects of boredom and idleness and stressed the development of healthy habits in daily life. The use of manual labor, education, exercise, arts and crafts, drama, music, reading, and the like was stressed. The cause of mental illness, if given attention at all, was usually considered to be a moral defect in character. Hence, perhaps, the name given to this type of treatment. As the reader may surmise, several of our founders derived their ideas about occupational therapy from moral treatment.

By the early 1900s a neuropathological etiology for some of the psychoses was fairly well documented and accepted. It was then assumed that all mental illness was caused by some type of neurological deficit. It was also assumed that, given sufficient time for skilled research, the hypothesized cause or causes would be found. Physicians became preoccupied with this research rather than with the patients' daily situation. Patients were left in the care of the least skilled of the hospital staff. There was also a pervasive feeling that, until the supposed neurological deficit was discovered, little could be accomplished in regard to patient care. These two factors led to a gradual decline of moral treatment. Patients came, in general, to be neglected and at times abused. The "back ward syndrome" slowly engulfed state hospitals.

By the early 1940s an entirely different etiology for mental illness gained dominance in the psychiatric community: unconscious conflicts due to faulty parent-child relationships were the cause of mental illness (7,46, 195,317,322,447,492,817,938). This was, rather simplistically stated, the psychoanalytic orientation to mental illness. This orientation began in the United States with Sigmund Freud's visit to this country in the mid-1930s. A number of psychoanalysts fled Nazi terrorism in the late 1930s and early 1940s and came to the United States. Through their work the psychoanalytic orientation gained popularity and widespread acceptance. The treatment of choice, thus, came to be psychoanalysis or psychoanalytic-oriented verbal therapy. The psychoanalytic orientation had minimal positive effect on the vast majority of psychiatric patients. Most patients were unable to participate in this type of treatment for it required a level of cognitive organization and verbal skill they did not possess. Further, there were very few physicians or other health professionals adequately trained to engage in this type of treatment. The overall negative effect of the psychoanalytic orientation was profound. Because the cause of mental illness was considered to be unconscious conflicts, and most patients were unable to participate in treatment designed to resolve these conflicts, there was nothing one could do. Further, the leaders in psychiatry were involved in the treatment of those privileged few capable of and financially able to participate in psychoanalytically-oriented treatment. This led to neglect of hospitalized patients and to the continued decline of anything that could be called treatment. The psychoanalytic orientation did not have any appreciable positive impact until the early 1960s, and then only in a somewhat diluted form.

The brief outline of the initial neurological orientation and psychoanalytic orientation points to an underlying conflict in psychiatry that continues to the present time. It is essentially a conflict over etiology, which is, of course, reflected in treatment approaches. In addition, there are a number of conflicts within each of these orientations. The major conflict, however, is essentially neurological versus the external environment. The question then is whether mental illness is caused by some type of neurological pathology or is caused by interaction in an environment that is not conducive to the development of flexible, adaptive behavior. Although the schism remains, in the current actual day-to-day treatment of psychiatric patients both approaches are usually used in combination.

In the neurological orientation, initially no great strides were made in finding the neurological deficits that were the cause of the schizophrenic, paranoid, or affective disorders: the major disorders for which individuals are hospitalized and/or receive extended treatment. Although disappointing, other attempts were initiated to provide relief for psychiatric patients. The first two types of somatic treatment that enjoyed considerable popularity in the 1940s and 1950s were insulin shock therapy and electroshock therapy (EST) (297,852). Although used extensively, neither had any lasting effect relative to the schizophrenic and paranoid disorders. A course of electroshock therapy was found to be effective for affective disorders, particularly those characterized by depression. Although the reason for the effectiveness of EST in relieving depression is unknown, it is still used in the treatment of depressive reactions that are unresponsive to psychoactive drugs.

The use of psychoactive drugs began in the mid-1950s (77,461,470,546,568). These various drugs have helped to diminish anxiety, depressive reactions, and the cognitive disorganization seen in the schizophrenic disorders. However, the neurophysiology that leads to their effectiveness is still in question. On the negative side, their use has often been abused, primarily by over- or undermedication of patients. Individual response to psychoactive drugs is highly variable, which complicates their prescription. Numerous side effects sometimes make psychoactive drugs dangerous or difficult for many individuals to tolerate. More positively, the major advantage of psychoactive drugs is that they tend to diminish gross pathological symptoms, thus making patients more amenable to environmentally oriented treatment approaches. Psychoactive drugs have made a marked contribution of decreasing length of hospitalization and have allowed many more individuals to live and work in the community, although often in a very marginal manner. Psychoactive drugs, as originally anticipated, have not led to the eradication of mental illness.

In the environmental orientation, a behavioral approach to treatment began to be used extensively in the middle 1960s (903,969,1037). This approach, primarily led by clinical psychologists, was essentially an application of operant conditioning; a theory of behavior formulated by B. F. Skinner. This theory, in brief, states that reinforcement—any event that increases or decreases the frequency of behavior—is the major factor that influences behavior. Thus, maladaptive behavior could be eliminated and a repertoire of adaptive behavior acquired through the judicious reinforcement of behavior. This type of therapy was used in the treatment of a variety of mental disorders but particularly with mentally retarded, mentally ill individuals who had been institutionalized for a number of years and with severely emotionally disturbed children. The approach was only moderately effective: the behavior acquired was not able to be sufficiently generalized to situations outside of the treatment setting. A continued high rate of reinforcement was needed to maintain the newly acquired behavior as part of the individual's usual repertoire of behavior. Such a reinforcement schedule is not usually available in the community. One of the advantages of the behavioral approach, however, was that staff become actively engaged with patients on a day-to-day basis.

The sociological approach to mental illness began in the late 1950s (87,126,437,489,490,581,859,1056). It had several strands of origin that came together in the community psychiatry movement of the 1960s. One thread was a reaction to the restrictiveness of the classic psychoanalytic orientation and to the questionable effectiveness of its widespread application to treatment. It was felt that the psychoanalytic orientation essentially viewed the individual outside of the context of culture and the various social systems that impinged on the individual on a day-to-day basis. Those with a sociological orientation also questioned the psychoanalytic contention that only very early childhood experiences were instrumental in the formation of the adult personality. From this concern many schools of thought, e.g., ego psychology, social psychology, neo-Freudianism, came into being.

Sociologists began to study psychiatric hospitals as social systems. Indeed, some of the writings of this period had the flavor of journalistic exposés (175,245, 348,367,838,926). However, they did fairly well document an important phenomenon: what appears to be irrational behavior on the part of patients who have been hospitalized for a long period of time is primarily an adaptive response to the situation they are in and not a symptom of mental illness. They found that the behavior of psychiatric patients is strongly influenced by intrastaff and staff-patient dynamics and not psychopathology. The major conclusion of various sociological studies was that environmentally oriented treatment could not take place in psychiatric hospitals until the social system of the hospital was altered to allow for more open communication, shared decision making, and self-direction on the part of the patients.

A third strand grew out of the concept of "therapeutic community" or "milieu therapy," as originated by Maxwell Jones in England and elaborated by others (216,257,489,490). This orientation was initially conceived in the context of working with individuals who would probably now be described as having antisocial personality disorders. It was later altered to some degree in order to make accommodations for the needs of patients in other diagnostic categories. The essential feature of therapeutic communities was the idea that day-to-day interactions between patients and staff and the problems inherent in people living, working, and playing together could be used as a means of helping patients acquire intrapersonal control and the interpersonal skills necessary for independent living. The characteristics of activities per se were not considered. They were primarily seen as a catalyst for altering interpersonal relationships. In other words, almost any shared activity would do. As originated and in its variations, this approach was highly verbal in nature.

The use of group-oriented techniques has had a fairly long history in psychiatry (474,604,1013). However, World War II provided the impetus for concentrated study of small group behavior. This research was generated by the need for massive numbers of highly heterogeneous individuals to work effectively and productively in small groups. It became almost immediately evident that small groups had a tremendous impact on individuals' behavior. Research relative to the structure and dynamics of small groups continued after World War II to the point that there is now a considerable body of knowledge regarding this phenomenon. Individuals concerned with the treatment of psychiatric patients began to manipulate and use the dynamics of small groups as a means of altering behavior. Emphasis, growing out of the analytic orientation, was on persuading people to look at and share their ideas and feelings: primarily those generated out of the immediacy of the here-and-now interaction of the group. These ideas and feelings were frequently related to past interpersonal experiences and current interactions that were taking place outside of the context of the small treatment group.

The sociological orientation to mental illness was also reinforced by the pragmatic experiences of the Korean War. In World Wars I and II, soldiers who reacted to the stresses of combat in a severely neurotic or psychotic manner were withdrawn from the combat zone, given treatment in military hospitals, and usually discharged from service. In the Korean War, another approach was initiated (601). Soldiers with stress reactions were treated within or at the periphery of combat zones and were immediately returned to their units. A significant proportion of these "temporary" war casualties successfully completed their tour of military duty. The rationale for this treatment approach was that the least distance, relative to space and time, between the stress situation and treatment, the more likely that the individual would be able to deal with the stress situation in an adaptive manner. Treatment on the whole involved the use of small verbal therapy groups made up of "temporary casualties" that were narrowly focused on the immediate reaction to combat stress. Emphasis was placed on ventilation of feelings, the catharsis of sharing, reassurance that one's reaction was neither atypical nor an indication of personal inadequacy, minimizing guilt, and reinforcing the individual's capacity to return to and cope with the stress of combat. Regardless of one's own personal feelings about this method of treatment in the situation of war, as indicated, it was highly successful.

The final major strand leading to the community mental health movement was the Burton-Hill Act of 1946. Because of the economic depression of the 1930s and the financial and manpower drain of World War II, there was an acute shortage of hospitals in the United States. The Burton-Hill Act allocated federal money for expanding or building community hospitals. To receive the money, a hospital had to meet several criteria, one being that the hospital have a psychiatric unit staffed to provide short-term treatment for up to three months. This was a revolutionary move in that, prior to this time, community hospitals had no psychiatric units and provided beds for psychiatric patients only if they were hospitalized under the guise of some other medical condition. These new units tended to be small, well staffed, patient oriented, and primarily concerned with acute care. Because such treatment facilities had never existed before, they were not burdened with tradition nor wedded to a particular treatment orientation. Moreover, the small size of the units and the type of patient population allowed for considerable flexibility and experimentation.

In summary, the strands of the sociological approach to mental illness were: reaction to restrictiveness and ineffectiveness of the classic psychoanalytic orientation, research in regard to the social dynamics of psychiatric hospitals, development of the idea of therapeutic communities, the extensive use of verbal group therapy, the situational approach to combat stress reactions during the Korean War, and the establishment of psychiatric units in community hospitals. The weaving together of all of the strands culminated in the Community Mental Health Act of 1963. This federal law mandated community-based treatment for the mentally ill and the mentally retarded. Community mental health centers, which provided direct services to individuals of all ages and families, were established. Short-term inpatient, partial hospitalization (day and/or night treatment programs), outpatient treatment, and follow-up programs were some of the major services offered. Because community-based treatment was defined as the most effective means of remediation, a massive effort was made to discharge the majority of patients in state psychiatric hospitals and institutions for the mentally retarded to the community. Community mental health centers were given the responsibility for providing the support services necessary to maintain these individuals in the community. The problems of drug abuse, so predominant in the late 1960s and early 1970s, also became the responsibility of the community mental health centers.

A natural extension of the sociological orientation was concern over the prevention of mental illness (165,166,202). Extending the idea of small groups as an instrument for therapeutic change, it was felt that these same ideas could be applied to the natural small groups that existed in the community: in the home, school, and work place. If these groups could be helped to function in ways that were mutually need-satisfying to their members, it was felt that there would be a marked decrease in the incidence and severity of mental illness. Thus, many mental health workers acted as consultants to various organizations and groups with the hope of preventing mental illness. There is little evidence to support the success of this undertaking; incidence of mental illness has not decreased since the 1960s.

The community mental health movement or structure for delivering services for the mentally ill and the mentally retarded is still very much with us today. As a movement, it has been somewhat effective. It has not, however, met all of the expectations that were gloriously described at its inception (85,717,958). But that is true for most movements. Community-based delivery of mental health services is the context within which much of the occupational therapy intervention relative to psychosocial components now takes place.

Occupational Therapy

The original philosophy of occupational therapy grew out of the humanistic orientation that was rapidly coming to an end at the time of occupational therapy's founding. Adolf Meyer, a psychiatrist who worked in a number of state mental institutions, is often considered to be the philosophical founder of occupational therapy. His philosophy was traditionally humanistic and his ideas regarding the care of mental patients was derived from the moral treatment approach. His influence on the profession came from two sources. Eleanor Clark Slagle, one of the founders of the profession, worked under his direction at Phipps Psychiatric Clinic in Johns Hopkins Hospital in Baltimore. Slagle was strongly influenced by Meyer and it was at Phipps that she began to formulate her ideas about the occupational therapy process. In 1922 Meyer wrote "The Philosophy of Occupational Therapy," which appeared as the lead article in the initial issue of the *Archives of Occupational Therapy* (678).

The first orientation of occupational therapy in psychiatry was derived from moral treatment, primarily as interpreted by Meyer and Slagle (678,904–907). Some of their major ideas were as follows. Mental illness is a problem in living that results in a deterioration of habits. The concept of habits used here comes from the nineteenth century idea of "clean habits" or "good habits." One was considered to have these habits if one was industrious, hard working, neat and clean, polite, self-controlled, emotionally restrained, moderate in all things, and essentially asexual. Personality was considered to be determined fundamentally by performance: the idea that you are what you do. The exterior persona was all important. Feelings were not supposed to influence behavior. If they did one did not have good habits. Good habits also entailed a balance between work, play, and rest. (It is from this latter idea that temporal adaptation, with a somewhat expanded definition, has come to be a part of the occupational therapy domain of concern.) To be occupied in some useful activity was seen as inherently good. This idea comes again from the nineteenth century belief that idle hands can essentially get one into all kinds of trouble. Activities were seen as a means for developing good habits. They were seen as having an organizing effect; organizing in the sense of a rhythm for one's daily life and in the sense of giving order to one's thoughts and actions. In the latter sense activities were seen as having a calming effect on the agitated and an energizing effect on the lethargic.

Slagle referred to her orientation to the change process as "habit training"—training in conduct, training in doing things in a socially acceptable way. To develop such habits she used arts and crafts, preindustrial work, unpaid employment in hospital workshops and grounds, table games, folk dancing, and active games in the gym and playing field. Activities were analyzed and synthesized along continuums of simple to complex, known to unknown, dull to interesting, and degree of concentration required. The interdependence of mental and physical health was emphasized. Good physical habits, e.g., eating, sleeping, exercise, and bathing regularly, were believed to lead to good mental health. A comprehensive approach was taken in terms of activities being planned for the patient's entire day. Such planning was essentially the responsibility of the staff, not the patients.

There were many favorable factors in this primitive, but discernible, frame of reference: the organizing effects of activities were recognized, socially acceptable behavior was required, a variety of activities were utilized, and there was concern about major facets of the human experience, e.g., activities of daily living, work, play, and rest, concern for the planning of the patient's daily life, and recognition of the importance of good physical health in the maintenance of mental health.

In a more negative light, moral treatment and, by extension, habit training were culturally bound to late nineteenth century middle-class values. This must have been particularly difficult for patients who did not share these values. Moral treatment was a celebration of the work ethic and in many ways was both oppressive and paternalistic. Habit training, as outlined by Slagle, was not oriented to helping patients return to the community. The goals of the change process were related to adaptation to the institution. Patients were not encouraged to be self-directed or to engage in any extensive problem solving. The internal emotional and affective experiences of the patient seemed to have been ignored. Finally, no apparent attention was given to helping the patient to develop interpersonal relationships of an intimate nature, even those of friendships.

As mentioned, beginning in the early 1900s, there was a steady decline in the belief that moral treatment was an effective means of assisting the mentally ill. The etiology of mental illness began to be seen as not due to the development of poor habits but rather to neurological pathology or unconscious conflict. Habit training and its theoretical rationale eventually came to be regarded as lacking in sophistication and efficacy. Only somatic treatment would cure the patient, for if the analytic approach was used for the patient unable to engage in psychoanalytically oriented treatment, nothing really could be done. About all one could do was to keep patients busy and to deal with their most obvious symptoms. Occupational therapy's response to this was to develop what this author refers to as the "symptomatic approach" to intervention (379,956,986). This was not considered to be a change process, for no real change relative to the patient's "basic problems" was anticipated. Rather, the symptomatic approach was essentially management, a type of intervention that has been previously defined.

William Rush Dunton, Jr., one of the founders of occupational therapy, wrote *Prescribing Occupational Therapy* in 1928 (251). This book describes the symptomatic approach to intervention. Essentially, he listed a large variety of psychiatric symptoms. For each symptom he outlined the characteristics of activities that would provide relief for the symptom. He then classified specific activities as to "their demands for attention, repetition, physical or intellectual effort, social factors, and criteria for rest, surprise or creativity" (251, p. 9). Dunton also described the interpersonal approach the therapist should use for each symptom. For example, for hostility, Dunton recommended activities that require gross, aggressive movements. The therapist is to set firm limits. For depression, initially stereotyped, repetitive activities should be followed by more stimulating activities. The therapist should be sensitive and supportive. For hallucinations, structured activities that require constant attention are recommended. The therapist should emphasize contact with reality.

The task of the occupational therapist, then, was essentially to match activities with patient's symptoms. Making the correct match between activity and patient was seen as the essence of the occupational therapy process.

Concomitant with this approach was a decrease in work as a therapeutic tool. Patients did continue to work in state hospitals but as a source of free labor and not for therapeutic ends. Much less attention was given to recreation/leisure activities, to temporal adaptation, and to a comprehensive approach to the organization of the patients' entire day. The negative aspects outlined relative to habit training continued.

The symptomatic approach has sometimes been described as "cookbook" occupational therapy. If one knew the patient's symptoms, and these were usually described by the psychiatrist in his prescription to the occupational therapist, then all one had to do is look up the "recipe." This may seem a delightfully simple approach to the beginning student and certainly one that would require far fewer hours in the classroom and in private study to learn. However, as effective as this approach might have been in managing symptoms, it rarely enabled the patient to develop skills needed for participation in the community. One of the reactions to this cookbook orientation in the following years was to articulate the occupational therapy process in relation to psychosocial dysfunction in a highly theoretical or abstract manner.

The review of the symptomatic approach has been somewhat negative up to this point. However, there are three major areas in which the symptomatic approach contributed to the development of the profession. First, the profession, at least in retrospect, accepted management as a legitimate part of the intervention process. The profession came to realize the activities, selected with care, could contribute to the relief of disruptive and uncomfortable symptoms. This was obviously of benefit to patients and, when occupational therapists returned to the change process, facilitated that process. The symptomatic approach encouraged occupational therapists to study the characteristics of activities in much greater detail. The process of activity analysis and synthesis was advanced to a far more sophisticated level than heretofore. Finally, the symptomatic orientation focused on the needs of individual patients. Habit training had been, to a great extent, an undifferentiated approach to the patient population. If mental illness was a state of having poor habits, then all patients had the same difficulty. Individualized planning for each patient was unnecessary. With the emphasis on matching patient and activity in the symptomatic approach, considerably more attention was given to identifying the needs and responses of each patient.

The psychoanalytic and sociological thinking of psychiatry began to have an influence on occupational therapy beginning in the mid-1950s. A new, more dynamic orientation was inaugurated at a conference in Boiling Springs, Pennsylvania. This conference, funded by the National Institute of Mental Health and sponsored by the American Occupational Therapy Association, was called to review and make recommendations regarding intervention relative to the psychosocial components of occupational therapy. Impetus for the conference grew out of dissatisfaction with the symptomatic approach: in particular, the use of arts and crafts to the exclusion of other activities, the lack of attention to the symbolic characteristics of activities, and minimal concern for the interpersonal relationship between patient and therapist.

Participants at the conference recommended that occupational therapists develop knowledge and skills in:

1. the use of self;
2. the use of groups and group techniques;
3. a more sophisticated use of activities;
4. creating a therapeutic milieu;
5. contributing to the psychodynamic formulation of patients' behavior through the use of personality, social, and skills evaluation;
6. developing treatment goals as supplementary to psychotherapy;
7. bridging the gap between community living and the hospital (1007).

Gail S. Fidler and Jay W. Fidler co-authored *Introduction to Psychiatric Occupational Therapy* (1954) and *Occupational Therapy: A Communication Process in Psychiatry* (1963), which dealt with areas similar to those considered at the Boiling Springs Conference (286,290). These two books had a marked impact on the profession and served as a basic textbook for several generations of occupational therapists. This more dynamic period in occupational therapy initially had a strong psychoanalytic orientation. In particular, it was influenced by the theories of Harry Stack Sullivan and Carl G. Jung. Later it was influenced more by the various aspects of the sociological orientation.

The following is a brief historical perspective of the Boiling Springs recommendations. The concept of "use of self" refers to the various interpersonal dynamics between therapist and patient, the impact these dynamics have on the intervention process, and the use of these dynamics in intervention. Prior to this time occupational therapists were aware that the attitude they displayed could influence a patient's behavior. Thus, the symptomatic approach suggested certain attitudes one should take when a patient exhibited certain types of behavior. But that was about all. There was little awareness of how the therapist's thoughts and feelings influenced interaction with patients. No attention was given to interpersonal dynamics between a particular therapist and client. As a matter of fact, there was not a great deal of concern about the patient's thoughts and feelings either. The importance of interpersonal relationships as part of the therapeutic process had yet to be recognized. Activities were essentially viewed as apersonal: a manipulation of the nonhuman environment. Activity analysis and synthesis did not take into consideration the interpersonal component.

With the recommendation to use oneself as a tool in the intervention process, occupational therapists became self-aware. They began to look at their own thoughts and feelings and those of their clients. They began to be concerned about nonverbal communication, transference and countertransference, and differences in cultural values. There was a lifting of the stringent rule to be impersonal and rigidly self-controlled at all times. Understanding oneself became an important part of being a therapist. Use of self became a legitimate tool of occupational therapy.

Use of self, in the long range view, has had an important impact on the occupational therapy process. In the short range, however, it had a profoundly negative impact on the profession. Occupational therapists stopped using activities! Not all therapists, of course, but a large percentage. The verbal interchange between therapist and patient came to be seen as the key to change. Activities were superfluous. In many settings it was nearly impossible to discern any difference between occupational therapy and the verbal therapy used by other members of the team. Occupational therapists became preoccupied with their new tool: not an unusual phenomenon. But their preoccupation was compounded and reinforced by the value system in psychiatric hospitals. Staff members who engaged in verbal therapy were accorded the highest status. Occupational therapists traded part of their identity, activities, for status. Also, not an unusual phenomenon.

The second recommendation, the use of groups and group techniques by occupational therapists, was emphasized by the participants of the Boiling Springs Conference. Since the beginning of occupational therapy, most intervention had taken place within the context of small groups. The majority of these groups were loosely knit aggregates, however, rather than cohesive productive groups whose members shared common goals. The recommendation was that occupational therapists should use the dynamics and therapeutic potential of groups as an integral part of the intervention process, not simply as the setting for essentially one-to-one intervention. Gail Fidler initiated the "new" use of groups by the introduction of "task-oriented" groups, a group that used activities and the therapeutic potential of small groups to help patients to communicate and discover their unconscious or unshared thoughts and feelings (289). The theoretical rationale for task-oriented groups was primarily psychoanalytic in origin. Fidler emphasized the use of activities in groups and contributed much to our understanding of the impact of activities on the dynamics of groups and the therapeutic potential of groups. Occupational therapists used task-oriented groups to some extent but there was a greater propensity to use groups as the basis for verbal intervention. The activity aspect of the group in many cases disappeared. There came to be little or no difference between groups led by occupational therapists and those led by other members of the health team. This state of affairs continued for some time. It was not until the 1970s that activities were returned to occupational therapy groups. At this time various types of groups proliferated using a variety of theoretical orientations. The concept "activity groups" was coined as an umbrella term to encompass these various types of groups, with six major categories of activity groups identified (711). From the initial recommendation for the use of groups in intervention, through the course of events outlined above, activity groups came to be one of the legitimate tools of occupational therapy.

The third recommendation was related to the use of activities. At the time of the conference, the use of activities had become essentially restricted to arts and crafts. The earlier use of a wide variety of activities for intervention had somehow been lost so that they were no longer part of the repertoire of current occupational therapists. Participants at the conference made a plea for returning to the use of a broader scope of activities. The psychoanalytic orientation, which was having such a profound impact on psychiatry in general, alerted some occupational therapists to the symbolic potential of activities. With the recommendation of the conference, occupational therapists began to study activities as a means for symbolic expression of unconscious or unshared conflicts, feelings, and ideas and as a means for gratification of infantile needs through the camouflage of the reality of the activity. An example of the latter is a patient and therapist regularly making and drinking chocolate milkshakes together. This activity, if properly designed, could satisfy a patient's infantile oral needs. The socially accepted nature of the activity may act as a screen, which in turn often allows a patient to gratify infantile needs without guilt or diminished self-respect. The Fidlers emphasized the importance of studying and using the dynamics of activities (289,290). They believed that an activity has inherent characteristics that elicit a typical response. When an individual responds in an atypical way to an activity, this is an expression of unconscious conflicts that are unable to be articulated on a verbal level. Finally, they believed that knowledge of the inherent characteristics of an activity would provide a key for understanding patient's unconscious ideation.

In 1960, *Nonhuman Environment* by Harold Searles was published (873). This book provided considerable documentation regarding the effect of the nonhuman environment on human development and on the way that we use the nonhuman environment as a means of relating to and dealing with the human environment. With the impetus provided by the Boiling Springs Conference, Searles' ideas were used to understand further the nonhuman aspects of activities and the potential psychological impact of the equipment and adaptive aids used in physical habilitation and rehabilitation. Although the nonhuman environment has been used by occupational therapists since the beginning of the profession, the phenomena had no conceptual label. But with its naming, it became almost immediately one of the recognized legitimate tools of occupational therapy.

A good deal of attention was given to the symbolic potential and dynamics of activities, both their study and use, as was recommended by the Boiling Springs Conference. However, the variety and breadth of its recommendations worked, for a time, at cross purposes. The idea of use of self overshadowed the rich and powerful possibilities of activities. Use of self was a new toy that did not lose its ability to fascinate for almost 20 years. It was only in the 1970s, during our search for uniqueness and unity, that occupational therapy returned to its original high regard for and use of purposeful activities. A balance, albeit somewhat unstable, was struck between the doing process and the interpersonal relationships that influence and are influenced by that process. The nonhuman and human components of activities were reunited.

The fourth recommendation of the conference was concerned with the therapeutic milieu. The idea of a therapeutic milieu or therapeutic community was defined in the previous section. The recommendation suggested that occupational therapists become involved in this orientation to treatment. Essentially, it was a natural orientation for occupational therapists, for it made use of the day-to-day activities that are an inherent part of people living, working, and playing together. In fact, in retrospect, one could wonder why occupational therapists did not formulate this orientation to treatment themselves. Be that as it may, occupational therapists had the skills to add another dimension to the therapeutic milieu. As developed by Maxwell Jones, the therapeutic community was essentially designed to help patients acquire intrapersonal controls and interpersonal skills necessary for independent living. Although occupational therapists could contribute to these goals, they also had the ability to assist patients in learning many of the task skills—the ability to manipulate the nonhuman environment successfully—which are an integral part of activities of daily living, work, and recreational pursuits. They also had the knowledge to assist patients in the area of temporal adaptation. In addition, occupational therapists had a relatively sophisticated understanding of the role of activities in all aspects of intervention and the ability to analyze and synthesize activities for the purpose of intervention.

Occupational therapists did, indeed, become a part of the therapeutic community orientation to treatment and in many ways made a significant contribution. Relative to the profession, the recommendation to become involved in the therapeutic milieu had a significant impact. With psychiatry's diminished interest in moral treatment and thus in the habit training approach of Slagle, occupational therapists had retreated from the daily life of the hospital ward: figuratively and often literally to the basement. By the mid-1950s occupational therapists had isolated themselves in their occupational therapy rooms to which patients came or were brought for one or two hours a day at the most. They did not see themselves nor were they perceived as part of the treatment team. With the Boiling Springs Conference recommendation and its reverberation through the profession, occupational therapists in great numbers emerged from their basement hideout, joined the daily life of the ward, and became a part of the treatment team—a place where, for the most part, they have stayed.

Closely related to the idea of involvement in the therapeutic milieu orientation was the Fidlers' conceptualization of the occupational therapy process as a laboratory situation. They used the term "laboratory" in the sense of a setting where one may observe, study, experiment, and practice, and where one can learn through experience. This is indeed an excellent way to conceptualize the occupational therapy process. In using the term "laboratory," the Fidlers did not intend that the occupational therapy process should take place in isolation from daily life. It was not a laboratory in the sense of a place insulated from and unrelated to the real world. Rather, it was the creation of a supportive environment for the learning of basic skills. The idea of occupational therapy as a laboratory experience has also been useful as occupational therapists have moved out of the hospital or clinical setting into the community.

The fifth recommendation of the conference was that occupational therapists contribute to psychodynamic formulations through the use of personality, social, and skills evaluation. The essence of this recommendation was that, by observing a patient's involvement in activities, occupational therapists could discern a great deal about the patient. On one level this was a good recommendation for it reminded and urged occupational therapists to study and use the tremendous amount of information that could be derived from observing an individual's participation in activities. In a very real sense this recommendation directed occupational therapists to engage in the evaluation process. Heretofore, occupational therapists had relied on the physician's prescription and essentially did not engage in any formal, independent evaluation of the patient. This may seem rather shocking to the current reader—how could one engage in planning intervention if one did not initially assess the patient's needs and ability to function. But such apparently was the case. Happily, occupational therapists eventually took this recommendation seriously and began to develop various means of assessment. This, however, did not happen immediately. Occupational therapists had not yet reached the necessary level of sophistication and self-confidence.

On another level the recommendation to contribute to the psychodynamic formulation through the use of personality, social, and skills evaluation was detrimental to the growth of the profession. It inhibited the profession in two ways: by maintaining the subservient role of the occupational therapist and by leading to a blind alley of projective techniques. In regard to the maintenance of a subservient role—latent in this recommendation was the idea that occupational therapists should, indeed, gather information about patients through observing their participation in activities. But occupational therapists were not to interpret this information (289,290,956). Essentially, it should be given in the form of raw data to the psychiatrist. It was the psychiatrist's responsibility to interpret the data, formulate the patient's psychodynamics, and arrive at a diagnosis. To its credit, this recommendation did encourage the occupational therapist to collaborate with the psychiatrist. Previously, occupational therapists had primarily been in the role of the recipient of prescriptions. So there was, indeed, some improvement in the suggested role of the occupational therapist. However, a peer relationship with the psychiatrist and other members of the treatment team was neither entertained nor anticipated at this time. Fortunately, this is no longer the case.

The second way in which this recommendation was detrimental was by leading occupational therapists to embrace the idea of projective techniques. This situation was in many ways a logical extension of consideration of the symbolic potential of activities and of the therapist's role in gathering information for the psychiatrist. In addition, the phenomenon of projective techniques—one of the legitimate tools of clinical psychology—was relatively new and very popular at this time. Two test batteries that made use of various art materials were developed, one by the Azimas and the other by the Fidlers (67,749). Interpretation of these batteries relied on the phenomenon of projection as a means of identifying intrapsychic content and discovering the psychodynamics underlying an individual's behavior. Both the Azimas and the Fidlers saw the information available from interpretation of the batteries as being directly applicable to planning intervention. But this is not what happened. Ignoring the idea that occupational therapists should not engage in psychodynamic interpretations, occupational therapists in fairly large numbers began to use these batteries and to make interpretations. Then the process stopped, arrested in midflight. Occupational therapists did not use the information for planning intervention. It may have been useful to someone on the treatment team, but certainly not the occupational therapist. What the occupational therapist did relative to intervention was independent of the data gathered from the batteries. The reason this was so detrimental to the profession was the massive numbers of hours, thought, and energy wasted by occupational therapists. There was obviously much to be done that may have been accomplished far sooner if so many occupational therapists had not wandered into this blind alley.

The sixth recommendation was to develop treatment goals as supplementary to psychotherapy. Much that was believed about the role of occupational therapists at this time is reflected in this recommendation. Latent in this recommendation is the belief that verbal psychotherapy was the treatment of choice. To their credit, the conference participants did not suggest that occupational therapists engage in the practice of verbal psychotherapy. Rather, their suggestion was that occupational therapists play a supportive role relative to verbal psychotherapy. Under the prescription and supervision of the psychiatrist, occupational therapists were to facilitate the expression of feelings and help patients to gratify needs symbolically or through sublimation. What occurred in the occupational therapy process was not discussed or explored within that context. Rather, the occupational therapist presented his or her observations to the psychotherapist. Together with the patient's report of the experience, the psychotherapist and patient discussed what had occurred in occupational therapy. This recommendation was detrimental to occupational therapy. It again placed the therapist in a subservient role relative to the psychiatrist and it dealt with only a constricted range of the occupational therapy domain of concern (290,956).

Although growth was inhibited, this recommendation eventually led to renewed study of the occupational therapy process. If occupational therapy goals could be supplementary to psychotherapy, then perhaps they could also be different than and to a great extent independent from the goals of psychotherapy. It is from this idea among others that occupational therapists began, over the course of several years, to define and guide the development of their own practice. It should be noted here that this process of separation from the dominance of verbal psychotherapy was facilitated by the recognition that many patients were unable to participate profitably in psychotherapy. There was a general search for new approaches.

The seventh and final recommendation of the Boiling Springs Conference was to bridge the gap between community living and the hospital. This recommendation anticipated the community mental health movement by several years and thus was quite farsighted of the conference participants. However, this recommendation did not become actualized until the mid-1960s when it was evident that psychoactive drugs would markedly decrease the length of hospitalization for most patients and the community mental health movement was initiated. At this time occupational therapy shifted from its preoccupation with intrapsychic process to facilitating patients' movement into the community. More emphasis was placed on developing skills in activities of daily living, prevocational preparation for work, and fostering recreational interests. Family interaction became part of our domain of concern. Occupational therapists began to move out of the shelter of inpatient psychiatric treatment centers into partial hospitalization programs, community-based programs of many kinds, and into private practice. The fifth piece of the intervention process, prevention, became accepted by the profession. The advent of the community mental health movement with its orientation toward short-term hospitalization also required occupational therapists to think through and redefine its priorities in intervention.

In retrospect, the Boiling Springs Conference and the writings of the Fidlers had a tremendous impact on intervention relative to the psychosocial components of occupational therapy. The conference and the Fidlers provided a sense of direction for the profession and brought it out of the stagnant period of the symptomatic approach. The effects are still being felt within the profession.

IN SEARCH OF IDENTITY

Although the rehabilitation movement, the recommendations of the Boiling Springs Conference, and the Fidlers' work contributed to the growth of the profession, there was still a sense of something missing. The profession began to be aware of a need for self-definition, a need to describe its uniqueness, to articulate what was generic to all areas of practice. The profession embarked on a search for identity. The process began in the late 1960s and continues to the present.

To describe this search it is necessary to return to the beginning of the profession and briefly discuss occupational therapy's relationship with medicine. In 1917 medicine was a respected profession but in no way the powerful organized institution it is today. Physicians, for the most part, were not well educated, there were few teaching hospitals, and medicine was primarily practiced out of an office in the physician's home. Specialization was rare; most physicians were general practitioners.

Although conceived within the matrix of medicine, occupational therapy originally existed somewhat apart from it. Relative to physical medicine, occupational therapists saw their role as facilitating convalescence, and thus not really concerned with disease or illness. In psychiatry, occupational therapists were involved in habit training. Their day-to-day work was seen as having little relationship to the role of a physician's, which was primarily administrative at that time.

The Flexner report of 1910, a study of medical education, and the rapid advances being made in medical research contributed to the reorganization of medicine and a marked increase in its status (292,304). By the 1920s physicians became better educated and medicine began to demonstrate its effectiveness in treating illness, a situation not particularly evident in the past. Medicine rapidly became the most powerful group among the various groups concerned with the delivery of health services.

Occupational therapy was one of many health-related professions that maneuvered for a position in the new power structure. Its place was tenuous at best. Occupational therapy was a very small, barely emerging profession that was still in its infancy. It was unsure of itself, and, by present standards, without a theoretical foundation. This is not to diminish the contributions occupational therapists made during this period. Rather occupational therapy, as is true of any emerging profession, was not altogether certain what it was about: it was a collection of good ideas and intentions. Occupational therapy was also primarily a women's profession. The subordinate position of women, and the need for male protection, was seen as the natural order of things.

As is typical in the situation described above, occupational therapy turned to medicine to ensure its recognition and an advantageous position in the power structure (443). Occupational therapy consolidated its relationship with medicine first by requesting that physicians prescribe occupational therapy. Therapists felt this would give some legitimacy to their intervention. Physicians, for the most part, agreed with this request. Although this ultimately placed occupational therapists in a subservient role to physicians, it apparently seemed worth the price. There was little question about the appropriateness of physicians' writing prescriptions for occupational therapists until the late 1960s.

As is probably evident to the reader, the prescriptive position of the profession was detrimental to its growth and development. With prescriptions, there was little need to define our domain of concern or theoretical foundation. There was little need for evaluation, intervention for the most part was based on the symptomatic approach, and there was little if any research. Carrying out prescriptions involves very little thinking (443).

Secondly, in order to consolidate its position, occupational therapy requested that the American Medical Association (AMA) undertake "inspection and approval of occupational therapy schools" (444, p. 13). The AMA agreed, and the accreditation of occupational therapy programs began in 1933. In conjunction with this responsibility, the AMA was given final jurisdiction over the "essentials" for basic professional education in occupational therapy. With physicians having such a large influence on occupational therapy education, the educational experience was bound to teach and reinforce subservience. It was in the best interest of medicine for occupational therapists to act as an aid to the physician. The responsibility of the AMA for basic professional education continues today.

By the 1960s, then, occupational therapy had been dominated and to a great extent defined by medicine for nearly four decades. It was in this context that a marked change in the orientation of the profession took place. Occupational therapy became self-conscious. The profession began to look at itself: what it was, where it had been, and where it should go (956).

There were several factors that contributed to this revitalization: with their involvement in the rehabilitation movement, occupational therapists slowly began to appreciate and understand the scientific method. If not researchers, they at least had to become good consumers of research. This was necessary in order to read and to understand the literature in this area of practice. Occupational therapists were becoming better educated. Some had master's degrees either in occupational therapy or related professions and disciplines; a few had doctorates. The 1960s was a time of great social change and the questioning of traditional ideas. It was inevitable that this spirit of inquiry would affect some members of the profession. Part of the social change that took place was the initiation of the women's movement. The movement affected many women who rapidly redefined their role in society and their position relative to men.

More strictly within occupational therapy itself there were three situations that brought occupational therapists together in a way that facilitated the fermentation of ideas.

In 1964 the American Occupational Therapy Association was funded by a Social Rehabilitation Service Grant to design and present a number of regional and national workshops (656,660). These workshops, held between 1964 and 1968, were concerned, as separate institutes, with supervision, group process, object relations, and education. Under the leadership of June Mazer, these workshops contributed to the theoretical understanding and clinical skills of hundreds of occupational therapists. In addition, the faculty for the workshops, drawn from all parts of the country, had an opportunity to work together over an extended period of time. As is often the case, this initimate and long-term association provided fertile ground for the development or consolidation of many ideas that were to influence the profession.

Following the workshops, a small group of faculty and invited therapists met in Albion, Michigan to attempt to integrate "a large number of divergent theories and thoughts to a specific framework which would include all aspects of the organism" (658, p. 451). This project, in addition, gave impetus to a special psychiatric section in the September-October 1968 issue of the *American Journal of Occupational Therapy* (18). Occupational therapists were invited to submit papers that described their theoretical orientation and its application in practice. Four papers outlining different orientations were selected for publication.

Secondly, during the 1960s, a group of therapists and students gathered under the leadership of Mary Reilly in Southern California. They began to examine the philosophy of moral treatment as expressed by Meyer and Slagle's work relative to habit training. This group, essentially, sought guidance from the "roots" or beginnings of the profession for concepts that would prove useful in giving the profession direction for the future. Several individuals from this group presented papers at a symposium in Boston. Given in 1970, this symposium was sponsored by the Maternal and Child Health Service of the Department of Health, Education and Welfare. The presented papers were subsequently published in the September 1971 issue of the *American Journal of Occupational Therapy* (20). Additional papers followed.

The third situation that allowed for a sharing of ideas was the theoretical and applied work of A. Jean Ayres. Many therapists became interested in her ideas in regard to perceptual motor function and, eventually, sensory integration. Common concerns brought these therapists together in a number of workshops, institutes, and informal gatherings. Ayres and her colleagues have published extensively in the *American Journal of Occupational Therapy* and other journals as well as having written several books.

A history of dependency on medicine, a better-educated membership, social revolution, and the opportunity for many therapists to share ideas and think together fostered the search for identity. The medical model became the first focus of concern. In accepting the protection of medicine, occupational therapy unconsciously accepted the medical model as being appropriate for occupational therapy. Therapists acted as if the medical model provided the foundation for practice despite the fact that there was no evidence to support this belief. As the term is used here, the structure of the medical model is similar to the structure of the occupational therapy model. The content, however, is very different. Much of the content of the medical model is unrelated to the occupational therapy process; much of the occupational therapy process is not reflected in the medical model. The legitimate tools of medicine, for example, are drugs, surgery, and conscious use of self. Occupational therapy shares conscious use of self as a legitimate tool with medicine. However, the medical model does not include the nonhuman environment (except for drugs), the teaching-learning process, purposeful activities, activity groups, or activity analysis and synthesis. The body of knowledge of the medical model focuses on various diseases, with no or little attention given to such areas of human experience as work and leisure. There is no mention of activities' potential for evaluation and intervention. The domain of concern of medicine is organized around the concepts of symptoms, pathology, and sequelae.

In the late 1960s occupational therapists began to realize that the content of the medical model was totally inappropriate for occupational therapy (23,484,486,616, 710,799). Whether this realization led to or was the consequence of the profession's search for identity is problematic; more than likely it was a circular rather than linear process. It was, however, the medical model that came to be the counterpoint in the search for identity. This search took three major forms or directions:

1. attempts were made to define the occupational therapy domain of concern;
2. the concept of frame of reference was developed (and a number of frames of reference formulated);
3. attempts to articulate a comprehensive theory for occupational therapy were initiated.

These forms are intertwined and not necessarily mutually exclusive. They are separated here for clarity and, retrospectively, in the process of the search, these forms were not always differentiated or even labeled. It is important to note that none of this happened easily; there was considerable conflict, and many of the issues raised at this time have by no means been resolved.

Several approaches were taken to define the domain of concern of occupational therapy. Prior to the late 1960s, occupational therapists concerned with physical disabilities described intervention relative to diagnostic categories, e.g., cerebral vascular accident, arthritis, spinal cord injury. With movement away from the medical model, occupational therapists began to identify intervention as being concerned not with diagnostic categories but with sequelae—the consequence of disease, injury, or deficit. They began to order these sequelae, eventually describing their practice as being concerned with motor functions, visual perception, some aspects of cognitive and psychological functions, activities of daily living, and, to some extent, work.

The situation in psychiatry was, however, somewhat different. With the number of theories regarding the cause and nature of mental illness, there was no common agreement about symptom, pathology, or sequelae. Thus, for example, hallucinations from a psychoanalytic point of view are symptoms, from a behaviorist point of view are pathology, and from a neurological point of view are sequelae. Thus, the situation was rather confusing for the occupational therapist: what were one person's sequelae was another person's pathology. Sequelae were not good focal points for ordering the domain of concern of occupational therapy relative to psychiatry. In addition, occupational therapists in psychiatry did not want simply to manage symptoms and were uncertain if they should or could be involved with altering pathology.

Occupational therapists in psychiatry thus took a different course. They began to identify their focus as being the development of basic skills that clients needed to function effectively in the community. These were ultimately defined as skills relative to cognitive and psychological function, social interaction, activities of daily living, and, again to some extent, work.

Neither of these major areas of specialization gave much attention to sensory integration, familial roles, play/leisure/recreation, or temporal adaptation. Work was not really considered that important either. Attention to these areas would come later.

The Southern California group proposed that occupational therapy alter its "initial perspective of patients from diagnostic labels to those of occupational roles of workers, student, housewife, retiree, preschooler" (652, p. 292). They referred to these roles as "occupational behavior." The group felt that healthy function rather than deficits, pathology, or sequelae should be the focus for intervention. Joan Rogers, somewhat later, described the relationship between disease (that could also read sequelae) and occupational behavior (820). A simplified version of her description is illustrated in Fig. 2–1. This figure suggests that some pathological conditions do not require intervention by an occupational therapist, and that some individuals who have no discernible pathological condition could benefit from occupational therapy intervention.

However, the Southern California group went even further in their proposal. They said that occupational therapy should be concerned only with play/recreation, work, and temporal adaptation. The performance components—motor function, sensory integration, visual perception, cognitive and psychological function, and social interaction—should not be a part of the profession's domain of concern. Many members of the profession, particularly those whose major focus of practice was on the performance components and activities of daily living, were horrified at such a proposal. Considerable controversy ensued and continues today.

King, and to some extent Ayres, took an entirely different approach to defining the focus of intervention (58,534). King states that treatment, which she defines as a reversal of the disease process, is implicit in the beginning philosophy and thinking of the profession. She

	No disease	Disease	
	Healthy person	Person with tonsillitis	No occupational behavior dysfunction
	"Empty nest" housewife	Person with spinal cord injury	Occupational behavior dysfunction

FIG. 2-1. The relationship between disease and occupational behavior.

feels that the profession's concern with sequelae is secondary and something to which we have devoted far too much time and energy. Occupational therapists should return their attention to pathology, in particular to pathology of the central nervous system. King believes that deficits in the capacity to integrate sensory stimuli is a major cause of most of the schizophrenic reactions, many developmental disorders, attention deficits, conduct disorders, and some disorders that are attributed to stress. She feels that occupational therapy should focus on these disorders: we should treat pathology of the central nervous system. Although King does not mention any position relative to the medical model, her orientation to pathology and treatment place the focus of intervention in far closer proximity to the medical model than therapists working in physical disabilities and psychiatry or the Southern California group.

Finally, and taking a somewhat different tack, the American Occupational Therapy Association (AOTA) Executive Board charged the Commission on Practice to form a task force to develop, among other things, a uniform terminology for reporting occupational therapy services. Completed and adopted by the Representative Assembly of AOTA in 1979, the report is, in part, an attempt to define the domain of concern of occupational therapy. The major categories used (with each having many subcategories) are (a) independent living/daily living skills, (b) sensorimotor components, (c) cognitive components, (d) psychosocial components, (e) therapeutic adaptations, and (f) prevention (29). The major problem here seems to be that the categories are on very different conceptual levels.

It would be nice to state at this point that the focus of intervention has been resolved in the profession. But that is really not the case.

The domain of concern, as outlined in Chapter 1, is to a greater or lesser degree drawn from the several orientations outlined above.

The second direction taken in the search for occupational therapy's identity was frames of reference. The term "frame of reference" was occasionally used in the occupational therapy literature prior to 1968 but it was never defined. It appears to have been used in the traditional dictionary sense of "a structure of concepts, values, customs, views, etc., by means of which an individual or group perceives or evaluates data, communicates ideas and regulates behavior..." (792, p. 563). The term was defined in the occupational therapy literature in 1968 in a more specific and narrow manner (658). The definition at that time was similar to but not identical with the definition given in the previous chapter. In their formulation, most frames of reference are only concerned with a small part of the profession's domain of concern and body of knowledge. Thus, their development grew more out of a need to give identity to one aspect of practice than to the profession as a whole.

It should be noted that frames of reference existed in the profession prior to 1968. However, they were not identified as such at the time of their development. They simply were not given any name at all. The first frame of reference relative to the psychosocial components of occupational therapy was habit training. This was an acquisitional frame of reference with emphasis on the learning of good habits. The symptomatic approach, the next recognizable orientation in occupational therapy relative to the psychosocial components, is not considered to be a frame of reference by this author. There is no evidence in the literature that anyone believed this approach to intervention would lead to change. It was designed to help clients to manage their most severe symptoms. This was a humane goal but it is not the change process. Habit training as a frame of reference is not used in occupational therapy today. The psychiatric community no longer accepts the idea that mental illness is the consequence of bad habits. But, perhaps more than that, the regimented, repressive, paternalistic flavor of habit training is no longer compatible with present day thinking.

The first frame of reference still in current use was analytical. It was developed by the Fidlers in the 1950s and is based to a great extent on the theories of Harry Stack Sullivan (289,290). It must be noted at this point that Gail Fidler's name has, over the years, become almost synonymous with the analytic approach to the change process. However, much of her work has a strong sociological orientation.

For occupational therapists working in psychiatry, the analytic orientation was predominant through most of the 1960s. Mosey in 1968 and Llorens in 1969 (both members of the Albion group) each introduced a broad based developmental frame of reference (616,703). Both of these individuals were strongly influenced by Ayres' work. It was Ayres who initiated the developmental orientation in occupational therapy. Mosey's and Llorens' frames of reference are referred to as broad based for they include many other areas in addition to sensory integration.

The 1970s saw a proliferation of frames of reference related to the psychosocial components of occupational therapy. Acquisitional frames of reference influenced by the behavioral approach in psychiatry became rather popular (236,355,438,482,606,641,740,896,948,990, 998). Most of these were based on the Skinnerean theory of operant conditioning. One was based on a wide spectrum of postulates derived from a number of learning theories (708). One additional analytic frame of reference, "object relations analysis," was added (705). The Southern California group formulated a number of frames of reference in regards to temporal adaptation, play, and work, with play, at times, being considered as preparation for the role of a worker (see Chapter 25 for references). These frames of reference, although primarily acquisitional, had strong developmental overtones. Finally, King proposed a frame of reference restricted to some schizophrenic disorders (533). It is concerned with sensory integration and is based on Ayres' work.

As mentioned, a given frame of reference only defines a small part of the profession's domain of concern. It was almost as if by studying parts of the profession, the whole would be revealed. This is, at best, a questionable assumption. Without some other encompassing structure, the profession would come to be defined by its collection of frames of reference. Frames of reference are important for the profession, but they alone can not define it. (As an aside, it is out of this concern that the occupational therapy model, as outlined in Chapter 1, and the idea of configuration, were developed.)

The articulation of a comprehensive theory was the third direction taken in occupational therapy's search for identity. A comprehensive theory organizes, usually around one or a few key concepts, the various theoretical systems that constitute the body of knowledge of a profession for the purpose of describing and affirming the holistic nature of its theoretical foundation and its practice. An adequate comprehensive theory for a profession is assumed to provide suitable guidelines for evaluation and intervention (532,677,685,885). Thus, proponents of a comprehensive theory for the profession do not consider frames of reference necessary. Comprehensive theories are also referred to as "grand theories" or "meta theories."

In addition to a search for identity, articulation of a comprehensive theory was motivated by two other factors. The profession was concerned with its unity as a group. As just discussed, there was a proliferation of frames of reference. There was also a movement at this time toward increased specialization in the profession. This movement was formalized by the American Occupational Therapy Association in 1977 with the formation of five special interest groups: developmental disabilities, geriatrics, mental health, physical disabilities, and sensory integration (22). The concern was that, with specialization, the wholeness or unity of the profession would be lost, that there would no longer be a basic sense of what the profession was as a holistic entity. It was felt that a comprehensive theory would provide a foundation for all areas of specialization and illustrate the elements generic to the occupational therapy process.

The other factor motivating articulation of a comprehensive theory is related to the perceived state of the profession's body of knowledge. Philosophers and sociologists concerned with such matters have stated that it has an organized body of knowledge (199,277,321,697, 776). Many therapists see our body of knowledge as being disorganized and in need of arrangement into some discernible pattern. A comprehensive theory was seen by some as a means of providing this order.

The group, which met in Albion, Michigan, attempted to formulate a comprehensive theory that used the concept of object relations as its nucleus (685). They made an effort to eliminate the dichotomy between mind and body and to place the individual in the context of the human and nonhuman environment, phylogenetic and cultural past, ontogenetic development, the social system, and the anticipated future. Emphasis was essentially on describing the nature of man in the environment. No attempt was made to describe the focus of intervention or theories basic to the intervention process. This ambitious, but embryonic system has not been further developed or refined.

The Southern California group divided on the issue of comprehensive theory. One faction maintained that play/recreation, work, and temporal adaptation was the essence of the occupational therapy process (20). They continued to study these phenomena and develop frames of reference. No attempt was made to formulate a comprehensive theory.

The other faction set about formulating a comprehensive theory, which they refer to as "human occupation" (521,522,524,525). In formulating this theory, they appear to be attempting to reconcile the original adamant stand of the Southern California group in regards to the focus of occupational therapy with the focus preferred by the majority of the profession.

The nucleus of human occupation is the individual, conceived of as an open system with three interrelated subsystems. The subsystems are considered to be hierarchical, with the higher governing the lower. Age and the demands of the environment serve as the context for viewing the individual.

The volitional subsystem is the highest level subsystem. Its function is to guide the individual's course of action and enact behavior. It has three parts: (a) personal causation, the individual's belief about the efficacy of action; (b) valued goals; and (c) interests.

The second subsystem, the habituation system, is concerned with actions that do not require conscious choice. It is made up of: (a) internalized social roles; specific roles of concern are not identified; and (b) habits, organized routines of behavior.

The function of the lowest level, the production system, is to produce action. It is made up of skills, actions organized to an end. These skills are: (a) social, (b) cognitive, and (c) physical.

The above is, essentially, the way the occupational therapy domain of concern is described in the theory of human occupation. The content is roughly equivalent to the domain of concern outlined in Chapter 1. The arrangement of elements and what that implies is, however, different.

There are four other major parts to the theory of human occupation. First, the individual is described as an open system in relationship to the environment. That is, the development and organization of the subsystems are affected by interaction with the environment. This interactional process involves a continuous cycle of: (a) input, information from the environment; (b) throughput, the way information is organized by the individual; (c) output, the behavior of the individual relative to the environment; and (d) feedback, information from the environment in regards to one's behavior.

Second, change in the individual over time, ontogenesis, is described as having two properties: (a) the various social roles that the individual is required or elects to participate; and (b) a three-stage process of exploring, competency, and achievement; energized primarily by the volitional subsystem, this three-stage process is repeated each time the individual faces a new situation or attempts a new activity.

Third the individual's interaction with the environment is described as either being characterized by benign or vicious cycles. A benign cycle describes adequate adaptation to the environment that is satisfying to the individual. A vicious cycle is the inability to meet the demands of the environment and/or to experience a sense of satisfaction.

Fourth, the essence of the occupational therapy process is "occupation." "Therapy must embody the characteristics of purposefulness, challenge, accomplishment and satisfaction that make up every occupation" (525, p. 778).

The above outline of human occupation presents only some of the highlights. Much of the complexity, by necessity, is omitted. This comprehensive theory is in the process of being developed. In its present form, however, it does have some deficits.

First, it does not appear to provide a structure for organizing all of the theoretical systems that have traditionally constituted the body of knowledge of the profession, e.g., symbolism, the unconscious, and psychodynamics, theories relative to how dysfunction is altered. Second, the evaluation process is not precisely described. Third, it is unclear where intervention should begin and the sequence of intervention, when there is deficit in more than one subsystem or the elements of a subsystem. Fourth, the dynamic theories presented—open systems and the three-stage process of exploration, competency, and achievement—do not provide sufficient guidelines for intervention. Fifth, in the case studies used to illustrate the application of human occupation, intervention is frequently based on theories not included in the comprehensive theory. Some of these deficits may well be eliminated as human occupation evolves.

Four other approaches to articulating a comprehensive theory for occupational therapy have been suggested. The nuclear concepts of these approaches are human growth and development (616,618,801), purposeful activities (220,288,291), the central nervous system (primarily the subcortical level) (534,856), and adaptation (465,535,547). None of these concepts have been developed and related to other concepts to such a degree that one could describe them as constituting a comprehensive theory. They may, in the future, be formulated in a more refined and systematic manner.

At the present time, occupational therapy does not have a comprehensive theory. However, the question that needs to be addressed is whether such a theory is desirable. Stated in another way, would a comprehensive theory satisfy the needs that motivate the search for such a theory in a way that would facilitate the growth of the profession.

In relationship to professional identity, a comprehensive theory may assist in consolidating the profession's sense of self. There is, however, the possibility that a comprehensive theory may require, indeed demand, a degree of loyalty to that theory that creative, divergent, independent thinking would neither be encouraged nor tolerated. This would strongly inhibit the adaptability and ongoing development of the profession.

A comprehensive theory that must account for wildly disparate phenomena—the situation in occupational therapy—is difficult to formulate. It may be simplified to the point that the complexity and richness of the phenomena are lost. It may be so intricate and labyrinthine that it is incomprehensible to any but the most dedicated scholar. It may be presented on such an abstract level that it verges on the philosophical. It may be so nebulous that it inhibits research or affords little guidance for practice.

If these deficits of a comprehensive theory can be avoided, such a theory may provide a sense of professional unity despite widespread specialization and differing points of view. If these deficits are not avoided, a comprehensive theory may provide an illusion of fundamental wholeness but serve no practical purpose.

The final question is whether a comprehensive theory would help to organize the body of knowledge of occupational therapy. Given one of the major functions of theory—the organization of knowledge—one might automatically respond in the affirmative (75,91,174,627, 720,780). However, the literature does not support such an immediate and automatic response.

There does not seem to be one logical way for a profession to organize its body of knowledge. It seems to organize its body of knowledge in a number of different ways, depending on the use to which the knowledge is to be put. The body of knowledge, for example, of occupational therapy might be organized for the purpose of basic professional education, advanced education, study in an area of specialization, understanding a particular age group, or formulating a frame of reference. Ideally, a profession develops different patterns of organization commensurate with the different purposes for which the body of knowledge is to be studied or used (776,777,917).

As the critique indicates, a comprehensive theory may not be the panacea that is attributed to it in its absence. One could also raise the question of whether the articulation of a comprehensive theory is worth all the time and effort that is currently being expended in the endeavor.

The search for identity is a journey not yet completed. There is still considerable disagreement about the destination and the best road to take. But perhaps it is good that the search, the journey, never ends.

To conclude this section, occupational therapy, through acceptance of and reliance on a medical prescription and AMA influence of its education, essentially allowed itself to be defined by medicine. By the late 1960s many occupational therapists found this situation intolerable and began to seek an independent identity. The search for self-definition was begun by many and took a variety of different forms. Although well on the way, the task is not completed. There is a sense, however, of separateness from medicine; prescriptions are a thing of the past. But a mature, coequal relationship with medicine has not yet been accomplished, at least not in relationship to the broader social system. In most states where occupational therapists are licensed, the law specifies that therapists cannot engage in evaluation and intervention without a referral from a physician (26,224,654, 1010,1032). A referral is a request by a physician for an occupational therapist to evaluate a client for the purpose of determining whether the individual is in need of occupational therapy intervention and what the goals of that intervention would be. It is the physician's responsibility to determine whether or not to advise the client to engage in occupational therapy intervention. This is the current legal definition of the relationship between medicine, occupational therapy, and the client. In actuality, occupational therapists often do engage in evaluation and intervention without a medical referral or with such a blanket referral that it is essentially meaningless.

Occupational therapists, in general, do not believe a medical referral is either necessary or acceptable. They see it as demeaning to the profession and to their professional integrity. There are attempts being made in several states to alter present licensure laws. Be that as it may, there is considerable positive distance between a prescription and a referral. With a referral, the occupational therapist, in collaboration with the client, determines the goals and means of intervention. This was not the case in the days of a prescription. The next step—society's recognition of occupational therapists as independent practitioners—is foreseeable in the near future.

SUMMARY

Part 1 has provided an overview of occupational therapy. The configurations, or component parts of occupational therapy—model, frames of reference, practice, data, and research—were described. The psychosocial components of occupational therapy were viewed in historical perspective. With this as background information, the stage for a more in-depth consideration of occupational therapy's domain of concern has, hopefully, been set.

Part 2

Domain of Concern

Part 2 of this text describes the domain of concern of occupational therapy as it relates to the psychosocial components of the profession. Attention is given to motor function and visual perception only in an effort to clarify and illuminate the other areas.

Each of the elements of the domain of concern is discussed as an entity outside the context of evaluation and intervention. Evaluation and intervention relative to these areas will be discussed in Parts 4 and 5 of the text. In general, each chapter includes a description of the area of human experience being addressed as it typically exists. Problems that an individual may encounter in a particular area are described only superficially, if at all. Thus, the focus of Part 2 is on function rather than dysfunction. Parts 4 through 6 of the text are addressed to dysfunction. This part of the text then is concerned with performance components, occupational performances, age (the life cycle), and environment.

3 Performance Components

This chapter is concerned with the performance components that constitute the psychosocial aspects of occupational therapy: sensory integration, cognitive function, psychological function, and social interaction. The aspects of human function included within the performance components have been drawn from the occupational literature. In the literature, performance components have been identified, labeled, and discussed from a variety of points of view. Thus, there is often considerable overlapping and compounding of concepts and different levels of conceptual organization. In addition, there is some disagreement about what is included within each performance component. An attempt has been made here to identify all major aspects of human function considered to be a part of the psychosocial performance components, and to organize and define them in a way that is compatible with the literature.

It is important to note that the terms used to label the various elements contained within each of the performance components are not necessarily analogous to the terms used to identify function-dysfunction continuums in various frames of reference. The areas addressed, however, are similar. Lack of parallel terms is primarily due to the use of various labels in the literature to denote the same general concept.

The performance components are discussed in this chapter in isolation from each other. However, as they exist in the individual they, of course, interact and in such a way that it is often difficult to identify the operation of any given process or skill. As described here it may seem to the reader that the divisions between the components are arbitrary. It is indeed difficult to discern where, for example, cognitive function ends and psychological function begins. The divisions made here between the performance components and the subcategories of the components are as much as possible based on the occupational therapy literature and the general body of knowledge relative to each of the areas under consideration.

The subcategories of the various performance components are quite numerous. They are presented in Table 3-1 to assist the reader in finding a way through the maze of concepts.

SENSORY INTEGRATION

The concept of sensory integration has evolved and changed since its first introduction in the occupational therapy literature (783,784). To give some order to the definition of sensory integration, this section is divided into three subsections—the processing of sensory information, definition and subcategories, and differentiation from other performance components.

The Processing of Sensory Information

On a very basic level, and simplistically stated, the central nervous system is concerned with the processing of sensory information in such a way that the individual can act effectively on the environment (148,255,739,961). Dynamically, the central nervous system translates sensory impulses into meaningful information and organizes that information so as to initiate an appropriate re-

TABLE 3-1. *Performance components*

Sensory Integration
1. Integration of tactile subsystems
2. Postural and bilateral integration
   a. Integration of primitive postural reflexes
   b. Mature righting and equilibrium reactions
   c. Ocular control
   d. Integration of the two sides of the body
3. Praxis

Cognitive Function
1. Attention, memory, and orientation
2. Thought processes
   a. Primary
   b. Secondary
   c. Tertiary
3. Levels of conceptualization
   a. Concrete
   b. Abstract
4. Intelligence
5. Factual information
6. Problem solving

Psychological Function
1. Dynamic states
   a. Needs
   b. Emotions
   c. Values
   d. Interest
   e. Motivation
2. Intrapsychic dynamics
   a. The conscious-unconscious continuum
   b. Psychodynamics
   c. Defense mechanisms
3. Reality testing
4. Insight
5. Object relations
6. Self-concept
   a. Identity
   b. Sexual identity
   c. Body image
   d. Knowledge of one's assets and limitations
   e. Self-esteem
7. Self-discipline
   a. Volition
   b. Self-control
   c. Self-responsibility and direction
   d. Dealing with adversity
8. Concept of others

Social Interaction
1. Interpretation of situations
2. Social skills
   a. Communication
   b. Dyadic interaction
   c. Group interaction
3. Structured social interplay
   a. Cooperation
   b. Competition
   c. Compromise
   d. Negotiation
   e. Assertiveness

sponse. The central nervous system, however, does not take in or register all available sensory data. Rather it acts as a filter, in that at any given time it selectively accepts and rejects specific sensory data. Data from a single sensory system (e.g., vestibular, tactile, auditory) may be processed in isolation. More typically, data from many sensory systems are brought together in such a way as to provide a multidimensional perspective of oneself and the environment.

The central nervous system can be roughly divided into three parts: the spinal cord, the subcortical areas of the brain, and the cerebral cortex. It is the latter two that are of concern here. The subcortical parts of the brain on the whole are involved with the processing of relatively gross vestibular, proprioceptive, and tactile information (58). Functionally, they are concerned with the survival of the organism, with the processing of information being not conscious and extremely rapid. Information is organized into relatively simple patterns that evoke responses of the entire body as a whole. The cortical part of the brain, in contrast, is concerned with the processing of more subtle and refined sensory data, including visual and auditory information. At this level processing tends to be conscious and less rapid. The organization of information is highly complex. Responses, based on more precise information, tend to be specialized, more discrete, and individualistic (58). It is generally believed that adequate processing of information at the subcortical level enables the individual to process information at the cortical level more effectively. This statement is not meant to imply, however, that the subcortical processing of information is basic to cortical processing. Development of skill in both subcortical and cortical processing begins at birth, if not before. Deficit at one level does not necessarily presuppose deficit at the other level. Please note that this definition is somewhat different from those proposed by Ayres and AOTA (55,433,434).

Definition and Subcategories

Sensory integration will be described here as a neurological process and not as an approach to evaluation and intervention. The distinction is made here specifically because "sensory integration" is the term used in occupational therapy to identify both a frame of reference and an area of human function. As previously defined, then, sensory integration is a subcortical process that involves receiving, selecting, combining, and coordinating vestibular, proprioceptive, and tactile (somatosensory) information for functional use. It is a dynamic process wherein "wholes" or gestalts of somatosensory information are formed, revised, or recombined in an infinite number of patterns to facilitate the planning and execution of interaction with the environment.

The location and function of the somatosensory receptors are as follows. The receptors of the vestibular system are located within the inner ear and the extraocular muscles and provide information in regard to the earth's gravitational pull and motion—of the individual and of the external environment. The receptors of the proprioceptive system are located within the muscles, joints, and ligaments and provide information about the relationship of body parts one to the other and their position in space. The receptors of the tactile system are distributed over all parts of the body and provide information about objects that come into direct contact with the body.

Sensory integration is a constant, ongoing process that takes place throughout the life cycle. The capacity to integrate sensory information is acquired over a period of years. It is not until around the age of 9 that a child acquires the capacity in its fullest or most refined sense. Development of sensory integration is stage specific; integration at one level is fundamental to integration at a higher or more complex level. There is, however, a good deal of fluidity. The sensory systems develop together from the beginning of life, although some may reach a mature level more quickly. It is the integration of these systems that is stage specific (58). Sensory integration can be divided into three major subcategories, with one of those categories being further subdivided (57,60,61).

Integration of Tactile Subsystems

It has been hypothesized that there are two tactile subsystems: (a) a protective system, which warns the individual of impending danger, and (b) a discriminatory system, which conveys information about the environment. The protective system is considered to be phylogenetically older, and therefore stronger. The discriminatory system is believed to have a checking or controlling function relative to the protective system. For adequate function, the two systems must be in balance so that the protective system is inhibited when the environment is safe for investigation and manipulation. Conversely, the discriminatory system must be inhibited when survival is threatened. Sometimes the two systems have never attained this functional balance and the protective system predominates. When this occurs, the individual is biased in interpreting a majority of stimuli as potentially dangerous and gives attention to many stimuli that others would consider to be irrelevant to the immediate situation. Deficit in this area is often referred to as tactile defensiveness.

Postural and Bilateral Integration

This subcategory is further divided into four areas. The first is integration of primitive postural reflexes, in particular the tonic neck reflex and tonic labyrinthine reflex. The tonic neck reflex involves extension of the arm toward the side to which the head is turned, flexion of the other arm, and a similar or opposite reaction in the lower extremities. The tonic labyrinthine reflex involves flexion of the arms and legs in the prone position and extension in the supine position. Mature righting and equilibrium reactions refers to flexibility in rotation around the long axis of the body (as in rolling), and automatic shifting of body weight to maintain balance. Ocular control refers to the eyes following visual stimuli in a smooth, fluid, coordinated manner and in coordination with each other and the capacity to cross the midline of the body visually. Integration of the two sides of the body refers to the ability to use both sides of the body together in a coordinated manner.

Praxia

This is the ability to execute skilled or nonhabitual motor tasks. Deficit in this area is referred to as apraxia.

Another area, "form and space perception," is often included as being a subcategory of sensory integration. Some individuals with difficulty in this area demonstrate deficits in the subcategories described above. When this is the case, intervention is directed toward enhancing integration of somatosensory input rather than direct training in the perception of form and space. Other individuals with problems in form and space perception do not demonstrate any difficulty in sensory integration. For the purpose of this text, this area of human function will be categorized as visual perception. Admittedly this is rather a gray area and will be discussed further in the last part of this section.

Individuals with sensory integrative dysfunction may have problems in one or more of the areas outlined above. The exact deficit must be determined through adequate evaluation. In general, however, individuals with sensory integrative dysfunction may exhibit some difficulties in the following areas. In the first area, hyperactivity and distractibility, the individual has difficulty sitting still and concentrating on the task at hand. Behavior appears to be disorganized and purposeless. In the second area, behavior problems, the individual's reactions are often atypical and thus may not be understood or accepted by others. There may be difficulty in coping with everyday stress or new and unfamiliar situations. In the third area, speech development, acquisition of language may be slow and there may be problems in articulation. In the fourth area, muscle tone and coordination, the individual may have low muscle tone and appear to be weak. There are often deficits in both gross and fine motor control, which leads to clumsy movements and difficulty in manipulating objects. In the fifth area, learning at school, the individual has difficulty in mastering reading, writing, and arithmetic.

Deficits in sensory integration have been studied primarily in relationship to children between the ages of 4 and 10 years who are suspected of being learning disabled. More recently, King and others have been investigating the possibility of sensory integrative dysfunction in relation to schizophrenic disorders.

Differentiation from Other Performance Components

There is some confusion in the literature in regard to differentiating sensory integration from some aspects of motor function and visual perception (784,785,856). Each of these components will be discussed briefly in order to clarify similarities and differences. Motor function, as previously defined, is the ability to use one's body to act effectively relative to the environment. The subcategories of motor function are: (a) range of motion, (b) strength, (c) endurance, (d) coordination, (e) muscle tone, and (f) reflex integration (960). It is the latter two subcategories that overlap with sensory integration. Problems in muscle tone (hyperactivity and hypoactivity) and defects in the integration of primitive reflexes, on the whole, are not believed to be attributed to difficulties in the processing of vestibular information—the key factor in sensory integration. Intervention in these areas is based on the work of Rood, Bobath, and Bunnstrom and involves the use of sensory stimulation, of an inhibitory and/or facilitory nature, and feedback from adaptive motor responses in order to normalize motor activity (732,960,1026). The terms used to label this type of intervention vary and include: sensory motor, neuromuscular facilitation, neurodevelopmental, and neurobehavioral. Some aspects of the work of Rood and Bobath have been incorporated into Ayres' frame of reference regarding sensory integration, but these are not the predominant features of this frame of reference.

Turning to visual perception, this performance component was previously defined as a primarily cortical process that involves the recognition, discrimination, and interpretation of visual stimuli relative to the tangible concrete properties of objects and events (183,506,692,815).

The subcategories of visual perception are: (a) visual figure-ground, the ability to select and attend to one aspect of the visual field while perceiving it in relation to the rest of the field; (b) visual discrimination, the ability to differentiate objects in the environment visually by their unique visual characteristics; (c) perceptual consistency, the ability to perceive objects possessing invariant properties such as shape, position, and size despite the variability of the impressions on the sensory surface; (d) visual memory, the ability to retain and recall what has been seen immediately or long term; (e) position in space, the ability to relate one's body to objects in space; (f) spatial relations, the ability to perceive two or more objects in relation to each other; and (g) visual-motor coordination, the ability to coordinate vision with the movements of the body or parts of the body (Jim Hinojosa, *personal communication*) (323, 324,587).

There are differences between visual perception and sensory integration. Visual perception is a cortical process whereas sensory integration is not. Visual perception does not involve the processing of gross visual sensations, which contribute to adequate equilibrium reactions, a subcategory of sensory integration. Visual-motor coordination involves the harmonization of vision and movement of body parts whereas ocular control is concerned with the visual pursuit of objects.

It has been hypothesized that the nature of visual perceptual deficits of developmentally disabled children are different from those of adolescents and adults who, through trauma to the brain, have acquired visual perceptual deficits. Discussion of this hypothesis is beyond the scope of this text. In general, however, intervention, regardless of causal factors or age, involves direct remediation of observed perceptual deficits with limited emphasis on underlying or related disturbances in other neural systems. Intervention is based on: (a) the principle that planned and controlled visual, as well as proprioceptive, tactile, and auditory sensory input, which elicits an adaptive visual-motor response, enhances visual perception; (b) principles of learning, with emphasis on those that relate to the provision of adequate cues, feedback, and opportunity for practice; (c) use of the client's residual capacities; and (d) the application of the above three postulates through the use of gross motor activities, paper and pencil and table top activities, and appropriate activities of daily living, prevocational and recreational activities (2,1035).

Intervention in the area of visual perception has been referred to variously as perceptual-motor training and perceptual motor therapy.

In addition to some of, at least superficial, similarities between visual perception and sensory integration, another reason for confusion regarding these two performance components is related to the history of Ayres' work (785). The early work of Ayres was concerned with visual perception. Feeling that remediation of visual perceptual deficit was not sufficiently effective in enhancing the function of learning disabled children, Ayres became involved with the study of the subcortical processing of the vestibular, proprioceptive, and tactile sensory input. She began to refer to this process as sensory integration. The movement from concern about visual perception to sensory integration was a fairly slow process. Some of Ayres' work which took place in this transition period did not make a sharp distinction between visual perception and sensory integration.

In conclusion, sensory integration, as a performance component, is different from motor function and visual perception. The latter are related to sensory integration as all of the performance components are interrelated but, like sensory integration, they are treated as distinct aspects of human function in this text.

COGNITIVE FUNCTION

As previously defined, cognitive function is a cortical process that involves the use of information for the purpose of thinking and problem solving. It is the process of perceiving, representing, and organizing sensory stimuli on the cortical level and essentially allows the individual to be oriented relative to dominant environmental features. The process often takes place on a conscious level but it may occur on an unconscious level. The subcategories of cognition follow.

Attention, Memory, and Orientation

The ability to focus in a sustained manner on one task or activity is referred to as attention (35,741). All stimuli are not given equal attention. Although a simplistic and not entirely accurate equation, stimuli that receive the greatest degree of attention tend to be remembered on a conscious level, stimuli given less attention are often remembered or stored at an unconscious level, stimuli that are not attended to do not become part of the individual's fund of information. Selective perception is regulated to some degree by the survival value of the available information. However, it is also influenced by the individual's interests, the value attached to the information, and the emotional gestalt in which the information is embedded.

A disturbance in attention may be manifested by "difficulty in finishing tasks that have been started, easy distractibility and/or difficulty concentrating on work" (35, p. 354). Any serious disturbance in attention will interfere with memory, orientation to the environment, and thinking. In addition, an attention deficit impedes adaptation to the environment because without adequate attention an individual is unable to carry out the required tasks of daily life. The term "attention span" is used to indicate the duration of an individual's ability to focus on a particular activity.

Memory is the retention and storage of information in such a way that it can be recalled (741). Representation refers to the manner or form in which information is stored (47). Information may be stored as exocepts, images, endocepts, concepts, or a combination of these. Exocept representation is memory of stimuli as an action or motor response. It can be illustrated by definition of the length of an object through the use of gestures or by memory of the movement necessary to tie a shoe. Image representation is the memory of stimuli in terms of an internal, pictorial quasi-reproduction. The modifier "quasi" is used to indicate that the image is not usually an exact reproduction of the stimulus event or object. Reproduction tends to be partial; some elements may not be included in the image. The expression, "I can see it in my mind's eye," describes perceptions remembered in the form of images. Whereas perceptions stored as exocepts are connected to specific stimulus experiences, images are able to be attended to without the presence of the corresponding stimuli.

Endocept representation is the memory of perceptions in terms of a felt experience. It is not a feeling (such as pleasure or guilt), although feelings are associated with an endocept as they are with all representations. Many persons experience endocepts in terms of bodily sensations. The expressions, "I have a gut feeling," or "I feel it in my bones," are often used to describe endocepts. Perceptions stored as endocepts are extremely difficult to communicate to others. Often the individual attempts to translate endocepts into images or verbal concepts that can then be communicated through some art form or the spoken word. However, endocepts invariably lose something in translation. The communicator feels the loss and may even state, "It is something like this but I haven't said it (or drawn it) exactly right." The ability to respond in an empathetic manner is probably based on endocept representations.

Concept representation is the memory of perceptions in terms of words. Concepts are words or phrases that label some similarity between seemingly varied phenomena. We tend to be most aware of concept representation for it serves as the means for much of our internal and external communication. Words have denotative meaning in that they stand for events, objects, and actions. They also have connotative meanings, however, in that they take on a variety of other interpretations, implications, or associations. Some of these may be emotional or affective in nature.

Information, then, may be retained in many forms. The form of representation is an important part of memory, but so is the duration (183,741,1021). To indicate duration, modifiers—long, short, and intermediate—are used in describing memory. Short-term memory refers to remembering events in the immediate past: an hour ago, this morning, yesterday. Memory of events in the distant past—10 years ago, in one's childhood—is described as long-term memory. Intermediate memory is pragmatically anything between short- and long-term memory. Stimuli that are represented in an exoceptual and endoceptual manner tend to be held in memory longer than stimuli that are represented in other ways. But this is by no means always the case.

There are many factors that account for the duration of memory, not all of which are understood. Some of the more important factors are: use, significance, degree of emotion associated with the stimuli, and the health of the central nervous system. Information frequently used by the individual and considered significant or important to the individual tends to be retained for a long period of time. Information associated with a high degree of affect or feeling (either negative or positive) also tends to be held in memory for a long period of time. However, such information may not be retained at a conscious level. Insult to the central nervous system—traumatic, chemical, or degenerative—often impedes memory temporarily or permanently. This may be related to short-term memory, long-term memory, or both. Individuals with organic mental disorders often have deficits in memory (35).

The last area included in this subcategory is orientation—the ability to locate one's self in one's environment with reference to time, place, and people (35). An individual who is disoriented demonstrates confusion about the date and/or time of day, where one is (place), who one is, and the identity of other individuals in the immediate environment. Disorientation is a severe deficit in memory and is a fairly common characteristic of some organic mental disorders.

Thought Processes

Thought processes or thinking refers to ways in which stored information is organized and processed—how it is combined, recombined, and manipulated (47). Information is rarely stored as isolated pieces of data. A piece of information tends to be integrated with other pieces of information to form meaningful wholes. These wholes or gestalts may be fairly stable or pieces of information may be separated from a gestalt and recombined with other pieces of information in an unlimited number of patterns.

There are three major ways in which information is processed: primary, secondary, and tertiary (47). Primary process thinking is characterized by disregard for formal logic. Temporal and spatial relationships are confused. One representation may fuse into others (condensation). Affect usually associated with one representation may become associated with another and/or one representation may come to stand for another (displacement). There is confusion regarding what is external and internal relative to the self. All events may be perceived as determined by the will of man or anthropomorphized forces (teleologic causality). Thinking cannot be reflected on after it has occurred. Primary process usually involves the organization of exocepts, images, endocepts, and denotative concepts. One representation often comes to stand for a whole aggregate of representations that have been grouped in some sort of a loose assemblage. Unconscious content, dreams, and fantasies are usually organized in a primary process manner.

Clinically, primary process may be seen in a phenomenon referred to as "loosening of associations." This phenomenon is described (35, pp. 361–362) as

> thinking characterized by speech in which ideas shift from one subject to another that is completely unrelated or only obliquely related without the speaker showing any awareness that the topics are unconnected. Statements that lack a meaningful relationship may be juxtaposed, or the individual may shift idiosyncratically from one frame of reference to another.

Primary process may also be evident in illogical thinking:

> thinking that contains clear internal contradictions or in which conclusions are reached that are clearly erroneous, given the initial premises.

Primary process thinking is characteristic of some of the psychotic disorders and often requires management.

In contrast, secondary process thinking is characterized by adherence to the rules of formal logic, attention to temporal and spatial relationships, lack of condensation and displacement, knowledge regarding what is internal and external relative to the self, reflectivity, and a search for the antecedent, physical cause of an effect (deterministic causality). Secondary process usually involves the organization of connotative concepts (although denotative concepts and images are occasionally organized in this manner as well). Secondary process is predominant in the organization of conscious and preconscious content. It is not a very stable process and is liable to disruption by experiences that arouse strong feelings.

Tertiary process thinking involves a combining of primary and secondary process organization. Mental content is subjected to primary process organization and becomes, in a sense, recombined or restructured. The newly organized content is then subjected to validation by secondary process organization. This is believed to be the essence of the creative process—a process leading to an end product that transcends the common responses of the individual's cultural group and brings about a desirable enlargement of human experience. It involves a temporary freedom from usual and ordinary secondary process organization. The creative product must, however, be compatible with secondary process; if it is not, the product is bizarre, not creative.

Primary, secondary, and tertiary process thinking are by no means mutually exclusive. In the course of a day most people probably engage in all three in various admixtures.

Levels of Conceptualization

Secondary process thinking can be viewed as being on a continuum from concrete to abstract. The polar ends of the continuum will be discussed here (47,302,985). Concrete thinking is characterized by concentration on one aspect of an object or event (centration), concern for the specifics or particulars of an item or thing without consideration of its relationships or classification, reaction to the immediate given object in the here and now, a reasoning sequence that moves from the particular to the particular, and concern for only the denotative meaning of objects. A person who thinks in a concrete manner would interpret the proverb "people who live in glass houses should not throw stones" in a literal manner with no concern for the other meanings the proverb might have (278,937).

In contrast, abstract thinking is characterized by decentration, cognitive or mental flexibility, the ability to apply concepts to a variety of related situations (generalization) and to classify objects in a number of ways, the capacity to perceive the viewpoint of others and to deal in the realm of the hypothetical. A person who thinks in an abstract manner might interpret the proverb stated above as "people who have done something wrong should not accuse others of the same wrong doing." Concrete thinking tends to be more typical of children whereas most adults are able to engage in at least some abstract thought. Degree of anxiety and intelligence are also factors that influence the ability to engage in abstract thinking.

Intelligence

Most definitions of intelligence in one way or another include three factors: the ability to deal with tasks involving abstractions, the ability to learn, and the ability to manage new situations. One succinct definition of intelligence is "the ability to undertake activities that are characterized by difficulty, complexity, abstractness, economy, adaptiveness to a goal, social value, and the emergence of originals" (268, p. 268). A more operational definition is "the individual's total repertory of those problem solving and cognitive-discrimination responses that are usual and expected at any given age level and in the large population unit to which he belongs" (268, p. 268). English, who provided this operational definition, continues by stating that

> the "usual and expected" response has been defined, by implication of test standardization, as one in which 65 percent to 75 percent of the given population are capable. What is thus usual and expected changes qualitatively as well as quantitatively with age and with the population;... intelligence level is measured by the proportion of the responses usual and expected in the population, that an individual manifests in a standardized sample of task-demand situations.... This definition leaves open the question of the organization of these responses. (268, p. 269)

Intelligence is an important factor in an individual's capacity to comprehend—the process of understanding the nature or meaning of objects and events; the process of knowing. It is the ability to grasp basic ideas. Individuals' capacity to learn is influenced by their general level of comprehension. It influences the rate of learning, the degree to which information or skills to be learned need to be broken down or separated into component parts, the ability to follow directions, and the complexity of tasks that can be mastered (376).

The majority of clients with whom occupational therapists work are of average intelligence. Persons who deviate from the norm at the high end of the continuum usually experience few problems in adaptation that are specifically related to intelligence. However, those who deviate toward the low end of the continuum do experience such problems. Thus, the remainder of this section defines mental retardation.

Mental retardation is characterized by "(1) significant subaverage general intellectual functioning, (2) resulting in, or associated with, deficits or impairments in adaptive behavior, (3) with onset before the age of 18" (35, p. 36). Operationally, individuals are described as mentally retarded if their general intellectual functioning as defined by an intelligence quotient (IQ) is 70 or below. Individuals with an IQ somewhat higher than 70 may be diagnosed as mentally retarded if there is a marked deficit in adaptive behavior. Conversely, individuals with an IQ somewhat below 70 may not be diagnosed as mentally retarded if there is no evidence of deficit in adaptive function.

Adaptive behavior, as used in the definition of mental retardation, "refers to the effectiveness with which an individual meets the standards of personal independence and social responsibility expected of his age and cultural group" (35, p. 36). There are several scales designed to measure adaptive behavior in a quantitative manner. None of these, however, are sufficiently reliable or valid to be used exclusively. Thus, considerable clinical judgment must be exercised in determining whether there is deficit in adaptive behavior. Mental retardation is sometimes, but not always, associated with other mental disorders and/or conditions that interfere with motor function. Most individuals, diagnosed as mentally retarded, need a variety of special services, including educational programs, protection, supervision, and financial support. Occupational therapists working with the mentally retarded are primarily concerned with increasing adaptive behavior and intervention relative to associated disorders and conditions. Meeting health needs, maintenance, and management are also a significant part of intervention.

Factual Information

Factual information is data about past and current events, the nature of people and objects, community institutions and resources, and requirements for self-maintenance. It refers to an individual's general fund of knowledge about the environment in which he exists and the social systems to which he belongs. It refers to an understanding about how things work, how to go about doing a particular task, how to get things done. Knowledge as used here refers to practical information as opposed to abstract knowledge that is not widely used in day-to-day interactions. It is concerned with survival. Examples of knowledge as used here are an understanding of how to shop for food, deposit and withdraw money from the bank, vote, follow a road map, find an indoor swimming pool, and get someone to repair a broken refrigerator.

The extent of an individual's general fund of knowledge is to some degree related to his or her level of intelligence, but the correlation is only moderate. It is more closely related to the individual's past experience in negotiating, using, and manipulating the environment. It is also influenced by cultural background, the degree to which an individual has lived in a sheltered environment, and the opportunity to be an independent, self-reliant, and self-directed person.

An individual may have a relatively broad fund of general information and not act on the basis of that information. This may be due to lack of skill or other emotional and/or physical limitations that impede adaptive use of the information. Lack of skill and other impediments are important, but not a part of factual information as defined here. Major deficits in general information are sometimes mistakenly attributed to some type of dysfunction in the psychological or social sphere. There may indeed be deficits in these areas but a deficit should not be assumed without assessment of an individual's general fund of practical knowledge.

Problem Solving

Problem solving is the process of selecting, planning, implementing, and evaluating a course of action that will adequately eliminate some difficulty encountered in the environment. As discussed here, problem solving refers to both difficulties encountered in the performance of a task or activity and difficulties encountered in coping with and handling situations in the wider environment (29). Problem solving may be overt as in the actual trial and error manipulation of objects or it may be covert. In the latter case, the individual determines the best course of action by thinking about various solutions or means of attaining a goal. In a manner of speaking, covert problem solving takes place in one's head whereas overt problem solving takes place on the table. Problem solving will be presented here as a sequential process: problem definition, identification of alternative solutions, decision making/goal setting, planning/organizing, and implementation. It is important to note, however, that problem solving rarely takes place in this direct, linear manner. More frequently the process is discontinuous, redoubled, and circuitous.

One component of problem solving—evaluation or judgment—is evident throughout the process. Evaluation involves critical analysis of the situation or information at hand, asscssing, appraising, and arriving at some conclusion as to the efficacy of a particular course of action. Judgment involves the same process as evaluation but also connotes an additional factor. One's judgment may be described as good or poor. Good judgment implies that a decision was made on the basis of common sense, with discretion and prudence; that it was made with wisdom.

Problem Definition

Problems that are not well defined are rarely adequately solved. Thus, the initial step in problem solving is to define the nature of the difficulty. Ideally, problems are solved in such a way that some action is implied if not called for. One of the major difficulties in problem definition is identification of the actual or substantive problem as opposed to a subordinate aspect of the problem or a problem tangential to the actual problem. Adequate problem identification has been described as the step that takes one halfway to problem solution.

Identification of Alternative Solutions

Subsequent to problem definition various solutions to the problem are formulated and entertained. The major difficulty encountered at this step is the lack of creative searching for solutions. Divergent or unusual solutions may either not be identified or, if identified, not considered. The range of possible solutions becomes constricted.

Decision Making/Goal Setting

Decision making is the process of selecting the best possible solution given the circumstances. Prior to selection, the pool of possible solutions is often narrowed, with the most improbable solutions being eliminated. The decision is then made from the remaining available choices. Decision making often involves a compromise in that the preferred solution may not be feasible in a given situation. Goal setting is usually subsequent to decision making and is a restatement of the decision in terms of what is actually to be accomplished. Goals are often set in relationship to time and the quality and/or quantity of what is to be accomplished.

Planning/Organizing

This phase of problem solving involves determining what needs to be done to reach the defined goal. Often a plan is devised that describes each sequential step to be taken. Planning involves some degree of organization: the setting of priorities; the scheduling of time; arrangements of people and things; ordering events; and seeing to it that resources, tools, and materials are available when needed.

Implementation

This final stage of problem solving involves carrying out the predetermined plan of action. Some of the important factors included in implementation are: working at a rate that is appropriate to the situation, giving appropriate attention to detail, neatness, and following the "rules" or specified directions if such is required. Of primary importance is the ability to follow through with plans so as to reach the desired goal. Lack of follow-through is probably the major reason goals are not attained. There are factors other than cognitive that impinge on follow-through. One of the major factors is psychological function, discussed next.

PSYCHOLOGICAL FUNCTION

Psychological function is the ability to process information from past events and information currently available from the environment in such a way as to view one's self, others, and one's life situation realistically.

The division between cognitive function and psychological function is, at best, a bit vague. Placing an aspect of human function in one area as opposed to the other is more by convention than by specific criteria. It appears, however, that aspects of human function identified as cognitive are fairly closely related to memory and intellectual capacity. In common usage, cognitive function is the ability to think and problem solve in a rational manner. On the other hand, psychological functions are influenced by and/or derived from the emotional, feeling part of the human experience. They are that element of the individual which, again in common usage, is seen as particularly "human."

Dynamic States

Dynamic states refers to needs, values, emotions, interests, and motivation. The term "dynamic states" is used to indicate that these aspects of the individual are often ever-changing and responsive to environmental influences. However, they are also often stable over a long period of time. The degree of stability may be one indicator of general mental health or optimal adaptation. This is not always the case; flexibility is also indicative of mental health and an asset in adaptation. There are also times in the life cycle—in particular adolescence and "midlife reevaluation"—when marked change in dynamic states is typical and supportive of continued growth.

Needs

Needs are inherent predispositions. Their existence or presence directs individuals to engage in activities that will sustain life (of the organism and the species), to be involved in the human community, and to maximize personal potential (193,268). Needs are considered to be inherent as opposed to learned or acquired. All individuals arrive in this world with the same collection of basic needs. In the process of development, these needs are elaborated and refined so that as adults, individuals may often describe their needs in a fairly idiosyncratic manner. Also, as adults, individuals establish various priorities relative to their needs. The satisfaction of a particular need, for example, may be seen as very important to one person but of far less importance to another.

Inherent needs have been described in a number of ways. Perhaps the best known systematic presentation is the one outlined by Maslow (648). He identifies a set of five basic needs and places them in a hierarchical structure. First are physiological needs, those needs that are basic to the maintenance of life, including the need for air, food, shelter, sleep, an optional amount of sensory stimuli and motor activity, and the release of sexually induced tensions. Second are safety needs, the need to be in an environment that is experienced as relatively free of harm-inducing elements: harm in both the physical and psychological sense. Third are love and belonging needs, the need to be loved and accepted because one is a unique and special person; to be accepted for what one is, not for what one has done or will do. Fourth are esteem needs, the need to receive respect from others for doing, for acting in relationship to the environment in a meaningful and productive manner; the need to be recognized for accomplishments. Fifth are self-actualization needs, the need to be one's self, to do and accomplish something of particular importance to one's self.

Maslow describes the above needs as hierarchical: that lower level needs, such as physiological and safety needs, must be satisfied before an individual can give attention to higher level needs such as esteem and self-actualization. However, there may be evidence of attention to higher level needs while the individual is primarily concerned with satisfying lower level needs.

To this list of needs most occupational therapists would add the need for mastery. This, as described by White, is the desire to explore, understand, and, to some extent, control one's self, other people, and the nonhuman environment (1014–1016). It is the need to be competent, to be the master of . . . something. If placed in the above hierarchy, the need for mastery would fall between love and belonging needs and esteem needs.

Needs were previously described as inherent. There are, however, learned aspects to needs. First, a person must learn what his needs are. Many people have a vague feeling of frustration because they are not satisfying one or several of their needs. Lack of satisfaction in this case is not due to environmental deprivation or deficit in ability. Rather a person does not know that a need is not being satisfied. For example, some people say they are bored when their real difficulty is that they are not satisfying their need for mastery. Second, after identifying what a need is, individuals must learn how to meet their needs in a socially acceptable manner: in an appropriate way, at the right time, in an acceptable setting. To learn how to identify and satisfy needs, an individual must experience both need gratification and an optimal amount of need deprivation. Optimal refers to a degree of need deprivation that allows the individual to be aware that a need is not being met, but not so much deprivation that strong negative feelings are experienced.

People meet their needs in a variety of different ways. A particular activity may satisfy one need for one person and a different need for another person. An activity may satisfy one particular need for an individual or it may satisfy multiple needs. In the latter case, the individual is likely to gain considerable pleasure through participating in that activity.

Health needs were previously described as inherent human needs which, when satisfied, allow an individual to experience a sense of physical, psychological, and social well-being. These needs are the same as the needs that have just been described. They were simply identified as "health" needs to differentiate such needs from those that arise from the consequence of physical or psychosocial dysfunction.

Emotions

Emotions are inner, subjective responses to need satisfaction and need deprivation (268). Similar to needs, emotions are considered to be inherent, not acquired or learned. Emotions arise not only from the objective degree of satisfaction and deprivation but are also relative to the person's view of the situation. Emotions are both positive and negative.

Positive emotions arise from or are responses to need fulfillment. They are described here as satisfaction, joy, liking, and love. Satisfaction is the response to need fulfillment that is considered acceptable by the individual. Joy is the response to an above average degree of need fulfillment. Liking is the response to a person, thing, or event that is associated with an acceptable degree of need satisfaction. Love is the response to a person that provides a much higher than average degree of need fulfillment. When love is experienced, the need-fulfilling aspect of the person becomes secondary. The person comes to be needed because he or she is loved rather than loved because he or she is needed. In order for positive emotions to be experienced, the individual must expect that need fulfillment will continue. One, for example, rarely feels liking for a person who satisfies love and belonging needs only on rare occasions.

Negative emotions are associated with need deprivation. They are here described as dissatisfaction, fear and anxiety, dislike, hatred, anger, and depression. Dissatisfaction is the response to need deprivation. Fear and anxiety are responses to anticipated loss of need satisfaction. Fear may be distinguished from anxiety in that the response is to "a consciously recognized and usually external threat or danger" (35, p. 354). Anxiety, on the other hand, is "the anticipation of danger, the source of which is largely unknown. . . . The manifestations of fear and anxiety are the same and include motor tension, autonomic hyperactivity, apprehensive expectations, vigilance, and scanning" (35, p. 354). Anger is the response to need deprivation when the individual believes that he has a right to need fulfillment. Dislike and hatred are degrees of negative feeling about a person or situation seen as need depriving or potentially depriving. Depression is a response to the loss of a need-fulfilling person, thing, or situation, or the response to the loss of a highly regarded personal attribute, capacity, social role, or life expectation. It occurs when the individual believes there is no substitute for what has been lost. Depression is characterized by lack "of interest or pleasure in all or almost all usual activities and pastimes" (268, p. 145).

Guilt and shame are also usually considered to be negative emotions. However, rather than being related to need deprivation, they are responses to an attempt to or actual fulfillment of needs in a manner that is unacceptable to the individual. Guilt is experienced when an individual acts (or thinks) in a manner which is contrary to his personal values regarding what is right or wrong. Shame is experienced when an individual acts in a manner that is unacceptable to a person the individual holds in high regard. The same act may arouse both guilt and shame.

As mentioned, emotional responses are inherent; they are not learned. However, learning is associated with emotions. One element that is learned or acquired is one's ideas about a situation. Through interaction in the environment, an individual comes to view a variety of people, things, and events as need satisfying or need depriving. An individual's ideas about and understanding of a situation will influence the type of emotional response evoked by the situation.

Emotional responses are an internal experience. Emotional expression is the outward manifestation of an emotional response. Emotional expression is learned. An individual expresses emotions adequately when the overt manifestation of emotions is sufficient to inhibit formation of an uncomfortable amount of internal tension and sufficiently controlled so as not to interfere significantly with current or future need fulfillment.

Closely related to the concept of emotion are the concepts of affect, mood, and feeling. Affect is "an immediately expressed and observed emotion." An emotion "becomes an affect when it is observable . . . as overall demeanor or tone and modulation of voice" (35, p. 353). A range of affect may be described as broad (normal), constricted, blunt, or flat. What is considered the normal range of affect expression varies considerably, both within and among different cultures. The normal expression of affect involves variability in facial expression, pitch of voice, and the use of body movements. Constricted affect is characterized by a clear reduction in expressive range and intensity of affect. Blunted affect is marked by a severe reduction in the intensity of affective expression. When affect is described as flat there is almost no sign of affective expression; the voice may be monotonous and the face immobile. Affect is inappropriate when it is clearly not congruent with what the individual is saying, or the reality of the situation. "Affect is labile when it is characterized by repeated, rapid, and abrupt shifts . . . without readily apparent reason" (35, p. 353).

> Mood is a pervasive and sustained emotion that, in the extreme, markedly colors the person's perception of the world. Common terms to describe mood are depression, elation, anger and anxiety. In the dysfunctional range mood may be described as dysphoric, euphoric, expansive or irritable. Dysphoric refers to a profound unpleasant mood such as depression or anxiety. A euphoric mood is an exaggerated feeling of well-being that is far beyond simply being very happy or cheerful. Expansive mood refers to lack of restraint in expressing one's feelings, frequently with an over-evaluation of one's significance or importance. An irritable mood is an internalized feeling of tension associated with being easily annoyed and provoked to anger" (35, pp. 363–364).

Feelings refer to ideas that are strongly influenced by emotions. There is an intimate association between the ideas and the emotion so that it is difficult for the person to differentiate or separate the two. In illustration, when an individual "expresses his feelings" one is not likely to hear a dispassionate presentation of objective facts.

Values

Values are the degree of worth ascribed to a person, thing, activity, or idea. The words right and wrong, good and bad, should and should not are statements of values (268). Values are described as being on a continuum: high positive, low positive, low negative, high negative. It is assumed here that an individual places some value on everything: thus there is no neutral point on the continuum. Although an individual may claim indifference to a particular person, idea, and so forth, this is rarely the case. However, individuals may not be aware of what value they have placed on a particular thing. The sum total of an individual's values is referred to as a system of values. The tendency to ascribe some degree of worth is inherent; the particular value assigned to a person, thing, activity, or idea is learned.

Values are acquired through direct experience and from persons or groups of persons who are important to the individual. Because of these two ways of acquiring values, and because values are acquired throughout one's life, an individual may have a value system that is not internally consistent. Thus, an individual may assign both a positive and negative value to the same thing. This is referred to as ambivalence or, in more common terms, as "mixed feelings." An individual's values are strongly influenced by the cultural environment in which the individual was raised or currently resides. These cultural values may be in conflict with the values of the wider culture or they may be in conflict with one's own personal values. In either case the individual may have some difficulty resolving or tolerating this situation.

Interest

Interest refers to a person, thing, event, or idea that concerns, involves, draws the attention, or arouses the curiosity of a person (268). Interests are those things that occupy an individual's mind, energy, and/or time. They may be of short duration or sustained for a long period of time. Interests often predispose an individual to engage in activities for their own sake and because of the pleasure derived from the activity. Interest does not, however, necessarily imply engagement or involvement. One can, for example, be interested in traveling but not have the time and/or financial resources to travel. One may be interested in physical fitness but never get around to establishing a daily routine that includes exercise. Most individuals have a variety of interests that they pursue. An individual who has few if any interests or does not pursue any particular interest either engages in little activity or in highly repetitive and stereotyped activity. Such an individual is said to have a poverty of interests.

Motivation

Motivation is "a specific hypothesized process that energizes differentially certain responses, thus making them dominant over other possible responses to the same situation. . . . it is the determiner of the direction and or strength of action or a line of action" (268, p. 330). This is only one of several definitions of motivation. Most definitions make use of two pivotal concepts: need and goal. Need in this case refers to a lack or deficiency in the person. Goal is described as the end result, "a state or condition which, when attained, brings to an end a direct course of behavior action" (268, p. 330). It is implied that the behavior or action is directed toward eliminating the need state of the individual.

Motivation has been described as being either intrinsic or extrinsic. Intrinsic motivation prompts a person to act on the basis of the satisfaction or incentive conditions that lie within or are obtained from the activity itself. Extrinsic motivation is "behavior controlled through the possibility of a reward or punishment external to whatever satisfactions or annoyances reside in the behavior itself: e.g., working for a prize rather than for satisfaction in the task itself." However, as English states,

> The distinction is by no means as absolute as it sounds. Any complex situation affords both extrinsic and intrinsic motivational elements. Moreover, a motivation at first extrinsic may come to be intrinsic: i.e., an activity first engaged in for outside satisfaction becomes itself satisfying (268, p. 330).

An individual may be aware of the factor(s) that prompt him to engage in specific activities. There is a consciously sought goal that the individual believes determines his behavior. Conversely, the individual may not be aware of the factor(s) that prompt his actions. This is referred to an unconscious motivation. Although a distinction is made between conscious and unconscious motivation, most complex activities are probably initiated and guided by both conscious and unconscious factors.

Intrapsychic Dynamics

Intrapsychic dynamics refers to the phenomena of conscious and unconscious, psychodynamics, and defense mechanisms (268). The term "intrapsychic dynamics" is used to indicate that the processes included in this category take place within the individual's mind, within the psyche. This is not to imply in any way that these processes are not influenced by the external environment: they are strongly influenced by other people and events. Dynamic refers to the fact that these are active processes that are usually in a continuous state of fluctuation or change.

Conscious and Unconscious

The conscious-unconscious continuum has been formulated to classify an individual's degree of attention to immediate external and internal stimuli, memory traces, and processes. For our purposes here these concepts will be further subdivided into conscious, preconscious, personal unconscious, and collective unconscious. Conscious is "a division of the psyche that includes those parts of mental life of which the person is momentarily aware" (268, p. 112). Preconscious includes those parts of mental life that are not in immediate awareness but can be recalled or focused on by the individual without undue effort.

Personal unconscious is a division of the psyche that includes those parts of mental life of which the person is not aware and is unable to become aware of directly without considerable effort. Unconscious has also been defined by the nature of its content. Two types of content are described: (a) formerly conscious ideas or processes that have been expelled (repressed) from the realm of the conscious; and (b) certain primordial and infantile wishes and impulses that have never gained access to the conscious realm (317,492,838).

Collective unconscious is "that part of the individual's unconscious which is inherited and which the individual shares with other members of the species" (268, p. 570). As described by Jung, the collective unconscious contains archaic memory traces that are common to all mankind and are not part of the personal experience of the individual (161,492). As used here, memory traces are not representative of past events. The individual is not born with remembrances of the collective history of the human race. What is hypothesized rather is the genetic transmission of ways of organizing information around common life experiences and ways of expressing these experiences. What is inherited then is the structuring potential of the central nervous system and not any specific information. The common life experiences that are organized and expressed in and through the collective unconscious are the major questions, changes, and anxieties with which mankind has been concerned throughout its history: birth, death, role transitions, youth, old age, leadership, fertility, hunger, disease, evil, afterlife, and cosmic forces, to name just a few. Archaic memory traces often emerge through and influence the formation of symbols, a process discussed in Chapter 10.

The unconscious, particularly the personal unconscious, has often been maligned as being the refuge for lethal forces and profoundly unacceptable ideas, best to be disowned or at least ignored. Regardless of one's particular philosophical or theoretical orientation, there is considerable evidence that there are ideas or thoughts and mental processes that occur outside one's immediate awareness. If the content and processes of the unconscious are considered to be bad or destructive, they probably will be experienced in that manner. It is thus probably wisest to think of the unconscious as neutral, as a natural phenomenon. Like all parts of nature, it can be used to further adaptation or misused to impede adaptation. The unconscious is only overwhelming when it is excluded from life.

Finally, there is a dynamic relationship between collective and personal unconscious, preconscious, and conscious. There is a continual flow of information between these arbitrary divisions of the psyche that affects and is affected by the individual's interaction within the environment.

Psychodynamics

"Psychodynamics" is a term used to identify systems for explaining behavior in terms of motives, needs, impulses, and so on (268). There are several different systems based on various theoretical orientations. The different systems will not be described here but rather focus will be on their common elements. A given system of psychodynamics attempts to explain the relationship between the individual's environment (past and present), mental life (process and content of the conscious, preconscious, personal and collective unconscious), and the individual's behavior. Systems of psychodynamics are also concerned with describing how conscious mental content becomes unconscious, the mechanisms for maintaining content in the unconscious, and how unconscious content influences behavior. Behavior sometimes appears irrational to an individual or an observer, i.e., not able to be explained by objective knowledge of the situation. A psychodynamic explanation of apparently irrational behavior gives meaning to that behavior by referring to hypothesized or identified unconscious content that is believed to motivate the behavior. Although a somewhat simplistic description, using a particular system of psychodynamics, an expert, given a gestalt of typical behavior, can fairly accurately predict the nature of the behaving individual's unconscious content. The converse is also true: given knowledge of unconscious content, an expert can fairly accurately predict an individual's behavior.

The common concepts used in almost all systems of psychodynamics are: conflict, repression, and defense mechanisms. Conflict is the "simultaneous functioning of opposing or mutually exclusive impulses, desires or tendencies" (268, p. 110). The discordance may be between opposed desires or between desires and prohibitions. One of the desires or the prohibitions may be conscious, but more typically the entire set of ideas that constitute the conflict is unconscious. The conflict in whole or in part may have been conscious at one time. However, it caused such a degree of anxiety that the individual "puts it out of mind" to such an extent that it is relegated to the unconscious. This process is referred to as repression: "the exclusion of specific psychological activity or content from conscious awareness by a process of which the individual is not directly aware" (268, p. 458). Repression is not only the exclusion of processes and ideas but also refers to maintaining this content in an unconscious state. Although unconscious conflicts are out of awareness, they continue to be expressed in the formation of symbols and in behavior. Unconscious conflicts are not unique to individuals who are described as having some type of neurotic or psychotic disorder. All individuals have a number of unconscious conflicts. The difference is in severity and the extent to which the conflicts lead to bizarre, stereotyped, or maladaptive behavior. Unconscious conflicts within a "normal" range give flavor to the individual. They contribute to making the individual unique, intriguing, and stimulating.

Defense Mechanisms

"Defense mechanism" is a term used to identify the various ways in which people maintain conflicts and other psychic content in an unconscious state. As used here, defense refers to "any activity, including thinking and feeling, designated to shut out of awareness any unpleasant or shameful or anxiety-arousing fact or one that threatens self-esteem." A defense mechanism

> is usually (if not always) unconscious—that is it is not intentionally acquired, and it operates automatically, without voluntary inception or control and without a conscious signal that it is operating. Its presence is betrayed by an otherwise unexplainable lack of relationship between the circumstances and behavior. Even quite unimaginative persons have ingenious defenses (268, p. 140).

Repression, previously described, is a defense mechanism and perhaps the most common. Other types of defense mechanisms are, to name a few: rationalization, projections, overcompensation, denial, reaction formation, alienation, withdrawal, emotional insulation, fantasy, projection, and sublimation. Defense mechanisms in their manifest form tend to express the nature of the unconscious conflict albeit in a disguised and oblique manner. In addition, the nature of some defense mechanisms allows at least partial satisfaction of suppressed desires or needs. Similar to unconscious conflicts, defense mechanisms are universal. All people engage in a variety of defensive maneuvers. They are a healthy means of dealing with intrapsychic content and facilitate adaptation. Indeed, an individual is severely disabled by a threatened or actual breakdown of a major portion of his or her defensive structure. Defense mechanisms are maladaptive only when they influence a major portion of the individual's repertoire of behavior.

Reality Testing

Reality is a difficult concept to define. Philosophically, reality as an independent entity does not exist. It is a phenomenon that exists only through the collective beliefs and values of a particular social system (95). It is not necessarily consistent, at least in its totality, between or across social systems or within the subparts of a social system. Reality has an elusive, ever-changing quality. Thus, an individual who is not a member of a closely knit, highly structured, primarily static social system is, throughout his life cycle, continually defining and redefining reality, that of the external environment and of his own inner world.

Reality will be defined in this text as if it existed as an independent concrete entity. Reality is "the actual environment objectively considered: the physical, the economic, and the interpersonal factors (including the 'real' attitudes and emotions of others) . . . the totality of that which can not be merely wished or thought away" (268, p. 242). Reality testing is the process of active experimentation to determine the nature of the environment and the conditions imposed by that environment on the individual's activities. It also includes assessing whether one's private, subjective ideas have any validity in the shared reality of the environment.

An individual with adequate reality testing has an awareness of the demands of the environment and makes adjustments in behavior to meet these demands in such a way that he ultimately secures satisfaction of needs. "When there is gross impairment in reality testing, the individual incorrectly evaluates the accuracy of his or her perceptions and thoughts and makes incorrect inferences about external reality even in the face of contrary evidence" (268, p. 242). Unshared conscious or preconscious content is often not subjected to reality testing. As such it frequently provides an inaccurate and inadequate guide for developing a self-concept or for interacting with the environment.

Insight

Insight may be defined either as a relatively permanent characteristic of the individual, as a state; or it may be defined as a process. As a state, insight is a "reasonable understanding of and evaluation of one's own mental processes, reactions, abilities; self-knowledge" (268, p. 264). It is a conscious understanding of the meaning and purpose of one's behavior. In clinical situations, insight is often used to refer to the degree of awareness or understanding an individual has in relationship to his own problems. It is the greater or less understanding of one's true condition when there is general evidence that one is in a state of physical or psychosocial dysfunction (278).

As a process, insight involves developing conscious awareness of the meaning or significance of pattern of interaction with people, things, or situations. It includes discovering the relationship between past and current events in one's own life and the relationship between one's own ideas or thoughts and the ways in which one interacts with the human and nonhuman environment. The process entails a considerable amount of self-observation and self-reflection and is usually facilitated by consistent and accurate feedback from others. The end result of this process, the gaining of new insight, may happen suddenly and be accompanied by a sense of surprise and wonder. On the other hand, it may be a gradual progression toward understanding unaccompanied by any profound emotional feelings.

Object Relations

The term "object relations" refers to the investment of emotions and psychic energy in objects for the purpose of satisfying needs (124,125,281,316,317,549,875, 876,923). There are several concepts that are used in the explanation of object relations. Objects are any human being (including the self), abstract concept, or nonhuman thing which has the potential for satisfying needs or interfering with need satisfaction. The individual seeks need-satisfying objects and attempts to eliminate objects that interfere with satisfaction. "Eliminate" is used here to describe the act of dealing with or manipulating interfering objects so that they no longer impede need satisfaction. The ways in which human objects satisfy needs or interfere with satisfaction are probably evident to the reader; it may not, however, be as evident in the case of abstract and nonhuman objects. Abstract objects are values or ideas. They are referred to as abstract because they are intangible and are typically given form through the use of language. Examples of need-satisfying abstract objects are value judgments regarding people, events, or particular actions; concepts such as democracy and peace; religious beliefs; ideas we have about what kind of person we are; and particular explanations regarding human behavior. Abstract objects may interfere with need satisfaction. Particular ideas that we have about ourselves, for example, may lead us to act in such a way that we are unable to satisfy our need for esteem. Examples of nonhuman objects that satisfy various needs are: food, toys, pets, a home, tools used in one's work, momentos of pleasant experiences, and gifts that one has received. Examples of nonhuman objects that may interfere with need satisfaction are dirty dishes, a broken appliance, a book that is difficult to comprehend, or street noises that interfere with concentration.

Drive is in many ways similar to motivation, which was defined earlier. (However, the concept of drive, not motive, is used in the theory of object relations.) Drive is defined as a person's active effort to seek need satisfaction and to deal with factors that interfere with satisfaction. Drives are conceptualized as being quantities of psychic energy that arise from the biological functioning of the organism. This energy is considered to be limited. Thus, it must be utilized in an economical manner if one is to satisfy all of one's needs. If excessive energy is utilized in satisfying one need, the individual is unable to satisfy other needs. Thus, he is less effective in adapting to the environment.

Two drives have been identified: libidinal and aggressive. Libidinal drive, plus an experienced need, activates the individual to seek objects that will satisfy that need. Objects that are need satisfying are said to be invested with libidinal energy; such an investment helps to ensure continual satisfaction of the need. There is, therefore, a dynamic relationship between an experienced need, libidinal drive, and the need-satisfying object. Aggressive drive is invested in objects that interfere with need satisfaction (44,621,699). It serves to focus the individual's attention on the need-inhibiting objects and to mobilize and sustain various behaviors that will be effective in eliminating the interfering object. Aggressive drive is here viewed as a positive energy utilized for creative adaptation to the environment. The investment of libidinal or aggressive drives in an object is referred to as the formation of an object-relationship. An object invested with libidinal drive is referred to as a libidinal object, whereas an aggressive object is a person, nonhuman thing, or abstract concept that has been invested with aggressive energy.

Aggressive objects do not necessarily have belligerent or antagonistic characteristics. That is, the objects in and of themselves are not destructive or injury producing. They are referred to as aggressive objects only because they are invested with an individual's aggressive energy. Elimination of aggressive objects as mentioned does not mean destruction of or injury to the object. It refers rather to removal of the object as an obstacle to need satisfaction. The individual's manipulation of aggressive objects is regulated by abstract libidinal objects (personal value system and/or the norms of his cultural groups). Libidinal and aggressive energy may be invested in the same object. For example, to a teenager, a mother may be said to be invested with libidinal energy because of her capacity to gratify the need for love. At the same time, however, she may also act as an obstacle to gaining esteem from peers. Similarly, different aspects of one's work may gratify one's need for esteem and present obstacles to one's need for self-actualization. This dual investment gives rise to ambivalence or incompatible feelings about a particular object.

When libidinal and aggressive energy are invested in objects we speak of attached energy. However, energy may also be free-floating, unattached to objects, which in itself creates a need: the need for investment in objects. Free-floating energy is normally utilized to satisfy more mature needs, or it may be expended in action. Energy usually comes to be free-floating through need satisfaction. It appears that a considerable amount of energy is utilized in the process of seeking satisfaction, and during the initial period of forming an object relationship. Once a relationship has been established and does indeed lead to need satisfaction, it can be maintained with less energy expansion. Free-floating energy may also be present when no objects are identified as appropriate for need satisfaction or the objects interfering with need satisfaction cannot be identified. This is usually only a temporary situation for the normal individual.

The objects utilized for satisfaction of a particular need often change over time. This seems to be a function of initial satisfaction, idiosyncratic elaboration of needs, normal development, and the demands of the social system. Thus, the need for love may initially be satisfied by the parents. This need may be gratified later in the life cycle by friends and one's spouse. Objects that satisfy the need for mastery are different during the adolescent period than during the period of initial vocational stabilization. Although bread and butter may satisfy a need for food, steak may well be preferred.

An appropriate libidinal object is an object that satisfies a need and is considered acceptable according to the norms of one's culture. An inappropriate libidinal object is an object invested with libidinal energy but not experienced as need satisfying and/or not considered acceptable by one's culture. An example of the former would be the attempt to satisfy the need for love by libidinal investment in a teacher who gives approval only for completion of class assignments. Investment in the idea of terrorism might be an example of the latter. Appropriate aggressive objects are the true obstacles to a libidinal object. Objects not causally related to difficulty in obtaining libidinal objects are inappropriate aggressive objects.

Substitute libidinal objects are less-preferred objects that nevertheless lead to partial need satisfaction. A man, for example, may spend time with friends when his wife is out of town. Substitute aggressive objects are not the true obstacles to need satisfaction, but their manipulation leads one closer to the libidinal object.

An individual who has mature object relations has selected appropriate and substitute objects that satisfy his needs in such a manner that he is able to attend to his need for self-actualization. His object relations are diffuse; a particular need is satisfied through investment in a number of different objects. Investment in libidinal objects is relatively continual and involves the total as opposed to a part of the object. An individual who has immature object relations (this is typical of a child) has difficulty selecting appropriate and substitute objects. He is primarily concerned with needs other than the need for self-actualization. His libidinal object relations may be discontinuous; he invests in objects only when they are in the process of gratifying a particular need. He may have limited object relations in that one or only a few objects are perceived as need gratifying, or he may invest in only a part of an object rather than in the total object. An example of the latter (part object relations) may be seen in hero worship. Particular qualities of the hero figure are invested with libidinal energy. Other more human qualities are ignored and even perhaps unknown.

Self-Concept

Self-concept is used here as an umbrella term under which other related concepts are subsumed. These related concepts are identity, sexual identity, body image, knowledge of one's assets and limitations, and self-esteem. Self-concept refers to how one views one's self as a person, one's sense of self, one's knowledge about oneself, one's beliefs in regard to the self, the emotions one associates with the self, and the value or worth ascribed to the self (290,671). In discussion of the concepts subsumed under self-concept there is overlap between some of the concepts. These concepts were drawn from the occupational therapy literature where the various concepts many times are used interchangeably.

Identity

Identity is a sense of self, who one is, and where one fits into a scheme of significant others. It is made up of one's constitutional givens, idiosyncratic needs, favored capacities, significant identification with and attachment to others, effective and successful defenses, and consistent and important social roles. It is, however, not simply a collection of attributes but rather something greater than the sum of its parts. When established, identity provides the individual with a sense of psychosocial well-being, of being at home in one's body, a sense of knowing where one is going, an inner assuredness of receiving recognition from those people in one's life who are seen as important (271,928).

According to Erikson, an individual's identity is initially established at the end of adolescence (271). Prior to that time Erikson describes the individual as being in a state of identity diffusion. This state of being typical in adolescence is characterized by uncertainty about who one is; one day the individual is thus and so and the next day something else. It is a period of trying on various identities or roles as in a movie or play. The formation of an initial identity is believed to be necessary for taking on the tasks and responsibilities of adulthood.

The establishment of an initial identity is an important factor in the developmental process, but that initial identity is rarely maintained intact for the rest of one's life. Identity changes as the individual progresses through the life cycle. The change may be a gradual one, with identity slowly evolving over time. The individual may not be aware of the change unless it is called to her attention by someone else. One may also become aware of a gradual change in identity through experiencing something located in the past. One, for example, may return for a visit to one's home town after an extended absence or attend a high school reunion 20 years after graduation. There is, in such cases, often the sense of a considerable difference in identity between now and then. In contrast to an evolving change, there may be a sharp break in the continuum of identity. The individual is acutely aware of this change and has a sense of being very different, of being a new person. A sharp and substantial alteration of identity may be preceded by a period of identity diffusion and/or a moratorium. The latter refers to a temporary cessation of usual activities to allow one time for reflection and decision making. A substantial change in identity may occur at a time of a major personal problem or at a turning point in one's life. It may take place in the context of career change or alteration in one's family life or it may be related to a particular age that is personally significant to the individual.

The dynamics of initial development of identity and alterations in identity are not altogether clear. It is felt that inherent within human beings is an urge for integration or homeostasis: that the individual seeks to become a whole, not remain a collection of parts. The development of identity is influenced by the feedback one receives from people who are significant to the self (671). Identity, however, is more than a reflection of others' ideas about who and what one should be or is. A person is, nevertheless, more comfortable if her identity is similar to and/or compatible with the identity ascribed to her by others.

An individual's identity influences the choices she makes in regard to her life. Choices are usually made to be consistent with one's identity and in turn solidify and support identity. Knowledge of another person's identity helps one to understand the individual and the choices the individual makes. Finally, prolonged identity diffusion after the time when an initial identity is usually established or between relinquishing an old identity and taking on a new identity leads to anxiety, confusion, restlessness, and a general sense of personal discomfort. It also leads to a sense of perplexity and bewilderment on the part of individuals with whom the person regularly interacts.

Sexual Identity

Sexual identity, a component of the individual's total identity, is often defined separately for clarity. Sexual identity refers to an individual's awareness of, feelings about, and interactions with others as a sexual being. The last characteristic, "interaction with others as a sexual being," essentially moves into the domain of social interaction. However, because the social component of sexual identity is so intimately related to one's personal sense of sexuality, the two will not be separated here.

Sexual identity is usually initially established about the age of four or five and is pregenital in nature. Major changes in sexual identity typically occur at adolescence and in young adulthood but changes may also occur at other times in the life cycle. An individual is said to have a mature sexual identity when he or she perceives his or her own genital sexuality as good and comfortably participates in sustained sexual relationships with others that are oriented to the mutual satisfaction of sexual needs. An individual who has attained full maturation of sexual identity experiences delight relative to the sexual aspects of his or her body and the body of others. One perceives the genitalia and secondary sexual characteristics as a source of pleasure for the self and a means of providing pleasure for others. He or she is aware of the periodic need for the release of sexual tensions and the needs of the other with whom he or she is sexually involved. The needs of both partners are taken into consideration and regulate the extent and nature of sexual interaction. Various techniques relative to seduction, sex play, and intercourse have been learned and are used differentially to bring about mutual satisfaction. Diminished need for release of sexual tension, if it should occur in oneself or one's partner, is accepted with minimal alteration in one's perception of the self or one's partner as a sexual being.

As outlined above, sexual identity refers primarily to genital sexuality. In the past, sexual identity also included those aspects of sexuality typically referred to as masculinity and femininity (287). Specific nongenital, sex-related characteristics were associated with being appropriately masculine or feminine as a part of one's self-concept and in interactions with others. Sex-related characteristics are now viewed by many people as being primarily culturally based, having little relationship to inherent sexuality. For the most part, characteristics formerly viewed as sex related are now considered more appropriately shared by both sexes. However, there is by no means total agreement on this issue.

Body Image

Body image, as one component of self-concept, is the visual image one has of one's body and the emotions one attaches to that image (862). It is the sense of what one looks like and how one feels about one's perceived physical appearance. Body image is initially established when the child comes to perceive his or her body as a holistic entity differentiated from the surrounding human and nonhuman environment. Through vestibular, proprioceptive, tactile, and visual stimulation initiated by the self and significant others, the child comes to perceive the body's parts as they exist in relationship to each other, and in space and as part of a totality. This process occurs through sensory integration, as previously discussed, and is often referred to as the development of body scheme (58). Body scheme is a subcomponent of body image.

Concurrent with and subsequent to the development of a basic body scheme, familial and cultural values, norms, and attitudes regarding the body and body parts are transmitted to the child. This information, usually accepted without much question by the young child, leads to further development and consolidation of body image. An individual's body image is, however, continually altered during the life cycle. Major changes typically occur during the grade school years as the child develops and compares his or her degree of physical coordination, strength, and endurance to that of peers. The period of adolescence requires adjustment to rapid physical growth and the development of secondary sexual characteristics: all of this being infused with strong sexual urges. The aging process requires further adjustment to changes in physical appearance, strength, and agility.

There are two elements to body image: perception or ideas and emotions. Perceptions or ideas refer to how an individual views his body in its parts and as a holistic entity. The individual may perceive his body realistically: i.e., in a way that is similar to how others view his body. Or the individual may have a very inaccurate or distorted view of his body. Most people invest a considerable amount of emotional feelings or energy in their body. These emotions may be either negative or positive, with the typical situation being a mixture of the two. An individual is usually more comfortable with himself if more positive than negative emotions are invested in the body. In addition, and typically, emotional investment is not evenly distributed to all aspects of the body. Particular aspects of the body are often considered more important and thus invested with more emotional feeling. Other components of the body are invested with less feeling and still other components may be essentially ignored. Although body parts are differently invested with emotion, it must be remembered that most people view their body as an integrated holistic entity (704,839).

Knowledge of One's Assets and Limitations

This refers to an individual's understanding of those things in which he excels, those things he is able to do with a fair degree of skill, and those things he is unable to do. Assessment and understanding are relative to gross and fine motor skills, attractiveness, intellectual capacity, social skills, past achievements, capacity in various social roles, and current endeavors. This component of self-concept also includes the degree to which one accepts assets and limitations. With identification of limitations, the individual may or may not be motivated to alter these aspects of the self. Acceptance of limitations implies that the individual recognizes that his personal limitations do not reflect total ineptness: that all individuals have some deficits. Knowledge of assets and limitations is part of one's self-knowledge and thus could probably be considered part of insight. However, the capacity for insight is a far more global and complex ability.

Self-Esteem

Self-esteem is essentially the evaluative component of self-concept. It is the degree to which an individual ascribes worth to himself. People who deem themselves worthy perceive the self as deserving of need satisfaction, recognition, success, and some part of the good life. Self-esteem refers to an overall feeling the individual has about herself and not to any particular aspect of the self.

Self-Discipline

Self-discipline as a general concept refers to an individual's capacity to manage himself in the conduct of his daily affairs. Included in the idea of self-discipline are volition, self-control, self-responsibility and direction, and dealing with adverse experiences. These concepts are not necessarily mutually exclusive.

Volition

Volition refers to the deliberate, conscious choice of a course of action, the power of choosing and controlling one's own actions (282). Volition is closely related to the concept of will and no distinction between these two concepts will be made here. The concept of volition stands in juxtaposition to both the idea that the individual is driven by internal, mostly unconscious forces and the idea that the individual's behavior is primarily influenced by factors that exist in the external environment. Volition adds a third element to the explanation of human behavior. The idea of volition implies that the individual has the capacity to be self-controlling and make decisions about how he or she will behave. No attempt will be made here to resolve these three different theoretical and philosophical positions. Suffice it to say that in all likelihood each of the three explanations for behavior is probably accurate to some extent. The balance or degree of influence of internal forces, environmental requirement or demands, and volition probably varies from individual to individual and is also probably situationally related. Volition is here simply described as one aspect of psychological function. It involves the knowledgeable consideration of the various alternatives and deliberate selection of a preferred course of action.

Self-Control

Self-control refers to skill in modifying present behaviors and in initiating new behaviors in accordance with situational demands. As commonly used, self-control includes inhibiting behavior that an individual perceives as being detrimental or destructive to one's self and to others. It also implies the degree to which the individual feels mastery over the self as opposed to being driven by external or internal forces that are beyond the individual's capacity to influence. A moderate degree of self-control is usually seen as optimal. Too little self-control leads to a feeling of not being master of one's self. Too much self-control has the connotation of lacking spontaneity and flexibility.

Self-Responsibility and Direction

This refers to the individual's recognition of himself as capable of and accountable for his own need satisfaction, establishing personal goals, and selecting a preferred life style. The individual recognizes that needs can only be satisfied through one's own efforts and not simply because one deserves need satisfaction. There is a sense of independence from others in that the individual realizes that he must make his own decisions about his life, and not rely on others to determine his goals. This is undertaken with full realization that others may neither approve of nor support one's decision. However, the individual also realizes there are certain obligations to others that must be met. The individual "owns" his behavior and realizes that he is answerable for the consequence of that behavior.

Dealing with Adversity

This refers to dealing with three specific areas of stress: success/failure, frustration, and anxiety (29). Success has only recently been recognized as a source of stress for many people. Success often has many hidden or unconscious associations that make it less than a pleasant experience. Some of the most common associations are that (a) the success is not deserved, (b) success involves too many additional responsibilities, or (c) success will lead to loss of friendship because of envy or jealousy on the part of others. An individual who cannot deal with success may not seek recognition from others, deliberately remain anonymous in the group, and, if successful, may ultimately turn the success into failure. In dealing adequately with success, the individual accepts the risk inherent in doing something better than others. In managing failure, a more understandable source of stress, an individual accepts the failure as being relative to one aspect of life experience, and accurately judges the degree, extent, and consequences of the failure. The person does not allow the failure to engulf her total self-concept. Some people fear failure even without any extensive experience with it. Such people, similar to those who have difficulty with success, tend to engage in very little risk-taking behavior.

Dealing adequately with frustration requires the capacity to tolerate delay in need satisfaction and/or a somewhat extended period of need deprivation. Adaptation is often facilitated by seeking out and temporarily accepting partial satisfaction through other activities. Frustration can also arise in the context of engaging in an activity or doing a task. This is a sense of impatience at delays and/or difficulty in solving presented problems. Many people develop strategies such as setting time limits for engagement in frustrating tasks, taking a break from the activity, planning an enjoyable task subsequent to completion of the activity, and so forth.

People's capacity to tolerate anxiety is extremely variable; some can endure a great deal, others very little. The capacity is also often influenced by one's current life situation. There are two common ways of adequately dealing with anxiety that may be used singly or in combination. The individual may move in and attempt to defuse or eliminate the anxiety-provoking situation. This may lead to a temporary increase in anxiety, which can be tolerated because of the foreknowledge that there will be a marked decline in anxiety subsequently. The other common adaptive way of dealing with anxiety is to engage in constructive activities that occupy the mind with other matters. The term "constructive" was chosen to differentiate these types of activities from anxiety-reducing activities, which are or are potentially destructive for the individual or others; substance abuse, promiscuous sexual activity, and violence come immediately to mind. Constructive activities do not directly affect the anxiety-producing situation. They do, however, promote an emotional calmness that in turn facilitates rational and productive problem solving.

Concept of Others

The last area of psychological function to be described is concept of others. Concept of others as used here refers to the ideas an individual has about other people. These ideas can be categorized as being: about people in general, about particular classes or types of people, and ideas about specific people significant to the individual (671,938).

An individual's concept of self strongly influences his concept of others. If the individual sees himself as unacceptable or unworthy, for example, he may view others in a similar manner. Or he may perceive others as being the opposite of the self: as highly acceptable and worthy.

Of primary importance in concept of others is whether the individual perceives others as basically trustworthy: as willing to share, provide assistance, not deliberately inflict pain or harm. When an individual sees others as trustworthy, the interpersonal environment is experienced as a safe place in which to interact. When an individual does not see others as trustworthy, he often develops additional negative ideas about others. They may be viewed as critical, hostile, competitive, seductive, and so forth. Finally, the individual may be uncertain about whether people are trustworthy. At times, the individual acts as if others are trustworthy, at other times as if untrustworthy. This often leads to an approach/avoidance manner of interacting that is usually thoroughly confusing to others.

The above discussion focused on perception of people in general. An individual may categorize all people as similar, with no distinctions made between classes or types, or the individual may have a differential concept of others. With a differential concept of others, people often make a distinction between those perceived as being in authority positions versus those seen as peers. Peers may be seen as relatively benign, whereas authority figures may be seen as controlling, detached, unsympathetic, and arbitrary. Aside from a distinction between authority figures and peers, an individual may classify people in a variety of other ways: race, religion, socioeconomic level, sex, age, and so forth. People within these various categories may be endowed with a variety of virtues and/or vices. Classifying people and attribution of specific traits to all members in that classification is referred to as stereotyping. Stereotype is "a relatively rigid and oversimplified or biased perception of... persons or social groups" (268, p. 523). Stereotyping is a relatively common phenomenon that can be highly detrimental to positive social interactions.

Ideas about specific people significant to the individual are important. Not only do they influence interaction with these people but these ideas often "spread" or are generalized to other people. This phenomenon is called transference: response to a person or persons in a manner that is similar to the way in which one responded to a significant person in one's past or current life experience (268). Transference will be discussed in some detail in Chapter 8. Suffice it to say here that a transference response can be confusing to the individual to whom such responses are directed.

As is probably quite evident to the reader, an individual's concept of others, whatever it may be, acts as a strong determinant of the way the individual approaches and interacts with other people. It is not the only determinant but an important one. Regardless of whether an individual has a generally positive or negative concept of others, this collection of ideas needs to be subjected to frequent reality testing. Without engaging in this comparing, assessing process, the individual's response to others may not be compatible or congruent with the reality of the situation.

With the description of concept of others, the discussion of psychological function is complete. As previously defined, psychological function involves intrapsychic process and content that are primarily influenced by or derived from the emotional, feeling part of the human experience. For the purpose of discussion, psychological function was divided into eight subcategories: dynamic states, intrapsychic dynamics, reality testing, insight, object relations, self-concept, self-discipline, and concept of others. Sensory integration, cognitive function, and psychological function, although strongly influenced by the external environment, are often thought of as internal processes. They take place within the individual. The last performance component to be discussed, social interaction, involves the individual much more directly in the environment.

SOCIAL INTERACTION

As previously defined, social interaction is the ability to engage with others in casual and sustained relationships individually and within the context of a variety of small groups. Anthropological and historical evidence indicates that human beings have always been social creatures. They have always existed within an aggregate or group of others. Indeed, survival for the first few years of life is only possible through the care of others. In later life it is only the rare individual who chooses to live outside of a community of others. Although occasionally difficult or painful, most people cannot imagine a satisfactory life without regular and intimate contact with others. Thus, the capacity to engage in social interactions is an important element of human experience. For purpose of discussion, social interaction will be subdivided into three parts: interpretation of situations, social skills, and structured social interplay (29).

Interpretation of Situations

Interpretation of the situation refers to an individual's capacity to be an astute observer of the social scene. It is a process that involves observation of people and social situations and assigning meaning to individuals' behavior and the interactions of people. A person skilled in interpretation is able to identify the needs, values, motivations, and emotions of other people fairly accurately. The individual is able to move into new situations and ascertain the expectations operant in the situation (587). The individual recognizes the reciprocal aspect of social interactions. Thus, the individual's own behavior is monitored in such a way that he is able to have a desired effect. This latter understanding is particularly important in engaging in social roles. Interaction in social roles—an identifiable reciprocal relationship between two or more people—requires an awareness of the purpose and meaning of the other's response and the monitoring of one's own behavior relative to that response. Interpretation of situations is similar in some ways to insight. Insight refers to an understanding of oneself, whereas interpretation of situations refers to understanding of others and the requirements of social interaction.

Social Skills

Social skills refers to the capacity to seek out others for the purpose of gaining assistance, fulfilling needs, or merely for the pleasure of being with others. It includes the ability to initiate, respond to, and sustain interactions with others in a way that is satisfying to oneself and others.

Communication

Communication is the process of transmitting and receiving information by means of words, tone of voice, facial expressions, and gestures from one person to another. It includes being able to listen to what another person is saying; to the message as well as to the meaning of the message. It involves being able to express one's emotions, feelings, needs, and ideas in a way that is both socially acceptable and comprehensible to the other person (104,770,841,860,938,996).

One factor that is particularly important in communication is the congruence between verbal and nonverbal messages. Verbal messages are the expression of feelings and ideas by means of words. Nonverbal messages are the expression of feelings and ideas through the use of tone of voice, facial expressions, gestures, and actions in the environment (290,382,786,841). When there is incongruence between verbal and nonverbal communication, the recipient of that communication tends to be thoroughly confused: the person is receiving two different and often conflicting messages. The recipient does not know which message to believe or respond to. Nonverbal messages, for the most part, however, tend to be the more accurate of the two. Incongruence between verbal and nonverbal messages is confusing for the transmitter also. Nonverbal messages tend to be unconscious, thus out of awareness of the individual. The transmitter may not know what message has been given. In addition, the response received by the initial transmitter may be far different from the transmitter anticipated. The communication process often degenerates into a meaningless interaction or is terminated. The ability to communicate comfortably and accurately is a highly valued skill in all aspects of daily life.

Dyadic Interaction

This is the ability to engage in meaningful interaction with another person. In its mature form it is the ability to participate in a variety of one-to-one relationships: friendships of various levels of intensity, intimacy, nurturing, and interaction with superiors and subordinates. Casual friendships are characterized by a feeling of liking, short-term and occasional engagement, and are often focused around a shared activity (181,811). The individual is not considered to be a central source of need satisfaction and, should the relationship end, there is minimal feeling of loss. At the other end of the friendship continuum, the relationship is characterized by a much stronger feeling of liking that at times may be described as love, engagement with the other individual is usually frequent and extended, and, although shared activities may be part of the relationship, they are secondary to simply being together. The individual is considered to be a central source of need satisfaction and termination of the relationship is experienced as a serious loss. As indicated, friend relationships are on a continuum, with any particular relationship at any given time somewhere on that continuum. Although discussed in relation to social interaction, friendship is considered to be one aspect of the occupational performance of play/leisure/recreation. It will be discussed more fully in that context in the following chapter.

Intimate relationships blend into the more intense end of the friendship continuum. An intimate relationship is conceived by both individuals as a partnership with a commitment to each other that is maintained regardless of adverse circumstances that may impinge on and create extraordinary demands within the relationship (271). The partners experience and identify the relationship as being characterized and supported by mutual love. There is a comfortable giving to and receiving from each other and a sharing of responsibility for all aspects of the relationship. There is a mutual trust and open communication. Although the relationship is intense, there is sufficient confidence, so that each partner is free to enter into other types of dyadic relationships. Intimate relationships frequently have a strong sexual component, which is viewed as an integral part of the relationship. This, however, is not always the case. Intimate relationships may or may not be found within the context of marriage.

A nurturing relationship is directed toward assisting another individual to grow and mature. It is characterized by giving attention, guidance, and love to another person (the individual receiving nurture) without the expectation of equal reciprocal need satisfaction (290,938). The relationship is, to some degree, unilateral relative to immediate need satisfaction. Satisfaction for the individual giving nurture may be delayed. It is essentially derived from the love and respect given by the other person during or subsequent to the process and in experiencing the growth of the other person. The relationship involves the giving of unconditional love or regard which respects the rights of the other person for self-direction and ultimate independence. Nurturing relationships properly conducted are time limited. The individual being nurtured is eventually expected to move out of the relationship with the approval and blessings of the individual giving nurture. The relationship between the individuals may continue but becomes one of friendship not nurture. Nurturing relationships occur (ideally) within the parent-child relationship, in some teacher-student dyads, and in the mentor-neophyte relationship. This latter type of dyad is found in work settings where a skilled and knowledgeable worker takes responsibility for helping a novice learn, grow, and advance in the world of work (821,888,932).

The superior-subordinate dyad occurs in many settings: work, school, leisure activities, the health system, legal and political systems, and so forth. Most individuals frequently find themselves as subordinate in an authority relationship, with some individuals also, at times, being in a superior position. A sound, authentic superior-subordinate relationship is characterized by open and clear communication; recognition of the rights, responsibilities, and expertise of each party; shared goals; concern for each other as individuals; respect; negotiation; and cooperation.

The relationships described above are only a sampling of the many dyadic relationships a person is involved in throughout the life cycle. In that sense they are only illustrative of dyadic relationships. On the other hand, friendship, intimacy, nurturing, and superior-subordinate relationships are basic and significant dyads for most people.

Group Interaction

Group interaction refers to the ability to be a productive member of a variety of small groups. It is the capacity to interact in such a way that the goals of a group are accomplished concomitant with satisfaction of personal needs and the needs of other group members (390,391,951). An individual skilled in group interaction is able to take on various roles in a group as such roles are called for in order to maintain the group as a viable entity. The collection of various types of interaction typically found in a mature, well-functioning group are referred to as membership roles. These roles, which make no sharp distinction between leader and follower, are often divided into two categories: instrumental and expressive. Instrumental roles are oriented to the selection, planning, and execution of the group task. Expressive roles, on the other hand, are oriented to the maintenance of the group as a group and the gratification of members' needs. At any particular time in a group, some roles are more necessary or important than at other times. What roles need to be taken at a given time will depend on the purpose of the group or where the group is in accomplishing a task or both.

Many of the interpersonal skills necessary for dyadic interaction are also required for group interaction. However, some additional skills are required: working and sharing with more than one person, being aware of multiple others and the dynamics of the group, toleration of a more extended delay in task accomplishment and need satisfaction, and the need to be more assertive. An individual usually interacts in a variety of groups—family, work, and leisure groups being the most common. Within each of these categories the purpose of groups will vary on a continuum from primarily task oriented to being primarily concerned with satisfaction of group members' needs. To function adequately in a group, the individual must be aware of the purpose of the group and particularize his repertoire of behavior so as to be an accepted and productive group member.

Structured Social Interplay

Structured social interplay refers to dyadic or group interactions that are formalized, at least to the extent that they have been identified and named. These interactions are cooperation, competition, compromise, negotiation, and assertiveness. Cooperation is working and acting together for a common purpose or benefit. It connotes active assistance and sharing with another person willingly and agreeably. Competition is contention or rivalry for supremacy, a prize, honor, or advantage. The struggle usually takes place between two or more persons or groups for an object desired in common, usually resulting in a victor and loser or losers. Between-group competition often calls for intragroup cooperation. Compromise is the settlement of differences by mutual concessions. An agreement is reached by adjustment of conflicting or opposing claims, principles, or ideas by reciprocal modification of demands. It may include the combining of two different alternatives or the ultimate solution may be quite different from either proposed solution. Compromise does not involve an individual or group giving up all of their demands or ideas and accepting the wishes of the other individual or group. That is capitulation. Negotiation is the process of dealing or bargaining with another in order to enhance one's position or advantage. The transaction takes place through direct discussion or through the assistance of a third party. Finally, assertiveness is behavior characterized by assurance and confidence. It usually involves putting oneself forward boldly and insistently in order to make a point or accomplish a given task. When used appropriately, assertiveness does not usually have the connotation of being a hostile interaction.

Each of these types of social interplay only occasionally takes place in a pure form or in isolation. More typically they occur in some combination, either taking place concomitantly or sequentially. Different social skills are required for each; an individual needs to have some facility for engaging in all of them. However, most individuals may be more competent in one type of interplay as opposed to another.

Social interactions—interpretation of situations, communication, dyadic and group involvement, and social interplay—are crucial components in being able to adapt to the environment. It is through social interaction that, initially, we are able to survive and ultimately able to gain pleasure from being with others.

SUMMARY

This chapter has outlined one aspect of occupational therapy's domain of concern: the psychosocial performance components of sensory integration, cognitive function, psychological function, and social interaction. They were presented as facets of human function, with only some interrelationships being identified. Various relationships between these facets will be described in more detail in subsequent parts of the text. Although somewhat lengthy, this chapter has only been addressed to one aspect of the domain of concern. The following chapter focuses on another aspect: occupational performances.

4 Occupational Performances

Occupational performances, one aspect of the occupational therapy domain of concern, are organized patterns of behavior through which an individual engages in and meets the demands of the environment. Occupational performances are subdivided into five areas: family interactions, activities of daily living, school/work, play/leisure/recreation, and temporal adaptation. The first four areas are generally referred to as social roles: family member, caretaker of the self, worker, and player. The other occupational performance, temporal adaptation, refers to the ability to organize one's time in order to fulfill adequately the responsibilities and enjoy the pleasures of one's required and/or desired social roles.

This chapter discusses the five areas of occupational performance. An introductory section provides an overview of the phenomena of social roles to set the stage for the discussion that follows.

SOCIAL ROLES

Social roles, a sociological concept, is used to identify an organized pattern of behavior that is characteristic and expected of the occupant of a defined position in a social system (73,191,199,203,207,360,457,611,671,697,764–766,823). A role exists only in relationship to a role partner; one cannot engage in role behavior in isolation. Some examples of roles are student-teacher, child-parent, husband-wife, therapist-client. As the examples indicate, one cannot be or act as a teacher without students, a husband without a wife, and so forth.

The duration of being in a role varies. One may play a role only briefly and periodically, as in being in the role of a complainant or of a customer. On the other hand, one may play a role for an extended period of time, being a parent or a worker, for example. The behavior required in long-term roles may vary markedly over time with one still essentially being in the same role. Thus, one may begin his worker role as a novice with little understanding of the job or responsibility. Later, one may be in a job position that is highly complex, demand a great variety of skills, and the taking of considerable responsibility.

The specificity of role behavior varies. In some situations, expected behavior is fairly strictly bound. Some examples are the role one plays at a religious service or as a chess player. Other roles are less strictly bound and played with a good deal of variation. There are only broad societal expectations with further delineation of roles by thc partners involved. Husband-wife and the role of being a friend are two examples. Traditional, fairly static social systems tend to define the roles of their members in a fairly strict manner with little variation tolerated. Less traditional, open, rapidly evolving social systems have less rigid definition of roles, allowing the role partners much latitude in determining how they will play their roles.

Role behavior is to some extent always dynamic, changing, varied, and being redefined. Role partners must continually accommodate their behavior relative to each other. Only in this way are the needs of each partner satisfied. Role interactions are experienced as a source of stress when this continual accommodation does not take place. If lack of accommodation is severe, the role partnership is likely to be dissolved. One way in which accommodation takes place is through "taking the role of the other." This is the process of imagining oneself in the role of the other partner. This helps the individual ascertain what the other individual's needs, motivation, and feelings are and the most appropriate response. The ability to take the role of one's partner enables the individual to participate in his role in a versatile and accomplished manner. Role partnerships are most satisfying and stable when the individuals are able to communicate with each other and have a shared system of values and expectations.

Most individuals are participants in a considerable number of roles simultaneously and throughout their life cycle. Some roles are seen as important; others are given little attention and engaged in without much thought. The roles to be discussed in this chapter—family member, caretaker of the self, worker, and player—are usually viewed as important by most people. There are, however, differences in the way that individuals rank these roles. For some, the role of family member is given first priority; others may identify their role as a worker as their most highly valued role. Important roles often form the nucleus around which the individual establishes identity. For this reason the loss of a major role is a serious threat to an individual's sense of integrity and requires major adjustment and adaptation.

Finally, social roles can be seen as being made up of two categories of behavior: task and interpersonal. Task behavior involves a doing process and usually entails manipulation of the nonhuman environment. Interpersonal behavior involves interaction with one or more persons and often includes the mutual satisfaction of social/emotional needs. For example, in the role of a secretary one is expected to use office machines; one is also expected to get along with co-workers and supervisors. Role disruption or alteration may occur if there is deficit in or loss of either task or interpersonal behavior. A saleswoman, for example, may be fired from her job not because she cannot do the required tasks but rather because she is unable to be responsive to customers. A severely disabled homemaker may have to give up many usual tasks but nonetheless can assist other family members by organizing, planning, and supervising their work in maintaining the home. The homemaker's role has been altered but in this case it has been retained.

Socialization is the term used to identify the process of acquiring a particular social role. Three important elements of this process are the neophyte (or learner), the setting, and agent(s). The neophyte, in most cases, engages in the socialization process because he desires the responsibilities, rights, and rewards that are contingent on full participation in the role. The individual is not a passive recipient in the learning process but rather plays an active part in mastering the expected knowledge, skills, and attitudes. At times the neophyte, in order to learn the desired role, places himself in a state of temporary need deprivation. This state arises from having to give up old ways of thinking, feeling, and acting. The process may require a change in life style with less time for family, friends, and recreational pursuits. The neophyte is also frequently in a dependent position. It is often others who define what is to be learned, when, and where the learning is to occur. The socializing agent frequently acts as gatekeeper, with the power to allow or disallow full participation in the desired role. Some need deprivation and dependency is tolerated because of the belief that the new learning will ultimately lead to an overall increase in need satisfaction. Although initially dependent, independence increases with the acquisition and successful use of knowledge, skills, and attitudes and recognition of competence by one's role partner(s) and peers.

Socialization can only occur in a setting in which the relevant behavior is elicited, evoked, required, permitted, and so forth. Practice must be possible, allowed, and encouraged. Feedback and reinforcement must be available from other individuals and/or from the outcome or consequence of behavior. Ideally, the setting is such that it arouses interest in exploring and the desire to master.

Agents are the individuals responsible for socialization. They are in almost all cases members of the social system in which the neophyte seeks membership. Ideally, the agent gives clear messages regarding expectations, offers support, and manipulates rewards and feedback to guide learning. The agent may be permissive at times, particularly at the beginning of the socialization process, with more strict standards set in more advanced stages. Ideally, the agent satisfies the neophyte's need for response, acceptance, approval, and recognition of a job well done. Again, ideally, there is a degree of affectual attachment between the agent and neophyte that is used to give added weight to rewards and feedback.

The socializing agent may be a role partner, a role model, a guide, or a group of others, or some combination of all of these. Using the example of learning to be a mother, the child, as a role partner, teaches a woman a good deal about the requirements of the mothering process. A woman's mother may act as a role model. Guidance in the mothering process may be provided by a pediatrician. A reference group is a group to which a neophyte wishes to belong. That desire motivates an individual to take on the values and behaviors of the group with the hope of being accepted as a full-fledged member. Continuing with the example, a new mother may identify the other mothers in the neighborhood as a reference group. She would thus monitor her behavior to conform to the expectations of that group. As the example indicates, several agents may be involved in the neophyte's learning of a particular role. There may also be different agents at different times in the process.

Some degree of conflict is inherent in the socialization process. The neophyte rarely wishes to fulfill all of the agent's expectations and most people are uncomfortable in a dependent position. Conversely, the agent may occasionally find the task of socializing time consuming and be impatient for more advanced or mature behavior on the part of the neophyte. The situation is ripe for conflict. Conflict, however, can and often does have a positive effect on the socialization process. It increases personal and emotional interaction. This may begin in anger but, if well handled, it can lead to increased understanding, a sensing of each other as unique individuals, trust, and even to affection. Through the conflict generated in the socialization process and the need to deal with it, the neophyte is also likely to learn something about how to deal with conflict in the anticipated role. Through the resolution of conflict, neophytes are able to perceive that they can have some, albeit small, impact on the social system. This tends to keep dependency at a tolerable level.

Finally, there is a process identified as anticipatory socialization. This is "a before the fact" trial period. The individual in a sense plays at the role but does not take full responsibility for the role. Some examples of anticipatory socialization are living with a possible mate prior to marriage, babysitting, going away to college, and summer jobs.

Social roles, to the best of our knowledge, have been the foundation for organizing interaction in the daily life of all communities (181). In the past, age and sex were the primary determinants of social roles, which were fairly strictly defined. Prior to the industrial revolution, an individual's various social roles tended to be integrated. Work, play, family life, worship, education, and so forth all blended together as part and parcel of community life. Life possessed a wholeness, with social roles being interrelated and complementary to each other. The cycle of the ecosystem that supported a community defined the rhythm of the community, its daily life and the seasons of the year. The time for work, play, and other activities was determined by the ecosystem and not the clock.

The industrial revolution disrupted the integration of social roles, leading to the present situation of role diffusion. Social roles are now compartmentalized and at times in conflict with each other. Work is separated sharply from other roles and undertaken in a particular place, at specific times, and amid work-specific relationships. Other social roles are excluded from the workplace and can only be fulfilled at hours other than those allotted to work. The workday has come to define the rhythm of the community. The clock has ascended to a position of extreme importance, making time a valued commodity.

With the above description of social roles, the socialization process, and the present situation of role diffusion and time consciousness, attention will now be turned to occupational performances. The discussion of family interaction, activities of daily living, play/recreation, and leisure will be general in nature. Additional information on how these roles are played through the life cycle will be outlined in Chapter 5. The reader is cautioned that this is a description of a part of the domain of concern. Evaluation and intervention will be discussed later in the text.

FAMILY INTERACTION

As previously defined, family interaction refers to nuclear, extended, and expanded familial roles in addition to (a) those relationships, dealing with the typical familial issues of intimacy, emotional support, sexuality, and child rearing, which are seen by the participants as being family-like in nature and (b) preparation for entering into new familial roles through such interactions as dating and courtship (171,253,254,274,375,449,687,766,854,868,888,891,1029).

The first social role that an individual is involved in is a familial role: the role of a child. It is an ascribed role in the sense that one has no choice in taking on the role; it is bestowed by the fact of birth. Although ascribed, an individual must learn the role of a child. Similar to the acquisition of other familial roles, it is learned through a process of socialization.

The family is apparently the first and thus oldest social institution. Although structured in different ways and often subjected to potentially destructive internal and external forces, it has endured through time. The family remains the single most significant social institution. It nurtures the young and provides support for the individual's interaction in the community.

Family, here, is defined broadly as a small social system made up of individuals related to each other by reasons of strong reciprocal affection and loyalties and comprising an identifiable household or cluster of households that persists over an extended period of time. Members enter through birth, adoption, marriage, or by being identified as a member of the social system by other members of the system and leave by death, mutual consent, or divorce. Divorce need not, however, terminate familial relationships. Members are not necessarily related by blood or marriage but have intimate relationships that they perceive as familial in nature.

The above definition was designed to account for a variety of relationships and life styles that are currently a part of our society. These include: cohabitation of unmarried partners of the opposite sex, homosexual partners, the individual who chooses to remain single and live alone, divorced partners, single-parent households, divorced individuals with or without children from former relationships who remarry, cyclical monogamy, and so forth. The issues that are typically familial in nature—intimacy, emotional support, sexuality, and child rearing—are similar whether one is a member of a traditional family or a participant in one of the relationships identified above.

Family structures are usually identified as nuclear, extended, and expanded. A nuclear family has traditionally consisted of a married pair with or without dependent children living in the same household. In our society, this family structure is usually viewed as the most significant and the one most responsible for typically family functions.

Increasingly, however, many nuclear families are organized around a single parent and one or more dependent children. The parent may or may not have been married, be separated, or divorced. The care and rearing of the child or children may be the sole responsibility of the parent in residence or that responsibility may be shared to a lesser or greater degree with the nonresident parent. Some children spend relatively equal time with each parent and thus essentially are members of two households. Single-parent families have not been extensively studied and there is little information about the effects of such a family structure on the individuals involved. From a review of the popular literature, however, the task of being a single parent is emotionally demanding and time consuming. The working single parent has particular difficulty in the area of temporal adaptation.

The extended family is made up of a variety of individuals of several generations related by blood, marriage, or mutual consent. Generally known as a kinship system, an extended family usually includes several nuclear families and single adults who live in separate households. The extended family remains viable in our society and, as will be discussed later, forms the matrix for many leisure activities (545,665,863).

An expanded family is made up of nuclear families and single adults, frequently of more than one generation, who have previously been related by marriage. The pivotal point or center of an expanded family is not the parental pair, as is the case in a typical nuclear family, but rather the children of the respective parents. The children are central in the sense of kin relationships which follow the line of natural parents. For example, an expanded family may be made up of a nuclear family consisting of two adults who had been previously married, two children from one of the previous marriages, and one child from the other, or two single-parent families consisting of the two now unmarried former spouses and their children. These are examples of fairly simple expanded families; others are larger and more complex. The relationships in expanded families are often intricate, obtuse, and demanding. The degree to which a given parent is involved with his or her child and an expanded family varies from none to considerable. As indicated in the definition of family, separation or divorce does not necessarily lead to departure from the family constellation.

Family interaction, regardless of family structure, is made up of a variety of roles. The most common familial roles are: grandparent, parent, spouse, child, sibling, aunt, uncle, various in-law relationships, stepparent or stepchild, unmarried partners, divorced spouses, surrogate parent, and preliminary or serious courtship roles. All individuals at one time or another play the role of a child. Other familial roles may be taken or acquired depending on life circumstances and choice. Most individuals, as adults, participate in a variety of familial roles.

The functions of a family are multiple. The first and historically the oldest is survival—of the species and of family members. The family takes primary responsibility for the care of infants and young children and food, clothing, and shelter for its members. Beyond physical survival of children the family is expected to provide a nurturing environment and an environment that leads to adequate socialization. The family is the initial socializing agent. It not only teaches the child how to take various familial roles but also teaches many of the skills necessary for being a caretaker of the self, worker, and player. The family is, in many ways, the representative of society. It helps the child learn the expected behavior and values of the broader social system.

In describing the family's function relative to development, developmental needs are sometimes described as being on two levels. First-order developmental needs refers to the acquisition or mastery of and adaptation to the environment and are typical of the period of growth and maturation in childhood and adolescence. Second-order developmental needs refers to transformations of status and identity of adult family members. The meeting of second-order needs frequently calls for reassignment or rearrangement of familial roles.

Traditionally, one of the major functions of the family was to regulate and structure sexual behavior. This function has diminished considerably with the advent of less restrictive sexual mores. However, it has by no means been lost. The family, to a great extent, is still responsible for imparting values relative to sexual behavior to children. What values should be imparted, however, is open to question. About the only point of agreement at this time seems to be that adolescents should use sufficient caution in their sexual activities to ensure that girls under 18 years of age do not become pregnant. Sexual activity of adults outside the family is primarily seen as a private matter, except in the case of sexual exploitation of children, prostitution, and in some cases pornography. Although there is considerable "casual" sex, most adult sexual behavior occurs within the context of spouse and partner relationships.

The last major function of the family is to provide emotional support. This has been described by some authorities as the major function of the modern family. A family, with adequate emotional resources, can give shelter, replenish energy, and provide guidance, which enables the individual to interact productively and with pleasure in the wider social system. Families often are a major component of an individual's support system.

The functions of families are compounded by two major issues: intimacy and power. Intimacy refers to a relationship that is supported by mutual love, trust, and open communication. It is a relationship that is often difficult to attain and is only maintained by attention, effort, and a willingness to compromise. Intimacy here refers not only to the relationship between spouses and partners but also to the relationship between parents and children. Power refers to control, authority, and influence. Each family has a particular power structure, which varies on a continuum from shared or equal to polarized in one family member. Power structures are often multidimensional, with a given individual having a great deal of power in one sphere of family life and limited power in another sphere. Power is related to and inherent in the sub-issues of dependence/independence, dominance, and compliance. Similar to intimacy, power is an issue that needs to be attended to by family members.

The life cycle of a family is characterized by a series of usual or normative events. Some of the major normative events are marriage, birth of a child, a child entering school, a child entering adolescence, the adolescent moving into adulthood and leaving home, birth of a grandchild, retirement, old age, illness, disability, and death. The families that make up an extended/expanded family may be at several different places in the family cycle. As a whole, the extended/expanded family may be dealing with and adjusting to a variety of normative events.

In addition, the family cycle may also be punctuated by paranormative events, which occur frequently but not universally. Some examples of paranormative events are miscarriage, the birth of a severely disabled child, marital separation and divorce, a marked change in socioeconomic status, and extrinsic catastrophe (war, famine, political or religious persecution) with massive dislocation of family units. Paranormative events place tremendous stress on a family and require considerable adaptation if the family is to survive as a viable unit. Paranormative events are particularly difficult for a family because, in most cultures, there are no ceremonial rituals to mark and support these events. There are no institutionalized patterns of responses available to family members or significant persons outside the family providing assistance and guidance for the family. This is not the case, however, with most normative events.

An individual and family are influenced by the multigenerational nature and history of the family. There is an endless chain of influences linking the developmental experiences of each generation, each individual. The influence is both longitudinal and horizontal. At any given time we are influenced by grandparents, parents, children, grandchildren, siblings, former and current spouses or partners, and in-laws. What family members have or have not been, what they are or are not doing, and various types of personal and family crises reverberate through the entire family social system—from the past, in the present, and on into the future. Particular interactions are strongly influenced by the family matrix in which they are imbedded.

Families are dynamic entities comprised of a variety of evolving patterns of interaction. Family patterns are sequences of behavior that can be thought of as a family's typical alliances and responses. Some of these patterns are fairly stable over time; others may be of a more temporary nature. The patterns of a family at any given point in its history relate to the combined and interacting needs of its members at that time. Patterns evolve in order to satisfy the needs of members. The health or adaptivity of a family lies in its capacity to develop patterns that are of such a nature and stability that they satisfactorily meet specific needs.

The appearance of a first-order developmental need of a child or adolescent sets in motion a sequence of events causing temporary disequilibrium of existing patterns. This ultimately leads to the rearrangement of elements and eventuates in a new, stable pattern that provides for meeting the new needs. The existing elements have been modified with no drastic change in the overall structures of the family. The appearance of second-order needs, on the other hand, often trigger an all-encompassing transformation of patterns, changing the entire constellation of the family.

One of the major social phenomena which has had and is having an effect on the family is the women's movement or, perhaps more correctly, the reevaluation and redefinition of sex roles. The traditional relationships between men and women—dominant/subordinate, independent/dependent—are in the process of being dissolved with a more egalitarian relationship being proposed. For women this has raised many family-related questions of whether to enter into a marriage, plan for a career or a less demanding position in the economic sector, have children, work during the early child-rearing years; and how to manage the combined responsibilities of child rearing, being the primary homemaker, and a career or job. For men, the redefinition of sex roles has called into question one of the pivotal factors of male identity: major financial responsibility for the family. Men are also being urged to become far more involved in parenting, to engage in household tasks formerly considered the responsibility of women, to be more comfortable in intimate interactions, and to be more open in expressing and communicating emotions. The evolving redefinition of sex roles has placed a good deal of stress on the relationship between spouses and heterosexual partners because neither men nor women have adequate role models to serve as a guide. Traditional role models, parents and the preceding generation of relatives, often can provide little guidance.

Our society is experiencing a fairly widespread reorganization of family units. Whether this will lead to healthier and happier family units is unknown at this time. However, it is known that this reorganization is traumatic for many people and may leave some individuals temporarily or permanently without an adequate support system.

The capacity to engage effectively and with satisfaction in familial roles is a skill to be nurtured within each individual ideally through interaction within the matrix of an effective family.

ACTIVITIES OF DAILY LIVING

Activities of daily living have been defined as all those activities that one must engage in or accomplish in order to participate with comfort in other facets of life. They are all those other things an individual must do to engage successfully in work, recreation, and family interaction. The list of these activities is seemingly almost endless, and they have been categorized in a variety of different ways. The following listing is most likely not complete and is provided for illustrative purposes only:

- *Personal hygiene:* elimination, bathing, grooming, dressing, dressing appropriately, washing, ironing, mending clothes.
- *Money management:* daily money transactions, banking transactions, budgeting, paying bills.
- *Shopping:* making lists for required items; shopping for groceries, clothes, personal items, and household goods; shopping for quality and best prices; keeping receipts, instructions, and warranties.
- *Meal preparation:* feeding oneself, knowledge of nutritional needs, meal planning, using kitchen appliances, using measuring and cooking utensils, cooking for self and household, cleaning up and maintaining order of kitchen, food storage.
- *Home:* locating and securing housing; furnishing and decorating; routine and major cleaning; minor household repairs; maintenance of household appliances; care of yard and lawn; utilities conservation; understanding of thermostat, circuit breakers, and water heater; home safety and security; community resources for household repairs.
- *Communication:* use of phone directories, use of telephone, writing personal and business letters, filling out forms.
- *Travel:* walking; using public transportation; using a map; buying, maintaining, and driving a car; securing a taxi or other forms of private transportation; traveling outside one's immediate neighborhoods and/or the city; safety precautions.
- *Health care:* appropriate use of medication, making and keeping appropriate medical appointments, taking care of minor illnesses, simple first aid, management of weight, engaging in exercise, adequate time for sleep, knowledge of contraceptive and venereal disease, wise use of potentially addictive substances (488).

Given such a lengthy list of activities of daily living, it is surprising that the psychological and sociological literature relative to this aspect of human experience is sparse (857,943). Much attention has been given to the other occupational performances, with activities of daily living rarely being mentioned except in relation to child development. One could speculate that this neglect is due to the fact that many activities of daily living have traditionally been the responsibility of women, thus, not of concern to the predominantly male scientific community. Occupational therapy, from its beginning, identified activities of daily living as being a significant part of human experience (635,678,783,960). Occupational therapy has traditionally been a women's profession. Thus, women's concern for this facet of life is not surprising. The following discussion is primarily based on common sense, conjecture, and what is available in the literature.

What may be an activity of daily living for one person, may be work or recreation for another. Driving a car may be work for the taxi driver, an activity of daily living for the individual going to a shopping center, and recreation for the sports car enthusiast. An individual's orientation may also influence how an activity is perceived. Weekly grocery shopping, for example, may be seen as an activity of daily living, whereas visiting a gourment food shop may be seen as recreation.

Difficulty in engaging in activities of daily living is more common than one would image. The degree of psychological or physical disability is not a factor here. There are many people who experience anxiety in contemplating calling for a doctor's appointment, finding and negotiating with a repairperson, shopping for clothes, moving to a new home, and so forth. This anxiety is often dealt with by prolonged procrastination, avoidance of the task altogether, or, with some loss of self-esteem, seeking the help of another person. People tend to be embarrassed by deficits in activities of daily living and are reticent in sharing this information. These hidden deficits tend to make the individuals perceive themselves as incompetent. In addition, they consume much time and energy in worry and in doing the activity in an amateurish manner, time and energy that could be used in a much more productive and satisfying manner.

Included here in the area of activities of daily living is the role of homemaker or homemanager (39,957). Traditionally such a role has been placed under the general heading of work. The work of a homemaker essentially involves taking responsibility for the majority of activities of daily living tasks of family members or other persons residing in a household. It involves doing and coordinating these tasks in such a way that they are accomplished at a given time and to the satisfaction of the homemaker and family members. Not including homemaking in the category of work in no way indicates that it is not a difficult and time-consuming responsibility, a job that requires a number of sometimes complex skills. Categorizing homemaking as a nonwork activity is also not meant to imply that it is a minor, not quite respectable activity. Homemaking is important, deserves recognition, and can be a highly rewarding activity.

Homemaking is not included under the general heading of work for three reasons. First, homemaking is structurally different from paid employment. This statement will be clearer after the discussion of work in the following section. Suffice it to say for now that homemaking is less confined to a specified period of time, does not require sustained complex interpersonal relationships, and is not necessarily isolated from other social roles. Second, homemaking as a lifelong alternative to paid employment is an endangered, quickly disappearing occupation. Most women work prior and subsequent to the child-rearing years. And a good number work through the child-rearing period. At the time of this writing, in the United States over 50 percent of women between 18 and 63 years of age are employed (736). The responsibilities of home management thus are typically shared among adolescent and adult family members. Although responsibilities are not always shared equally, it is inaccurate to ignore the household maintenance role responsibilities of each family member. Third, individuals who live alone or with friends are homemakers. This appears to be a little-recognized phenomenon.

Activities of daily living can be a source of conflict within a family and for individuals. In regard to a family, many households no longer have a fulltime homemaker. Yet someone has to do the shopping, cooking, cleaning, repairs, and so forth. Families are confronted with organizing and sharing household chores in a somewhat equitable manner. As there are no traditional guidelines or role models, conflicts are almost inevitable as family members negotiate with each other (108,491,855).

In regard to individuals, historically there has been a link between gender and some activities of daily living. Some men, therefore, are uncomfortable ironing and mending clothes. Seeing to the repair of the car, patching the cement walk, and renegotiating a loan at the bank are often new responsibilities for a woman. Men and women sometimes see the performance of traditionally opposite gender tasks as being a threat to their sexual identity. There is also, at least initially, often a feeling of incompetence relative to performing such tasks. This in turn can lead to a diminished sense of self-esteem.

The capacity to engage in activities of daily living is an important, although frequently unconscious, part of an individual's identity. It indicates to one's self and others that one is capable and competent, in control of the situation, able to negotiate the environment, and independent. The ability and parental permission to engage in various activities of daily living are minor benchmarks in the developments of children and adolescents. These increments toward adulthood are praised and shared with relatives and friends. In the adult years, the ability to engage in activities of daily living is for the most part given little attention and taken for granted, and is, hence, an unconscious part of identity. It is often only through temporary or permanent decrease or loss of the ability to engage in activities of daily living that their significance becomes apparent. An acquired disability often leads to a deficit in the ability to carry out activities of daily living. When this occurs the individual's identity is often altered as he sees himself as less competent and less independent. Individuals who, because of physical or psychological deficits, have never mastered many activities of daily living often feel incompetent and dependent on others.

SCHOOL/WORK

As previously defined, school/work refers to the various social roles involved in being a student and in being a participant in remunerative employment. Work is a major, complex area of human experience. For many people, it is a significant component of identity and thus reverberates through all aspects of the individual's interaction with the environment. Because of the complexity of work, discussion here is divided into nine areas: definition, work and society, structure and characteristics of the work setting, work and the individual, stress in the workplace, the work cycle, work-related deficits, women and work, and the student as a worker. The vast majority of the literature in regard to work is based on the study of men in the economic sector. It is important for the reader to remember this bias in considering the following discussion.

Definition of Work

Work is an instrumental activity, carried out by human beings, which involves a struggle with the environment for compelling material reasons: physical survival, social survival, and rewarding social status. It is any formal activity that prepares one for or involves earning a living: being a student or remunerative employment. It is limited by time, place, and structural organization (168,192,459,727,743,872).

In order to provide dimension to the definition, some key concepts will be discussed. "Instrumental" is that with or by which something is effected, the means, to serve some purpose. The function, or purpose, of work is to ensure survival of the individual, the social system, and ultimately the species. As an instrumental activity, work is not undertaken because it is intrinsically satisfying, although that may be the case for some people. Rather, work is considered to be the means to some end.

"Struggle with the environment" refers to two aspects of work. As a struggle, work involves labor, toil, and drudgery; it involves applying one's self with industry. Although many people would not use these adjectives to describe their work experience, in general, there are few who would say these elements are entirely absent from it. Second, work involves exertion or effort directed toward producing or accomplishing something relative to the environment. It involves mastery or planned alteration of the human and/or nonhuman environment.

Work is limited by time, place, and structural organization (142). Work occurs in defined time. There is a temporal space, a time for work. Individuals are usually able to delineate at any specific time whether they are or are not working. Work is limited in place: the school, factory, store, office, or field. Work may extend or take place out in the wider environment but it has a central place of origin. At times an individual's major place of work is the home. In this case an area or a part of the home is usually designated as the workspace. Such a designation tends to facilitate organization and maintains distinction between family or personal activities and work. Work for the most part has a particular structural organization with defined roles, responsibilities, and privileges. This aspect of work will be discussed later in this section.

The role of being a student is included with the role of worker for several reasons. Being a student is an instrumental activity that entails mastery of the environment. The needs motivating the student are similar to those motivating the worker in the economic sector. The activities of a student are limited by time, place, and a structural organization similar to that of work. The tasks and interpersonal skills acquired in the classroom and related areas are directly applicable to the work situation. Academic level achieved and major focus of study have a fairly direct bearing on participation in the world of work. Although school here is described as preparation for remunerative employment, it should be noted that factors outside the realm of school influence occupational choice and career patterns, and that formal education is also designed to develop knowledge, skills, and attitudes that are not necessarily related to work.

The play of children has been closely linked with work in the occupational therapy literature. There seem to be three major reasons for this close association. The first is related to the varying meanings of the term "occupation," which has been defined as (a) "one's usual or principal work or business, especially as a means of earning a living," and (b) "any activity in which one is engaged" (792, p. 996). Occupational therapists seemingly have merged these two definitions and thus refer to play as the work of children. Second, some occupational therapists with a strict developmental orientation believe that an individual needs to learn how to play prior to learning how to work. The third reason play has been so closely associated with work in the occupational therapy literature is that the activities of play or recreation—games, sports, craft activities—are frequently used as the vehicle for teaching skills that are basic to work: cooperation, following directions, attention to detail, and so forth.

The play of children is not included here in the general category of work. This choice was made for several reasons. The psychological and sociological literature concerned with play is quite broad in its perspective. On the one hand, play is seen as an activity with its own functions and structures, which differentiates it from other spheres of human experience. On the other hand, play is seen as the means for acquisition of any number of human capacities, essentially all of the performance components. It is also seen as preparation for all of the major adult roles. Finally, the general literature emphasizes that, although the activities of play are used extensively in early elementary education, formal education is also a process of weaning a child from play to an attitude of industry and discipline. For these reasons play is not classified as work. Survey of the general literature seems to relate play more closely in structure and character to the recreational/leisure sphere of human experience. Thus, it is categorized in that manner in the text. It is so placed with full recognition of the imperfections of all systems of classification.

Work and Society

Work is one of the major structural components of a society and one of the bonds that holds the members of society together (142,479,727). Beyond procreation and the nurture of small children, work provides for the survival, maintenance, and growth of a society. It is a precept of all societies that adults should be involved in a productive role in some sector of the society's social system. Consequently, training for work occurs in all societies.

Because of the importance of work, societies develop a set of values and beliefs about work that serves to regulate and influence work and to place work in relationship to other aspects of the society. Although there are many facets to the work-society relationship, only three will be discussed briefly here: the place of work in the social system of a society, the worth ascribed to work, and who should work.

In most of Western society, the economic sector is seen as an "intermediate zone" between the nation/state and family/individual (142). The state determines the broad economic structure of the society: being placed somewhere on the overlapping continuums of socialism-capitalism, controlled-free economy. The economic structure, whatever it is, broadly defines the norms of the workplace. This has meaning to the individual primarily as it impinges on his or her work. How people are treated at work—wages, working conditions, opportunity for advancement, self-determination—has a profound influence on their attitudes toward society. Conversely, who and what an individual is as a person will influence his choice of work and his interactions in the work setting. In turn, the kind of work an individual does has a powerful influence on defining his own and immediate family's place in society. The latter occurs because society makes a differentiation between occupations relative to prestige. Varying degrees of worth are assigned to the types of work existing in a given society. The prestige assigned to an individual's occupation influences, to some degree, the individual's investment in his job and his self-esteem.

A great worth is ascribed to work in the United States. This phenomenon is sometimes referred to as the work ethic. It arose from the Reformation, which occurred in Europe in the sixteenth century. Prior to that time, most types of work were not held in high regard. For a variety of reasons, work came to be regarded as the means to salvation during the Reformation. The byproduct of work, wealth, was defined as good because it meant that one was acceptable in God's eyes and well on the way to salvation. This belief about work existed at the time of the Industrial Revolution and was used by society to encourage people to change their work behavior (e.g., move into the factories) so as to provide the numbers and types of workers needed to support the revolution. The work ethic has at this time, for the most part, lost its religious connotation. However, it has not lost its strength as a belief. In the United States to work is good, a measure of one's worth. Individuals who do not work are accorded very little value. The reason why one does not work may temper that valuation but does not alter it substantially. The adult who does not work, consequently, has considerable difficulty maintaining self-esteem at an adequate level.

All known societies have defined work responsibilities by sex and age (181). At the time of the Industrial Revolution, with the economic sector being removed from the home, women at first were not expected to engage in that sphere of productivity. It became apparent fairly soon that was not a wise idea. Because of their inferior status and docile nature, women would work for lower wages than men. The Industrial Revolution, in order to prosper, needed cheap labor. In addition, the economic structure at that time was such that a man could rarely support a family on the salary he earned as a factory worker. Thus, not surprisingly, the mores of society changed. It was fine for women to work if their salary was needed to support their family and if they stayed in low-paying, nonsupervisory positions. These beliefs and values about women's place in the economic sector have changed only in a minor way since the Industrial Revolution.

Age is the other major criterion used by society to define work responsibilities. Until the late nineteenth and early twentieth centuries, appropriate age for involvement in the economic sector was broadly defined: from the age of 7 or 8 years (in the lower socioeconomic classes) to the point where one was no longer physically able to work. Neither child labor laws nor laws regarding retirement as we know them today existed. For humanitarian and economic reasons, society's views about age and involvement in the economic sector have changed. By the 1930s laws were enacted to exclude children from work until the age of 16 years. This was done to protect children from exploitation and the unhealthy aspects of many work settings. These laws were also encouraged by workers in the fairly accurate belief that child labor was responsible for the low wages and/or unemployment of some adults. The retirement age was set at 65 years both because it was felt that older people deserved a few remaining years free from work, and to make room in the labor market for the ever-increasing population of young adults (155). The decision to place the age of retirement at 65 was somewhat arbitrary. At that time, 65 was considered quite old and the life expectancy for an individual of that age was very short. The use of age as the criterion for retirement was far easier than attempting to define in measurable terms whether an individual was physically and mentally capable of working at a particular job.

At the present time there is little evidence that American society will change its ideas about when youth should be free to enter the economic sector. However, the age at which individuals can legally be required to retire has recently been raised to 70 years. Eligibility for and the amount of money paid in Social Security benefits are under critical and urgent review, with marked curtailment in view. Consequently, it is likely that many individuals will not be able to afford to retire before the age of 70 years. American society is questioning its ability to support financially its growing population of nonworking individuals over the age of 65 years. The ramifications of this phenomenon are unknown, for society and for the individual. However, there is likely to be a greater effort to maintain elderly people in the economic sector and a greater recognition of the contributions able to be made by this age group. This, given the high value placed on work in our society, may well enhance the status, identity, and life satisfaction of individuals over 65 years of age.

Structure and Characteristics of the Work Setting

The work setting, as is true of any social situation, has a twofold aspect: extraindividual and intraindividual. The extraindividual component refers to what exists, what is real, and what, through consensual validation, is believed to be the nature of the situation. The intraindividual component refers to what the individual perceives as being real, as existing. Ideally, for the individual, the two components are relatively congruent with each other. If there is wide divergence, the individual is likely to have difficulty in a work setting. This section is primarily concerned with the extraindividual aspect of work.

The formal structure of work is a defined pattern whereby a number of individuals are linked together to perform specialized roles as part of a team effort (207,276,348,727). These roles are performed according to certain social rules, made by specially designated persons, which prescribe how one is to relate to others in the hierarchical structure, the time and place of such interaction, and the desirability of contained cooperation.

In the formal structure, individuals are often linked together through an intermediary system of machines or technology and written communication. The connection between people then is often not direct as in a face-to-face interaction. Indeed the interpersonal aspect of work may be highly diffuse and distant in time and place. There is frequently an impersonal quality to the manner in which individuals are linked together.

Within a particular work setting and within an occupation, there is a variety of worker roles: general worker, foreman, middle management, specialist, top management, to name just a few. Each occupation has its own taxonomy of roles, which if complex, are usually organized in hierarchical and horizontal systems. Various roles are established and compartmentalized to provide ease in learning and performance. Viewed over time, an individual's work experience may be characterized by the learning of a variety of new work roles, including task and interpersonal components.

Work settings are bound by and maintained by a set of formal rules that, to a great extent, define the situation. Responsibilities, rights, and privileges are prescribed. The rules define the goals, the tasks to be performed, and how these tasks are to be accomplished. These rules are usually made by others, often without any consultation with the individuals who must act within the context of the rules. The merit of this system of establishing rules is not being addressed here. What is important is that work settings, like any social situation, are characterized by rules. Without such rules there would be chaos with little task accomplishment. The individual, in order to be a worker, must learn how to behave within a system of rules.

Time is an important aspect of the work setting. One must begin work at a given time, work for a prescribed period of time, and a certain amount of work or a task must be completed in a specified time. Clients, supervisors, even friends, can only be related to at specific times at work.

Finally, relative to the formal structure, the place of work is public in character in a way that is not found in other major social roles. There are only degrees of privacy, with much of one's work open to scrutiny by others.

The informal structure of work includes all those aspects of the setting that are not provided for in the written policies, rules, and organization charts (207,276,348,727). Founded on natural, loosely organized work groups, it essentially fills in the gaps left in the formal structure. Relationships that are formed have a personal quality rather than being prescribed by the organizational chart; communication tends to be more egalitarian. The informal structure allows the individual to bypass formal procedures and alleviates some work monotony.

The major function of the informal structure, in contrast to the task orientation of the formal structure, is to satisfy social-emotional needs. It assists an individual to establish and maintain a personal identity within a large organization and provides an opportunity for the individual to utilize special personal skills and abilities. Within the formal structure an individual may have little prestige or status. This is often not the case in the informal structure where the criteria for acceptance, recognition, and respect are far different. A person's position in the informal structure, regardless of what it may be in the formal structure, contributes a good deal to the individual's feeling of self-worth. The informal structure permits the individual to have some control over the work situation. It diminishes the individual's sense of alienation and powerlessness, which one often experiences relative to the formal structure. The informal structure provides many non-monetary rewards for the individual's effort within the work setting.

The culture of work consists of the traditions, customs, laws, rituals, details of dress and grooming, style and content of speech, rewards, and routines associated with the workplace (142,168,727). Each society has a general culture of work that is accepted by most of its members. Some examples of the general work culture in the United States are arriving at work on time, showing a degree of respect to one's supervisors, and appropriate dress for a job interview. In addition, there is a culture particular to most occupations and many work settings. Wearing white coats in a laboratory, the jargon of professions or disciplines, and graduation ceremonies are examples of particular cultural patterns. Part of the process of becoming a worker entails learning the general and particular customs of the workplace.

Work and the Individual

The above discussion about the structure of a work setting said little about the individual in that setting. This section, then, will deal with the individual: the personal requirements for being a worker, what work means to the individual, and social relationships within the context of work (949).

In order for an individual to take on the role of a worker, she or he must have some degree of mobility and manual dexterity, the capacity to comprehend and follow directions, and the ability to perform a task (727). The individual's grooming, dress and style, and content of speech must be within broad socially defined limits. In interpersonal relationships, the individual must relate to peers, subordinates, and superiors in a manner appropriate to a work setting and accept (or appear to accept) various systems of customs and beliefs. In short, an individual needs to possess certain prerequisite skills and abilities: the individual must act and look like a worker. This description of capacities necessary to enter into the world of work is general in nature. It does not include specific skills needed for a particular job. The refined skills of a given occupation are built on the basic work skills just described.

Paid employment usually results in a sense of achievement, independence, freedom, and security. A particular job, however, does not always lead to the feeling state just described. For some people work is highly satisfying, a primary activity, and the major source of personal identity (142). Other people may experience their work as a singularly stultifying and frustrating experience. There are, of course, many points on this continuum.

Satisfaction with one's work is closely related to why people work (120). There appear to be three major reasons: money, satisfaction of esteem needs, and gratification of the need for mastery. These reasons are by no means mutually exclusive. people who are motivated by money may be concerned with being able to afford the ordinary things of life: food, clothing, shelter, and maybe a little extra for something special. Closely related to this reason for working is the desire for financial security. Some people may take a somewhat lower paying job if it offers the guarantee of continued work and a reasonable income after retirement. Other people motivated by money are more concerned with the accumulation of wealth and the life style and prestige afforded by wealth. Esteem needs motivate an individual to work because they want to be recognized by family, friends, and the wider community as being a productive member of society. Associated with this motivation for working is the satisfaction derived from recognition and respect from co-workers or from members of one's occupational group. Finally, some people work because they enjoy the challenge: to gain knowledge, to understand, to master.

Individuals tend to be satisfied with their work if the rewards are commensurate with the expectations and aspirations that attracted the individual to the job in the first place (120). Although an individual may have an overall degree of work satisfaction, there is also usually a sense of differential satisfaction. Thus, an individual may assess her job relative to specific aspects: supervision, working conditions, opportunities for personal development, material benefits, the organization as a whole, and so forth. One's general degree of satisfaction then will depend on the satisfaction derived from these various aspects of work, and the weight one gives to each of these areas.

The degree to which one's role as a worker influences identity varies. Even for individuals dissatisfied with their job, the idea of being able to work, of being a worker, is an important part of their identity (142). However, the identity of such people is also greatly influenced by familial roles and recreational activities. Individuals who perceive their work as being very important and satisfying are often shaped, regulated, molded, even assimilated by their work. Their work, occupation, profession becomes the central core of their identity. The importance of work to identity becomes evident when an individual is not working, because of an acquired disability, economic circumstances, or forced retirement. The loss of the work role tends to diminish the individual's capacity for self-determination; income is reduced or gone entirely; the status and social relationships that accompany a work role are lost. The individual's identity may well be traumatized. Identity redefinition must often take place before a person is able to regain a sense of self as an individual and a sense of one's place in the community.

The work setting, in addition to being an important factor in identity, presents a complex set of interpersonal relationships (168,727). Indeed, for many people the interpersonal aspects of work may be the most challenging element of the work situation. A worker is often required to relate to a heterogeneous assortment of people in the context of a variety of relationships: peer, supervisor-subordinate, service provider-client. Each of these types of relationships requires a different set of behaviors that must be executed with skill and self-assurance. Complexity is compounded by the need to switch from one set of behaviors to another very quickly. In addition, one person vis-à-vis the worker may be, in the course of one day, a peer, a supervisor, and a client. Thus, in many work settings the individual needs to have a wide, flexibly organized repertoire of behavior.

Interpersonal relationships in a work setting may provide stimulation or succor. In either case they may lead to a consciousness of similarity that forms the basis for an informal work group. Such a group may energize, excite, and provide incentive for exploring new ideas or possibilities, or it may console, reassure, give understanding. Regardless, an informal work group often provides for considerable need satisfaction. Work relationships, on the other hand, may be anxiety provoking and/or exasperating. In this case the individual often attempts to maintain a formal, distant relationship and participates in informal work groups in a perfunctory manner, if at all. The pleasure of intimate work associations is not available to this individual: at least not within the context of the given work setting.

Finally, the situation of work may be the impetus for the development of friendships: a place to find friends or friendship may be fostered out of the common shared experience of work. Friendship here is differentiated from collegial relationships, the latter being relationships, of varying degrees of importance to the individual, which are primarily centered on common work interests. Friendships on the other hand, may grow out of common work interests but extend into a sharing of personal and family oriented recreational activities.

Stress in the Workplace

A stressor is any event that severely disturbs or interferes with the normal physical, mental, or emotional equilibrium of an individual. A stress reaction usually occurs when the individual perceives the stress-inducing situation as being one that is not amenable to alteration by the typical adaptive responses available to him at that time. Stress will be discussed here only in relation to work. It may arise, however, in any sphere of human experience. Situations that cause stress, unless they are of a catastrophic nature, vary from one individual to another. Stress in the workplace is described in the literature as having two sources: the work situation itself and the expectations, conflicts, and anxieties the individual brings to the work situation (479,890). One of these sources may be the predominant cause of stress or, more likely, the two sources interact to produce a stressful situation. These two sources will be described separately in the following discussion.

It is important to note that there is a difference between stress-inducing situations and ordinary hard work or heavy responsibility. The latter do not, in and of themselves, usually cause stress. One of the major sources of stress in the workplace is considered to be in the structure of the work setting. The typical structure of work is often characterized by authoritarianism, powerlessness on the part of the worker, and the treatment of human beings as means to an end. Such a structure is viewed as being incongruous with the wider social system, which emphasizes democratic decision making, personal choice and responsibility, and the treatment of human beings as total entities. Work comes to be viewed as meaningless, limiting relative to personal autonomy and mobility, and not compatible with satisfying many personal needs.

Shorres discusses this source of stress in relation to middle management (890). He states that modern American corporations dehumanize those that give allegiance to them. Organizational structure is said not to be pyramidal, but rather to resemble an onion with power resting in the middle, like a maze. The individual never knows who is really in a superior position, or whom or what to believe. This leads to a feeling of always being in error, causing a state of constant fear, or complete, demeaning obedience. In addition, corporations dominate employees and encourage them to identify their self-interest with that of the company. Such identification does often occur, leaving the individual in a state of pervasive anxiety. The company not only has the power to fire the individual, but also to destroy the person's sense of self.

The situation of the blue collar or unionized worker is seen by Shorres as far better. Because of the union, work rules and expectations are well defined. Grievance procedures and regularly scheduled contract negotiations are publicly conducted. Further, the individual is not expected to give his total being to the company, only his hands for a defined period of time. Others do not see the situation of the blue collar or unionized worker in such an advantageous light. Union officials are not necessarily trusted. They are often seen as serving their own interests or those of management, leaving the worker a powerless pawn.

Jacques conceptualizes the stress emanating from the workplace somewhat differently (479). He describes stress situations as those in which a person finds himself either (a) being held accountable for completing tasks that cannot be completed because of inadequate resources or inconsistencies in the organization, or (b) being held accountable for tasks that are either too difficult because they are beyond the capacity of the individual or too easy because the level of work is far below the individual's capacity. Given these situations, the individual is likely to feel frustrated, inadequate, or bored.

Finally, stress may arise from the nature of the occupation itself. There are some occupations considered deviant by the wider social system (727). Others, although in general not considered deviant, may require engagement in activities that violate social norms and/or the law. Some occupations involve dirty, disagreeable, or dangerous tasks; others require a demeaning, subservient posture relative to superiors or clients. All of these situations may arouse feelings and ideas about the self that are at variance with the individual's identity.

The expectations, conflicts, and anxieties the individual brings to the workplace are the other source of stress to be discussed here (479). First, an individual's capacity to work may be impaired by the absorption of energy in internal conflicts. This leaves little energy available for dealing with unexpected demands and situations. Thus, even minor incidents may be experienced as stress. Second, all individuals have to come to terms with the primitive fears of early childhood arising from being incompetent, helpless, and dependent on others for survival and need satisfaction. The degree to which an individual has resolved these fears will influence the person's ability to deal with the reality-based uncertainties and insecurities of the workplace. Third, the individual may have such high expectations for his own performance, that he takes on too many or too difficult tasks, a set of responsibilities that could be accomplished only by the most extraordinary person. Fourth, if work is by far the largest factor in the individual's identity, any problem or difficulty that may arise at work may be seen as a threat. Finally, the individual may not have an adequate support system: others, within or outside the context of work, to whom he can turn for advice, reassurance, and comfort. In such a case, work problems are often not dealt with on a day-to-day basis but allowed to grow unchecked into stress-producing situations.

Individuals often tolerate a high degree of symptom-producing work stress if the status and prestige of the job and/or the financial reward is sufficiently high. There are also other people with a seemingly personal, destructive component who are easily and repeatedly seduced into stress-inducing situations, and who stay in these situations past the point where there are actual symptoms of stress. People have considerably more difficulty with stress if they see the problem as being within themselves rather than the organization. It becomes even more difficult if the individual is, indeed, not adequate for the job. Work-related stress, similar to other types of stress, can lead to a variety of physical and emotional problems, which in and of themselves can lead to additional stress.

Work Cycle

The work cycle is a continuous process, following a sequence of characteristic stages loosely connected with chronological age (183,345,939). It is a developmental process that extends from approximately the age of 6 years to retirement. It includes the acquisition of basic work skills (task and interpersonal), initial and subsequent occupational choices, formal training or education for a specific work role, on-the-job socialization, movement within an occupation, and withdrawal from the workplace. Although the work cycle follows a sequence of typical stages, it is influenced by the interplay of factors within the individual and environmental factors. Personal factors influencing the work cycle are sex, age, race or nationality, physical condition, appearance, intelligence, education, personality or temperament, abilities (both general and specific), and interests. Whatever the constellation of attributes described above, they are likely to qualify an individual for a number of occupations in which he or she is able to succeed and gain satisfaction. A characteristic pattern of attributes, however, is more appropriate for some occupations than for others.

Environmental factors that influence the work cycle are parents, partners, significant adults, peers, geographical distribution of industries, state of the economy, regional manpower needs, social class and financial position of the family, and its willingness to be mobile in the pursuit of work. Environmental factors change over time and may have a positive or adverse effect on the unfolding of an individual's work cycle.

The portion of the work cycle that has been studied most extensively is the period that leads up to initial occupational choice: the first 10 to 15 years of the cycle. This part of the cycle is divided into three stages: fantasy choices (6-11 years), tentative choices (11-17 years), and realistic choices (17-early 20s). Initial occupational choice is considered to be the outcome of compromise at each stage. The process is considered to be somewhat irreversible wherein earlier decisions tend to reduce the degrees of freedom available for later decisions. It is increasingly more difficult to reverse the investment in time and effort. If reversal or return to an earlier stage does occur, the individual may experience a temporary sense of failure and insecurity. Initial occupational choice is also limited by the individual's failure to perceive the existence of certain occupations or, without due consideration, finding certain occupations objectionable or unacceptable, too unattainable, or requiring too great an expenditure of time, money, and effort. Accurate information about a variety of occupations and knowledge of one's self are considered to be factors of considerable importance in selecting an occupation that will be congenial with one's aptitudes, interests, and values.

The other period of the work cycle that has recently been given some attention is the period of reassessment (35-50 years). At this time the individual pauses to contemplate, and plan for the remaining years of his work cycle. A career change of some magnitude may occur. It appears that, if a new occupation choice is made, the process leading up to that choice is somewhat similar to that just described for initial occupational choice, the difference being a shorter time span and usually considerably more knowledge: of occupations and of the self.

The work cycle is guided by a socialization process, which has been previously described. A few additional comments are necessary. Socialization is affected by a matrix of social experiences initially channeling development toward a general worker role. Subsequently, socialization is directed toward development of attributes specific to a particular occupational role. The latter, more specifically focused socialization is concerned with the acquisition of knowledge, techniques, occupational values, and ideology and "tricks of the trade." It is important to note that socialization occurs throughout the work cycle. It is as operant in the final stage of departure from the work cycle as it is in the formative stages. A more complete discussion of the work cycle is provided in Chapter 5.

Work-Related Deficits

Problems related to taking on the role of a worker have been studied extensively by Neff (727,728). He has categorized these difficulties in three different ways: deficits arising from inadequate early socialization, common behavioral patterns of individuals who have marked difficulty in the workplace, and the work problems of individuals who have a recognized disability. These categories are not mutually exclusive; any given individual may fit fairly easily into more than one of the described categories.

Deficits arising from inadequate socialization are threefold. The individual may not have internalized the precept of society that people are expected to play a productive role in the social system. The subculture of work is simply unknown or unrecognized by such an individual. Not only is the idea of work alien but the individual has not acquired the basic task and interpersonal skills necessary for the work role. Second, the individual may have internalized society's requirement for productivity, but within the context of a deviant subculture. The individual is willing and able to work, but in an occupation society considers to be illegal, immoral, or both. Finally, the individual may have only partially internalized the worker role but remains in conflict regarding some aspects of the role. Conflicts often center around relating to peers and to authority. The individual may have difficulty controlling certain needs for intimacy or privacy or have difficulty meeting the standards imposed by others.

Neff identified five common behavioral patterns associated with marked difficulty in the workplace:

1. A major lack in work motivation with a high negative value being placed on the work role;
2. manifest fear and anxiety as a response to the demand to be productive;
3. a general response in the work setting characterized by open hostility and aggression;
4. marked dependency;
5. a profound degree of social naiveté.

Although not identified as a particular pattern, in addition to the above, people who have difficulty in the work setting may be impulsive, withdrawn (apathetic), and/or self-deprecatory.

Individuals with recognized disabilities may be handicapped relative to work in three ways. First, there may be impairment or limitation of certain functional abilities and aptitudes that are required for specific kinds of work, e.g., mobility, manual dexterity, intelligence, cognitive organization. Second, there may be difficulty in coping with the negative and aversive feelings that one's disabilities arouse in others. Third, the disability may have arrested, distorted, or blocked the development of task and interpersonal skills basic to the worker role.

Although Neff feels that many individuals with work-related deficits can learn to become workers, he also realistically states that some individuals may never be able to work or only be able to be employed in a protective environment such as a sheltered workshop. Being a worker is a very important social role. People can, however, lead satisfying lives without being a worker.

Women and Work

As mentioned in the introduction to this section, there is little research about women in the worker role. It is presumptuous to say that the ideas about work outlined above apply equally to women. Until more information is accumulated, one can only tentatively suppose that many of the ideas do apply to women as well as men. Some exceptions documented in the literature, at least to a degree, will be discussed here (79,96,171,234,455, 478,855,872,888).

The general socialization process for women is different from that of men. Most women are socialized to the role of spouse and parent first and to that of being a worker secondarily, the opposite being true for men (727). Society's assumptions and priorities are quite clear. Men are responsible for providing financial support for home and family. Women are not expected to be competent in the workplace; men are not expected to be competent in familial roles. This set of values is in the process of changing, but that change is not particularly marked. Women in the world of work are not really taken seriously (872). They are useful and welcome in the marketplace, but only in low paying, low level positions; their first commitment is to children, husband, and home; they are only temporary workers. The fact that a woman is successful and satisfied with her job is still noted, with bewilderment, in the national news media (171).

With socialization to the worker role being secondary, many women, not surprisingly, have difficulty in being a worker. They have problems with seeing themselves as a worker; being a worker is less central to their identity. They have problems with being assertive, particularly in relationship to men. Women have difficulty in dealing with the impersonal nature of the work setting, placing a higher value on emotionally integrated personal relationships. They tend to be less comfortable with competition, preferring a more open and collaborative work climate. Women often have problems in leadership/administrative positions, particularly in the areas of setting goals and priorities for themselves and others, delegating responsibility, time management, objective and critical assessment of subordinates and superiors, and applying negative sanctions. Finally, women, being to a degree outsiders, see much that is ridiculous, affectatious, and petty in the workplace. Men may not take women in the workplace seriously, but there are many women who have difficulty taking some of the mores and customs of the workplace seriously (673).

Although now illegal, women continue to be discriminated against in the work setting (117). Discrimination occurs on two levels: economic and genital. Economically, women are in the lowest paying, often least skilled jobs, and have considerable difficulty in advancing beyond this position. This is not entirely the fault of the workplace. Many women enter the world of work with minimal training or skills. However, little is done on the job to provide training or opportunities for appropriate socialization. There are other women, well qualified to advance to higher levels of an occupation, who are neither encouraged nor allowed to do so. It is true that some women do not want the responsibilities and often heavier workload of more advanced positions. However, this is not always the case. In a situation where both a man and a woman are equally qualified for an advancement, the man continues to be more likely to get the position. Discrimination is, however, more subtle than simply who is selected to fill a job opening. It occurs primarily in the socialization process that takes place in the work setting. A woman is often not given the opportunity to participate in the matrix of experiences that are, in part, designed to prepare one for more advanced positions (888). Women are less likely to be given a special project or problem to handle, to gather with coworkers and supervisors at a bar after work, or to go on a business trip with the boss. It is in these situations that a good deal of socialization for advanced positions takes place. In addition, women are much less likely to have mentors to guide and assist them in continued learning and to champion their progression in the work setting. Women are unlikely to have mentors because most people in superior positions are men. Thus, there are an insufficient number of women mentors. Men often prefer not to enter into a mentor-neophyte relationship with a woman. There is always a sexual element present, which adds a complicating element to the relationship. This may cause some problems for the participants in the relationship, and/or nonparticipants may raise questions about the possible sexual nature of the relationship.

Sexual harassment or genital discrimination is another problem women sometimes find in the workplace. Harassment may take the form of supposedly humorous comments related to women's anatomy or stereotyped "feminine" characteristics, seeking a sexually based relationship, or the demand for sexual intercourse. This may occur in the casual daily activities of the factory or office, or it may take place in the context of preferential treatment or job advancement. Such harassment is not particularly surprising. Neither men nor women have been socialized to participate in mixed-sex work groups; they do not know how to deal with the issue of sexuality. People, for the most part, have not learned how to relate to members of the opposite sex outside the context of family interactions and couple-related activities. Traditionally, men have been socialized to view women primarily as sexual beings; women have been socialized to use sexuality to gain recognition, acceptance, and favors. Given this traditional socialization, it is actually a wonder that there are not more sexually related problems in the workplace than there are. Nevertheless, the burden to define and maintain the limits of sexuality in the work setting is often placed on women. Women are most often blamed if these limits are overstepped. The myth of the seducing woman and innocent foolish man is still thriving in the workplace (171).

Turning to another issue, women often find themselves in conflict vis-à-vis work and the demands of child rearing. This is particularly true of women who are strongly motivated to pursue a career. There are several questions that must be addressed by women, which, incidentally, are rarely addressed by men. The first is whether to have children. If a woman decides to have children or a child, the next question is when. The options are essentially (a) to have children prior to beginning a career, or (b) to become somewhat settled in one's career and then have children. If one takes the first option, there may be considerable delay in career preparation or in beginning a career. If one takes the second option, there may be a temporary interruption in one's career either in actuality or in the time and energy one has to devote to one's career. The final question that must be addressed is whether to work while one is raising young children. These are all difficult questions, with different consequences, for familial roles and one's role as a worker.

Finally, the work cycle of women is likely to deviate from that of men (872). Differences in the socialization process have already been mentioned. A woman's work cycle is likely to be punctuated with delays and interruptions. There are often less frequent promotions and the occupational level attained may be lower than that of a man with comparable skills. There is a tendency in our society to believe that for women to be really accepted and in the workplace, that their work cycle should mirror that of men. The modern work setting and the male work cycle are intertwined, developed together and influencing each other. The work cycle of women, although still in flux, does not mesh well with the current design of socialization and progression in the workplace. A compromise of some type does seem in order.

The Student as a Worker

School is the primary formal learning situation in our society that prepares the individual for entry into the job market (183,271,400,587,669,727). It serves to wean the child away from fulltime play and the family. It forms the bridge between the home and the wider community. Graduation from high school or college is referred to as a commencement: the beginning of adulthood, of being productive. Graduation signals to the individual and to the community that the person is ready to move into the world of work. In addition, a high school diploma or college degree is prerequisite for entry into many occupations.

The structure and interpersonal demands of school are similar in many ways to those of the workplace. However, at least initially, there is some flexibility and tolerance for individual differences. Learning tasks are relatively simple, often couched in play activities. As one progresses through school, learning tasks become increasingly structured, complex, and demanding: relationships with teachers and administrators often become more impersonal.

Motivation to engage in formal learning tasks is similar to that of work to some extent. Initially, however, the child is often motivated by love and acceptance needs. It is only later that the individual makes the connection between school and work and thus the connection to money. As the association between school and work becomes stronger, the individual's studies often become more directed and goal oriented.

Essentially, the individual's purpose for being in school is to master task and interpersonal skills basic to being a worker. In addition to gaining command of academic subjects, the individual learns to follow directions, organize and implement a task, perform disliked tasks adequately, accept judgment on the basis of performance, function within the confines of an externally imposed time schedule, be punctual in attendance, and groom one's self and dress in an appropriate manner. Interpersonal skills such as accepting the authority of the teacher, behaving differentially and appropriately in the classroom, informal interactions in the lunchroom and on the playground, and how to engage in cooperative and competitive activities are also learned. Individuals deprived of usual and typical school experiences have considerable difficulty in taking on the role of a worker.

Some students have difficulty coping with the demands of the school setting. This may be due to a physically disabling condition, intellectual impairment or other cognitive deficits, emotional problems, or various types of learning disabilities. A child who is not able to perform adequately in school has a good deal of difficulty maintaining an adequate self-image. Aside from the fact that most failure experiences are difficult to cope with, the child does not have a large store of past success experiences to refer to as does the adult. Beyond the child's familial role, she has few other roles to use as a source of satisfaction and focal point for organizing an adequate self-image. Children who do poorly in school are likely to act out their frustrations in a number of different ways and to demonstrate a markedly low self-esteem. In the future, such individuals often have difficulty in the workplace.

In summary, work is a major, complex area of human experience. It is a significant component of identity and thus reverberates through all aspects of the individual's interaction with the environment. Work is an instrumental activity, carried out by human beings, which involves a struggle with the environment for compelling material reasons: physical survival, social survival, and rewarding social status. The work setting has both a formal and informal structure that demands specific behaviors on the part of the individual. Although work can be highly satisfying and rewarding, it can also be a source of stress. Individuals' work-related experiences are organized in a work cycle: a developmental process following a sequence of characteristic stages loosely connected with chronological age. It extends from approximately six years of age to retirement. The work cycle of women differs in some respects to those of men, and women encounter some additional problems in the workplace. Students are considered to be in preparation for their roles as productive workers, the school offering socializing experiences, which enable the individual to learn task and interpersonal skills basic to the work role.

PLAY/LEISURE/RECREATION

Play/leisure/recreation (PLR) is that sphere of solitary or shared human experience engaged in for the purpose of amusement, relaxation, or self-actualization. The formation and maintenance of various types of friend relationships are an important part of this aspect of human interaction. Play/leisure/recreation glorifies interests, caters to needs, flatters capacities, and blends reality and fantasy. It includes rituals and ceremonies, spontaneous play, games, sports, hobbies, contemplation and conversation, literature and the arts, and voluntary participation in the affairs of the community. It contributes to personal satisfaction and growth, provides an outlet for emotions, joins individuals together in friendships, and is one of the major bonds that unifies a community and a society (131,132). The totality of PLR is a universal activity found in every known society and cultural group. Children play; adults find time for leisure, engage in solitary pursuits, or join together in recreational activities.

As a sphere of human experience, PLR is often defined in the negative, primarily in terms of being a nonwork activity. It is a nonwork activity but, in part, shares some of the characteristics of work: effort, concentration, serious intent, and so forth. Defined by differentiation for the purpose of this text, PLR are those activities that one engages in outside the time spent in activities of daily living, familial responsibilities, and work. That is not to say that PLR activities do not take place within the context of familial interaction and the workplace; they do. In addition, some activities of daily living are treated or engaged in as PLR activities. The lines then between these four spheres of human experience are not set or impervious. There is an intermingling that enhances all spheres and promotes a sense of integrated personal identity (131,132,181,192,762).

Play/leisure/recreation activities may be solitary or shared. As a solitary endeavor they are undertaken and enjoyed alone, often providing relief from the demands of human interaction. As a shared endeavor they form the matrix for and sustain friendships. It is primarily in this sphere of human experience that one relates to nonfamilial others on a personal level marked by mutual affection.

There is a component of PLR that is not often found in the other three major spheres of human experience: the not real, the pretend, fantasy. It is found particularly in children's play, in literature, and the arts but it is also a component of many of the other aspects of PLR. Reality and fantasy are combined, fused, harmonized to produce experiences not found in conventional interactions in the "real" world.

Participation in PLR is considered to be a social role. The ability to participate is acquired through a socialization process. It is not usual to think of children learning how to play; infants seem to engage in playful activities spontaneously. This is true, but only if the environment is designed to elicit and facilitate play-like activities. As the infant grows older, some limits are set and particular kinds of play are encouraged and discouraged. The importance of socialization becomes increasingly evident as the child begins to share play activities with others and learns games and sports.

The significance and centrality of one's role as a player varies between individuals and at various times in the life cycle. It is a sustained social role that begins in early infancy and continues until near or at the time of death.

This section is divided into three parts: play, games, and sports; leisure; and recreation. This separation is made with the understanding that these overlap and are intertwined. There is, nevertheless, something different about each aspect. Play, as in the primary activities of early childhood, is more spontaneous, unstructured, and fantasy laden than activities usually described as recreational. Games and sports are "played," but they have externally imposed rules. Leisure as an entity is usually described in terms of time: the period when one is free from work, other employments, and social obligations. Recreation is usually described in terms of various types of activities and has the connotation of being a part of adolescent and adult experience. One would, for example, rarely speak of the recreational activities of a three-year-old child, or for that matter the leisure time of a three-year-old. The division, although arbitrary, is made.

Play, Games, and Sports

The play of early childhood, fairly freestyle games, formal games, and sports can be seen as being on a rough continuum related to the life cycle.

Play

Play is an activity in which there is a high degree of choice and a lack of constraint from conventional ways of handling objects, materials, and ideas. It provokes laughter, pleasure, and enjoyment but is, at times, taken very seriously. There is a special quality to play activities that occurs prior to participation in games with externally imposed rules: prior to the age of six years. This is also the age at which most children enter first grade. Daily life comes to be divided fairly distinctly between the time of school and a time for play. The discussion here, then, will focus on the play of the preschool child (305,394,418,602,669,684,902,977,1002). The school-age child continues to engage in preschool play but begins to participate in a number of other, more complex PLR activities.

In the literature, play has been conceptualized in a variety of different ways. It has been categorized by: (a) activities, e.g., toys, games, books, television; (b) types, e.g., imitation, exploration, movement; (c) function, e.g., the development of organizational skills, problem solving, practice of adult roles; and (d) age, the typical play behavior at a given point in chronological age.

Each way of categorizing has its particular purpose. Of concern here are the process and function of play, with activities used primarily for illustrative purposes. Areas to be discussed are theories of play, types of play, deficits in play, and play as an attitude.

Theories of play are multiple and varied (669,684). Through the ages many scholars have been interested in the phenomenon of play. They have asked the question, "What is it for, what is its purpose?" Plato and Aristotle saw play as the way in which children prepared for the productive responsibilities of adulthood. The idea of play as the means whereby children practice and perfect skills needed in adult life has continued to this day. In the seventeenth through the nineteenth centuries, various other theories of play were suggested. Play was seen as the way in which the child used up surplus energy. Others simply considered it as the expression of childish imagination and ideas. Stanley Hall and his associates put forth a recapitulation theory of play. Children were seen as repeating the evolutionary chain from animals to modern adults—reenacting in play the interests and occupations in the sequence in which they occur in prehuman animals and primitive, prehistoric man. Evidence for this was the child's early interest in water play—manifestation of our aquatic ancestors; interest in climbing—manifestation of our relationship to primates; interest in hunting, fishing, and being in groups—manifestation of primitive tribal life. This theory is no longer generally accepted.

The eighteenth and nineteenth centuries saw a growth of concern about childhood and education. Children were no longer seen as little adults, but rather as being different and worthy of study in their own right. Teachers were urged to take into consideration children's natural interests and stages of development. This educational reform culminated in the work of Froebel, who insisted that young children learn best through spontaneous play (605). He stressed the importance of play in early academic learning. In the twentieth century, Susan Isaac brought this idea further and emphasized the value of a rich and free environment as an aid in learning (469). She identified three kinds of play as being important: (a) gross motor activities, which helped to perfect bodily skills and muscular control, (b) play with objects and toys, which prompted children to ask questions and develop reason, and (c) imaginative play, which satisfied frustrated desires and relieved inner tension. Imaginative play was also seen as a bridge for intellectual development, where a child passes from the symbolic meaning of things to active inquiry into their real construction. In this same vein, more recently, the International Council for Children's Play defined the purpose of play as a means of facilitating (a) physical development and bodily health, (b) emotional stability and mental health, (c) intellectual growth and learning, and (d) friendliness and cooperation between children.

There are three more specialized theories of play that are currently viewed as relevant. A psychoanalytic theory of play was outlined by Sigmund Freud (317). In this theory play is seen as a manifestation of, and guided by, the pleasure principle. The wishes and conflicts of each developmental stage are reflected in children's play either directly or by substitute or symbolic activity. Unpleasant events are repeated in play because repetition reduces excitement and may enable the child to master the disturbing event by bringing it about, rather than by being a passive recipient. Anna Freud and Melanie Klein emphasized the symbolic meaning of play and used this as the basis for understanding and treating emotionally disturbed children. They formulated the idea of play therapy.

Arthur Jersild developed a theory in regard to imaginative play (481). He stated that this type of play promoted the learning of social behavior, provided an outlet for forbidden behavior, and was a means whereby the child could express his interests. He felt that imaginative play eventually takes the forms of day dreams, which in turn may facilitate problem solving. Jersild was particularly interested in the phenomenon of imaginary playmates. He felt that such playmates provided companionship and that, at times, they were endowed with virtues the child did not have. On the other hand, imaginary playmates may be endowed with antisocial behavior and may be placed in the position of a scapegoat.

Piaget viewed play both as a manifestation of and a vehicle for the development of cognition—the capacity to engage in logical thinking (302,773). He viewed the play of infants as the process of changing incoming information to suit the child's requirements, with no concern for the reality of the stimuli. As children grow older their play demonstrates a more accurate representation of reality; it becomes increasingly constructive and adapted to reality. At that point, Piaget states that play, as such, ceases. It is replaced by activity controlled by collective discipline and codes of honor: by games with rules.

There are various types of play; four will be briefly described here: exploratory and movement play, fantasy and make-believe play, imitative play, and social play (684). Exploratory and movement play is a response to stimuli, especially new or different stimuli. It involves the continuum of looking, listening, manipulating of the infant to the running, jumping, throwing, and rough and tumble play of the older child. There are three facets to exploring and movement play that are repeated in endless variation: (a) exploration as a reaction to novel stimulus patterns, (b) manipulation, which itself produces changes in stimuli, and (c) repetition and repetition with variation, which serves to integrate the experience with the rest of the child's repertoire of skills. Repetition with variation is often less a function of the degree of novelty than of the complexity and number of skills the child possesses.

Exploratory and movement play changes over time, as the child becomes more mature. It increases as the child becomes capable of more varied activities and thus can impose more change on the environment. This is followed by a decrease as fewer events and skills are novel, and those that are novel are mastered very quickly. Finally, there is a waxing and waning of this type of play. As the child becomes capable or aware of specific activities, these are explored, practiced, mastered, and ultimately integrated into the child's repertoire of behavior. When they have been fully explored, the child moves on to something new and more challenging.

Exploratory and movement play seems to arise out of the human organism's "bias" toward novelty and mastery. A monotonous environment usually gives rise to discomfort, irritation, and attempts to make the environment more interesting or stimulating. A child seems to thrive best in an environment where there are a variety of sounds, sights, smells, tastes, and things to touch, and freedom to explore. As important as novelty is, it is best if presented in the context of the familiar. This reduces fear and overexcitement, which hinders perception and integration. The inherent desire to master or be competent can be seen on two levels: physical and cognitive. The child spends considerable time mastering body movements and the surrounding physical environment. The newly bipedal child's preoccupation with walking and the concentration addressed to the removal of shoes are examples of physical mastery. Cognitive mastery is the intellectual understanding of stimuli: the why, the what, the how. It involves classifying, coding, and organizing events into manageable units, which in turn facilitates taking in additional information. What an individual knows already is boring. What is perceived as too complicated, however, is equally tiresome. Unexpected variations on a theme are what seem to attract.

Fantasy and make-believe play involves the processes of imagining and pretending. It begins when the child uses patterns of behavior developed in response to one set of objects as a response to a new set of objects. The child "pretends" that the old and new sets are similar. Patterns of behaviors then are used out of their original context. A child, for example, may manipulate her father's nose as if it were a door knob, expecting the father to open his mouth. Later real objects are no longer needed, as in throwing a non-existent ball. The child will imagine himself as all sorts of interesting characters involved in a variety of harrowing or pleasant adventures. A set of dominoes becomes an army; a panda is given a birthday party.

Children's conscious involvement in fantasy and make-believe play is thought, at least in part, to be due to less than a mature grasp of secondary process thinking. Thinking is still governed by primary process, with its confusion regarding temporal and spatial relationships, condensation, displacement, lack of formal logic, and ill-defined difference between what is real and not real. This interpretation of the genesis of fantasy and make-believe play is supported by the decrease in this type of play around the age of seven or eight years. By that time children are able to engage in a good deal of secondary process, albeit concrete, thinking. Children's thinking about objects, people, and events has become sufficiently skilled to dispense with the props of objects and actions. Make-believe play, to a considerable extent, is replaced by daydreaming. Make-believe play does, however, continue for some children into adolescence.

In addition to the previously presented ideas of Freud and Jersild about fantasy and make-believe play, other purposes or functions have been ascribed to this type of play. It is felt that such play contributes to the development of self-awareness, imagery skills, verbal skills, emotional awareness and sensitivity, flexibility, and creativity. It is felt that children who engage in appropriate amounts of fantasy and make-believe play are more secure and happier than children who are either deficient or primarily involved in this type of play.

Imitative play involves activities that reproduce or mirror events in the same way and sequence as they occur. It is encouraged by considerable contact with adults, older children, and a generally rich environment. Imitation may not be exact, often including a good deal of variation on a theme. The child essentially identifies with another person and plays the role of that person in a realistic kind of way. There is many a father, for example, who has observed his child faithfully reproduce his parental role, a cogent experience. At around six or seven years of age, there is a marked decrease in imitation play; the child now engages in covert, internal thinking about people and events: overt action is no longer necessary.

One of the major functions of imitative play is thought to be a sort of rehearsal of adult roles. Closely related to this function is the development of the capacity to take "the role of the other," an important factor in any role relationship. The child also distills out of his imitated interactions various rules and sanctions that are a part of social interactions. Imitative play is often derived from a situation that impressed the child. The function of such play is to assist in understanding, integrating, and storing that impression, to remember because it was a happy experience or to lessen the anxiety of and exert some control over an unhappy experience.

The last type of play to be discussed here is social play. Social play begins in early infancy and is initiated by adults. The child responds by about the age of six weeks with a smile, the first truly social response in the child's repertoire. By seven months the child is an active participant in social play with adults and, in fact, initiates such play. The child's interest then slowly turns to other children, starting initially by simply observing their behavior. There is a stage-by-stage process by which the child becomes more involved with other children and learns to be a participant with them in shared play. These stages will be outlined in Chapter 5. The development of social play is initially facilitated by adults who take pleasure in such play. Later it is enhanced by the presence of supportive adults and the availability of children of a relatively similar age. The function of social play is readily apparent. It is the beginning of the development of social skills: of learning how to interact with a variety of others outside familial interactions.

Four types of play and the function of each have been outlined. It should be remembered, however, that these types of play are not mutually exclusive. They blend together and may rarely be seen in their pure form. In watching a child involved in a given play interaction, one may observe two, three, or all four kinds of play intertwined. The probably universal children's activity of "playing house" is a good example.

Up to this point the importance of play, both as a source of satisfaction and as the means whereby the child learns many skills necessary for adult life, has been outlined. The child, then, who does not play or plays only within a narrow range is at a marked disadvantage. Deficits in play are found in a variety of children (74,363,681). The physically handicapped child is often unable to explore and manipulate the nonhuman environment and frequently lives within a restricted human environment. The child who is unable to organize stimuli at the subcortical level, or at the cortical level, or who is intellectually impaired, is often unable to make any sense out of the environment; it appears a jumbled, chaotic mess. Without assistance, such a child is not able to impose order. The child who lives in an emotionally deprived situation, in a ghetto, or an impoverished rural area often lives in a monotonous, unstimulating environment. But more important, such a child is frequently primarily concerned with survival. Preoccupation with survival obliterates play. Children who do not play live in a restricted world circumscribed by their environment's deficit.

The immediate response of children who do not play is as varied as the reasons for deficits in play: they may engage in disruptive behavior, withdraw, become overly dependent, be reduced to self-stimulation, develop bizarre and repetitive patterns of behavior. These perfectly natural responses nevertheless compound the problem. They set up another barrier to engaging in meaningful, pleasurable play. These children fear failure and rejection: the inherent need to master and be competent lies buried under frustration and past defeats.

Children who do not play come to adulthood ill prepared. They lack task and interpersonal skills, have no sense of their place in the world, feel unable to effect change on their environment, do not know what to expect, or what is expected. They are basically naive, and often angry.

Beyond being an activity, play is an attitude (418,602). Children play, seemingly with a great deal of joy. Play, regardless of its various functions, appears to be engaged in for its own sake, because it is pleasurable. Serious activities, in contrast, deal with taking care of bodily needs, dealing with external facts, or are concerned with specific practical ends. But play is more than an activity of children. It is an attitude, a way of relating to the environment. As such, it permeates the daily activities of some individuals. The play element is operant in those individuals who experience the joy of mastery and approach tasks with a glint of joviality in their eyes. It is seen in the individual who does not take a good deal of the human experience entirely seriously.

Playfulness is also reflected in a particular type of cognitive style characterized by flexibility and spontaneity. The individual is able to draw on previous knowledge, play with existing ideas, and relate them to new facts. It is the ability to rearrange the familiar and the capacity for distancing that frees the individual from being bound by social stereotypes and traditional ways of thinking. It is the ability to engage in divergent thinking.

A playful cognitive style fosters creative thinking in the arts and in science. In being able to play with ideas, the individual is able to shed new light on the human experience and advance our scientific knowledge of the universe. A playful cognitive style enables an individual to enjoy humor and wit for themselves, and as a means of relieving tension and some of the drudgery of life. The individual realizes that dealing with serious matters is not always helped by taking the matter seriously. A playful attitude brings excitement and zest to living. It is one of the delightful characteristics of being human.

Games and Sports

Games and sports begin to replace preschool play at about the age of six years (902). Previous to that time, a child or a small group of children frequently make up their own rules to give some structure to how a game should be played. The rules, however, are made up for that moment of play; the game may be played in an entirely different way the next time. Rules are flexible and a change may be negotiated during the game. When the child begins to engage in games with externally imposed rules, he or she essentially enters the world of adult-like games and sports.

Caillois differentiates the sphere of games and sports from other spheres of human experience—family interaction, activities of daily living, and work—on the basis of six criteria (157). Games and sports are: (a) free, not obligatory; one can choose to participate or not to participate; (b) separated, circumscribed within space and time that is defined and fixed in advance; (c) uncertain, the course cannot be determined or the results known beforehand; there is some latitude for innovations left to the player's initiative; (d) unproductive, neither goods, wealth, nor services are created; (e) governed by rules, ordinary laws are suspended; players participate under conventions that are established for the purpose of the game; and (f) make-believe, a new reality, different from that of daily life, is operant during the period of play.

Games and sports, in addition to play, have been viewed as a phenomenon that serves to bond social units (181,801,811). In such a scheme, play is seen as taking place with intimate partners serving to integrate the individual into such associations. Games take place with peers and serve to integrate a locality, neighborhood, or ethnic community. Sports take place with people from different districts, social classes, and ethnic backgrounds. They serve to integrate entire communities in nation-state or international units.

Although games and sports may have a role in maintaining social units, they have also been described as being important in developing and maintaining skills needed for daily interaction in a social system. Team games and individual and competitive team sports require the adherence to a set of rules that are externally imposed by the nature of the game or sport. Through involvement in games, the individual must act within certain constraints that govern socially acceptable behavior in a particular situation. There is a need to relate to, share, and cooperate with peers, as well as dealing with an adversary and competitive interactions. A differentiation must be made between fair and foul play. Sports and games that require physical skill call on the individual to be independent, self-reliant, and to take responsibility for one's self. One gains a sense of being master of one's own body.

Games of strategy require the individual to attend to the motivations, thinking, feelings, and behavior of others. One essentially must take the role of another person, an important skill in the acquisition of any new social role. Games of chance require the individual to recognize and deal with the fact that there are events over which one has no control. They help the individual to maintain a human perspective in the face of the unknown, ungovernable, the supernatural. Conversely, there is exhilaration in trying to beat the odds and winning through no real efforts of one's own. Solving various types of puzzles is quite the opposite of games of chance. It provides an opportunity for individuals to see themselves as a causal agent. In solution of a puzzle, there is a sense of being in control of the situation at hand.

In conclusion, play, games, and sports serve as sources of personal enjoyment, help to form social bonds, and facilitate the development and maintenance of a variety of skills.

Leisure

Although the physical body must be nourished, protected, and sustained, and children raised, the individual pursues and endeavors to attain something more. The individual seeks meaning in life, ideals for which to strive. The individual seeks physical and emotional health, a degree of freedom, self-knowledge, to be wanted by and useful to others, and to find one's place in the universe. This takes place or is accomplished to a great extent within the context of leisure (37,131,132,157, 181,219,501, 608,762,811).

Leisure is derived from the Latin verb *licere*—to be permitted. Now it is usually defined as a time when one is free from family and other social responsibilities, activities of daily living, and work. It is characterized by a feeling of comparative freedom and self-determination. The individual has a range of choices: limited to some degree by availability of facilities, the individual's knowledge of opportunities, time, money, and the opinions of others as to what constitutes desirable use of leisure time. The latter is not decisive but taken into account. Freedom of choice implies there is something from which to choose, and that the individual is capable of making a choice. Choice and involvement in leisure activities are motivated by enjoyment and personal satisfaction.

Leisure is sometimes thought of as simply a means of providing a compensatory balance relative to activity of daily living/work/family responsibilities. This is not wise, for it demeans the importance and richness of leisure. Thus, here, leisure will be treated as a complete entity, not as an adjunct to other aspects of human life and social order. A universal phenomenon, leisure exists in desperate poverty and in economic affluence. Involvement in leisure is particularly human and demonstrates our wonderful capacity for finding the occasions and recalling or inventing the ways of not being useful. Much of leisure is spent within the matrix of small groups, which are characterized by open expression of feelings and mutual affection. As such, leisure serves to establish and sustain intragroup bonding.

Until recently, the society seemingly most concerned with leisure was that of the ancient Greeks. Leisure was considered a way of life that enabled men to develop and express all sides of their intellectual, physical, and spiritual nature. Education was directed toward this end. The concept of leisure class was not those who did not work, but those whose overall life possessed a wholesome, leisurely character. The purpose of work was to attain and support leisure. The Greeks felt that without leisure, there could be no culture: arts, letters, scholarly pursuits, sports and games, religion, and the orderly conduct of community affairs. This philosophy of leisure is not entirely accepted in our society today, but is often held up as the ideal for which we should strive.

Recreation is a part of leisure. The term is derived from the Latin verb *recreare*—to create anew or to refresh after toil. Recreation takes place during leisure, but it is a narrower concept best approached and understood through the notion of play—activities socially recognized as being divorced from the serious business of living. Leisure, the broader phenomenon, takes in the whole of nonwork and other obligations where individuals are free to choose. It can occur in settings that have not been constructed purely for recreational purposes, e.g., the family, educational settings, and religious institutions. Recreation as a phenomenon depends on the prior existence of leisure time.

A differentiation will be made here between leisure and recreational activities. Again the distinction is somewhat arbitrary and is based on the degree of seriousness with which the activity is approached. These "nonrecreational" leisure activities will be discussed at the end of this section.

The amount of leisure time currently available to individuals seems to be the source of some controversy in the literature (181,608,811). Comparison is often made to pre-industrial society. It is sometimes assumed, with little hard evidence, that the majority of time in pre-industrial society was devoted to work, to basic survival. This is probably not the case. Hunting and gathering societies do not spend the majority of their time in the search for food but rather enjoy a good deal of leisure. Pre-industrial Western European society, being agriculturally based, was primarily regulated by the cycle of planting and reaping. There was little work to be done in the winter. The large number of religious holidays and festivals is well documented. The other point of comparison is in relationship to the working hours of the late nineteenth and early twentieth centuries, when the workday was indeed long, often with only one day a week free from work, and no vacations. There probably was very little leisure. Improvements in technology and unionization have led to a gradual decrease in the workday and workweek.

Proponents of the idea that we have more leisure time now than ever before present the following evidence. People are living longer. Although people work more hours in their lifetime, the ratio between hours worked and nonworking hours has changed: nonworking hours have expanded more in comparison to hours worked. Smaller families have increased the leisure time of women. There is a growing leisure market—legal and illegal (e.g., drugs, pornography). People are spending more time (and money) on entertainment, sports, travel, and vacations away from home. Finally, it is said that people are, in general, bored and do not know what to do with all of the leisure time they do have. Proponents of this point of view sometimes become rather emotional on the subject, suggesting a crisis at hand. They feel that a vast majority of the population is not prepared to enjoy leisure time. This position is taken usually on the assumption there will be a marked reduction in work hours in the immediate future.

Proponents of the idea that we have less leisure time now than in the past present a different point of view. Their basic premise is that leisure time remains a scarce commodity. They point to the fact that since World War II there has been no major reduction in the workweek. People in management and the professions seem not to have benefited from the modest decline in the workweek, often spending more than eight hours per day in the workplace and bringing work home for the evening and weekends. Many workers attend school for the purpose of job advancement; others hold more than one job or work overtime. It appears that this generation of workers spends more time in traveling to and from work than other generations.

Linder, in *The Harried Leisure Class*, presents an interesting thesis (608). He defines leisure as consumption time: a time to spend what we earn. Rather than having excessive free time, he feels there is less than sufficient leisure time. If there is a leisure class, it is troubled by repeated incursions and burdened with problems and cares. Linder states that economic growth and affluence lead to an increase in the buying of consumptive goods and an increase in the cost and decrease in the quality of services. People have bigger homes, more appliances, and increasingly complex recreational equipment. These goods require service and maintenance. Individuals either have to pay for these by working longer hours or taking care of these goods themselves. In either case, they have less time for leisure. Because of the desire for more leisure time, individuals decrease their time spent in eating, sleeping, and exercise. This in turn minimizes the enjoyment of leisure, with the net result of a harried leisure class. Although written somewhat tongue-in-cheek, Linder makes an interesting point: in pursuit of leisurely consumption, we lose the leisure.

Finally, there is another school of thought that holds that the amount of leisure time is not the issue; rather, it is how we use that time (131,132). The work ethic and its ramifications are seen as the culprit. The stresses of the workplace leave people exhausted, so they have neither the energy nor inclination to engage in any but the most passive leisure activities. The status attached to work and income encourages women with leisure time to enter the world of work. The attitudes of the workplace are brought to leisure: compulsivity, activities as the means to an end, externally imposed conditions, considerable anxiety, high degree of time consciousness, and avoidance of self-actualization. Leisure is seen as too much to do and not enough time. Anxiety is generated by the decisions to be made; activities that are not as time consuming are selected, and activities managed or packaged by others are chosen so as not to waste precious time.

Whether individuals have more or less time for leisure is probably not as important as how they spend the time they do have. Whether one is able to choose freely, and gains satisfaction from the chosen activity, is probably more significant than the factor of time.

Leisure and society are closely related. Leisure cannot be well understood outside the society in which it takes place (501,811). Leisure both contributes to a society and is influenced by that society. In general, leisure is believed to enhance the well-being of a society as a whole. It assists in integrating the community, provides an outlet for feelings of rivalry and celebrates socially significant occasions. More specifically, leisure is considered to be closely related to the cultural life of society. Culture here refers to the arts, letters, scholarly pursuits, sports and games, religion, and the orderly conduct of community affairs. The exact relationship between culture and leisure is questionable: is a society's culture shaped mainly by leisure, or is the reverse a more accurate statement? What is known, however, is that the study of leisure activities tells us much about the basic themes and values of a society.

It has been well documented that culture depends on leisure and the nature of that leisure for its existence and sophistication. Leisure and the culture it engenders are related in direct proportion to the advance of industrial technology or level of productivity. Culture is influenced by how many people a society can support who are not directly involved in productivity and how these people use their time. People not needed for the physical survival of the society may engage in making war, or they may contribute to the enhancement of the culture. If a society wants and can support artists, priests, and athletes, it will have them.

Society frequently attempts to control leisure or conversely to use leisure as a means of control. The most obvious evidence of control is in relationship to what activities, by law, will be permitted. In order to have a viable society, as opposed to anarchy, leisure activities must be contained within a framework of law. Thus, in our society there are laws that govern such possible leisure pursuits as drugs, sex, and violence. More indirectly, there is evidence that the political and industrial sector act so as to encourage uses of leisure that are compatible with their vested interests and that support an existing or desired social order. Examples of this are evident in totalitarian states' control of youth activities. Leisure activities are also used as a means of stifling discontent, as opposed to dealing with the underlying problems. A classical example of this process is the Roman circus. Closer to home, it is evident in the building of recreational facilities in a seriously economically depressed ghetto. On the other hand, societies also build libraries, parks, and athletic facilities that are available to all, including the economically disadvantaged. Although social control of leisure does exist in our society, it is relatively lax. Leisure activities are persistently susceptible to change: fads and fashions rise and fall.

The value system of a society is concerned with the major activities of its members. As mentioned there are those who feel people in our society are dominated by awareness of the clock. The value placed on time, that time be used to give a high yield, prevents relaxed enjoyment of leisure. In addition, there are a number of value judgments in our society about what is good leisure. It should be used constructively and creatively, not as an escape or passive entertainment. Leisure activities should have a strong spiritual base, contribute to health, develop creativity, enhance appreciation of art, literature, drama, nature, and the scientific world, and promote service to others. Roberts' comment on the proper use of leisure is cogent:

> Doing something with one's time tends to be regarded as meritorious. Doing nothing in particular is often considered a reprehensible waste of time. Having a hobby, developing an interest and playing in a sport are regarded as worthwhile uses of free time that deserve public patronage. Sitting around being entertained, drinking and watching television are less likely to be commended as arts deserving sponsorship and cultivation . . . [the condemnation of popular leisure activities is] often propagated by people who view their own taste as superior. (811, p. 101)

There are many factors that influence leisure. Leisure is free from many of the constraints imposed by the workplace. Nevertheless, leisure behavior is shaped by an individual's present circumstances and past history (181,811). Leisure activities may be solitary in nature, but more typically they take place within the context of a group. People organize leisure time around experiences they value, building on the social relationships that surround them. Social relationships are the key processes that link leisure to the wider social system. Regardless of the particular society, leisure is consistently the arena where intimate bonds are established and maintained. It is organized around friend and kin relationships. The quality of leisure depends more on the quality of relationships than on the nature of the activities engaged in or the availability of community facilities. It appears that the demand for leisure facilities is as much a demand for environments that will support interpersonal relationships, as a demand for a place to pursue specific activities.

In addition to the desire for social intercourse, leisure is influenced by an individual's age, gender, marital status, education, and work. A person's place in the life cycle affects particular uses of leisure. Adolescents, for example, often use leisure time to gain new experiences, a variety of experiences, and to experiment with various identities. Individuals who are retired, on the other hand, may see leisure as a burden of too much time, or as finally enough time to pursue an avocational interest. Major junctions or points of transition in the life cycle are a time of "unfreezing," which affects leisure. Usual activities are often discarded, new and different activities explored, and frequently, with some amazement, found interesting. Leisure activities typical of various stages in the life cycle will be outlined in Chapter 5.

In all known societies, gender, in conjunction with age, has been a primary factor in influencing social roles. This is true in the individual's role as a player, as it is in other social roles. Although there is a loosening of gender-activity ties in our society, they have by no means been broken. The typical sports and games of the grade school child tend to remain gender related. Few boys play with dolls; few girls play football. When their children reach adolescence, parents tend to be more concerned about how their daughters, rather than sons, are spending unstructured leisure time outside the home. Girls are likely to be more accountable for their time and restricted in their choice of activities.

Married women's leisure activities outside the home tend to be engaged in with their spouse or within the family group. This appears to be so whether a woman is primarily a homemaker or employed. Married women rarely go out alone with friends for a social evening. Daytime leisure activities for women who do not work are either engaged in alone or in the company of other women, typically within the local community. For unemployed women with young children, the family often becomes the only base for establishing a social network. Thus, an extended kinship system can greatly enrich a woman's social life. The absence of such a system tends to restrict leisure activities to home and nuclear family. Even when a woman's responsibility for young children is diminished, the general pattern of leisure activities remains much the same. Women tend to have a smaller number of friends than men. These friendships, however, tend to be more intimate and emotionally richer than those of men. Women usually belong to a smaller number of voluntary groups than men, but the amount of time they devote to these groups is equal to that of men.

For men, the roles of husband and father seem to be less extensive and demanding. Their job serves as a source of social relations, and they are better able to maintain contact with friends during evening hours and weekends. As with women, the neighborhood is a source of social relationships. Men, however, are less restricted to neighborhood or family. The social network of men tends to be spread over a wider base, leading to a wider range of leisure interests. Men tend to have more friends than women and belong to a greater number of voluntary groups.

Although gender is a relatively strong determinant of leisure companions, it is less influental of leisure activities. This is a relatively recent but marked phenomenon. With the connotation of play, society has become less stringent in gender-activity delineation. Leisure has become the arena for enjoying the prerogatives and challenges of typically opposite-sex activities. Women in the voluntary sector chair committees, raise funds, and determine the expenditure of various organizations. They may also take up carpentry and become knowledgeable supporters and fans of various organized sports. Men feel comfortable in exploring the culinary arts, doing needlecrafts, and spending Saturday working in a residence for retarded children. Gender can be blurred in the sphere of leisure in a way that is less acceptable in the "real" world of other social roles.

Marital status seems to have a rather profound effect on leisure. Research relative to marital status and leisure is primarily based on studies of men. Their extrapolation to women thus is primarily conjecture. Unmarried individuals under 30 years of age spend most of their leisure time in social activities that are oriented to being with friends and meeting new people. There is a courtship, mating aura that surrounds many leisure activities. Little leisure is spent with family members.

Unmarried individuals over 30 years of age find most of their peers are married. After the first year or two of marriage, people tend not to spend leisure time with single individuals. There is a mild social taboo against such contact; single people somehow threaten the integrity of marriage or partnerships. Thus, for unmarried individuals there tends to be a gap in currently available companions and former life styles. This void is usually filled with activities: doing things, rather than in social intercourse. Activities selected either do not require companionship or generate their own interest group. More time may be spent in solitary activities, or there may be considerably more time spent in leisure activities with family members. The latter is fairly common for individuals who live in close proximity to siblings who have children. Spending leisure time with nieces and nephews becomes an enjoyable experience. It appears that only in the absence of social relationships that otherwise fill leisure time does pursuing specific interests become the focus of leisure activities.

Marriage marks the main break with the adolescent and postadolescent leisure style. Interest becomes focused on activities with one's conjugal partner rather than a wide circle of friends. Leisure activities are centered around the home with children, other adult family members, and a small circle of friends. Time spent with casual friends and in social pastimes far removed from home decline sharply. Home, family, television, and the immediate neighborhood form the martix for leisure. The above comments are relative and juxtaposed with the earlier comments related to gender. Both men and women become, with marriage, more home and family centered relative to leisure. This change in focus seems to be more profound with women than with men.

Although not as influential as age, gender, and marital status, education does have some effect on leisure. People with more education tend to spend more time with friends outside the home. Formal education into the early twenties enlarges individuals' personal social network, making them less dependent on family members. College education not only helps to broaden one's contacts, but contributes to the development of social skills. When an individual marries, however, the variations education explains are marginal.

In the past, the study of leisure was primarily seen as an adjunct to the sociology of occupations. Work was seen as the central influence on how people spent their leisure time. Work does influence leisure but age, gender, and marital status are more important variables. There is wide variation in the use of leisure among individuals in the same occupation and the same activities are popular among individuals in diverse occupations.

There are, however, some relationships between work and leisure. For individuals whose work is dangerous or disagreeable, there is often a sharp demarcation between work and leisure. Leisure is used as a distraction or way of escaping from the unpleasantness of work. Other people are essentially indifferent toward their work. It is neither seen as tremendously rewarding nor as particularly distasteful. Such people regard work and leisure as simply being two different parts of their life. They are seen as different types of experiences that provide different satisfactions. Finally, there is a pattern in which work extends into leisure. This pattern, referred to as occupational communities, involves the development of shared viewpoints, attitudes, values, and social relationships. These communities seem to arise when work is intrinsically satisfying and emotionally isolating, or unusual hours isolate individuals from other companions. A good deal of time is spent with colleagues, talking shop, attending meetings, and so forth. People who participate in occupational communities have a wider social network and spend more time away from home, family, and television. When occupational communities do develop they have a considerable impact on leisure.

Income does have some influence on leisure simply because many leisure activities are expensive. People with a low income tend to spend more time watching television and socializing with friends and family. People with higher incomes participate in more activities. People at different income levels have many of the same interests, but there are numerous, subtle variations in how these interests are pursued. Many individuals, for example, like to take vacations away from home and enjoy participation in sports. Where people take vacations and what sports they become involved in are influenced by income.

The nonrecreational leisure activities to be discussed here are fairly limited in number: religion, education, and volunteer community activities (131,132).

Leisure and religion have always been closely related. It is within this matrix that human beings have celebrated the great events of the life cycle and seasonal changes. Most religions have used ceremonies, song, dance, and feasts as a means of celebrating. In addition, in more modern times, churches and temples have been concerned about the leisure needs of their members, often sponsoring a variety of recreational activities for them. Religion and leisure have much in common; they both can contribute to the growth of the individual, provide a chance to achieve balance and perspective, allow one to express inner desires, and recognize the supreme worth of the individual. Religion can also be in conflict with some leisure pursuits. Ideas about personal enjoyment and religious devotion may not always be compatible. Religion has often been used to hold in check overindulgence, excesses, and hedonistic attitude, which are possible within the context of leisure.

In the previous section, education was discussed as similar to and as a preparation for work. For a good deal of the population, education remains principally a competition for credentials. However, for many adults continuing education has become an enjoyable way to spend leisure time (212). They derive pleasure from the opportunity to meet people, acquire new knowledge, and develop various skills. There is a chance to explore and to gain a sense of mastery. Leisure education may be community-based or be located within an institution of higher learning, thus providing a good deal of variation in terms of breadth and depth. Advanced industrial societies can afford education for other than economic returns. The growth of leisure means that education can be extended beyond its purely vocational relevance.

Volunteer community activities, perhaps more than any other leisure activity, relate the individual to the broader social system. It is also an activity that is essential for the maintenance and well-being of most communities. Volunteer community activities include, for example, working for a political candidate, sitting on the school board, visiting the homebound, coaching a little league team, tutoring a student, organizing a protest meeting, planning a block party, and so forth. Many people find volunteer community activities intrinsically rewarding. They also often derive considerable satisfaction from being able to make a direct contribution to the welfare of others. Involvement in the community provides an opportunity to meet a variety of people and to broaden one's circle of friends. It is a leisure activity that is particularly suited to the needs of homemakers who are not employed and individuals who are retired.

Leisure is a time free from work and other responsibilities. It is the time in which one has an opportunity to engage in what is traditionally referred to as recreational activities.

Recreation

Recreation was previously described as being derived from the Latin verb *recreare*—to create anew or to refresh after toil. It refers to those activities that are socially recognized as being divorced from the serious business of living. Some of the most common recreational activities are briefly outlined below. Three points, however, should first be noted.

There is a clear distinction between professional and amateur recreational activities. The individual who participates in professional sports is working, not playing. One's involvement as a spectator and follower of professional sports is recreation. Participation in amateur sports is, of course, recreation. The same is true for the arts. An individual who makes a living, or attempts to make a living, in the arts or as a craftsperson is engaged in an occupation, not recreation. As an avocation or hobby, many people play a musical instrument, write poetry, or build furniture. But such activity is viewed as recreation by the individual. Admittedly there is a fine line between occupation and avocation. An avocational pursuit may be approached with considerable discipline and dedication. It may be consuming of time and energy. It may be an important focal point of identity. Avocational pursuits, however, are not recognized by society as work; they are not considered to be productive: one is only considered to be "playing." Thus, avocational pursuits rarely provide the social status that is derived from being a worker.

It is important to note that there is strong evidence to support the idea that what surrounds the activity is far more important than the activity: the activity is secondary (181,811). Solitary activities are often engaged in to gain temporary relief from interpersonal interactions. The activity per se may be irrelevant. What is more significant is the purpose the activity is selected to fulfill. The activity may be chosen to block out the activities of the day, to occupy the mind with less personal, less demanding or trivial matters, or to escape the real momentarily. On the other hand, activities may be chosen to facilitate contemplation, and to give one the opportunity to review the affairs of the day and plan for tomorrow. In regard to shared activities, attraction to and satisfaction derived from an activity are more related to whom one is with, than what one is doing. It is very often the person or people with whom the activity is shared, not the activity, that accounts for the degree of pleasure.

Finally, recreational activities, similar to games and sports, are sometimes viewed as the means whereby an individual acquires certain skills. These skills have been identified as those that are needed for (a) manipulation of the nonhuman environment; (b) interacting with the human environment; (c) managing events that are unforeseen or unusual; and (d) dealing with the issue of values. Certainly, the development of skills in these areas is one of the major tasks of childhood and adolescence. Basic abilities are probably acquired by the beginning of adulthood. There is likely to be some variation, nevertheless, in the degree and extent that one needs a particular skill at any given time. Therefore, the purpose of many recreational activities in the adult years may well be the refinement of basic skills, the development of more advanced skills, and the maintenance of skills not currently required in daily life. Finally, one might hypothesize that, given the satisfaction derived from recreational activities, there is inherent pleasure in learning and exercising the skills necessary to deal with the four areas outlined above.

The recreational activities outlined below are by no means considered to be inclusive. In addition to games and sports, previously discussed, the following are common recreational activities.

Doing nothing is not often recorded in research reports, thus it is very difficult to say how much time is actually devoted to this activity, or non-activity. The variation between people is probably considerable. It would seem highly unlikely that people are engaged in activities during all of their leisure time. With the connotation of time as a valuable commodity, doing nothing may be construed by some as being a waste of time. In that we know very little about doing nothing, it seems inappropriate to imply that doing nothing is a negative activity. It may be that such an activity, in moderation, may provide a respite from demands and have an organizing quality as one moves from one activity to another.

People spend a good deal of leisure time in conversation. If there is an activity involved, it tends to be secondary and primarily facilitative in nature. Conversation takes place in the context of social gatherings in the home, adolescent haunts, and in bars and restaurants. Conversation is such a pervasive part of leisure that individuals who lack basic social skills are at a distinct disadvantage.

Television is by far the most popular recreational activity (811). It is also one of the recreational activities that has been roundly condemned. The excessive violence, explicit sexuality, unreality, and mindlessness of some television programming have been widely discussed. It is also good to realize, however, that television is a powerful source of information that has vastly increased the knowledge base and social awareness of a good portion of the population. More importantly, perhaps, is the fact that television is a shared family activity. Most television watching is not solitary but takes place in the company of others. Television can often facilitate a sense of camaraderie and a feeling that one is part of a community with others. The weekend football games, for example, may be an important source of conversation for the better part of the week.

Physical exercise has become an increasingly popular activity. Widespread discussion of physical fitness has emphasized the importance of regular exercise for maintaining both physical and mental health. Americans have taken to the gym, playing fields, and roads in great numbers.

Involvement in nature through camping and hiking provides much pleasure for many people. For some it may be the challenge, for others the opportunity to be out of a city and breathe fresh air; for still others it may be the chance to reconnect with a part of the nonhuman environment not found near home. Silence and solitude may also be an important factor contributing to enjoyment (131,132).

Many people find reading, whether it be newspapers, magazines, novels, poetry, or nonfiction, a tremendous source of pleasure. They read to gain knowledge, to share in the comedy and tragedy of the human experience, to be inspired, for entertainment, to escape. Individuals who devote a considerable amount of leisure time to reading consider newspapers, magazines, and books to be close companions.

Avocational pursuits or hobbies are a major source of recreation for many people. They may include arts and crafts activities, gardening, or collecting something of particular interest. Hobbies are very often solitary activities, but they may also become shared through participation in associations devoted to a particular activity and/or sharing the end result of the activity with others. Through engagement in many avocational pursuits, the individual often comes to understand and appreciate aesthetics. One is also in a position to make normative judgments to evaluate what oneself and others are able to do or produce.

Participation in the arts, directly or vicariously, is a way of expressing and sharing ideas and feelings. Involvement in music, dance, drama, the cinema, photography, painting, and sculpture is one means of experiencing kinship with others—those whom one is with now and those distant in time and place. Two of the arts, music and dance, are important to all age groups. They tend, however, to have particular significance to adolescents and young adults, and are often used as a means of generating group solidarity.

In conclusion, although only a few have been mentioned here, recreational activities are seemingly endless in number and variety. They grow out of the free play of young children. When undertaken in a playful manner, recreational activities can be a great source of need satisfaction. Concomitantly, they are the means whereby a number of skills are learned, refined, and maintained.

Deficits in leisure and recreation are fairly common. Leisure may seem a luxury to be coveted, savored, and enjoyed if only one would suddenly be given a sizeable sum of money. But it is rarely perceived as such to those who have leisure thrust on them: the unemployed, the underemployed who are only working parttime, the aged, the retired, the ill and disabled, the mentally retarded (181,526,822). There is no pleasure in enforced leisure. It is very difficult to substitute leisure and recreational activities for work. As mentioned, work gives a status in the community that can rarely be attained through avocational pursuits. In our society, work precedes leisure, which in turn is usually seen as a reward for fulfilling a useful role in society. Lack of work tends to reduce the individual's capacity for self-determined behavior and, consequently, diminishes self-esteem. For those in a position of enforced leisure, recreational activities may not be an adequate solution. They do, however, make life more bearable.

On the opposite end of the spectrum are those people with little or no leisure time: some students in higher education, executives, people just starting out in a demanding career, individuals who hold two jobs, working single parents with young children. True, some of the these people do not want leisure time, but for many there is little choice in the matter (608).

The amount of time available for leisure activities, however, is only one of the problems related to leisure. Some people feel that recreational activities are bad and that one really ought to be "working" at something all of the time. Other people do not know how to play; life is very serious, and there is no sense of being playful. Individuals who lack basic social skills often have difficulty participating in anything but solitary recreational activities. Others are so deficient in one or more of the performance components that they are unable to participate in typical and usual recreational activities. Some individuals have such difficulty in leaving their home that choices in recreational activities are severely limited. For any variety of reasons, people may engage repeatedly in the same recreational activities long after these activities have ceased to be enjoyable or need satisfying. Finally, some communities do not have a sufficient number or variety of recreational facilities. This latter situation is particularly difficult for adolescents and young adults who seek recreation outside their home.

The problem of the amount of time available for leisure activities serves as a bridge into the last occupational performance.

TEMPORAL ADAPTATION

Temporal adaptation is not a social role, but rather refers to the ordering of social roles in a time dimension (155,519,578,608,626,734). More specifically, temporal adaptation refers to the ability to organize one's time in such a way as to fulfill the responsibilities adequately and to enjoy the pleasures of one's required and/or desired social roles. Its relationship to the other occupational performances is hierarchical. Temporal adaptation becomes a focus of concern only after an individual has acquired the rudiments of two or more social roles.

Of fundamental importance in understanding temporal adaptation is the concept of time. Time is a universal dimension and an inescapable boundary of human existence. As such, it guides and structures experience and activity. Time is a limited resource that is irreversible and irreplaceable. Each individual has a limited but unknown amount of personal time to give and receive love and to accomplish life goals. Until the very end of the life cycle, the time allotted is undisclosed. It is this unknown aspect of personal time that gives time a mysterious quality, a force that compels one to action or a burden that stretches seemingly to infinity. It is precious in joy, insufficient for work, and unwelcome in sorrow.

Perception of time is a particularly human characteristic. Inherent in the human condition is knowledge of the past, the fleeting moment of the present, and anticipation of the future. Each individual is influenced by a historical past, which is transmitted through family and other social institutions. One also has a personal past made up of events and experiences unique to the self. Man draws on his past experiences as an information source for future action. He projects himself into the future, planning events, and setting goals that may not be realized for days, months, or even years.

Perception of time is influenced by one's place in the life cycle. The infant perceives time in relation to bodily needs. The young child must learn about time as an external factor, with the hours of the day regulating certain activities. Time often seems so long: the wait for a promised trip to the park seems never ending. The young adult sees time in two somewhat incongruous ways. Everything must be experienced, be done now. On the other hand, time stretches into infinity: there is more than sufficient time. In the middle years comes a sense of one's mortality, a sense of time running out. Life goals and plans are often reconsidered in this perspective. Another change in perception of time frequently comes with old age. There is a resolution of the fear of time running out and an appreciation of the present.

Time may be perceived as linear but also as cyclical. The movements of the solar system and the seasons of the year have marked time in all known societies. The study of nature's cycles has been of utmost importance in human societies: when to gather, when to hunt, when to plant crops. Human life itself is cyclical: birth, the flowering of adulthood, death; the menstrual cycle; sexual arousal and satiation. Each day has its own cycle of work, gathering for meals, leisure activities, and sleep. There is a rhythm, a regularity in cycles of time that becomes a part of most individuals. It gives structure to the familiar, the routine, the predictable. Cycles have an organizing effect on the individual. Disruption of regular cycles, of daily routines, often leads to a sense of disorientation and confusion, a feeling of being unsettled, of being in a somewhat chaotic state.

Temporal adaptation is learned. Each person is born with an internal rhythm that is partially species-specific and partially idiosyncratic. The latter may be altered to some degree by cultural influences, but it remains operant. For example, some people need more sleep than others; some people do their best work in the morning, others late at night. Idiosyncratic internal rhythm is, to a degree, altered and temporal adaptation acquired through the socialization process. Each society gives a particular value to time, and has sets of ideas about time. With some flexibility, a society defines expected behavior relative to time, e.g., when one mows his lawn, eats breakfast, and meets friends for a drink. Through socialization the individual learns about, and how to adapt to, the temporal framework of society. Further, a society socializes its members to organize their use of time relative to social roles. Daily life is divided into specific time segments when one is expected to engage in one role, as opposed to another. A 13-year-old student, for example, goes to school from nine to three o'clock, spends time with friends in the late afternoon, has dinner with family members, studies in the evening, maybe watches a little television, and takes a shower before retiring. Societies also have a temporal framework for different periods in the life cycle when individuals are expected to participate in various roles. Our society, for example, does not condone motherhood at 15 years of age, or becoming a father at 65 years of age.

Within the general constraints set by the social system, an individual's use of time is influenced by needs, values, and interests. On the basis of these, the individual determines priorities and decides how much time will be allotted to specific activities. Based on priorities, the individual sets goals within the context of time: short-term, medium range, and long-term goals. Plans are made as to how one will reach these goals. Daily patterns of time use are influenced by such goals and plans. As needs, values, and interests change during the life cycle, so does the individual's priorities. Thus, one's daily pattern of time use will also change. If adjustments are not made, the individual is not able to reach newly set goals; there is not enough time.

The adaptive use of time is characterized by control, the right amount of control. Organization of time ideally is neither too tight (i.e., compulsive, overorganized, preoccupied with time), nor too loose (i.e., indifferent, disorganized, lazy). Adequate control over time allows one to engage in necessary and desired activities and to be flexible and spontaneous. Experts in time management suggest that adaptive scheduling of time is based on conscious awareness of one's priorities, knowledge of one's own internal rhythm, and awareness of when various role partners are available for and receptive to interaction (578,626). Ideally, time is scheduled to reflect priorities but with sufficient time for essential activities (eating, sleeping), routine tasks, interruptions, and dealing with unforeseen problems. Scheduling should be sufficiently loose so as to accommodate to different times of the year and special situations. A daily routine with some flexibility is generally comfortable for most individuals. A need-satisfying routine is believed to contribute to the maintenance of physical and emotional health.

Temporal dysfunction may occur in any number of life situations, both normal and pathological. Perhaps the most common disturbance in temporal adaptation occurs with change in social roles. The student entering a demanding graduate program must rearrange routines to make more time for study. The new mother must adapt to the internal rhythm of her infant. The woman returning to employment must adjust to the nine-to-five schedule of the workplace. The retired individual no longer has the structure of work to organize time. The loss of a role partner, particularly a spouse, can lead to a sense of an intolerable future.

Temporal dysfunction may arise from physically disabling conditions. The person with severe motor impairment may require considerably more time to perform activities of daily living than unimpaired individuals. They may not be able to maintain a pace of life typical for their age group. Individuals with acquired disabilities may have to give up their role as a worker, many tasks associated with familial roles, and usual recreational activities. It may be difficult for them to find new, suitable activities. People with chronic illnesses may have complex, time-consuming regimens to carry out to prevent physical deterioration. Family members of disabled individuals also may find themselves in a state of temporal dysfunction as they attempt to cope with change in their social roles and life situations.

Deficits in temporal adaptation are also associated with psychosocial dysfunction. Individuals who are mentally retarded may have difficulty ordering events in time, have little control over when they engage in daily activities, or be unable to make plans for the future. Individuals with organic mental disorders, either degenerative in nature or substance induced, may be disoriented relative to time. They may be unaware of current time (day, week), or the sequence of past events may be confused. This phenomenon is also seen in some schizophrenic disorders. Individuals with affective disorders (manic or depressive) may disregard time or be unable to conceptualize and plan for future time. Anxiety disorders are sometimes characterized by rigidity in daily routines, severe procrastination, or difficulty in setting reasonable priorities relative to social roles.

In conclusion, temporal adaptation involves the ordering of tasks and personal interactions in time. It gives structure to the satisfactory fulfillment of social roles. The capacity to organize time in an elegant manner allows us to take the responsibilities of and enjoy being a family member, caretaker of the self, worker, and player.

5 Age: The Life Cycle

Age is the third part of the occupational therapy domain of concern. As such it gives perspective to an understanding of performance components and occupational performances: it provides an additional dimension. Age is always taken into consideration in the evaluation and intervention process. In the application of developmental frames of reference, age becomes the focal point for assessment and designing activities for change. In the application of analytic and acquisitional frames of reference, age serves as a backdrop to understanding the client's capacities and limitations. Meeting health needs, prevention, management, and maintenance can only be effective if dealt with in the context of age. There is much that is different about an individual at 6 months, 5 years, 13, 25, 50, and 70. It is to these differences that this chapter is addressed, and to the recognition of similarities.

Age is the temporal determination of the life cycle. Cycle has the connotation of the recurrence over a period of time, of certain events being repeated in the same order and at the same interval, of a sequence of changing states that, on completion, produce another state identical to the original one. Human life has been described as cyclical for in the life of each individual there is a repetition of events that has occurred in the life of all other members of the species since the origin of the species. There is a cyclical repetition to human life as each generation is born, nurtures the young, and dies (171,531). Within the life of each individual there is a recurring need to deal with the universal issues of trust, intimacy, personal adequacy, aggression, reality, sexuality, dependency, independence, and loss.

The life cycle of the individual is described as beginning with conception and ending with death. Within that period of time, an individual is confronted with various life tasks that need to be mastered. An individual must, for example, learn to walk, communicate, accept and give love, be productive, and face death. In a general sense, the tasks are set. The manner in which one masters these tasks is variable: influenced by genetic endowments and life circumstances.

This chapter is essentially an overview of the psychosocial components of the individual life cycle. Other aspects will only be discussed as they relate to and impinge on psychosocial components. As an overview, this chapter is not an in-depth outline of human growth and development. Rather it is a summary of various theories, with primary focus on the social roles of family interaction, activities of daily living, work, and play/leisure/recreation. Temporal adaptation will be considered in conjunction with each age level. To give sufficient background for evaluation and intervention, the initial mastery of sensory integration and cognition will also be outlined. This chapter is primarily organized around age levels. The three final sections focus on divorce, chronic illness/disability, and death. These are separated from age because they are phenomena that exist or occur irrespective of age and impinge on all age groups.

INTRODUCTION

As one of the parameters of our domain of concern, occupational therapists study human growth and development for several reasons (222). One reason is as a way in which to understand clients. Regardless of their particular difficulties or problems, understanding is increased by knowledge of where a client is in the life cycle and the developmental tasks with which they are immediately concerned. An individual's age may also be instrumental in how he reacts to dysfunction. A particular life stage may be one of the major factors in causing dysfunction.

Irrespective of a client's current age, occupational therapists need information about clients' past life experience. Such information provides many clues to clients' current responses and how they are likely to respond in the future. How an individual has approached and dealt with developmental tasks in the past tends to influence his approach to and handling of future developmental tasks. Individuals carry the experiences of their past with them: we are who we are to a great extent because of our many past experiences. Knowledge of human growth and development helps the therapist to identify pivotal events in the process. Knowledge of how a client dealt with these events contributes to understanding of the client.

Occupational therapists also study human growth and development to facilitate the establishment of rapport. People interact in a number of different levels, one of them being the perspective of age. Simultaneously, an individual relates to others from the point of view of her own age, from a place in the life cycle, and from the social events that shaped her generation. In illustration, a person in her 30s tends to view life differently than an individual in her 40s. But there is more than a difference in 10 years of life experience. The 30-year-old is a child of the 1960s, the 40-year-old of the 1950s. These were very different decades in terms of the social events that occurred. In addition, it is difficult for a person to remember the perspective they had at a younger age. Thus, when individuals of different ages attempt to relate there is a dissimilarity in perspective. The generation gap is a real phenomenon. Study of human growth and development helps one to bridge that gap, although it can never be eliminated entirely.

Finally, occupational therapists study human growth and development to facilitate self-knowledge: a crucial factor in the conscious use of self. Such study helps to answer the questions of who I am, why am I the person I am today, how will I change in the future. Curiosity about the future is a part of human nature. In knowing something about the future one is able to identify the tasks ahead. Knowledge of and anticipatory preparation for future events tend to decrease anxiety and facilitate mastery. One comes to have a sense of "How can I grow and change" rather than being propelled by unknown forces.

Although sometimes used interchangeably, three concepts of human growth and development (265,362,400, 733,840) need to be defined for clarification. Growth is the increase in the size of an individual of body parts as measured by increased weight, volume, or linear dimensions. It is primarily influenced by heredity, hormonal activity, and nutrition. Maturation is the unfolding, elaboration, or progression of a bodily structure or inherent capacity. One speaks of the maturation of the central nervous system or of cognitive functions. Maturation has the connotation of being a continuing process that begins at conception and ends at death. Development is the progressive behavioral changes that occur between birth and death. It is the acquisition of new behavior and the relinquishment of old behavior. Development, although influenced by growth and maturation, is primarily dependent on experience, on interactions within the environment. Development is essentially dependent on learning. The occupational therapy process is not directly concerned with enhancing growth. It is concerned with facilitating maturation and with promoting development. For ease in discussion, the term "development" will be used in this text as an umbrella term, unless a distinction needs to be made between growth, maturation, and development.

Structurally, human development has been conceived in a number of different ways. Development is described as horizontal and longitudinal (616,618). Horizontal refers to the development of a variety of abilities or skills at the same time. Thus, for example, one can speak of the typical development level of a three-year-old child in the areas of motor function, vocabulary, relationship with peers, and so forth. Longitudinal refers to development over time. It is the description of one area of human function from initial emergence to full flowering or full course. Piaget's description of cognitive development is an example of an apogee approach; Erikson's description of psychosocial development is illustrative of taking an aspect of human function through its full course.

Within the context of horizontal and longitudinal development, progression is sometimes described as linear, spiral, and/or marked by stages or crises (271,339,888). Linear development is progression with the connotation of an increase in some function or capacity. An increase in an individual's general fund of knowledge would be an example of linear development. A spiral pattern of development can be conceptualized as a helix: winding about on an axis in continually advancing planes. The continuous return to and reconciliation of universal issues and periods of equilibrium and disequilibrium are examples of a spiral pattern of development. Development marked by stages is a stairlike pattern, with each step being the addition of behavior that is qualitatively different than the behavior evident at the previous stage. An example is the development of motor skills; sitting, standing, walking, and so forth. Crises, as used in developmental theories, is similar to how it is used in literature. It refers to points in a sequence of events at which the trend of all future events, for better or for worse, is determined. Crisis is used in the sense of a juncture or turning point, not in the sense of an emergency. Crises are normative events, such as marriage, the birth of a child, or retirement.

There are four characteristics of human development that seem to hold true regardless of the particular area of development being discussed (58,222,339,362,912). These principles are:

1. Development is orderly, predictable, sequential, and cumulative. People are unique and have a number of individual differences. Nevertheless, most development follows a particular pattern. These patterns may arise from the common biological substratum of all individuals or it may be imposed by the social system in which the individual exists. Development is considered to be cumulative in that past experiences and capacities acquired influence the individual's present and future development.

2. Each individual develops at a different pace and differentially in various areas. There are general normative periods when typically an individual gains a particular skill or ceases to exhibit a specific kind of behavior. In general, these normative periods are fairly broad, giving wide latitude to what would be considered typical development. There is probably more variation in the pace of adult development than in that of a child. Development is differential in that horizontal development tends to be uneven. An individual may develop very rapidly in one area and much more slowly in another. It is only when the variation is extremely wide that development is considered to be atypical.

3. At any particular time, an individual may place particular emphasis on one aspect of development to the exclusion of others. Thus, for example, a graduate student may concentrate on academic studies to such an extent that she is little concerned with the development of an intimate relationship. Emphasis is usually time limited, with some correction in balance taking place later.

4. Development tends to follow a general-to-specific pattern. Thus, for example, initially a child's social interaction with peers may be undifferentiated. Subsequently, the child develops a more discriminate repertoire of behavior, varying interactions with particular friends or in particular situations. This pattern can also be seen in typical courtship behavior, where the individual dates a number of possible partners before selecting a particular mate.

These four characteristics of development interact with each other to form variety of changing patterns.

There is one other tendency in development that cannot really be identified as a characteristic in that it does not hold true across all areas of human function. The term used to identify this tendency is "critical period"—a time when, if a particular sequence of events does not take place, the individual more than likely will always experience the consequence of one or more developmental deficits (316,912). The first trimester of prenatal development is considered to be a critical period for the formation of body structures. If language is not acquired by the age of five years, the individual is likely to have a serious language deficit in the future (334). These are the two critical periods that are well-documented in the literature. As our understanding of human growth and development expands, other critical periods may be identified.

The scientific study of the life cycle is fairly recent (155,265,497,531,733). Historically, study was initiated relative to childhood. It began in the early nineteenth century and appears to have been motivated by society's increased concern for children in general. This was a period marked by social legislation for the protection and welfare of children and state support of at least a few years of education. Children in school were a readily available population for study. Research relative to infant and early childhood development did not begin until somewhat later. The next phase of the life cycle addressed was adolescence. This began in earnest in the 1920s and 1930s. Again, the availability of a "captured" population was a factor. More and more adolescents were continuing their formal education in high school. The 1950s and early 1960s saw the beginning of research relative to the aged population. Gerontology—the study of individuals over 65 years of age—was primarily motivated by the rapid increase in this segment of the population. It was not until the early 1970s that scientists turned their attention to the population between 18 and 65 years of age. It should be noted that there were pioneers who began study of the various phases of the life cycle prior to the dates specified above.

There seem to be two major reasons for the interest in the middle years of the life cycle being so delayed. The scientific community in general seemed to believe nothing really significant happened between adolescence and old age. Psychoanalytic theories were particularly influential in this regard, for they emphasized the importance of early childhood experiences in shaping adult behavior and responses (317). The other reason is related to the age of active scientists: 30 to 55 years of age. It is far easier to study people who are distant in some way from oneself. This distance allows the scientists to place a psychological barrier between themselves and their subjects. Such a barrier permits one to treat subjects as if they were somewhat a little less than human. There is a natural tendency not to want to examine oneself or one's kind too intently. The dictum "to know thyself" has only recently been heeded by individuals in the human sciences. Because of the history outlined above, research relative to aging and particularly the middle years of the life cycle is somewhat sparse and not as well documented as research in the areas of childhood and adolescence. It also tends to be biased toward the white, middle-class segment of the population.

There are several methods for studying human development, each with something distinct to contribute and each with some limitations (58,497,531,733). Study of animal behavior has contributed to knowledge of biological growth and maturation and to some extent to an understanding of social behavior. Human behavior studied in experimental situations has contributed primarily to the understanding of how people form and interact in small groups. As with animal studies, the conclusions drawn from studies in experimental situations are and should be limited relative to generalization. Longitudinal studies involve observation of the same individuals over a period of time. There are many advantages to this type of study, for each individual essentially serves as his own control. The major disadvantage is that longitudinal studies are very expensive and a considerable number of subjects, for one reason or another, drop out along the way. Cross-sectional studies involve the observation of groups of individuals at different ages at one time. These studies are far less expensive than longitudinal studies but they may also be situationally biased. The latter refers to the influence of broad social events on a particular generation: the economic depression of the 1930s and the social unrest of the 1960s, for example. The difficulty here is in separating out what is particular to a given age and what is specific to the social situation which they collectively experience. It has been documented, for example, that individuals over 65 tend to be more conservative than adults of a younger age. However, what is not known is whether this is a typical phenomenon of aging or related to their coming of age during the 1930s. Cross-cultural research is one way of minimizing the situational bias of cross-sectional research. It also contributes to an understanding of the effect of different social systems on the developmental process.

Study of the life cycle, or one facet of human development, has occurred in the biological sciences, medicine, psychology, sociology, and anthropology. The various orientations have provided a multidimensional perspective for understanding of the developmental process. There are as a result many theories, with no one theory which accounts for every aspect of the developmental process. The variety of theories also offers alternative explanations for various types of behavior. One theory may seem to "explain" a given person's behavior better than another theory. Occupational therapists should be conversant with the major theories of development. The overview to be presented in this chapter is an integration of a variety of theories. It is essentially presented to give a holistic view of the psychosocial components of the occupational therapy domain of concern. As an overview, it is not meant to replace an in-depth study of human development.

Human development is often considered to have three dimensions: biological, psychological, and sociological. These components are considered to be interdependent to the point that it is difficult to address any aspect of the life cycle without considering all three. For clarification, the biological components are heredity, physical growth, and maturation, which includes the aging process, illness, and death. All of these will be briefly discussed in the following sections, except for heredity. Genetic endowment determines to a greater or lesser degree an individual's physical appearance, including rate and extent of growth and physical maturation. It influences basic personality characteristics and various capacities and skills. Heredity also predisposes one to various illnesses and is a factor in determining the course of one's aging process and the age of one's death.

The psychological components have been previously discussed except for learning. Learning is a process wherein behavior

> originates or is changed through reaction to an encounter situation provided that the characteristics of the change . . . cannot be explained on the basis of native response tendencies, maturation or temporary status of the organism (e.g., fatigue, drugs, etc.) (427, p. 17).

Learning is discussed in more detail in Chapter 9.

The sociological components are social roles, the socialization process, and cultural influences. The first two components have been described previously. Cultural influences refers to the social structures, pervasive ideas, values, norms, and expectations that are accepted and shared by a particular social system. Cultural influences have a large impact on shaping the given potential of the individual. Chapter 6 will, in part, be devoted to a discussion of this area.

With these introductory remarks, the next several sections of this chapter will be devoted to a brief description of various age levels.

PRENATAL DEVELOPMENT AND THE NEONATE

The development of the fertilized ovum into a thriving, active infant able to sustain an independent life is an awesome phenomenon (468,843,912). It is the period of most rapid growth and maturation, taking approximately 266 days. The changes that occur in the remaining portion of the life cycle, although exciting and amazing, pale in comparison. Briefly, the course of events is as follows.

First, the germinal period comprises the first two weeks of prenatal growth. During this time there is continuous and rapid cell division, with some differentiation. It comes to an end when the mass of growing cells is fully implanted in the wall of the uterus.

The embryonic period, which lasts eight weeks, is characterized by the formation and differentiation of the various structures and organs. Approximately one month after conception, arm and leg buds are differentiated from the cellular mass. The details of the head, rudimentary eyes, ears, mouth, and brain are able to be observed. The brain shows some primitive specialization. The heart, liver, kidney, and stomach, although rudimentary, can be seen. The embryo is between one-fourth and one-half inch long. By the end of the second month, the features of the face are distinct and covered with skin. The arms have recognizable fingers and thumb. The legs, which grow more rapidly than the arms, have differentiated knees, ankles, and toes. All organs of the body are formed and functioning, including the endocrine system. The heart is beating regularly and steadily, electrical activity of the brain is evident, and muscles are innervated.

The fetal period starts at the third month after conception and is marked by the beginning formation of bone cells. By the end of the third month there are additional refinements of the extremities and facial features. The palate and lips are formed. Sexual differentiation has occurred. The fetus is active, being able to kick, turn, open and close its hands, move the thumb in opposition, and open its mouth.

The fourth, fifth, and sixth months are a time of continued growth and refinement. At the beginning of this period the fetus is about six inches long and weighs about four ounces. By the end of this period the fetus is 12 to 14 inches long and weighs approximately 1½ pounds. In these three months there is increased spontaneous activity with apparent periods of sleep and wakefulness. In the sixth month, the eyelids begin to open and close and there is lateral and vertical eye movement. Eyelashes and brows are formed. Taste buds have developed and there is evidence of a marked grasp reflex. The respiratory system is still very immature. At the end of the sixth month breathing patterns at best are irregular. Survival outside the womb is sometimes possible with extraordinary measures. Because of breathing difficulties and consequential oxygen deficit there is some risk of brain damage for infants born this prematurely.

In the seventh, eight, and ninth months there continues to be considerable growth. The various body systems mature to the point of being able to sustain independent life safely. During the seventh month the cerebral hemispheres grow rapidly, folding over and covering the more primitive portions of the brain. Specialized responses are now possible. The immunity system also matures. At birth, the neonate is usually between 19 and 22 inches and weighs between 5½ and 9½ pounds.

The course of prenatal development outlined above is typical and, with minor differences, invariant. However, it is influenced by genetic inheritance and environmental factors. The information transmitted by the genes determines the differentiation and growth of the fetus. Genetic deficit of one type or another can contribute to defective growth or malfunction of organs. There are some aspects of dysfunction that are a direct result of genetic inheritance.

Environmental factors influence prenatal development through the mother. The impact of these influences varies relative to type, intensity, and time of impact. The first trimester (12 weeks) is the most critical period of gestation, for this is the time of differentiation and formation of organs and body structures. Major environmental factors include drugs and other agents ingested by the mother, maternal nutrition, exposure to roentgen rays, exposure to viruses and bacteria, and the Rh compatibility of the parents. The influence of the emotional state of the mother on the development of the fetus is unknown. The folklore of many cultures attests to the longstanding belief that there is a marked and direct relationship. Research has not supported this belief except to the extent that emotional health influences the physical health and behavior of the mother. A woman who feels emotionally stable and secure is far more likely to inhibit ingestion of potentially harmful substances, eat properly, and get a sufficient amount of exercise and rest. The availability and regular use of prenatal care facilities is also an important factor in maternal health.

On leaving the warmth and security of the womb, the neonate is almost immediately confronted with major adaptive tasks. Adjustment must be made to a drop in body temperature, an external mode of nourishment, and a redirection of oxygen flow. These adjustments are typically made in a matter of hours.

The neonate is born with the ability to respond to and interact with the environment. Within the first few days of life the neonate is able to see within a range of 8 to 12 inches and appears to prefer complex patterns to more simple ones. There seems to be a definite preference for an actual human face, or a picture of one, over other visual stimuli. The neonate can detect changes in temperature, distinguish tastes, smell and discriminate between odors, localize sounds, and show preference for certain sounds and volume. The vestibular and tactile systems are relatively mature, with the neonate showing a preference for rocking or other slow rhythmic movements, warmth, light touch, and a reasonable amount of pressure. Motor activity is primarily reflexive; nonreflexive activity is gross and random. Three oral reflexes—rooting (turning the head towards the point of oral stimulation and opening the mouth to grasp the nipple), sucking, and swallowing—are well developed in the full-term neonate and ensure adequate nourishment. With the responses outlined above, the neonate begins extrauteral development.

INFANCY TO ONE YEAR OF AGE

Although development is not as rapid as during the prenatal period, the first year of life is marked by considerable change (11,74,339,667,912). The infant's behavior is strongly influenced by a number of reflexes, those present at birth and those that appear at various times after birth. These reflexes, which foster the development of many skills, eventually disappear or are integrated into the infant's repertoire of behavior.

Motor development is characterized by (a) a cephalocaudal pattern, progressive control and coordination from head to foot; and (b) a proximal-distal pattern, progressive control and coordination of body parts closest to the spine to those that are farthest away. Following these patterns, and aided by reflexes, the infant acquires head control and, sequentially, the ability to roll over, sit, crawl, stand, and, by the end of this period, is often able to walk alone or with assistance.

Sensory Integration

Sensory integration during the first year of life is characterized by three stages (58). The first stage is the integration of the tactile subsystems (0–3 months). The infant develops an adequate balance between the protective and discriminatory subsystems such that a differentiation between injurious and noninjurious tactile stimulation is possible. This integration is believed to take place as a result of the physical maturation of the nervous system and through the tactile stimulation arising from the handling, fondling, and caressing of the infant by his parents. General tactile stimulation also helps the infant to experience the skin as the physical boundary of the self, a primary source of security and the beginning of the development of self-concept.

The second stage is the integration of primitive postural reflexes (3–9 months). The tonic neck and tonic labyrinth reflexes are sufficiently integrated that the infant is able to move in patterns that are the opposite from the reflex patterns. Integration is only beginning at this time and these reflexes still may be elicited, particularly if the infant is tired. Complete integration will not occur until around six or seven years of age. The infant now simply has the ability to act outside these reflex patterns.

The third stage involves the mature righting and equilibrium reactions (9–12 months). Maturation in this area is the result of the integration of vestibular and proprioceptive information. This leads to the development of various postural reactions, such as rolling over, sitting, and taking a position for crawling and to the ability to shift body weight automatically to maintain balance. The infant now experiences the gravitational pull of the earth in a positive manner. This gives rise to the sense of knowing where one is and how one is moving in space. There is a feeling of stability relative to earth, a great source of security.

Cognition

There are four stages of cognitive development in the first year of life (141,302,774). In the first stage, the infant uses inherent behavioral patterns for environmental interaction (0–1 month). The inherent behavioral patterns of concern here are sucking, grasping, crying, gross bodily movements, and recognition of and attention to visual and auditory stimuli. Although these responses are inherent, they appear to become more refined through environmental interaction. By the end of the first month the infant is able to locate the nipple with some facility, has a strong grasp and sucking response, cries and is stimulated to cry when he hears another baby cry, moves body parts in a vigorous manner, and attends to visual and auditory stimuli with considerable interest.

In the second stage, the infant acquires the ability to interrelate visual, manual, auditory, and oral responses (1–4 months). The inherent behavior patterns mentioned above that lead to pleasurable consequences tend to be repeated and consolidated into new behavioral patterns. Typical patterns the infant develops are: anticipatory sucking in response to visual, positional, or auditory cues; more active looking and the ability to follow objects in motion; more active listening and seeking the cause of auditory stimuli; smiling response to the human face; vocal responses when alone and in the presence of others; evidence of intentionality in thumb sucking; anything placed in the hand is usually visually inspected and brought to the mouth; anything placed in the mouth is grasped; attempts to grasp objects in visual field; and imitation of actions that are a part of behavioral repertoire (does not imitate new actions).

In the third stage, the infant attends to the environmental consequences of actions with interest, represents objects in an exoceptual manner, experiences objects, acts on the basis of egocentric causality, and seriates events in which he is involved (4–9 months). Attention to environmental consequences of actions refers to the repetition of motor acts that influence the surrounding environment: the first active exploration of the world. Prior to this time the infant's attention has been primarily directed toward his own body or the very near environment. The infant now intensely studies, manipulates, and rotates objects. Experimental actions are directed toward objects. The infant engages in a good deal of attention-getting behavior and repeats actions in order to reproduce it in others. Exoceptual representation—memory of stimuli in terms of the action response to the stimuli or actions directed toward the stimuli—is evident by the infant's ability to initiate an appropriate motor response to unfamiliar objects that are similar to objects in his usual environment. An infant, for example, may attempt to drink from a goblet even though he had never seen that type of drinking vessel previously. Such behavior also indicates a primitive idea of class and classification. With exoceptual representation, the infant, in addition, has some recognition that the intensity of a given act will influence the intensity of the results.

The ability to experience objects refers to capacity to recognize that objects have some permanence. With development of this capacity the infant anticipates the ultimate position of a moving object from observation of its trajectory, searches for objects lost in the very immediate past, and recognizes an object when only a part is seen.

Action on the basis of egocentric causality refers to the belief that one's own actions are completely responsible for the response of other people or objects. There is a quasimagical quality about this type of causality as, for example, turning away from the mother to induce a funny expression on the mother's face. The intentionality of the mother is not recognized. The actions or gestures used are not directly related to the response desired. Egocentric causality is not always entirely replaced by a more advanced type of causality and may continue into adulthood. This can be seen in the gesture of knocking on wood to avoid the occurrence of an unwanted event.

The ability to seriate events in which the infant has been involved refers to a primitive idea of before and after relative to events in which the infant's own actions have been a part of the sequence. When this learning has taken place, the infant indicates displeasure or confusion when the regular sequence of events is not followed. If, for example, the child is usually sung a song before the light is turned off at bedtime, there is likely to be a good deal of protest if a song is not produced.

In the fourth stage, the infant is able to establish a goal and to carry out intentionally the means, recognize the independence of objects, interpret signs, imitate new behavior, apprehend the influence of space, and perceive other people or things as partially causal (9–12 months). The infant is able to establish a goal prior to action and select and imitate actions deliberately, which will lead to that goal. The goals of concern here are simple and immediate as are the means. For example, the infant in the desire for sustained attention may continually drop toys off the tray of his highchair. An observer of this action receives an impression of unequivocal intentionality; fallen toys were not due to clumsy movements on the part of the infant.

Recognition of the independent existence of objects refers to the understanding that objects exist in their own right and are not dependent on one's manipulation or visual perception. The infant realizes that objects hidden from his sight continue to exist. In understanding the independent existence of objects, the infant also comes to recognize his existence as independent from others. This is an important step in that the infant begins to perceive himself as being differentiated and separated from his parents. This process continues for many years. Differentiation at this time is primarily concerned with physical separateness.

Interpretation of signs refers to anticipation of future events on the basis of a current event. The sequence of events must be familiar to the infant. An example of this aspect of cognition is the child moving toward his stroller when he sees his mother taking his jacket out of the closet.

With the capacity to imitate new behavior, the infant is able to observe simple behavior that is not a part of his repertoire and to imitate the behavior or behavior that is structurally analogous. For example, the infant will try to cut his food with a knife or attempt to make a noise like the bark of the family dog.

Apprehension of the influence of space is more exploratory behavior at this time than an integrated ability. What occurs at this stage is an active study of differences in size, shape, perspective, and changes in objects resulting from different positions of the head. Objects are looked at from many different directions and a good deal of time is spent in attempting to fit objects into other objects and in defined spaces. The infant, for example, will try to fit various toys through the bars of his crib, manipulating them in several directions to see if he can get them through the bars.

In perceiving objects as partially causal, the infant realizes that other people or things may be somewhat responsible for an effect, but believes the cause and effect relationship is set in motion by his actions. The true volition of other people is not recognized. An example of recognition of partial causality is the child pointing to a desired toy out of reach with the expectation the toy will be brought to him. This is one step beyond the quasimagical gestures used to cause events.

Family Interaction

The infant essentially comes into the world as an asocial or presocial being (167,281,310,316,544,632, 716,923). All libidinal energy is invested in the self: a state referred to as primary narcissism. The infant's first developmental task relative to family interaction is to establish an intimate relationship with his parents. This process, bonding or the formation of a primary object relation, requires the joint interaction of infant and parent. Intimate bodily contact, which occurs in context of feeding, bathing, dressing, and frequent and regular cuddling, caressing, and fondling, is one of the major factors in promoting the infant's emotional attachment to his parents, and the parents' attachment to the child. It is also prompted by the parents' providing predictable, continuous care in which unpleasant stimuli are relieved and pleasant stimuli presented.

The infant, through positive reactions to the parents, contributes to the bonding process. At approximately one month of age the infant begins to smile at people. Smiling is indiscriminate in that he does not just smile at his parents or other familiar people. However, smiling does help to cement the bond between the parents and the infant. The parents experience the smile as a reward, which promotes contact with the infant. The infant also responds in a positive way to parents by ceasing to cry when picked up, cooing, watching the parent, and showing pleasure when being fed, played with, and cuddled.

The infant's formation of a primary object relationship takes place over the course of about nine months. At about three or four months of age, the infant begins to recognize his parents and forms what is described as a discontinuous object relation. This, however, is considered to be a "partial" in that the infant does not perceive the totality of the parents, their assets, limitations, needs, and so forth. Libidinal energy is invested in that aspect of the parents which "loves and takes care of me." The establishment of a primary object relationship at around nine months is often evident in "stranger anxiety." The infant begins to withdraw from unfamiliar people and may cry or become upset when one or both parents leave the home for a period of time. The degree of stranger anxiety varies considerably from one infant to another. It appears to be less in infants who have been exposed to a number of people and temporary absences of parents.

The establishment of a primary object relationship is the foundation for the development of basic trust—confidence in and certainty of the essential integrity and goodness of others. It also forms the foundation for future interactions on an emotional level and for comfort in exploring the wider environment. The acquisition of trust is the first stage of psychosocial development as described by Erikson.

By seven months of age the infant has become a much more social being, preferring the company of others to solitude. By nine months the infant has become an active, accepted part of the family constellation, knowing and responding differentially to each parent, siblings, and familiar relatives. The infant appears to have a sense of belonging to the family.

Between 9 and 12 months the infant becomes considerably more active, crawling and sometimes walking at this age. The increased mobility and exploration of the home environment can be a source of danger to the infant, and often to things in the environment. The infant begins to hear the word no and feel the sting of a slapped hand. The discipline process has started and will continue for several years. Although now the occupant of a specific family role, socialization has essentially just begun.

Also at this time the infant begins to invest aggressive energy in external objects. Previously, aggressive energy had been primarily manifested in crying and expressed in a diffuse and undirected manner. Now aggressive energy is invested in specific objects. Object choice may not be very accurate, however, and the infant's ability to manipulate aggressive objects successfully is very limited. The infant expresses his anger by biting, hitting, throwing objects, stomping his feet, occasional temper tantrums, and engaging in forbidden activities. Parents, people seen as rivals for the attention of parents, and things that the infant cannot successfully manipulate are the major objects perceived as need frustrating and it is these objects that are now invested with aggressive energy. The socialization process in the coming few years will shape both the expression of anger and behavior used to deal with need-frustrating people, situations, and things.

Activities of Daily Living

Activities of daily living for the infant center around establishing rhythmic daily patterns and eating (11,334, 400,714). Initially, the infant spends the majority of his time sleeping, waking usually only when hungry. The degree of structure imposed on the infant's internal pattern relative to eating and sleeping varies in our society from fairly rigid to permissive, a middle course being the most typical. With growth and maturation, periods between eating are lengthened and more time is spent in wakeful activity. By nine months the infant is eating three major meals a day, with periodic snacks and sleeping approximately 10 hours at night, with a nap period in the afternoon and sometimes in the morning. The remainder of the day is spent in play.

For most infants the sucking response is active at birth. The bottle or breast is usually the major source of nourishment for the first two or three months. Soft foods are introduced at this time as well as fruit juices. The variety of soft foods requires both physiological and psychological adjustment on the part of the infant.

By nine months the infant is usually weaned from the bottle although may enjoy a bottle prior to bedtime at night. He is able to drink from a cup or glass but is likely to need some assistance. Foods that require some chewing have been introduced by this time and the infant is able to finger feed independently. Although the child may attempt to use a spoon, very little food is accurately placed in the mouth. It is, however, placed in many other locations.

Play

The first behavior that may be classified as play is the looking and listening of an infant that begins shortly after birth (334,714,758). Crib mobiles, for example, are a source of seemingly endless fascination. The first toy of an infant is his own body, which is studied with considerable interest. By three or four months the infant moves toward, touches, and handles objects. Most objects are explored with his hands as well as his mouth. Up until about the seventh month, the infant plays with only one toy at a time. After seven months the infant is able to coordinate the use of two toys. Until 10 months the infant treats all toys and materials alike. Differentiation in handling and manipulation begins at about this time. Initially the infant plays by himself, needing only colorful and varied objects to look at and explore. By around five months the child begins to enjoy social play initiated by adults or older siblings. The infant initiates social play with adults by nine months, enjoying such games as peek-a-boo and patty-cake. Imitation is an important part of play at this time. At one year of age the infant may observe other children playing but makes no attempt to join in. Play is limited to solitary activity and interaction with adults.

ONE TO THREE YEARS OF AGE

Between one and three years of age the child gains considerable mobility, learning how to walk and run with stability and ease (11,74,339,667,912). Auditory perception becomes much more refined. This, in conjunction with the development of praxis, leads to a rapid increase in language comprehension and the acquisition of speech. From a vocabulary of about five words at one year of age, by three years the child has a fairly large vocabulary and is able to construct simple sentences. Visual perception also becomes much more refined, in particular visual figure-ground and position in space. The elaboration of auditory and visual perception is associated with a decrease in distractibility and an increase in attention span. The relationship here is probably reciprocal rather than cause and effect. Finally, although still highly dependent on family members, by three years of age the child enjoys being with other children.

Sensory Integration

There are two stages of sensory integration development, which takes place between one and three years of age (58). The first stage is the integration of the two sides of the body, the acquisition of a body schema, and the development of gross praxis (1–2 years). With integration of the two sides of the body, the child is able to cross the midline visually and manually and to use both sides of the body together in a coordinated manner. The child is able to engage in activities that require the use of both hands and feet, using them jointly or in a reciprocal, cooperative manner. The child acquires an accurate body scheme—an awareness of each body part, the relationship of one body part to another, and what movements each body part can make. The child is able to experience her body, where it is and what it is doing, without looking at it or touching it. An accurate body scheme allows the child to develop gross praxia—the ability to engage in unfamiliar gross motor tasks. At first considerable attention and consideration is given to these tasks; later the child performs these tasks with ease and little need for attention to them. Performance has become automatic. With development of this level of sensory integration, the child's actions become more coordinated, organized, and purposeful. One senses the child's physical control over her body.

The second stage of sensory integration development is the development of fine praxia (2–3 years). The refinement of visual perception and good gross motor planning allows the child to develop fine praxia. Fine motor planning, also referred to as eye-hand coordination, involves the use of visual stimuli as the basis for directing the movements of the hand and fingers. But such direction is not possible unless there is considerable stored information about the way in which the hand moves and the effects of gravity. Thus, there needs to be a constant organized flow of information from the visual, vestibular, proprioceptive, and tactile systems and from previous stored information. Good eye-hand coordination allows the child to pick up small objects, manipulate objects with precision, and eventually to write. With the development of fine praxia, the child has acquired the basic elements of sensory integration. These elements will be further refined until about the age of 9 or 10 years.

Cognition

There are three stages of cognitive development between one and three years of age (47,141,302,774). The last stage begins at the age of two and continues to be more refined until five years of age.

The first stage involves the ability to engage in trial and error problem solving, use tools, perceive variability in spatial relations, seriate events in which one is not involved, and perceive the causality of other objects (12–18 months). Trial and error problem solving is the active manipulation of objects to bring about a desired result. Goals are able to be reached by new and unfamiliar means. This is a readily observable skill and can be seen in the child attempting to get the rings in order on a stack toy. Tool use involves the manipulation of one object by application of another object rather than the hand. It can be observed, for example, in the child's use of a spoon or using a stick to retrieve a ball that has rolled under the couch. Perceiving variability in spatial positions refers to the realization that spatial positions are not fixed. Learning is illustrated by the child going around the table to get a toy car that has been pushed to the opposite side. If the most direct or obvious route to a desired object is blocked, the child is able to figure out and use an alternative route. The trajectory of an object is no longer as important as the final resting place of the object. The child is now able to remember the order of a simple sequence of events (seriate events) through observation of these events rather than through direct participation in the events. The child, for example, may repeat three or four actions after observing another person perform these acts in a given sequence. This forms the basis for considerable imaginative play, a major activity of this age group. In acquiring the ability to perceive the causality of objects, the child loses her sense of impotence; she recognizes others are causal. In addition to recognizing the effects of gravity, the child perceives herself as the recipient of the causal activities of others. The child now realizes her actions or willing an event does not account for all the events in the immediate environment.

The second stage involves the ability to represent objects in an image manner, to make believe, to infer a cause given its effect, to act on the basis of combined spatial relations, to attribute omnipotence to others, and to perceive objects as permanent in time and place (18 months–2 years). Image representation is memory of stimuli in terms of an internal pictorial quasirepresentation. With acquisition of this skill the child is able to engage in covert trial and error problem solving. The child can think about how an object should be manipulated rather than actually manipulating the object. The child is now able to remember actions of another person and imitate these actions several days later. The relationship between pictures of objects and real objects becomes understood.

Make-believe is the reenactment of familiar events by using inadequate objects and treating them as if they were adequate. The child, using a block as an electric razor and shaving like Daddy is make-believe playing. There is a differentiation between the pretend and the real event. The child knows the shaving is not actual. The ability to distinguish between the real and the not real becomes more highly refined with further development. However, it is at this point that the basic ability is acquired.

To infer a cause given its effect refers to the recognition that familiar inanimate objects do not act spontaneously. When apparently spontaneous movement does occur, the child is either able to identify the cause or engages in activities likely to lead to identification of the cause. The child, for example, will run to see who is playing the music box. The child also, unceasingly, asks the question why.

In attributing omnipotence to others, primarily the parents, the child believes that others control natural phenomena (for instance rain, or the growth of flowers) and that others know what the child is thinking. This seems to be a stage necessary for the child to clearly understand that he or she is not omnipotent. This is a stage where parents or caretakers are seen as tremendously powerful.

In perceiving objects as permanent in time and place, the child comes to understand the temporal and spatial relationships of objects. The concept of time as independent from familiar daily routines is beginning to be recognized. Judgment of space and mass is more refined. Ice cream cones melt very quickly on a hot day, for example. The child's conscious thought processes show far less evidence of condensation and displacement: a major step in the development of secondary process thinking.

Cognition at the third stage is characterized by the ability to represent objects in an endoceptual manner, to differentiate between thought and action, and to recognize the need for causal sources (2–5 years). Endocept representation is memory of stimuli in terms of a felt experience. It is similar to some extent to motor planning, which in a sense is memory in terms of motor acts. Endocept representation is an elusive type of memory. The only reason it is described as being developed at this stage is that adults often recall experiences from this age in the form of endocepts. The child at this age does not have the verbal capacity to communicate endocept memories. However, it may be a part of the ability to engage in make-believe and fantasy. There is some question of whether the capacity to remember in an endoceptual manner is necessary for full maturation of cognitive ability. There are many adults who seemingly have no difficulty in cognitive function who are unable to describe any endoceptual memories.

Through recognizing the need for causal sources, the child comes to understand there is likely to be an identifiable cause for every effort. At this age, however, the cause ascribed to an effect may be idiosyncratic and not necessarily the cause and effect relationship considered acceptable by the child's cultural group. In attempting to limit the number of unknowns in the environment, the child engages in defining and organizing the causal relationship of events.

Family Interaction

The major task for the child between one and three years, using Erikson's taxonomy of the stages of psychosocial development, is the acquisition of a sense of autonomy (271). This is a sense that one is independent, self-governing, and possessing the freedom to determine one's own actions. This autonomy is obviously relative, for the child continues, in actuality, to be quite dependent on caretakers. Autonomy only begins at this age, with the child developing a sense of physical separation from parents, mastery over her own body, and a sense of having some control over the external environment. The converse of autonomy is shame and doubt, a lack of self-assurance and a feeling of humiliation at being small and dependent.

With increased mobility the child ventures out to explore the environment and to test the limits of the self and the environment (72,281,310,316,632). Behavior is characterized by periods of voluntary leaving and returning to caretakers. In leaving, the child initially likes to have the caretaker in full sight. Later the child is comfortable knowing where a parent is and that he or she is readily available. The child voluntarily returns to caretakers to check to make sure they are still there, for solace and reassurance, and as a source of security when injured, frustrated, or tired.

Although usually approached with much bravado, temporary separation is not necessarily easy for many children. The movement toward independence is sometimes facilitated by a "transitional object." This may be a small blanket, a favored stuffed toy, or some variation on that theme. The transitional object may be taken along in exploration of the environment. In such a case it is often left to drop as the child is caught up in the excitement of an activity. The child frequently cuddles with the transitional object when frustrated or unhappy. It is often taken to bed, particularly at night. At this age sleep may have the connotation of being alone, of a separation from all that is familiar and real.

The child becomes increasingly sure and adament about likes and dislikes, what is desired and what is not wanted. Although these ideas are not usually very consistent over time, at the moment they are firm and widely proclaimed. The child also wants to do things for himherself, to be independent, to be "grown up." The tenacity of these ideas and actions is often referred to as oppositional behavior. Such behavior usually reaches its peak between two and three years of age. This period has been referred to as the "terrible twos" and is punctuated by frequent and explosive "no" and "I want." Oppositional behavior seems to facilitate a sense of autonomy as the child defines the self by contrast to compliance and conformity.

The task of parents is often one of setting limits. The first priority is usually the safety of the child who is frequently reckless in exploration. With little knowledge of her capacities and limitations, the child does not tend to be self-protective. The second priority is helping the child to acquire patterns of behavior that are acceptable within the context of the family and neighborhood. Consistency of expectations and firm but gentle discipline are imperative in this aspect of the socialization process.

The child makes many forward strides in independence and self-control. However, this age is also characterized by periods of regression to more primitive, infantile patterns of behavior. This typically occurs when the child is overtired, frustrated, or placed in situations where demands are too great.

Although still needy of parental support, the child increasingly sees others as need fulfilling: siblings, other persons in the home, grandparents, a favored aunt or uncle. The child also sees nonhuman objects as need fulfilling. This includes not only transitional objects but preferred toys, perhaps the family dog, new shoes, mother's camera, and peanut butter sandwiches. In the language of object relations, the child transfers some libidinal energy from the primary object to other objects. The child shows particular delight in seeing and interacting with these objects and demonstrates possessive behavior toward them. The child's libidinal object relations are now described as being semi-diffuse. The child is able to satisfy his or her needs through investment in a number of different objects. Object relations are not totally diffuse because the parents continue to be the predominant and most important libidinal object.

Activities of Daily Living

Between the ages of one and three, the child is assisted in mastering bladder and bowel control. This is usually accomplished by the age of three, with occasional accidents at night. The child also masters the task of using a spoon and fork. Some children are able to use a knife by the age of three, whereas others may not be able to do this for another year or so. Many children go through periods of being a finicky eater but slowly learn to eat the foods typical of the family diet. Table manners must be learned, and that eating is not a time for play; foods, although interesting to explore, are not toys. Socialization relative to the eating habits and rituals usually takes place in the context of family meals. The opportunity for imitation of parents and older siblings is important. The child begins to assist with dressing and undressing, bathing, and putting away things. Greater independence in undressing usually occurs first with continued assistance often needed for over-the-head garments. In dressing the child does not attend to the necessities of whether a garment is right side out or on backwards; shoes only by chance are put on the right foot. Although cooperative in being washed, the child sees bathing as play and a time for attention from parents. By the age of three the child knows how to pick up and put away toys. However, this task is rarely done without prompting and is usually most successfully carried out with guidance and assistance from a sibling or parent (334,400,714).

Play

There is a marked increase in the variety of play activities at this age (684,716,770). Initially the child enjoys water and sand play and any activity that involves fitting or placing one thing inside another. Forms and spatial relations are of considerable interest, as are different textures. Simple toys that can be put together and taken apart are enjoyed by the age of two. With increased stability in locomotion, movements relative to sitting, standing, and walking become the object of games. Pull and push toys, wagons, and eventually scooters and tricycles allow for experimenting with gross motor skills. Outdoor play is often preferred, at least for part of the day. If circumstances permit, by the age of three children begin to acquire a large number of cars, trucks, airplanes, dolls, stuffed animals, and sets of blocks. These toys, explored in reality, are often also used as the basis for make-believe play. Imaginative play begins at about 18 months of age. By three years the child is able to combine an elaborate medley of events. However, ideas seem to be juxtaposed in a fairly idiosyncratic manner. At about 14 or 15 months of age, if not before, the child begins the long process of learning how to draw. Initial efforts involve scribbling, with no attempt to form figures; the marking of the paper is pleasurable in and of itself. Later the child becomes preoccupied with getting recognizable shapes on the paper. Simple geometric shapes and the human figure seem of most interest at this age. The child enjoys looking at picture books, being read to and told stories, and watching television. These activities are not only entertaining but also provide ideas for and stimulate make-believe play. Cartoon characters on television as well as people in the child's environment serve as the basis for considerable play that involves imitation. Television programs like *Sesame Street* perhaps contribute to some cognitive development at this age, but much of what the child seems to learn is primarily rote memorization and imitation.

Up until the age of two years, the child's play tends to be solitary or with parents or older siblings. The child remains initially somewhat fearful of adult strangers. If allowed to initiate contact at her own pace, however, the child will become friendly, and will approach and invite the adult to be a play partner. With children of approximately the same age, the child is more likely to be an observer or, if placed in close proximity, essentially ignore her peers. At about the age of two, the child begins to engage in parallel play: playing comfortably in the presence of other children. Although there is minimal sharing, there is an obvious awareness of each other and mutual stimulation. By the age of three play continues to be parallel but there is some sharing of toys and one child may imitate the play activity of another child. The children may all be engaged in the same activity such as block building but there is no attempt to engage in a joint effort. The three-year-old child knows she is not to hit another child, throw things, or take another child's toy without asking permission. However, these rudimentary social rules often still need to be enforced by an adult.

THREE TO FIVE YEARS OF AGE

The physical growth of the child becomes slower now than it was prior to this time. During the years three to five new skills are added but it is also a time of skill consolidation. The child's behavior comes to have more of a quality of being planned and better organized.

Cognition

This period of development involves refinement of the last stage of cognition outlined in the previous section. The reader is referred to that section for review.

Family Interaction

By the age of three years, the child's initial sense of autonomy is established (72,281,310,316,632). He has some idea of selfness and of the degree to which he is allowed to determine his own behavior. The parent-child battles and struggles are over. The child has become more "civilized"; the parents' sense of vigilance and being on guard is relaxed. There is a period of quiescence, with family life being more peaceful. This is admittedly only a lull prior to another period of rapid development.

At the age of approximately three years the child becomes aware of sexual differences. Prior to this time differentiation between the sexes was seen primarily as a matter of dress and role behavior. Now the child becomes aware of the anatomical differences. With this awareness the child develops the idea of being a definite sex. There is considerable interest in the genitals, one's own and other people's. The child may raise a number of questions, be concerned about not having or losing a penis, and engage in sexual exploration with playmates. The child also usually discovers the pleasure one can derive from self-stimulation; masturbation is a fairly common activity, particularly when the child is bored or tired. These sexual concerns and activities assist the child in learning about his sexual nature, which in turn provides the basis for development of a sexual identity. The socialization process, ideally, provides accurate information about sexual differences and guides the child in learning appropriate pregenital sexual expression. What is considered appropriate is strongly influenced by family values and those of the neighborhood. Typically, in our society, a child learns, for example, that genital exploration with playmates and public masturbation are not acceptable. More symbolic expression, toy guns and frilly dresses, is usually considered appropriate.

In conjunction with sexual concerns and activities, the child often goes through a period of attachment to the parent of the opposite sex and some feelings of jealousy and rivalry toward the parent of the same sex. This is traditionally referred to as Oedipal behavior. The parent of the opposite sex is the recipient of considerable attention and rewarded with compliant behavior. The child engages in activities and develops skills that please the opposite sex parent. This is often behavior that is traditionally considered to be gender related, e.g., the little girl may engage in rigorous gross motor activities or go fishing with her father; the little boy may assist his mother in the kitchen and help out with caring for a younger sibling. This aspect of Oedipal behavior not only contributes to the development of sexual identity, it also helps the child to learn something about traditional opposite gender role behavior.

The parent of the same sex is not treated with the same deference accorded the opposite sex parent. The same sex parent may be ignored or disobeyed. The child may engage in behavior which he or she knows the parent finds irritating, and may attempt to hurt the parent's feelings. However, the child is often in considerable conflict about this behavior. On the one hand, the child may just as soon wish the parent was out of the way. On the other hand, the child loves the same sex parent and realizes the dependency on that parent. The conflict goes even deeper. At some level there is realization that the idea of an exclusive life with the opposite sex parent is an impossibility.

The child's struggle with the Oedipal situation takes place in the family arena, in dreams, and in wakeful fantasies. Nightmares, fascination with monsters of all sorts, and a preoccupation with violence are common at this age. Resolution of the Oedipal situation comes slowly. It is essentially brought about through a process of reality testing. The child comes to realize that his infantile effort to separate the parental pair is not going to be successful. Love for and dependency on the same sex parent win out over wanting the demise of that parent. The child comes to accept the incest taboo, one more step in the socialization process, acquiring the values of the social system. By the end of the Oedipal period, the child has reached the stage of pregenital sexuality. He perceives his sexuality as good, acceptable to others, and a source of pleasure. He is also aware that direct genital behavior is unacceptable in this period of the life cycle and that overt expression must be held in abeyance until a more appropriate time. The child comes to realize that love can be shared between family members, that exclusivity is neither desirable nor possible in a well-functioning family. There is a beginning awareness of family dynamics and patterns of behavior that facilitate family cohesiveness and solidarity.

By five years of age the struggle for autonomy is a thing of the past and the Oedipal experience for the most part resolved. This allows the child to direct his energies to engaging in activities for the pleasure derived from them rather than to assert his autonomy or to define a sphere of unquestioned privileges. Erikson refers to this process as the development of initiative. Initiative is characterized by a vigorous, self-confident mode of behavior, a loving, relaxed manner of interacting, a sense of directionality, and fairly good judgment. Erikson describes the opposite of initiative as guilt—guilt in relation to sexual desires, the wish for the elimination of the same sex parent, and other contemplated or actualized interactions with the environment. Such guilt often interferes with selecting and initiating a course of action and deriving pleasure from activities. The child is hesitant in his approach to the world and lacking in self-confidence.

In the context of experiences outlined above, the child internalizes the values and norms of the family and wider social system relative to what is and is not appropriate behavior. Prior to this time, the child's behavior has been primarily regulated by parental edict, a fear of parental anger, or the desire to please the parents. Now the child has come to accept various ideas of what is right and wrong as his own. The child has invested libidinal energy in appropriate abstract objects and in so doing has learned to control aggressive drive or behavior. On the basis of internalized values and norms, the child is able to make judgments about acceptable methods of dealing with aggressive objects. The child is more accurate in identifying aggressive objects, able to invest aggressive energy in these objects, and realizes that, on the whole, nonhuman objects should not be destroyed nor people injured. This process is often referred to as the development of a superego.

Activities of Daily Living

Between the ages of three and five, the child learns to manage elimination independently. He acquires the ability to dress and undress without assistance, except for back closings and perhaps tying shoes. The child is able to wash his hands and face, brush his teeth, and bathe by himself. Adult prompting and supervision, however, are often necessary. The child's standards of cleanliness frequently are not as high as those of his parents; being clean and neat is not one of the child's major priorities. The extent to which the child is asked to take responsibility for household tasks varies from family to family. However, by the age of five years the child is capable of picking up his bedroom in a passable manner, assisting with simple meal preparation tasks and table setting, feeding the dog, emptying waste-baskets, dusting the more obvious surfaces of furniture, watering the plants, sorting socks, and so forth. Performing the above outlined tasks may not always be done willingly or with much style. However, engaging in such activities helps the child to acquire some sense of responsibility and participation in the affairs of the family. The task component of the role of being a child is beginning to be learned (334,400,714).

Play

Hopping, skipping, jumping, and throwing are now within the child's capacity. These activities are enjoyed for their own sake and incorporated into a variety of play activities (11,74,339,912). Rough and tumble play is enjoyed with peers and adults. A basic sense of bodily security and object consistency enables the child to experiment with new physical sensations derived from twirling and playing with double vision. With the development of more refined eye-hand coordination, the child enjoys coloring, cutting with a scissors, and drawing. The capacity to reproduce accurately geometric shapes, the human figure, and everyday objects is greatly increased. Play in this age period is characterized by elaboration and making activities more difficult. There is a great deal of pleasure derived from and pride in accomplishment. Make-believe and imitation flower into the enactment of many-faceted events, which are now more conventionally ordered (684,716). The relationship between reality, pretense, and fantasy is clearer to the child providing a more secure base for make-believe activities. Playing house, going shopping, killing the bad guy, and imitating parents' work tasks take place repeatedly, with many variations on the theme. Dressing up is incorporated in these activities as the child takes the role of mother, father, superman, policeman, doctor, and a variety of television characters. The child is often involved in making things: necklaces, paper and paste constructions, snap together models, and so forth. Building with a variety of different types of blocks becomes much more complex, creative, and elegant. Although most construction activity is guided by imitation and creativity, the child is able to follow two- or three-step verbal, demonstrated, and pictorial directions.

Television continues to be a part of the child's play activities. Programs such as Sesame Street and The Electric Company often become part of the child's daily routine. These programs help the child to learn basic concepts, letters, and numbers. They also stimulate the ideas that are used as the basis for other play activities. Cartoons are still enjoyed but the child also becomes interested in other kinds of programs. Network "specials," various series on educational television, news programs, and the enactment of traditional childhood stories give the child a broader perspective of the world outside the home and neighborhood. Television now becomes less of a solitary activity and more a social activity shared with family members.

By the age of about four years, the child has moved from parallel play to the ability to engage in project group interaction (684,770). Such interaction is characterized by a child's involvement with others in a short-term task that requires some shared interaction, cooperation, and competition. The task is seen as paramount and there is minimal sustained interaction outside the task. The child is still preoccupied with exploring and testing to determine whether or not peers can be trusted. The child remains egocentric in the sense that he moves in and out of a task on whim. Interest in an activity promotes engagement with others, but with loss of interest the child simply leaves. Peers are approached to assist with a task and the child usually gives assistance when requested by a playmate. There is a dawning sense that one must help others if one is to receive help from them. The child has a more refined idea of the rights of others and the proper playground and playroom etiquette.

A child between the ages of three and five years is often in a daycare program or nursery school. Such a setting encourages the acquisition of group interaction skills, provides stimulation for engaging in a vast variety of activities, contributes to the refinement of gross and fine motor skills, and enhances cognitive development. A child who is not involved in some sort of a structured group experience may initially find himself at some disadvantage at the beginning of kindergarten. Daycare programs and nursery school facilitate play. They are not designed or intended to promote the development of academic skills; they are preparation for this aspect of development.

The beginning of friend relationships occurs at this time. The child makes friends with particular playmates, spending time with them, playing together, and visiting their homes. These first friend relationships are casual in nature and focused around shared activities. They tend to be fairly easily disrupted and are minimally concerned with need satisfaction. The child's friendships are important to him but less significant than family relationships. The child's major source of emotional satisfaction and support comes from the family. Friends are, for now, simply someone to play with.

FIVE TO ELEVEN YEARS OF AGE

These are the first school years when the child makes the initial transition from being a child protected in the home environment to participation in the wider community. School serves both as the bridge to and preparation for that participation. Physical growth is relatively slow. However, there continues to be refinement in gross and fine motor coordination and an increase in strength and endurance.

During the first part of this phase of development (5–7 years), it is believed that differentiation between the two hemispheres of the brain takes place, each taking on specialized functions (58). There continues, however, to be considerable communication between the two hemispheres. Without this, the specialized functions of the brain would not be coordinated. There would be a sense of splitting, of some activities being totally divorced from others. With differentiation and specialization, specific capacities begin to be governed by each hemisphere. It is believed that the left hemisphere is concerned with understanding and using language, with speaking, listening, reading, writing, and the use of formal logic. The right hemisphere is concerned with nonverbal perception, with interpreting tactile input, spatial relations, and understanding and appreciation of the visual arts and music. It is also believed that the right hemisphere is responsible for the intuitive capacities and dealing with emotional issues. The above description of function is in relationship to a person who is right-handed. For a person who is genetically left-handed, the specialization may be just the reverse.

Differentiation and specialization of the hemispheres also leads to hand and eye dominance. With the development of dominance, the fine motor skill of one hand becomes increasingly refined and one eye leads when the two eyes work together in binocular or depth vision. For example, the latter allows the child to be more proficient in hitting and catching a ball. At this time the child is also able to discriminate between right and left on an experiential level and not by using external clues as, for example, a small scar on one index finger. Right-left discrimination on a more fundamental level involves the ability to perceive a horizontal sequence and to identify the difference between reversed images. This is prerequisite to learning how to read and write since these activities involve the ability to scan written lines consistently from left to right and to tell the difference between letters (e.g., to distinguish between the letters b and d).

Without hemispheric differentiation, the two halves of the brain tend to develop similar functions, with none being developed well. The child will not acquire dominance. Both hands or either hand will be used for fine motor work but dexterity will not be as highly developed as the child who has acquired dominance. Lack of eye dominance results in continual alteration of the lead eye, causing difficulty in binocular vision. With lack of differentiation the two sides of the body will not work well together. The body does not seem to "fit together" and appears to be uncoordinated. Finally, inadequate differentiation and/or communication between the hemispheres may lead to overspecialization. One hemisphere becomes hyperdominant, the child becoming overly specialized in the use of language or the use of nonverbal perception. This leads to a deficit in processing some types of sensory information and organizing certain adaptive responses.

With adequate hemispheric differentiation and specialization, the child is able to organize letters and numbers. This ability is essential for adequate performance in school, the major task of this stage of development.

Cognition

Between the ages of six and seven years the child develops the ability to represent objects in a denotative manner, to perceive the viewpoint of others, and to decenter (47,114,302,774). Denotative representation is memory of stimuli in terms of words that stand for and name objects. The word is perceived as part of the object or equivalent to it. In acquiring this aspect of cognition the child's use of language becomes more accurate and she is able to read at age level. In addition, the child is aware of higher and lower levels of classification, is able to form classes on the basis of similarities, and is able to add or subtract classes to form superordinate and subordinate classes. The ability to classify is important for it allows the individual to organize and deal with a large mass of information and considerable detail.

The ability to perceive the viewpoint of others refers to coordinating one's own perceptions with those of others. The child is now able to take the role of others on a higher cognitive level; she can think about what the other person might want to do or how the other person might respond in a given situation. This is different than previously when the child could only take the role of another through imitation. The child also comes to realize that her own point of view is only one of many possible points of view. Contemplation of various ways in which a person or event might be perceived is comfortable. The child no longer takes egocentric, inflexible points of view.

Decentration is the process of distinguishing several features or characteristics of an object. The child is able to take a balanced view of all aspects of a person, object, or event and to use this information in thinking and making judgments. The child no longer focuses on the single outstanding characteristic of an object or is concerned only with surface phenomena. Attitudes and actions become far more flexible.

Family Interaction

The difficulties of living within a family constellation are now, to a great extent, a thing of the past (72,316, 343,632). The child enjoys being a family member and is well aware of its privileges and responsibilities. There is, for the most part, a comfortable interaction with members of the immediate extended and expanded family. Freed from much conflict, the child has the capacity to give love in an open and affectionate way. She is able to care for younger siblings and cousins. She begins to be aware of her parents' needs and frustrations and is able to give some support and comfort. The child is aware of family dynamics and usually uses them to foster family peace and solidarity.

With the child's increased independence in personal care, there is less intimate contact between child and parent. This is a gradual physical distancing process that varies considerably between children, some wanting more physical contact than others. There is also a difference in the amount of physical contact typical of a particular family. At the younger end of this age group there is still some hugging and caressing during the day and the child still enjoys cuddling when being read to. At the older end of this age group there is often only a perfunctory kiss before leaving for school and at bedtime. However, there still may be some physical contact—head on a parent's lap or an arm around the shoulder—during shared television viewing.

Although the child has internalized many of the family's values, there is still some reliance on the parents for reinforcement of those values and guidance in acceptable behavior. There are occasional times when the child loses her temper, disobeys family rules, teases and argues with siblings, and talks back to parents. Depending on the severity of these infractions the child may be reprimanded, sent to her room for a cooling off period, denied television watching, suffer a reduction in allowance, or have some privileges taken away for a period of time. When there is a clash between the values of the family and that of the peer group, the family's value system usually prevails. This is not always the case in the next period of development.

The child enjoys participation in family activities but there is also a decreasing amount of time spent with family members. School, friends, lessons of one kind or another, and perhaps sleep-away camp draw the child outside the family circle. There are times that it appears, at least to the parents, that home is simply a base for operations in the external environment. Food, bed, clean clothes, and a telephone sometimes seems all that is needed for sustenance. This is, in fact, not the case. The child continues to receive the major portion of her emotional support from the family. The gradual change is in the amount of contact needed for the maintenance of that support, not in the need for support per se.

Activities of Daily Living

As in family interaction, there is a gradual increase in independence and responsibility in activities of daily living (335,400,714). Care of the self comes to include cutting fingernails, washing one's hair, and combing and brushing it neatly, and selecting appropriate clothes for specific activities. The child comes to have rather distinct ideas about type of hairstyle and preferred type of clothes. In our society, seemingly regardless of cultural subgroup, girls in this age period are somewhat more concerned about dressing and grooming than boys.

Increased development is also seen in the child's capacity to use the telephone. Initially learning how to answer the phone correctly, the child learns to carry on a conversation, dial the phone independently, find a number in the phone book, and use the phone as a means of social interaction. A similar sequence of events is seen in independence in travel. The five-year-old child is generally accompanied to school or carefully placed on the school bus. Later the child is able to handle increasing freedom in traveling about the neighborhood. The acquisition of a bicycle facilitates mobility and allows the child greater speed and range. The child may be permitted to use public transportation. The extent of freedom the child has relative to travel is often dependent on the safety of the community and the various distances that need to be traveled.

The child, somewhere in the middle of this period of development, usually begins to receive an allowance. This may be a specific amount of money per week or based on defined household tasks the child is required to perform. What expenses are to be covered by the allowance varies as does the amount of money received. The child's allowance is the first experience with money management: whether to spend or save, how to set priorities in regard to what will be purchased. During this period, the child begins to develop an idea of the worth of money, family values in regard to money, and the role money plays in daily life in the family and in the wider community.

In the home, the child is often given more responsibilities for household tasks and is increasingly capable of carrying out such tasks. Most children are required to make their own bed and care for their own room. A good many children go through cycles of tolerating considerable disarray in their room to wanting everything meticulously in its proper place. By the middle of this age period, children are usually able to make their own breakfast and lunch and contribute substantially to the preparation of dinner. By the age of 11 years a child is frequently capable of preparing a simple meal for him- or herself and other family members. Other household tasks a child may be involved in are going to the store to pick up items for a parent, yard work, shoveling snow, helping with cleaning and maintenance chores, cleaning up, doing the dishes, and laundering clothes. Although the child is capable of doing many household tasks, organization so as to accomplish a number of tasks simultaneously is difficult. The child also needs supervision relative to performing tasks when they should be performed and maintaining an acceptable quality of performance. The number of household tasks required of a child is influenced by the cultural group to which the family belongs and whether one or both parents work outside the home.

School/Work

Entrance into formal schooling is a big event for most children (271,335,400,555,587,669,684,714,716,758, 770). It is usually anticipated as a sign that one is "growing up" and as such is a benchmark in the life cycle. The child may experience some initial anxiety but this is usually overcome in a matter of days. The transition from being a preschooler to being a student is facilitated by both the human and nonhuman environment. Parents indicate their pleasure that the child is in school, are interested in the child's daily experiences, proud of her achievements, and available for emotional support and occasionally consolation if the need arises. Teachers in the lower grades are usually relatively permissive and understanding of differences in developmental levels and readiness for the demands of the school situation. The nonhuman environment facilitates transition by the child bringing home objects made and work accomplished which can be shared with family members. Favored toys, mementos from trips, and small pets may be brought from home to share with the teacher and classmates. These interactions help to bridge the gap between home and school.

The other major transition that occurs at this time is movement from being primarily a player to becoming a worker. School demands a new way of interacting with the environment. It requires sustained concentrated effort with externally imposed demands and limits. It involves work. Regardless of how much the child enjoys school, by at least the age of six years the child is aware of the difference between play and school work. The transition takes several years. In kindergarten and first grade, play is used as the major vehicle for accomplishing the goals of the academic program. Although there is some time for free play, most of the play activity is structured and guided to teach specific concepts and skills. Gradually there is less play and more emphasis on specific learning experience. There is still a good deal of physical activity involved but the information to be learned is readily apparent to the child. Finally, the child is required to sit quietly and concentrate on academic subjects that entail no gross physical activity. The trip from the sand-and-water table to the desk has been accomplished. The transition, then, from play to work is movement from physical action on the environment, to the imposition of structured thought, to the deemphasis of action. This pattern is used, primarily, because it follows or mirrors cognitive development.

The demands of the school situation are multiple. The basic skills of reading, writing, and mathematics must be mastered, refined, and used. By the age of 11 years the child also has acquired a working knowledge of biology, the physical sciences, history, and the social sciences. The child has usually been introduced to the arts, although an appreciation of aesthetics is not yet well developed. The 11-year-old child has acquired a large fund of knowledge and is able to apply it in understanding her immediate environment and the world beyond family, school, and community.

With school the child is introduced to a more strict interpretation of time (519). As a preschooler, the child's daily life was primarily regulated by a biological clock: the cyclic need for food, sleep, and activity. Although there were some external limits imposed by the timing of family activities, these were defined to some extent by the child's own internal rhythm. The situation changes with entrance into school. The child must be up, dressed, and in school by a specified time. In school, activities are regulated by the clock; they begin and end at a specific time. School work and assignments must be accomplished in a given period of time. Tests, often by the second grade, are timed. By the third or fourth grade the child is likely to have homework. Thus after school and evening hours must be planned to allow sufficient time for out of school assignments. The child not only must become time conscious, she must also learn how to budget time. Initially, given outside assistance, eventually the child must internalize the time demands of the school environment. This is usually accomplished by 11 years of age except perhaps in relationship to homework. This may still be an area where parental guidance is necessary.

Another demand of the school situation is to conform to external standards and expectations. Collectively this is often referred to as the development of good study habits. Some of the demands and expectations are: attention to the teacher and to a specified task, neatness and accuracy, following directions, taking responsibility for the work assigned, organizing work and one's efforts, using resource materials and the library, communicating verbally and in writing, working independently, seeking help when needed, and being able to comprehend, recall, integrate, and apply learned concepts. The development of study habits begins in kindergarten. They are usually mastered at least on a fundamental level by the age of 11 years. Without such mastery the child is ill prepared for the requirements of more advanced academic work.

The social demands of the school situation are also considerable. The child must learn how to engage in the social interactions that are an inherent part of the student role. First, the child needs to be able to relate to and accept the authority of the teacher. To a preschooler all authority is seen as being invested in her parents. Initially, the child may view the teacher with some suspicion, as an extension of the parents, omnipotent, or someone who limits and interferes with one's freedom, or any combination of these attitudes. Through interaction with teachers and reinforcement from parents, the child usually comes to trust teachers in general and feel that their actions are motivated by concern for the welfare of students. In conjunction with the development of trust, the child learns to accept direction from teachers in a positive and cooperative manner. The manner in which the child has dealt with the authority of her parents will influence her relationship with teachers. The relationship with teachers, in turn, will influence how the individual relates to other authority figures in the future.

The school setting requires a capacity for differential interaction, depending on the situation. Different responses are expected in the classroom, lunchroom, and playground. In the classroom, the child must learn how to work with others in a shared task which is externally imposed, work without interrupting others, and participate in class discussions. In the lunchroom the child must be able to engage in conversation, sit quietly, and eat in, at least, a somewhat socially acceptable manner. On the playground the child must be able to follow the rules of the game. One of the essential values the child acquired during this age period is a respect for the rights of others. The child's relationship with peers will be discussed in more detail in the following section.

As mentioned in Chapter 4, vocational development begins at the age of five or six (183,345,939). The first phase, which continues to about the age of 11 years, is referred to as the fantasy stage. The child, often prompted by adults, contemplates what she will do when she grows up. Over the course of these years the child arrives at a number of possibilities. These choices are usually influenced by the status, glamour, or adventure associated with a particular type of job and by the child's life experiences. The child who has a chronic health problem, for example, may want to be an occupational therapist or a physician. The child who has just been to the ballet may want to become a dancer. The work of one's parents is not a major influence at this time. The child often does not understand the jobs of her parents unless there is a highly visible quality to their work. The work of a photographer is, for example, sufficiently concrete for the child to understand; the work of an accountant is not. The other reason parents' jobs have little influence on vocational choice at this age is that children rarely see anything particularly glamorous about their parents' work. Occupational choice at the fantasy stage is made with little regard for the outcome of that choice. There is no concern about the skills or qualifications required. Choice is only centered on the pleasant or exciting aspects of the job.

Play/Leisure/Recreation

In this area of human experience the child is also going through a period of transition (72,555,632, 684,716,770). There is still involvement in typical preschool play activities, an elaboration of some of these activities, and many new interests. Life comes, rather abruptly, to be divided into a more adult-like rhythm of work, play, and rest. The sphere of games with rules is joined and becomes comfortable.

The child continues to enjoy play that involves physical activity. With persistence, growth in strength, endurance, and coordination, the child is able to engage in increasingly more demanding and complex activities. In this age group the child is likely to enjoy rough and tumble play or "wrestling," tag, hide and seek, climbing trees, jumping rope, swimming, riding a bicycle, ice and roller skating, riding a skateboard, skiing, and so forth.

Most children remain interested in drawing. It is a means of communication that is very useful prior to gaining facility in expressing ideas in writing. The child becomes interested in perspective and concerned about composition. Drawings become elaborate and very detailed. Many drawings are action oriented and/or are meant to illustrate a sequence of events. Toward the end of this age group, the child often becomes interested in drawing cartoons.

Make-believe activities continue to be devised and acted out until about nine years of age. The child plays with dolls, fights the never-ending battle between cowboys and Indians, and takes many odysseys through outer space. At the age of nine the child begins to lose interest in acted out make-believe. Cognitive capacity has increased to the point that the child can think about objects, people, and events without the props of concrete action. However, this by no means marks the end of fantasy. The child daydreams, enjoys the fantasy in books and television, and plays various games of strategy which have a strong element of fantasy.

Interest in construction remains dominant and becomes more elaborate. Blocks of various kinds and sets of basic structural components (e.g., Tinker Toys, Legos, Capsila) are formed into complex objects and structures. Human figures are often included in the play associated with the objects constructed. The child frequently enjoys putting together models, doing so with great care and attention to detail. The child begins to explore various arts and crafts such as woodworking, making puppets, craft stick construction, decoupage, sewing, and other needlecrafts. In the context of construction, many children become interested in the mechanics of things, their toys, and household objects. Taking apart things, figuring out how they work, and putting them back together becomes a very enjoyable activity. The exploration of household objects may, however, cause some parental concern.

As mentioned in the discussion of family interaction, children in this developmental phase derive great enjoyment from being with playmates. Although a child may have a few special friends, being with a group of playmates is of primary importance. Friendship still remains at the casual level and specific "special friends" may change every three or four months. The child is not yet capable of sustained, nonfamilial emotional involvement. Although the child enjoys some solitary leisure time, she usually prefers to share activities with playmates.

Two different stages of group interaction take place at this age level. The first stage involves the ability to participate in an egocentric-cooperative group (5–7 years). Egocentric-cooperative groups are characterized by group members selecting, implementing, and executing relatively long-term tasks through joint interaction. The child's interaction in the group is characterized by enlightened self-interest: the awareness that one's rights will be respected only through respect for the rights of others, that one's needs for recognition and to be judged as adequate will only be met through meeting this need in others, and that to be accepted by the group one must act in an acceptable manner. The child learns to be cooperative in group interaction because of her own needs, not for the sake of task accomplishment or for altruistic reasons.

Egocentric-cooperative groups are centered around specific activities. They provide for satisfaction of esteem and mastery needs but not for satisfaction of love and belonging and safety needs. These latter needs continue to be met within the context of the family. Participation in egocentric-cooperative groups provides an opportunity to gain experience in cooperation and competition, sportsmanship, leadership and other group membership roles, identifying group norms and goals, and how to respect the rights of others. After successful completion of this stage of group interaction skill development, the child knows how to satisfy her esteem needs and those of others in a group situation. The child also sees herself as a person who is able to participate in groups and as a person who has a right to belong to groups.

The second stage involves the ability to participate in a cooperative group (9–12 years). A cooperative group is characterized by homogeneous membership and mutual need satisfaction. The group is usually made up of children of the same sex and relatively the same age. This is the typical "gang" of pre-adolescence. The group has an exclusive quality that is not found in the previous stage of group interaction skill development. Members of the group recognize with some pride that they are group members. There may be some fringe members made up of younger children or children who are not yet capable of participation in this type of group. Group members tend to be somewhat secretive and want a degree of separateness and privacy. They may have a special meeting place, a particular badge of membership (e.g., hair style, tee shirts, ring), and use code words or a shared jargon. Although the group may form around a common interest, the group is not primarily concerned with an activity or task accomplishment. Rather the purpose of the group is to be with each other, to share ideas and confidences, and to feel accepted by a small nonfamilial group without an authority figure. Within the context of a cooperative group, the child learns to express positive and negative feelings in a group and to meet group members' needs for safety and love and belonging. The group facilitates the development of social consciousness, a sensitivity to the needs of others, and a sense of loyalty. The child learns to care about a group of others for, at least some, unselfish reasons. Participation in a cooperative group is the first major step in breaking away from dependency on the emotional support of the nuclear family.

In addition to play activities, the child's leisure time is usually well occupied. Reading often becomes of considerable interest to the child. Although not entirely giving up fantasy stories, the child also enjoys stories about characters similar to her in age and life situation. The child also comes to enjoy biographies, adventure stories, history, and books about how things work. Many children are involved in a variety of lessons: piano, dancing, tennis, gymnastics, art, and so forth. The child participates in many shared family activities, with the child now being more active in selecting activities and in contributing to the success of the activity. Common family activities are trips to zoos, museums, and historical sights, camping and hiking, attending religious services, entertaining relatives and friends of the family, cook outs, family vacations, and watching television. The latter not only serves as the nucleus for family interaction, it also augments the child's formal education. News and science programs are often watched with considerable interest. The child's understanding of current events is frequently quite sophisticated by the age of 11 years. Organized groups with adult supervision are usually available in the community. Most children belong to one or more groups such as scouts, little league, school clubs, and groups sponsored by religious organizations. Summers may include day or sleep-away camp experiences. Organized groups help the child to develop social skills, expose the child to a variety of activities she might not explore on her own, and sometimes introduce the child to the idea of service to the community.

In the area of recreation, the child begins to be involved in games with rules and sports. Although she may find rules confusing at first and inhibiting to activity and self-expression, the child at about the age of six or seven years begins to enjoy formal games. There is often a good deal of delight in the chance to win, the skill of playing, and the challenge of following the rules. The child learns to accept defeat with some degree of graciousness, sharpens skills through competition, and comes to understand that cheating is unacceptable. Some of the games children enjoy at this age level are cards, board games, chess, softball, kickball, soccer, football, volleyball, and basketball. Team sports are particularly enjoyed at the more advanced end of this age group.

Erikson refers to this time in the life cycle as the age of industry (270). He uses industry in the sense of the application of one's efforts to the completion of a task. The task may be in the area of school or play, but wherever, it involves steady and persevering diligence. The child learns to win recognition by producing things, by being productive. Erikson also uses industry to refer to learning the fundamentals of technology: how to handle the utensils and tools used by adults. In the process of doing things with and beside others, the child begins to understand sharing, the division of labor, and the work norms that regulate interaction in the child's culture. The converse of industry is inferiority. The child who fails to master the skills expected in school or in recreational pursuits or who fails to receive recognition from her peers and parents feels markedly inadequate and doomed to mediocrity or failure.

Finally, by the end of this age period, the child has a fairly accurate idea of her assets and limitations (74). The child comes to understand what she is able and not able to do. Limitations are accepted with perhaps some desire to alter these limitations and attempts to do so. The child recognizes at the same time that some limitations do not reflect total ineptness; she has a dawning recognition that all individuals have deficits that must be accepted. The child is proud of her assets and attempts to refine them and capitalize on them. Assessment of assets and limitations is relative to skill in using the body, in both a fine and gross manner, physical appearance, intellectual ability and achievements, social skills, and interests.

ELEVEN TO EIGHTEEN YEARS OF AGE

The part of the life cycle between 11 and 18 years of age is, in our society, referred to as adolescence. The term comes from the Latin verb *adolere*—to grow, to mature. Adolescence is a time of considerable growth, maturation, and development in all areas. Adolescence is the bridge between being a child and being an adult. The end of adolescence is recognized as the age of majority in most Western societies: the age when the individual has the legal rights and responsibilities of being an adult.

Puberty occurs during the initial period of adolescence (11,505,555,912). This is the term used to demarcate the time when a youth is first capable of sexual reproduction. Pubescence is the period of about two years which precedes puberty.

The chain of events involved in adolescence is initiated in the hypothalamus, which triggers the pituitary. The pituitary gland modulates and coordinates the activity of the endocrine and nervous system, which leads to the many physical and psychological changes of the adolescent period. Prior to pubescence, the growth and maturation of the sexes is fairly similar both in rate and kind. This is not the case in adolescence. Pubescence begins earlier in girls, starting at about the age of 11 years; for boys it begins at about 13 years of age. There is considerable variation within the sexes, genetic differences and environmental factors (e.g., nutrition, climate) seemingly being responsible for this variation. The nature of the physical changes that occur is, obviously, quite different. The sexes come to be clearly differentiated relative to body size, body contour, and secondary sexual characteristics.

Briefly, the physical changes that occur in adolescence are: (a) acceleration and then deceleration of skeletal growth; (b) altered body composition as a result of skeletal and muscular growth, together with changes of the quantity and distribution of fat; (c) development of the circulatory and respiratory system, leading, particularly in boys, to increased strength and endurance; and (d) the development of gonads, reproductive organs, and secondary sex characteristics.

Physical growth in adolescence often occurs in one or more spurts and usually continues for a longer period in males. Rapid acceleration in growth is frequently accompanied by temporary periods of decreased endurance and incoordination. The youth may tire more easily and may need more sleep than usual. Previous smooth and skilled gross motor movements may appear to be lost for a period of time as the youth becomes acclimated to his new stature and strength.

Endocrine activity leads to the maturation of primary sex characteristics and the growth of secondary sex characteristics. Maturation of the ovaries, fallopian tubes, uterus, and vagina constitute the development of primary sex characteristics in girls. In boys it is marked by maturation of the testes, penis, and the organs that transmit sperm from the testes to the penis. The growth of pubic and axillary hair are two secondary sex characteristics that occur in both males and females. The other secondary sex characteristics are, for girls, the development of breasts and increased width and depth of the pelvis. For boys, there is an increase of facial and body hair and a deepening of the voice. Menarche, the first menstrual period, traditionally marks puberty in girls. However, a girl may conceive prior to menarche or not be capable of conception for some time after menarche. Menstrual periods tend to be somewhat irregular at first and accompanied by a degree of discomfort. The attainment of reproductive capacity in boys is not marked by a particular biological event. However, fairly reliable signs are the pigmentation of axillary hair and the onset of nocturnal emissions—ejaculation during sleep. Puberty leads to increased genital excitement and a new sexual urgency.

Adolescence is often a time of emotional turmoil. Emotional lability, frequent and marked mood changes, is common. Emotions and feelings are intense during this period and are often expressed accordingly. The adolescent often experiences a sense of pent-up energy and feelings of restlessness.

The physical and emotional changes just described influence all aspects of development in this phase of the life cycle.

Cognition

Between the ages of 11 and 13 years, the youth attains the most mature stage of cognitive development (47,141, 302,774). This final stage involves the ability to represent objects in a connotative manner, to use formal logic, and to work in the realm of the hypothetical. Connotative representation is memory of stimuli in terms of words that are consciously perceived as only labels for a classification of some common characteristic. The youth is now able to think on the abstract level and deal knowledgeably with theoretical material. He is able to understand the nature of theory and its relationship to observable phenomena. The capacity to classify becomes far more sophisticated and the youth is able to order events or objects easily in a variety of different ways. The youth's thinking becomes more flexible and there is increased appreciation of the multiple meaning of words. With this capacity, the youth is able to understand philosophical principles, more subtle forms of humor, and read poetry and other forms of literature with greater comprehension, discrimination, and pleasure.

The use of formal logic is the ability to maintain one promise during a reasoning sequence, to reflect back on a reasoning sequence, and to base conscious thought and action on deterministic causality. The latter refers to assigning sufficient and accurate causes to events. Formal logic is a process and not a specific conclusion. What is logical in one culture may be illogical in another. The premise taken as the point of departure for a reasoning sequence is influenced by the ideas of one's cultural group, as is the definition of sufficient and accurate causes. In order for a person to be said to be using formal logic, the premises selected and causes given for events must be compatible with those of his culture. The statement, for example, that wearing a pod of garlic around one's neck will protect one from getting the common cold is considered quite logical in some cultures, but not others. In acquiring the ability to use formal logic, the youth is able to identify and return to the original point of departure during a reasoning sequence and recognize and correct contradictions in logic in his own and others' reasoning process.

The realm of the hypothetical refers to that which is future, unknown, conjecture, or open to speculation. The individual capable of hypothetical thinking is able to engage in consideration of that which goes beyond the immediate here and now of current interactions, to imagine "what might be," to perceive both the obvious and the subtle, to deal with the idea of chance and probability, and to solve problems by isolating all of the possible variables and relationships and, through experimentation and logical analysis, determine which of these is validated by the present data.

With the development of this last stage of cognition, the individual has all of the skills necessary to engage in secondary and tertiary process thinking. Although the capacity is present by about the age of 13 years, it may be several years before it matures to its fullest. Maturation is dependent on the youth's life experience, particularly those related to formal education. Not all educational systems foster the maturation of this capacity. Although this is considered to be the last stage of cognitive development, it is important to realize that the individual will continue to accumulate a considerably greater fund of knowledge.

With the capacity to use formal logic and work in the realm of the hypothetical, the youth frequently applies this manner of thinking to questioning ideas and beliefs, those of his family and of the wider social system. He becomes interested in religion, politics, ethical considerations, and moral judgments. He seeks answers for the problems of society. The youth becomes concerned about the future, his own and that of the world in which he lives.

Family Interaction

Family relations during the adolescent period are rarely peaceful (113,200,242,332,344,555,718,758,770). Discord between youths and their parents is commonplace. The youth's self-concept and sexual image are in a state of upheaval. There is a search for who one is, for identity. There is a need to redefine one's familial role from being a child to being, if not an adult, then something quite close to that desired role. There is a need to reform the child-parent bond from the ancient puerile one to the adult familial bond of affection and mutual respect. These considerable tasks are accomplished within the context of the family and with peers. Although somewhat difficult to separate, only the familial portion of the struggle for adulthood will be discussed in this section: the place of peers in this struggle will be discussed later.

The adolescent period is often, in part, likened to the struggle for autonomy of the two-year-old child. There is the same need for definition of self and for redefining one's relationship with parents. Partially, this is accomplished by turning away from the family to peers for emotional support and guidance, an option not available to the two-year-old. The adolescent has a strong sense of ambivalence toward his parents. On the one hand he wants to be separate from them, allowed to make decisions on his own, and in general be permitted to manage his own affairs. On the other hand the adolescent wants to be able to rely on his parents when he runs into trouble and wants them available for support and guidance when he feels this is necessary. Typically, there is oscillation between these two positions as there is in much of the adolescent's behavior. At times the youth will act in a mature and competent manner; at other times he will act foolishly with apparent disregard for the consequences of his actions.

Within the family, the struggle for identity, for autonomy, for adulthood usually focuses around several common issues. The adolescent is likely to raise questions about the parents' values, religious and political beliefs, and life style. These questions are raised for a variety of reasons. They are of interest to the youth in and of themselves as he attempts to sort out his own values and beliefs. They are also raised to engage in an argument. This provides an opportunity to practice and consolidate newly developed cognitive skills. Out of the anger and frustration of internal turmoil and parental constraint, the adolescent may simply want to provoke the parent. A good argument serves this purpose well. Arguing then may simply take place for the sake of arguing.

Parents may object to the adolescent's friends or peer group. They may feel the youth is spending too much time with the peer group to the neglect of his studies or family responsibilities. Or they may object to the activities in which the peer group engages. Such things as style of dress and hair, taste in music, preferred dances, political activities, and so forth are of concern to some parents. Almost all parents, however, are concerned about their child's possible use of drugs and alcohol. In experimenting to define himself, the adolescent frequently finds these parental concerns irritating and evidence that he is being treated like a child. Although often wanting some control, the adolescent objects to the setting of limits.

A similar situation arises in regard to sexuality. The new and strong sexual urges of adolescents seem to demand release. Although some satisfaction may be gained from masturbation, the adolescent usually wants to explore his new found sexuality more fully. The universal incest taboo focuses sexual exploration outside the family constellation. The parents usually, and again legitimately, have some concerns about genital exploration. Even if not openly discussed, the sexuality of the adolescent influences parental-adolescent relationships. Closely related are the issues of pregnancy and contraceptives. Restraints on recreational activities that may lead to sexual exploration are usually more severe for girls than boys in most families and cultural groups. However, this does not mean that restraints are absent in the case of boys. Imposed limitations are, on the one hand, welcomed by the adolescent, for they provide controls the adolescent may not be able to impose himself. On the other hand, they are unwelcomed for the reasons mentioned above.

Other common points of conflict revolve around such issues as use of the family car, responsibilities for household tasks, participation in family leisure activities, and money. The adolescent may want the family car too frequently, not wish to do household tasks, show little enthusiasm for family leisure activities, and want to spend more money than the family wishes to provide or is able to afford. Through dealing with these and the above-mentioned issues, the adolescent comes to develop some sense of autonomy relative to family and parents. This is a gradual process and, periodically, a rather unpleasant process for all parties involved.

One factor that impinges on the struggle for autonomy is the emotional lability and intensity of the adolescent. This not only makes the adolescent uncomfortable but tends to confuse parents. They are often not quite sure what the adolescent is feeling, nor for that matter is the adolescent. Emotional lability and intensity can make any discussion and sharing of differences a difficult process. At times the adolescent may be calm and reasonable; moments later there may be tears or shouting. Stormy scenes are usual. In order to deal with his feelings the adolescent frequently seeks privacy away from family members. He may retreat to his room seeking solace in music, reading, a hobby, or just thinking. Although the family may consider this behavior unusual, and allow it to become a source of conflict, it does provide a respite for both adolescent and family.

Toward the end of adolescence the youth often "falls in love." Although this is rarely the beginning of a permanent partnership, the relationship provides relief from many family tensions and helps to resolve whatever issues remain relative to autonomy. The adolescent becomes so involved with another person that the struggles within the family become far less significant. He experiences a broadening support system and the feeling that someone else understands. Through participation in this romantic liaison, the adolescent thinks that he should be more responsible, be more like an adult. In this situation, the thought often leads to behavior. Although not necessarily autonomous, the adolescent feels more of a sense of being his own person.

Activities of Daily Living

By the end of adolescence, the individual has learned most of the basic survival skills for living independently (171,400). Although he may not know how to perform specific activities, he has the cognitive, motor, and social skills necessary to learn these activities very quickly.

Throughout this period, the adolescent becomes increasingly independent in travel. In many communities, the bicycle is the major mode of independent travel at the beginning of this age period. By 12 or 13 years the adolescent is allowed and able to travel fairly far afield. He is able to use public transportation alone and by about 14 years of age learns how to use a map regarding routes and to read time tables. In some areas a motorcycle may replace a bicycle, allowing greater freedom and mobility. By the age of 15 or 16 years, the adolescent is able to plan and make the necessary arrangements for a trip outside the city. However, he may need some guidance in securing tickets, making reservations, and attending to small details. The hallmark of independence in travel for many adolescents is learning how to drive a car. A driver's license is a coveted badge of maturity.

During this age period, the adolescent masters the basic skills of communication. By the age of 11 years he is quite capable of using the telephone: excessively in the view of some parents. By 13 years of age he is able to write a decent thank-you letter, maintain an ongoing correspondence with a friend or family member, and cope with the forms and directions of mail order purchasing. The adolescent in our society has also often learned to use a computer as a means of communication.

With the onset of pubescence, the adolescent frequently becomes somewhat preoccupied with personal self-care. Beyond regular bathing, the adolescent gives a great deal of attention to nails, hair, and skin care. The face is regularly checked for blemishes and the changing contours of the body are frequently explored in the bathroom mirror. Girls learn how to shave their legs and axillary hair, to put on make-up, and to use sanitary napkins or tampons properly. Boys must master the art of shaving facial hair. The adolescent also becomes interested in clothes. The unisex uniform of sneakers, jeans, and tee shirt, although not replaced, is augmented with a variety of other clothes and accessories. Clothes take on considerable importance as a means of identification with peers and as a means of role experimentation (271). They are at times treated more like costumes than daily wearing apparel. By the age of 14 years most adolescents are able to select appropriate clothing for themselves with occasional parental guidance. They usually shop for their own clothes by about the age of 16 years, being accompanied by a parent only for the purchase of special or relatively expensive items. The adolescent also gains skill in clothes maintenance. They are able to determine when clothes need to be washed or sent to the cleaners, how to read and follow the directions for the care of various articles of clothing, attend to minor repairs, and polish shoes. The time spent on grooming, clothes, and dressing is considerable. The time spent in the bathroom alone may be a source of amusement or frustration to family members. However, this preoccupation serves a very useful purpose. It allows the adolescent to adjust to and become comfortable with his new body. It also provides an opportunity for the adolescent to try out a variety of self-images: of what he wants to be, of how he wants to look, and what visual messages he wants to give about himself to other people.

By the age of 12 the adolescent is usually given an allowance that is to be used to cover such things as transportation to school, school lunches, contributions to church or temple, and some recreational expenses. The allowance may be supplemented by income derived from other sources, such as babysitting for neighbors and doing special household chores. But regardless of the source or size of income, the adolescent begins to learn how to manage money. By the beginning of this age period he has some sense of the worth of money relative to what it will buy and he is able to make change and determine if the change he has received is correct. Given some income and the responsibility for paying specific expenses out of that income, the adolescent acquires basic skills in setting priorities and budgeting money. With rarely enough money to spend and much to buy, the adolescent begins to search out where a desired item can be purchased at the least cost. After some experience he realizes that the quality of the item must also be taken into consideration. The adolescent has acquired the rudiments of comparison shopping. In addition, by early adolescence many youths have a savings account and have learned the necessary procedures for depositing and withdrawing money; adult assistance, however, may be needed in carrying out the process. By the end of adolescence, most youths have had experience in cashing a check, and some may even have their own checking account. In the course of adolescence, experience in the purpose of and how to use banking facilities is usually acquired.

The adolescent is frequently given increasing responsibility in performing household tasks. The major difference in this age period aside from quantity is that the adolescent is given whole rather than assigned parts of tasks. The adolescent, for example, is not asked to empty the bathroom waste basket and wash out the sink. Rather he is given the responsibility for cleaning the bathroom, of determining what needs to be done and doing it. Specific details do not need to be spelled out. In regard to meal preparation, the adolescent is able to make up a list for grocery shopping and make the necessary purchases. There is an increasing capacity to make dishes that require multiple ingredients, refined preparation of food, and exact timing. The adolescent also acquires the ability to prepare a meal made up of several items and have them all ready at the required time.

Finally, the adolescent is increasingly able to manage his own time. The external clock has been internalized so that less prodding is necessary to ensure his attendance to the constraints of time. Left to his own devices, the adolescent will usually accomplish what needs to be accomplished in a span of time. Admittedly, the adolescent may leave things to be done at the last moment and set time priorities that are disconcerting to parents and teachers. But the external clock has become sufficiently integrated that, in the final hour, all that needs to be done is usually accomplished.

School/Work

At about the beginning of junior high school or seventh grade, the educational system demands the mastery of more complex academic material (587). The adolescent continues to be involved in obtaining a fund of knowledge but there is a new requirement to use knowledge from a variety of sources to arrive at a conclusion. The ability to integrate knowledge in this manner is heavily dependent on the attainment of the last stage of cognitive development. There is also an increased demand for independent study, with only general guidelines from teachers. Considerably more homework is required. The acquisition of knowledge is now almost entirely dependent on reading, except for the laboratory sciences. The capacity to read with a fair amount of speed and good comprehension is imperative. The adolescent is also usually required to do a considerable amount of writing. The ability to select and organize information, to present it in a logical sequence, and to follow the rules of spelling, grammar, and punctuation must be mastered. Tests become a far more serious matter, with the adolescent fairly quickly coming to realize their significance. Some degree of test anxiety is rather common. More pressure frequently is put on the adolescent for excellence in academic performance. This pressure comes from family, school, and peers and is often internalized by the adolescent. There is more emphasis on grades as the measure of one's performance in the academic setting. Classmates often compare grades and evaluate each other to some degree on grades received. In some school settings, there is considerable competition for grades.

The school setting does offer other opportunities for learning and demonstrating competence through a variety of extracurricular activities. However, because these activities are not, strictly speaking, required, they will be discussed in the section on leisure/recreation. Academic achievement remains, for most students and their families, the major task to be accomplished in the school setting.

The situation of the school changes in the adolescent years. No longer organized around a classroom group with a designated single primary teacher, students move from class to class with different classmates in each class. Courses taken may change each semester and there is often a number of electives to be selected. The adolescent must accommodate to a variety of teachers, a larger number of classmates, and a greater degree of impersonality. Many large schools are unable to provide a secure environment for students. In such schools, the adolescent must take responsibility for his own physical safety and the protection of his personal belongings; he must become street wise. Most high schools are essentially bureaucratic in structure, involving many levels of authority, specialized avenues of communication, a large number and variety of regulations, and official forms and documents. The adolescent must gain some skill in negotiating this bureaucratic system in order to manage his life in the school setting adequately.

Adolescence is a time of more active engagement in the world of work (183,345,939). Starting at the beginning of this period the youth may begin to babysit, have a paper route, and do odd jobs for relatives or neighbors. Motivated primarily to earn spending money, the adolescent begins to learn something about the responsibilities of the workplace and relationships with a work supervisor. He also learns something about his skills and interests. By approximately the age of 16 years, the adolescent is likely to have a summer job of one sort or another and perhaps an afterschool job. This, the first "real" job, adds to his knowledge about work and himself as a worker. He also learns about applying and interviewing for a job and relationships with co-workers. Although money is a strong motivational factor, the adolescent often looks for a summer job that will be fun, interesting, or an opportunity to learn something new, or, ideally, all of these. In reality, the adolescent may have to settle for a job that is low paying and less than stimulating.

Through experiences in a variety of jobs with a variety of supervisors, by the age of 18 years the adolescent is able to enter into a "peer authority" relationship. Such a relationship is characterized by a realistic perception of a supervisor's expertise and power relative to oneself. The sense of authority as being omnipotent is gone. The adolescent comes to see his supervisor as similar to himself except for the supervisor's position in a given situation, and usually his greater knowledge and skill. He is comfortable in interacting with supervisors and recognizes the distinction between relating to a supervisor in the context of work and in the context of nonwork activities. The adolescent has the beginning ability to judge the appropriateness of directions given and to act on the basis of that judgment.

In regard to vocational choice, the adolescent enters into the second stage: tentative occupational choices. This stage is divided into four phases: interest, capacity, values, and transition.

In the interest phase (11–12 years), the adolescent begins to realize he will be required to make a decision about a future job. Choices are now based on personal interests: hobbies, new subjects in school, and particular areas of fascination (e.g., astronomy, marine life, cars). The adolescent becomes interested in and wants to know more about his parents' occupations and those of adult relatives. Parents' suggestions about a possible future occupation for the adolescent are elicited.

In the capacity phase (13–15 years), the adolescent begins to realize that interest is not sufficient, that skills are also important. This recognition prompts the youth to investigate the prerequisite skills necessary for particular occupations. At the same time the adolescent directs his attention to looking at his own capacities and seeks feedback from teachers and parents about them. It is around this time that the adolescent begins to make some decisions about whether he will go to college, seek some type of vocational training, or if he is more interested in an occupation where training is essentially on the job. These decisions usually influence the remaining course of study the adolescent will undertake in high school. The adolescent comes to realize education has a role to play in preparation for work and in helping to make future career decisions.

In the value phase (15–16 years), the adolescent, based on his value system, tries to determine which of his various capacities and skills he might want to apply to an occupation. With this in mind, he compares these capacities and skills and his interests to a variety of known occupations. From this process he selects a range of occupations suited to his abilities. He then assesses the kind and degree of satisfaction in very personal terms, such as income, will it satisfy his interest in helping others, will he be able to apply his mathematical skills, and so forth.

In the transition phase (17–18 years), the adolescent is confronted with the realities of impending decisions in regard to work. With this as an impetus he begins to look at the hard facts: opportunities available, status, opportunity for advancement, working conditions, length and nature of preparation, real financial return, and so forth. By this phase, the adolescent may seek summer jobs in an occupation that he might select for a career. This allows him to investigate first hand the occupation and himself in that occupation. If a job is not feasible in a possible desired occupation, the adolescent may participate as a volunteer in the setting where the occupation takes place.

Leisure/Recreation

Peer groups become increasingly important in the adolescent period (113,200,242,332,555,718,758,770). They are often seen by the adolescent as being more significant than any other aspect of his life. Peer groups form the base of support for the process of redefining familial relationships and developing a new sense of autonomy. The conformity apparent in adolescent peer groups serves to bind the group together, thus enhancing its function as a base of support. Conformity and its correlate, peer pressure, are sometimes viewed as a negative factor in the adolescent's development. However, this is probably only the case when the values and activities of the peer group are markedly deviant from those of the society in which it exists. The majority of peer groups serve as a positive force in the developmental process. Initially made up of one gender, as in the discussion of cooperative groups, adolescent peer groups become heterosexual by about 14 years of age if not sooner. These groups will be described further in the last part of this section.

In regard to group interaction skill, the final stage of development occurs between 14 and 17 years of age. This stage is characterized by the ability to interact in a mature group: a group where there is a balance between task accomplishment and the satisfaction of group members' needs. Mature groups typically have a heterogeneous membership and no sharp distinction between leader and follower roles. Although there may be a designated leader, in a mature group, leadership-follower functions are shared by all group members. This type of group was discussed in Chapter 3 in the section on social interactions. Mature group interaction skill is essentially the coming together of the skills acquired in egocentric cooperative groups and cooperative groups. In mastering this stage of group interaction skill, the adolescent is able to be comfortable in heterogeneous groups and take those instrumental and expressive roles that are required for adequate group function at any particular time. Interaction in mature groups is most evident in the adolescent's participation in extracurricular activities. Adolescent social peer groups are usually not mature groups. They are sexually heterogeneous but they tend not to be task oriented. A task or activity may serve as a nucleus for group interaction but the activity per se is not particularly important. Any number of activities would do. The purpose of the adolescent peer group is to give its members an opportunity to be together and to provide emotional support.

By the age of 12 years, the majority of adult leisure and recreational activities have been learned. As mentioned, the adolescent continues to enjoy solitary activities (e.g., reading, listening to music), using them both as a means of relaxation and of gaining control over emotions that temporarily seem out of hand. From previous exploration of arts and crafts, the adolescent often develops a serious interest in a particular hobby, such as sewing, painting, or stamp collecting. These may be solitary pursuits, or in part shared with others. Most adolescents enjoy physically demanding activities. These provide an opportunity for release of pent-up energy and relief from feelings of restlessness. They also give adolescents an opportunity to become accustomed to their new bodies and regain lost gross motor coordination. The new sense of social awareness frequently leads the adolescent into community activities. This interest may take the form of service, such as volunteer work in a psychiatric hospital or helping to raise money for the renovation of a local historical landmark. The interest, on the other hand, may take a more political form, such as collecting petitions for state gun control or protest demonstrations against the threatened closing of a child daycare center. Concern about religion may prompt the adolescent to become involved in groups associated with a church or temple. These groups, in addition to providing spiritual guidance, often serve as a place for meeting peers with similar interests and as a base for community service.

Extracurricular activities take up a good deal of leisure time for many adolescents. Large junior and senior high schools sponsor any number of activities both to develop nonacademic skills and to promote the appropriate use of leisure time. Some common activities include student government, school newspapers, drama groups, music groups of various sorts, debate, photography club, and competitive sports.

Friend relationships during the initial part of adolescence remain on the whole casual. This is true except for a particular relationship with one or two other peers. Known as a chum relationship, it is characterized by mutual trust, sharing of confidences, and minimal competitive interaction. This is an emotionally charged relationship in which the other person is experienced as being extremely important to the self and the needs of the other person are felt as being equal to the needs of oneself. A chum relationship is usually shared with one or two members of the same sex. It may occur with a member of the opposite sex but this is unusual and complicates the relationship with sexual issues. An example of a chum relationship is the adolescent who has spent the entire school day and after school hours with his friend and then needs to be on the phone with him for two hours in the evening. There seem to be endless things to discuss and ideas to be shared. Parents and other casual friends are excluded from these relationships and their approval is neither actively sought nor desired. Chum relationships provide a sympathetic source of comfort when the adolescent is experiencing difficulty with parents or with the larger peer group. It is a relationship in which the adolescent learns to perceive and meet the needs of another person on a one-to-one basis, to experience his own humanness, and to feel compassion for and empathy with another person. Chum relationships are not mature friendships. They have an intensity, preoccupation, and jealous possessiveness not found in mature friendships. Chum relationships usually only occur in this phase of the life cycle. They provide the formation for future love and friendship relationships. Chum relationships usually draw to a close about the age of 14 or 15 years, when heterosexual relationships become increasingly important.

The second stage of sexual identity, the ability to accept sexual maturation as a positive growth experience, is acquired primarily through leisure activities with peers. Beginning about 14 years of age, the adolescent starts to enjoy, in fact is eager to participate in, heterosexual activities. These activities, in addition to several of the ones previously mentioned, often include concerts, parties, dances, and simply hanging out at local gathering places. Initially there is a good deal of teasing, fooling around, and some rough and tumble play as the adolescents become accustomed to interacting in nonsupervised heterosexual groups. Dating usually begins around this time although there is considerable variation in the time of dating and patterns of dating from community to community and between adolescents within a given community. Typically, dating activities begin with casual pairing at a group activity. A sort of "when Mary and John are at the same activity they are together a lot." Contact outside the context of a group activity is minimal. This advances to asking or being asked to accompany someone to a previously scheduled formal or informal group activity. At about 16 years of age, identifiable couples emerge from the group. This often marks the first experience of falling in love. The couple spend considerable leisure time together and often are invited to the outings or celebrations of each other's families. Interaction between the couple continues, however, to take place mainly within the context of group activities or activities with another couple. There seems to be safety in numbers and comfort in not having to spend too much time alone together. Group dating also provides an opportunity to learn appropriate couple interaction from peers. This is an important part of the socialization process that will eventually culminate in the formation of partner relationships. Couple relationships tend to be temporary, with occasional rather intense relationships being interspersed with more casual ones. This gives adolescents an opportunity to know a number of individuals of the opposite sex, to begin to define the kind of individual they might want as a partner, and to learn more about themselves. Through the formation of a number of couple relationships and group dating, the adolescent discovers something about the differences between the sexes, the chemistry of attraction—mysteries that will continue to be studied through the life cycle, and never solved.

Sexual experimentation is typically a part of adolescent peer interaction. Partially in fantasy, partially in reality, from holding hands to intercourse, the adolescent attempts to come to terms with genital sexuality. Initially, sexual fantasies tend to be fairly romantic and nonspecific; as the adolescent matures, they become more genitally oriented. Fantasies are likely to focus at first on the unattainable, e.g., television idols, rock stars, parents of friends, and teachers. Later, fantasy is focused on particular individuals in one's peer group. The sex play of adolescence, kissing, petting, necking, gives the youth an opportunity to explore his own sexual feelings, to learn something about control of sexual impulses, and to experiment with his capacity to arouse. It also helps the adolescent to understand the sexual feelings and responses of the opposite sex. The sex play of adolescents usually does not provide for the release of sexual tensions nor is it necessarily a part of sharing an intimate relationship. Intercourse between adolescents may or may not serve the same function as sex play; it may or may not provide for the release of sexual tension. The social pressures, both condemning and condoning sex play and intercourse, often put the adolescent under a great deal of stress, with accompanying feelings of guilt and inadequacy—certainly not the best circumstances to explore newfound sexual urgency and to establish one's sense of genital identity. Nevertheless, by the end of this phase of the life cycle, most adolescents have acquired the ability to accept sexual maturation as a positive growth experience. The adolescent sees himself as a genitally mature individual, able to control sexual impulses, and experiences himself as being sexually attractive and desirable.

EIGHTEEN TO TWENTY-FIVE YEARS OF AGE

The major question of this period of the life cycle is, "What am I going to do with my life?" In answering that question, the individual is making the first major life decisions about the future. The decisions focus around the issues of career choice and marriage: what kind of occupation to pursue, whether to get married and to whom. These decisions seem particularly large because the individual often sees them as the making of definitive plans for the rest of her life. Although these decisions are important and will be influential relative to the distant future, they are not as totally deterministic as the individual perceives them to be at this time.

The corrollary to "What am I going to do with my life?" is, "Who am I?" In answering this question, the individual establishes her initial or first identity (271). As previously defined, identity is a sense of self, of who one is and where one fits into a scheme of significant others. It is made up of one's constitutional givens, idiosyncratic needs, favored capacities, significant identification with and attachment to others, effective and successful defenses, and consistent and important social roles. In the attempt to establish identity, the individual may take a moratorium from the usual responsibilities of life. Some individuals, for example, take a year or so off before getting their first "real" job, or between college and graduate school, or they may drop out of school for a few years.

Family Interaction

This and subsequent sections in regard to family interaction will be subdivided into discussion of various familial roles (171,319,593,888). Up to this point in the life cycle the individual may have had several familial roles, e.g., sibling, grandchild, nephew, but the most important role has been that of child relative to parents. During this age period, the individual frequently takes on an additional role, the partner role.

In relationship to parents, this is a time of separation: physical and psychological. Physical separation may take place through various periods of transition. The individual may travel, go away to college, take a temporary job outside the city, and so on. However, the individual returns home for fairly extended periods: one still has a bedroom. Although transitory, these physical moves away from home give the individual some idea of what it is like to be on one's own without daily parental contact.

The major step in physical separation is moving into one's own home, making a home for oneself. Typically this involves moving into an apartment—alone, with a friend, or with a partner, to which one may or may not be married. Although one has one's own home, the move from the parental home is not necessarily complete. Many of the individual's personal belongings may remain in the parental home. There tends to be considerable contact with parents, e.g., regular telephone calls, stopping over for dinner, spending Sunday together. There may also be periodic returns to the parental home: between moves from one apartment to another, vacations, when the individual gets sick, and so forth.

Physical separation from parents may be delayed because of health or financial reasons or because it is customary in one's culture to remain with parents until marriage. This makes establishing an independent life more difficult. The individual needs to find her own space and time removed from daily family activities. This is often accomplished through agreement with parents that the individual is not expected to be with the family regularly for meals, can determine her own time for returning home in the evening, is not required to engage in as many household tasks, and the like. These types of agreements allow for the distancing necessary at this point in the life cycle.

Psychological separation from parents begins during this period. It is, however, by no means completed at this time. With the struggle for autonomy over, the individual begins to de-idealize her parents. Parents come to be perceived more realistically as being neither all right nor all wrong. This change in perception leads to the individual's having a great deal more confidence in her own judgment. The individual begins to be more comfortable in making personal decisions about future plans and life style. The individual comes to realize that her values and ideology or world view do not have to be congruent with those of her parents. Although not necessarily agreeing with parental values and life styles, the individual comes to have respect for them.

In relation to partners, there are two issues of concern: sexual identity and the formation of partner relationships. These two issues, although closely related, will be separated here simply for ease of discussion.

The stage of sexual identity usually attained in this period of the life cycle is the ability to give and receive sexual gratification. This aspect of sexual development is acquired through both autoerotic and shared sexual experiences. It involves a time of exploration, now definitely genital, in which the individual becomes aware of her own response pattern: what is arousing, what leads to pleasure and satisfaction. At the same time, the individual becomes aware of the response patterns of others: how they differ from and are similar to one's own. In attaining this stage of development, the individual is cognizant of her sexual needs, the quality and quantity of her sexual responses, and the stimuli that maximize her ability to respond and be satisfied. The sexual needs of others are recognized and there is appreciation of the varieties in sexual responses. The individual is able to use various techniques for satisfying herself and others and is able to vary techniques according to the needs and desires of the sexual partner. Intercourse comes to be seen as a way of expressing affection and love and as a means of satisfying physiological needs. The development of this aspect of sexual identity may occur in the context of a partner relationship or in the context of various couple relationships. It can usually only be learned, however, with sexual partners between which there is mutual respect and affection.

A partner relationship, as used in this text, refers to a sustained relationship characterized by love and respect. It may or may not be an intimate relationship; it may or may not exist in the context of marriage. To clarify, some partners have a satisfying relationship with each other but it is not intimate in nature; partner relationships may exist outside marriage and/or cohabitation.

In this phase of the life cycle, the individual usually continues to be involved in a variety of couple relationships while in the process of seeking a partner. Typically one or more partner relationships have been established by the end of this period. If more than one, they are usually serial in nature, monogamy remaining a relatively strong societal norm.

The formation of a partnership is typically preceded by courtship. In the process of courtship, individuals become increasingly knowledgeable of each other, explore their capacity for love and their love for each other. Courtship is also usually the time of getting to know each other's family. Family response to an intended partner varies. Even if the response is highly positive, a period of becoming acquainted and accommodation is necessary. The same, of course, is true for the intended partner. The family constellation must be expanded and altered to allow for the entry of a new member.

In the formation of a partnership, the individual must learn to engage in the give and take necessary for the maintenance of the relationship. Adaptations and adjustments must be made to the other person's use of time, leisure interests, friends, value system, current priorities, and moods. Partners must learn to deal with their conflicts: engaging, disengaging, negotiating, resolving, and continuing the relationship. They must also learn how to tolerate essential differences in opinion. Additional adjustments are necessary in learning how to live with another person. The close proximity of cohabitation brings up the issue of privacy, needing to be alone, and the time that will be shared together. The idiosyncratic habits, likes, and dislikes of each partner bring up the issue of what behavior can and cannot be tolerated. Other issues that need to be dealt with are the division of household tasks, how money will be spent, time for family and in-laws, and so forth.

At this time in the life cycle, entering into a marriage is expected social behavior in most cultures. It is during this period that most people marry for the first time. Aside from general social expectation, there may be an internal urge to get married and considerable pressure from family and friends. The individual then is confronted with the decision of whether to marry. Marriage may be seen as an impediment to preparation for or pursuing a career. The individual may wish to marry but not be able to find a suitable mate. The question then is whether to enter into a convenient marriage with an unsuitable mate or to wait. For women there is the issue of marriage and family versus career. As this brief outline suggests, there are often many conflicts around decisions regarding marriage.

Activities of Daily Living

Learning to take care of oneself, independent from parents, is one of the major developmental tasks of this age period. There is much that the individual must now do on her own. Financially, the person may still be dependent on parents or earning a salary or some combination of these. If still dependent in whole or part on the family, the individual must make arrangements with the family in regard to the amount of money, what it will be used for, and when and how the individual will receive the money. Regardless of the source of income, the individual must learn to budget money and stay within that budget.

Health care is another area of concern. One must purchase health insurance, find a physician, make regular visits to the dentist, ophthalmologist, and so forth. The individual needs to learn how to care for herself when she is ill and decide if medical attention is necessary.

The individual must take care of her own clothes: buying, cleaning, and keeping them in repair on a regular basis. An apartment must be found, sometimes several times during this period. It must be furnished, decorated, and cleaned regularly. Home repair must be done or the individual must find someone to take care of it. One must shop for and prepare food with some attention to a nutritious diet. Finally, in regard to transportation, the individual for the first time may buy a car and learn to take responsibility for its maintenance.

School/Work

In regard to vocational development, this is the stage of realistic choices (183,345,939). It has three phases:

exploration, crystallization, and specification. Having already chosen a narrow band of jobs or fields, in the exploration phase the individual looks more closely at the intellectual and/or physical requirement within the band. Crystallization occurs when the individual feels she is in possession of a sufficient amount of information about herself and her potentials to make a firm decision about a particular career. Specification is the process of actually selecting a specific occupation. A particular specialty within the occupation may, however, not yet be determined. This stage of vocational development may occur while the individual is in school or while she is working. The first job that one takes is often not what will eventually be the individual's final choice of vocation. This is true for most people, the exception being individuals who have engaged in baccalaureate or graduate study to prepare for entry into a particular occupation.

For many people, college is seen as a situation that will prepare them for a broad spectrum of vocations. While in college, the individual may consider the possibility of graduate school. The questions that individuals often ask are whether they have the intellectual capacity, are able to tolerate the delay, and whether they can afford it. School tends to be taken more seriously as the individual enters professional studies. This is true regardless of whether professional studies are at the undergraduate or graduate level. The individual gives priority to professional studies, seeing liberal arts as irrelevant and a waste of precious time. Within professional studies, students tend to give lip service to the importance of theoretical knowledge but are primarily concerned about practical application. The individual usually studies diligently but is also impatient to get out into the real world.

Individuals who do not enter a four-year college program may go to a junior college for the purpose of vocational preparation, attend a free-standing vocational school or program, or they may immediately enter the job market. In the latter case the individual may serve a formal apprenticeship, participate in a structured on-the-job training program, or simply pick up the necessary skill on the job from more experienced workers.

Regardless of the length or type of preparation or previous work experience, an adjustment period to one's first fulltime job is often necessary. There are expected codes of behavior to learn, many more specific task skills to acquire, and interpersonal relationships to understand and establish. The individual is now, regardless of her own inclinations, a worker. There may be feelings of great excitement or a sense of being trapped in a nine-to-five routine, seemingly for the rest of one's days. An individual may be any place on this continuum. There may be considerable commitment to one's first fulltime job or it may be seen as temporary, a time to gain a clearer idea of what one wants to do, or to gain experience for future vocational pursuits. By the end of this phase of the life cycle, however, most men have accepted the worker role and made it a part of their identity. This is not necessarily true for many women.

Leisure/Recreation

Many of the activities enjoyed in the adolescent period continue to be enjoyed in this phase of the life cycle. Active and spectator sports, dancing, music, and "hanging out" are common leisure time activities (181,811). There is often a seeking out of the unusual or the exciting. Activities such as television, hobbies, and reading tend to be of less interest at this time. Most leisure time is spent out of the home: one's own or that of one's parents. Activities with one's family of origin are curtailed except for special family occasions such as birthdays and anniversaries, religious holidays, and national holidays.

A good deal of time is devoted to conversation: a continuing process of sorting out values, defining life goals, and sharing experiences. Individuals in this age group tend to be, in part, quite serious about life. They feel that the decisions they make now are irreversible and therefore require a good deal of serious consideration. Their solemnness and sense of dealing with weighty matters also come from their lack of life experience. They have yet to experience and come to understand much of the comedy and tragedy of human life. One sometimes gets the feeling that they are playing at being adults and have not quite learned the role.

One of the leisure/recreational tasks of this age group is to find a compatible group of friends (593,888). High school friends tend to be left behind as the individual prepares for a job or begins to work. New friends may be made in college, but these too are left behind on graduation. Individuals who move out of town to begin a new job have particular difficulty in becoming a part of a circle of friends. The continued popularity of single bars attests to this difficulty.

Nevertheless, most leisure activities in this age group take place with friends. The groups formed tend to be heterosexual—concerned with finding partners and courtship interactions. Although partners may spend some leisure time alone, initially they may continue to be involved in group activities. Interaction with a group tends to delay intimacy, a developmental task of the next phase of the life cycle, and interaction with other partners provides role models that can facilitate the consolidation of partner relationships. It is also comforting to know that difficulties in one's own partnership are very similar to the difficulties experienced by other partners.

TWENTY-FIVE TO THIRTY-FIVE YEARS OF AGE

In this period of the life cycle, there are two counterpoised issues: the urge to build a firm structure versus the urge to explore and experiment; and intimacy versus isolation. These are related issues but sufficiently different to discuss separately (271,272,593,888).

The urge to build a firm foundation is the desire to put down roots, to create a stable life for oneself, to settle into the business of being adult. The converse, the urge to explore and experiment, is the desire to remain free from many adult responsibilities, to finish the business of growing up, to be sure that all possibilities have been glimpsed or experienced and weighed. These two positions are reflected in family interaction and work. The individual may decide to get married, start to raise a family, buy a home; or the individual may decide not to marry, if married, to get a divorce, or postpone having children. In the area of work, the individual may settle into one occupation and set career goals; or the individual may repeatedly change jobs from one occupation to another, or continue to stay in graduate school.

Intimacy refers to a deep emotional commitment in interpersonal relationships. Intimacy is founded on and emerges out of a clear and secure sense of identity. The individual now has the capacity to commit herself to concrete affiliations with others and the strength to abide by such commitments. There is a willingness to fuse aspects of one's identity with that of others without fear of loss of selfness. The capacity for intimacy is reflected in partner and friend relationships, and in the nurturing of children. Isolation is the avoidance of intimate experiences, often out of fear one may loose a tenuous sense of personal identity. People are seen as somewhat dangerous, with the possibility that they may encroach on one's "territory." There is a sense of not wanting to be involved, a fear of closeness. The inability to establish intimacy and fear of isolation may lead the individual to submerge or lose oneself in another person. Whatever sense of identity one may have had is encapsulated and set aside. This phenomenon may also occur because of cultural values and social pressures. Submerging oneself in another may make one feel comfortable in some ways, but the price is high, and one's situation basically insecure. This is a situation that has been somewhat typical for women in our society.

Family Interaction

Financial independence from parents is usually gained in this phase of the life cycle (96,171,234,319,593,888). The individual becomes self-supporting or relies on a partner for financial support. Financial assistance may, however, be sought in emergency situations or extraordinary events, such as buying a house. Emotional independence increases, resulting in less frequent contact with parents. The individual may continue to seek advice from parents but does not see their advice as a direct expectation. Firm relationships with in-laws are established, with the individual being accepted by and feeling a part of her partner's family of origin.

During this phase of the life cycle, some individuals make a decision not to enter into marriage or to live with a partner, at least for the foreseeable future. Such an individual makes life plans for herself independent from partner relationships. Similar to her counterparts with partners, the individual often buys a house or condominium with the intention of establishing a permanent home. There is a sense of settling into a preferred life style. Such an individual may or may not have sexual partners or children. The individual is likely to have mature intimate friend relationships.

Partner relationships now tend to move to an intimate level. Such a relationship is characterized by deep trust, open communication, and a commitment to a long-term relationship. Love matures into an enduring emotion, rather than the excited state of "being in love." It becomes the foundation that allows the partnership to endure internal and externally imposed conflict and stress. At this point, there are few illusions about one's partner. The other's assets and limitations are well known and, if not appreciated, at least accepted. The idea that partnerships are not maintained by the excitement of love is fully recognized. The partners realize they must work and strive on a regular basis to ensure the continuation of their relationships. Compromise becomes an accepted part of daily interaction. Intimacy by no means, however, results in a conflict-free relationship. The most common major issues at this time are whether to have children, the sharing of child rearing and household tasks, and child discipline.

Some of the conflicts faced primarily by women relative to having children and work have been outlined in Chapter 4. There are, however, many concerns regarding child rearing, shared by both men and women. Some of these concerns are (96,171,947): (a) Can I really perceive myself as being a parent; can I incorporate that role into my sense of who I am?; (b) Do I know how to be a parent?; (c) I do not like the thought of the grubby parts of the job (e.g., getting up in the middle of the night, changing diapers); (d) The fun stops; what will I be missing?; (e) I will really have to become an adult; (f) It is an awesome responsibility; a parent is something you can never stop being, the one choice and commitment where there is no backing out.

Although these concerns are paramount in the decision to have a child, they continue during the period of pregnancy and postpartum adjustment. The whole idea of being a parent does not really strike one until the individual is in the role of parent.

Pregnancy is a time of wonder, physical change, and some degree of anxiety (171,378,504,912). For a planned child, the discovery of pregnancy is a joyous event for the women, partners, and extended family—a time for celebration of the renewal of the life cycle. The physical changes of pregnancy are multiple and include absence of menstruation, morning sickness, abberations of appetite, tiredness, increased frequency of urination, breast changes, and abdominal enlargement. Perhaps the most exciting physical event is quickening, the first movements of the fetus. Slight at first, they become stronger as pregnancy advances. The feeling of life gives reality to the pregnancy and the impending birth of a child.

The psychological adjustment to pregnancy is not always comfortable. There may be emotional liability marked by periods of irritability, moodiness, and attacks of weeping. These emotional anomalies are probably due to hormonal changes, and, like morning sickness, usually disappear after the first trimester. There are, however, many fears that may continue throughout pregnancy. There are fears about the self. Physical changes may cause the women to feel unattractive and raise concerns about whether her body will ever return to its former shape. Pregnancy sometimes brings about a decrease in sexual interests, which may give rise to questions about current and future relationships with one's partner. There may be fear of the pain of labor and delivery and concern about being competent in this process. There may be fear of death in childbirth. The woman may have fears about the child: will she miscarry; will the child be stillborn; will the child be normal. These fears and concerns are seemingly quite common and not evidence of an unusual state of affairs.

During the period of pregnancy, fathers often share the same fears as those outlined above. Some men may experience a decrease in sexual interest in their pregnant partners, but this is fairly rare in a good partner relationship. Some men, in their anxiety, tend to be oversolicitous or seemingly insensitive and unsympathetic. Many men feel they are somehow being left out of this event—to the relief of some and the consternation of others.

Parents of the partners are usually overjoyed with the fact of pregnancy. At this time, a woman often feels a closer bond with her mother and mother-in-law, seeking advice and support from them. Pregnancy and childbirth, to some extent, alter parent-child relationships. Through procreation young adults often feel they are confirming their masculinity or femininity; that they are able to do what their parents have done; that they have fulfilled a responsibility to parents. Parents tend to see their children in a new light; they have proved they are responsible adults. These perceptions often lead to a new feeling of mutual respect and a feeling of being more coequals.

The postpartum period is usually one of considerable joy: the child is safely delivered; the anxieties of pregnancy are over; there is a sense of personal accomplishment (378,912). However, this is also a period of considerable adjustment. Physically, there is an initial tiredness. A vaginal discharge lasts for three or four weeks. Initially, there is some vaginal discomfort. For women who plan to nurse their babies, milk appears 60 to 72 hours after delivery. Regardless of whether a woman is nursing, there tends to be some breast soreness for a few days. Menstruation begins four to eight weeks after delivery, but there is considerable variation, especially for women who are nursing. The uterus returns to its usual shape and size in about six weeks. Intercourse may be resumed after six weeks.

Physical adjustments are in a sense minor in comparison to some of the other adjustments that need to be made (171,761,947). Newborn infants are demanding of time and energy, and their demands must be met regardless of the hour and circumstances. This requires a new life style that may be difficult for parents to accept. For parents with their first child, the tasks of infant care must be learned and mastered. Change in life style and the tasks of infant care often require a marked change in routines and usual daily events. Temporal adaptation is often severely strained.

The demands of the infant often place a strain on the relationship between partners. Either may feel he is being pushed aside by the other partner and the infant. There may be feelings of jealousy and rejection. These feelings can be exacerbated if, indeed, one parent attempts to form an exclusive relationship with the infant and precludes the other partner from the relationship. The needs of each parent in the postpartum period must be given considerable attention if the adjustments, so necessary in this period, are to be made successfully.

Establishing a love relationship with an infant is not an automatic process. Parental love is not an inherent response; it is learned and grows over time. The initial emotional response to an infant is basically concern for survival of this helpless being. Love comes later as the child begins to respond. Because of the myth of inherent mother love, women who are aware that initially they do not experience love may feel considerable guilt. It is through this process of learning to love that parents begin to acquire the ability to nurture. A nurturing relationship, as previously described, is directed toward assisting another individual to grow and mature. Learning to give nurture continues for parents essentially through the adolescent period, if not beyond.

Postpartum adjustment is often particularly difficult for fathers. A man has few but traditional role models for being the father of an infant. The father role in our society has been seen as providing support for the mother. He is supposed to relieve the mother occasionally from some chores, serve as her contact with the outside world, and reinforce the fact that she is a good mother. This role is no longer considered acceptable in many parts of society, and in many families. Without proper role models, however, the father is often very uncertain as to what to do with this tiny being who he suspects might break. Learning to be an active participant in the parenting process from the beginning is a frightening experience for many men. For fathers who have taken on the challenge of learning, however, the rewards have been great.

Postpartum depression for a woman is not an unusual occurrence. It is characterized by feelings of being overwhelmed, not being able to cope, with sadness, lethargy, and periodic crying for no apparent reason. It is probably more common than realized, and is often hidden by playing the socially accepted role of the joyful new mother, or ascribing the feelings to the usual postpartum tiredness, physical discomfort, and preoccupation with the infant. There is no agreed on cause of postpartum depression. Some of the contributing factors seem to be hormonal change, conflict about being a parent and becoming an adult, and the often considerable alteration in life style and temporal adaptation. The ways in which a woman has reacted to and coped with stress in the past also are influential in her response to the postpartum period. Postpartum depression usually lifts after about three months. It is only occasionally that the depression is sufficiently severe, that medical or some other nonfamilial assistance is sought. Familial assistance usually includes support, help with infant care, some assistance in time management, and arranging regular periods of time for the woman to be free from responsibilities and able to pursue her own interests.

Child rearing is one of the major familial tasks in this phase of the life cycle. Previously, this process was explored primarily from the child's point of view. The shift now is to the perspective of the parent. Within a nuclear family, the issues of child rearing must be worked out between the parents and with the child. In a single-parent family, many of the decisions regarding child rearing must be made and implemented by the individual alone or in conjunction with the nonresident parent (545,863). The extended or expanded family may serve as a resource for information, guidance, and a source of support. On the other hand, they may be an interfering, nonsupportive element that can cause considerable difficulty for everyone involved. The need for support in child rearing is a very important factor. Whether it be from the partner, family, or friends, adequate support allows the individual to make decisions with some degree of confidence and reinforces the implementation of those decisions. Adequate support also provides the individual with a reasonable perspective: the universality of the struggles, the recognition that in the course of events each phase will pass, and the sense that the process is best undertaken with a degree of playful humor.

The cornerstone of child rearing is the provision of an environment that is characterized by love, acceptance, security, consistency, and enjoyment. Such environments do not come into existence out of good intentions, but rather are an ongoing effort on the part of parents. It is within the context of the pervading tone of the familial environment, as just described or one of lesser quality, that the issues of child rearing are addressed (171,947). Some of the major issues are: (a) the behavioral expectations for the child in the home, neighborhood, and school, and the timetable for changes in expectations; (b) how discipline is to be handled and who is responsible for that discipline; (c) the academic, religious, moral, and sex education of the child; (d) setting aside sufficient time to be with the child for play, recreation, and quiet times for talking; (e) dealing with sibling rivalry; (f) how to raise a child in a pluralistic society that is characterized by gender stereotypes, prejudice, and violence; (g) guiding the child's selection of friends. For working parents, finding, coordinating, and supervising child care on a daily basis, and in the event of child illness, school holidays, and the like; (h) the degree to which the child should be consulted in decisions regarding family matters and the child's participation in decision making; (i) negotiating and resolving conflicts of all kinds, including those that lead to the alignment of one faction of the family against another; (j) parental privacy and time to be alone with one's partner and to engage in personal interests and pursuits.

These issues are not resolved once, but continue to be reconciled repeatedly, as the child progresses through the phases of the life cycle.

The issues outlined above may make child rearing seem a great and formidable task. Indeed it is. But the rewards are beyond measure: the joy in watching a child grow, the fun, companionship, sharing, being a part of another life as it unfolds, being a guide. All of this and more is worth the hard parts. It is an experience that cannot be recounted in word.

Activities of Daily Living

In the process of establishing a firm foundation for the future, the individual is often required to give considerable attention to financial matters. Budgeting now often includes a partner and a child or children. Typically, this is the time when people buy their first homes and become seriously involved in dealing with financial institutions. There is often a concern for and an attempt to save money for the future education of children. Home, life, and additional health insurance may be obtained.

Household tasks often now become more of a chore. There is a sense of not playing house anymore. Many previous tasks, enjoyed in leisure, now simply must be done. With the birth of a child or children, the quantity and quality of household tasks change. Responsibility for these additional and new tasks needs to be assigned or reassigned between partners.

Whether children are involved or whether the individual is focusing on the development of a career, this is the most stressful time in the life cycle relative to temporal adaptation (103,108,491,593,879,888). Time becomes a more valued commodity, of which there never seems to be a sufficient amount. There is often a nagging sense of "how is it all going to get done." Skill in elegant time management, if it is ever to be acquired, is usually attained in this phase of the life cycle.

Work

At this point, the individual has, usually, completed her preparation for an occupation and begun what is seen by her as her life's work (183,272,872,939). Trial periods of various sorts are over. The role of a worker has taken a firm place in the individual's identity. The individual wishes to see herself and be seen as successful in this facet of life. From a more general approach to one's chosen occupation, the individual has often selected a particular area of specialization. For many individuals there is an attempt to find and establish a relationship with a mentor (593,888). A mentor is able to enhance one's knowledge and skills, give guidance, provide support, and in general smooth the way for promotion and career advancement.

It is during this period that the individual sets career goals. These may be long-term goals, with the idea that this is what one wants to accomplish before one has completed the work cycle. Or more limited goals may be set, with a comprehensive statement of this is what I want to accomplish or be by a given age. For individuals who perceive themselves as seriously involved in a career, this is a period of establishing oneself. Work becomes a paramount concern. One is willing to work exceptionally hard for long hours. There is a willingness to put aside temporarily recreational activities, the cultivation of friendships, and even family matters. In striving for a particular goal, the individual maintains a singular focus. Individuals less seriously involved in a career may also work long hours at this time. Concerned primarily about money and the expense of raising a family, they often work overtime or have a second job.

Work now provides a structure: for daily life and for future plans. The individual also develops a perspective of work somewhere on the continuum of being a major preoccupation to "it's a living." Work is given a place in the context of daily life and in the scheme of one's life plan. A balance of some sort is struck between work and the individual's other goals and responsibilities.

Leisure/Recreation

The leisure/recreational activities of this age group are as was described in Chapter 4 (171,181,811). For married couples, there is a marked reduction in social life outside the home or neighborhood. More time is spent with one's partner, alone, or with one or two other couples. Recreation is family centered with one's own children, other neighborhood families, and, if close by, members of one's extended family. Leisure activities tend to be more sedentary and passive, with less involvement in active sports.

This is the time in the life cycle when the individual is likely to have the least amount of leisure time. Work, child rearing, and household tasks take up a considerable amount of time. This leaves neither time nor energy for relaxation or pursuing special interests.

Mature friendships begin to develop at this time. As previously defined, these are relationships characterized by a strong feeling of liking that at times may be described as love, and by frequent and extended periods of engagement. Although shared activities may be part of the relationship, they are secondary to just being together. Mature friendships can also tolerate some distance in time and space. However, there tends to be fairly regular and frequent contact by letter or telephone. The individual now has the capacity to respond on an emotional level without jealousy or loss of sense of self. The relationship is considered important, and time and effort are expended on its maintenance. It is not, however, dealt with as a major preoccupation. In this phase of the life cycle, in our society, mature friendships are usually formed with persons of the same gender. They are thus insulated from sexuality and the process of forming partnerships. Later in the life cycle, with greater sophistication in sorting out sexuality from the other aspects of interpersonal relationships, individuals are more capable of forming mature friendships with persons of the opposite sex. Mature friendships provide an opportunity to give to others, and to receive love and support. They give a dimension to life that is not found in other relationships.

THIRTY-FIVE TO FIFTY YEARS OF AGE

This period in the life cycle is marked by a time of reassessment (155,171,493,593,888). This is a time of reevaluating one's marriage, career, values, goals, choices already made, and what is often seen as stereotyped social roles. This is sometimes referred to as midlife crisis: a turning point that will affect the course of one's future life. It is a time to make decisions about the future; to continue with the status quo or make a change in direction; to maintain one's identity or to seek a new identity.

The exact reason for reassessment during this period is unknown, but one factor appears to be the confrontation of aging and death. The physical changes of aging become evident in oneself and in one's peers (155,504,912). Some of the changes include graying; loss of hair; decreased skin elasticity, leading to wrinkles; decreased muscle tone, stamina, and strength; the effects of gravity on the body over time, resulting in changes in the contours of the body; decrease in visual and auditory acuity; and menopause. These changes bring about a sense of loss of youth—a sense that one cannot escape the aging process; that one will not always be youthful; that one is not immortal.

Death becomes a reality at this time in the life cycle. It becomes a factual entity that must be dealt with, and no longer denied. The physical changes of aging contribute to this realization. Other factors are the awareness that in all likelihood one has lived more than half of one's allotted years, the aging of one's parents, and sufficient life experience to recognize the fragility of life and the true meaning of the life cycle.

Resolution of the midlife crisis takes many forms. Initially and understandably, there is a sense of panic. Usually only temporary, such panic motivates the individual to engage in the reassessment process. There is sometimes an attempt to recapture lost youth, a flight into the myth of happy and carefree adolescence. One may decide to get divorced, change jobs, or treat one's self to a long-deserved indulgence. Many individuals become extraordinarily self-centered, concerned about their health, and preoccupied with making decisions for the future. A moritorium during this period is somewhat common. It may involve a leave of absence from work, or moving out of the family home for a period of time, or it may involve a more mild suspension of usual activities.

This period in the life cycle has been likened to adolescence, both in the turmoil involved and in the search for identity. Like adolescence, the conflicts and concerns do get resolved, although admittedly sometimes with considerable pain and discomfort. But it is a time when one has the opportunity to reassess, to rework identity, to make changes, and to set new goals.

Erikson has referred to this time as the period of establishing generativity (271,272). By generativity he means the mature desire to generate and regenerate objects, products, ideas, and the like. It is the desire to take care of the young and planet earth, so as to assure the next generation life and strength. It is a sense of wanting in some way to leave this world a better place than at the time of one's own birth. This is an expression of altruism, not self-exaltation. Generativity is manifested through being creative or productive, nurturing, teaching, being a mentor, concern for the environment, serving others, and the like. According to Erikson, lack of generativity leads to stagnation, the latter being characterized by self-absorption and a state of personal impoverishment.

Family Interaction

In this period of the life cycle, the individual's perception of his parents changes (151,171,319,593,888). Emotional separation finally occurs, and the individual attains "filial maturity." With this maturity, the individual gives up the view of his parents as the ultimate providers of safety. He is now ready to assume full authority and responsibility for himself. The individual also discovers that he is alone. This is aloneness in the existential sense that, regardless of family and friends, we are ultimately alone. No one can fully understand, share our experience, or protect us from being hurt. No one can shield us from death. Filial maturity is most likely attained through the recognition of parental aging and their impending death.

Through emotional separation, parent and child establish a new relationship based on mutual respect and love, rather than on generational position and dependency. It is at this time that parents and children are able to establish a mature friend relationship, a relationship based on equal positions. This by no means implies that the special bond between parents and child is broken. The bond with its collection of positive and negative shared experiences and feelings is broken only after the death of parents and adequate mourning for their death. The period between the development of filial maturation and the death of one's parents is often a special time of new understanding and appreciation of each other that was never previously possible. It is frequently remembered with a good deal more fondness than some other times in the parent-child relationship.

This period in the life cycle usually marks the end of fertility for women. This is not true for men, many of whom are able to father children into their 70s or 80s. For women who have no children, this is the last opportunity to make an active choice (96,171,234,319,888). The decision, which may have been put off time and time again, can no longer be avoided. This realization usually becomes a significant force in the middle and late 30s. For many women, at this time, there is a resurgence of the ideas that children are a significant means of self-fulfillment and the unique task of women: to be fertile, to reproduce, to follow one's biological destiny. For some women, there is a feeling of emptiness and a sense of a desolate yawning future without children. Often there is a sense of the need to nurture with the insistent question of "What am I missing?" The factors taken into consideration in the decision not to have children in the past are often still operant. There are two elements, however, that are likely to be somewhat different. A woman in her middle and late 30s is likely to be far more capable of integrating her role as a partner, her career aspirations, and motherhood than is a younger woman. Partner relationships are likely to be more secure and the woman has, if typical, established a firm foundation in the occupation of her choice. Motherhood, although naturally disruptive, can usually be managed with some elegance. The other component that is different is the urgency of the decision and the emotional factors that accompany the ticking of the biological clock. For women then, this is indeed a crisis in the literary sense, a turning point of some significance.

Menopause is the period of natural cessation of the menstrual cycle (155,171,396,912,1003). It is usually marked by irregular menstrual periods prior to the cessation of menstruation. Biologically, a woman is considered to be postmenopausal after she has not had a menstrual period for one year. The absence of menstruation is related to the disappearance of functional follicles in the ovaries. There seems to be a hormonal decline at the gonadal level because the sex-related pituitary hormones continue to be produced. Menopause in other primates does not occur until near the end of the life cycle.

Menopause has not been studied in any depth by the scientific community. The following information must be read as tentative findings only.

Cessation of menstruation usually occurs between 40 and 50 years of age, although it may occur earlier or later. The age of onset of menopause is unrelated to the age of menarche or the number of pregnancies. It appears to occur earlier in women who are unmarried, those who smoke, and those who typically react to stress with weight loss and amenorrhea (the absence of menstruation).

There are several physical changes that may accompany menopause. It is important to note that these changes do not occur in all women. The following are the most reported physical changes. There may be erratic function of the vasomotor system, which leads to periodic episodes of flushing, feeling warm, and perspiration. The vaginal wall may atrophy and secretions that lubricate the vagina may decrease. This may lead to pain during intercourse, which is easily eliminated by lubrication with cream and continued regular stimulation of the vagina. There may be urethra and bladder irritation due to their being less cushioned by the atrophied vaginal walls. This may lead to a burning sensation during urination and increased urinary frequency. Erratic function of the vasomotor system and urethra and bladder irritation are temporary conditions that disappear in a relatively short period of time.

There are some psychophysical experiences that may accompany menopause. Similar to most of the physical changes mentioned above, these experiences are also temporary. The most common of these experiences are emotional lability and irritability, waking anxiety (i.e., waking up in the middle of the night in an acute state of anxiety for no apparent reason), lassitude, fatigue, headaches, and short memory lapses. These symptoms tend to be sporadic, and there is some question of whether they are due to hormonal changes per se, or the psychological reaction to menopause. The hormonal change is not really significant as to the amount produced. Hormone therapy may be useful on a very temporary basis. However, such therapy is quite controversial, as it may contribute to the development of cancer. The best treatment is generally believed to be the continuation or resumption of satisfactory sexual activities.

The social and psychological meaning of menopause is often far more significant than the actual physiological changes. Some of the common feelings and ideas women may need to deal with are: (a) evidence of the fact that one is aging; that an irreversible change has taken place; (b) that one's body is no longer good for anything; (c) in no longer being able to bear children, one's usefulness in life is over, there is nothing left; (d) femininity is lost, and thus one is no longer attractive; (e) fear that one will be rejected by one's partner and/or men in general; (f) the belief that one should not have any sexual desires and that if one does, this is decidedly abnormal.

Psychological response to menopause seems to be determined by the life history of the woman relative to her sexual identity, capacity to deal with change, and the psychosocial structure of her family. The number of women who experience difficulty with menopause is unknown. It has been reported as being approximately 10 percent, but this, for many reasons, is not a particularly reliable figure. Unless there are serious psychological problems, there is no decrease in sexual desires or interest in sexual activities. Biologically, there is no change in a woman's pattern of sexual response after menopause (105,155,285,650). A good many women respond to menopause in a highly positive manner. One need no longer be bothered with the inconvenience of menstruation and, perhaps more importantly, with worry about contraception.

Many women in their 40s appear to go through a sort of metamorphosis, which is sometimes referred to as "delayed blooming." Such women experience an increased interest in sexual activity and far more pleasure in this activity. They also appear to have a sharp increase in self-confidence and are more able to be appropriately self-assertive. There is no physiological reason for this metamorphosis, but there are good psychosocial and cultural reasons. Change in sexual interest and response is probably due to lessened concern about child care. Time and energy are freed to be reinvested in sexuality. After menopause, a woman need no longer be concerned about becoming pregnant, a worry that may have inhibited sexual interest and response. The factors that cause women to be more confident and assertive are related to accomplishment or having proved one's competence. In our society women are supposed to conceive, give birth, and raise children. Women who have done so feel they have accomplished the task society expects of them. Women, with or without children, who are involved in a career, have by their 40s more than likely become established. They are confident in their capacity to be productive in the world of work. They also often feel they have managed well or excelled in a domain previously reserved for men. Women in their 40s tend to be more comfortable with themselves than at any other previous time in the life cycle. This is, of course, a rather sad commentary on the typical environment our society provides for the development of women.

Although there is no physiological change in the sexual response pattern of women in this period of the life cycle, this is not the case for men (105,155,285,650). There are several changes that men experience at this time: it takes longer to obtain an erection, there is more control over ejaculation, the volume of seminal fluid is reduced, orgasm begins to be experienced in a shorter one-stage period compared to two or more stages in earlier life, and there is a physiologically more extended refractory period (the time between erections). Men occasionally experience the same psychophysical reactions outlined above relative to women. Such experiences appear to be less common for men, but again there are no accurate statistics.

Western society's ideas about sexual expression are still based on the myth of male genital superiority—the ideal for men being short refractory periods and rapid ejaculation. The physiological changes at this time can lead to a good deal of psychological turmoil and concern. Because men are often ill informed about sexual matters (as are women), they often believe they are becoming impotent, in which case they sometimes do. Sexual interest and arousal have far more to do with emotional states than with hormones. The hormonal changes in men, similar to women, are at the gonadal level, with only a slight decrease in the amount of sex hormones being produced. Men, indeed, are quite capable of sexual intercourse, which now may be more easily prolonged and ultimately more satisfying for the two people involved.

This time in the life cycle marks the acquisition of the final stage of sexual identity. This is essentially the ability to accept the physiological changes that occur at this time. It is the capacity to accept altered sexual responses, if these are evident, continued enjoyment of genital sexual activities, and continued perception of the self as a desirable sexual being.

The time of reassessment and possible role and identity change has a profound effect on a partner relationship. Each partner must be sufficiently secure in his own sense of self to allow the other partner to grow as he sees fit, or not to grow. Ideally, growth and change occur together and in a complementary, compatible manner. If not, one partner may be threatened or, apparently, simply lose interest in the other partner. The adjustments and adaptations in a partnership are often as difficult as those made at the time of initial formation of the partnership and the beginning of cohabitation. They may be more difficult, in that the excitement of being in love and the initial sexual intoxication is not there to cushion conflict. On the other hand, the long-standing intimate love in the relationship and sexual compatibility may serve as an adequate buffer. Although a partnership may be terminated at any point in its existence, this period is one in which disruption often occurs.

Many women who have never been employed or have not been employed for a number of years enter the job market at this time. Women, particularly if their children are still fairly young, may experience considerable guilt and ambivalence. Such feelings may put additional stress on the partner relationship. Some men feel threatened by their partner being employed (103,171,888). A woman's identity and thus typical manner of behaving may be radically altered. Out of necessity, there is frequently a change in the partner's life style and daily routines. The responsibility of being the family breadwinner is a very important part of some men's concept of self. Thus, their identity may be threatened by an employed partner. Conversely, some men feel that a working partner lessens some of the burden of being the sole source of financial support. The family may be able to afford a few luxuries that were not possible previously. This may ease the tensions that surround a woman beginning to work outside the home.

Some men, particularly those who are a little older than their partners, may feel envious. Women may have the choice of working or not working, and of what type of work they would like to do. Men do not as frequently have these choices. As mentioned, women at this place in the life cycle have greater self-confidence and more available energy. They have an enthusiasm for life, a sense of adventure, and a willingness to experiment that many men do not have, and therefore covet.

The sexual differences between men and women at this time in the life cycle may cause difficulties. Men, with their concerns about potency and their lack of experience with assertive women who are actively interested in sex, may draw away from or reject their partner. Men who do so often turn to younger women who are more naive in sexual matters and less demanding. Women, with their concerns about their desirability and more comfortable with the male sexual response pattern of short refractory period and rapid ejaculation, may turn to younger men to reinforce their continued attractiveness and for sexual satisfaction. Sexual readjustment of partners is often necessary at this time—a sometimes difficult task with all of the other adjustments that may be occurring at the same time.

In this phase of the life cycle, the individual's children tend to be adolescents. Adolescents have been discussed relative to the child's perspective. Extrapolation to the parent's perspective is probably fairly easy, and thus will be only briefly reviewed here. The adolescent's position relative to the parents is one of challenge. The adolescent confronts the family with new ideas, language, mannerisms, and values. In the panorama of human life, this confrontation serves as a bridge between the new and the old generations. In the immediacy of family interaction, it can be disconcerting and troublesome. The stance of the adolescent, in the eyes of the adolescent, is one of being a member of the loyal opposition. The question parents have is in regard to how loyal. The adolescent is preoccupied with testing authority, but complicates the matter by vacillating between childish behavior and acting very much like a responsible adult.

Common issues parents must deal with between themselves and with the adolescent have been previously outlined. Relative to these issues, the major questions and concerns of parents are (171): (a) whether to take something seriously or to let it pass lightly; (b) is a new interest a passing fancy, an inappropriate trend that needs to be nipped in the bud, or something that ought to be incorporated into family life; (c) whether the adolescent's relationship to a new friend or group is superficial, or the relationship should be evaluated for its possible effect on the adolescent and impact on the family; (d) how much the family can afford to support what the adolescent wants (e.g., emotionally, relative to time, financially); (e) when is the adolescent seeking independence, and when does he or she want limits set; (f) when to give direct guidance and when to let the adolescent learn on his own.

These questions and concerns reverberate through the daily life of parents of adolescents. They are addressed, but never resolved with any degree of finality until the end of adolescence. They will be raised again tomorrow, next week, the following month, and two years from now.

The degree of difficulty between parent and adolescent varies considerably (171,947). It is dependent on a good many factors, the major ones being the past relationship between parent and adolescent, the degree to which there is open communication, and the flexibility of the parent in dealing with change. The family that is secure and takes care of itself is the one best able to deal with the adolescent transition. The individual who is aware that this too is a time of reassessment for himself is in a position to be empathetic to the turmoils of adolescence. It is also helpful if the individual is able to remember his own adolescence with some degree of empathy for the person he was at that time. The capacity to roll with the punches and to be eager to learn something from the next generation is also helpful. In conjunction with some of the characteristics described above, parents survive their children's adolescences through periodically reminding themselves that the storm will pass and by enjoying the company of the child during pauses in the turbulence.

Activities of Daily Living

In the area of financial matters, the individual may be quite concerned with saving or arranging support for his children's education. It is also the time when the individual begins to think about planning financially for retirement.

Considerably more attention is given to self-care than was often evident during the last period of the life cycle. This occurs for two reasons: physical evidence of the aging process and change in identity. With recognition of the aging process, the individual becomes more concerned about health and physical appearance. The individual may spend more time in food preparation, taking note of the caloric, salt, and cholesterol content of various foods and chemical additives. There is interest in not only maintaining an adequate weight, but in eating foods that will impede the development of cardiac and circulatory problems. Junk foods no longer have a prominent place on the kitchen shelf. Meals are often prepared "from scratch" with considerable care. The individual also often becomes concerned about exercise, developing a daily or weekly routine. Such exercise may be directed toward general physical fitness or toward altering body contours. Evidence of aging also prompts more attention to grooming, particularly for women. Washing one's face quickly, running a comb through one's hair, and throwing on a pair of jeans and a shirt no longer seem sufficient. Wrinkles appear with regularity. Considerably more attention is given to care of one's complexion, the application of makeup, and wardrobe.

A change in identity almost inevitably dictates a change in physical appearance. There is a need to have congruence between the ideas one has about the self and the image one projects to others. An identity change is usually accompanied by a period of identity diffusion; the individual may try out a variety of different images. One may change his hairstyle, grow a moustache or beard or shave them off, and select a new style of clothing and accessories. All of this takes time until the desired physical appearance becomes a natural and spontaneous part of the self. In the meantime, one may spend a considerable amount of time in front of the mirror.

With the growth of children, household tasks usually are shared somewhat more equally among family members, thus putting less burden on any one individual. However, if a woman returns to work at this time, there often needs to be a reshuffling of household tasks. Men (and children) frequently must take on additional and unfamiliar tasks, an experience not often greeted with eagerness and delight. In addition, the individual may be required to take over some activities of daily living for aging parents. These may be relatively simple tasks such as making sure a parent makes an appointment to see the dentist, or more complex such as assisting parents to sell the family home and relocate in a new residence.

Work

For those individuals who have had a mentor, this is a time of separation (593,888). Such a separation may be accompanied by some degree of conflict over values, goals, or means. Conflict facilitates breaking the dependent bond, but may lead to feelings of guilt and remorse. On the other hand, many separations take place amicably. Regardless of the way separation occurs, it often results in the sense of being cut off to make one's own way. A reliable source of support and security is felt to be lost. The relationship between former mentor and neophyte usually becomes one of respected peer and colleague. Their work relationship may continue to be close, or both may feel more comfortable with a somewhat separated work life.

In separating from one's own mentor, the individual may take on the role of mentor himself. This nurturing role, an important aspect of generativity, is essentially learned through having been a neophyte who was guided by a mentor. If one has never been in such a role relationship, becoming a mentor is somewhat more difficult. Role behavior must be learned in the context of the relationship and through observation of other mentors. There are, however, some individuals who are not yet ready to become a mentor. Such individuals may perceive the younger generation of workers as rivals for their positions. They are not inclined to teach them the knowledge and skills necessary for advancement.

Reassessment relative to work takes many forms (593,888). Some individuals see this time as the last chance to strive for previously determined work goals. Others decide that goals set earlier are no longer particularly important and settle back to enjoy the position they now have. Still others decide to do something entirely different. A career change may involve movement into an entirely different occupation, or the individual may stay in the same occupation but take on a different job or position. An example of the latter is a scientist, who has been primarily an administrator, deciding to give that up and go back to the laboratory. Deciding on a career change is a difficult decision to make and it takes considerable courage. Often there is the idea of returning to a simple life relative to work, of moving closer to nature or to the basics. The problem with this orientation is that what one thinks one is returning to may be idealized or romanticized, far from the reality of the situation. In a career change there is much new knowledge to be acquired and skills to be learned. There tends to be considerable and legitimate fear of failure and the question of what do I do then. There is the sense of burning one's bridges and facing an uncertain future.

Many women return to being employed at this time (96,103,171,872). The process, and reaction, of a particular woman is often dependent on the time she has been unemployed and the support she receives from her family. Women are in various situations. They may be returning to a former career, entering the general work market with some or very few skills, or starting a new career. For many women, school may come first. This cushions the return to the world of work; the hours are somewhat flexible and it can be done on a parttime basis. The woman may complete a desired level of education, replace obsolete skills, or gain the knowledge and skill necessary for a new occupation. In addition, the school situation helps a woman to become familiar once again with interacting in a nonfamilial, authority-controlled, bureaucratic setting.

Within the work setting, many women have lost their seniority; others must start out in the lowest of positions. In entering a new environment, there are many new tasks and interpersonal skills to be learned. For a period of time a woman may feel inept and incompetent. Many women are accustomed to making decisions for themselves and others. They are often not in a position to do that in a work setting. The knowledge gained from life experience is frequently neither appreciated nor rewarded.

There are two common conflicts women experience relative to returning to work. One is primarily family related. A woman may want to work yet feel her children still need her at home during the day. On returning to work she may experience some degree of anxiety and guilt. The other conflict is related to societal pressure and expectations. From many sectors of society women get the message they are wasting their time at home being a mother and that having a job is an exciting, rewarding experience. The life of a working woman has been glorified in the mass media. Thus a woman often comes to feel that she really ought to work. Once working, the woman is confronted with the reality of work; one is frequently in a low position, not taken seriously, and involved in very boring, sometimes demeaning work. It is nothing like the woman was lead to expect. Yet, because of social pressure, it is difficult for a woman simply to walk away and take up her former way of life. She believes, often quite correctly, that many people would consider such behavior as, if not weird, at least extraordinary.

Leisure/Recreation

The leisure/recreation pattern is similar as that outlined in Chapter 4. For married couples, with some exceptions, leisure activities remain primarily family and neighborhood based—but more in the company of adults rather than a mixture of age groups (811). Children are now of an age where they are inclined to spend time with peers away from parental involvement. There are of course still many activities that parents and adolescents do enjoy together.

Because of the decrease in and equalitarian sharing of household tasks, individuals frequently have more leisure time than in the preceding age period. This permits involvement in some additional leisure activities. It is at this age when many individuals become involved in the community. This is often motivated by a sense of generativity: the desire to make the community work and be a better place for their children (271,272). Individuals may engage in political activities, join service organizations, or participate in volunteer activities. Such individuals feel a responsibility for their community and experience themselves as being very much a part of the community.

For some individuals, part of their leisure time may be related to work. They may entertain and be entertained by work colleagues and share other recreational activities with them. Often such leisure interactions are motivated by interests other than simply enjoyment. They may be used as a means to get ahead, as an opportunity to talk to the right people and to make contacts, as a way of returning favors, or as evidence that one belongs to an important clique. Engaging in such activities may be very satisfying or it may be seen as a duty one cannot afford not to perform. In the latter case, these activities should probably be classified as work, not leisure.

Some individuals become interested in creative pursuits or in the development of craftsmanship. For the first time there may be sufficient time and inclination to take up a hobby. Such interests are another example of generativity.

FIFTY TO SIXTY-FIVE YEARS OF AGE

It is in this period of the life cycle that many individuals reach their full potential in many facets of life, e.g., creativity, love, friendship, leadership. In the arts, sciences, government, media, and the economic sector, people in this age group are in command, wield power and influence, set norms, and make decisions (155). For more ordinary mortals it is a time of integration, of feeling more relaxed and in control of oneself and the situation at hand. This does not mean that the world stops or that there are no problems to be confronted and solved. It simply means that through a collection of life experiences many people have gained sufficient wisdom to deal with life's problems more objectively and with less inner turmoil. There is more acceptance of the inevitability of the life cycle and one's place in it. Although not particularly appreciated, there is a less panicked approach to physical aging (593,888).

There is a good deal more self-acceptance and self-confidence in this period. With this sense of self, the individual is more comfortable in recognizing parts of the self that have been hidden or denied. Jung refers to this as the acceptance of the shadow side (493). He associated the shadow side with opposite gender characteristics: the anima being the feminine side of men and the animus being the masculine side of women. He felt that men became more nurturing and caring and women became more assertive. This is probably a cultural artifact but nevertheless the phenomenon is sufficiently evident to be noted. Moreover, the idea of the emergence of the shadow side is also evident in nongender facets of life. There is a feeling of no longer needing to pretend, to one's self or others. One is able to enjoy assets without false modesty and accept limitations with humor and grace. The individual expects others to accept her, not despite limitations, but with limitations—these being as much a part of one's self as one's assets. With the acceptance of one's own failings and imperfections, the individual has a far greater capacity for empathy and compassion.

Family Interaction

It is in this period of the life cycle that there is often an experience of role-reversal between parent and child (105,155,171,497,531,733,888). Parents often become dependent on their children for financial and/or emotional support. The individual must often care for parents through a long terminal illness or give the care that any aged person needs. This role reversal is frequently uncomfortable for the parent and for the child. Aged people, like anyone thrust into a dependent position, can be difficult to get along with. They are sometimes rigid in their thinking and cantankerous in their ways. The individual is bound to experience some anger both at the parent and the responsibility imposed by the parent. This anger is usually followed by considerable guilt, which does not help the situation.

The death of each parent is a wrenching experience. It is made more difficult if the parent-child relationship has not moved through the usual cycle described in this chapter. If the cycle has been aborted, if the issues of love, dependency, control, and respect have not been addressed, then death brings an unnatural closure. Engagement in and completing the mourning process become far more difficult. It is through adequate mourning that the individual finally forgives the real or supposed transgressions of the parents.

This discussion is brief by design because there will be a section on illness and death at the end of the chapter.

With children grown and out of the home, partners often have more time for each other. This can be a time of rediscovery of each other, a process of becoming reacquainted, a deepening of love. The physical aging of the partner is accepted and accommodated, if necessary. This can also be a time of discovering there is nothing there—that somehow, out of the awareness of either partner, the relationship has been emotionally terminated.

Each partner's recognition and acceptance of his shadow side may cause some conflict. However, the nature and intensity of this conflict are rarely comparable to that which occurred relative to the reassessment of the previous period. For intimate partners, the nature of a partner's shadow side is not a particularly great revelation. Although actions based on the discovery of an unknown part of the self may be somewhat disconcerting to a partner, they are usually adjusted to after a period of time.

In regards to children, this is the time of disengagement. The role of being a parent becomes one of assisting the child into adulthood, and letting go. In the process of launching children into adulthood, the individual must deal with many issues: (a) allowing a child to make his or her own decisions, knowing when to give advice and when advice is not wanted; (b) accepting a career choice and life style; (c) seeing a child enter into serious sexual relationships, giving guidance judiciously; (d) accepting the child's choice of partner and taking the new individual into the family; (e) keeping out of the conflicts of the younger generation but being available with nonjudgmental support; (f) dealing with a child's prolonged financial and/or emotional dependency; (g) having a child return home because of personal problems or divorce; the return may include grandchildren; (h) seeing one's child as an adult and establishing a relationship of mutual adulthood rather than parent and child.

Through resolving these issues, the individual masters the capacity to engage in the nurturing process. The final phase, the ability to withdraw when the other individual (the child in this case) is able to function independently, is completed. Difficulty in accomplishing this final stage can lead to withdrawal of support prematurely or to a tenacious holding on. Neither strategy is helpful to the child, the parent, or their relationship.

When the last child leaves home there is often a sense of loss, a feeling of there being a great void. Sometimes referred to as the "empty nest" experience, it is particularly difficult for women who are not employed or who have few interests outside the home. It is an experience, however, shared by both mothers and fathers and is very real. The individual has in a very profound way given up a major social role—being a parent—and the home truly feels empty. As with any significant loss, there is need for a period of mourning and readjustment.

With the loss, or more accurately the major alteration of one social role, the individual often takes on a new one: that of being a grandparent (560). Although the individual may be delighted with the reality of a grandchild, she may not be tremendously pleased with the prospect of being a grandparent. Such a role sometimes has connotations of being old and not quite altogether competent. Although pleased, the individual may have some difficulty in integrating this new role into her sense of self-identity. The age at which one becomes a grandparent and the personal meaning attached to being a grandparent will influence the ease with which this role is assumed.

The way in which an individual plays the role of a grandparent varies considerably. The social parameters for this role are far less strict in our society than those for many other social roles. An individual's style of being a grandparent is not necessarily reflective of his feeling about being in that role. Some of the common styles of grandparenting are: (a) the fun seeker, one who enjoys play and adventure; (b) a surrogate parent; (c) the reservoir of family lore and wisdom; (d) a somewhat distant figure who arrives only on holidays and family occasions; (e) a friend. Most grandparents combine two or more of these styles to form their own unique relationship with a grandchild. Styles of grandparenting frequently change over time, being influenced by the current personal needs of the individual, the needs of the grandchild, and the dynamics and situation of the grandchild's nuclear family.

An individual sometimes enjoys the grandparent role more than she enjoyed the role of being a parent. She is free from the day-to-day responsibilities of child rearing and only occasionally, for example, needs to attend to the tasks of changing diapers and quieting a restless child in the middle of the night. With somewhat less involvement of self, the individual is comfortably able to experience pride in a grandchild. There is less concern about the child growing to fulfill one's own unconscious goals. Love for and interaction with a grandchild are less burdened by the doubts and anxieties of being a parent.

With a good relationship with one's own child and with one's grandchildren, the rewards of being a grandparent are considerable. The individual gains a sense of biological continuity in the reality and development of the grandchild in a way that cannot be experienced in the abstract. The individual feels emotional self-fulfillment and a vicarious sense of accomplishment. There is a good deal of satisfaction in being able to teach and guide a grandchild and help out in various other ways.

Being a grandparent is not always, however, a happy experience. The conflict with self-identity has been mentioned. Other difficulties may cause the role to be seen as more a burden than a source of satisfaction. Some common difficulties are: (a) the style of being a grandparent preferred by the individual may be different from what is expected or acceptable to one's own child; (b) the individual and her child may not agree about behavioral expectations and methods of discipline for the grandchild; (c) the parent of the grandchild may try to exploit the relationship between grandparent and grandchild by requesting an excessive amount of financial support or child care on the part of the grandparent; (d) the relationship between the individual and her own child may be so strained that no relationship between grandparent and grandchild is ever established or only established in a very tentative manner.

In being a grandparent, the individual acts as one more bridge between generations. It is, like most familial roles, influenced by the past, by current needs and expectations, and by the future.

Activities of Daily Living

With children out of the home, there is a decrease in household tasks. The number of tasks may not diminish but the quantity of the tasks does. There are fewer clothes to wash and not as much food to prepare for meals. Partners settle into a routine of task performance.

Conflict over the division of tasks that occurred in the last age period is now usually over resulting in a relatively equitable sharing of tasks. The family home, particularly if it is large, may be sold. The individual or partners must find a smaller house or apartment. Convenience of location is usually taken into consideration, the individual no longer feeling she must live in the suburbs for the sake of the children. The new home is often located closer to the place of work, near a shopping center and a church or synagogue, and convenient to public transportation. Retirement, formally a vague future situation, is now much a reality. The individual makes financial plans for retirement in order to maximize available retirement income. A serious plan for saving money may be initiated. There is often considerable concern about being able to live comfortably on a reduced, fixed income.

The individual may become responsible for many of her parents' activities of daily living. Travel is sometimes difficult for an aged person. The individual may need to assist parents in banking matters, shopping, and getting to a physician's office or clinic. If a parent needs assistance with personal care, the individual may attend to this herself or make arrangements for someone else to do this. When one parent dies, the other parent may need considerable assistance with financial matters and living arrangements, and considerable emotional support. Some individuals have a parent come to live with them. In addition to the psychological adjustment of another person, and a parent, living in the home, the sharing of household tasks may need to be realigned. Two women living in the same home is particularly difficult, especially in relation to the traditionally women's domain of the kitchen. The issue of territoriality must be addressed and somehow resolved. When, for whatever reasons, a parent who is unable to live alone does not live with a child, other arrangements need to be made. The individual may be responsible for locating a suitable protective environment or extended care facility for the parent. This is not only an emotionally difficult decision to make, it is a time-consuming task. In addition, the parent usually needs assistance in moving out of his/her home, disposing of some of the objects that have accumulated over the years, and making the necessary financial arrangements.

Work

There are three major responses to work in this phase of the life cycle: satisfaction, fear of retirement, and bitterness (593,872,888,939). Individuals who experience satisfaction feel they are finally doing what they always wanted to do, that they are doing their life's work. There is a sense of peace and contentment rather than striving to get ahead. The pace of work tends to be steady and productive without necessarily being spectacular. Realistic goals are set for what the individual would like to complete prior to retirement. The individual has a sense of accomplishment and experiences this time as a period for reaping the rewards of past efforts. In the work setting, the individual is usually given considerable respect and others look to her for guidance and advice. The individual has a sense of the past in regards to the work setting and is able to assist younger workers in putting current happenings into historical perspective. Others often see the individual as the guardian of the ethics, norms, and traditions of the work setting. With retirement more of a reality, the individual is often able to accept the role of a mentor more easily. In such a role the individual is able to groom others to take over one's work, to build on what one has accomplished.

Some individuals contemplate retirement with a good deal of dread. They see it as the end—not just the end of their work cycle, but the end of everything important in life. Often these are individuals who have made their worker role central in their sense of identity. The individual wishes to keep all the power which she has and acts to maintain that situation. One of the methods used is to make oneself as indispensable as possible—not sharing knowledge and skill or maintaining an idiosyncratic manner of accomplishing work tasks that is difficult for others to comprehend. Such an individual is not likely to enter into the role of a mentor or prepare successors. The individual tends to be highly critical of others, seeing them as incompetent. New ideas are feared and viewed with a good deal of suspicion. The individual may set unrealistic goals for herself and at times for others in the work setting. The pace of work continues to be high but not necessarily productive. In essentially denying retirement, the individual often makes herself and co-workers unhappy, if not miserable.

Some individuals feel bitter about their work experience. For a number of reasons they may not have accomplished the goals that they set for themselves. They may attribute this lack of success to themselves, but more typically it is attributed to the work situation. It is, of course, more comfortable to assign the cause of failure to a source external to the self. However, there may be a considerable truth in their perceptions. Indeed, they may have been treated unfairly and without consideration or sensitivity. Whatever the case, the individual feels beaten by the system, defeated by factors outside her capacity to control. Such an individual has little interest in work and tends to do a slipshod and superficial job, even sometimes sabotaging others' efforts. The individual's major preoccupation is counting the days until retirement.

Regardless of the individual's attitude toward work, there is a tendency not to seek overtime work, bring work home, or have a second job. During the last few years of the work cycle there is usually a period of deceleration, a decrease in productivity, and a withdrawal of emotional investment in the work place and in one's role as a worker.

Leisure/Recreation

This is the time of psychological preparation for retirement (155,593,811,888). Although not attended to by all individuals, such preparation facilitates adjustment to the end of the work cycle and the beginning of considerable leisure time. Anticipatory socialization for the role of being a retired worker takes several forms. The individual often thinks about what she is going to do on retirement, what daily life will be like, what activities will be undertaken, where she will live. The individual may talk to or spend time with persons already retired. If the individual can afford to do so, she may take longer than usual vacations to get a feel for what it will be like not to work. Experimentation with a variety of hobbies and other leisure activities is common. Indeed, there is now usually sufficient time to develop new interests and to explore possibilities for retirement.

Individuals in this age group, freed from many family responsibilities, often spend more time traveling. There is a desire to see more of the world, to free one's self temporarily from the restrictiveness of the known and the usual. Travel is also sometimes motivated by the sense of, if not now, then maybe never. There is an awareness that health and mobility problems may impede travel in the future. The individual continues to enjoy participation in various sports, although participation may not be so vigorous. There tends to be less interest and active involvement in community affairs, particularly for individuals who have moved into a new community or anticipate leaving the community on retirement. Involvement in activities associated with religious institutions may decrease, although attendance at religious services does not necessarily change. Close friends become more appreciated and one has a greater sense of their importance in one's life. More leisure activities are now shared with friends. On the other hand, privacy also becomes more important for some individuals. They become increasingly comfortable in solitary activities, enjoying time alone with their thoughts and favored activities.

More leisure time may be spent outside the home now than previously, but leisure activities do continue to be family oriented. Family activities are now likely to include the extended family of one's parents, grown children, and grandchildren. The organization and preparation for holidays and family celebrations often become the responsibility of individuals in this age group. This may not, in total, be viewed as the most pleasant task. But ultimately, considerable pleasure is usually derived from such activities. In being given, and taking, responsibility for family occasions, the individual is seen as the keeper of family customs and traditions.

SIXTY-FIVE YEARS OF AGE TO DEATH

There are many biological theories about aging, about the changes that take place in the body, which eventually leads to deterioration and death (155,497,531,733,912). None of these theories have been verified. The search continues for the key that will reveal this biological mystery. However, there are some things known about aging and aged persons. The first part of this section will be concerned with presenting some information about this final stage of the life cycle. Areas to be briefly discussed are: demographics situation, myths regarding aging, physical changes and health, and changes due to one's place in the life cycle.

About the Aged Person

Statistics about a particular population may be somewhat dry. Nevertheless they do provide a perspective not available in other forms. Demographic information on the aged population includes all people over 65 years of age. This is the traditional, albeit arbitrary age of retirement initially specified in the 1880s social legislation of Bismark in Germany. It continues to be used for social purposes, e.g., demographic research, age of retirement, eligibility for benefits, and the like. The age 65 has little relevance to an individual's capacity to function, general health, mental ability, psychological adaptability, or creativity (155).

The available statistics indicate that there are approximately 72 million people in the United States over 65 years of age (155,737). Of these, 95 percent are living in the community, the other 5 percent residing in institutions of one kind or another. Over two-thirds of the elderly are women; thus, there are about 143 women for every 100 men. Most elderly men are married; most elderly women are widows. These gender differences are due to women living longer, to the fact that wives tend to be younger than their husbands, and that men have more opportunity to remarry. It is far easier for a man to find a partner in this age group simply because there are more unattached women available. Women are three times as more likely to live alone than are men. This is an important statistic because it documents the high probability that many women will spend the last years of their lives living by themselves. This is rarely taken into consideration in the socialization process. Twenty-five percent of the elderly are poor, if one uses any realistic standard. Many others are living on a reduced income. Retirement income tends to be fixed, which is devastating in times of inflation. Poverty or relative poverty and living alone are probably the two major social problems of the elderly.

There are many myths regarding aging. They have come into being through folklore and from misinterpretation of research findings. The following are some of the common myths (155).

One myth is that chronological age determines the aging process. There is a vast variation in physiological, psychological, and social aging. There is a reality to chronological age, but one's "age" is primarily determined by physical health and by where the individual is in the psychological life cycle. This phenomenon is evident in the folk saying, "You are as old as you feel."

Another myth is that all old people are senile. Senility refers to a cluster of behaviors characterized by a tendency to live in the past, difficulty in making decisions, intellectual impairment, negativistic behavior, forgetfulness, lack of concern about others' feelings and attitudes, and an apparent lack of any interpersonal needs. One may indeed see these characteristics in some elderly people, but they are more often due to depression, grief, and/or anxiety than to nerve cell atrophy. The latter is a consequence of arteriosclerosis, a natural biological component of the aging process.

That old age is a time of tranquility, a time of serenity, when the individual enjoys the fruits of his or her labor and is content to be in a rocking chair, is another myth. The elderly, in fact, have many developmental tasks to accomplish and few are content with inactivity.

Some people believe that old age is a time of disengagement, that the elderly person is disinterested in others, the world and wishes to retreat into himself. He does not care how others respond to him. On the contrary, most elderly people are actively interested in others and in current events. The elderly are in need of considerable emotional support.

Another myth is that the elderly are resistant to change; that the elderly cannot learn, and do not want to learn or adapt. Response to change depends more on previous experience and life-long ways of adapting than anything inherent in the aging process. Elderly people do tend to be somewhat more conservative but this again is probably due to socioeconomic influences of the past and current pressures, not to the aging process.

Finally, some feel that aging is a myth. There is really nothing to the aging process, thus elderly persons should behave as if they were young.

In all myths there is an element of truth. It is important to focus on the kernel of truth and not give credence to the whole myth.

The aging process is marked by a large number of physical changes (155,531,597,912). The time when these changes begin to occur and the extent of the change are strongly influenced by heredity. These heredity-related changes are referred to as primary aging. Secondary aging is physical change associated with life circumstances, care of the body, stress, trauma, and disease. The aging process, in general, results in a decrease in the function of the various systems of the body. Briefly some of these changes are:

1. Respiratory system—loss of efficiency and a reduction in vital capacity.
2. Skeletal system—structural changes leading to a reduction in height, a stooped posture, stiffening of the joints, loss of teeth, and osteoporosis (loss of calcium resulting in fragile bones which are fairly easily broken; much more common in women than in men).
3. Nervous system—atrophy of the brain cells which decreases reaction time and may or may not impair cognition. (Intelligence quotient scores increase until the 20s and then level off. Speed of reaction does decrease but judgment, accuracy, and general knowledge tend to increase with age.)
4. Sensory system—decrease in auditory acuity so that the human voice often sounds muffled and droning (tends to lead to social isolation, because of difficulty in communicating, which in turn can lead to decreased reality testing and suspiciousness). Decrease in visual acuity characterized by difficulty adapting to sudden changes in light intensity, the need for a high intensity of artificial light when that is the only light source available, and difficulty with near vision. Decline in smell and taste leading to less interest in and enjoyment of food (this coupled with dental and gastrointestinal problems can result in malnutrition, which in turn leads to a decrease in all areas of function). Decrease in tactile perception, particularly of heat, cold, and light touch, and in response to tactile stimuli. Decline in vestibular and kinesthetic perception compensated for by a change in gait pattern, which is slower and provides a wider walking base.
5. Muscular system—structural changes leading to atrophy, hypotonia, weakness, and decline in the ability

to respond rapidly and effectively in an emergency situation.

6. Cardiovascular system—thickening and calcification of the arteries, excessive deposits of starch-like material in the vessels, progressive increase in the peripheral resistance to blood flow, decline in cardiac output at rest, and decrease in the cardiovascular system's capacity for responding to extra work.

7. Urinary system—decrease in filtration rate and an increase in urinary frequency.

8. Gastrointestinal system—changes which result in digestive problems, impairment in absorption, and constipation.

9. Skin and subcutaneous tissues—decrease in skin elasticity and resilience leading to wrinkles, skin discoloration and wart-like growths, loss of hair pigmentation, atrophy of gums, atrophy of subcutaneous tissue leading to difficulty in regulating body temperature and less protection against trauma, decrease in sweat and oil glands leading to dry skin.

10. Reproductive system—as previously described, some slight decrease in hormonal level; interest, desire, and capacity continue until death.

Health problems are a fact of the aging process. Approximately 85 percent of the population over 65 years of age have a health problem, with many individuals having more than one chronic condition (105,155,913).

The major primary diseases or conditions of the elderly are depression, acute and/or chronic organic mental disorders, glaucoma, cataracts, Parkinson's disease, degenerative joint diseases, rheumatic arthritis, osteoporosis, cerebral vascular conditions, cerebral vascular accidents, diseases of the circulatory system, emphysema, cardiovascular-renal disease, cancer, and diabetic mellitus.

The primary orientation to the health of the aged has been indifference and neglect. It has also been the medical treatment of choice. Medicine has taken two approaches to care of the elderly. One approach is simple: to tell individuals their health problems are due to the aging process and they must learn how to live with that fact of life. The other approach is to inundate the individual with a variety of medications, without taking into consideration the heightened sensitivity to drugs, which is characteristic of the elderly individual. Adverse reaction to chemotherapy is common in the aged population.

Medicine's typical interpersonal interaction with the elderly is to behave as if the individual is incompetent. More is often explained to a child than to an elderly individual. Few physicians take the time to make the refined diagnosis necessary to determine specific treatment and closely follow the effects, intended or unintended, of that treatment. Few people in medical institutions are concerned with assisting the elderly individual in understanding his problems and giving him sufficient information so that he can make an informed decision in regards to a course of treatment. Few people care. It is not an exaggeration to say that the delivery of health services to the elderly in this country is a national disgrace.

Physical changes and health aside, the elderly individual's place in the life cycle has considerable influence on his world view and behavior (155,272,493,497). The individual's perspective comes from the experience of having lived a long life and the imminence of death. Even in the circumstances of rapid social and technological change, the individual often has a sense of the fundamental essence of the human condition. Human beings will love and hate each other; children will be born and people will die. There is altruism and the capacity to be inhumane; the life cycle will continue. The individual has seen it and experienced it before. His reaction to world events is from the perspective of long-term familiarity. He is not surprised and, at times, perhaps is a bit cynical. Aged individuals often see their current task in life as the sharing of their accumulated knowledge and experience with the younger generations. They have a historical perspective not available to the younger generations. They are the caretakers of the tradition of a family, a community, a culture, a society. Although wisdom is not defined by experience, but rather how one uses that experience, many elderly people are very wise.

The individual's place in the life cycle tends to cause some change in perspective and to arouse certain interests and concerns. For many individuals there is a change in the sense of time. There is a resolution of the fear of time running out: an end to the sense of panic about time. The individual comes to value time in the immediacy of the here and now. Life comes to be lived in the moment, the present time of today. The past may be interesting to consider and explore; a source of comfort; or to be ignored. The future is known.

The individual often acquires a sense of elementality: the capacity to sort out the important from the less important. The elemental components of life are identified: the supernatural; the mysteries, wonder, and power of nature; love and friendship; the birth and growth of a child; human touch. Elementality makes perception more acute, even with diminished sensory reception. Color, shape, tone of voice, and tactile exchanges are noted with new appreciation and understanding.

With an intimate sense of the life cycle in its entirety, many individuals develop a new or renewed interest in philosophy, religion, history, art, and literature. These are the elements of a cultural heritage which speaks most directly to the totality of human experience. With the vantage point of age, exploration of these resources becomes an enjoyable experience or new discovery.

Concern about leaving a legacy is almost a universal interest. A legacy, something handed down from the past, provides a sense of continuity, giving one the feeling of being able to participate in life even after death. The desire to leave a legacy has various motivations: not wanting to be forgotten, wanting to give of oneself to those who survive, wishing to remain in control or influence what happens in this world after one's own death. The latter may be implemented through a will that sets strict limits on how money or property is to be used and/or describes prerequisite behavior for gaining control of money or property. A legacy may take other than economic forms. It may include one's children; those to whom one has given help or taught; the products of one's work; and treasured objects such as jewelry, furniture, the family Bible, and so forth. Concern about leaving a legacy is one means of taking account of one's life, of determining what has been worthy in that life, what one has given or is able to give to future generations.

Erikson has described the task of this period of the life cycle as the development of integrity (271,272). By this he means the acceptance of one's life as something that was and had to be and giving meaning to the life that has been lived. In the process of developing a sense of integrity, the individual accepts the triumphs and disappointments of his life, tries to make of his life a coherent experience that forms a link in the chain of generations from which one received and to which one has contributed. The process of establishing integrity puts the individual in a vulnerable position as it requires a review of one's life, a clear look at what one has and has not accomplished, the ways that one has given and denied need satisfaction to others. Through the development of integrity, one gains a sense of personal dignity, and becomes reconciled to one's death. The opposite of integrity is despair: the feeling that one's life has been nothing and thus one is nothing; the feeling that the time is now short, too short to attempt to start another life, to accomplish something. The individual feels self-disgust and often has a profound fear of death.

This period of the life cycle involves considerable learning. The individual must identify, understand, and find use for what he has already attained in a lifetime of learning and adapting. The individual must learn to conserve his strength and resources when necessary and to adjust in the best way to those changes and losses that occur as part of the aging experience.

Family Interaction

With the onset of retirement, partners have considerably more contact with each other (105,127,155,171, 285,497,531,650,733). Initially, there is the question of what do you do with each other all day, together. A different pattern relative to time spent together and time apart has to be established. Both partners need to develop a new routine, identify interests to be pursued, and coordinate these with one's partner's preferred routines and interests. If one partner does not do this, the other partner may feel that he must give up his own interest to entertain the partner or follow her momentary whim. This is likely to cause dissension and anger at being used. A woman who has never worked may find her husband taking over chores and decision making that she has seen as her prerogative and territory. Household tasks and responsibilities need to be redefined.

Both men and women fear the death of their partner. Thoughts of the void that will be created and the loneliness without one's partner are extremely uncomfortable, particularly if they are not shared. Many individuals have never lived alone, having gone directly from their parents' home into a home with a partner. They literally do not know how to cope without a partner. Aside from the idea of being alone, the individual may lack skill in many activities of daily living. This adds to the fear of one's partner dying.

During this period of the life cycle, one partner is often required to care for an ill or disabled partner. This task can be enormous, time consuming, and restrictive in terms of one's own life. Although such care is usually given willingly out of love, it also can give rise to considerable anger and guilt. Anger arises from the feeling of what right does this person have to demand my time and attention. Guilt arises from the feeling that I love this person, I should want to take care of her; it is wrong to be angry and it is socially unacceptable to talk about how I feel. Thus, the individual frequently carries a psychological burden in addition to the physical and emotional care of his partner.

With a compatible partner, enjoyable sexual relationships can continue until death. What can cause some difficulty in sexual relationships is the illness or disability of a partner. Both partners may fear sexual intercourse due to the effects of exertion or because of pain. This fear often leads to a lack of desire and sexual relations may cease altogether or only occur sporadically. However, with adequate knowledge about the illness or disability and positions that will minimize discomfort, many partners are able to continue satisfactory sexual relationships. This requires some degree of open communication because it involves exploring, perhaps for the first time, alternative ways of giving and receiving sexual gratification.

The death of a partner, for many people, means the end of interest in sexuality. This appears to be a cultural artifact having nothing to do, obviously, with any biological factors. Many groups in our society believe that elderly individuals, particularly if they are not married, have no interest in sex. This is especially so in the case of women. The individual, thinking that interest in sex is somehow abnormal, loses interest and desire. Other individuals who continue to be aware of their sexual needs but have no partner may find release of sexual tensions and relaxation through masturbation. However, such activity may be accompanied by some degree of guilt, feeling that masturbation is wrong, unnatural, and the like. Many people have never explored the sexual pleasures that one can give to oneself.

Relationships with children, whatever else they may be, are often characterized by some degree of dependency. The role reversal that may occur at this time is often more difficult for the parent than for the child. For many individuals, dependency on one's children is somewhat of a disgrace, a sign of weakness, and a situation to be avoided if at all possible. Being dependent after all of the years of helping a child to be independent is very difficult. Having to ask for and accept help with any degree of grace is a hard task to master. Request for emotional support is often accompanied by the stated or unstated feeling that, "I have no one else to turn to," and the plea to "accept me as I am at this time." Financial support is often the most difficult to request. There is the feeling of taking away from one's child money she would use for herself and her children. Accepting one's child as caretaker in activities of daily living particularly relative to self-care may be experienced as demeaning. The extent to which the individual is able to ask for and accept help comfortably is influenced by his ability to accept the inevitability of dependency and the past parent-child relationship.

In this period of the life cycle, the individual is often more accepting of the role of grandparent. The individual's style of being a grandparent may be as it was previously or the style may change. There is need to adjust to grandchildren's growth and development and perhaps adjust to their different world views. Because of the grandparent's position in the life cycle, the individual is often able to accept, understand, and give counsel in areas where parents cannot. The individual may be able to fulfill a very important familial role—transmitting the mysteries of life, the unknown rather than the absolutes.

Activities of Daily Living

Individuals' attitude toward and ability to engage in activities of daily living will depend to a great extent on their health. For some individuals this may be the first period in their life when they have had sufficient time to enjoy activities of daily living (154). For some of them, for example, meal preparation and yard work, may now become more of a leisure activity than an activity of daily living. For some individuals, familiar activities of daily living may provide a source of comfort and stability when many other facets of their life are changing.

If the individual moves to a new place of residence, there is the need physically to create a new home. Although it may be quite difficult to leave the old home, making a new home can be a source of much pleasure. The feeling of being able to have things just as one would like may be a new experience. There is time to give attention to small details.

With the onset of health problems or simply a decrease in function due to the aging process, performance of activities of daily living may become increasingly difficult. Conservation of strength becomes a necessity. Many individuals become far more efficient relative to motions and the expenditure of energy than they had been in the past. Accomplishing tasks may take much longer than previously, leading to a considerably greater period of the day being spent in performing activities of daily living. It may be more difficult to bathe, dress, prepare meals, travel, and shop. Frequent rest periods may be needed. The individual may have to decide that some tasks are simply not worth the time and energy they consume. Meal preparation may become more complex if the individual is on a special diet. Some elderly individuals give little attention to maintaining an adequate diet. This may lead to malnutrition, which as mentioned, can result in additional health problems.

Safety relative to activities of daily living may become a major preoccupation. With sensory and motor deficits, the individual may fear falling or injuring himself in other ways. This is true both within and outside the home. Leaving one's home can also be a fearful prospect. Many elderly people, because of low income, live in unsafe neighborhoods. The possibility of getting robbed and injured is very real. The individual's home is known territory; the external world may be difficult to cope with. Elderly people often become easily disoriented, especially in new settings or situations, and fear they will not be able to respond adequately.

Individuals who have lost a partner and are living alone have particular difficulties. Activities of daily living that were previously shared must now be done by oneself. This often greatly diminishes pleasure in the performance of tasks. Eating a meal or shopping, for example, when previously shared, now becomes simply a chore. In addition, there are often unfamiliar tasks, previously the responsibility of one's partner, that must now be taken care of by oneself. The individual is likely to feel inept and incompetent in performing these tasks. In doing them, one is also reminded of their lost partner.

Activities of daily living that center around the home and involve personal care, nevertheless, are highly significant for elderly persons. It is an area where they can feel self-sufficient and in control of the situation. Even if they occasionally need outside help, the individual has a sense of place in which they can do as they please.

Work

For most individuals this period marks the end of the work cycle (105,155,497,531,733). Whether an individual should be required to retire at a particular age, be it 65 or 70 years of age, is a social, economic, and political question that will not be discussed in this text. The fact is that most people do retire in this age period: some voluntarily, others nonvoluntarily. Retirement is accompanied by a change in an individual's power, status, and the loss of the daily structure provided by work. This change may be anticipated and accepted with a good deal of pleasure or, on the other hand, it may be a catastrophic blow to one's sense of identity. Individuals who have a positive attitude toward retirement have usually done a considerable amount of "psychological work," to prepare themselves for the changes that come with retirement. The alteration of power and status are accepted; plans for the retirement years have been made. Other individuals have a highly negative attitude toward retirement. Their job or being a worker has been central to their identity and retirement may well be perceived as a personal insult. They are not comfortable with the loss of power and status and they have not planned for the future. Such individuals may experience a sense of panic in the initial period of retirement and a severe loss of self-esteem.

Regardless of one's attitude toward and plans for retirement, there is still a feeling of entering the unknown. This perception is certainly reality based, as the great majority of individuals have spent a good part of their adult lives working. The structure and routine of work is deeply imbedded into the rhythm of daily life. A period of adjustment is inevitable. It takes varying amounts of time to settle into a new pattern of daily life that is comfortable and that truly feels a part of the self. The individual also has the task of finding use for the knowledge and skills that he has attained up to this point in his life. This search takes place, typically, in the leisure sector.

Leisure/Recreation

What use to make of one's time, the development of a daily routine, and how to satisfy one's various needs through leisure activities are the developmental tasks of this age group (105,155,171,497,531,733). Money is an important factor, for to some extent it will influence the life style that the individual fabricates for himself. Travel, a move to a warm climate, participation in public forms of entertainment, and the like require an adequate income. Without sufficient funds, an individual's choices as to how to spend leisure time are somewhat restricted.

Most individuals develop a routine, often structured around activities of daily living, which includes a variety of activities: a mixture of active and sedentary pursuits, some with friends and/or partner, some alone. Many individuals once again enjoy participation in the affairs of the community. This allows for the use of knowledge and skills previously acquired or it provides an opportunity to develop new skills. Individuals in this age group who appear to be most satisfied with their lives are those who have particular interests they pursue with diligence. The interest per se makes little difference. What is important is the satisfaction that such an interest provides. Individuals who have no significant interests often appear to be adrift and without purpose. They sometimes seem to be marking time until they die.

Friends continue to be important, in particular old friends. They have seen the individual at his best and worst, given support when needed, and shared many experiences with him. The death of a close friend is traumatic, leaving a void that is difficult to fill. New friends are hard to find, and establishing intimate friend relationships requires the expenditure of considerable energy that may not be available. Individuals who have retired usually seek friends among other retired people. Friendships formed in the work setting tend to dissipate over time if the friend continues to be employed. The individuals find over time that they no longer share common interests and concerns. Women, again, tend to have mostly other women as friends. Involvement with family members usually continues as it was in the previous age period.

As the aging process progresses, the individual comes to be more restricted in leisure activities. Difficulty in leaving the safety of one's home limits social interactions and involvement in out-of-home activities. With sensory deficits, television, reading, using the telephone, sewing, and some craft activities become difficult if not impossible. This is often a time of loneliness and boredom. Attachment to and care of familiar objects may become quite important at this time. They serve as an aid to memory and provide a sense of comfort, security, and continuity. It is these loved objects that will be passed to the next generation.

Death, the final point of the life cycle for the individual, will be discussed in the last section of this chapter. Two other factors that influence the life cycle, divorce and illness, are described in the interim.

DIVORCE

The vast majority of people living today are affected directly or indirectly by divorce (171,269,270,460,531, 545,593,665,863,888). One out of four marriages is terminated in such a manner. One may be affected by the divorce of one's parents, oneself, one's child or children, and the divorce of intimate friends. Divorce may affect an individual at any time during the life cycle. Its impact is considerable and, at least temporarily, disruptive. The life cycle and the developmental tasks inherent in the cycle, however, do continue. Divorce often makes the accomplishment of these tasks more difficult, but the tasks remain to be mastered.

Divorce is one common life cycle event for which there are no rituals or rites of passage. Nonparticipants, as much as they care, have considerable difficulty relating to the process of divorce. There is no tradition of expected behaviors and responses that a nonparticipant can draw on to guide her interaction with participants in divorce process. This frequently leaves participants without adequate support. There is a sense of social aloneness of doing something outside the normative structure of the social system. This feeling arises from the lack of social rituals and occurs regardless of the evident frequency of divorce.

Divorce is a complex social phenomenon, the legal decree being only a moment in the course of events. Because of this complexity, this section will be divided into three parts: the process, postdivorce adjustment, and the remarried family.

The Process

The process of divorce seems to be easier the younger one is and if there are no young children involved. This is not to say that it is not a traumatic event. It simply appears that postdivorce adjustment is somewhat less difficult. The length of the marriage is also a factor.

The causal factors of divorce are probably as numerous as the number of divorces. Actually, focus on the question of causal factors is unproductive; it is like asking someone why they feel in love. In addition, the problem stated by the partners is rarely the real reason, whatever that reason may be. Essentially divorce occurs out of long-standing conflicts that cannot be resolved. Some common sources of conflict are sexual difficulties, overinvolvement in work or child rearing, financial disagreements, relationship with in-laws, and the uneven growth of partners. Communication breaks down to such point that the conflicts cannot be negotiated or reconciled.

The dominant spouse is usually the one who seeks the divorce. In the process one spouse is often portrayed as having engaged in some inexpedient or unsavory behavior or to be in a general state of dysfunction. Which spouse is portrayed in this manner usually depends on the perspective of the individual describing the situation. For participant and nonparticipant alike, it is convenient to have someone to blame. Placing blame seems to help to bring coherence to a situation that is frequently inexplicable. Although it maintains ambiguity, the actuality of the situation is that both parties are responsible and neither is at fault.

The emotions that surround divorce are considerable. In the extreme, there may be such negative feelings, so intense and experienced to such a degree, that the individual believes that her autonomy cannot be maintained with frequent contact with her spouse. There is a feeling of not wanting to be in the same vicinity as the spouse or to talk with the spouse even by telephone. More specifically, some of the emotions commonly aroused by divorce are anger, feelings of abandonment, a marked decrease in self-esteem, and guilt. These emotions not only occur around the time of divorce but may continue for an extended period thereafter.

The two major issues that need to be negotiated in the process of divorce are financial arrangements and relationship with children. In regard to financial arrangements, the couple's economic resources must be divided in some sort of equitable manner. This includes the residence, household objects, cars, and savings. It also includes what, if any, ongoing financial support is to be provided by one spouse for the other. Alimony per se seems to be a dying institution. However, some time-limited support may be provided for a spouse who is not currently self-supporting. At least partial financial support for a child is usually given to the parent who has legal custody of the child.

Child custody has traditionally been awarded to the mother. Although this is still usual, it is not uncommon for fathers to seek and be granted custody. More recently, joint custody has become a prevalent means of defining the parents-child relationship. In such an arrangement, both parents have equal responsibility for making any major decisions that will affect the child. Joint custody is often regarded as the preferred way of dealing with the issue of child custody. It is only viable, however, if the parents are able to resolve their differences to such a degree that they are able to put the welfare of the child first—not a particularly easy task of the emotional atmosphere of the divorce process. Regardless of custody arrangements, the issues that are usually of major importance are child financial support, responsibility for making decisions relative to the child, and the time the child will spend with each parent.

There is considerable difference between legal and emotional divorce, the latter often occurring two or three years after the former. The time between legal and emotional divorce will here be referred to as the postdivorce period. It is usually only within this period that the conflicts, emotional reactions, financial arrangements, and relationships with children are truly worked out and resolved. The postdivorce period ends only with their resolution.

A child is profoundly affected by divorce. It is also good to remember, however, that a child is also profoundly affected by living in a household where there is chronic conflict and/or a poverty of communication. Parents who remain married for "the sake of the children" are rarely doing them a favor. It appears that children have the most difficulty in dealing with divorce between the ages of 4 and 12 years. Prior to the age of 4, the child seems to have little idea of what is happening. There is an egocentric quality that seems to protect the child. After the age of 12 years, the child has a sufficient sense of autonomy and mastery to feel less dependent on the solidarity of the parental pair. The child by this age is also able to grasp some of the reasons for the divorce, if not understanding, at least able to accept it as another fact of adult life. Aside from age, the child's reaction is also influenced by the intensity of her emotional attachment to each parent and the degree of conflict between the parents. Another important factor is the extent to which the child is the focus of the parents' emotional struggles. The child caught in the middle for whatever reasons is likely to be deeply hurt. The child's reaction to divorce usually includes most or all of the following: difficulty in comprehending, anger at one or both parents, feeling of insecurity, anxiety, a temporary period of regression and/or a delay in developmental progress, guilt growing out of the belief that she is somehow responsible for the divorce, denial, and the fantasy that the parents will be united in marriage once again. The postdivorce period of children, similar to adults, is often quite lengthy. The child's adjustment is strongly influenced by the relationship between the parents in the postdivorce period. The adjustment is relatively easy if the parents are able to maintain respect for and friendly relationship with each other. The same is also true for the divorced couple.

An individual's parents' reactions to divorce is important. Their response can either make the individual feel more guilty and unworthy or it can help the individual feel that a reasonable course of action was selected given the situation. Ideally, parents remain uninvolved relative to the issues and maintain a neutral nonjudgmental attitude toward both parties. This is often difficult, as parents themselves may feel that the divorce is a reflection of some deficit in how they raised their child. This difficulty is compounded by parents, quite naturally, not wanting their child to be hurt or in pain. An individual needs emotional support from parents particularly in the postdivorce period. One way this is often provided is through giving additional assistance with child care for at least a period of time.

Postdivorce Adjustment

Regardless of whether the individual lives alone or forms a single-parent family, there are common problems in adjusting. The period of adjustment lasts from two to four years, the length of time not always being recognized by participants and nonparticipants alike. There may initially be a sense of freedom and a state of mild euphoria. This usually passes fairly quickly and is replaced by the reality of being alone without a partner. The task at hand is essentially to create a new life. The stability and structure of work are particularly useful during this period. Individuals who are not working at the time of divorce not only lack the sense of order work provides but they also must often go through the process of looking for a job and adjusting to a work setting. Many individuals need to find a new residence and to make a new home for themselves. There may be a sharp decrease in financial resources. It is more expensive to live alone and, where children are involved, essentially to maintain two residences. Being alone, even if one has children, is a difficult adjustment. It can at times be a frightening experience to realize there is no one who will be there in time of need; there are periods of loneliness, and a serious lack of emotional support.

The individual with children has additional problems in adjustment. The parent who does not have child custody and who is severely limited in the time allowed to spend with the child may become depressed and/or angry, feel rejected, and experience a general sense of incompetence. Being with the child may initially be extremely painful because the sense of loss is reexperienced at each parting. The task of establishing a new relationship with the child is very difficult for such a parent. The parent with full custody of a child and minimal relationship with the former spouse often experiences a marked increase in responsibility. There is no one with whom to discuss various situations; decisions about child rearing must be made alone. In addition, such individuals often are required to take on increased responsibility for financial matters and decisions.

Divorced parents are required to deal with the emotional reactions of their children while they are attempting to deal with their own reactions. There is sometimes the tendency to become overinvolved with one's child. This is often due to loneliness, feeling that one has to make amends for the divorce, or believing that one must be both mother and father. Overinvolvement, if it continues for a long period of time, can lead to an emotional bond between parent and child so intense that age-appropriate separation from the family is delayed. The child, particularly an only child, may feel such a degree of responsibility for the parent that the child believes he must stay home and care for the parent. Between parent and child of the opposite sex, the emotional bond may result in a resurgence of the Oedipal conflict in the child and sexual interest in the child on the part of the parent.

On the other hand, the individual may not give sufficient attention to the child. The individual may become so caught up in self-adjustment that he or she is unable to focus on the needs of the child. Insufficient attention may also be due to the pressure of time. The individual who is working, taking care of a home, and raising one or more small children alone is a very busy person. There is often simply not enough time to spend with a child. The child may feel neglected and express that feeling in a variety of ways designed to get additional attention.

Regardless of personal inclinations, a parent must maintain some kind of communication with the other parent. The relationship with the other parent must be fostered without allowing one's own feelings to get in the way. Without adequate communication, children are often put in the position of relaying messages and/or may use the situation to play one parent against the other. If a relationship with the other parent is not fostered, the child may be caught between love for both parents or develop extreme animosity toward one parent. Divorced parents must also adjust to the fact that a child may periodically show marked preference for one parent as opposed to the other. This behavior is fairly typical of preschool children and adolescents regardless of the marital status of parents. It is, however, sometimes more difficult for a divorced parent to understand and adapt to this temporary favoritism without feeling hurt and rejected.

The divorced parent must determine the way in which relationships with the opposite sex are to be handled with the child. The parent must figure out an appropriate way to deal with the fact of sexual activity: to what extent it will occur in the home with the child present, whether to spend the night away from the home with a sexual partner, how and what aspect of these matters will be discussed, and so forth. This may be particularly difficult with adolescents who are in the process of exploring and regulating their own sexuality. The divorced parent must also determine how and to what extent a child will be involved in one's social activities. In conjunction with this decision, the parent must decide what kind of relationship one's child should have with the individual with whom one is currently involved. The seriousness and anticipated length of the relationship are usually a factor in this decision.

For most divorced individuals there is at some point the need to reenter the single world. Married friends, if the friendships persist after divorce, are often occupied with family and other married friends. The individual is often cut off from his or her former social network and relationships. The individual needs to find compatible people with whom to share leisure activities. If many former friends are lost because of the divorce, new, intimate friendships need to be formed.

The other reason for entering the single world is to find sexual partners or a partner with whom one can form an intimate long-term relationship. For a time, many individuals experience little sexual desire and have no interest in dating even casually. It is as if they are exhausted from the process of divorce and preoccupied with the other aspect of adjustment in the postdivorce period. Somewhat numb, the individual feels little or no sexual desire.

Other individuals appear to need to prove to themselves that they are still sexually desirable. Such individuals may become involved in a number of sexual relationships that are fairly indiscriminate and very short term. This way of dealing with self-doubts is fairly common and usually limited to a short period of time. For individuals initially numb, this may be the first phase of reentry into intimate, extended sexual relationships.

Eventually the individual settles down to a more serious approach to finding a new partner. The problems are considerable. Externally the difficulty is finding people one might consider for a partner. Single bars have become somewhat of an institution. But the idea let alone the actuality of going to a singles bar is not acceptable to many people. Participation in a variety of leisure activities, the work setting, friends, and luck are the usual sources for finding prospective partners. Another external problem is finding the time and the financial resources for dating and courtship. This is a particularly significant factor for the individual responsible for a single-parent family.

Internally, the difficulty is often the person's self-concept. Many individuals feel emotionally scarred, impaired in some way, not good enough to maintain a relationship. Failure, as divorce is frequently perceived, does not enhance self-confidence. The individual often lacks skill in the intricacies of dating, feeling clumsy about the whole process. There is often the experience of being an adolescent once again.

Dating both casually and seriously is an important part of postdivorce adjustment. It allows the individual the time and experiences that heal old wounds and promote the reformation of an accurate and adequate self-concept. Individuals tend to associate happiness and self-worth with finding an intense emotional involvement with another person. There is some validity to this idea, but attempting to do this before an adequate period of adjustment can cause serious problems. Individuals who move from one marriage to another without any or a very short period of adjustment often find themselves with the same conflicts they encountered in their previous marriage. Although the second marriage may be successful and satisfying, it may initially be the arena for working out a number of personal issues.

For many people, the period of postdivorce adjustment is a time of tremendous growth. An extremely painful period, it nevertheless provides an opportunity for reassessment and a moratorium of sorts. As this period comes to a close, most individuals feel they have a better sense of who they are, what they want, and where they are going. There is a feeling of now being ready to set priorities and to get on with the business of living.

The Remarried Family

According to the available statistics, about 75 percent of the people who are divorced remarry. There are probably many more who form long-term partnerships but do not necessarily marry. Remarriage often marks the end of the postdivorce period. As such, it is a time of considerable self-confidence, a time of looking toward the future to a new, more satisfying life. But as with all new endeavors, there is much to be learned and new problems to solve. The individual needs to establish or redefine a considerable number of relationships. The first and probably primary role interaction that must be organized into a functional unit is that between the two new partners. It is on this relationship that many, if not most, of the other multiple relationships will hinge. In addition to the typical issues involved in establishing any partnership, previously divorced partners have other concerns. The partners may bring children into the relationship as well as long-term, established patterns of interacting and considerable life experience. In regards to children, the partners must come to some decisions about behavioral expectations and discipline and how this responsibility is to be shared. New ways of interacting with a partner must be learned, and old ways unlearned. The adjustment of the new partners may be compounded by their being at different places in the life cycle. This may be because of differences in age or it may be due to a differential pace in approaching and mastering developmental tasks. The difficulty in understanding someone at a different place in the life cycle, previously discussed, may make mutual adaptation somewhat more difficult.

The reaction of children to remarriage is influenced by age, their own postdivorce adjustment, and the extent to which they know and like the new partner. Some children are comfortable with their parent's remarriage. They are pleased to see their parent happy and more content; they feel a greater sense of security and stability in the home and they may feel less pressure to provide emotional support for their parent. On the other hand, some children have an adverse reaction to the remarriage of their parent. They may believe their privileged position has been usurped and, indeed, this may be a very accurate perception. This may lead to feelings of rejection, jealousy, and anger. The fantasy of one's parents remarrying must be given up. The child may be concerned about whether the new stepparent will insist on a change in her relationship to one or both of her natural parents. If the partner brings children into the new family, the child must establish relationships with stepsiblings. This is particularly difficult for a child who has had no siblings.

The individual's relationship with his or her child or children will change with the addition of another adult into the family constellation. The intimacy of the relationship may be diluted to some degree and there may be less time for the parent and child to be alone together. The parent has to work out how to deal with situations where the needs of the child and those of other family members cannot be met simultaneously. If the partner brings children into the marriage, another set of role relationships must be established. The individual, in conjunction with the partner, must determine the most appropriate role in relationship to the child: surrogate parent, friend and advisor, a somewhat distant figure, and so forth. Definition of the stepparent role will also be influenced by the role which the natural, nonpartner parent plays in the child's daily life. Establishing and maintaining an appropriate stepparent role is a delicate operation that requires continual thoughtful vigilance. Indeed the role may never seem as spontaneous and straightforward as the parent role relative to one's natural child.

In forming an expanded family, new relationships often need to be established with former in-laws and with one's previous partner. The former partner may have some negative feelings about the marriage of the previous spouse. This is particularly true if the individual has not remarried or formed an intimate partnership. Negative feelings may arise from the fact of the marriage itself, from dislike or disapproval of the former spouse's new partner, or concerns about the effect of the stepparent relationship on the individual's own relationship with his or her child. The individual must also establish compatible relationships with her partner's former spouse and with her new in-laws.

A remarried, expanded family is a complex, ambiguous system. It has many nuclei and uncertain parameters. There is a continuing desire for the resolution of ambiguities, an event that is unlikely to occur. Flexibility and the capacity to live with unknowns are definitely an asset.

CHRONIC ILLNESS/DISABILITY

Chronic health or functional problems are a very real part of the human experience (6,76,406,664,728, 847,865, 899,935,981,1041). They may begin at birth or at any point in the life cycle. They may be relatively mild, such as hay fever or astigmatism, or very severe, such as paraplegia or schizophrenia. They may be physical or emotional or a combination of both. Chronic illness/disability may not seriously affect the life cycle; on the other hand, it may cause developmental delay or disrupt the life cycle entirely, as in the case of severe mental retardation and neurological impairment. Although the life cycle may not be seriously disrupted, it may be much more difficult for the individual to master developmental tasks and to attain and maintain a preferred life style. Chronic illness/disability affects not only individuals but also their family. It is a personal problem as well as a social problem.

Response to Chronic Illness/Disability

Chronic illness has been defined as

> all impairments or deviation from the normal which have one or more of the following characteristics: are permanent, leave residual disability, are caused by nonreversible pathological alterations, require special training of the patient for rehabilitation, may be expected to require a long period of supervision, observation or care (935, p. 1).

By this definition, an individual who is physically disabled is chronically ill. Many physically disabled people do not see themselves as ill, nor should they. The term "chronic illness" will be used here as an umbrella term to include all chronic health or functional problems. As the definition indicates, chronic illness refers to a relatively serious health problem. It will be used similarly in the text. However, it is important to remember that even minor chronic health problems can be a factor in the development of interests and in the decisions one makes in regards to life style.

For the purpose of clarification, chronic illness can be contrasted with acute illness, which is a brief, sudden, and severe illness. Terminal illness, on the other hand, is the final illness prior to death. It may be the final phase of a chronic illness or it may be a condition arising from some other source. All chronic illnesses are not terminal, although chronic illness may be a factor in the onset and course of the terminal illness. Terminal illness will be discussed in the final section of this chapter.

There are two types of chronic illness: acquired and developmental. An acquired chronic illness is a condition that occurs after approximately 21 years of age. A developmental chronic illness is a condition operant from birth or acquired prior to 21 years of age. The use of the age of 21 years to distinguish between acquired and developmental disability is relatively arbitrary, although now defined by law. The essential difference is in the individual's capacity to function in a relatively autonomous manner prior to the onset of the illness.

Chronic illness may be thought of as having three phases: acute, rehabilitation/habilitation, and chronic. The acute phase is the initial onset and/or a brief, sudden, and severe exacerbation of a chronic condition. The rehabilitation phase is a concerted effort on the part of the individual, usually with the help of others, to regain former capacities or to learn to live and work with remaining capacities. This phase occurs typically in acquired chronic illness. The habilitation phase is the acquisition of the ability to function and to learn to live and work with whatever capacities one is able to acquire. This phase is part of a developmental chronic illness. The chronic phase is a relatively stable period of continuing illness, with emphasis on the word "relatively."

The course of a chronic illness, the phases that occur, vary with the particular individual and the nature of a condition. Some illnesses such as hypertension rarely have an acute initial onset, whereas a cerebrovascular accident does have an acute onset. Conditions such as schizophrenic disorders and arthritis tend to have acute periods of exacerbation, whereas acute phases are less likely to occur in chronic organic mental disorders and learning disabilities. Some conditions with acute phases are also characterized by periods of remission, a diminution of some of the disabling effects of the illness. Remission is particularly common in some neuromuscular conditions such as multiple sclerosis and in collagen diseases such as lupus erythematosus. The rehabilitation/habilitation phase may never occur in any formal way, as is often the case with some forms of cancer. It may occur formally only once, such as with an individual with a leg amputation. It may be a long ongoing process, which is often true for children with cerebral palsy. Finally, it may be periodic; chronic anorexia nervosa and spina bifida are two examples. The typical course of a chronic illness will affect the developmental process. A pattern of continually repeating acute phases in childhood, for example, is likely to be detrimental to mastering age-appropriate developmental tasks.

An individual's reactions to and/or problems encountered are different in the various phases of chronic illness. In the acute phase, whether it be initial or the result of exacerbation, the individual is usually in a high state of anxiety. He is concerned about his physical or mental condition, about what is happening to his body or what is going on in his mind. Primary anxiety is compounded by the setting of most acute care: a hospital. Confined to bed or to a restricted area, the individual may experience severe sensory deprivation. Such deprivation often leads to a feeling of not being in contact with a known reality—a very scary experience. Temporal orientation may be seriously undermined. The environment, human and nonhuman, is strange; there is nothing familiar to provide support and a sense of order. The individual is often in severe pain and/or receiving high doses of medication. Both situations tend to increase disorientation and thus anxiety.

The meaning of the illness to the individual will also influence his response to the acute phase. For some individuals, taking on the sick role involves becoming the passive recipient of the care offered, accepting medication and medical procedures without question. At the other end of the continuum, the individual may see the sick role as one in which a person takes an active part in determining what medication will be taken and which medical procedures are best for him. Such an individual will seek information and raise many questions about the daily regimen. The way the individual participates in the sick role is also influenced by the degree to which he trusts and respects the medical system. He may see it as a sophisticated, competent system dedicated to maintaining his health and well-being or he may view it from essentially the opposite perspective. The sick role will be discussed in more detail in Chapter 6.

On a somewhat more personal level, the individual may be angry; why did this have to happen me? He may experience shame and guilt, feeling the illness is his fault and/or feeling that because of his illness he is neglecting his responsibilities to others. On the other hand, the individual may be rather content to be ill or at least in the hospital. The individual may see the hospital as a safe place where he can receive more skilled care than he could at home. Or the individual may be glad to be out of the anxiety-producing external environment, free from the conflicts and responsibilities inherent in that environment.

The individual's responses in the acute phase tend to be less extreme as his medical status stabilizes and as he becomes acclimated to the hospital setting. The diminution of extreme responses allows the individual to become somewhat more comfortable and able to take a more objective view of the reality of his illness and the environment.

The habilitation phase, because it is so closely related to age, will be discussed in the next part of this section. The rehabilitation phase usually begins after the initial acute phase or after a marked change in the individual's functional status. This change may be negative or positive. Response to the first rehabilitation phase will be discussed here because aspects of this response, perhaps in a milder form, often occur in most rehabilitation periods.

An individual's response to the rehabilitation phase will, to some extent, be influenced by the nature of the disability, its severity, and the possible duration. One of the major tasks of the rehabilitation phase is for the individual to recognize and accommodate to his disability. This is a long-term process and does not usually occur all at once. Recognition and accommodation may at first be fairly superficial. As the individual becomes more aware of the nature of his disability and what it means relative to his capacity to function, there is another period of recognition and accommodation. This process may be characterized as periods of gain in understanding, a plateau, and so forth. As mentioned, the process is typically quite long and may extend well into the chronic phase, or it may never be completed. Fear, anxiety, and anger are experienced frequently and intensely throughout the process.

Each individual adapts or attempts to adapt to chronic disability in his own way. The following is, however, a typical sequence of events. Initially the individual is in a state of shock and is generally numb, a feeling of being suspended in time and place. Next there is often denial that there is really anything seriously the matter; recovery is expected and one will be able, very shortly, to return to life as usual. This is followed by some acknowledgment that one does have a chronic illness that will require an alteration in life style and perhaps anticipated future goals. With this first acknowledgment, the individual's defense mechanisms are often activated. Regression, dependency, overcompensation, withdrawal, and projection are common defensive maneuvers. After a period of time these maneuvers usually prove to be ineffectual as the individual is repeatedly confronted with the reality of his situation. This leads to further acknowledgment, now with a fuller realization of the loss that has been sustained. A period of mourning for the loss frequently takes place accompanied by some degree of depression. This is a time of grieving for what could have been, for the privation and forfeiture of some dreams and plans. With successful completion of at least some mourning, there is further acknowledgment of disability. Finally the individual begins the process of making the adaptations necessary to resume the life cycle, to get about the business of living once again. This sequence is not necessarily the same for everyone nor, as mentioned, is it necessarily linear.

The process of adapting to chronic illness seemingly cannot be rushed or substantially altered. An individual can be supported in the process by others and given some guidance, but essentially the task belongs to and is the responsibility of the individual. Perhaps the two most misunderstood parts of the process are denial and the use of other defense mechanisms and mourning for lost function. Defensive reactions and maneuvers are not pathological. They are a healthy and normal response to a traumatic and stressful real situation. Just as the body has typical remedial responses to physical trauma, so does the psyche. Defense mechanisms protect the individual from being overwhelmed by painful reality before the individual is able to deal with that reality. They give the individual time to adjust at his own pace. Defensive reactions are only pathological when they are extreme or last for an exceptionally extended period of time.

Mourning for lost function allows the individual to put away those things of the past that can no longer be. The process of mourning will be discussed in the last section of this chapter. Suffice it to say here that the grieving process needs to happen and ultimately facilitates adaptation.

An individual's response to chronic illness is influenced by factors other than the nature of the disability, its severity, and possible duration. Age is one factor that will be discussed. Three of the other major factors are the individual's predisability adjustment, cultural influences, and his family's reaction. In regards to adjustment, the individual's degree of age-appropriate maturation in the various areas of human function is an important element. Also important is the extent to which the individual has a clear idea of his predisability assets and limitations and the ways in which he has coped with adversity and stress in the past. The individual's identity relative to the nature of the disability is also important. If the disability has a serious impact on one's body image, significant social roles, or important life goals, the individual's reaction is likely to be more severe. Thus an individual who prizes cognitive function may have a less profound reaction to a disability that limits physical activity than an individual who has a strong preference for active sports and games. On the other hand, the individual who prizes cognitive function may have difficulty adjusting to a condition requiring medication that interferes with clear thinking.

The individual's cultural background is likely to influence his response to chronic illness in a number of ways. In any culture there are norms, standards, and typical points of view. Some of these related to chronic illness are: (a) how pain is tolerated and feelings expressed; (b) what is considered physically attractive and what parts of the body or human capacities are believed to be most important; (c) disabilities that are considered acceptable and those that carry a degree of social stigma (e.g., hypertension versus alcoholism); (d) the degree of deviation from the norm permitted without rejection; (e) attitude toward the medical/rehabilitation system; (f) the way in which the patient or sick role should be played; (g) the value placed on self-reliance, work, and intimate relationships.

The influence of cultural background on chronic illness and all aspects of human experience will be discussed in greater detail in Chapter 6. It has been mentioned here to give an added dimension to the understanding of response to chronic illness.

Family reactions, whatever they are, will influence an individual's response to chronic illness. Specific reactions will be discussed in some detail below. Suffice it to say for now that the more supportive, accepting, and flexible family members are, the more likely the individual will be able to adapt to disability. The family can do a good deal to facilitate the individual's adjustment but it cannot perform that task for the individual.

During the rehabilitation phase of chronic illness, the individual is confronted with a variety of issues or concerns. For many people the paramount concern is the degree to which they will be able to be independent. For such individuals, the idea of being dependent is associated with loss of autonomy and being incompetent. Another concern is whether, given my disability, people will still respect, like, love me. This is a particularly important issue for individuals who have had self-doubts in this area prior to the onset of the chronic illness.

Sexuality is paramount for some individuals (100,263, 370,814). The questions often raised are will I be sexually desirable to others, will I be able to participate in sexual activities, will I be able to satisfy my partner, will I feel sexual desire, and will I be able to be satisfied sexually. These questions may not be raised initially because the individual may not feel any particular interest in sexual matters. This often happens when the onset of the illness has been acute and sudden or when the majority of energy is being expended on survival and regaining basic capacities. On the other hand, they may be of immediate concern because the individual experiences a lack of sexual desire. Regardless of when these questions are raised, they are of considerable importance.

The initial social role given first priority is usually self-care. The individual wishes to be as independent as possible in basic activities of daily living. One's role as a worker and the familial roles of parent and/or partner are second in priority. Leisure/recreation is often not given much consideration until the end of the rehabilitation phase or the beginning of the chronic phase. The same is often true relative to temporal adaptation.

The specific concerns outlined above are juxtapositioned with the individual's awareness, at least at some level, of the physical and psychological task ahead—in many cases a task of great enormity. The question of what is going to happen to me, will I be able to manage is always there.

The rehabilitation phase is rarely a smooth uninterrupted path toward adaptation. It is typically marked by a number of pauses, setbacks, and digressions. These interruptions frequently cause an increase in anxiety and activation of defensive maneuvers. Some of the events that cause interruptions are problems within the family that may or may not be related to the individual's illness, change in relationship with family members and friends, financial concerns, variation in the rate of progress, a new recognition of the degree of one's disability, anticipated discharge from the hospital or rehabilitation setting, return to the community, and problems confronted in developing a new life style. These interruptions cannot be avoided. The individual must deal with each of them as they arise, in whatever way possible at that moment in time.

It is important to remember the tremendous amount of energy expended in psychological adjustment to chronic illness, regardless of whether the disability is primarily physical or psychological in nature. There is usually less than the optimal amount of energy available for the other aspects of the rehabilitation process. The individual who has a schizophrenic disorder, for example, and the individual who has suffered severe burns both have much to learn and work to do in the rehabilitation phase. In addition, however, they are expending energy just keeping themselves together and figuring out what needs to be done in the future. It is also important to remember that the individual hurts and that he is scared. At any given moment he may want to crawl into a hole or rail at the world—somehow, any way to escape the pain.

The line between the rehabilitation and the chronic phase of illness is vague at best. It is often arbitrarily drawn at the point when the individual returns to the community after hospitalization or a period of time in a rehabilitation setting. However, there is considerable overlap between phases.

Within the chronic phase there are many tasks to be dealt with. The majority of these tasks are ongoing—resolved for a period of time perhaps but rarely solved. As the individual continues in the life cycle, these concerns will be repeatedly addressed.

Carrying Out Prescribed Regimens

This must often be done to prevent medical and psychiatric emergencies and/or to control symptoms. The individual must learn how to carry out the regimens and have enough self-discipline to carry them out in the designated manner and frequency. The time necessary to do this needs to be made a part of the individual's daily routine. Many regimens are both complex and time consuming.

Management of Medical and Psychiatric Emergencies Once They Occur

Many emergencies cannot be prevented regardless of how carefully the individual maintains prescribed regimens. In a sense the individual and family must always be prepared to act quickly and effectively in case of an emergency. A plan may need to be devised and an attitude of vigilance sustained.

Adjustment to Change in the Course of the Illness

The course of the illness may be characterized by a relatively downward trajectory or it may be marked by alternating periods of exacerbation and remission. New adjustment must be made to accommodate for increase or decrease in the capacity to function. The individual who experiences occasional remissions may, during these periods, come to believe that the remission is permanent. This may occur regardless of how well he is informed about the nature of his illness. In such a situation the individual may experience rather severe depression and anger when the illness goes into a phase of exacerbation.

Dealing with the Physical Environment

The individual who is physically disabled must often be concerned about appropriate housing, special transportation, the high cost of artificial aids, and difficulty in getting adequate and prompt repairs. For individuals with motor impairment, a decrease in energy, or neurological deficits, the physical environment of the home may need to be reorganized to allow the individual to function as independently as possible. Ideally this is accomplished in such a way that it does not unduly interfere with the life style or function of other family members. The physical environment will be discussed more fully in Chapter 6.

Funding to Pay for Treatment or to Manage Despite Partial or Complete Loss of Employment

Individuals sometimes must adjust to living on a severely reduced income with concomitant alteration of life style. This may lead to feelings of anger or self-pity. If reduced income affects other family members, the individual may experience a considerable amount of guilt. The individual may also need to learn how to secure funds from various public sources. This can be a highly complex process requiring mastery of skills in assertiveness, negotiating, and being persistent.

Reestablishing Social Roles

The individual in conjunction with family members may need to redefine his family roles, giving up some role tasks or taking on different tasks. The individual may not be able to work or engage in many favored leisure activities. With any extensive change in social roles, alteration in the individual's sense of identity is also usually required.

How to Deal with the Illness Publicly

The way in which the individual manages his illness relative to the public will depend to a great extent on the degree of stigma attached to the condition. One of the major questions is to conceal or reveal the condition to others, and to what others. The individual may wish to disguise the condition, for example, by using a cosmetic artificial hand rather than a hook on some social occasions. He may minimize the significance of a symptom or the seriousness of the condition through reassuring others that it is nothing or by the use of humor. The individual may devise ways of temporarily eliminating the handicapping element of his condition, for example, by going off a restrictive diet at parties or while on vacation. Some individuals deal with their illness by publicly announcing the illness and attempting to change the public's knowledge and attitude toward that illness.

How to Deal with Others' Responses to Clearly Visible Chronic Illness

The individual must learn how to accept and/or respond effectively to such behavior as staring, rejection, intimate personal questions about the illness or the effect it has on his life, intrusive offers of or actual assistance, and the message that one is incapable of decision making, thinking, and planning independently or of understanding communication. In dealing with such behavior, the individual must learn how to keep his, often legitimate, anger under control and how to understand prejudice.

Attempts to Normalize Both Interactions with Others and Style of Life

Despite chronic illness, most individuals want to interact with others in ways that are typical within their shared social system. In the work setting, for example, the individual may not want special considerations or privileges. Although the individual may need to alter his life style, he usually tries to keep alterations at a minimum in order to maintain his own sense of having a typical life style. The individual may, for example, prefer not to use various types of adaptive equipment, feeling they interfere with the style of life he desires.

Prevention of or Learning to Live with Social Isolation

The individual may not work and/or have difficulty participating in a variety of leisure activities. Means must be found to maintain contact with friends and relatives who do not live in the individual's home. Interests that do not involve continuous interaction with others may need to be developed.

Readjustment of Temporal Adaptation

The individual may find he has too much time, e.g., no longer employed, or too little time, e.g., physical limitations make activities of daily living very time consuming. New routines and scheduling may be required. The individual may need to adjust to potentially fragile patterns of temporal arrangements because of the typical course of his illness, i.e., exacerbations and remissions or frequent medical or psychiatric emergencies.

The tasks and concerns inherent in chronic illness require the individual to learn to care for and take care of himself. The individual must develop the ability to be mindful and considerate of himself without becoming self-preoccupied.

The Factor of Age

The age of onset of chronic illness is not only a major factor in how the individual responds to the illness but it also influences the individual's ability to master developmental tasks. Some of the effects of age are as follows.

The developmentally disabled child may, initially, have a poor nurturing experience. The essential child-parent bond may form very slowly because of the child's atypical responses, the parents' shock and sadness relative to the disabled child, and the frequent and protracted separations that may occur because of medical problems. Once formed, the bond may be exceptionally strong. (This aspect of chronic illness will be discussed further in the last part of this section.)

The preschool disabled child may take longer to assert himself and to develop the sense of autonomy that is usual by the age of three years. Age-appropriate activities of daily living may not be mastered at the usual time. The child may not engage in the play activities typical of the preschool child. The degree of self-control that most children have attained by the age of five years may not be evident. These developmental delays may be due to overprotection on the part of the parents or the child's physical or cognitive deficits or a combination of the two.

The child's awareness of his illness, of being different from other children, usually comes about slowly over a period of years. The gradualness of the process, however, does not necessarily make it less painful. As the child gains increasing awareness, there may be periods of rebelliousness, withdrawal, regression, and the like while the child struggles with a very uncomfortable reality.

Prior to beginning school, the child may have some idea of differentness. It is with entry into school, however, that the child is confronted with a reality that can no longer be concealed by family or clinic personnel. The nature of one's disability may be impressed on the child by repeatedly being excluded from many activities. The child comes to realize that a disability is significant. Although consideration and special privileges may be given, this more often than not leads to rejection on the part of other children. Benign acceptance of being different is not typical of children; the child learns about the capacity of human beings to be inhumane and cruel. The chronic aspect of the illness comes to be recognized with a concurrent diminution of the hope for a cure. One begins to settle for pragmatic solutions and the work entailed in their implementation. Just prior to adolescence, the child has usually attained the emotional readiness to see his condition as part of himself and hesitantly begins to incorporate it into his sense of self and his plans for the future.

The extent to which the child's early education takes place in a sheltered environment is likely to influence the child's awareness and acceptance of disability. The phenomenon of "mainstreaming," the education of a disabled child in the least restricted environment, is relatively new. There is more belief and hope than research documenting the efficacy of this type of education. Whether a child's ultimate adjustment is enhanced by early education in a regular classroom as opposed to a sheltered setting is unknown. There is evidence to suggest that movement from a sheltered environment to a regular classroom can be quite traumatic. The process of adapting to the new school setting may, at least temporarily, impede academic and social learning.

The disabled adolescent and young adult, in addition to the usual developmental tasks, has other concerns and issues that must be dealt with. The child may be ill prepared for the onset of adolescence because of diminished opportunity for a variety of experiences; or adolescence may be delayed for the same reason. Many disabled children are socially immature, somewhat naive about the world, and lacking in basic practical knowledge.

The physical changes leading up to puberty may result in actual deterioration in the adolescent's physical condition either permanently or temporarily. This may be due to the typical course of the illness or to the physical growth that occurs at this time. Peers may become more acutely aware of the adolescent's differences so that he may be or feel that he is being excluded from even more activities than previously. The disability itself may preclude certain activities that provide social status and feelings of competence, for example, dancing, athletics, and driving an automobile. The emphasis on physical attractiveness, so common in the adolescent period, may cause the individual to feel that he is ugly and unlovable. Sexual maturation with its concomitant problem of impulse control may be particularly difficult for the socially immature disabled adolescent. The individual's previously accepted affectionate behavior may no longer be considered "cute" or acceptable to others. Leaving school may be a shock since realistic preparation for the role of a worker and for an occupation may have been inadequate. The handicapped youth is often ill prepared for all adult social roles.

The developmentally disabled individual often experiences an extended habilitation phase, which usually begins with recognition of the illness and continues until the individual has progressed to the acquisition of the major adult social roles or until no further marked change can be anticipated. As in all chronic conditions, the individual usually maintains involvement with medical services of one kind or another. Habilitation differs from rehabilitation in many respects. The initial trauma of adjusting to the illness and required change of life style is absent. The individual has a minimum of past experiences on which to build. In addition to dealing with the sequela of the illness, typical of both the habilitation and rehabilitation process, habilitation is much more focused on developmental tasks. The individual involved in habilitation usually has a much greater degree of dependence on family members, both physically and psychologically.

The individual's involvement in formal habilitation may be episodic or continuous; it may occur in a clinical setting, either on an inpatient or an outpatient basis, or it may occur in a residential setting or within the context of a special or regular school. The individual's response to the habilitation process, at any given time, is influenced by past experience with the health delivery system and the individual's current interests, developmental issues, and psychological state. The individual may fear interaction with "strangers" or unknown procedures; he may be uncooperative and in general difficult to engage or even tolerate. On the other hand, he may be more than willing to investigate something new and different, be cooperative in participating in suggested activities, and be full of humor and good will. Or he may be all of the above within a matter of days, if not hours.

The response to an acquired disability from late adolescence onward is much as was described in the discussion of the rehabilitation and chronic phases of illness. The factor of age is an overlay on this response. The late adolescent and young adult tend to be concerned about how the illness will affect the attainment of all of their hopes and dreams—all that has been untried, not experienced, not lived. In particular, the individual is concerned about marriage, being able to have a family, being able to work. A relatively young individual may have had little experience with adverse conditions or a serious loss. Thus his capacity to cope with difficulties and problems may be neither tested nor refined. On the other hand, the younger individual is usually relatively physically healthy, often appears to have an unlimited amount of energy, and does not yet have a firm life style. Therefore the individual may be able to address the problems presented vigorously and with considerable flexibility.

The older person who acquires a chronic illness tends to be concerned about how he will be able to care for his family and if he will be able to continue to work. If the condition is associated with the aging process, the individual is directly confronted with the fact of his aging and the reality of death. In addition to the acquired chronic condition, therefore, the individual is faced with other issues that need to be addressed. Having more life experiences, the individual may have already seen the end of some dreams and hopes. He may have developed effective coping mechanisms that can be brought to bear on the presented problems. On the other hand, he may find it more difficult to change a settled and comfortable life style. The individual in the 35 to 50 year age group may see the onset of a chronic illness, in retrospect, as a fortuitous opportunity. Such an individual may experience the event as an occasion to review life goals, to set new priorities, and to rearrange his life. The advent of an acquired disability may be seen as a second chance and the opportunity to make a new start.

For the elderly individual the onset of chronic illness may be viewed as the end of life. The fear of death, no longer latent, may now become a preoccupation. The illness may be an addition to other chronic conditions and interrelated with the aging process in general. The individual may feel helpless and extremely vulnerable. There may be loss of hope as the individual recognizes the irreversibility of the condition. The fantasy that the chronic illness will somehow go away, often used by a younger individual, is less likely to be available to the elderly person. The feeling of one's body changing and the body monitoring which starts in middle age may now become more pronounced. For the elderly individual chronic illness menas more visits to physicians, more and longer hospital stays, and a more lengthy period of rehabilitation. The individual may, in turn, be annoyed, worried, or bored by the various routines and procedures. The elderly person is more prone to the side effects of drugs. Dizziness, loss of appetite, weakness, nausea, dulling of consciousness, and the sedating effect of some medication may be particularly demoralizing for the elderly individual. Side effects may lead to a sense of disorientation, confusion, and a feeling of not being able to cope with even minor problems. The individual may perceive his capacity to function as far more seriously impaired than objective data suggest. The former in many cases is far more important than the latter.

Although age is a factor in response to chronic illness, it is important to remember that there are other factors that influence the individual's reaction and capacity to adjust. Relative to age, response may be based more on where the individual perceives he is in the life cycle or developmental tasks mastered and those yet to be addressed rather than on chronological age. It is also important to remember that age-specific tasks continue. They are not suspended but rather impinge on and affect all phases of chronic illness.

Family Interaction

The first reaction of a family to the chronic illness of one of its members is usually shock and disbelief. Initially the family is usually capable of coming together to deal with the practical tasks inherent in the situation. With the relief of the immediate emergency, the family may disorganize for a period of time. There then tends to be a slow recovery and a reorganization of the family. The post-acute illness organization may be different in that familial roles may be restructured, particularly relative to tasks and responsibilities. The various reactions and course of events, tasks, and concerns outlined relative to the individual also occur within the family. This is true for all three phases: acute, rehabilitation/habilitation, and chronic. Essentially the family goes through the same phases as the individual.

The family's response is, of course, influenced by the degree and type of disability and on whether the individual is likely to return home. The structures the family has for dealing with internal stress are also a significant factor. Of primary importance is the degree to which family members are able to support each other. The internal support system may or may not be augmented by the extended and expanded family and the family's external support system. The individual's role in the family is also important. It has been found, for example, that a family in which the mother becomes disabled is more likely to become seriously disorganized and slower to reorganize than if the disabled individual is the father. Depending on the nature of the disability and the individual disabled, some family interaction patterns are likely to be more strained than others. Severe arthritis of a mother may, for example, cause strain in her sexual relationship with her partner. It may not cause any difficulty in the relationship with her two sons. However, it is important to note that strain in one family interaction pattern is likely to cause strain on other patterns. The place of the family in the family cycle is also an important factor in the response to chronic illness.

Although the family may be considered as a unit, it is made up of individuals. Each family member will respond in his or her own way. The response will be affected by age, sex, personality, and so forth. A family member's response will also be influenced by the relationship to the disabled individual, parent-child and partner relationships usually being the most significant.

There are several issues and tasks that the family or a family member must deal with. Some of the major concerns follow.

Resolution of Anger and Guilt

Anger at the disabled individual for disrupting one's life is an extremely common response. It essentially takes the form of the rhetorical question, "How could you do this to me?" Disruption may be in the form of serious alteration in life plans and expectations or relative to the necessity of taking on more responsibilities. The young adult, for example, who is raising a family may find a disabled parent a tremendous financial and emotional burden. Feelings of anger are usually soon followed by guilt over having such feelings. Unshared and unresolved anger and guilt can be extremely disruptive to ongoing family relationships.

Making a Life for Oneself Apart from the Disabled Individual

This task is particularly important for the primary caretaker of the disabled individual—be it a child, partner, or parent. There is a tendency for the primary caretaker to make the disabled individual the center of his daily life and future plans. Motivated by a misguided sense of love and a good deal of guilt, such an orientation is extremely detrimental. It leads to further anger and guilt on the part of the caretaker and places a considerable burden on the disabled individual. In addition, it makes the caretaker less effective in his task.

Providing Physical Care

This may become the responsibility of the family or of one family member. If this is not possible because of the severity of the disability or because no family member is willing and/or able to take on this responsibility, the family must make arrangements for this care. Outside help may be found to enable the individual to stay in the family home. Finding such help is often difficult, as is keeping a helping person for a long period of time. There is likely to be a good deal of turnover in personnel. Finding and teaching a helper to care for the individual can be a time-consuming task. Having a nonfamilial person in the home also may cause difficulties in family relationships. If the disabled individual cannot be cared for in the home, arrangements for institutional care of one kind or another must be made.

Assisting the Disabled Individual to Be as Independent as Possible

This is closely related to the issue of physical care. The more independent the person is able to be, the less are the demands placed on other family members. The individual is also more likely to be able to stay with the family. The two major impediments to helping the individual to become self-sufficient are feelings of sympathy and guilt and family member lack of knowledge of how to assist the individual toward independence. In addition, many times, it just seems easier for a family member to do something for the individual. It often takes less time and the family member does not have to experience the struggle of the individual as he attempts to carry out a particular task.

Giving Support to the Chronically Ill Individual

The major support needed is emotional, although financial support may be necessary also. In providing emotional support, the family must communicate feelings of love and acceptance and assurance that they will meet present and future legitimate needs. Support, it must be noted, does not mean smothering or treating the individual as if he were incompetent. The task of giving continuous emotional support can be greatly facilitated by teaching and/or encouraging the disabled individual to meet the emotional needs of other family members. This can only occur, however, if family members turn to the disabled individual for need satisfaction.

Maintaining the Individual's Role in the Family

This is important both during the habilitation/rehabilitation and the chronic phases. Adjustment to chronic illness is greatly impeded if the individual begins to realize that he has no functional part in the affairs of the family. The individual's role in the family becomes that of "the handicapped member"—hardly a satisfying role, or one that will encourage the individual to reengage in the mastery of developmental tasks. The majority of disabled individuals are able to fulfill the interpersonal aspect of role performance; the task aspect might need to be altered. A father, for example, may not be able to play catch with his daughter but he is still able to provide the love and guidance that are part of the parent role. The individual who is unable to work may compensate for lack of that social role by taking responsibility for additional household tasks. When the role performance of one individual in a family changes, the role performance of all family members is likely to be altered to some degree. This will necessitate adjustment for everyone involved, adjustment that may take a good period of time to accomplish.

Changes in Life Style

Change in family life style may be due to an alteration in the family's financial situation. There may be a decrease in income or part of the family income may need to be spent on the care of the disabled member. The nature of the individual's illness may preclude various recreational and leisure activities the family had previously enjoyed together. The individual's disability may be such that he needs considerable rest and a calm environment. Younger children's exhuberant activities may need to be curtailed and older children may only occasionally be allowed to invite friends to their home.

Adjustments in Temporal Adaptation

Typical family routines may need to be altered to accommodate the disabled individual. Meals, for example, may be served earlier, later, or take a longer period of time. Time may be required to take care of the disabled individual. If and when hospitalized, arrangements must be made for visits. This is particularly time consuming if the individual is hospitalized some distance from home.

Finding and Using Community Resources

Similar to the individual, the family or a family member may need to become skilled in negotiating for available funds and resources.

The Developmental Task of Family Members

Age-specific tasks continue regardless of whether there is a disabled member. Parents must attend to the developmental needs of all of their children. They cannot afford to concentrate the majority of their attention on one child or on a partner. Similarly, children ought not to be given responsibilities that are either beyond their capacity to carry out successfully or that interfere excessively with their school work or leisure time activities.

The above discussion related to the reactions and concerns of families to a chronically ill family member was general in nature. The next portion of this section will deal with more specific issues.

The Chronically Ill Child

Families with a chronically ill child have some additional difficulties not covered in the general discussion (153,814). The parents of a child who is obviously different at birth experience shock and grief almost immediately. Other infants seem to be somewhat deviant at birth or shortly thereafter. Problems may be suspected but their nature and extent are not evident until somewhat later. It is often difficult to pinpoint infant abnormalities during the early months. Differential diagnosis in young children is a formidable task, particularly when the child has multiple disabilities. Many parents spend considerable time, money, and energy seeking a definitive diagnosis and treatment for a child who does not seem to be following a normal pattern of development.

The chronically ill child presents young parents, who often have had little child rearing experience, with many problems. It is a test of their ability and their capacity to adjust in the face of great difficulty. Infants who are not healthy often respond in ways that do not elicit a positive response in parents. They may be minimally responsive, not nurse properly, engage in continual and intense crying, become rigid on contact, have abnormal reflex patterns, struggle against being held, or exhibit other unusual behavior. The child may be in a physically unstable condition and there may be realistic concern about the child's survival. There may be a long period of separation before the child is able to leave the hospital and/or the child may be repeatedly hospitalized during the first months of life.

After the initial shock, parents may experience a sense of great sadness. They often feel angry, embarrassed, a revulsion for the child, and guilty in that they hold themselves personally responsible for the child's deficits. They may be uncertain about their worth in that they have produced a less than perfect child. Consequently, they may question their capacity to care for the child and to engage in a nurturing relationship. This, obviously, is not an ideal situation for fostering the formation of the child-parent bond. Parents of chronically ill infants initially have considerable difficulty in feeling love and affection for their child. The bonding tends to occur somewhat later than is the case between a healthy child and parents.

In addition to the difficulties described, the parents must deal with the response of family members and friends. Their response may be negative or they may simply not know what to say or do. The usual patterns of visiting, religious ceremonies, and family celebrations associated with birth may not occur or be strained at best. Thus the social rituals marking a significant occasion in the life cycle are not properly observed. For the parents there is a sense of emptiness and a feeling they have participated in a non-event.

The physical care of a disabled child is often an anxiety-provoking, time-consuming, and physically demanding task. Parents may be uncertain about how to position the child for ease and comfort in feeding, dressing, and bathing. There may be complex prescribed regimens to follow and emergency procedures to learn. Adequate information, guidance, and support may not be available. Parents may be uncertain about how to play with the child, fearing both a negative response from the child and that they will somehow harm the child. Enjoyment of the child may be limited simply because so much time and energy is involved in physical care.

The parents of a child with a chronic illness are faced with many tasks in addition to those typical of child rearing; or the tasks are made more complex because of the child's illness. Some of these tasks follow.

Physical Demands

As a severely disabled child grows older there are increasing physical demands. This is particularly true if the child is unable to walk, dress, and feed himself and take care of his elimination needs independently. The physical demands are also great when a child must be constantly under observation. This occurs particularly in the case of children who are destructive of the self or the environment or who do not have the cognitive ability to maintain their own safety. The physical demands of parenting are often one of the major factors in deciding to place a child in some type of a protected environment.

Coordination of Services

Finding adequate services for a child is sometimes very difficult. This is particularly true if the child's diagnosis is questionable, if the child has multiple disabilities, and/or if the family lives outside a large metropolitan area. The child may need services provided by a variety of different sources. The parents must establish good communication with a large number of service providers, including the school system. It is usually the parents who must take the responsibility for maintaining some degree of cooperation, order, and communication between the various institutions providing services. The parents must either provide or arrange for transportation for the child. This is particularly difficult if both parents work or if there are other young children in the family. Because finding and coordinating services is such a problematic task, many families are very hesitant to move to a new location, even if this would be financially advantageous for the family. Appropriate schools, habilitation facilities, and other necessary services may not be available. The mobility of the family may be severely limited.

Being a Therapist

Many disabled children are placed on a home program with the expectation that the parents will act as therapists. It is questionable whether this is a particularly wise plan. Mixing the roles of therapist and parent may be detrimental to the child-parent relationship. This is particularly true when the therapeutic maneuvers are painful, seriously resisted by the child, and/or time consuming. The parent is put into the position of insisting that the child do something he does not want to do. This is in addition to the typical discipline all parents must impose. The child may come to see the parents as rigid in their demands and unsympathetic to his needs. Therepeutic maneuvers become one more source of conflict between parent and child. The time spent in therapeutic activities may be far better used in playing with and enjoying the child. On the other hand, parents may have little choice in the matter. The child may need daily periods of therapeutic activities. It may be both too demanding of time and energy and too expensive to bring the child to a clinic every day. Daily home treatment by a therapist is prohibitively expensive.

Public Reaction

Parents must find some way to deal with other people's response to their child. As previously mentioned, people often react with a good deal of insensitivity if not negativistically to individuals who look or act differently. Parents must also help the child to understand these reactions and to respond appropriately to them. It also helps if both parents and child can somehow develop a relatively thick skin.

Dependency versus Independence

One problem in helping a child to develop an appropriate degree of autonomy is the reality of the child's dependency on the parents. For example, a child who cannot dress himself is dependent. Parents must find areas where the child can be independent. The other problem is related to parental concerns. Out of fear for their child's safety some parents may unduly restrict the child's activities. There is a fine, often difficult line to draw between what is probably safe and what may be dangerous. The child's developmental needs must be taken into consideration as well as the precautions arising from his illness. The parent must often legitimately act as a protective, assistive, controlling agent far beyond that required by the parent of a healthy child. This leaves far less room for the child to establish a sphere of autonomy.

Discipline

Closely related to the development of autonomy is the matter of discipline. It is difficult for many parents of chronically ill children to set and maintain firm expectations regarding appropriate behavior. This difficulty may be due to one of two factors or a combination of both. It is difficult to discipline a child who is sick. There is a natural tendency to set less strict limitations, to be more lenient, to feel sorry for a child burdened by deficits. On the other hand, chronically ill children sometimes have a good deal of difficulty controlling their behavior due to emotional problems, neurological impairment, or mental retardation. Discipline of such children requires considerable firmness, patience, and fortitude. An undisciplined child disrupts a family and limits the child's opportunity to interact in the community. Not setting and maintaining firm expectations is ultimately detrimental to everyone involved, including the child.

Motivation

Parents of disabled children must often be concerned with motivating their children to engage in activities in which the child may not perceive any immediate intrinsic reward. It is easy for a child to lose interest when the end goal of mastery is such a distant possibility. Children are likely to become bored, anxious, and rebellious. Withdrawal from various activities is not unusual. Motivation must somehow be maintained relative not only to the habilitation process but also to activities of daily living, school, and potential recreational activities. As may be obvious, the parents also must find the means to maintain their own motivation and to combat the realistic tendency to become discouraged.

Sexuality

In regard to masturbation, the distinction between privately acceptable versus publicly acceptable behavior may be difficult for the blind, retarded, or emotionally disturbed child to understand. Excessive masturbation is not uncommon and may be entirely unrelated to sexuality. The child may masturbate because of physical irritation (e.g., tight underpants, skin rash, brace straps rubbing the genital area), to gain attention, because he is bored, and so forth. It is particularly important that disabled children be prepared for the physical changes and increased sexual desire of puberty. Parents may be so concerned about whether their child will ever be independent that it takes priority over the question of sexuality. Chronically ill children may be so restricted in their experience with peers that the considerable amount of sexual information gained from that source may not be available to them.

Contraceptive issues must also be addressed. The use of chemical birth control agents may be contraindicated because of the documented or questionable interaction between such agents and the medication being taken by the individual. The nature of the individual's illness may also increase the risks related to the use of chemical birth control agents. Mechanical contraceptives may be contraindicated where there is loss of genital sensation or when motor dysfunction (e.g., paralysis, spasticity, and athetoses) interferes with convenient and effective use. Intrauterine devices (IUDs) have some side effects, and can be pulled out or expelled. Mechanical contraceptives and IUDs cannot always be used effectively by individuals who are mentally retarded or by individuals who are impulsive, emotionally labile, sexually promiscuous, and the like.

Sterilization of mentally retarded and emotionally disturbed individuals who are not considered able to be responsible parents is a matter of some controversy. In its favor, it eliminates the concerns parents or other caretakers may have about the individual becoming pregnant or impregnating a woman. The children of individuals who are mentally retarded are likely to be of low intelligence due to hereditary factors or the lack of a stimulating home environment. These children may become a burden to society. Retarded and emotionally disturbed individuals who are sterilized are able to move more freely about the community without supervision. It also makes living in a group home more feasible. Sterilization may allow the individual to share sexual satisfaction and affection with a solicitous partner. Involuntary sterilization, on the other hand, is considered by some to be a violation of human rights. In some states it can only be done if approved by the courts and/or a board of independent medical examiners. The decision to seek sterilization for one's child is a very difficult decision for many parents to make.

The rearing of a child with a chronic illness puts a great deal of stress on the parental pair. The major burden of care frequently falls on the mother. With the father presumably away at work all day, the mother must deal with the day-to-day problems alone and frequently unassisted. Because of continuous close contact, the mother is prone to become overly involved with the child, having little life or interest of her own. She may be angry that she is unable to work or have more leisure time and that she is carrying the major responsibility for the child. Finally, she is likely to be very exhausted. The father, away all day, may not be particularly involved in the child's rearing or in the habilitation process. In the evening the home situation may not be particularly comfortable, with a tired and perhaps angry wife and a child that needs extraordinary attention. This stressful situation may disrupt the partner relationship. The individuals may stay in the same household and go their separate ways or the partnership may be dissolved.

Fewer individuals who are developmentally disabled marry than individuals who are not disabled. Whether a disabled individual marries is to a great extent dependent on how he perceives himself physically, esthetically, and socially. Another factor is his and his family's attitudes toward the whole idea of a person with his type of disability getting married. The individual may or may not have been raised with anticipation of a future marital role.

There are no statistics available on whether disabled individuals tend to marry other disabled people or people who are nondisabled. When married, however, they face the same problems and issues as the abled. For two individuals who are severely disabled, marriage may be of greater significance because they are not able to participate in a variety of other social roles. The question of whether to have children is somewhat more complex for disabled individuals. One factor that must be considered is whether the parent's disability is genetically linked and the probability of children inheriting the disabling condition. The potential parents must decide whether they want to take the risk of having a disabled child. This risk has been considerably reduced by medical advances relative to the monitoring of the developing fetus and the option of abortion. Other factors to be considered are whether pregnancy may in any way exacerbate the woman's condition and whether the partners feel they are physically and emotionally capable of rearing a child.

Acquired Chronic Illness and Sexuality

The last part of this section will outline the relationship between acquired chronic illness and sexuality: an important aspect of family interaction (100,263,370,694, 814). The onset of a chronic illness is likely to have some effect on the sexual relationship between partners, at least temporarily. A person who is in pain or feels ill and debilitated is often not particularly interested in pursuing sexual activities. The sense of loss, accepting the chronic nature of the illness, and adjusting to disability also lead to a diminished interest in sexuality and capacity to engage in sexual activities. With the onset of a chronic illness, the individual's sexual identity and his self-esteem may suffer a severe blow. Such a situation is very detrimental to satisfactory sexual relationships. It is important to remember that there is often a wide discrepancy between the sexual function of the individual (what he is actually able to do) and the individual's current feelings about his sexual capacity and desirability.

During the rehabilitation phase, as mentioned, the individual is often preoccupied with whether he is a lovable person. The partner may also be concerned with whether she will be able to love this person. If the individual has become physically altered in any way, there is often a feeling of shared vulnerability when clothes are shed. The partners must face the deformity and related problems, if any, together. Changes in familial roles and the conflict inherent in such change may interfere with the intimate sharing of ideas and feelings. The newly ill individual may be so wrapped up in his own needs, losses, and frustrations that he is unable to attend to the needs of his partner. The partner in turn may experience this as indicative of rejection. In addition, the healthy partner may be preoccupied with anger and guilt and also be mourning her partner's loss. For both partners there is often the fear that sexual intimacies may cause further injury. This is true even in cases where the disability bears no particular relationship to the sexual act. The above fears, worries, and preoccupations can markedly interfere with sexual adjustment, at least for a period of time.

Above and beyond the psychological factor, there are some chronic illnesses that functionally limit some sexual interaction. The disability apparently studied the most relative to sexuality is spinal cord lesions. The level of the lesion and whether or not it is complete are an important factor. Because of sensory loss, few men or women experience orgasm. Whether a man experiences orgasm seems to be dependent on the intactness of sensations associated with the muscle contractions of ejaculation. Both men and women can be sexually aroused by tactile stimulation above the level of the lesion. For men there is a high degree of impotence and sterility. However, many men are able to attain an erection. The fertility of women is not affected. At the time of injury the menstrual cycle may be interrupted but usually returns in about six months. A woman can become pregnant and have a normal delivery. A catheter or bowel and/or bladder incontinence may complicate sexual activities but they do not in and of themselves prohibit intercourse. Individuals with spinal cord lesions continue to have strong sexual urges. These are sometimes fulfilled through fantasy and dreams, with satisfaction being similar to the type of satisfaction experienced before the trauma. The individual may experience fantasy or phantom orgasm. This is done apparently through mentally intensifying an existing sensation from some neurologically intact portion of their body and reassigning the sensation to their genitals. Empathetic gratification can also be experienced when the partner achieves orgasm.

Other chronic conditions have been less well studied. The following information, however, has been fairly well documented:

- Cardiovascular insult—It is usually suggested that the individual wait for 8 to 12 weeks before resuming sexual activities; no other sexual problems exist.
- Cerebrovascular accident—May be some weakness but no other difficulty.
- Prostate surgery—With the most common type of surgery (transurethral resection), function usually re-

turns but ejaculation is retrograde into the bladder. With extirpation of the prostate, the capacity for erection is lost but orgasm is still possible.

- Urinary surgery or colostomies—For men the situation may vary from full capacity for erection and orgasm to complete impotence. Women are far more likely to experience orgasm.
- Diabetes—There is a decrease in the secretion of pituitary gonadotropin, which affects the erective responses in men and leads to sterility due to retroflux ejaculation into the bladder. This usually occurs quite early in the course of the illness. The decrease in gonadotropin in women leads to an absence of orgasm, but this usually occurs much later in the course of the illness. Sexual interest continues and remains constant for both men and women.
- Muscular dystrophy—Does not affect sexual functioning directly except for cosmetic changes.
- Multiple sclerosis—May lead to impotence or ejaculatory difficulties but appears to cause no problems for women.
- Hepatic and renal disorders—Diminished sexual interest, particularly in the acute phase because of fatigue, lethargy, and despondency. There is a deterioration in sexual function after development of uremia, which often continues even after treatment.
- Pulmonary diseases—Low physical endurance may cause some difficulties.
- Arthritis—Joint inflammation and degeneration may lead to diminished motion and pain in hip joints.
- Alcoholism—Impotence may continue even after years of sobriety due to peripheral nerve damage. Women appear to have no sexual difficulties.
- Depression—Often a significant decrease in sexual interest and activity.
- Chemotherapy—Depending on the medication, may lead to a decrease in sexual interest for one or both sexes. Men may experience impotence and inhibited ejaculation. Women of child bearing age must also be concerned about the effect of medication on the fetus. The relation between medication and chemical contraceptives has been mentioned previously.

In conclusion, illness is a part of the life cycle and has a profound effect on that cycle. It can never be dealt with as an abnormal or atypical phenomenon. It is a part of life, a part of the human experience—as is death, the last moment in the life cycle of an individual.

DEATH AND LOSS

Death and loss cannot be separated from life. For the individual, one's own death is always there at some point in the near or far future. The death of others influences the individual throughout the life cycle. Loss—of a dream, of a friend, of a treasured object, and so forth—is a relatively common experience for everyone. Death and loss can only be accommodated through adequate grief and mourning. Without such an experience, death and loss remain a pernicious factor that may have a negative effect on the individual's future adaptation.

The Meaning of Death

Death, the one certain event in the life cycle, has multiple interpretations (504,620,689). These interpretations vary from one culture to another and according to the circumstances of the death. Because of the unknowns that surround death—when it will occur and what happens after life—it is an event shrouded in mystery, awe, and considerable anxiety.

Death is an individual experience, but beyond that it is a biological, psychological, and social event. It is biological in the sense that it is the end of life as we know and understand life to be. The life-sustaining functions of the human body cease. Death is psychological in the responses it engenders: fear, anxiety, rage, grief. It is psychological in its effect on the individual: anticipation of one's own death and dealing with the death of others. Death is a social event for it has an impact on the social systems of the family, community, and at times the nation. Death is the loss of one member in the social system and it is evidence to all of the fragility of life and the mystery of death. For these reasons and to comfort those who grieve, death has traditionally been surrounded by many social customs and ceremonies. In many cultures the events surrounding death have been quite elaborate. Although varied in form, they are typically designed to honor the dead individual, to facilitate mourning, and to reaffirm life and the life cycle. The social events surrounding death in industrial Western society are far less elaborate than those in other cultures. There are many reasons for this, chief among them probably being emphasis on the secular and rational and general avoidance of the reality of death.

The meaning of death to an individual is, ultimately, a very personal matter. It is, however, often some combination of or variation on a number of themes. The following are some of the common meanings of death.

- It is not a part of me—The individual interprets death as something that happens to someone else, not to herself. Even in the face of a high probability of death, the individual feels she will be untouched; her luck will hold. This evasionary way of thinking, the denial that death will occur except in some very distant future, is extremely common. It seems to allow the individual to be free of a threat or some sort of contamination. It is a way of defending against the anxiety of death, permitting the individual to continue life untroubled.

- It is an active force—Death is seen as an entity that has an existence of its own. It is seen as attacking its victims. There is the sense of not having any control over its capricious choice. This meaning of death often occurs in the context of accidental death, violent death, and the death of a young person.
- It is a passive factor—Death is seen as a culmination of a process which is the individual's life. It is seen as the natural course of events, inevitable and thus understandable.
- It is a mythological being—Death takes the form of an animal or a creature which appears in human form. As such it is found in folklore, literature, dance, the visual arts, and waking and sleeping fantasies. In medieval Europe, death was often represented as the grim reaper: a human skeleton with a scythe over his shoulder. Death has also been symbolized as a pale horse, an angel, a gay deceiver. The dance of death is sedate; death is so powerful, extreme movements are not needed.
- It is the great leveler—All individuals, no matter how prominent or powerful, will die. In death, even the most humble are equal to the great.
- It is the great validator—In death the individual's worth is judged. This evaluation may be seen as the prerogative of the living. Or it may be seen as taking place in the hereafter, where one is rewarded for good and punished for evil.
- It is symbolic—The death of an individual or individuals can take on a meaning which is far greater than the death itself. Individuals may die for a cause, such as those in Northern Ireland who died in a hunger strike. The deaths of Martin Luther King, Jr., John Lennon, and the Holocaust had and have tremendous symbolic meaning.
- It unites—In death the individual comes once again to be with those she loved.
- It separates—Death brings a relationship to an end. The loved one is no more; the survivor is left alone.
- It is the ultimate problem or the ultimate solution—Death is there to be faced over and over again, to be reckoned with, reconciled to; it pervades all of life. Conversely, death will bring peace, cessation to the struggle; it will be a welcome end to life.

Very closely related to the meaning of death is the interpretation of what happens after death. Similar to the many meanings of death there are many interpretations of afterlife. Afterlife is probably most commonly thought of as an altered state of being. As such it may be characterized in several ways.

- Life as usual—Afterlife is considered essentially to be similar to life in this world. The individual is the same after death but in another world and faces similar crises and challenges as in life.
- Perpetual development—Afterlife is the process of evolving into a higher state of consciousness. Death is only one step in continued development.
- Cycling and recycling—Afterlife is only a temporary state of being. The individual after a period of time will be reborn as a human being or some other form of life.
- Enfeebled life—There is continued existence after death but the individual does not do very much of anything. This belief, whether the individual was in heaven or the underworld, was typical in ancient times and is still quite dominant today.
- Waiting—Initially afterlife is a period of waiting for the final judgment: an unspecified time when all human beings will be evaluated. Subsequently everyone will proceed to their ultimate destination or condition.

In contrast to a state of being, death by some people is considered to be a state of nonbeing or actually no state at all. Afterlife in any form does not exist. Death is the endpoint of a biological process. There is, however, a good deal of medical and legal controversy about when death actually occurs.

Death is most commonly thought of as taking place in the more advanced stages of the life cycle. As such, death is usually referred to as occurring from natural causes. But death from "unnatural" causes is also fairly common. Killing, accidents, disasters, and suicide are part of the human experience. Cultural groups assign varying degrees of positive value to human life and consequently have various norms regarding the taking of human life. Killing of one kind or another may be condemned, condoned, or treated with indifference. Cultural groups, therefore, have different attitudes toward capital punishment, war, systematic killing for political or religious reasons, terrorism, murder, abortion, access to sufficient nutritional supplies, poor sanitation, safety precautions in industry, and the like.

Most individuals have difficulty making sense of accidents and disasters: fire, flood, earthquakes, hurricanes, household accidents, and transportation casualties. It appears far easier to seek to blame others rather than seeing them as random events or blaming oneself. Warning-predicting-preventing systems or methods may be inefficient for several reasons: individuals prefer not to leave disaster prone areas, have a sense of personal immunity, interpret death from disaster or accidents as only happening to those who ought to be punished, or individuals are unwilling to be inconvenienced. The avoidance of the idea of the possibility of death as described above is in itself a statement about attitudes toward death. Basically it could be interpreted in two different ways: that death is too anxiety provoking to consider or that people do not hold their life in very high regard.

Suicide is the form or means of death that is probably the most laden with emotional overtones. It is rarely treated with indifference by any social system. In various societies at various times suicide has been considered to be sinful, a criminal act, a sign of character weakness, evidence of mental illness, honorable, and a rational alternative to pain and suffering. In his classic study of suicide, Durkheim attributed rates of suicide to various types of relationships between the individual and society. He felt that there were four relationships that lead to high rates of suicide:

1. Deficits in society's control over the individual;
2. Excessive integration of the individual into a society that condones suicide;
3. The individual suffers a rupture in his relationship to society;
4. Society is oppressive and blocks individual fulfillment.

Durkheim took a sociological approach to suicide (620). Other explanations have been based on philosophy, interpersonal problems, or intrapsychic conflicts. It is probably safest to say that suicide has no simple causes that can be easily established.

A particular individual's reasons for committing suicide are varied. In a successful suicide, the reasons, obviously, can only be surmised. Some of the common reasons are believed to be: a desire for reunion with loved ones, a means of finding rest and refuge, a punishment to others, and a self-imposed penalty for failure. It is believed that many suicides were a mistake, never intended to be carried through to completion. It is also believed that many deaths that appear to be accidental may well be disguised suicides.

There are numerous myths about suicide which are common in our society. Some of these myths are: a person who talks about suicide will not acutally take his or her life, only specific classes of people take their own life (e.g., the poor, the rich), only depraved or mentally ill people commit suicide, the tendency to commit suicide is inherited, suicide is related to the weather or cosmic influences, suicide can be prevented, or suicide can only be prevented by a psychiatrist or a mental health facility. Myths regarding suicide and the emotional overtones of suicide have contributed to our lack of understanding of this phenomenon. They have also made suicide perhaps the most difficult form of death for family members and friends to deal with adequately.

Death tends to have different meanings as the individual advances through the life cycle (504). Interpretations of death are highly culture-bound. The meanings of death relative to the life cycle to be outlined here are derived from studies in industrial Western society. Children do think about death even at a very young age. It is a frequent theme in childhood fantasy as the child tries to figure out the meaning of death. Between the ages of three and five years, death is seen as a continuation of life but on a reduced level. It is seen as temporary and in many ways analogous to sleep. Ideas of departure and separation as in a person going away are common. In a more negative vein, children in this age group think of death as a lonely, scary experience. There is considerable focus on the coffin. They feel it would be boring to be in a coffin and express fears about not being able to get out of the coffin and of being buried alive. To children between five and nine years of age, death is seen as a final irreversible event. They frequently represent death as a person or some animate being. Many believe that by killing this personification that death will not occur. The idea that death may be eluded is also common.

After the age of nine years, children perceive death as personal, universal, and inevitable but on rather an abstract level. Adolescents and young adults frequently romanticize death: dying of a mysterious illness, dying for a cause, or departing in a blaze of glory. Their fantasies often include the idea of dying young, sometimes as a way of punishing parents or peers or as a manifestation of the fear of growing up or growing old. Death becomes more real as the individual advances through the life cycle. The personal realization of death comes at a different point in the life cycle for each individual. Death frequently begins to be used as a measure of time between 40 and 50 years of age. The idea is often expressed in "given the amount of time I have left, I would like to. . . ." The individual feels that she would like to have a particular experience or to try something new. There is also the idea that it makes no difference what others will think for it will not matter after death. In the advanced period of the life cycle or in terminal illness, the individual on the threshold of death comes to terms with life.

Death is the endpoint of life for an individual, but that is only one aspect of death. For most individuals death punctuates the life cycle, as we are periodically forced to adapt to the death of loved ones, those we admired, assassinations, the trauma of war, and natural disasters. The death of a loved one is often seen as important, sometimes more important than one's own death. Death is also viewed as the affirmation or renewal of life. This is exemplified perhaps best in the death of a national leader. In England, for example, the death of a king is announced with the proclamation, "The King is dead; long live the King."

In conclusion, it is only through understanding the meaning of death to another person that we are able to comprehend their grief and assist in their mourning. It is not wise to assume that what death means to oneself is similar to what death means to another person.

Terminal Illness and Dying

In essence, dying is not a time-limited event that begins shortly before death (105,127,154,155,171, 272,497,531,570,733,771,849,853). Rather is begins from the moment of birth. Aging is a slow process of dying. Dying, however, as a time-limited event usually begins with a somewhat more clearly defined point of onset. Pragmatic modes of defining onset are: (a) when it is recognized by medical personnel that nothing more can be done to preserve life; (b) when those significant to the individual realize death is imminent; (c) when the individual accepts at some level (i.e., cognitively or emotionally) that she is dying.

These various modes of onset do not necessarily occur at the same time. Some individuals know they are dying long before it is recognized by others. Other individuals do not accept their death as occurring in the near future even in the face of massive amounts of evidence.

The factor of differential onset raises the question of whether individuals should be told they are dying. There are essentially two schools of thought. Some people believe that whether the facts should be communicated to the individual is dependent on the individual's ability to tolerate such information. It is, however, difficult to determine if an individual is able to deal with the fact of her dying. Another criticism of this approach is that the individual may be well aware of her imminent death. If others pretend unawareness, the individual is left alone not only to deal with her dying but with the lack of a shared reality. On the other hand, some people believe an individual should be told immediately that it is quite likely that she will soon die. In recommending this approach, proponents feel that if an individual is not prepared to recognize she is dying, her defense mechanisms will come into play to protect her from unacceptable information. They believe that by telling the individual about her impending death that she is able to prepare for death in an environment of shared reality. Critics of this orientation feel that an individual's defense mechanisms may not protect her and that she will be overwhelmed by information she is not ready to hear. These two different points of view have not been reconciled but the latter seems to be currently somewhat more accepted.

There is no typical or usual reaction to dying. Some people, for example, who accept the fact of their death, systematically withdraw from previous activities and relationships. Other people who also accept the fact of their death make no changes in their daily routines and interpersonal relationships. They appear to perceive death as the end of a life which they will pursue as long as they can. Response to imminent death is influenced by the individual's age, sex, ethnic background, interpersonal relationships, personality, and life style. Essentially, the individual dies as she has lived. Response is also affected by the specific disease and the type of treatment. The degree of pain, discomfort, and disfiguration that occurs during terminal illness is often a significant factor. Many people are more concerned about those who will remain after their death than they are about their own death per se. Others welcome death as a release from pain and struggle. Finally, individuals' reactions are closely related to whether they have resolved their life experiences and problems and whether they feel they have made a contribution to others during their life.

Kubler-Ross describes five stages of dying (570):

1. Denial of death;
2. Anger and rage at the injustice and unfairness of one's own death;
3. A bargaining stage in which the individual attempts to make a deal with God or fate in return for life (this is eventually seen as futile);
4. Depression and preparatory grief over the loss of life and loved ones;
5. A level of acceptance is reached with a quiet expectation of death and a lessening of interest in the outer world including loved ones.

Although these appear to be fairly typical stages, not all individuals go through all of them. In addition, the process is not necessarily linear in that the individual may repeatedly return to earlier stages.

A family's reaction to terminal illness of one of its members is in many ways similar to that described above relative to the individual. There are frequently feelings of anger toward the dying person for leaving family members. Guilt is also common not only relative to feelings of being angry but also derived from the feeling that one somehow should have done more to prevent the terminal illness. Terminal illness brings about a fairly large change in a family's life style. This is true whether the individual is at home or in some type of institution. This alteration is seen as temporary, which in many ways makes it more difficult to deal with than the change in life style that will occur after the individual's death. The latter, seen as a far more permanent change, is a goal to work toward. The temporary nature of terminal illness leaves the family, sometimes almost literally, in a state of suspended animation. Many developmental and ordinary daily tasks are given little attention, with the family's energy being focused on the dying individual. A long terminal illness often leaves the family drained of emotional resources.

Family members are often involved in anticipatory grief and mourning in preparation for the individual's death. This is considered to be a healthy process that facilitates expression of grief and the work of mourning subsequent to death. The only drawback in engaging in anticipatory grief and mourning is that such a process naturally involves the withdrawal of some emotional energy from the dying individual. Thus, it is possible that family members will not be emotionally available to the individual at a time when they are needed the most. It is during terminal illness that family members go through the process of saying goodbye to the dying individual. This is usually accompanied by a sharing of memories both good and bad, the resolution of old conflicts, and forgiveness for real and imagined past transgressions. It is good to remember that anticipatory grief and mourning and saying goodbye are very exhausting undertakings.

During the terminal illness of a family member, children in the family often do not receive the usual amount of parenting. With parents preoccupied, children are also often not given the support that they need for dealing with their own emotional responses. The feeling of deprivation that they experience may lead to a period of temporary regression and/or developmental delay. Older children may have to take increased responsibility for care of younger children and household tasks. These responsibilities may be far beyond what the child is truly capable of doing in a competent manner and he may therefore feel inadequate. Increased responsibility may generate not only anxiety but a good deal of resentment toward the dying individual and the parent.

One of the major tasks of the individual during terminal illness is the "work of dying." This includes not only dealing with feelings about one's own death but also laying ghosts from the past to rest—cleaning house so to speak. A part of this process involves the resolving of old conflicts: those within oneself and those in relationship to other people. The work of dying often takes place within the context of a life review: a process of examining and contemplating the past events and circumstances of one's life. Such a process usually arouses the full spectrum of human emotion. It is for this reason that people speak of the work of dying, for it is a task that requires much time and energy.

Many individuals, at one time or another, contemplate their preferred way of dying: the cause and the when, where, and with whom of their death. Some individuals, for example, may say they would prefer to die after their children are grown and independent or after they have completed what they define as their life's work. Some people wish to die suddenly, whereas others would prefer to linger sufficiently long to say goodbye to family and friends. Some people say they would like to die at home, whereas others may prefer to die in a hospice-type setting.

Such speculation, just outlined, usually takes place when the individual is in the peak of health. However, the terminally ill individual ought to have some say in how she will die. The individual's own preferences and life style should be taken into account, if not given priority. Some people suggest that the individual formulate and write a living will. This is done at the beginning of the terminal illness and outlines what kind of care the individual would like to receive. It usually includes a statement about acceptable drugs, the use of extraordinary means to prolong life, and euthanasia. The latter is a complex moral and legal issue that is just beginning to receive the attention it deserves. A living will is meant to ensure that the individual has input into the total pattern of care and that her intentions will be respected.

Most people in the United States die in a medical institution, a place where there tends to be more emphasis on physical care than emotional concerns. The term "dying trajectories" is often used to identify the duration and process of the individual's passage from life to death. It refers to how everyone expects a particular individual's situation to develop. Certainty and time are important dimensions. Ideally knowledge of these factors helps the staff to organize their time and the tasks that need to be performed, and to deal with emotional issues: the dying individual's, the family's, and their own. A lingering trajectory, the individual not dying as soon as expected, usually does not produce disruption in an institutional environment, although it may be very hard on the individual and the family. In an expected quick trajectory involving the emergency room and intensive care unit, the medical system is at its best. Change is radical and swift, calling for an active response. The majority of medical personnel are comfortable in coping with death through activity. An unexpected quick trajectory not anticipated by the staff often leads to an emergency atmosphere. There is the danger of making a poor decision under time and emotional pressure. A wrong action may be taken or definitive action may be delayed. There is the question of obeying all of the traditional rules and procedures or doing what might save the person's life. The individual's perceived social value may influence the actions taken. In both expected and unexpected quick trajectories, the medical staff usually has little time to provide support for family and friends. Regardless of the trajectory, many staff members have a good deal of difficulty in discussing impending death with the dying individual. Although there have been some recent changes for the better, there is still considerable reticence on the part of staff. The individual's need for emotional support continues throughout the dying trajectory. Even when apparently unconscious, it is believed that most individuals maintain some degree of mental alertness to the very end of life.

A situation or setting that is conducive to the work of dying, which takes the individual's wishes into consideration and is supportive of the individual, family, and friends, has several characteristics. Care is focused on the remission of symptoms, control of pain, and the relief of anxiety. The environment provides security, protection, and ample opportunity for the individual to be with other people. Caretakers, family, and friends are enabled to truly be with the individual. The capacity of others to listen to the individual and to communicate comfortably is fostered. In addition to open communication, the nonverbal communication of touching, a great comfort to most individuals, is emphasized. There is ample opportunity for leave taking. Family and friends are encouraged to be with the individual in a private situation not only while the individual is living but also when she is newly dead. The family is given the opportunity to discuss dying, death, and related emotional needs with the staff. Caregivers have adequate time to form and maintain personal relationships with the individual and the family. The individual is given an opportunity to experience her final hours in a way that has personal meaning. A mutual support network among the staff, which includes both the technical and emotional dimensions of working with the terminally ill that helps them to provide more adequate care, is an important part of this type of setting.

The above description of a situation that is conducive to dying in essence describes the hospice movement. The term "hospice" refers to a place of shelter and comfort. Although a hospice may be a place, it is more than that. It is philosophy and means of providing care for the terminally ill. The individual as well as the family is actively involved both in the necessary decisions and in providing emotional support. If the individual and family so desire, the individual may remain in her home as long as feasible or until death. Hospice staff provide the necessary support and assistance to allow the individual to die in her home if that is what is desired.

Loss

Loss is a state in which the individual is deprived of something of importance for which there is no hope of recovery (607,849,886). Death is only one type of loss. Although perhaps considered the most significant, there are many other losses to which the individual must accommodate throughout the life cycle. An individual may experience bereavement from the loss of: (a) a loved one through divorce, miscarriage, rejection, or geographical separation; (b) a nonhuman object such as a pet, a home, a treasured piece of jewelry, a family heirloom; (c) a social role through retirement, the loss of a job, a child no longer needing nurture, an individual no longer needing protection and guidance in a work setting; (d) an anticipated or expected event such as a promotion, a good grade, vacation, hopes and dreams for the future; (e) a part of one's physical self such as a body part, sensation, diminished sight or hearing, motor or cognitive function, diminished athletic ability, the ability to bear children, sexual potency, youth.

It is sometimes forgotten how serious the above-mentioned events are and that they can lead to a reaction of grief. An individual's response may not be understood because the observer is unaware of the seriousness of the loss that has been sustained. Indeed, the individual may not be aware of the significance of the loss and therefore unable to account for her feelings or behavior. The degree of grief and the mourning required will vary with the severity of the loss. Severity can only be determined by the individual and not by any external measure. What is experienced as a great loss to one individual may be a relatively minor unpleasant event to another. The degree to which the loss is related to the individual's sense of identity, the degree of emotional investment in the lost person, object, or experience will determine the intensity of the grief response.

Grief and Mourning

Grief and mourning are the natural responses to loss (105, 127, 154, 155, 171, 497, 504, 531, 733, 849, 853, 886). Grief is a state of physical distress and severe mental suffering. There is the experience of sharp sorrow and painful regret. All spheres of function are likely to be affected, with increased vulnerability to all of life's hazards. Mourning is the manifestation of sorrow and includes the process of accepting and adjusting to the loss.

Grief and mourning overlap with each other. The typical sequence of reactions occurs in four phases. First, there is a feeling of numbness, with an inability to recognize or accept the loss. Next, there is a shock of reality as the enormity of the loss begins to penetrate the individual's awareness. Physical, psychological, and behavioral responses follow. Some common physical reactions are a feeling of emptiness in the stomach, weakness in the knees, feeling of suffocation, shortness of breath, a tendency to sigh deeply, insomnia, digestive disturbances, and anorexia.

Typical psychological reactions are a sense of unreality, sadness, despair, impotence, feelings of being abandoned and rejected, helplessness, low self-esteem, and feelings of inadequacy and loneliness. The individual may become obsessively preoccupied with loss or act as though the loss were temporary or had not occurred. As in the case of chronic illness, the individual may experience considerable anger and guilt. Anger may be directed at the individual who dies, the individual supposedly responsible for the loss, and/or at the seemingly uncontrollable forces that caused the loss. There is often an experience of rage and a desire for revenge. Guilt may arise from the feeling that one has no right to be angry, from the idea one did not do enough to prevent the loss, or from the fact that one survived. There are frequently alternating periods of anxiety and longing for return to the situation prior to loss, as well as periods of depression and despair.

Some behavioral reactions that often occur are irritability, distractibility, disorganization of usual patterns of response, aimless wandering, difficulty or inability to engage in social roles, and disinterest in social interactions.

Finally, there is adaptation in which the individual accepts the reality of the loss and begins to find ways to fill the void by identifying with a new life style and people.

The duration of grief and mourning is dependent both on the severity of the loss and the adaptive capacity of the individual. There is also variation in the time that it takes for the individual to pass through each phase. The process is often not linear as the individual may, particularly under additional stress, regress to a previous stage. In the case of significant loss, acute grief usually lasts for one to two months, the mourning period for six months to a year. A more extended period of mourning is not, however, uncommon. There is a difference between social and emotional recovery. Social recovery refers to the individual's capacity to reengage effectively in social roles and usually occurs prior to emotional recovery. Emotional recovery refers to the withdrawal of emotional investment in the lost phenomenon and reinvestment of that energy in other phenomena. This is a much slower process and often takes an extended period of time.

The death of a loved one leads to a variety of reactions. There is frequently the desire to recover or resurrect the dead person. The knowledge that this is irrational does not, initially, diminish this desire. On the other hand, the individual may wish to preserve the image of the loved one as if the dead person were still alive. This effort to enshrine often takes the form of keeping things just as they were before the death of the loved one. The dead person's personal belongings are left in place and holiday rituals of particular importance to that individual may continue to be carried out. This way of dealing with loss may also include avoidance of new contacts that might replace the role of the one who died. Another fairly common way of dealing with the death of a loved one is by idealizing the dead person: he could do no and never did any wrong; she was a perfect person in every way. Such an appraisal usually becomes more realistic as the individual begins to adapt to loss.

Death of a spouse, particularly after a long marriage, is perhaps the most difficult loss to sustain. For an elderly person, loss of a spouse is probably the crucial factor in predicting decline or breakdown in function both physically and emotionally. Individuals who have had an opportunity to prepare themselves for the loss of their mate usually are better able to reorganize their lives during the ensuing months. Men tend to keep their feelings to themselves and make a more rapid social recovery than women. However, their emotional recovery is slower. When a spouse or partner dies, the surviving individual, in addition to dealing with grief and mourning, usually has many practical decisions to make. Some of the decisions that must be made are where to live, what to do about the family home and possessions, how to dispose of the spouse's personal effects, and what kind of contact to maintain with the spouse's relatives. There are often new financial and domestic responsibilities to learn as well as new social roles to establish. If there are young children, the remaining spouse must take on sole responsibility for their rearing. Dealing with loneliness is often a major problem, particularly for an individual who has had no experience in living alone at any time in her life. The feeling of being alone includes fear for one's physical survival in a world that is frequently seen as threatening and uncertain. In loneliness there is also the fear of emotional isolation. This is not the fear of being unable to relate but the reality of not having anyone with whom to relate. In many cultural groups there is the belief that one should be independent and "do for oneself." This frequently compounds the problem of loneliness.

For young children the death of a parent is a very difficult experience. Their reaction to the loss is similar to that described in the four phases of grief and mourning. Additional stress often occurs because the child is not likely to have the full attention of the remaining parent for a period of time. This leads to lack of emotional support for the loss and to an interruption of the normal interaction patterns necessary for growth and security. More attention is often given to the grief of the spouse than to the child. There seems to be an assumption that the grief of the child is less and/or that he will somehow adapt. The child, thus, is often left in a state of severe anxiety with no one to whom to turn. For an adolescent, the death of a parent may interfere with achieving independence through the usual route of criticism, rebellion, and increased interaction outside the family. When there are younger children the adolescent may be put in the position of parental surrogate. The adolescent may be expected to provide the major source of emotional support for the remaining parent. Plans for continued education may be disrupted due to financial constraints. These demands may not only be made by the family but they may also be strongly reinforced by the cultural group.

The death of a child is frequently perceived as a major tragedy. The death appears out of place in the life cycle: untimely and irrational. In addition to grief and mourning for the loss of the child, parents often experience another loss. Children frequently become important to the emotional functioning of the family as an extension of the parents' hopes and dreams. Thus, parents have not only lost a child, they have lost many of their expectations for the future. If the child has no siblings, the loss is further compounded by the parents' loss of a major social role; they are no longer parents. Parents may blame themselves for the child's death or they may blame each other. In the latter situation there may be so much anger that the marriage or partnership may be terminated. Siblings may feel that they must make up for the loss of the child. They may be put into the position of having to be exceptionally docile and obedient or they may be urged to fulfill the expectations the parents had for the dead child. If the child has committed suicide, the family as a whole may not only experience considerable guilt but they may also feel a great deal of shame.

Mourning as it extends into time becomes less intense. However, passing the milestones of each year, holidays, anniversaries, birthdays, and so forth remains difficult for a long period of time. The first year is particularly traumatic. As mourning becomes less intense, anxiety frequently increases. It is aroused by the individual's awareness of the adjustments and new learning that must occur. The degree of anxiety is proportionate to the task at hand, resources available, and the chance of failure. Resources in terms of knowledgeable guides and emotional support are probably the most crucial factors.

The process of grief and mourning occasionally does not take place in a typical fashion. It may be delayed so that the individual initially does not seem to be bothered by the loss. The individual continues her usual activities and does not experience any particular sense of sadness. It is only some time much later that the person experiences grief and begins the process of mourning, which then takes its normal course. This seems to be a natural kind of delay and seemingly benign in its origins and consequences.

Grief and mourning may, on the other hand, be delayed apparently out of fear of engaging in the process. The individual may engage in a variety of activities and seemingly always must be busy doing something at all times. On the other hand, the individual may acquire some physical illness that excuses her from her usual activities. In this case, somatic complaints are used as an initial substitute for mourning. Those who first fear grief and mourning in most cases eventually begin the process after a period of time.

For some individuals the mourning period is unusually prolonged. This phenomenon seems to arise from considerable ambivalence in regards to the loss. If the loss is relative to a beloved person, for example, the individual may have considerable negative feelings in regards to the lost person that have never been resolved. The lost person is often endowed with highly favorable characteristics, with unfavorable traits being completely forgotten.

Some people never seem to mourn properly. Although there is evidence of good social recovery and a fair amount of emotional recovery, there is some aspect of mourning that has not been accomplished. Some of the milestones of each year continue to be abnormally difficult. There are occasional situations that remind the individual of the loss which she finds particularly hard to deal with. The individual, indeed, may live with unfinished mourning throughout her life. Finally, there are some people who do not mourn because they cannot focus their sadness on the loss. Either they cannot identify the loss or they engage in denial—of the loss itself or of the significance of the loss. Such individuals are highly prone to recurrent depression.

Difficulty in mourning is by no means entirely a personal matter. There are few mourning rites in industrial Western society. In addition, the norms of society do not encourage a display of emotion, talking about loss, or temporarily disengaging from usual activities. If one must mourn it should be done in private. Mourning is not considered to be a communal event. There is the belief that the individual should pull herself together and continue daily life with a "business as usual" attitude. Thus not only is mourning not particularly socially acceptable, it is also something that many people do not know how to do. As with the majority of human activities, one must learn to mourn: to mourn productively and with resolution. In other societies, the ability to mourn seems to be acquired through participation in the rituals and customs of mourning which are embedded in the fabric of the culture. In such social systems, the individual has role models, personal experiences with others who mourn. Mourning is seen as a natural part of life.

SUMMARY

This chapter focused on the life cycle from conception to death. It was organized to emphasize the major social roles of the human experience. The idea of a cycle was recurrent: the cycle of work, the cycle of the family, and so forth. The cycle of one life as it evolves is important, but so is the life cycle as it occurs from generation to generation. It is through understanding of recurrent cycles and the individual's place at a given time in these cycles that we come to appreciate the complexity and richness of each individual: the past, this moment in time, and something of the future.

6 Environment

The environment is here defined as the aggregate of phenomena that surrounds the individual and influences his development and existence. It includes physical conditions, things, other individuals, groups, and ideas. One of the philosophical assumptions of occupational therapy is the belief that the individual can neither be understood nor assisted toward a more adaptive mode of behavior without consideration of the environment: past, present, and future. It is assumed that the individual does not exist in a vacuum but that he is continually affected by and is affecting the environment. It is assumed that no aspect of human function, social roles, and growth and development is immune to the influence of the cultural, social, and physical environments.

The idea that the individual cannot be understood outside the context of his environment is by no means new or unique to occupational therapy. It has, to the best of our knowledge, been a part of the belief system of all cultural groups and it is one of the basic tenets of most health professions and social science disciplines (472,672,940). The concept of the individual in environment has received particular attention since the early 1950s. It was at that time that the construct of general system theory became popular (122,136,145,582,595,941, 983,984). Developed as a structure for organizing knowledge, the purpose of general systems theory was to identify systematic theoretical constructs that would describe the general relationships of the various aspects of the empirical world. Two approaches not necessarily mutually exclusive to the organization of knowledge have been suggested:

1. To select general phenomena that are common to many different parts of the empirical universe (e.g., equilibrium, differentiation).
2. To arrange empirical fields of study in some form such as a spectrum or hierarchy based on the complexity of the organization of their basic units (e.g., individual, family, group).

It was felt that the organization of theories in some systematic kind of way would facilitate interdisciplinary communication, help to identify the interrelationship of empirical phenomena, and guide research toward gaps that might become evident. The concept of general systems theory was a response to the proliferation of highly specialized fields of scientific study. By the 1950s advances in knowledge had been so great that scientists were able to master only a very small portion of their field. Even scientists in the same discipline had become so specialized that they had difficulty communicating with each other. There was a similar situation relative to interdisciplinary communication. It was felt that the systematic organization of theories would remedy this situation. General systems theory was also seen as a means of compensating for the reductionism that is an inherent part of science. Reductionism refers to the division of phenomena into small manageable units for the purpose of in-depth study. Thus, for example, scientists study the nervous system and the skeletal system as separate entities rather than taking "the nature of the human organism" in its totality as a basic unit of study. General systems theory was not proposed as an alternative to reductionism but rather as a way of emphasizing the interrelationship of the component parts of various empirical phenomena. Formulation of a systematic organization of theories is not an attempt to establish a single self-contained "general theory of practically everything" that would replace all the particular theories of the various disciplines. Rather it is the attempt to find a level of somewhat common discourse between the highly specific that has little meaning and the general that lacks any substance.

Although no widely accepted general systems theory has been developed, discussion of this idea led to a greater recognition and/or reaffirmation of the holistic nature of the individual and the interrelationship of the individual and the environment. The latter relationship is often referred to as an open system—the influence of the environment on the individual and the individual on the environment.

With that brief digression, the last portion of the parameter of the occupational therapy domain of concern is the cultural, social, and physical environment of the individual. As previously defined, cultural environment refers to the social structures, values, norms, and expectations that are accepted and shared by a group of people. The social environment refers to the matrix of people with whom the individual presently relates and to those people he will need to relate to in the future. These people may be family, friends, acquaintances, coworkers, fellow residents, and individuals who are in control of and/or provide services. Physical environment refers to the availability of adequate food, clothing and shelter, and the material surroundings in which the individual lives or is likely to live in the future. The latter includes such things as possible architectural barriers that may impede the mobility of the physically disabled individual, the complexity of the environment that may cause difficulty for the cognitively impaired individual, ambiance, the degree of physical safety, and the opportunity to be surrounded by nonhuman objects that have personal meaning to the individual.

It is generally felt that the individual's past and present environment accounts for a considerable portion of his ideas and behavior. Much of the significant variation in individual human behavior is considered to be derived from differences in the culture and structure of the groups to which the individual belongs, and to his status and position within those groups. This is not to negate the importance of genetic endowments and psychological states and processes that mediate the group's effect on the individual. It should be remembered that the cultural, social, and physical environment is not a mold that forms its members into duplicate copies. There is always a great variety and range of personalities and behavior in even the simplest environments. Nevertheless, the environment is a significant factor in an individual's definition of a situation. The individual tends to react to the meaning of information as it is perceived by his cultural and social environments and not necessarily to the "objective" facts of the information as they are discernible to others.

The individual's environment is taken into consideration both in the evaluation and intervention process. Relative to evaluation, function and dysfunction can only be defined in reference to the individual's environment. A 21-year-old woman who was unable to prepare a meal would be considered to be in a relatively severe state of dysfunction in one social system, whereas lack of such skill would not be considered at all unusual in another social system. The same could be said of almost all aspects of performance components, occupational performances, and one's mastery of developmental tasks. It is only through understanding of the individual's environment that the therapist is able to make some determination of whether an individual is in a state of function or dysfunction.

Goal setting for intervention, in particular the change process, is influenced by the individual's future environment. The concept of "expected environment" is used to refer to the individual's anticipated place of residence, social interactions, activities, and so forth subsequent to the termination of intervention. It is through some knowledge of expected environment that the individual and therapist are able to set reasonable goals. The man, for example, who intends to return to his job as a salesman will need to acquire greater skill in interpersonal communication than a man who is a night watchman.

In selecting activities for intervention, the individual's past and present environment must be taken into consideration. In helping an individual develop cognitive skills, for example, collating, making a macrame belt, or writing a simple computer program may all be suitable. Which of these activities would be appropriate is likely to be dependent on the individual's past and present environment.

The degree to which environment is the focus of intervention varies. The social and physical environment may be of primary concern in prevention, meeting health needs, and maintenance. It may be of less importance in management. In the change process attention to the environment is veritable. The therapist rarely tries to change an individual's values or ideas that are a traditional part of his cultural background. A person who is trying to learn how to function effectively in a community that consists of members of his own cultural group does not need someone to begin raising questions about the mutually shared values and ideas of his cultural group. Rather he needs someone to help him learn how to live within the limits of these values and ideas. There are, however, a few occasions when a therapist is concerned with helping an individual to change his culturally based values and ideas. The individual's values and ideas may be so different from those of the broader community that they interfere with his need satisfaction and/or the rights of others. This may be the case, for example, when the individual belongs to a deviant criminal subculture. On the other hand, the individual may, because of immigration, be thrust into an entirely new culture. Such an individual may need some assistance in adapting to the folkways and mores of the new culture. When adaptation to a new culture is the focus of the change process, great care is taken to respect the values and ideas of the individual's culture of origin. A somewhat more complex situation arises when the individual's culture equates disability with social incompetence and/or defines specific disabilities in a highly negative manner. Intervention relative to this problem and those described above will be discussed in Chapter 28.

In the change process the individual is often assisted in developing skills appropriate to relating to his present social environment or he may be helped to move into a different social environment. The social environment itself, particularly the family, may become the primary focus of intervention. Finally, the individual may need assistance in adapting to the physical environment. Emphasis is then on helping the individual to develop skills in problem solving and dealing with the stress and frustration arising from an inadequate physical environment. Alteration of the physical environment may also enable the individual to function more adequately.

The environment, then, is a part of the parameter of the occupational therapy domain of concern because knowledge of the individual's environment: (a) facilitates understanding of the individual; (b) helps to define the individual's areas of function and dysfunction and to set goals; (c) assists in selecting appropriate activities for intervention; and (d) may become the primary or secondary focus of intervention.

There is considerable overlap between the cultural, social, and physical environments. However, to provide some structure for the discussion to follow, this chapter will address each of these areas separately.

THE CULTURAL ENVIRONMENT

The subject of culture is very complex and one of major concern both to anthropologists and sociologists. It will by necessity only be introduced here with the hope that the reader will explore this topic in much greater depth elsewhere (244,419,441,467,475,548, 561,566,735,933,942).

Definition

Culture is a set of shared understandings held in common by members of a group. These understandings may be categorized as:

- Descriptive—agreements about the nature of the universe and its contents, e.g., God created man, the earth is round, and illness is caused by natural phenomena.
- Procedural—agreements about how things should be done, e.g., driving on the left side of the road, respect for the elderly, and eating three times a day.
- Ethical/aesthetic—agreements about what is desirable, beautiful, and good, e.g., being married, pierced ears, and giving to charity.

The culture of a group is the sum of its morally forceful understandings acquired through learning and shared by the members of that group. The concept of culture, it should be noted, is concerned with the understandings that members of the group hold in common, not the ideosyncratic ideas of individuals. Although culture shapes the lives and thoughts of the group's members, many cultural understandings are not a part of conscious psychic content. The unconscious element of many aspects of culture make it a phenomenon that is somewhat difficult to share with people who are not members of the culture. The unconscious aspect also makes cultural understandings powerful behavioral influences.

The above definition of culture refers to the nonmaterial aspects of culture. It does not include, for example, homes, clothes, food, tools, weapons, or religious articles. Although it is often difficult to separate the material and nonmaterial aspects of culture, the nonmaterial is of primary concern in this text. In addition, as used here, culture does not refer to behavior. Behavior has a voluntary component that is frequently missing from shared understanding. For example, an individual may violate a shared understanding by his behavior but still accept it as an important belief. People's shared understandings about what group members should and should not do may or may not be acted on by the members at a given time. This, however, does not change the cultural prescription.

Culture is not a monolithic structure that all group members possess equally. It is incompletely shared, even in a fairly simple culture. Understandings are frequently distributed among subgroups, the most common divisions being age and gender. However, everyone in one subgroup is clearly aware of what is expected of members of another subgroup. This helps to link the subgroups together and makes it possible for members of the various subgroups to communicate and interact comfortably. Not all shared understandings affect everyone. There are usually only a few cultural prescriptions that are deemed appropriate for all group members under all circumstances.

The shared understandings of a culture are not simply an aggregate of disconnected common beliefs. A culture is organized in a relatively coherent and consistent manner. Cultures tend to be organized around a small nucleus of ideas from which other understandings are derived and which dictates the relationship between understandings. One of these meta-understandings in industrial Western culture, for example, is the rights of the individual versus the rights of the state. The organization of a culture also defines which understandings are more or less important, which are general or specific, and which go together with which others. The structure of a culture designates where, when, and with whom an understanding is operant. Cultural organization is not always constant. Violence, for example, is generally abhorred in our culture but nonetheless glorified. The parts of a culture, on the other hand, may be internally consistent but not necessarily compatible. Thus the norms that influence the business world and family interaction have continuity but they are not always in accord with each other.

Culture is a necessary part of the human experience. Without culture, indeed, there would be no human experience. Because of our evolution and biology, there is no known alternative to shared understandings. They contribute organization and techniques for dealing with the physical environment, provide for the continuation of the species, and ensure the satisfaction of basic human needs. Culture is both the primary human adaptive mechanism and the foundation for social life. There are several key concepts used in the description of culture. They are briefly defined below.

Status is the social position or rank of an individual or group in relationship to another or others within a social system. Individuals or groups who have a given status, whether it be assigned or acquired, are expected to behave in a manner congruent with the specific cultural understandings relative to that status.

Social structure refers to the system of relationships between the constituent groups of a social system. It is the way in which the various groups are organized relative to each other.

Norms are shared attitudes or understandings of what is legitimate or normal behavior for a given individual in a given situation. They are the ways in which one is expected to behave under prevailing circumstances. Certain individuals are expected to follow some norms more rigidly than others, e.g., priests or lawyers. However, there is often a great gap between the ideal and the actual patterns of a culture. Norms have been divided into two categories: mores and folkways.

Mores are norms that are considered to be vital to the survival of the cultural group. Two examples are: mothers should provide for the physical and emotional needs of their children, and one should not question the basic tenets of one's religion.

Folkways are norms that one is expected to follow but they are not considered to be compulsory. Two examples are: men should step aside to allow a woman to pass through a door first, and a 7-year-old child should respect his elders.

Sanctions are the means by which a culture ensures that the norms of a culture are maintained in everyday interaction. They are what the group does to support the continuation of its shared understandings. Essentially, rewards are given for conformity to normative behavior and punishment meted out for nonconformity. Positive sanctions include approval, monetary gain, and an increase in status. Negative sanctions include disapproval, social ostracism, and, in extreme situations, removal from the cultural community. The term "sanction," when used without a modifier, usually refers to a negative response to nonconformity. Lack of compliance with mores usually leads to a more severe negative sanction than lack of compliance with a folkway, although this is not always the case. Positive sanctions, at least on the behavioral level, are more likely to be given for conformity to folkways than mores. An individual is so much expected to follow the mores of his culture that no particular reward is considered necessary. Sanctions, especially negative sanctions, tend to be differentially applied, depending on the status of the individual.

The acquisition of culture accrues through learning. This process, usually referred to as enculturation, involves the learning of the language, traditions, values, conventions, and symbolic meanings of a culture. The norms of a culture are transmitted from one generation to the next or to an adult who has recently joined the cultural group. Eventually, the shared understandings of one's culture are internalized so that conformity to norms is primarily regulated by intrinsic factors as opposed to the external sanctions of the cultural group. The process of enculturation is similar to socialization, involving the use of rewards and punishments, modeling, and interaction with role partners.

Although passed from one generation to the next, culture is a vital and dynamic force that is always in the process of evolving. The rate of change varies from one culture to another, but there is always some degree of change. The continuity of a culture may be altered in a quantitative or qualitative manner. A new element may be added with very little change in other elements of the culture. Such an addition tends to be relatively minor. The addition of a more significant element often modifies many other elements of the culture. Such a change may call for a relatively major revision in the organization of the culture. A quantitative change might, for example, be the introduction of a new fashion of clothes. The changes in gender-related behavior and the relationship between men and women that is now occurring in industrialized Western society are an example of a major qualitative cultural change. Alteration in a culture, whether technological or of a social nature, may invoke the introduction of an entirely new principle or a new application of a known principle to a new situation. The introduction of computer technology is essentially an example of both types of cultural change. It was originally a new principle which is now being applied in many sectors of our society.

Culture change may come about through internal or external factors. Internal change may be the result of technological inventions, climate alteration, population pressures, or cultural fatigue. The latter factor appears to have been one of the causes of the social upheaval of the late 1960s and early 1970s. As is frequently the case, this involved the younger generation questioning or abandoning part of the culture's shared understandings. However, the persistent continuity of culture can be seen in this process. The younger generation continued to be influenced by the culture, albeit in a negative manner, by being strongly against many of the norms of the culture. A social revolution of this sort tends to be self-limiting as the younger generation matures and returns to many of the more traditional values and conventions of the society. However, residual changes may persist in the culture as, for example, in this case a greater tolerance for differences in life style and less trust of government officials.

A culture is influenced by external factors in three major ways. In the process, referred to as acculturation, a borrowing of cultural traits takes place between two societies living in continuous first-hand contact. In the United States, for example, a modification of Mexican food has become quite popular, whereas Mexico has developed a liking for fast food establishments. In the process of diffusion, a culture trait or cluster of traits is adopted from a culture with which the adopting culture has little contact. The influence of African art on nineteenth century Western European art is an example of diffusion. As in the case of acculturation, diffusion involves selective borrowing; only certain traits are chosen in preference to others. Some of the major factors influencing selection are novelty, utility, or prestige attached to the particular trait. In the process of assimilation, one society abandons its own culture in favor of the culture of a neighboring or a conquering cultural group. This occurred to a great extent, for example, to the Jewish community living in Germany prior to World War II. Assimilation, it should be noted, is not the same as the merging of two cultures to form a culture different from either of the parent cultures. This is an extreme form of acculturation. An example of this is what is now referred to as Anglo-Saxon culture. Similar to acculturation, there are degrees of assimilation.

Although cultures are always in the process of evolving, there are times when the change is so rapid that members of the culture have great difficulty in adapting to the change. This is particularly true when the change is accompanied by a loss of agreed-on norms. The culture becomes disorganized, often resulting in a sense of confusion and loss of direction on the part of cultural group members. Rapid cultural change also tends to put a considerable strain on the relationship between generations with a sense of discontinuity of shared life experiences. This is a phenomenon that is fairly common for cultural groups that have immigrated to the United States.

As mentioned, although culture has a powerful influence on the individual, it does not form each individual to an exact facsimile of every other individual in the culture. Clyde Klucholn makes this clear in his statement to the effect that every man is in certain repects like every other man, like some other men, and like no other man (548). In addition to genetic differences, no two individuals have exactly the same life experiences. The elements of a culture do become part of the individual's personality, but not all components of personality are elements of the culture. Although the culture prescribes much of an individual's behavior, it by no means prescribes all behavior. There are nevertheless common personality traits shared by members of the same culture despite individual differences. This alikeness is produced by similar childhood socialization and shared understandings not directly affecting child rearing. Thus, scientists often speak of a model personality type characteristic of a particular cultural group.

Up to this point, cultural groups have been discussed as if they existed in a fairly pure form in some degree of isolation from each other. Although this is true in some cases, it is not true in pluralistic societies like the United States. Pluralistic societies tend to include many cultural subgroups that have shared understandings that are different from those of the larger social system. Examples of cultural subgroups are the extremes of social class, ethnic groups, and some occupations. Cultural subgroups usually occupy different positions of power and prestige relative to the dominant culture. In addition, the lack of shared understandings frequently leads to problems of communication between the various subgroups and between subgroups and the dominant culture. Difference in power and prestige and communication difficulties often cause misunderstandings. Although no panacea, knowledge of cultural differences can facilitate interaction with members of various cultural groups.

Social class, particularly in the United States, is primarily determined by a combination of level of education, amount of income, and occupation (963). It is such a common concept that it needs no further explanation here. The culture of the health professions, here considered an occupational group, will be discussed in the last part of this section. The concept of ethnic group may need some definition. For the purpose of this text, ethnic groups are defined as a collectivity within a larger society having real or reputed common ancestry, memories of a shared historical past, and a culture organized around one or more symbolic elements seen as the epitome of their sense of common identity (284,395).

There is considerable intra-ethnic and inter-ethnic group variation. The following are some of the factors that influence those variations.

Homogeneity

This refers to the degree to which members of a given ethnic category have a set of shared understandings. Membership in a given ethnic group is often defined by the dominant culture. The larger social system may place individuals in one ethnic group who do not experience a strong sense of cultural identity with other members of the group. This occurred, for example, in the white Anglo-Saxon Protestant majority in the United States placing all Italian immigrants in the same ethnic group. People from Northern and Southern Italy did not perceive themselves as sharing much of a common cultural heritage.

Significance

This refers to the range of social situations in which ethnic identity is expressed. For some the shared understanding permeates many aspects of daily life. For others ethnicity may be evident on certain days of the year or in the context of joint political or philanthropic endeavors.

Region of Residence

Many ethnic groups at the time of their immigration or shortly thereafter took up residence in various parts of the country. Because of the different experiences available, the cultural evolution of each regional group may be rather dissimilar. An individual raised in an Irish Catholic enclave in Minneapolis, for example, may not have all of the same cultural understandings as an individual raised in a similar situation in Boston.

Generation

Some ethnic groups experienced the majority of their immigration several generations ago, whereas others are fairly newly arrived. In the latter case, new members from the ethnic group's place of origin are often continually being added to the group. Newer groups are less likely to have been involved in the acculturation process relative to the dominant culture. The same is true for an individual. A third generation member of an ethnic group is more likely to share some of the cultural understandings of the dominant culture than a first generation member of a cultural group.

Social Class

Ethnic groups as a whole and individual members who have attained upper socioeconomic status tend to be similar across ethnic groups. In other words, ethnic differences tend to be diminished. The group or individual's cultural understandings are more related to class than ethnicity. This is not the case relative to a lower socioeconomic position. Although sharing some cultural understanding relative to class, the majority of shared understandings are related to membership in a particular ethnic group.

Degree of Association

The extent to which an ethnic group is isolated or maintains distance from other cultural groups will influence the extent to which it adheres to shared understandings. The same is true for an individual. Interaction with members of other ethnic groups tends to dilute shared cultural understandings.

Degree of Assimilation

Many of the factors outlined above relate to the extent to which an ethnic group or individual has been assimilated into the predominant culture. With total assimilation, the group and the individual lose all sense of ethnic identity; they become part of the predominant culture. This may happen very quickly, more slowly, or not at all. However, much of our knowledge of cultural influences is unconscious. Many individuals, for example, may see themselves as being part of the predominant culture; the shared understandings of their ethnic group have been long set aside. However, in a situation of considerable stress, the individual may respond more on the basis of cultural understandings shared by members of his ethnic group than on the understandings of the culture in which he professes membership.

The relationship between the individual, his ethnic group, and a predominant cultural group has perhaps best been expressed by E. V. Stonequist's concept of the "marginal man." This concept was developed to identify the individual who stood between and essentially straddled two cultures. With figuratively one leg on each side, the individual is torn because of a loyalty to and a sense of identity with both cultures. This is a position not to be envied because the individual often feels alienated from both cultures—a person without any shared understandings. In a pluralistic society this is not an uncommon state of existence (933).

The understanding of a culture different from one's own is no easy task. The intellectual orientation of cultural relativism is usually considered to be the most useful approach. Cultural relativism is an orientation that assumes that behavior of members of a group can be understood only within the context of the culture of that group. A pattern of behavior can only be considered relative to the individual's culture. Thus the question is, how would the individual's behavior be assessed by members of his own group? For this reason it is necessary to know the shared understandings of the individual's culture. Cultural relativism as an intellectual tool is very different from a scale for evaluating cultures or as an instrument of moral judgment. Neither evaluation nor judgment is implied in the concept of cultural relativism. It is simply an intellectual orientation used for comprehension of the behavior of people from groups with cultures dissimilar to one's own.

The development of a sense of cultural relativism is hampered by the common human trait of ethnocentrism. Ethnocentrism is an orientation to the understanding and evaluation of people, the way they act, what they believe, and what they value, according to the culture of one's own group. Ethnocentric biases lead the individual to believe that the shared understandings of his own culture are universally correct. In encountering different patterns of behavior in another culture, the individual tends to see them as erroneous. He regards his own culture as superior. The behavior his own culture has taught him to believe is immoral or strange, he sees as immoral and strange when exhibited by members of another cultural group. Even when cultural divergence is recognized intellectually, the individual may believe that the "different" behavior of a person from another culture is due to lack of adequate moral character, stupidity, or personal weakness. Ethnocentrism is such a common phenomenon because most of our knowledge of the world is gained through direct experience in our culture of origin and through the observations and reports of other members of our culture. In gaining knowledge this way, there is no awareness of alternatives. We are oblivious to the alternative categorizations, values, and behavioral modes that our particular culture excludes or neglects. As mentioned, much of the shared understandings of one's culture are unconscious. Thus individuals who live in a culture are the least aware of the characteristics of that culture. They sincerely believe their norms are an inherent part of adequate and appropriate human interaction.

The understanding of, bringing to conscious awareness, the tenets of one's own culture is one step in developing a sense of cultural relativism. One means of gaining such knowledge is by being submerged in another culture for an extended period of time. In addition to learning about a culture different from one's own, it helps the individual to become aware of his own cultural understandings. The attempt to rid one's self of ethnocentric biases is probably an impossible task. All that one can reasonably hope to do is to become aware of at least some of one's biases and try to suspend them when attempting to understand an individual who comes from a culture different from one's own.

In addition to ethnocentrism, understanding individuals from another culture is made more complex by the tendency to perceive others in a stereotyped manner. A stereotype is an oversimplified and standardized conception, usually invested with emotion, of the traits held in common by a social group. A whole complex of characteristics may be attributed to an individual on the basis of membership in a cultural subgroup. Because of seemingly inherent cognitive processes, individuals tend to classify. Thus the tendency to stereotype is a cross-cultural trait. One therefore must be continually on guard against stereotype thinking. The outline of the factors which influence inter- and intracultural variations was an attempt to mitigate the tendency to perceive individuals and ethnic groups in a stereotyped manner.

Areas of Cultural Differences

The process of socialization is universal but the method of teaching and the content of what is taught vary. The variations are innumerable. Only some of the major areas of cultural difference will be outlined here. The references for this section provide far more detailed discussions. This section is designed merely to sensitize the reader to the concept of cultural differences (51, 134, 139, 169, 235, 284, 329, 349, 395, 437, 480, 603, 809, 1004, 1020). The following are some of the major areas of cultural variation.

The Inherent Nature of the Individual

Some cultures believe that the individual is basically good and that happiness can be attained in this world. Other cultures believe that the individual is inherently bad or at best quite imperfect. Happiness should not be expected in this world. Rather the task of the individual is to act in prescribed ways so as to ensure his happiness in the next world.

The Relationship of Human Beings to Nature

Nature may be seen as the ultimate giver of sustenance for survival and therefore something that should be treated with awe and respect. Other cultures see nature in a far less benign manner. It is either viewed as more powerful than human beings or something that should be studied and controlled.

The Individual's Relationship to Other Individuals

Appropriate relationships in most cultures are prescribed on the basis of status, social role, age, and gender. The latter includes the relationship between men and women and the appropriate behavior and activities for each of the sexes. The degree to which and what other people are to be trusted is also prescribed. In addition, the extent of formality in interpersonal relations varies.

Language

Some cultures have their own language; others share a common language with other cultural groups. When a language is shared, the given culture may have its own dialect or accent. There may be differences in idioms and in the denotative and connotative meaning of many words and phrases. To a considerable extent, language structures thought processes. This is particularly apparent in the way in which phenomena are categorized and at the advanced level of abstract thinking. Even if an individual speaks the language of another culture fairly well, his cognitive processes may continue to be influenced by his native language.

Religion

The extent to which a culture believes in supernatural beings and forces and the importance of these beliefs in daily life vary. There is also considerable difference as to whether the supernatural is loving and merciful or strict and vengeful and how one communicates with the supernatural. When religion is an important factor in a culture it provides explanations for human situations (often through myths), promotes group solidarity through shared experiences, and key religious themes influence a wide sphere of cultural understandings. This situation is not true in more "secular" societies where religion plays primarily a ceremonial role.

Family Relationships

Family interaction is a complex phenomenon that includes many elements. Some of these are: child rearing practices; the way in which familial roles are carried out; the importance of the nuclear family versus the extended family; prescribed behavior and rituals relative to courtship, marriage, birth, and divorce; the power structure within the family; and the extent to which the family is central in relationship to the other aspects of the individual's life. This is, of course, only a partial listing of the areas included in family relationships.

Work

Some cultures consider work very important and equate it with that which is right and good. Other cultures consider work a necessary evil, something to be avoided or at best tolerated so that one may enjoy the other aspects of life. In such a case it is not considered central to identity.

Ways of Expressing Needs and Feelings

Individuals in all cultures learn how to express their needs and feelings in a way that other members of the group can understand and accept. The manner of expression, however, is subject to much variation cross-culturally. Two continuums of variation are degree of directness and forcefulness of expression. Included in this area are when, where, and with whom it is appropriate to discuss various subjects and the words used in such discussion.

The Group Versus the Individual

In some cultures the group, whether it be the family or an aggregate of peers or co-workers, is considered to be the most important unit. What the group decides is good and one is expected to go along with the decision of the group. In a culture with this orientation, competition between group members is usually not acceptable. It may, however, be encouraged between groups. Other cultures see the individual as the all-important unit. They feel that each individual should and must succeed or fail on his own merit. Cooperation, when it occurs, tends to be self-serving and competition is the most common mode of interaction.

Time

Some cultures are rooted in the past: traditional ways of thinking and acting are the best. Such groups take a dim view of change and give little attention to the idea of progress. Other cultural groups are primarily concerned with the present. They feel the past is unimportant and the future is unknown, so it is best to enjoy and live in the present. Still other cultural groups are future oriented. Saving money, ultimately raising one's own or one's children's status in society, and being recognized as having made a contribution to the community are examples of a future-oriented group. Such a group also tends to believe that change and progress are important to the welfare of the group. The rhythm of life also varies from one culture to another. It may be based on the day, the seasons of the year, or the entire life cycle. Time may be an important commodity one should not waste; it may be considered impolite if not immoral to be late. Other cultures are much more casual about time. Being someplace at a specified time is not considered to be of any particular importance.

Age

Most cultures define a variety of responsibilities and privileges relative to age. Concern about an individual's age and attitudes toward the aging process vary. Some cultures see the older person as having considerable knowledge and wisdom—qualities that are not found in children and young adults. Old age is defined in some cultures by the number of years one has lived. In other cultures it is defined relative to the individual's ability to function in an independent manner. An aged individual is treated with a good deal of respect and caring by some cultural groups. Other groups treat the aged person as obsolete and a burden to society.

Dying and Death

There is a considerable variation in regard to the openness with which dying and death are treated and the rituals that surround this aspect of human experience. The same is true in regard to grief and mourning. A variety of cultural ideas related to death were discussed in Chapter 5.

Food

Most cultural groups have a preferred diet and do not find other kinds of food particularly palatable. In some cases they will simply not eat such food, even when the supply of traditional foods is quite short. Some foods may have a symbolic meaning and are eaten only at special times. Other foods may be forbidden entirely. Fasting or the limited intake of food for a period of time is a common practice in some cultures. In many cultures, food and the activities that surround the preparation and eating of food are invested with considerable meaning and emotion.

Acceptance of Individual Differences

There is considerable variation in the degree to which a culture will accept an individual who deviates from what is considered normal. Deviation may be relative to physical appearance or behavior. Some cultures are able to accept quite pronounced deviation in some areas but not in others.

Reason and Literacy

Some cultures prize logical reasoning and refined problem solving, whereas others feel that a far more subjective and emotional approach is best. Literacy and education may or may not be considered important or they may be only considered important for some members of the cultural group.

Historical Heritage

Some ethnic groups are extremely proud of their cultural heritage and see themselves as being somewhat better than other ethnic groups. Other groups have the reverse attitude. When a cultural group is in a position of being a minority, they may see this as a serious liability or it may be of little concern. Attitudes toward other cultural groups vary from feelings of kinship, to indifference, to hate. Stereotyping often plays a part in these attitudes as well as historical relationships with a particular group.

Political Ideology

In most cases a cultural group is not totally liberal or conservative. They may take a different stance, depending on the particular issue. Some cultural subgroups are more concerned about political issues and active in political affairs than are other subgroups.

Health and Illness

Although occupational therapists do not use the medical terminology of health and illness, it will be utilized in this section. The reason for this is that research regarding cultural differences relative to perceived states of physical, emotional, and social well-being or the lack thereof has been primarily formulated in medical terms. The ideas to be discussed here are not directly related to the practice of occupational therapy. They are, however, sufficiently related to be of considerable importance to the occupational therapist's understanding of the relationship between the individual and his cultural environment (244, 348, 395, 472, 475, 672, 727, 764, 925, 940, 1050).

States of health and illness and the causes of such states are, with some exceptions, culturally defined. Reaction to disease and pain and to the treatment provided is bound up with a whole system of beliefs and values that influence people to respond and behave in a distinctive manner. There are many unknowns regarding the relationship between culture and health. However, from what is known, there is little question that a relationship exists.

The "rational, scientific" concept of disease is a comparatively recent development in history. Prior to that time and in many cultures to this day, illness and injuries had a vast number of meanings. Minor injuries and ailments whose causes were visible and obvious and the consequences not likely to be lethal were resolved with natural means. Beyond this point an indisposition was scary, perhaps deadly if untreated and perhaps of a mortal nature anyway. In some cultures the only "natural" death was one caused by warfare, violence, or accident. Even some cultures did not believe that, for the question was why did one individual die as opposed to another. Chance in many cultures is not considered a sufficient explanation for anything, let alone death. Typically, when an individual was in physical pain, in mental anguish, or in danger of dying, the cultural group sought help from specialists who had knowledge beyond that of the rest of the members of the group. Such an individual was held in high regard and in many cultures was invested with power believed to be derived from supernatural forces. The power of the healer to a great extent was felt to be derived from his special relationship with the supernatural, which allowed him to use magic. Simply stated, magic is the formula of doing the right thing at the right time, using the proper objects, and saying the right words. Magical practices are based on empirical data: not necessarily gathered in what might be considered a scientific manner, nevertheless it was based on observation. Once a practice proved its superior excellence, it was endowed with a kind of force and power of its own.

The above description may seem at first glance to be the practices of a very primitive culture. There are, however, some striking similarities between the description and scientific medicine. A physician is contacted when the individual decides that his condition is sufficiently serious that he needs expert advice and help. Physicians have high status and are endowed with considerable power to heal that may not necessarily be warranted. The power ascribed to physicians is evident in the documentation that placebo medication is sufficiently effective that it is far above the level of chance. We expect the physician to have a stethoscope ready at hand and to conduct a physical examination in a certain fashion. If this does not occur the individual often feels that he has not been given proper attention and may question the competence of the physician. Words continue to be endowed with some magic as the student reader may recognize in his concern for knowing the right words to say in particular clinical situations.

Scientific medicine, legitimately granted recognition for what it has accomplished, continues to be a litany of unknowns. One question previously mentioned is, when is an individual healthy and when is he sick. The point where health ends and disease begins is arbitrary at best. There are some signs, although not universally accepted, of obvious good health and obvious disease. It is all that is in between that is questionable. A state of health tends to be defined in the negative: the absence of any evidence of disease or disability. What the individual perceives as illness is not always brought to the attention of a physician nor is what is brought to his attention always conceded by him to be illness. The factors that govern the individual's assumption of the sick role are largely unknown. (The concept of sick role will be discussed in the section on social environment.) Much more needs to be known about people's criteria for perceiving, acknowledging, and describing their own disordered function and behavior. One survey of people in the United States and Great Britain indicates that out of a population of 1,000 adults in a one-month period, 750 will experience an episode of illness (as reported by the individual), 250 will consult a physician, and 9 will be hospitalized. The study showed that there was no relationship between the severity of the condition and whether a person consulted a physician or was hospitalized (672).

In the area of psychosocial function, the terms "adjustment" or "adaptation" are often used: used as if their meaning were unequivocal. This is not necessarily true because they have been used to cover all of the responses of the organism to external factors irrespective of whether these factors are classified as healthy or morbid. Although social approval and disapproval play a large part in deciding what should be called social maladaptation, it does vary according to the group that expresses the approval or disapproval and the situation in which the behavior occurs. Forms of behavior that an outsider might identify as maladaptation may enjoy social approval, at least for a period of time, by a section of society. Some examples that come immediately to mind are the artist half-starving in his loft and an individual taking an unpaid leave of absence from his job in order to "find himself." Thus the criteria for healthy functioning are not primarily social. It is a misconception to equate ill health with social deviation or maladjustment. There is a great deal still to be learned about the cultural and situational factors that lead to different modes of expressing symptoms of psychological distress. It is also unknown under what conditions expression of psychological distress becomes evidence of an underlying deficit in the individual's capacity to function in an adequate manner.

A relationship between cultural dislocation and health has frequently been suggested. Hinkle's study of this relationship led to the following findings (432). Cultural dislocation, accompanied by social change and a change in interpersonal relations, may result in a significant negative alteration in health if: (a) the individual perceives the change as negative in relationship to his immediate past situation; (b) the individual has a preexisting illness or susceptibility to illness; or (c) there is a significant change in the individual's activities, habits, ingestants, exposure to disease-causing agents, or in the physical characteristics of his environment.

In the absence of any of these factors, an individual was not likely to experience any negative change in health. Individuals who did not respond as predicted in the presence of the three factors mentioned were described as people who have a capacity to experience cultural change and personal deprivation without a profound emotional or psychological response. No data were presented to account for this difference in response to cultural dislocation.

The purpose or functions of medical intervention appear to be similar across almost all cultures. These functions are to (a) prevent and cure disease, (b) reassure and allay anxiety, and (c) assist the individual to adjust to the behavior demanded by his culture. The latter may take the form of modern day psychotherapy or positively sanctioning participation in the sick role for a period of time.

Although the functions of medical intervention are similar, the means used and the shared understanding surrounding health and illness are not. Thus the cultural background of the participants in intervention is very important. In a highly stratified and pluralistic society there are likely to be considerable cultural differences between health professionals and lay members of the society. This frequently happens when the health professional and the patient have different cultural backgrounds. It also can happen, however, when the health professional and the patient were reared in the same cultural group. The education received by health professionals in industrialized Western society is such that they are socialized into a culture quite different from that of their origin. This "medical culture" has many common understandings that are often not held by members of other cultural groups. The health professional and the patient each are likely to interpret the other's behavior in terms of his own values and beliefs, making for difficulty in communication and comprehension.

To illustrate some of the cultural differences between the health profession and the lay public, some of the shared understandings of the health profession are outlined below. It should be noted that, as is true with any cultural group, not all of the understandings to be mentioned are shared by every member of the cultural group.

First, it takes full responsibility for establishing what phenomena are considered to be disease, what the causes of particular diseases are, how to determine a diagnosis, what means should be used for treatment, and when a disease is in remission or has been terminated.

Second, it tends to see the patient as the passive recipient of services. This characteristic and the first one place medical professionals in a position of authority. Thus the patient is made to feel that his own experience of his illness is incorrect, irrelevant, and/or inferior. His own ideas and opinions are seen as insignificant.

Third, it perceives illness as a biological phenomenon that precludes or severely inhibits attention to the personal and social concerns that patients and families bring into the medical situation. By focus on the biological phenomena of disease (deviation from the norm of measurable somatic variables), the cultural, social, and psychological constructions of the problem by the patient and family are virtually excluded. In many cultures psychological stress, worry, strained interpersonal relations, and unfavorable environmental and living conditions figure prominently among the multiple etiological factors that are used to interpret and understand illness. This is in contrast to the predominantly biological parameters of the situation as conceived by the health professions.

Fourth, it provides little education for health professionals in regard to cultural, social, and psychological components of illness. Thus medical personnel are ill equipped to deal with this aspect of the patient's problem. This is all the more serious when the patient and health professional have different cultural origins.

Finally, it interprets disease primarily as "person centered," temporally bounded, and discontinuous. The former leads to a tendency to exclude family and friends from the intervention process and/or to be minimally concerned with their worries and problems. The latter leads to perception of disease as an acute phenomenon; the patient is expected to recover or die. It also promotes a discreet and segmented approach to intervention that requires only an episodic focus on the patient.

Until health professionals are conscious of their own cultural biases in approaching illness, they are unlikely to attend to the views of laymen regardless of their cultural background or to comprehend the importance of laymen's views in the shared enterprise of dealing with acute episodes and the long-term process of chronic conditions.

The culture of the health professions can perhaps be best perceived in contrast with the shared understandings of other cultural groups in regard to health and illness. Prior to looking at some of the areas of cultural differences, it should be noted that there are ethnic differences in disease rates. The factors that appear to account for some of these variations are access to medical treatment, genetic predispositions, adequacy of nutrition and housing, degree of exposure to pathogenic agents, and ethnically patterned pathogenic cultural standards or behaviors (e.g., the use of alcohol and the high ingestion rate of certain types of foods). There is, however, much that remains unknown about the factors that account for variation in ethnic group disease rates. The sampling methods used have also been questioned; much of the research has made use of subjects who were hospitalized or making regular clinic visits.

In addition to disease rates there are several other cultural differences between ethnic groups.

Techniques for Health Maintenance

This area includes the degree to which an ethnic group is concerned about such things as regular visits to a dentist and medical checkups, pre- and postnatal care, preventative immunizations, cleanliness, adequate diet, regular exercise, home safety, and the care of minor ailments. This area is particularly important in terms of the extent to which the cultural group will respond to information about preventative measures and self-care.

Presentation of Complaints Regarding Illness

There are many ways in which symptoms are differentially perceived, evaluated, and acted on, or not acted on. Whether an individual allows his symptoms to rise above the threshold of mild complaint depends on the way in which he perceives illness and on what he thinks is the appropriate response to illness. Three factors seem particularly important in determining illness.

The first factor is the location or nature of the symptom. Cultural groups become alarmed about different symptoms, e.g., pain, impotence, gastrointestinal problems, weight loss, fever, respiratory problems. The second factor is the duration and intensity of the symptom. Some cultural groups expect the individual to respond immediately to the symptom; others feel no action is called for unless the symptom persists for a long time or is extremely severe. The third factor is the social effect of the symptom in terms of interference with valued social activities or the fulfillment of role responsibilities. In this case expected behavior may be to attend immediately to a symptom that interferes or it may be to ignore the symptom and stoically carry on with one's usual routine. There are also cultural differences in the way in which symptoms are presented. Many cultural groups have a particular vocabulary for describing symptoms that may not be understood by an outsider. On the other hand, the words used may be understood by the listener but he may ascribe a very different meaning to the words. The expression, for example, "I have a nervous stomach," could have a number of different meanings. Symptoms may be presented in a very circumspect manner. The most serious symptom, as perceived by the individual, being presented last, for example. The individual may be obviously vague about complaints related to aspects of the body that are not openly discussed in his culture; problems related to elimination and sexual matters are common areas of difficulty. In some cultures emotional concerns and psychological distress tend to be expressed as physical or somatic problems.

Pain and Discomfort

There are cultural differences in the definition of what is painful. If an individual expects to feel only minimal pain, then that is likely to be his experience. The degree of pain and discomfort experienced in childbirth is one example. Response to pain varies from one culture to another. Individuals who are members of some cultures express pain in a volatile and highly emotional manner; others may simply deny the existence of pain. When there is a strong positive motivation, people will undergo extraordinary pain without complaint. Attitudes toward pain may differ. Some individuals simply want relief; others are more concerned with the meaning of pain relative to their future health.

Relationship to the Culture of the Health Professions

There is considerable variation in the extent to which different cultural groups make use of modern medical personnel and facilities. Many cultures feel that the vast majority of illnesses will respond to home remedy and that medical attention should only be sought when the condition has reached severe proportions. Some cultures have their own providers of health care who may be consulted prior to, in conjunction with, and/or following involvement with modern health professionals. There are differences in knowledge about biomedical categories of disease and conceptions about the causes of disease and illness. Some cultural groups, for example, accept a psychological interpretation of various illnesses; others do not. Information about therapeutic resources and how to find and use them also varies. There are differences in understanding the expectations of the health professions' culture. The individual may or may not know how to give a medical history, describe his problem, request specific services and information, and so forth. The individual's culturally influenced response to the medical situation is likely to be evident in his general style of interaction: his attitude toward authority figures, response to members of the opposite sex, reactions to the age of various health professionals, ways of expressing emotion and asking for help, expectations regarding the behavior of personnel, understanding of terms used, and response to an explanation of his diagnosis and suggested methods of intervention.

Adherence to a Therapeutic Regimen

Some cultures consider following treatment advice evidence of responsible behavior; others do not. There are differences in the degree to which the individual will raise questions and want explanations. Some individuals are accepting of medication and other procedures; others are reluctant and mistrustful. Adherence to therapeutic regimens in a medical situation does not necessarily indicate that the regimen will be followed at home. The individual's response in the home setting is far more likely to be influenced by his cultural background than response in a medical setting. At home the individual often feels far more comfortable following the tenets of his culture than the strange ideas and values found in the medical situation.

This section has not dealt with the shared understandings of any specific cultural group. The reason for this omission was to minimize the possibility of responding in a stereotyped manner to members of a given group. It is suggested that the therapist explore the shared understandings of the various cultural groups with which he or she interacts regularly. This can be done through an exploration of the literature. But perhaps a far better way is to discuss the norms, values, and ideas of a particular culture with members of that culture.

THE SOCIAL ENVIRONMENT

Culture is an important factor in understanding an individual and as a consideration in the evaluation and intervention process. The social environment in which the individual lives is also important (474,672,940). There are components within the social environment that, influenced to some extent by culture, are essentially cross-culture phenomena. There are, for example, age and sex patterns relative to illness. Children are more susceptible to infectious disease, adolescents tend to sustain more physical injuries, older adults are prone to cardiovascular conditions. Women tend to become depressed in their forties whereas men are more likely to become depressed in their late sixties and early seventies. Men take more health risks than women, seek medical care less readily, are less expressive about illness, and are more stoical when in pain. Socioeconomic status influences the way in which a state of illness is articulated. Individuals, for example, who have less formal education, live in a rural setting, and have a low income are more likely to express psychological distress through the presentation of physical symptoms. Although people classify illness within the tenets of the common lore of their culture, among the most educated classification is closest to that of contemporary medicine.

The next section addresses a more in-depth discussion of four social factors that are cross-cultural.

Social Networks

Social networks are a web of voluntary relationships that make up an individual's primary social environment (197, 940). They delineate the nature of the environment to which the individual is exposed, provide emotional and,. at times, financial support, and place constraints on behavior. All people within an individual's social network do not necessarily know one another and each of these people may have her own network of social relationships with others.

Social networks can be placed on a continuum from close to loosely knit. In a close-knit social network, most of the people know each other and interact with each other independent of the instigation of a particular individual. The network tends to be geographically contained in terms of a neighborhood or community. Members of the network have a sense of in-group identification and feelings of belonging and frequently are members of the same ethnic group. They tend to consider the ideal relationship between people who live nearby to be one of mutual interdependence and material assistance. Close-knit social networks also establish rather strict norms relative to acceptable behavior. This may have one negative aspect. The individual frequently feels there is no escape from actual or supposed surveillance by kin and neighbors. Such a perception, which is often quite accurate, encourages conformity, lack of individualism, and susceptibility to social control through gossip. There is then a trade-off between shared understandings and social support and the requirement for complicance with accepted customs.

Individuals who live within a loose-knit social network tend to be physically mobile. They frequently have many different sets of social networks, with work or professional associations often being the most close knit. Physical proximity is not associated with social proximity. A formal attitude is taken toward people who live close by. Individuals with a loose-knit network tend to seek emotional satisfaction and social support in a less direct manner and have more varied types of needs. They experience less dependency on the extended family and may have only occasional contact with them. Stress is placed on material and social self-sufficiency of each household. They depend on persons dispersed over a wide area for friendship, the sharing of mutual interests, and emotional support. Social controls are based on many factors other than those exercised by local residence. For an individual with a loose-knit social network, there is a trade-off between greater autonomy and less immediate support. Such individuals also must learn to live in a matrix of different and often conflicting values and expected modes of behavior.

The type of social network an individual has is influenced by personal choice as well as the social attributes of occupation, place of residence, class, sex, birth rank, and size of family of origin. The structure of one's network may vary over time, depending on mobility, marital status, and one's progress through the life cycle. Individuals who frequently move from one place of residence to another, who are divorced or widowed, or who are elderly tend, at least temporarily, to have a loose-knit social network. The sense of social uncertainty and loneliness that results from leaving a contained network where every nuance of social behavior was understood is often severe. This is particularly true for individuals who are not working or who are homebound. The experience of dislocation is less severe if the new place of residence is perceived as physically better, if the new neighborhood is similar to the old relative to class and ethnic background, and if neighbors tend to be accepting of new residents. Irregardless of these factors, however, it may take considerable time for the individual to establish a new network that is and is perceived as supportive as the former network. The old neighborhood is likely to be seen always, in may ways, as the ideal place of residence.

Family Structure

Family structure can be a source of considerable support for an individual or it may have a negative impact on the individual. The latter will be briefly discussed first.

There are several family patterns that are considered to be detrimental to the individual. These patterns are seen as either being a causal factor in the development of dysfunction or as inhibiting the further growth of a disabled individual. The patterns may occur singly or in some combination. One pattern that has been documented as being fairly common is physical abuse. Wives, children, and elderly people are sometimes subjected to beatings or deprivation of food. Serious permanent injury or death is not uncommon. Although the abuse may be ostensibly physical in nature, it takes little imagination to comprehend the tremendous psychological component to such abuse.

Inhibition of development is another pattern. For any number of reasons the family may not foster acquisition of functional patterns of behavior or independence. This may happen, as was mentioned previously, with the developmentally disabled child or the individual with an acquired disability. However, it may also occur relative to an individual who has no discernible disability. The pattern may be seen in situations where children and adolescents are prohibited from engaging in the usual and typical activities of their age group, where wives are discouraged from pursuing their own interests, and when elderly people are treated as if they were senile and incapable of making a serious decision.

The pattern of giving mixed messages occurs when family members say one thing and act in a way that is contrary to their statements. One example of mixed messages is when a father advises high standards relative to sexual activities for his daughter and at the same time behaves in a very seductive manner toward her. Mixed messages are also apparent when behavior in the home is not congruent with behavior in the wider community. A mother, for example, may portray herself as a loving and concerned parent to friends and relatives and be incapable of giving any kind of affection to her children. A pattern of mixed messages leaves the recipient totally confused and markedly ambivalent toward the sender. The individual is essentially left without any clear idea in regard to expectations or the sense of a shared reality.

The last pattern to be discussed is referred to as scapegoating. A dictionary definition of a scapegoat is "one who is made to bear the blame for others or to suffer in their place." As patterns of family interaction, scapegoating may take two somewhat different forms. One subpattern involves the definition of one family member as inadequate, sick, or deviant in some way. Because of the tremendous pressure toward conformity to family expectations, the individual usually acts in the prescribed manner. The other subpattern is that one family member bears all of the wrath or "transient madness" of another family member, usually a parent. The function of these patterns is to maintain the apparent stability of the family and to protect family members from recognizing that there are seriously defective interaction patterns within the family. There is typically a conspiracy of silence surrounding such patterns; indeed, for the most part they are unconscious. The scapegoat, if aware of the pattern, may hesitate in making any statement about the situation for fear of disrupting the family or of making matters worse than they already are. She often believes that by behaving in the prescribed manner or by absorbing the irrational behavior of the parent, she is taking responsibility for holding the family together—a perception that is often quite accurate. Evidence for the existence of patterns of scapegoating is apparent when the scapegoat leaves or is taken out of the family situation. The family usually either selects another scapegoat or becomes highly disorganized. The individual who is the scapegoat tends to develop a number of behavioral patterns which, although functional within the family, are dysfunctional in interactions outside the family setting. Most individuals who have been scapegoats do not trust other people, have difficulty in accepting affection, are uncertain as to what is "real" in any situation, are hypersensitive to interpersonal dynamics, and have a decidedly low self-esteem.

The supportive strength of families in the presence of stressful situations, illness, and disability is dependent to a great extent on the types of social networks in which they are embedded. It is also dependent, however, on several other factors. One factor is the structure of the family, which essentially varies along two continuums: disorganized to stable, and rigid to flexible. A family that is stable and relatively flexible is usually able to provide the best kind of support for an individual. The family's financial situation is also a factor. Families in financial straits usually cannot allocate economic resources for the care of a disabled individual. In addition, long working hours and worry about money often leave little energy for giving emotional support. A small family is often less capable of providing support than a larger family. In a larger family, responsibilities for a disabled member can be shared among members so that one individual does not have to bear all of the burden of care. A small family is sometimes able to draw on the resources of members of the extended family. This can only occur, however, when there is an extended family available and they are willing to provide assistance. A family's place in the life cycle may mitigate against providing assistance. A woman, for example, with three young children may only be able to provide minimal assistance to her brother who has recently sustained a severe spinal cord injury. The ability of the family to engage in open and honest communication is another important factor. This is not an all or none phenomenon. There may be generally good communication but with some areas being discussed far less freely. Thus there may be weak or strained links in the family's communication system. The family's means of dealing with stress in the past is a major indicator of how they will deal with illness or disability and the extent to which they are able to provide support. Finally, the place where the family and its various members are in adjustment to the individual's condition and the degree of anger and guilt will influence capacity to give support.

Although the family can provide a tremendous amount of support, there are times when it is detrimental to the individual, the family, or both for the individual to remain within the family setting. The care of the individual may be so extensive and pervasive that the function of the family is severely disrupted. This may be the case, for example, with a severely retarded and multiply handicapped individual, an autistic child, or an individual who needs a highly complex medical regimen to maintain life. An individual's personality structure and/or disability may be such that she makes such excessive demands that the family is in a constant state of turmoil accompanied by considerable anger and guilt. Although there are times when such interaction patterns can be altered through outside assistance, there are other times when this cannot be accomplished. There are situations when there is no family member able or willing to provide the care and support that the individual needs. This is particularly likely to occur at the two ends of the life cycle: the young child and the aged individual. At times the family is quite able to give support, but the individual's further growth may be enhanced by living outside the family home. The young adult, for example, who is mildly or moderately retarded, multiply handicapped, or emotionally disturbed may be able to become far more independent living in a group home of some sort. When the family pattern of interaction is essentially pathogenic, as described previously, it is often wisest to remove the individual, at least temporarily, from this potentially destructive environment. This is usually only considered after efforts to alter the family structure have failed. The recommendation for an individual to leave the family home is not made lightly or without due consideration of a number of possible alternatives. This area will be discussed further in Chapters 29 and 30.

The Sick Role

A sick person has a special position, a social role, with implicit rules and privileges (348,472,672,727, 764,940). The conditions under which sick privileges are confirmed vary between cultures, families, and social situations. The latter refers to participation in the sick role, for example, at home when one has a mild cold but not taking this role while one is at work. Criteria for being permitted to play the sick role are bound up with cultural and familial norms and values which define being sick as opposed to malingering and hypochondria. These norms and values, as well as financial resources in some cases, determine whether one may legitimately take a sick role.

The sick role in the presence of acute illness, although varying somewhat from one culture to another, usually takes the following forms: (a) the individual is exempt from usual social responsibilities; the extent of exemption is dependent on how serious the illness is considered to be by the group; (b) the individual cannot help herself and must be cared for by others; (c) being sick is regarded as a misfortune; it is assumed the sick person will desire to get well and, in fact, is under an obligation to do so; or (d) the individual should seek competent help and cooperate in the process of getting well.

If an individual attempts to take the sick role when the group does not consider this to be justified, he or she is often accused of being lazy, simply attempting to avoid responsibility, or emotionally disturbed (not, it should be noted, mentally ill). An individual who does not assume the sick role when it is deemed necessary is subject to negative sanctions, considered to be a fool for taking such risks, and, at times, seen as a menace to herself or others. Individuals who do not assume the proper partner role relative to the sick person, e.g., be sympathetic and act as a caretaker, are also subject to negative sanctions.

Traditionally, according to the norms of the health professions, the individual in the sick role was expected to cooperate by being passive, resting, and doing what one was told to do without question or explanation. For some lay individuals these traditional expectations are no longer considered to be valid. They desire to be more active participants in making decisions about their medical care and request extensive information so as to be able both to understand and to make informed decisions. Some health professionals consider this to be rather deviant behavior, preferring the more traditional definition of the sick role.

The expectations of passivity and so forth as part of the sick role are not considered to be compatible with the habilitation/rehabilitation process. Rather active participation and questioning are felt to be necessary for the process to be successful. This may cause some confusion for an individual who is used to taking the traditional sick role.

The sick role seems to be less often condoned relative to emotional problems as opposed to physical illness. This is particularly true in the case of affective and anxiety disorders and disorders characterized by substance abuse. Individuals who are, for example, depressed or anxious are sometimes thought to be malingering or are simply told to "pull themselves together." In either case, they are denied the sick role. Paranoid, schizophrenic, and organic mental disorders are more likely to lead to the individual being defined as sick. As with all illness, mental disorders are defined by the culture. The manifestation of mental disorders is also strongly influenced by culture. Conversion disorders (loss of physical function as an expression of psychological conflict or need), for example, was quite common in nineteenth century Europe and the United States. It is now a fairly rare diagnosis. The extent to which certain patterns of behavior are defined as mental disorders is, to some extent, also influenced by the tolerance of the culture for diverse behavior.

The above discussion of the sick role is primarily related to the behavioral expectations of an individual who is in the acute and habilitative/rehabilitative phase of illness. A chronic sick role only occurs in cultural groups where there is technology allowing a number of chronically ill individuals to survive, an economy to support unproductive individuals, and a system of values that insist they should be cared for. These factors have only been relatively common in the past hundred years. Thus, the chronic sick role is far less well defined than that of the behavior expected in acute illness.

Cultures have treated chronic illness when it occurs in a variety of ways. When the illness is endemic to the group it is often not defined as illness. Malaria in some underdeveloped countries is an example of such a situation. In some cultures the person is given a variety of special privileges but is not expected to play the role of a worker, spouse, or parent; essentially she is expected to act like an invalid. Other cultures assume the individual will engage in any activities that she is able to master with no particular privileges or limitations prescribed.

Being bedridden has long been recognized as a role in Western industrialized society. However, there is ambiguity in regard to people who are up and around and able to hold a job. They seem all right and therefore may not be defined as ill. Families often experience difficulty in according them the necessary relief from normal obligations warranted by their condition. On the other hand, they may not expect them to take a reasonable amount of responsibilities.

In some cultures, the chronic sick role offers a prolonged escape from everyday responsibilities and for this reason some people may prefer this role despite the disadvantages of disablement and unemployment that it entails.

There are those people who take on or prolong the sick role as a means of coping with stress. For such people, the symptoms presented are frequently of no special consequence but rather seem to establish the legitimacy of taking the sick role and of forming a relationship with a helping person. Often physical symptoms are presented, at least initially, because the individual's culture may define such symptoms as more acceptable than evidence of emotional distress. Symptoms of physical illness, on the other hand, may be presented well beyond the usual normal course of the illness. This serves to maintain the sick role for an extended period of time. Such symptoms are often due to emotional distress. Misattribution of this sort may occur because of the similarity of the symptoms. Continued complaints of fatigue and weakness, for example, may follow the apparent clinical termination of a debilitating disease. This may actually be evidence of depression or anxiety. Information about possible sources of the individual's symptoms provided in a sympathetic and supportive way often helps to avoid attributional errors and new reasons for anxiety on the part of the individual. This is far better than blanket reassurance that provides no alternative framework for the individual to understand her symptoms. Reassurance that does not take into account the individual's assessment of the threat that she faces, whatever that threat may be, serves only to mystify and undermine the individual's confidence in the therapist. Approaches that facilitate the individual's coping efforts are far more useful.

Community Resources

Community resources here refers to special agencies and organizations that are concerned about the health and quality of life of chronically ill or disabled individuals and their families. These may be directed and staffed by trained personnel, by concerned citizens including chronically ill and disabled individuals and their families, or by both. Some examples of the services provided through community agencies are specialized medical care, habilitation/rehabilitation services, financial support and/or the provision and maintenance of equipment, home health care personnel, day programs, home visits, meals delivered to the home, temporary fulltime care, vocational counseling, training centers, support groups, family and/or individual counseling, residential homes, social and recreational activities, and so forth.

The extent to which such resources are available in a community varies. There is also considerable variation in the degree to which they are utilized by individuals and families. Important factors are knowledge of these resources and the capacity to use them wisely and well. As mentioned, it often takes considerable social skill to locate, become connected with, and receive optimal service from community resources. The ability to negotiate is particularly important. Other factors influencing use are the individual's and family's financial situations, cultural values regarding the use of such resources, personal preference, the severity of the individual's condition, the nature of the individual's social network, and the structure and dynamics of the family.

All of these factors seem to be interrelated. Limited financial resources and severity of the individual's condition lead to a greater use of community resources. Cultural and personal values that place emphasis on self-sufficiency and, if necessary, reliance on members of the immediate family mitigate use of community resources. Individuals and families who have a close-knit social network make less use of community resources. In the absence of a close-knit network, a family in trouble is likely to need considerable assistance from social agencies and for a long period of time. There seems to be an inverse proportion between the degree of support a family is able to provide and the need for and use of community agencies. An individual is often likely to turn to community agencies when there is change in the family structure such as death of a member, marriage, divorce, change in residence, or the illness of another family member.

Knowledge of and helping individuals and families to make optimal use of community resources are an important function of the occupational therapist. Not only do community resources provide valuable practical assistance but they also help in minimizing a sense of isolation and the anxiety that is aroused by the feeling that one is alone with nowhere to turn for help.

THE PHYSICAL ENVIRONMENT

Although the cultural and social environment strongly influences behavior and the individual's capacity to adapt to external and internal stress, the physical environment also plays a role. This section discusses the physical environment as it impinges on the psychosocial capacity of the individual. The nonhuman environment, a more general category that includes the physical environment, is discussed in Chapter 7. Discussion here will be limited to more immediate kinds of responses to the physical environment.

The first concern that most people have about the physical environment is in relationship to adequate food, clothing, and shelter. What is adequate may be defined by one's culture and social network. There is, however, a fairly universal level that is considered below subsistence. Existence at such a level for any period of time is not only detrimental to physical health but to the individual's psychological well-being. Malnutrition and the diseases related to poor sanitation and the extremes of temperature are debilitating. In such a condition the individual is more susceptible to stress and less able to adapt. When individuals are primarily preoccupied with providing at least subsistence food, clothing, and shelter they have little energy for coping with emergencies and unexpected contingencies. The new situation is viewed as a catastrophic event rather than a problem that must be addressed and solved. A sense of disorganization and a high level of anxiety or depression are likely to occur. The individual's physical and emotional resources have been stretched too far. This is particularly likely to occur in the absence of an adequate family structure and/or a close-knit social network.

In addition to adequate food, clothing, and shelter, the physical environment is distinguished by ambiance: the mood, character, quality, and tone of the atmosphere. Individuals' sensitivity to ambiance varies. Some people do not really seem to care what they eat, how they dress, or where they live as long as they perceive it as adequate in satisfying their particular needs. Others might define the situation as drab, sparse, and lacking in any real comforts but this is totally immaterial to the individual involved. Some people, on the other hand, are highly sensitive to the ambiance of their physical environment. They feel uncomfortable, out of sorts, and even anxious or depressed if their environment is not perceived as suitable according to their definition. There are, for example, individuals who prefer living in a neat, well-ordered environment. Other people prefer a less structured environment with belongings simply somewhere in the vicinity; orderliness is not considered a high priority. Living in an environment that does not have a compatible ambiance can be a source of stress. This is particularly important to remember when an individual is not in his usual environment, for example, when he is in a hospital or extended care facility.

The lack of physical safety is another factor that can lead to emotional distress. Threats to physical safety may be present in the work place, school, on the street, or in one's home. The latter two sources of threat to safety were discussed relative to elderly individuals but they can also cause concern for any age group. Children and young adults often do not feel safe on the streets or other public places and the likelihood of one's home being robbed is quite high in many parts of the United States. Women have an additonal threat to their safety: rape. Many women, with good reason, feel they are in a highly vulnerable position, and must be continually on guard against such an event. Rape itself is an extremely traumatic experience, with frequently profound psychological repercussions. The feeling that one is unsafe can lead to a chronic state of anxiety. Additional energy is needed to manage such anxiety. This leaves less energy to cope with other aspects of daily life.

Physically disabled individuals may experience limited range of motion, decrease in strength and endurance, uncoordination, loss of use of one upper extremity or one side of the body, blindness, deafness, and the necessity to use a wheelchair, crutches, cane, or a walker. Such disabilities impede adequate and competent interactions in relationship to the physical environment. The environment becomes filled with barriers that may be found in public places, at home, or in the workplace (635,636,960).

Some common architectural barriers are stairs, curbs, raised thresholds, the height of water fountains and public telephones, heavy and revolving doors, toilet stalls, public transportation, and the structures of supermarkets, theaters, and restaurants. In the home the individual may be faced with too narrow hallways and doorways, inadequate kitchen and bathroom design, difficulty in reaching light switches, inadequate telephone equipment, and so forth. In addition to the barriers found in public places which may make accessibility to the workplace difficult or impossible, the design of the workplace may present other barriers. Architectural barriers cause a great deal of frustration for a disabled individual. They limit independence and diminish the individual's sense of competence and mastery. They may make it very difficult or impossible for a person to work or to participate in many recreational activities. The individual may, essentially, be confined to the home for long periods of time. Such a situation is not conducive to good mental health. A sense of boredom, isolation from others, and poor self-esteem are common. This in turn may lead to anger, depression, and other signs of emotional distress.

The complexity and lack of order in the physical environment may cause difficulty for individuals who are deficient in the areas of sensory integration, visual perception, orientation, intelligence, and problem solving. Unable to comprehend or structure the physical environment adequately, such individuals often have a chronic sense of confusion and disorientation. Anxiety and withdrawal are common responses.

The opportunity to be surrounded by objects that are perceived as attractive and that have personal meaning is another important facet of the physical environment. The need to be surrounded by and dependent on functional aids and adaptive equipment may be experienced as most unpleasant. Movement into a sheltered environment may necessitate giving up treasured objects. That which has personal meaning is replaced by utilitarian objects that feel quite foreign to the individual. Neither of these situations is conducive to a general sense of need satisfaction.

CONCLUSION

The environment—cultural, social, and physical—is one of the parameters of the occupational therapy domain of concern. Similar to occupational performances and age, it is taken into consideration in evaluation and intervention. The individual can only be understood and assisted when the therapist has knowledge of the client's past and present environment and some idea about the client's future expected environment.

Part 3

Legitimate Tools

As discussed in Chapter 1, legitimate tools are one part of a profession's model. They are the permissible means by which the practitioners of a profession fulfill their responsibility to society. It is through the use of its tools that a profession attempts to achieve its goals in meeting specific needs of society. Although the legitimate tools of a profession may change over time, at any given time, members of a profession are expected to use only those tools that are currently defined as legitimate for the profession. When a practitioner uses other tools he or she may be negatively sanctioned by members of the profession, by society, or by both.

Perhaps more than any other part of a profession's model, a profession holds its legitimate tools in high regard. They come, for many, to represent or symbolize the profession. This probably occurs because tools have a more tangible quality than a body of knowledge or domain of concern, for example. The stethoscope of the physician; the blackboard, chalk, and pointer of the teacher; the loom and leather craft supplies of the occupational therapist are legitimate tools frequently used to symbolize these professions. Granted such symbols are stereotypes and also usually out of date. Nevertheless, they are important for they serve both to identify and as a means of communication. Legitimate tools are often the most obvious and concrete point of articulation between the profession and society.

The legitimate tools of occupational therapy are the nonhuman environment, conscious use of self, the teaching-learning process, purposeful activities, activity groups, and activity analysis and synthesis. Each will be discussed in this part in some detail.

7 The Nonhuman Environment

The term "nonhuman environment" refers to all aspects of the environment that are not human. Prior to discussion of the nonhuman environment as a tool it would seem expedient to focus on it as an entity in its own right. This chapter is divided into two parts: the nature of the nonhuman environment and the nonhuman environment as a tool.

THE NATURE OF THE NONHUMAN ENVIRONMENT

Harold Searles' name is almost synonomous with the concept of the nonhuman environment (873). His text on the subject is considered a classic; it is suggested that the reader explore the book in its entirety. Here three aspects of Searles' text will be outlined: (a) the way in which the nonhuman environment facilitates normal growth and development, (b) the nonhuman environment as a possible source of anxiety, and (c) the ways in which constructive interaction with the nonhuman environment can be impeded.

Facilitation of Development

One of the first tasks of the infant is to differentiate between the self and the environment. Much has been written about the differentiation process relative to the human environment. For example, the child at some point comes to distinguishing the difference between herself and her mother. But in order to see the self as truly human one must also identify basic differences between what is human and what is not human. Through stimulation by the nonhuman environment and self-stimulation, the infant begins to perceive "the me versus the not me" or what is external to the self as opposed to internal to the self. Through interaction with various components of the nonhuman environment the child begins to identify those characteristics that are unique to being human. This process continues through life and, in some ways, is never really completed. An illustration of this is the tendency to attribute human feelings to favored pets or plants.

The nonhuman environment contributes to one's sense of security. It tends to be more stable and predictable than the human environment. Periodic changes in the nonhuman environment do occur but they are likely to be rhythmic in nature: day and night, the seasons of the year. In addition, the nonhuman environment often provides a continuity of experience as one moves through time and space. For example, the custom of offering a visitor food and something to drink is not only something one is taught to do as a child but it is a custom common to most of the cultural groups one is likely to encounter in adult life. The nonhuman environment provides a sense of security in a physical manner, e.g., the lock on one's door, the telephone in case of an emergency, a flashlight when the electricity fails. The nonhuman environment also provides security in a symbolic manner. A classic example is the transitional objects of a child. Whether it be a frayed blanket or a stuffed animal, these are significant and important objects that contribute to growth. But even as adults, individuals have nonhuman objects that symbolize a security-giving person or situation. For example, many young adults, when leaving their parents' home to establish a new home, take some special object with them that is carefully kept and guarded.

The nonhuman environment offers an opportunity for self-understanding. Love, tenderness, nurturing, sadistic or selfish impulses can be directed toward the nonhuman environment with some degree of safety. For example, a child learns much about his capacity to nurture by caring for a puppy; an adult in moments of anger or frustration may throw pillows, slam down books, or break a tennis racket. Such activities provide an opportunity for the individual to become consciously aware of these feelings and impulses. In addition, the individual, hopefully, comes to recognize that these emotions are good, acceptable, and a controllable part of the self. Some of the individual's assets and limitations may be tested through interaction with the nonhuman environment. Manual dexterity, problem solving, tolerance for ambiguity, and the ability to give and receive love are some examples that come to mind.

Similar to gaining self-understanding relative to the nonhuman environment, one can also gain greater understanding of others. Observation of another person's interaction with the nonhuman environment gives the observer considerable information about that person. Individuals tend to express feelings more freely and honestly toward the nonhuman environment than toward the human environment. Although a precise relationship cannot and should not be made, there is often some relationship. For example, an individual who is cruel to animals may not be someone whom we would want as a friend. The individual who asks before looking through one's bookshelves may arouse a very different response.

The nonhuman environment facilitates the initial development of all performance components as well as their maintenance. Some of the examples given above have emphasized the relationship between the nonhuman environment and psychological functions and social interaction. It is important to remember, however, the significance of the nonhuman environment in relationship to sensory integration, visual perception, and cognitive and motor function. In the early years a child is exposed to a vast variety of sensory stimulation from the nonhuman environment: sounds, textures, shapes, smells to name only a few. These stimuli provide the impetus for development of sensory integrative skills. It is through manipulation of nonhuman objects that the child often begins to conceptualize and learn about relationships—for example, balls are for throwing, cups are for drinking, only so many blocks will fit into a pail. Motor development is enhanced through interaction with the nonhuman environment. Watching a child learn how to go up and down stairs provides ample evidence of this relationship. However, it is not only initial development but the continued development and maintenance of these functions that is facilitated by the interaction with the nonhuman environment. As noxious as it occasionally is, the nonhuman environment presents us with sensory stimuli that must be integrated. Our continued need for cognitive stimuli is evident in the current popularity of games of strategy. We use such activities as jogging, swimming, and racketball to maintain motor function.

The nonhuman environment enhances the quality of life. This is particularly evident in our use of tools and various technologies. For example, most homes in the United States have running water; food is available at the local supermarket and various means of transportation get us fairly quickly to distant locations. These conveniences, so to speak, allow more time to engage in other activities that may be far more rewarding than, for example, fetching water from a well. Various tools and technologies have freed the individual to devote more time to interpersonal relationships and activities that satisfy self-actualization needs.

Similarly, in many respects, the nonhuman environment can be a source of pleasure, enjoyment, and relaxation. A walk on a quiet beach in the early evening, reading a good book, and listening to classical music are experiences which many people regard as special. We treasure and enjoy many of our possessions, e.g., our home and its furnishings, a worn bathrobe we wear after a long day's work, a wall hanging we bought while visiting a foreign country. All these, too, enhance the quality of our life.

Finally, relative to growth and development, the nonhuman environment provides relief from the human environment. There are times when the individual needs to be away from other human beings. In the healthy individual this is a periodic and temporary need for withdrawal. During this time the individual has an opportunity to relax, sort out feelings and ideas, make plans, and recoup energy. After such a period of withdrawal the individual feels refreshed and ready for further productive interaction with the human environment.

The Nonhuman Environment as a Source of Anxiety

Interaction with the nonhuman environment offers many opportunities for positive growth and development, as briefly outlined above. However, the nonhuman environment may also be a source of anxiety. This occurs in two different ways. One is that there appears to be a desire to be nonhuman versus a fear of regression to being nonhuman. Individuals tend to glorify that which is nonhuman. They perceive the life of plants and animals as being stable, free from anxiety and stress, without responsibility. Thus, we use such expressions as "free as a bird" and "cool as a cucumber." Conversely, individuals fear return to an infantile state of nondifferentiation from the nonhuman environment. There is something innately horrible in the contemplation of not being able to think, to talk, to move. The deep response we have to the statement "She is alive but will always be a vegetable" is one indication of fear of becoming nonhuman. It does not matter if one knows the individual being discussed, the response is one of fear of loss of one's own humanness. Involvement with the human environment is occasionally unsatisfying, leading to the desire to escape and become part of the nonhuman environment. In turn this leads to a fear of regression. Thus a conflict situation is established—a situation that can possibly cause considerable anxiety.

The other source of anxiety relative to the nonhuman environment also arises out of a conflictual situation. On the one hand, individuals appear to have a desire for oneness with the universe, and on the other hand, a desire for a sense of humanness and individuality. This is the existential conflict of the wish to be part of and similar to others and the wish to be unique and different from all other objects, whether they be human or nonhuman. Relative to the first wish, individuals seem to feel a sense of unity with the nonhuman environment. This may be a conscious or unconscious feeling. Intellectually we know of our origin and phylogenetic development from that which is nonhuman. But even prior to the articulation of the theory of evolution our relationship to the nonhuman environment was expressed in myths, literature, dance, and the visual arts. To make things a bit more complex, individuals in Western society have pretty much disowned all that is perceived as "animal" in the human species. Thus, for example, euphemisms are used to speak of defecation and the natural odors of the body. Conversely, individuals in Western society seem to be preoccupied with individuality. There is a somewhat realistic fear of being faceless in a faceless crowd, of being identified as only a number. Thus the idea of the common nature of all individuals and the foundation of that nature in the nonhuman environment is sometimes threatening to the individual living in urban modern Western society.

Impediments to Constructive Interaction with the Nonhuman Environment

The nonhuman environment facilitates growth and development but also may be the source of some natural tension. However, neither of these situations will occur if constructive interaction with the nonhuman environment is impeded. There are several factors that may cause this to happen. First, the individual may be overly concerned with the nonhuman environment. This may occur because excessive demands are made by the nonhuman environment or because of its threatening or ambivalent nature. An example of excessive demands is the young girl who must take responsibility for most of the cooking, cleaning, and laundry for a large household. This child has little opportunity to experience the nonhuman environnment as a source of pleasure or an area for exploration. The nonhuman environment may seem threatening or ambivalent to an individual who subsists in the cultivation of a small plot of land. If this land is in an area where there are recurring floods and drought, the individual may view the nonhuman environment as an unfriendly and uncontrollable force.

An individual may not be comfortable in interaction with the nonhuman environment because efforts to do so are received with disfavor by significant others. This may, for example, occur in a situation where a parent forbids a child to climb trees, roller skate, or learn to ride a bicycle for fear the child might be injured. Although such a child may come to experience pleasure in reading or playing the piano, one part of the nonhuman environment is not being fully utilized for growth.

Conversely, excessive need to use the nonhuman environment to gain approval from others may impede constructive use of the nonhuman environment. For example, a child may perceive that his worth is measured by the grades he receives in school or his skill on the basketball court. Such an individual is not using the nonhuman environment to facilitate well-rounded development but as a means to gain acceptance.

The human environment may seem so threatening to the individual that she or he uses the environment as a means of unhealthy escape. This is different from the use of the nonhuman environment mentioned earlier. The nonhuman environment can serve as a periodic and temporary means of withdrawing from the human environment. This is not the situation being discussed here. The individual literally uses the nonhuman environment as a relatively permanent refuge from the human environment. For example, an individual may become preoccupied with a hobby that does not require any interaction with others, or an individual may become engrossed in the paperwork of her job to the exclusion of interacting with other people in the work setting.

Adequate use of the nonhuman environment may be impeded because the individual has come to see himself as a nonhuman object. This usually occurs because the individual has been treated as if he were nonhuman by significant others. This may occur, for example, when a child is raised by parents who are preoccupied with and take great pride in their collection of antique clocks. The child may well perceive that to get any attention it may be far better to be more like a clock than a huamn being. In many work situations, the individual is made to feel like a nonhuman object by management. The expression "I feel like a cog in a wheel" is a reflection of this kind of experience.

Finally, constructive interaction with the natural nonhuman environment may be impeded by technological advances that have placed a distance between the individual and nature. This is particularly true of people who live in large urban areas. Steel and concrete, the sounds of traffic, noxious odors, and air pollution are far from grass and trees, the sounds of crickets, the smell of wet earth, and clean air. When a friend tells a city dweller she is going to the country for a long weekend, there is likely to be at least a momentary feeling of envy. The need for periodic contact with nature persists in even the most confirmed urban inhabitant.

The ways in which an individual has perceived and used the nonhuman environment in the past and the way in which he now perceives and uses it are important for the occupational therapist to understand. If an individual fears the nonhuman environment or views it primarily as a means for escape from the human environment, the occupational therapist may initially have some difficulty in engaging the individual in evaluation and intervention. This is by no means an insurmountable problem, but comprehension of the individual's position is necessary for the development of adequate rapport.

THE NONHUMAN ENVIRONMENT AS A TOOL

As a tool, occupational therapists view the nonhuman environment as an entity to be mastered, an aid to facilitate participation in occupational performances, and as a vehicle for assisting in the development of performance components. Each of these facets will be discussed separately.

In order to be able to function and adapt, the individual must have some capacity to master the nonhuman environment. Mastery refers to the knowledge and skill necessary to use and control the nonhuman environment to such an extent that one is able to engage in required and desired occupational performances. For individuals who are disabled in some way, mastery refers to the capacity to manipulate the nonhuman environment to the fullest extent possible given the objective fact of their limitations.

Without age-appropriate mastery, the individual is at a disadvantage (1014–1016). For example, the person who is not able to cook, balance a check book, or drive a car frequently becomes dependent on others for these tasks or somehow organizes his life so that these tasks are unnecessary. Such dependency often requires a number of compromises that the individual ultimately may find distasteful. Organization of life experiences to avoid unmastered tasks often leads to restriction of activities and further impoverishment in experience.

There are two major consequences of lack of mastery. First, the individual often feels inept and incompetent and thus has a less than optimal level of self-esteem. Second, the individual uses excessive amounts of energy in dealing with or avoiding dealing with the nonhuman environment, energy that is not then available for engaging in other aspects of the human experience.

There are several reasons why an individual may not have mastered the nonhuman environment.

Lack of opportunity. The individual may have lived in such a sheltered environment that he was unable to have the experiences necessary for acquisition of the required knowledge and skills. Such a situation is sometimes induced by parental restrictions. This often occurs in the case of the individual who is developmentally disabled or in family situations where the individual is for whatever reason not expected to or prohibited from gaining competence relative to the nonhuman environment.

Preoccupation with the human environment. In this situation, mentioned previously, the individual experiences the human environment as such a threat that minimal attention or energy can be directed toward mastery of the nonhuman environment.

A marked change in one's life situation. This may occur in the case of an acquired disability, inadequate preparation for a change in social roles, such as becoming a parent, death of a partner, divorce, or moving into a new environment, e.g., a young adult living alone for the first time or movement into a new cultural group.

Secondary gain. This refers to the gratification received from lack of mastery of the nonhuman environment such as dependency, control of other individuals, attention, special privileges, and exemption from some responsibilities. Lack of mastery because of secondary gains may be indicative of difficulty in social interaction or low self-esteem.

Individuals tend to be embarrassed by lack of mastery of the nonhuman environment, particularly in relationship to activities of daily living. This is an important factor to remember in evaluation. Intervention in this area involves designing experiences that enable the individual to gain mastery of the nonhuman environment to the extent to which that is possible. Experiences are designed based on knowledge of the aspects of the nonhuman environment that need to be mastered and principles of the teaching and learning process.

As a tool, the nonhuman environment is used as an aid to facilitate participation in occupational performances. This entails the use of an object in order to perform activities in a more adaptive or functional manner, either in the here and now or relative to the future. Some of these aids (634,636,960), primarily in relationship to motor tasks, are: (a) static or dynamic splints, which may be protective, supportive, and/or corrective in their purpose or used to substitute for absent motor power; (b) mobility aids such as wheelchairs, equipment to facilitate transfers, crutches, canes, walker, and automobile adaptations; (c) adaptive equipment such as devices to enhance energy conservation, communication, hygiene and grooming, dressing, feeding, meal preparation, task performance in the workplace, and recreational activities; (d) prosthesis or artificial limbs.

Concerns about selection, design, fabrication, fitting, and training in the use of such aids is outside the scope of this text. What is important here is the individual's acceptance of and adaption to these devices. The occupational therapist takes into consideration the effect that devices have on the individual's concept of self, in particular body image, and the individual's sense of the appropriateness of devices. For personal or cultural reasons, the individual may object to devices. They may be seen as unacceptable for cosmetic reasons or because the individual feels that he can manage far better without their use. Devices may be unacceptable because the individual is expected to be dependent by his cultural group or because he enjoys the position of dependency. Individuals who come from a cultural background in which there is a fascination with all kinds of mechanical devices and a premium is placed on self-sufficiency may have less difficulty in using adaptive aids.

The individual's feelings about the nonhuman environment, particularly that part which is constructed of metal and plastic, is an important factor. The individual may feel that such objects are not natural and thus foreign and alien to the self. There may be a feeling of revulsion at having such objects close to the body or of being dependent on such objects. An individual, for example, may reject a metal cane but readily use and take pride in a well-crafted oak walking stick.

The nonhuman environment as an aid to facilitate occupational performances is also important in regard to activities that are less dependent on a motor component. Nonhuman objects can be used to enhance activities of a more psychosocial nature. The arrangement of the nonhuman environment and the importance of being surrounded by meaningful objects have been mentioned previously. Some examples of additional aids are a detailed schedule of each day's activities for the individual who is extremely anxious or confused, written and/or pictorial directions for maintenance regimens (medical, functional, or relative to equipment), a weekly plan of activities for individuals who have difficulty in the area of time management, a pet of some kind to combat feelings of loneliness and uselessness.

In addition to the practical importance of nonhuman objects, they also may serve as an aid to function in a symbolic manner. The concept of symbolism will be discussed in Chapter 10. Suffice it to say for now that a symbol is anything that has special complexity of meanings in addition to its conventional and obvious meaning. Any of the above-mentioned aids may serve to facilitate function through their symbolic meaning as well as their practical purpose. A detailed daily schedule of activities, for example, may help the confused individual to know where he should be and what he should be doing. But it may also be important because it reminds the individual that there is someone who cares about him and understands his current dilemma. The symbolic as well as the practical aspect of an aid to function is always taken into consideration.

Finally, the nonhuman environment is used as a vehicle for assisting in the development of performance components. Vehicle is used here in the sense of a means for accomplishing a purpose. The important word here is means rather than end. The individual does not interact with the nonhuman environment so as to gain mastery. Mastery is secondary if significant at all. The nonhuman environment as a vehicle can also be differentiated from its role as an aid to function. As an aid, the nonhuman environment is essentially a supplement to insufficient resources. As a vehicle, the nonhuman environment is used to help the individual to attain the necessary resources. Some examples may clarify the nonhuman environment's role as a vehicle to enhance function. A platform swing or large beach ball may be used to develop adequate equilibrium reactions. Problem solving may be enhanced through figuring out the best way to beat an opponent in a simple game of strategy. Following a given pattern to make a reed basket may be used to develop reality testing. Group interaction skills may be enhanced through participation in a softball game.

CONCLUSION

In the occupational therapy process, the nonhuman environment is most frequently used in conjunction with the human environment. It is combined with the human environment to form an activity that is suitable for evaluation or intervention.

8 Conscious Use of Self

Conscious use of self, simply stated, is the use of oneself in such a way that one becomes an effective tool in the evaluation and intervention process. This chapter will explore many elements that are a part of or in part constitute conscious use of self, and how the neophyte begins to acquire the use of this important tool. The acquisition of conscious use of self is an ongoing process, more deeply understood and used with more skill but never completely mastered even by the most skilled clinician.

DEFINITION AND COMPONENT PARTS

Conscious use of self, as previously defined, involves a planned interaction with another person in order to alleviate fear or anxiety, provide reassurance, obtain necessary information, provide information, give advice, and assist the other individual to gain more appreciation of, more expression of, and more functional use of his or her latent inner resources. Such a relationship is concerned with promoting growth and development, improving and maintaining function, and fostering a greater ability to cope with the stresses of life (290,312,337,536,790). Conscious use of self may be differentiated from spontaneous response to another person. Spontaneous response is typical of daily interaction with most other people. Such a response is often unconscious or subconscious in the sense that the individual does not preplan what messages will be communicated. Conversely, conscious use of self involves considerable forethought relative to the nature of a particular message and how that message is best conveyed to another individual. Conscious use of self does occur and is important in some aspects of daily life. However, it is imperative in the evaluation and intervention process.

Conscious use of self includes but is greater than rapport and the art of practice. Rapport is a comfortable, unconstrained relationship of mutual confidence between two people. It is a relationship established out of perception of the other as a unique, knowledgeable person who is worthy of respect and love. It is based on perception of the other as a total human being: an individual with a past, present, and future, including social roles, personality characteristics, idiosyncratic traits, assets, and limitations. It is a relationship perhaps best described by Martin Buber, paraphrased as, I bring to you all that I am and I accept from you all that you are (144). Establishing and maintaining rapport is both a simple and complex undertaking. It requires much of the therapist but the rewards, in turn, are great.

In working with clients it is good to remember that some of them may be ambivalent about establishing rapport with anyone. For any number of reasons the client may have difficulty beginning and maintaining reciprocal relationships of any kind. The need for such social relationships is inherent; if they are absent, the desire for them is activated. However, the client may fear establishing rapport because of marked difficulties in past relationships; he or she usually does not want to repeat these experiences. The client may have been rejected and hurt frequently enough to have learned well how to reject others. The client's ambivalence arising out of the desire for and fear of establishing rapport puts a heavy burden on the therapist. He or she must then play the more active role and take major responsibility.

The art of practice has been defined as an interpersonal experience which diminishes the isolation of the individual; which reaffirms the power of the mind, body, and spirit; which assists the individual in discovering meaning in existence. It is instrumental in fulfilling the universal need for individuality, and for a sense of kinship and relatedness to others (114,174,630,696,712). In the experience of art there is a sense of identification with others, with the human condition. There is a feeling that someone, at last, understands and is able to give substance to one's own unique ideas and concerns. In this experience the individual has a sense of his or her own singular potentiality and participation in the comedy and tragedy of human life.

The art of practice is difficult to describe. It has an elusive quality; the actions and feelings inherent in the process are not easily translated into words. For clarification, however, it is not the skilled application of scientific knowledge or a global sense of caring about and wanting to help others. The skilled practitioner is able to make fine discriminating choices of appropriate scientific knowledge and professional skills applicable to the individual problems presented by clients. Skilled practice is the ability to ask the right questions, to select suitable evaluative tools, and to design intervention strategies to meet the current needs of each client. All of this, however, can occur in an atmosphere in which the client is treated without feeling, and treated as something subhuman at best. Discriminate use of knowledge may be combined with the art of practice, but the skilled application of knowledge per se is not art.

A person may wish to be of assistance to others who are experiencing difficulty in functioning. This is a noble intention and often one of the major reasons why one elects to become a member of a health profession. But such an intention must be shaped into disciplined action. It is not sufficient simply to "help others." In fact, such help may be more detrimental than instrumental in enhancing function. To elaborate, there is considerable difference in feeding a person and helping a person to learn how to eat independently. The latter mode of interaction is far more beneficial to a client. Even that, however, is not art. One can be a systematic and sympathetic practitioner. Practice, however, only becomes art when a therapist is able to transcend sympathy and translate empathy into a process that brings the individual to a state of renewed sense of self and a deeper understanding of one's place in a community of others. Through the art of practice the therapist helps individuals to know and use their potential, to accept their limitations and discover their strengths, to appreciate their individuality, to grow in their relatedness to others, to love, to play, and to find purpose in life.

However, the establishment and maintenance of rapport and application of the art of practice per se are not likely to enhance a client's ability to function in the community. This is not to say that these areas are unimportant. They are very important if not crucial. They are, however, only the foundation for the building, not the building itself. Conscious use of self is the manipulation of one's responses to assist a client. Depending on the situation, the therapist may be supportive, permissive, accepting, cajoling, strict, demanding, or some variation on these themes. The particular response called for on a given occasion will depend on the current needs of the client and the frame of reference being used for evaluation and intervention process.

The conscious use of self also involves a sensitivity to one's personal response to the client (98,818,866). In other words, "How does the client make me, as a therapist, feel; what am I experiencing?" This information is valuable for it assists in assessing the client's feelings, which may not be openly expressed. The therapist, through a personal response, experiences whether the client is feeling comfortable, wants to express positive feelings, is anxious, decidedly hostile, or is acting as if the therapist is the client's nurturing grandmother. With this information, the therapist is able to meet the client's specific needs and to help the client express feelings more directly.

Conscious use of self involves manipulating one's responses to assist the client in gaining or maintaining function. It involves experiencing and understanding the client's various messages. Conscious use of self may be used in one-to-one interaction, in interaction with a group of clients, or with those others significant to the clients. The means by which a therapist makes effective use of the self may vary from one situation to another. However, typically they include verbal dialogue, gestures and facial expressions, and "touching with care" (464).

There are a number of qualities or characteristics that allow the therapist to use himself or herself as a tool (91,93,94,98,266,311,313,818,866). Some of these follow.

A Perception of Individuality

This is a recognition of the individual as indivisible, as an integrated whole and not a collection of parts or systems. A person cannot retain human qualities if divided or reduced to abstract elements. Even to speak of the "mind, body, and spirit" denies individuality. It is true that in study we divide to understand more clearly.

For effective practice, however, the therapist integrates the various subsystems and comes to know the client as an individual. The therapist is not concerned with encouraging a child to use both hands, assisting an individual to explore feelings, or helping a patient wash her face. Rather the practitioner is concerned with the whole: hands, feelings, and face belong to an individual. Each client, although sharing much in common with others, is perceived as special, unique, different from all other people—and indivisible.

Respect for the Dignity and Rights of Each Individual

This respect is maintained regardless of the individual's past or present circumstances or possible future potential. Such a philosophical orientation is often adhered to in the abstract but not always sustained in daily interactions with clients. It is indeed difficult to respect the dignity and rights of individuals who are severely retarded, who have abused a child, or who reject any involvement in the intervention process. It is the master practitioner who reaffirms the dignity and rights of each client in the context of all interactions with the client.

Empathy

Empathy involves entering into the experience of another individual without loss of one's own sense of separateness as a unique and different individual. Empathy is the ability to feel the pain and joy of another person, fully realizing it is not one's own pain and joy. To be separate from but with another individual requires a sense of relatedness to the human condition in all of its manifestations and a sense of one's own singularity. The separateness of empathy is important for it allows the therapist to solve problems, to make sound judgments, and to interpret with objectivity. The togetherness of empathy is important, for it allows the practitioner to be open to the feelings, ideas, and values of the client.

Compassion

Compassion is a feeling of deep sympathy and sorrow for another person who is stricken by suffering and misfortune. It is accompanied by a strong desire to alleviate the pain or remove the cause. The ability to be kind and gentle in manner and word regardless of the situation comes from the internal experience of compassion.

Humility

Humility is the modest sense of one's own importance. The therapeutic situation is no place for arrogance, an attitude of superiority, excessive pride, or exaggerated sophistication. A sense of humility is fairly easy to attain when one remembers the limitations of one's own knowledge and knowledge in general. The ability to apologize with sincerity for acts of commission or omission grows out of an appropriate sense of humility.

Unconditional Positive Regard

Unconditional refers to concern for the client without any restrictions, limitations, qualifications, or modifying circumstances. Positive regard includes acceptance, respect, concern, and liking for the individual as a human being. Acceptance, however, should not be equated with agreement or approval. There are times when the therapist does disagree with the client and disapproves of his or her behavior. Such reactions, when they occur, are restricted to the issue of contention or a specific aspect of behavior. The reaction is not allowed to spread so that it becomes one's reaction to the client as a holistic individual. Unconditional positive regard is a global attitude; disapproval and the like are particular in nature. It allows the therapist to be accepting even under trying conditions of hostile and uncooperative behavior. Unconditional positive regard also includes a nonjudgmental stance on the part of the therapist. It is not the therapist's prerogative to make a moral judgment about the client's thoughts or actions. These kinds of judgments, if they occur, be they negative or positive, are concealed from the client. Subjective, personal feeling of a judgmental nature should not be permitted expression.

Honesty

It appears that in the long run it is best to be straightforward, candid, and truthful. With this stance there is a far greater possibility of developing trust. Honesty is also a means of showing respect for the client's intelligence and capacity to deal with the realities of life. Being honest is often much more difficult for the therapist than it is for the client to accept the information offered. The therapist's capacity to be honest is frequently reflected in the degree to which the client is straightforward in interactions with the therapist.

A Relaxed Manner

A therapist who is tense, worried, or anxious is going to have little success in establishing any kind of relationship with a client. The habit of leaving all other concerns aside except those specifically related to the client one is with at the moment allows one to be truly with the client. Being or giving the appearance of being rushed is also detrimental to establishing a relationship. A reasonable amount of time should be set aside for one's interaction with the client. Although the therapist may be very busy and feel that he or she has insufficient time to fulfill all responsibilities, this is the therapist's problem and not the clients'. The therapist who is always rushed and in a hurry also acts as a very poor model relative to temporal adaptation.

Flexibility

The ability to modify behavior to meet the circumstances of the moment or the needs of a particular client is a great asset. An overly rigid approach to such things as scheduling, acceptable behavior, and adherence to one's point of view is not usually appreciated by the client. One of the most effective factors in all types of intervention is the client's favorable expectations. The therapist, then, should be prepared to modify his or her approach, within limits possible, in order to meet the expectations of various kinds of clients. Subsequently, the rapport that is developed frequently leads to modification of a patient's expectations in a more therapeutically useful direction.

Self-Awareness

Self-awareness is the ability to recognize, with a reasonable degree of accuracy, how one reacts to the outside world and how the outside world reacts to oneself (15, 648,818). Self-awareness implies not only knowledge about the self but also the capacity to make changes in the self that will lead to more effective interactions with clients. There are several reasons why self-awareness facilitates the intervention process. With self-awareness one tends to be more at peace with oneself. Intrapsychic conflicts are able to be resolved or accepted as a normal part of being human. A state of peace or relative equilibrium frees energy that can be used to deal with the client's problems. There is greater ability to be open to the responses of others. Self-awareness allows the individual to experience the feelings of others both subjectively and objectively. It is only in this way that the feelings of others come to be accurately perceived. A tendency to deny a particular feeling in oneself often results in denial, misinterpretation, or a judgmental attitude toward a similar feeling in others. Faulty evaluation becomes highly probable. Self-awareness leads to recognition of the needs of the self. With such recognition, the individual is able to seek need gratification more accurately and to tolerate delayed gratification so that it does not interfere with client care. Attempts to gratify personal needs through the process of client care drastically impede the effectiveness of intervention. Finally, self-awareness permits the individual to change inappropriate attitudes and behavior. Such change is not possible, or is highly unlikely, unless the individual knows what needs to be changed.

Humor

Although somewhat of an extreme statement, there is probably nothing worse than a therapist who lacks a sense of humor. The ability to recognize the incongruities or peculiarities present in a situation and facility in perceiving and expressing what is amusing and comical in human nature, including one's own, are an important asset for a therapist. There are, of course, times when humor is not appropriate. However, some levity, a lightness of mood and spirit, can often make a difficult situation or experience tolerable. Humor used in a genial and mellow manner is an important component of conscious use of self.

Acquisition of the above-mentioned characteristics, at least to the student reader, may seem to be an awesome task. Indeed, their acquisition is no simple matter and, as mentioned, not ever really attained. These characteristics are what the therapist strives for, not what he or she possesses in their entirety.

The Ideal Relationship Between Client and Therapist

Occupational therapy is considered to be a collaborative process between the therapist and the client. It is a shared relationship in which both client and therapist have rights and responsibilities. Briefly, the client has the right to be treated as a unique individual and to receive the benefits of the occupational therapist's knowledge and skill. The client has the responsibility of participating in the planning and implementation of a program of intervention. In turn, the therapist has the right to receive respect from the client if such respect is earned and to fair remuneration for the application of his or her skills and knowledge. The occupational therapist has the responsibility of acting in an ethical manner and participating in the mutual planning and implementation of a program for intervention with the client. Collaboration has the connotation of sharing, of doing with, not doing for or doing to. It is truly a mutual process.

Collaboration, however, is not necessarily limited to the relationship between the client and the occupational therapist. The therapist also has the responsibility to collaborate with other individuals who are concerned with the welfare of the client. These other individuals may be family members, close friends, employers, teachers, or members of the health team. The issue of confidentiality is, of course, important in this aspect of collaboration.

Occupational therapists usually work as a member of a health team. On first contact, the therapist explains this working relationship to the client. The essence of this explanation is that the therapist will share all information regarding evaluation and intervention with other team members. This information includes not only specific facts, but personal thoughts and feelings the client expresses. With the client's understanding of this aspect of confidentiality, the relationship between therapist and client becomes a contract. Thus, for example, when a client says, "I want to tell you about this but do not tell my physician or social worker," the therapist's response comes out of the previously made contract rather than personal feelings or loyalties. The therapist's response is quite simple: "If you do not want to share this particular information with your physician or social worker, then do not share it with me."

Confidentiality and collaboration between the therapist, client, and those significant to the client other than members of the health team is somewhat more problematic. Important variables to consider are age, comprehension on the part of the client, and the understanding of significant others. Two rather simplistic examples may be helpful. It is very important for the occupational therapist to establish a collaborative relationship and share information with the parents and teachers of a mildly retarded 5-year-old child with perceptual problems. A 16-year-old girl who is paraplegic may feel far more comfortable discussing her concerns about sexuality with a therapist, knowing that the therapist will not share this information with her parents. Collaboration and confidentiality cannot be reduced to a formula. The therapist's ethical code, good judgment, and wisdom eventually must serve as the guide for being a responsible therapist.

COMMON ISSUES AND RESPONSES

In clinical practice there are many issues and responses that occur. Some of the more common ones will be outlined in this section. The discussion is brief, as it is presented primarily to alert the neophyte to the issues and responses and not to give detailed information about how to solve these areas of possible difficulty. When faced with many new situations, the beginning therapist often believes that his or her ideas and reactions are unique to him- or herself. This is particularly true when the therapist feels isolated and has inadequate supervision. This section, then, is presented to reassure the neophyte that his or her reactions are neither indicative of incompetence nor particular to him- or herself. Therapists are made over a long period of time; they are not born.

Some of the common issues and responses that arise in a clinical setting follow (91,93,94,98,155,266,290, 311,313,464,817,818,866).

Attitudes

Attitudes are a disposition, feeling, or position toward persons, ideas, or situations that are relatively set and of a long-term nature. Many attitudes come from the shared understandings of one's cultural group; others are idiosyncratic to the individual. Some attitudes not conducive to effective interactions with clients are briefly outlined below.

Individuals often respond negatively to severe illness or disability. There seems to be an almost inherent fear reaction to major deviation from the norm, to disfigurement, to the inability to manage the very basic tasks of self-care. This fear seems to arise from a primitive rejection of that which is strange, which has an unknown quality. Differentness is often equated with that which is ugly, which in turn is equated with that which is ominous, evil, and malevolent. People seem to react spontaneously to a physical deformity or bizzarre behavior by the thought of "this could happen to me." There is a tendency to withdraw as if the differentness were somehow contagious. It is difficult for people to feel a sense of kinship with an individual who overtly is "not like them." They, thus, often assume that the individual does not have the same needs and desires that they do. Negative attitudes toward those who are physically deformed or who exhibit bizarre behavior are particularly prevalent in cultures characterized by considerable superstition and in cultures that put a high premium on physical perfection and logical thinking.

Feelings of hostility are another fairly common response to disabled persons. This arises from the belief that disabled persons are too much of a burden for society, that they do not contribute to the general good but rather are placed in the privileged position of not being required to work. In addition, they are seen as being too demanding in regard to their special needs. At best it is felt that disabled individuals should be content with whatever sustains the level of maintenance the society as a whole is willing to provide and that they should stay out of sight and out of the mainstream of society.

Negative reactions to individuals with emotional difficulties are compounded by the belief that it is the person's own fault. Some people feel the individual is malingering and that he or she should "pull him- or herself together" and get about the business of functioning in a responsible manner. On the other hand, if emotional difficulties are not thought to be the fault of the individual, then it is often believed to be the fault of the parents—a belief, incidentally, that has been fostered by modern psychiatry and to some extent by the mass media.

There are four common ways in which therapists deal with the fear aroused by severe illness and disability and the guilt they tend to have regarding their feelings of hostility. First, the therapist may deny the trauma and severity of the client's situation. Response to the client is then characterized by "well, it happened, but life must go on." This is the "stiff upper lip" approach to the problems of the client. Second, the therapist may essentially make the client into a nonperson by maintaining a psychological distance from the client and experiencing no personal or emotional involvement. One manifestation of this orientation is to label a client by the condition, such as a "hemi" or a "quad." The client's name and thus identity becomes singularly irrelevant. The third way of dealing with a negative reaction to disability is to become overly sympathetic. The therapist feels so sorry for the client that appropriate intervention is not initiated, limits are not set, and expectations are essentially nonexistent. This response often occurs with children but it is by no means limited to that age group. Finally, the therapist may deal with the trauma of severe illness and disability by engaging in and attempting to act out a rescue fantasy. In this response, the therapist again engages in denial and believes that he or she will help the client not just to return to life as usual but to a life far better than prior to the onset of illness or disability. Such an attempt is, except in rare instances, doomed to failure and leaves both the client and therapist feeling inadequate and markedly disappointed. In using a rescue fantasy as the basis for intervention, the therapist is attempting to use the client as a means of retreating from his or her own feelings and the reality of the client's situation. The same, of course, could be said for the other common means of dealing with severe illness and disability.

Another important set of attitudes the therapist brings to the clinical situation are those relative to age. As previously mentioned, the gap between generations and even age groups is a very real phenomenon. The greater the difference in age, the more difficult it is for the therapist to understand the client or for the client to understand the therapist. The therapist can only bridge the gap through an intellectual and emotional understanding of the life tasks and concerns typical of various age groups. Attitudes, however, usually precede understanding and interfere with the development of understanding. Attitudes toward three age groups are of particular importance: the aged, children or youths, and clients similar in age to that of the therapist.

In the clinical setting negative attitudes toward the elderly are relatively common. They arise from a number of sources. First, the therapist may come to the clinical setting with the idea that aged individuals are senile, rigid in thought and manner, prone to rambling speech that is irrelevant, old fashioned in morality and skills, and, on the whole, difficult to get along with. Second, working with elderly individuals may stimulate the therapist's fears of aging: of becoming old, unattractive, less competent, dependent, unloved, in pain, alone. Third, elderly people may remind the therapist of his or her own parents and thus arouse conflicts about the relationship with his or her parents that have not been reconciled. Fourth, the therapist may feel he or she has nothing useful to offer because older people cannot change their behavior, or their problems are due to untreatable conditions. Fifth, the elderly client will die soon, therefore the therapist is wasting skills that could be better used to help those who may possibly have a long, productive life ahead of them. Sixth, the client may die, leaving the therapist to feel his or her knowledge and skills are nothing in comparison to a far greater, inevitable force. Seventh, working with the elderly may give rise to the therapist's fear of death: his or her own and those of his or her parents. Finally, colleagues may be contemptuous of the therapist's interest in and efforts to assist the elderly, indicating it is a waste of time, or that the therapist is preoccupied with death, or fearful of meeting more important professional challenges.

Overcoming negative attitudes toward the elderly, from within, from colleagues, and from society, is no easy task. Therapists who are unable to deal with negative attitudes toward the elderly often move to a clinical situation where there is a younger population and a greater feeling of hope for the long-range future. This is regrettable, but nonetheless understandable. A therapist who is uncomfortable in a particular clinical setting should not be there. It is not conducive to the development of rapport or the continued growth of the therapist. For some therapists, it takes considerable time before they are truly comfortable in being a therapist with elderly individuals.

One common attitude toward children is that they are essentially little adults: that they think and respond exactly like adults. Another common attitude is that they are very different from adults: that they do not have the same feelings and needs as adults. These conflicting beliefs are often held by the same individual. Interaction with a child then becomes selective, depending on what attitude is operant at the moment. The therapist, for example, may assume that a young child will feel bad if he or she hurts the feelings of another child. This is frequently not the case, as young children do not have the same capacity to put themselves in the place of another person or to empathize. On the other hand, the therapist might assume, for example, that a young child cannot comprehend death. Thus the child's impending death is not discussed with her. Consequently, the child is not given the opportunity to express her fears and to come to terms with the reality of her own death. The attitude that children are in some ways like and in some ways not like adults is frequently not based on any kind of factual information. It is rather based on a set of beliefs about what children should be like, how they should behave, and what they should know about.

Another common belief about children is that they are particularly precious and the primary resource of society. Thus the reaction to a child being severely ill or disabled or dying is often one of profound horror. It is a more intense feeling than the individual is likely to experience in the case of an adult. This sense of horror is derived from the idea that the child has not yet had a chance to experience life. Here is an unlived life, potential that will never be realized. It seems such a waste, so unjust. There is in this attitude a good deal of romanticism in regard to what the child's life would have been like. There is rarely the idea that a child who struggles to overcome many obstacles may be a more knowledgeable and skilled adult than if never having faced such challenge.

Attitudes toward clients in one's age group are often strongly tinged by identification. The therapist has a tendency to believe that the client's values, beliefs, and expectations are like his or her own. This is due to similarity in age, differences in cultural background being somehow ignored. In addition, because of identification, the therapist has a greater tendency to experience the phenomenon of "there but for the grace of God am I." The therapist feels that it is only some supernatural force, or luck, or chance that has kept him or her, so far, from being in the place of the client. These thought processes are illustrated by the young therapist who begins working with a 25-year-old woman who was severely injured in an automobile accident. For several weeks thereafter the therapist drives his car with considerable attention and caution.

There are various attitudes toward using touch as a means of communication. Some therapists feel that it is unseemly to touch another person for the purpose of showing affection or giving reassurance. This attitude may be one of the shared beliefs of the therapist's culture; it may be derived from equating touching and sexuality, or it may arise from the feeling that touching invades the privacy of the self and the client. Attitudes about touching may be positive in general but negative in particular. The latter is exemplified by hesitation and difficulty in touching skin that has been burned or is severely scarred in some other way, is wrinkled, or that does not seem to be particularly clean. There is often a feeling of revulsion and a desire to withdraw.

Attitudes toward a client's sexuality may be somewhat negative. This may be due to one or several factors. The therapist may feel uneasy about his or her own sexuality, lack knowledge about sexual matters, be unskilled in dealing with casual flirtation, or experience discomfort in discussing sexual issues. Negative attitudes are also influenced by cultural myths and taboos relative to the sexuality of children, the elderly, disabled individuals, people who are mentally retarded, and psychiatric clients. In general, these shared understandings are that people in the categories mentioned are either asexual or they should be asexual.

Communication

A collaborative relationship is dependent on adequate communication: the giving and receiving of information (104,410,841,842,860,996). Rapport cannot exist if communication is not reciprocal or if it is unclear to either the client or the therapist. As mentioned previously, one area of difficulty is incongruence between verbal and nonverbal communication. The words an individual says may not match the tone of voice, posture, gestures, or facial expression. This causes considerable confusion. Being somewhat more primitive and less subjected to conscious control, nonverbal communication tends to be more accurate than verbal communication when there is a discrepancy. On the other hand, nonverbal communication tends to be a more universal language and can often be used fairly effectively when the therapist and client do not share a language that both of them have mastered. It should be noted, however, that there are some cultural differences in nonverbal communication.

Some clients speak in a highly idiosyncratic manner. Their communication may be characterized by blocking, circumstantiality, confabulation, articulated delusions, distractibility, flight of ideas, grandiosity, illogical thinking, incoherence, loosening of association, perseveration, poverty of content, and so forth. The therapist needs to listen attentively, with perseverance, in order to comprehend the latent meaning of the client's communication. Considering such language, in part, as symbolic rather than literal and treating it as a symbolic puzzle to be solved may help the therapist to identify what the client is trying to communicate.

The client and therapist, although they speak the same language, may use a quite different vocabulary. This may be due to cultural, class, or regional differences. The therapist's vocabulary should be regulated by the client's capacity to comprehend the words being used. If a word that is not in the client's vocabulary needs to be used, it is defined and explained carefully. Use of the patient's vocabulary is sometimes helpful but this should not be carried to extremes.

Dependency

All persons have some dependency needs. The extent of the dependency need varies according to the maturity of the individual but the need is never absent. With rare exceptions, clients are initially dependent. This may be a primary feature of their difficulty, or it may be the result of injury or disease. Whether the dependency is excessive or realistic to the situation, it must be gratified. It is usually only through gratification of these needs that the client is able to move in the direction of independence.

Three problems frequently arise relative to dependency. The therapist may be uncomfortable with the task of satisfying dependency needs, particularly when the needs are defined as being excessive. This may be due to the therapist having dependency needs that are not being met or a cultural background that emphasizes the importance of being self-sufficient. Regardless of the cause, the consequence is often a demand that the client be more independent than he or she is willing or able to be at that particular time.

On the other hand, the therapist may derive considerable satisfaction from gratifying clients' dependency needs. In its extreme form, the therapist may maintain the client in a dependent position long after this is either necessary or useful. In this case the therapist is using the intervention process to satisfy his or her own needs, a situation that is always detrimental to the client.

The third common difficulty relative to dependency is more related to the client. Some clients appear to be unable to express or accept gratification of dependency needs. This may be due to the individual's cultural background or it may be the result of the belief that if one lets down one's guard even temporarily and admits to dependency needs, one will become permanently dependent. Nevertheless, the client does need to receive gratification of dependency needs. The therapist, in such a situation, attempts to satisfy these needs symbolically or in a manner that is not consciously recognized by the client.

The therapist's need for dependency cannot be satisfied in interactions with clients. However, these needs do require gratification elsewhere. Without such gratification, the therapist is unlikely to be able to function adequately in the intervention process. Some ways in which these needs may be gratified will be discussed later in this chapter.

Expression of Feelings

In any relationship between two people, including that of client and therapist, anger arises from time to time. Anger is typically due to need frustration, which may have occurred in the relationship or in some other situation. Anger that comes from outside the relationship but that is expressed in it can be detrimental. Anger that arises within the relationship is usually functional because it serves to identify and helps to eliminate need frustration. In the client-therapist relationship, the therapist initially accepts the client's anger, attempts to eliminate causitive factors, and eventually helps the client to eliminate these factors by him- or herself. The therapist's anger that arises in the relationship may sometimes be expressed. The appropriateness of such expression is dependent on the situation and capacity of the client. A client, for example, may be quite able to control certain offensive behavior but for whatever reason is not doing so at the moment. An expression of mild anger on the part of the therapist might well be appropriate in this situation. The judicious expression of anger can be a useful tool. The therapist should avoid expression of anger that originated outside the client-therapist relationship. The therapist also avoids expressing anger in a hostile manner or in a way that antagonizes or humiliates the client. Hostile remarks on the part of the therapist frequently initiate a cycle of hostility-counterhostility, which is, to say the least, not productive.

Many therapists find it difficult to express positive feelings. This is seemingly a characteristic of the dominant culture in the United States. Therapists are often hesitant to express feelings of liking and affection for clients. There is the belief that somehow this type of behavior would be "unprofessional" and out of keeping with being objective. There is no evidence to indicate that the expression of positive feelings is detrimental to the client-therapist relationship.

Constrictions relative to the expression of positive feelings seem to be a factor in minimal attention being given to clients' capacity to demonstrate positive feelings. There is, on the other hand, much concern about helping clients to express negative feelings of one kind or another. The influence of cultural beliefs on the choice of intervention goals is quite evident in the situation outlined here.

Another influence of culture can be seen in the discomfort many therapists have in the presence of intense emotional expression. If expressed, emotions should, it seems, be demonstrated in a restrained manner. The exuberance of adolescence, crying, overt expressions of grief, a good angry verbal battle, and hearty laughter are not often found in clinical settings. When such expressions do occur, there is a tendency to minimize them. Therapists seem to want people to stop crying or fighting, and respond to laughter as if it were an unusual event.

Burnout

This phenomenon has received much attention of late (150,318). "Burnout" is traditionally the term used to describe a fire that is totally destructive of something, or of that which exhausts. It is the latter meaning that most closely fits the more current use of the word. A therapist who describes himself as burnt out is essentially saying that he or she has no more emotional or physical energy left for dealing with the demands of a particular clinical setting. Burnout is most likely to occur in working with those who are severely retarded and multiply handicapped, individuals with chronic schizophrenic disorders, individuals who reside in continuing care facilities, and terminally ill clients. Burnout seems to occur from the actual demands of the job, the frustration and feeling of impotence because one cannot do more, and the lack of a sense of accomplishment because there is so little evidence of positive change. Burnout can be avoided to some extent by setting more realistic expectations, adequate support systems, and job enrichment of various kinds. Therapists who stay at a particular job after burnout has occurred tend to be indifferent toward clients or deal with them in a rejecting or punitive manner. In either case, they seem only to go through the motions of intervention. Unless burnout can be dealt with in the job situation, it is probably best for the therapist to work with another population, at least for a period of time.

Overinvolvement

Overinvolvement refers to the tendency to become preoccupied with or fully absorbed in the problems of one's clients to the point that it engages all of one's emotions and interests. The overinvolved therapist tends to lose objectivity and eventually effectiveness as a therapist; he is also a good candidate for burnout. Although overinvolvement does occur, it tends on the whole to be self-correcting, particularly with good supervision. It diminishes as the therapist becomes more self-assured, has experienced both success and failure in the clinical setting, and becomes more aware of the dominant role the client plays in the intervention process. Other strong interests outside the clinical setting also help to diminish overinvolvement. Fear of overinvolvement is often a more important factor than overinvolvement itself. Because of the fear, some therapists take a detached, unemotional stance relative to clients. This is just as detrimental, if not more so, to the intervention process and the continued professional growth of the therapist. It should be noted that overinvolvement is not caring deeply, being concerned about one's clients, and occasionally spending a good part of an evening trying to figure out how to deal with the problems of a particular client. That is being a good, committed, and probably effective therapist.

Transference and Countertransference

Transference is an unconscious psychological process characterized by a response to a person in a manner that is similar to the way in which one responded to a significant individual in one's past life. It seems to maintain congruence with past experiences and minimizes the fear or uncertainty involved in interacting with an unfamiliar person. An example of transference is responding to all persons in an authority position as if they were one's father. Transference is a fairly common phenomenon and is not something that just occurs in a clinical setting. It is one of the defense mechanisms and, in a mild form, is by no means pathological in nature. Transference is used in the change process when that process is based on an analytical frame of reference. Its use will be discussed more fully in Chapter 21. Transference is not used when the change process is based on other frames of reference or in the other types of intervention. Transference on the part of clients is inhibited by the therapist acting and responding as a total three-dimensional person. This includes sharing ideas and feelings and a part of one's daily experiences with the client. Transference is less likely to occur if the therapist allows the client to see him or her as a unique and special person with distinct characteristics.

Transference does occasionally occur on the part of the therapist. It is most likely to take place when a client reminds one of a family member, e.g., grandparent, parent, sibling, or child. Transference inhibits the capacity of the therapist to interact with the client based on that particular client's needs. The therapist can monitor the possibility of transference on his or her part by questioning whether the relationship with any client is markedly different from that with other clients. Two good clues are if the therapist feels an unusual amount of liking for a client or finds him- or herself frequently impatient with a particular client.

Countertransference is an unconscious cognitive process characterized by a response that is expected and desired by an individual who has formed a transference relationship with oneself. The individual acts as if, for example, she was the person that the other individual would like her to be or has decided she is. The functional purpose of countertransference is unknown; it is probably based on the human tendency to act on the basis of others' expectations. An example of countertransference is the male therapist taking a fatherly role toward the young client who acts as if the therapist were her father. Although a therapist may have difficulty in inhibiting the client's formation of a transference relationship, a countertransference response should be avoided; it in no way enhances the patient-therapist relationship.

Giving Advice

With a few exceptions, it is generally not wise to give advice to a client. The forces for change in behavior, in general, come from within the individual and not from some outside agent. The therapist's task is to help the client view his or her problems in a new perspective so that the forces for change may be released. When given, advice is often not followed for a variety of reasons. The client may feel that the recommended course of action is not appropriate. Although the advice may seem sound to the therapist, it may not be compatible with the client's style of interaction. On the other hand, the client may ignore advice as a means of maintaining a sense of independence and integrity. The client may feel that being told what to do indicates the therapist thinks he or she is incapable of self-knowledge and of working out his or her own solutions. When the client follows the advice, the client may experience a temporary sense of relief but has learned little and undue dependency may have been encouraged. When the suggested course of acting does not work, the client usually feels that he or she is not responsible—the therapist is.

There are times, however, when it is wise to give advice. This is particularly true when the client is confused, not able to make a decision or paralyzed into inaction by anxiety or depression. Withholding advice in these situations would be both inhumane and detrimental to the intervention process. The client frequently views the advice as an indication of caring and concern on the part of the therapist. Once started on a reasonable course of action in terms of dealing with the problem, the client frequently feels an increased sense of comfort, safety, and personal integration. With this as a base, the client is often able to move forward in solving problems independently. When giving advice it is good to remember that the recommended action should be well within the current capabilities of the client and congruent with the client's behavioral style.

Giving Information

Providing information is different from giving advice. It takes two forms which are not necessarily mutually exclusive: giving factual data and outlining the consequences of a particular course of action. In giving factual data, it should be remembered that there seems to be an inverse relationship between the amount of information given and the amount understood and remembered. Thus, only a little information should be given at one time. Information should also be given in a form that is comprehensible to the client. It is frequently better to err on the side of too simple rather than too complex. If appropriate, information given verbally should also be given in a clearly written form.

In outlining the probable consequence of a particular course of action, the therapist provides that information which will assist the client to decide whether or not to take the given course of action. The therapist might, for example, outline for the client possible consequences, both negative and positive, of returning to school. It is then up to the client to make a decision regarding school. As few clients respond well to scare tactics, any possible negative consequences of a particular course of action are best presented in a factual, nonemotional manner. In giving information as with giving advice, it is important to determine if the client is asking for information, advice, expressing an attitude or feeling, or something else entirely.

Giving Reassurance

The giving of genuine reassurance is designed to restore the client's confidence in him- or herself. It can be given directly through a simple honest statement that there is nothing to be concerned about. It can also, and at times more adequately, be given in a less direct manner. It can, for example, be given through touch. The provision of information can be reassuring when the information is correct, given at the time it is wanted, and provided by someone the client trusts. Reasonable limit setting can provide reassurance by giving structure to a situation and thus reducing anxiety. Reassuring a relative can in turn provide comfort to a client. The quiet presence of a trusted person in times of overwhelming fear, e.g., before surgery or during a psychotic episode, can provide real reassurance.

Sometimes reassurance is given for the wrong reason. Reassurance may, for example, be given when a client is registering a complaint, talking about a problem, or expressing negative feelings. The therapist's response of reassurance essentially serves to deny the importance of the issue being raised by the client and/or classifies it as trivial. In giving this kind of pseudoreassurance, the therapist frequently begins to discuss irrelevant material to distract the patient. All of this may make the therapist feel more comfortable but it certainly does not help the client, or the client-therapist relationship, in any way. The therapist is engaging in avoidance. The client is led to believe, often rightly, that the therapist does not understand or want to understand.

Individual Therapeutic Style

During the first year or so of practive the therapist develops his or her own therapeutic style. There is no such thing as a right or wrong style. One therapist, for example, may be quite strict about what behavior is or is not acceptable, another may use a considerable amount of humor, and still another may keep clients up to date on the mystery story he is reading. Each of these therapists may be very effective even when working with the same type of client group. What is important is not the style per se but the extent to which the therapist is comfortable with the style. It has to fit the therapist in such a way that it becomes a natural part of the self—not something one puts on at the entrance to work, but something spontaneous. An effective therapeutic style is one that seems natural to the therapist and is sufficiently flexible to meet the varying needs and expectations of clients. An individual therapeutic style is developed through trying out a variety of different modes of interactions with clients: keeping those that feel right and seem to work, discarding those which do not, and never being afraid to try out a new mode of behavior. Although one may have a basic therapeutic style, similar to personal identity, it develops and changes over time.

In conclusion, this section has outlined some of the common issues and responses that arise in clinical practice. The therapist learns to deal with these issues and responds in an adequate manner through involvement in supervision and participation in support systems.

SUPERVISION AND SUPPORT SYSTEMS

The continual process of becoming a therapist is no easy task. It probably cannot occur without participation in an adequate support system. Without such a system, the therapist's professional growth is likely to be inhibited. This, in turn, usually leads to inadequate and outdated evaluation and intervention, stagnation, and quite possibly to professional burnout. A support system in this context refers to a combination of interactions that seem to assist in and sustain the development of continued professional competence. Supervision is one aspect of a support system and probably, at least for the beginning therapist, one of the most important components of the system.

Supervision

Supervision is an ongoing collaborative process between a supervisor and supervisee directed toward continued professional growth of the supervisee (1,27,258, 286,351,421,702,721,1027,1034). It is directed toward increased effectiveness in the application of therapuetic principles in the day-to-day care of clients. The ultimate goal is to enable the supervisee to engage in evaluation and intervention solely on the basis of the client's needs. This goal is attained through the process of integrating theoretical knowledge with appropriate affectual responses. The major goal of supervision can be broken down into the following subgoals:

- To develop a sense of professional identity, including acceptance of the standards and values of one's professional group;
- To increase theoretical knowledge;
- To develop intellectual curiosity;
- To solve problems in an organized and analytic fashion;
- To make accurate decisions in a reasonable amount of time;
- To be objective, flexible, and independent in thought and action;
- To develop self-awareness and make changes in behavior on the basis of such awareness;
- To cultivate individual abilities;
- To apply theory to practice.

Understanding of theoretical material and appropriate emotional responses are interdependent elements of any effective interaction with clients. To attempt to separate them ultimately leads to inadequate if not inappropriate intervention. Theory and feelings cannot be disconnected in the intervention process nor can either stand alone. The application of theoretical principles by themselves does not lead to greater adaptation on the part of the client, and neither does intervention based on the therapist's spontaneous emotional response to the client. Theoretical principles serve as a guide to action. Through reference to theory, the therapist selects the activities that will most effectively help the client move to a state of function. The therapist's feelings must be such that they facilitate accurate perception of the client's situation, the selection of appropriate theoretical principles, and suitable responses to the client.

The supervisory process takes a variety of forms or, more accurately, variations on a major theme. In general, it involves an initial phase, which is concerned with assessment of the supervisee's learning needs. This is a collaborative process involving mutual sharing of evaluative findings. Evaluation is concerned with identifying what the supervisee needs to learn and how this might be learned best given the learning style and personality of the supervisee. Some of the areas of focus in evaluation are: (a) areas of knowledge and specific skills in which the supervisee feels competent, those in which he or she feels incompetent, and those which he or she would particularly like to master; (b) the methods of learning that the supervisee finds most comfortable and productive; (c) possible sources of anxiety, the supervisee's typical ways of dealing with anxiety, and the capacity to master anxiety; (d) capacity to engage in problem solving; (e) flexibility in dealing with clients' needs; (f) ability to function under pressure and in ambiguous situations; (g) willingness to look below the surface behavior of one's self and others; (h) the ability to engage in a collaborative relationship.

The above information may be compiled through the supervisee's submitting information about past professional experiences, an autobiographical sketch, and an outline of perceived learning needs and style of learning. In addition, the supervisor may draw on information found in the supervisee's academic records, reports from previous supervisors, and letters of recommendation. This and other information that seems pertinent is shared in an interview, with the purpose of identifying the supervisee's strengths and the areas where specific help is needed.

The supervisee and supervisor then come to some agreement on the goals to be attained and a plan for reaching these goals. The more specific the goals and the plan, the easier it will be to implement the plan and ultimately to judge the degree of learning that has occurred. The plan is a working outline for supervision and is subject to alteration when circumstances warrant. The plan may be changed, for example, if the supervisee achieves the initial goals, when additional assignments require the mastery of more knowledge or new skills, or when the plan proves to be inappropriate for the supervisee.

Although supervisory plans vary from situation to situation, usually covered are the supervisee's assigned responsibilities including the nature of the client load and the type of care required, theoretical material to be integrated, skills to be developed, and the teaching techniques to be employed in supervision. Goal setting and the plan for supervision must be established through collaboration between supervisee and supervisor. Without collaboration there is frequently a feeling of confusion on the part of the supervisee and the absence of needed motivation. The process may be doomed to failure before it even begins.

Supervisory meetings usually take place once a week, with more frequent meetings perhaps being needed initially or during times of particular difficulty. The primary focus of the meetings is on interaction between the supervisee and clients. The supervisee comes prepared to discuss specific aspects of various cases or one client may be discussed for a number of weeks. Some supervisees and supervisors find it helpful if a written report of the material the supervisee wishes to discuss is given to the supervisor prior to the meeting. When, for example, one client is to be discussed, the supervisee may write a summary of the client-therapist interaction that took place during the previous week. If the meeting is to be concerned with consideration of evaluation, data and preliminary interpretation may be submitted to the supervisor prior to the time of the meeting. Written reports (a) encourage bringing information and feelings to a conscious, verbal level: the only level which permits sharing to take place; (b) allow for thoughtful consideration and critical analysis of the situation; (c) provide an ongoing record of client evaluation and intervention and the supervisee's growing facility in working in this area; (d) allow for further identification of problems in learning; and (e) help the supervisee and supervisor prepare for supervision prior to the actual meeting.

Clients are the primary focus of supervision unless some factor within the supervisee is perceived as interfering with the evaluation and intervention process. One or several factors may be causing difficulty. The supervisee may, for example, lack some particular knowledge and/or skill, deny or distort some of the client's behavior, or experience negative feelings toward the client. When a particular problem is identified, the focus of supervision shifts from the client to the supervisee. The nature of the problem is explored and the supervisee and supervisor, together, discuss various ways in which the problem may be eliminated.

Evaluation of the supervisee's learning takes place throughout the supervisory process. Periodically, however, it is often formalized and one supervisory meeting is devoted entirely to joint evaluation. Evaluation is relative to the goals set for a particular period of time and is based on criteria that are clearly understood by both parties. Together the supervisee and supervisor determine what goals have been reached and the extent to which movement has taken place relative to other goals. The supervisee also gives feedback to the supervisor regarding the supervisor's role in facilitating the supervisee's professional growth. This mutual interchange allows for the necessary alterations and adjustments that will further enhance the supervisory process.

Within the general framework outlined above, several different techniques may be used. The type of technique chosen will depend on the nature of the material to be learned and the various ways of learning that the supervisee finds most useful. Supervision, similar to other learning processes, tends to lead to some anxiety on the part of the learner. This is especially true in the initial phase. The supervisor and supervisee do not know each other well and if the supervisee has just moved into a new work situation, there is added stress that tends to increase anxiety. To minimize anxiety, the supervisee should receive support and satisfaction of legitimate dependency needs. A positive working relationship between the supervisee and supervisor is all important. Initial focus on tasks that the supervisee has mastered also gives security. In addition, a clearly defined structure for the daily responsibilities of the supervisee and for the supervisory meetings decreases anxiety. The need for structure usually diminishes as the supervisee gains a feeling of confidence and trust.

The relationship between the supervisor and the supervisee is a valuable tool for learning. The support, permission for the expression of feelings, praise, and criticism given by the supervisor greatly enhances the learning process. Because of the close relationship and frequent contact between the supervisor and supervisee, transference on the part of the supervisee sometimes occurs. At various times the supervisee, for example, may relate to the supervisor as an authority figure; a representative of the opposite sex; a particular age, ethnic, or religious group; a critical judge; or an all-knowing, all-powerful individual. The supervisee is helped to perceive the supervisor more realistically. The transference relationship is not explored to its causal source. It is discussed to help the supervisee to put the transference into perspective, to make changes in behavior, and to understand the transference relationships of clients. All interactions between the supervisee and supervisor, it should be noted, are not influenced by the transference process. For example, the supervisee's reaction of anger, in a given situation, may be appropriate in terms of the behavior of the supervisor.

In addition to the relationship between supervisee and supervisor, several other techniques are used to facilitate learning. The supervisor may give specific information to the supervisee or identify sources of information. A reading list or periodic assignment of an article or book is quite usual. The material must, of course, be appropriate to the current learning needs of the supervisee. Too little or too much information leads to anxiety, a sense of disorientation, and dependency.

The supervisor may use a Socratic method of teaching. Through asking questions, the supervisor stimulates thinking and helps the supervisee integrate and use knowledge in a productive manner. The questions are such that the supervisee arrives at conclusions in a logical manner. The supervisee's understanding of the process of how he or she arrived at a conclusion is as important as arriving at a specific conclusion.

Demonstrations and use of audiovisual aids such as tape recordings, films, and closed circuit television are another effective technique. Through demonstration, the supervisee is able to observe a competent therapist make use of various professional skills. Evaluative techniques, for example, may be demonstrated prior to the supervisee's use of the techniques. The advantage of audiovisual aids is their reproducibility. The material can be gone over several times or explored from several different perspectives. In a film, for example, the supervisee may at different times observe nonverbal behavior, verbal responses, interaction with the nonhuman environment, or human interactions. A tape recording of an interview or a group meeting may be replayed to compare initial impressions with later impressions and to identify interactions that were previously not noted.

The use of role playing gives the supervisee an opportunity to experiment with new skills prior to their use in client-therapist interactions. Common problems that may arise in management or the change process can be explored first in a relatively safe environment. Role playing gives the supervisee practice in thinking through problems and making decisions regarding appropriate responses in the immediacy of the situation. The need to integrate emotional and factual information may be demonstrated and practiced. By taking the role of the client, the supervisee may develop greater skill in empathizing with various types of clients. In the client role, the supervisee may experience the impact of the therapist's behavior on the client.

The reflective thinking that accompanies keeping a diary is sometimes a useful method for exploring feelings. This is a diary about the feelings one experienced, not what one did in the course of the day. Contemplation of feelings takes some practice. Some people ignore their feelings. Simply looking at their behavior, they ask themselves why they behave in a given manner. Reasons for behavior are filed away in the individual's mind ready to be given forth at a moment's notice. This is an intellectual process frequently unrelated to feelings. Often, too, the reasons are not accurate. They may be acceptable to the individual but not very useful for gaining self-knowledge. It is usually only through exploration of feelings that the causes of one's behavior become known. Newly discovered aspects of the self cannot usually be completely accepted or integrated unless they are validated by another person. The process of diary-keeping and periodic review of the diary may lead to increased self-knowledge. Through sharing this new self-knowledge in supervision, the accuracy of the knowledge can be determined. Validation helps avoid the possibility of perceiving aspects of the self inaccurately. The sharing of this kind of information in supervision is only possible if the supervisee sees the supervisor as accepting, trustworthy, and perceptive.

Supervision may take place in a one-to-one situation or in a group setting. Decisions regarding the type of supervision that would be most appropriate is based on preference and the learning needs of the supervisee, time constraints, and the number of supervisors available. Group supervision is particularly useful when supervisees are working with clients in a group setting. The interaction that takes place in the supervision group can provide many examples of group dynamics and typical problems that occur in any kind of group.

There are several advantages to group supervision. Although the supervisor is still considered to be the "export," all group members are encouraged to consider and present their ideas about the particular situation or problem under consideration. This places the supervisee in a less dependent position, and he or she is able to gain satisfaction from giving help to peers. The group tends to stimulate interest in learning and maintenance of high standards of performance. The support and warmth provided by the group tends to diminish anxiety and often allows for more freedom and risk-taking behavior. The sharing that takes place in a group allows for the expression of many points of view. Group members come to understand that there is more than one way of looking at and solving a problem. They become aware of the problems other supervisees must handle and thus feel less alone in the work of being a therapist.

Although there are several advantages to group supervision, there are also some disadvantages. In a group, discussion often shifts from one topic to another. This may be a means of avoidance but it is also a natural phenomenon that is nondefensive in nature. The number of clients that can be discussed are reduced because of time limitation. Similarly, one client usually cannot be discussed over a period of several group meetings. At times there is hesitancy on the part of some group members to expose their work. Such an individual is often able to blend into the group in such a manner that hesitancy is not noticed. A group frequently tends to avoid conflict or the discussion of "unpleasant" material. Unless the group understands the function of constructive criticism, this very important learning tool may not be used. Avoidance of criticism is particularly common in relationship to a group member who is perceived as less skilled than the majority of the group or who appears to have a relatively poor self-concept. Group supervision sometimes leads to less intense self-examination. The group may demand less self-awareness or the individual may not feel secure enough in the group to engage in the process of examining his own feelings and responses. Many of the problems in group supervision can be corrected if the supervisor and supervisees are aware of the possibility of their occurring.

Learning to become a therapist, initially and continually, is an anxiety-provoking business. Excessive anxiety may give rise to various patterns of behavior that serve to reduce anxiety. These may become evident in the process of client care and/or in the supervisory process. Before discussing some of these relatively common patterns of behavior, it is important to note that many therapists may experience little anxiety. Such individuals use protective measures to regulate tempo and amount of learning. These are constructive and necessary measures to facilitate integration of new knowledge and skill. The capacity to use protective measures is an asset. The therapist who does not experience any particular anxiety should not automatically think that there is something amiss.

Common patterns of behavior or problems that may arise in the supervisee's interaction with clients are:

- Making judgments on the basis of too little information;
- Poor interpretation of the information available;

- Faulty evaluation of the client's major areas of difficulty;
- Inappropriate or unclear goals;
- Lack of understanding of the steps needed to attain the stated goals;
- Identification with the client to the point that the therapist feels helpless like the client;
- Difficulty in understanding the client's ambivalence;
- Intellectual understanding, but minimal emotional understanding;
- Assumption of the role of the well-intended parent who can rechannel the client's life into a more satisfying mold;
- Concern with theoretical aspects of the client's situation without interest in the client as an individual;
- Refusal to become involved with the client or to engage in a meaningful relationship.

Some problems that may arise in the supervisory relationship are:

- A submissive attitude toward the supervisor with no attempt to make the supervisory process one of mutual exploration;
- Fear of being judged;
- Statements of inadequacy and a plea for pity as an attempt to ward off any criticism;
- Inability to identify problems in client care with the expectation that it is the supervisor's responsibility to define problems;
- A desire for the supervisor to give information, think through problems, and make all decisions;
- Complaints that supervision inhibits spontaneity and effectiveness in client care;
- Skepticism regarding all suggestions offered by the supervisor;
- Refusal to accept constructive criticism;
- A negative attitude toward looking at one's own feelings and the belief that self-knowledge is an irrelevant part of being a therapist;
- Confusion between personal therapy and supervision.

There are several different ways that the supervisee may be helped to deal with problems that arise in relationship to clients or in the supervisory process itself. The method used depends on the supervisee and the nature of the problem. The supervisor may provide an opportunity for the supervisee to gain additional knowledge and skill. Their relationship may allow for the release of feelings, which tends to reduce internal tension and enables the supervisee to take a more objective, analytical approach to the situation. The situation may be objectified by focusing attention on the client rather than the supervisee's problem with the client. Temporarily eliminating the demand for self-examination allows the supervisee to deal with his or her own feelings at a rate that is comfortable. As in the method above, this also helps the supervisee to become aware of ways that may be used to help him- or herself and others explore an emotionally charged situation.

The supervisor may provide information about the client's behavior and usual reactions to this type of behavior, discuss a problem he or she encountered that is similar to the supervisee's problem, or universalize the problem through teaching a psychological principle. This, in turn, helps the supervisee to feel that his or her response to the situation is a normal, human reaction. The supervisee may be helped to identify his or her behavior and the feelings provoking the behavior. Sometimes it must be pointed out to the supervisee that there is some problem in the interaction with a client. Self-appraisal by the supervisee is requested. This method encourages the supervisee to take responsibility for understanding and dealing with his or her personal reactions.

Sometimes the problems in learning demonstrated by the supervisee arise out of poor supervision as opposed to the supervisee's difficulties per se. In other words, the supervisor may have problems in fulfilling the role of a supervisor. Some difficulties that a supervisor may experience are:

- Failure to orient or poor orientation of the supervisee to the supervision process;
- Inadequate assessment of the learning needs of the supervisee;
- Poor planning of supervisory sessions;
- A desire to evaluate and engage in intervention with the client by remote control;
- A need to have the supervisee remain dependent;
- A judgmental attitude;
- Difficulty in gaining the supervisee's trust;
- Fear of the expression of strong feelings by the supervisee and the temporary diffusion that may accompany such expression;
- Perception of the supervisee as fragile;
- A desire for the supervisee to use the same therapeutic style as oneself;
- A tendency to push the supervisee and to demand more of him than he is currently capable of doing;
- Lack of confidence in oneself as a therapist or a supervisor or both;
- The need to provide answers or a feeling that one has all the answers.

Supervision is a collaborative process with the supervisee being an active participant. When the supervisee perceives a problem in supervision, it is his or her responsibility to discuss the problem with the supervisor. This frequently helps the supervisor to identify behavior on his or her part that is interfering with productive supervision. It is not the responsibility of the supervisee to help the supervisor to modify behavior. This task should take place outside the supervisee-supervisor relationship. However, the supervisee does have the responsibility of fulfilling the very human needs of the supervisor for acceptance, respect, appreciation, and so forth, as well as for giving positive feedback. As in any interpersonal relationship, such behavior makes the supervisory relationship far more satisfying and productive.

How one becomes a good supervisor is beyond the scope of this text. Only a few comments are in order. One must learn to be a supervisor just as one must learn to be a therapist. Competence in client care does not automatically indicate one has the knowledge and skill needed by a supervisor. Candidates for a supervisory position should receive proper training, which includes the mastery of didactic material as well as practice of supervision under skilled guidance.

Support Systems

Supervision, as mentioned, is only one aspect of a therapist's support system, albeit a very important part. It is generally agreed that students and beginning therapists need supervision. When they cease to need supervision is an unanswered question. Certainly one of the main goals of supervision is to promote independent function. However, we currently lack objective criteria by which one may judge the supervisee's capacity for independent function. This is usually decided by the supervisee and supervisor together on the basis of their collective judgment. Another means for dealing with continued professional growth after discontinuation of formal supervision is peer supervision—another aspect of a support system.

Peer supervision may be contrasted with formal supervision in that no one person is designated as supervisor. Two or more therapists with relatively similar knowledge and skills meet regularly to discuss particular problems encountered in client care. Each person takes joint responsibility for presentation of material and helping others to think through problems, gain new knowledge, and develop new skills. Peer supervision is oriented to discussion of clients for whom the therapists are responsible for the purpose of immediate and direct application. It provides an opportunity for therapists to work out specific problems in client care. Peer supervision is particularly useful because it diminishes the sense of "aloneness" felt by many therapists who function relatively autonomously. It contributes to the maintenance of professional standards. It ensures more adequate client care and it allows for the sharing of new concepts and ideas. This type of supervision requires the participants to take considerable responsibility. However, the therapist who is considered able to function without formal supervision is also a therapist who is able to accept responsibility for his or her own and others' continued professional development.

Consultation may be another aspect of a therapist's support system (27,128,229,261,471,477,495,586, 659,682,779,974). Securing consultation is a way of gaining advice and counsel from a person in regard to a specific problem in a defined area—advice and counsel the individual is free to accept or reject. Its purpose is to add to and enhance the knowledge and understanding of the person seeking help in order to solve a particular problem. Assistance is given through a professional relationship. The function of the consultant is to help others to help themselves. The consultant is usually a person who has specialized knowledge and skill as well as a broad general background in the area of concern. Of particular importance is the consultant's objective point of view, which helps one to perceive problems in a nonemotional manner.

Consultation, as it is being discussed here, is concerned with helping the therapist to be more effective in working with a particular client in the here-and-now. The difficulty may be the therapist's lack of theoretical knowledge and skill or problems in establishing and maintaining a good therapeutic relationship or both. Consultation may also be used to assist in solving organizational problems, establishing departmental goals or policies, and so forth. Although of considerable importance, this type of consultation is outside the scope of this text.

Whereas supervision, either formal or peer, is a long-term, ongoing process, consultation is not. It is a temporary relationship that usually entails only one or two meetings. The therapist may seek consultation from another occupational therapist or from a member of a different profession. The consultant may or may not be associated with the same facility as the therapist.

The success of the consultation process is dependent as much on the therapist as on the consultant. Prior to seeking a consultant, the therapist defines the problem as completely as possible. On the basis of this definition, the therapist selects an individual who has particular knowledge and skill in this area. After securing the services of a consultant, the therapist provides him or her with all of the information that may have a bearing on the situation. The therapist ideally is open to all of the suggestions made by the consultant and rejects none without due consideration. The therapist actively engages in problem solving with the consultant. This is a mutual process in which the therapist takes equal share of the responsibility. Perception of the consultant as someone who will solve all problems is detrimental to the consultation process. The problem can never be placed in the hands of the consultant; it is and remains the problem of the therapist. The ultimate decision reached and implementation of the decision are likewise the responsibilities of the therapist. The therapist should feel free to accept or reject the advice of the consultant. However, rejection of suggestions because of a wish to appear independent or superior and acceptance of suggestions because of feelings of inferiority or fear of retaliation on the part of the consultant should be avoided.

Consultation is a collaborative, interpersonal process. Both therapist and consultant take responsibility for establishing a good working relationship. Trust, respect, and acceptance of each other are important. Each of the participants have human needs that require gratification. Interaction should be such that both therapist and consultant perceive the entire experience as satisfying and growth producing.

A therapist's support system may include in-service education (212,215,243,252,422,448,551). This is usually a regularly scheduled program, within an institution, concerned with learning new knowledge and skills that may ultimately be used in client care. It should not be confused with supervision or consultation, for these interactions are oriented to helping the therapist deal with the problems of individual clients with whom the therapist is presently working. In-service education is particularly useful in helping therapists keep up with the rapidly expanding theories and techniques pertinent to client care.

Planning and implementation of in-service education are the responsibility of everyone who will be participating. To be successful, the program must be relevant to the work of all participants. Common interests and the areas in which participants feel a particular deficiency need identification. This is sometimes difficult when participants are members of different professions. Compromises are sometimes necessary. There should be some degree of general agreement if the experience is to be profitable and supportive.

The group setting of in-service education is usually a positive factor. The interplay between participants tends to facilitate learning. The group provides a sense of security, which often allows people to be more comfortable in admitting ignorance and knowing they are not alone in that ignorance. Sharing differences of opinion and testing out tentative ideas are facilitated in a group setting.

In-service education is conducted by someone with expertise in a particular area. This may be one of the regular participants or someone who is not a member of the group. Ideas and opinions from an outsider often stimulate thinking and help participants consider issues from a different perspective. Learning is facilitated by participants testing out the ideas presented in their work with clients. If this step is ignored or avoided, the ideas presented by the expert become "interesting information" that remains irrelevant to client care.

Professional meetings, workshops, and study groups are other components of a support system. Professional meetings and workshops usually provide an opportunity to meet with therapists from a wide geographical area. Professional growth is enhanced by the opportunity to gain new knowledge, share problems, and develop and maintain colleague relationships. The therapist often returns home with a greater sense of kinship with others in the profession and a lesser sense of being isolated and alone. Study groups are made up of therapists who meet regularly to consider particular topics of mutual interest. They differ from in-service education in that participants are often from a number of different facilities and there is usually no designated expert. Participants gain information through a search of the literature and other sources and share and discuss this information with each other. Particular clients are usually not discussed except perhaps to illustrate the topic under consideration.

Many therapists find that a major portion of their support system exists within the informal structure of the facility in which they are employed. The importance of the informal structure in a work setting was discussed in Chapter 4. The informal structure helps the therapist maintain a personal identity and satisfy personal and emotional needs. The role of the therapist requires the individual to provide for the needs of others without expectation of reciprocal need satisfaction. There is thus, in metaphorical terms, a drain on the emotional resources of the therapist. These resources can only be replaced by need gratification, which comes from outside the direct client care situation. The informal structure, if properly constituted and utilized, can provide much of this needed gratification. Therapists should be aware of how to gain need satisfaction within the informal structure and, in turn, how to provide need satisfaction to other therapists. Lunch hour, gatherings in the staff lounge, and the moments before and after a formal meeting are important periods of time for replenishing one's capacity to give to others.

The final aspect of a support system to be identified here exists outside the therapist's work role. It exists within the therapist's social network, in the capacity to participate in and derive satisfaction from other social roles and in the ability to maintain adequate temporal adaptation. The therapist who takes care of his or her physical needs, spends time with friends, has a variety of recreational interests, and enjoys familial interaction is likely to have the energy and ability to make good use of him- or herself as a therapeutic tool.

9 The Teaching-Learning Process

The teaching-learning process has been a tool of occupational therapy since its inception. From its beginning, occupational therapy has been concerned with teaching various activities as a means of relieving boredom and anxiety, restoring strength and endurance, and facilitating a healthy balance between work, play, and rest. Over the course of the years the profession's domain of concern has broadened. Occupational therapists, however, continue to teach activities and, perhaps more accurately, they are involved with teaching clients those skills that are necessary for living in a community of others.

As a tool, however, the teaching-learning process was, for some period of time, rarely mentioned in the occupational therapy literature, simply not discussed in professional circles. The major reason for this hiatus seems to have been concern for professional identity. As mentioned, in the 1950s and early 1960s, occupational therapists were concerned with self-definition. In so doing they wanted to disassociate themselves from the image of being teachers of arts and crafts. This was commendable because, although occupational therapists do at times teach arts and crafts, this is only a small part of practice. In the process of clarifying their role, however, occupational therapists jettisoned the teaching-learning process, discarding more than was really necessary. Occupational therapists did not stop using the teaching-learning process; they just stopped discussing it in any public forum. Occupational therapists emphasized being a "therapist." This helped to align them more closely with medicine, still a major concern, and to distance them from technical-level occupations. Being a therapist carried much more prestige, and was much less clearly defined. The unknown aspect of being a therapist lends it some mystery and a little magic—far better than the prosaic ordinariness of being a teacher. To be a therapist, then, was somehow better than "helping clients to learn."

Approximately 12 years ago, occupational therapists began once again to recognize publicly the teaching-learning process as one of their legitimate tools. Two major factors that contributed to this new recognition appear to have been (a) a marked increase in self-worth and self-awareness on the part of occupational therapists, and (b) the health profession's acceptance of B. F. Skinner's theory of operant conditioning as one means of bringing about change in behavior. This latter factor led to the realization that learning was a part of the therapeutic process, and respectable. Occupational therapists began to look at their practice to identify those aspects that were primarily based on one or more theories of learning. This gave rise to a number of acquisitional frames of reference.

AN ORIENTATION TO LEARNING AND THEORIES ABOUT LEARNING

With the above brief comments about this somewhat mistreated tool, a few definitions may be useful. Teaching is the process of "instructing by precept, example or experience" (792, p. 1457). It is the process of facilitating the acquisition of knowledge, skills, and attitudes. Learning is a process wherein there is a "change in a subject's behavior to a given situation brought about by his repeated experience in that situation, providing that the behavior cannot be explained on the basis of native response tendencies, maturation or temporary status of the organism (e.g., fatigue, drugs)" (427, p. 17). Stated from a somewhat different perspective, we say that a person has learned something when he does something one day that he was unable to do the day before; or that he does something differently from the way he did it the day before. The change in behavior that occurs as a result of physical maturation, some physiological deficit or imbalance, or damage to the central nervous system is not considered to be learning.

Learning is a process that can be perceived only through a change in an individual's verbal or nonverbal behavior. It takes place within a person. A teacher can only design a situation that he or she believes will enhance or facilitate learning; the learner does the actual learning. It is very difficult to make someone learn something if he or she does not want to learn it. Learning can be forced only when the teacher has total, life-and-death control over the learner's environment. Obviously this is neither the usual nor a desired situation in occupational therapy. The client-learner is free to learn or not to learn. This is one of the client's basic privileges. A therapist can only help a client want to learn through the design of appropriate learning situations.

The term "teaching-learning process" is used here to indicate the close relationship between the teacher and the learner. An individual can and does learn much without the aid of any formal or informal teaching. It is only in those situations when the individual is unable or unlikely to learn without assistance that a teacher of one sort or another is required. Thus, the tool of teaching-learning is used or applied only when an individual is unable to acquire independently those skills that are necessary for successful participation in a community of others.

Psychology, the study of human behavior, is the major discipline concerned with the examination of learning. Many theories of learning have been developed which are in whole or part addressed to the following questions (427):

1. What are the limits of learning (differences in capacity, who can learn what, change in capacity with age and so forth)?
2. What is the role of practice in learning?
3. How important are drives and incentives, rewards and punishments?
4. What is the place of understanding and insight versus trial and error?
5. Does learning one thing help the individual to learn something else?
6. What happens when one remembers and when one forgets?
7. Is there one or several kinds of learning?

During the period 1930–1950, the time when most learning theories were developed, it was felt that neurophysiology had very little to offer that was relevant to the understanding of learning. The major psychological theories of learning were never intended to describe the specific, actual events that occur in the nervous system. The tactics of psychologists were those of descriptive behaviorism supplemented by intervening variables such as motivation, needs, drives, and so forth. The scientific question was whether a theoretical system provided an adequate explanation, description, or prediction about learned behavior. The internal structures involved and changes in these structures were considered irrelevant (193,416,427,429,452).

Neurophysiologists were not satisfied to leave matters at that level, wishing to discover more about the relationship between the nervous system and learning (163, 408,409,416,889,922). The physiology of the receptors and effectors (muscle action) is not usually considered relevant to the study of learning. Their normal functioning is an important but not a sufficient condition for learning. Neurophysiologists are, thus, concerned primarily with the central nervous system—the brain in particular. The questions they have addressed are related to what structures and processes are involved, how is information stored and retained, can other structures be substituted when the original ones are unable to function properly, what changes during learning, how does learned information persist, and what destroys it.

The neurophysiological study of learning is relatively new. What has been discovered at this point is the role of the hypothalamus in motivating behavior and the paramount importance of the reticular activating system in arousal. Memory is considered to involve a relatively permanent physical or structural change in the nervous system, which has been labeled encoding. The persistence of memory or retention is a function of the degree of persistent neural activity relative to the experience. The latter is not entirely supported by research. Neurophysiologists have also contributed to the understanding of the different functions of the right and left hemispheres of the brain. Neurophysiology may eventually provide important information about the learning process, but at the present time it does not offer much in regard to how learning takes place.

This leaves us then primarily with psychological theories of learning. All individual theories are imperfect in that they fail to describe all types of learning with equal validity. There is presently no unified or comprehensive theory of learning, although the search continues. In the interim, occupational therapy, similar to other professions that utilize the teaching-learning process as one of their tools, must make use of whatever knowledge is available. One course of action is to restrict oneself to one theoretical position; another is to select from the collective knowledge those ideas that seem to be of value relative to one's particular situation (777,917). Occupational therapy has, in part, taken the former. Thus, there are some frames of reference based exclusively on operant conditioning. Occupational therapy has also taken the route of selecting from the collective knowledge in regard to learning. It is this approach that will be discussed here: an approach referred to as principles of learning.

PRINCIPLES OF LEARNING

Principles of learning are a collection of generalizations that have been distilled from various theories of learning (427). They consist of summarizations of empirical relationships that have been fairly well verified or have a reasonable amount of empirical support. Many of them, however, have not been stated with sufficient precision to be considered "laws" of learning. Drawn from many theories, the various principles of learning are, in a large part, compatible with the major theories of learning. The principles of learning relevant to the occupational therapy process follow.

1. *Learning is influenced by the individual's inherent capacities, current assets and limitations, age, sex, interest, and past and present culture group membership.* One inherent capacity that must be taken into consideration is the intelligence of the client. This does not mean the therapist must know the client's exact intelligence quotient. The therapist determines in a general way how intelligent the client seems to be, and how slowly or how rapidly the client seems to learn. If the client seems to be below average intellectually, the therapist may find it necessary to use more simple words in talking with the client and select activities that are compatible with the client's abilities. This is also important when working with a client of above average intelligence; complex activities that involve considerable cognitive skill are often more appropriate for such an individual.

Another important inherent capacity is energy level. This does not refer to hyperactivity or hypoactivity, but energy level in the normal range. There is wide variation in the amount of vigorous physical activity a person seems to need. Some people tire after only a small amount of physical activity, whereas others' capacity for sustained improvement in a high level of physical activity is seemingly almost boundless. Similarly, some people can sit for a long period of time doing an intricate task or participating in lengthy emotional discussions, whereas others respond to such situations after a period of time with restlessness and apparent disinterest. They essentially respond with the implied or overt statement of, "I have to get out of here and *do* something." Although such a response may be motivated by wanting to avoid the situation, it may also be that the person simply cannot tolerate being physically inactive for a long period of time.

Other factors included under the heading of "inherent capacities" are general physical health, previous or current damage to the nervous system, how well a person is able to see and hear, loss of sensation, degree of coordination, and the like. Difficulties in any of these areas are taken into consideration in planning intervention.

Current assets and limitations refers more specifically to what the individual is and is not able to do. It is related to previous learning relative to performance components. Learning of a specific task or interaction cannot take place unless the individual has the prerequisite motor skills, sensory integrative capacity, perceptual ability, cognitive and psychological functions, and social interaction skills. In designing an activity, the individual capacity in the area of performance components must be taken into consideration. Assets and limitations also refers to specialized abilities or talents the individual might have and particular deficit such as lack of any athletic skills.

Another reason why it is important to take a client's assets and limitations into consideration is that people learn more easily if they are encouraged to do the things they do well in conjunction with learning something new. Through knowledge of a client's assets, the therapist is better able to design an activity that makes use of these assets to facilitate learning in other areas.

An individual's age must be given sufficient attention. It is not always age per se that is important but what activities people think are appropriate for various age groups. Some people feel that only children use finger paints, that middle-aged women do not roller skate, and that only old men play cribbage. Set ideas about relationships between age and activities are usually not dealt with in intervention unless a client has such a narrow view of what activities are appropriate for his age group that he is unable to satisfy his needs. The therapist respects clients' ideas about age and appropriate activities and seeks out activities that they believe are suitable to their age. This is not to say, however, that the therapist cannot gently encourage clients to try some activities to which they originally responded with, "That's kid stuff," or some variation on that theme.

Adolescents and young adults, as an age group, often have special activities they enjoy. For many, the special activities of this age group serve as a source of identity and as a way of setting themselves apart from the older and younger generations. Adolescents and young adults often learn more easily in a situation that makes use of activities that are currently popular in the youth subculture. It is helpful if the therapist keeps track of this rapidly changing scene.

There has been considerable change in many groups regarding what activities are appropriate for women and men. The women's movement has altered many people's thinking about sex-specific activities, both in the family and in the wider community. However, not everyone's ideas have changed. Some still believe strongly in the difference between activities suitable for women and those suitable for men: the idea of "women's work" and "men's work." Given the current situation, the therapist should be sensitive to the client's feelings about engaging in activities traditionally thought of as being "feminine" or "masculine." Ideally one creates an environment in which clients feel comfortable engaged in any activity, regardless of its gender connotations.

Difficulties arise in intervention when a person is not interested in the activity being used to enhance learning. Some people, for example, are interested only in activities that have a useful end-product. Others are interested in activities that have a creative aspect. Still others do not like activities that involve competition. The more interested a person is in an activity, the more likely that person is to learn what the activity was designed to teach.

Culture, as an important factor in understanding a client, was discussed in Chapter 6. In relationship to the teaching-learning process, an individual's cultural understandings and beliefs about specific activities must be taken into consideration. Learning is enhanced if the activities used in intervention are seen as relevant by the individual's cultural group. In addition, cultural understandings affect response to elements of an activity. Food preferences and the meaning of particular foods, for example, are strongly influenced by an individual's cultural background. Thus, the cultural aspect of food needs to be taken into consideration in planning activities that involve food preparation and/or eating.

2. *Attention and perception influence learning.* Attention is the ability to process some part of incoming sensations and to ignore others. There are several internal and external factors that influence attention. The individual, for example, may be preoccupied with a variety of thoughts, paying little heed to what is going on around him. There may be several happenings in the environment that compete for the individual's attention. Learning does not occur, or it does not occur in an optimal manner, if the individual is not attending to the learning task. The therapist, then, must attempt to ensure that the individual suspends preoccupying thoughts, at least temporarily, and attempt to make the environment minimally distracting. Gaining the patient's attention is usually facilitated by designing an activity that is of particular interest to the client.

Perception as used here is the interpretation of selected sensations in the light of past experiences. It is an internal analysis that allows the individual to make sense out of the world and assign meaning to experiences. Perception is influenced among other things by the intactness of the nervous system, by habits of thought acquired in one's cultural group, and by personal ideas and ways of structuring the environment. A client's perception of a learning situation may be similar to that of the therapist, or it may be very different. It is necessary, then, for the therapist to determine how the client is perceiving the situation. If the client perceives the learning experience much differently than the therapist, learning may occur, but it may not be the learning that the experience was designed to facilitate.

3. *The learner's motivation is important.* Motivation is an internal process that spurs an individual on to satisfy some need. There is considerable variation in regard to the source of motivation. Theories vary on a continuum from biological, to psychological, to sociological. Biological theories consider motivation ultimately dependent on physiological needs, such as hunger, thirst, and protection from the extremes of temperature. Psychological theories closely related to biological processes ascribe primary motivation force to sexuality in all of its manifestations and to aggression, the urge to destroy oneself, other people, or objects. Other psychological theories, less closely related to biological processes, ascribe primary motivation to the need for love and affiliation; innate curiosity, which is manifested in exploration, manipulation, and the search for knowledge; the desire to fulfill one's potential; and the need to master and be competent. Sociological theories focus on the importance of social pressures as the source of motivation. Sociologists usually recognize more basic sources of motivation, but consider these insignificant compared to the demands made by the shared understandings of a cultural group. Regardless of the particular theory, all of the sources of motivation mentioned above are here considered to be primary in nature. They become elaborated and refined in many ways so that eventually they become fairly idiosyncratic to each individual.

Another source of motivation, somewhat aside from the continuum outlined above, is the individual's level of aspiration. This refers to a person's goals or objectives and their expectations in regard to their capacity to meet these goals. An individual's level of aspiration is influenced by his self-concept, in particular that aspect of self-concept related to what the individual believes he is able and not able to do. The concept of self-fulfilling prophecy is relevant to understanding the relationship between level of aspiration and learning. The individual who has high expectations for himself and believes he will meet these expectations is likely to gain a good deal from relevant learning experiences. The individual with low expectations is likely to gain far less from the same experience. An individual's expectations, thus, appear to be quite influential in the motivation that an individual brings to a learning situation.

Motivation is a factor that is within an individual. The therapist, in order to facilitate learning, attempts to determine a client's source of motivation. With this information, the therapist is able to design purposeful activities that will tap these sources. Thus the client's own potential for learning is made available. It is sometimes assumed that the therapist is responsible for motivating a client. This is not necessarily true. The therapist is responsible for designing appropriate learning experiences based on his or her understanding of the client's source of motivation. That is all. The client is ultimately responsible for determining what learning experiences he or she will engage in, and what he or she will gain from the experiences.

4. *Learning goals set by the individual are more likely to be attained than goals set by someone else.*

What is to be learned must be seen as relevant by the client. As mentioned, occupational therapy is a collaborative process. The client and the therapist together set the goals for intervention. This is true for the long-term goals of the entire intervention process as well as for short-term goals set along the way. Goal setting by the client focuses attention on what is to be learned and gives the client a sense of responsibility for and participation in the intervention process. Setting goals in collaboration with a client will be discussed in more detail in Chapter 17. The point to be made here is that the client's learning will be enhanced by participation in the goal setting process.

5. *Learning is enhanced when the individual understands what is to be learned and the reason for learning.*

One way of assessing whether this principle of learning is being adhered to is to talk with clients after a session in occupational therapy. If the majority of clients are unable to say why they were participating in the session, or what they expected to gain from participation, it is fairly safe to guess that the full potential of the occupational therapy process is not being utilized. Minimal learning takes place if a person does not know what he is supposed to learn or why he is being encouraged to learn something new.

Ideally, the therapist demonstrates or at least describes in detail what he or she expects the client to learn. Further, the therapist explains how learning this particular skill, information, or value will lead to the previously set goals. For example, one way of helping people learn how to participate in a nurturing relationship is to encourage them to care for plants or an animal of some kind. If the client does not understand how the nurturing demands of plants and animals relate to his desired goal of participating more in the care of his infant daughter, he will probably feel that the activity is meaningless. Some of the major points—"What do I get in return?" "Who is going to take care of these nonhuman things while I am away for the weekend?" "They certainly are demanding and take up a lot of my time"—will never be brought into focus because the client does not understand the purpose of the activity. The therapist who asks, "What would it be like if I were in a situation where I was supposed to learn something but did not know what or why" is well on the way to understanding this principle of learning.

A subpart of this principle is that learning with understanding is more permanent and more transferable than rote learning or learning by a formula. For example, a young woman who is going to be living away from her family for the first time may be helped to learn how to make up a budget. A sample budget may be used to facilitate learning. If the client merely follows the outlined budget with little idea of what the categories mean or why a specific amount of money is allotted to each category, she is unlikely to use a budget when she moves into her own apartment. Much time was wasted, both by the client and the therapist, and no real learning took place.

6. *Learning is increased when it begins at the individual's current level and proceeds at a rate that is comfortable for the individual.*

The principle is probably self-evident but it does need to be emphasized. One of the major mistakes therapists make is to assume clients are able to do things they are really not able to do. Intervention is sometimes begun at a point far above the client's level of function. For example, a client who is not able to maintain any interest in what is going on around him is not going to be able to participate in an active game of volleyball. Rather, he may need a one-to-one situation in which the therapist makes a concentrated effort to maintain the client's attention. On the other hand, a therapist may begin intervention at a point far below the client's current level of function. The client, in this case, is very likely to become bored, and so is the therapist. Adequate evaluation greatly limits the possibility of beginning intervention at a level that is incompatible with the client's current capacities.

There are limitations in the amount of learning that can take place at one time. Failure to attend to this factor may lead the therapist to expect too much from the client in a specific time period. When these expectations are not met, both the therapist and client are likely to be disappointed. Such disappointment can be avoided by the therapist's identifying realistic expectations relative to the quantity of learning that is likely to occur in a given span of time.

The knowledge, skills, and attitudes a client needs to acquire may take a long time to learn. The rate of learning may be very slow, and at times it may appear as though no learning is taking place. Clients may go through periods in which it seems there is no change, and then suddenly begin to learn again. Some individuals appear to need a hiatus in learning to integrate and consolidate what they have already learned before they are able to go forward in the learning process. The difficulty is in trying to determine whether a client is experiencing a hiatus, whether there is something in the intervention situation that is interfering with learning, or whether he or she just cannot advance any further in that particular area. Sometimes the only thing a therapist can do is wait and see, make some changes in the learning situation, and wait some more.

It should not be assumed that all clients learn slowly. Many advance very quickly in the development of desired abilities. If not prepared for such movement, the therapist may retard the client's growth and extend the time of intervention beyond what is really necessary.

7. *Active participation in the learning process facilitates learning.* This learning principle is central to occupational therapy. Verbal therapies often involve discussion about problem areas and difficulty in doing. Occupational therapy encourages clients to act in order to discover the nature of problem areas and to attempt to make necessary changes within the immediate situation.

Active participation refers to two related ideas: learning through discovery and learning through doing. Discovery learning or techniques involve gaining knowledge of or insight about something previously unknown or unseen through active involvement in a here and now situation. Discovery learning experiences need to be carefully designed. If they are not so designed, they tend to be characterized by a pooling of collective ignorance, which in turn leads to frustration, feelings of insecurity, and a lack of learning. If well designed, they tap the individual's curiosity and desire to explore, and enhance learning.

Learning through doing refers to gaining knowledge and skill through involvement in a learning experience where one is required to act, to engage. Some examples of learning through doing are a client's taking charge of the bulletin board in order to begin to develop a sense of responsibility, making a link belt as the first step in acquiring task skills, playing checkers as a means of acquiring the ability to be competitive, and collating hospital forms to develop work habits. Active participation means that an individual is fully there in the learning situation. He is not being taught; he is learning.

8. *Reinforcement and feedback as the consequence of action are important parts of a learning experience.* What happens after an individual has done something strongly influences whether or not he or she is likely to repeat the behavior. If the act leads to need satisfaction, it is likely to be repeated; if it leads to need deprivation, it is not likely to be repeated. The term "reinforcer" is used to designate any event that increases the frequency of a given act. A reinforcer is something that is ultimately need satisfying. Some common reinforcers are approval, respect, a sense of mastery, a feeling of accomplishment, money, and food.

Behavior that is not reinforced tends to drop out of a person's repertoire of usual behavior. A client, for example, may always have received attention and sympathy when she complained of vague aches and pains. If the people in the client's immediate environment stop giving her attention and sympathy when she complains, but instead give her approval for other things she does, the client is likely to stop talking about her aches and pains. This is not only an example of eliminating a type of maladaptive behavior, but it is also an example of differential reinforcement. Differential reinforcement is the process of giving reinforcement for one kind of behavior and not giving reinforcement for another type of behavior.

It is generally felt that punishment or other need-depriving events should not be used in the intervention process. One reason for this belief is that punished behavior does not seem to drop out of a person's repertoire of behavior; he only gives up the behavior in those circumstances where he is likely to be caught. Another reason is that fear of punishment or need deprivation can be so severe that a person may stop trying to learn. For example, a therapist who makes critical remarks to clients in a discussion group may find that the clients eventually refuse to discuss anything at all. If a person knows he is going to be punished if he makes a mistake or does not always live up to the expectations of others, he is likely to try to avoid the situation entirely. Positive reinforcement, then, is considered to be more effective than negative reinforcement.

In the initial stages of learning, the individual often needs a considerable amount of reinforcement. Less reinforcement is usually needed later on in the process, although some reinforcement is always necessary if the behavior is to be maintained in the individual's repertoire. Ideally, movement from frequent to infrequent reinforcement is gradual. Abrupt changes in the amount or frequency of reinforcement may interfere with the learning process.

One of the major concerns of the therapist is finding what will work as a reinforcer for a client. Not all clients respond to attention and approval. This is particularly true for clients who are extremely withdrawn or depressed. Candy, gum, or cigarettes sometimes serve as reinforcers for clients who presently seem to be experiencing only very primitive needs. As intervention progresses, the therapist slowly substitutes less concrete reinforcement, such as approval or attention. Reinforcement used in intervention is ultimately designed to be similar to the kind of reinforcement that is available in the community. It should be remembered that new behavior must eventually be performed in real life situations to provide real life reinforcements. If this does not occur, the behavior is likely to be very quickly lost from the individual's repertoire.

Learning in many areas is enhanced by feedback: knowledge of the results of any behavior. It is the information one receives about the way one's behavior affects other people or things. Reinforcement is somewhat similar to feedback as it can be a good source of information regarding one's behavior. If, for example, an anticipated reward is not received for one's behavior, the individual is likely to look at his behavior to ascertain why the reward did not occur; what did he do wrong? Feedback, however, usually provides more information. It tells the individual something about why his behavior was or was not effective. It confirms adequate or adaptive behavior and provides the basis for correcting faulty behavior. Feedback allows for the testing of behavior. This is the process of trying something provisionally: through feedback, the individual is able to decide whether to accept as his own or reject a particular behavioral response.

Considerable feedback about behavior can be derived from the nonhuman environment, particularly when there are objective criteria to determine the success of the end-product. If, for example, a child is building a windmill out of Tinker Toys using a picture on the box as a guide, the child is able to tell if her windmill is constructed in a manner similar to the one illustrated on the box. The child is also fairly readily able to see where an error might have been made. In regard to the human environment, many times a person does not know how his behavior affects others. He needs information about what people think and feel about his behavior. The actions and responses of others frequently provide nonverbal clues about the effect of behavior. But reading these clues is often difficult. Thus it is useful for other people to give feedback verbally. Individuals also need information about how they are doing in a learning situation. "Am I doing all right?" "Is this right or wrong?" These are common questions of any learner. Answering these questions, even if they are not asked directly, provides the learner with valuable information.

9. *Learning can be enhanced through trial and error, shaping, and imitation of models.*

Trial and error is responding to a new situation with a variety of goal-directed acts. The motivated learner keeps trying until finding something that works. Trial-and-error responses may be overt and visible to an observer or they may be covert in that the person thinks about various courses of action. Individuals are more likely to engage in trial-and-error learning if they are in a setting where mistakes and false starts are seen as a normal part of the learning process. There should also be plenty of time to work things out. Trial and error involves figuring things out for oneself rather than being told: a learning style preferred by many people.

One common way of learning is through shaping: a process whereby successive approximations of the desired behavior are reinforced. Successive approximation refers to increasingly more accurate attempts to do something correctly. A toddler learning how to walk and feed himself are good examples of successive approximation. The process of shaping may be illustrated by a therapist's helping a client to learn how to make his bed. At first the therapist gives approval or some other reinforcement for any attempt at making the bed. Later, approval is given only if the sheets and blankets cover the bed. Still later, the therapist gives approval only if the sheets and blankets are straight on the bed with no wrinkles. Finally reinforcement is given only when the bed is completely and neatly made.

Imitation is responding to a new situation by copying the behavior of another person more or less accurately. Learning is accomplished vicariously through observing another person making a skilled response. The crucial factor in imitation is good models. Faulty or inadequate models lead to faulty learning. In a treatment center, for example, a staff that is not able to express emotions adequately or resolve conflicts among themselves is going to have a difficult time helping clients to develop these skills. Models for imitation are usually selected by an individual for two reasons: he likes and respects the other person and wants to be like him, and/or he sees that the other person's behavior is effective in getting what he himself wants. Incidentally, much of the socialization process is considered to be imitative in nature. A cultural group is the reservoir of the most successful responses that the group has found to deal with particular kinds of situations in the past. Through imitating these responses, the individual acquires the traditional ways of acting and thinking, which are part of his culture.

10. *Frequent repetition or practice facilitates learning.*

It is rare for an individual to develop a complex skill by practicing the skill only a few times. The behavior implicit in the skill has to be repeated many times in order for it to become really part of the person. It takes considerable repetition before a skill is so well learned that one can apply the skill automatically without having to think about it. The skills that clients hope to learn are very complex and, unfortunately, they are not always given enough time to practice them. Clients are sometimes discharged before they have had enough time to integrate new learning. An individual, for example, may learn to function fairly well in a protective and supportive ward group. When discharged, however, that person may have considerable difficulty participating in the complex groups found in the community. The importance of practice also points to the desirability of there being extensive learning situations available for clients. Clients usually do not learn well if they only receive help with their learning one or two hours a day. This is not to say that clients do not need time to integrate learning and for relaxation; they do. But in many treatment centers, clients spend far too much time in meaningless activities or doing nothing.

Practice in different situations encourages generalization and discrimination. Generalization is the ability to apply what was learned in one situation to another appropriate situation. Discrimination, on the other hand, is the ability to determine what is appropriate behavior for one situation as opposed to another situation. Together, generalization and discrimination are the ability to match behavior to the situation. Practice in different situations helps a person learn what behavior to use in a variety of different circumstances. Generalization can be facilitated, for example, by encouraging a client to apply newly learned task skills to all tasks he is asked or required to perform. Helping a client to realize what tasks require considerable attention to detail and what tasks demand much less concern for detail is an example of how a therapist may enhance a client's capacity to discriminate.

11. *Planned movement from simplified wholes to more complex wholes facilitates integration of what is to be learned.*

This principle is a synthesis of two common learning theory postulates. One of these postulates is the idea that learning is enhanced by moving from the simple to the complex. The other postulate contains the idea that individuals perceive and give meaning to experiences by their characteristics in toto and not by considering an unorganized aggregate of the parts. An example of application of this postulate is helping a client to use a public transit bus in the context of getting ready to go somewhere, getting there, and engaging in some pleasurable activity at the end of the journey. Just taking a bus ride for the sake of learning how to use public transportation is breaking an activity into meaningless parts.

In designing a learning experience, the therapist analyzes what is to be learned. This is done in terms of graduated levels of complexity of what is to be learned and meaningful whole, which constitutes the totality of that which is to be learned. In teaching a client to be self-sufficient in taking care of her need to eat every day, for example, the therapist determines the knowledge and skills necessary to carry out this activity and which tasks are more or less complex. Initial learning may take place in the context of the therapist and client preparing a simple soup and sandwich lunch together. The idea of basic nutritional needs may be introduced later when the client is ready to take responsibility for planning the menu for the client and staff Saturday brunch. Skills in this case are being learned in a simple to complex sequence, each step being imbedded in a recognizable whole.

12. *Inventive solutions to problems should be encouraged as well as more useful or typical solutions.*

There are few problems that have only one solution and few activities that must be performed in one specific way. Thus the learner should not be led to believe that there is only one right way of doing things. Rather a good learning situation promotes the idea that there are a number of ways of performing a task in a successful manner and many modes of relating to people in a given situation. This is not to say that typical ways of dealing with things and events are never suggested; they are. Many of the clients involved in occupational therapy are not able to engage in any sort of creative problem solving. Simply learning the usual ways of dealing with people and things is difficult for them. They need help in learning how to function, not in developing creative ways of functioning. This is particularly true of individuals who are of below average intelligence, who have neurological deficits, and who have been hospitalized for a long period of time.

On the other hand, there are clients who can profit from learning in an atmosphere that encourages divergent thinking. They can gain much from the opportunity to consider a variety of ways of accomplishing a particular task. As a matter of fact, they often arrive at solutions that are far better than the possibilities considered by the therapist. Inventive solutions can be arrived at if there is a willingness to consider situations from many different directions. On the other hand, there needs to be some structure, some sense of orderliness and consistency, as well as general values about what is right and wrong. Structure with flexibility is perhaps a good way to describe a beneficial learning situation.

13. *The environment in which learning takes place is an important factor.*

The atmosphere of the learning situation has a strong influence on the satisfaction the individual gains from a learning experience as well as what is learned and how well it is learned. A calm, organized environment, for example, tends to facilitate learning, whereas a hurried, disorganized environment does not usually do so. The characteristics of the learning situation should always be taken into consideration. Some major elements to consider are whether the situation is cooperative or competitive; whether the general tone is authoritarian, democratic, or laissez faire; and whether the individual is learning in a solitary situation or within the context of a group. Certain kinds of learning may be enhanced by a given atmosphere; other learning may be impeded in the same atmosphere. The learning of work habits, for example, may be facilitated if the environment is somewhat authoritarian. An authoritarian environment is not likely to be useful in learning how to make decisions for oneself. In addition, some individuals learn more easily in one type of environment as opposed to another. Some people, for example, are more comfortable learning alone, whereas others prefer the company of other people.

14. *There are individual differences in the ways anxiety affects learning.*

Some people learn best when they are moderately fearful or anxious. Anxiety seems to motivate this type of person to engage in the enterprise of learning. Other people can learn only if they are relatively free of anxiety. Even a moderate degree of fear seems to make them feel disorganized and unable to learn. Some people, for example, can only study for an exam the night before, whereas others are more comfortable preparing for the exam throughout the semester. Similar responses can be seen in a group of clients who have a specific date on which they must leave the treatment center. Some work steadily at eliminating their problem areas throughout their stay. Others seem to idle away their time doing little to find solutions to their problems in functioning until the last few weeks of their stay. The therapist attempts to identify the optimal level of anxiety for each client and to regulate the learning situation accordingly. Decrease in anxiety is fairly easy to obtain through providing an adequate amount of support and reassurance. Raising a person's level of anxiety is somewhat more complex. The therapist is often tempted to threaten a decrease in need satisfaction or need deprivation. This comes very close to threatening punishment as a means of facilitating learning. As mentioned, it is probably best to avoid punishment in the teaching-learning process. The therapist, then, must be inventive in trying to help a person who needs to be moderately anxious in order to learn. It is generally agreed that a very high degree of anxiety interferes with learning. Only a very few people are able to learn when they are in a state of extreme fear. About the only thing most people are able to do in a high-anxiety situation is to try to find a way out of the situation.

15. *Conflicts and frustrations, inevitably present in the learning situation, must be recognized and provisions made for their resolution or accommodation.*

Conflict may arise between the therapist and the client in regard to the goals or means of intervention. As in any intimate relation it may occur over minor matters that are somewhat extraneous to the actual process of intervention. The client on the other hand, may experience internal conflict. She may, for example, be ambivalent about the goals of intervention, wanting to attain the goals and being fearful of being able to or expected to function on a more advanced or mature level. Frustration is an inherent part of many learning situations. The individual, by placing herself in the position of a learner, is essentially saying that she does not know something or how to do something and that she needs help. In this statement, an individual's needs for security, independence, and mastery are often not initially met. Unmet needs give rise to feelings of frustration. Frustration may also come from the intervention process itself; the learning may take longer than the client had expected or be more difficult than anticipated.

Perhaps the most important word in this principle is "inevitable." Conflict and frustration are inherent components of most learning and particularly the learning that takes place in intervention. It is important that the therapist accept the inevitable rather than blaming him- or herself for being insensitive, inept, lacking in knowledge, and so forth. It is also important that the therapist help the client to realize the inevitability of conflict and frustration; without such realization, the client is likely to have feelings similar to those of the therapist.

The signs of conflict and frustration are multiple but some common ones are withdrawal, generalized anger, a conscious or unconscious attempt to alter the learning situation to avoid intimidating elements, resistance, and denial. Resolution and accommodation may occur when the therapist makes some changes in the learning situation. However, such a unilateral solution is often not as successful as the client and therapist working together to determine how the situation can be made more comfortable without substantially altering the goals and appropriate means of intervention.

16. *There needs to be continuity between the learning situation and the experiences for which the learning constitutes preparation.*

The therapist can help a client function in the treatment setting, but it is far more important that the client be able to function in the community. Thus, the therapist's efforts must be focused on designing learning experiences that will help the client transfer what is being learned in intervention to daily life in the community. By far the best way of ensuring transfer of learning to community interaction is for the client to be in the community while participating in the intervention process. If a client is able to go home in the evening or on weekends, is able to go out shopping during the day or have dinner with friends in the evening, or is only able to go out for a walk or sit in a nearby park, the client has an opportunity to try out new behavior. Difficulties in using newly learned skills or not knowing whether one response is better than another can be talked about while the situation is real and fresh in the client's mind. Clients who remain in treatment centers for long periods of time without any contact with the outside world have no way of knowing if they have really acquired new knowledge, skills, and values; neither does the therapist. Intervention is taking place in a vacuum. Many clients learn how to function in a treatment center, but remain totally inept at functioning in the real world. Clients must have an opportunity to try out new ways of acting in an unsheltered situation. If they do not, the sheltered situation may be a hindrance to rather than a help in furthering their growth.

CONCLUSION

The principles of learning outlined above are not rules, but rather ideas to be considered when the therapist is thinking about what he or she can do to help a client learn to function in a more adaptive, satisfying manner. Principles of learning do not answer the question of "how in my situation, with this client." They do not say what will work best, or of the appropriate emphasis or balance. One principle may be of considerable importance for the learning of a specific client and less important for another. Part of being a therapist is to find out what will help each client to learn.

10 Purposeful Activities

Purposeful activities have been a part of occupational therapy since its inception. In the course of using purposeful activities, occupational therapists began to learn far more about the potential of activities for restoring and maintaining function. With this recognition, the study of activities was initiated. Research, primarily qualitative in nature, has focused on the nature of activities and the way in which activities can be used to facilitate evaluation and intervention. These two foci of research are related but somewhat different in orientation. In studying the nature of activities, occupational therapists consider activities as a phenomenon to be explored in its own right. The assumption is that one cannot understand or use activities as a tool until their inherent properties are known. The other focus of research has been related to designing activities for evaluation and intervention. Although it would seem logical that the first focus of research would precede the latter, this has not always been the case. But then, this is not unusual in the study of any legitimate tool. In medicine, for example, through the ages many drugs have been effectively used without full understanding of their inherent ingredients or properties. The nature of activities will be discussed in this chapter. The way in which activities are used to facilitate evaluation and intervention will be discussed briefly in the following chapter and in more detail in Parts 4 and 5.

Purposeful activities, considered by many to be the major legitimate tool of occupational therapy, have been defined in a variety of ways. In this text purposeful activities are defined as doing processes that require the use of thought and energy and are directed toward an intended or desired end result. Purposeful activities may be contrasted with random activities, which are undirected and without a predetermined goal. They also may be contrasted with "busy work" or mindless repetitive tasks designed primarily to keep one physically occupied and out of mischief.

An activity is usually not considered purposeful unless the reason for engaging in the activity is apparent to the doer. The purpose of the activity may be related to the process, as in using an activity to minimize anxiety, or related to the end result, as in the learning of a particular skill. The individual's perception of the purpose of an activity is influenced by the shared understandings of his culture. If the individual's culture does not see an activity as being relevant to its values and needs, it is unlikely to be viewed as relevant by the individual.

An activity is also not considered to be purposeful if an individual is coerced into participation. This does not mean, however, that the individual's participation in an activity must be entirely voluntary for the activity to be considered purposeful. A child's participation in classroom activities, for example, may not always be voluntary.

The end result of a purposeful activity is planned or hypothesized by the individual. It may not be attained, but that does not negate the purposefulness of the activity. The end result of a purposeful activity is not necessarily a tangible finished product. If there is a product, it may be far less important than the process out of which it was derived. For example, one may be pleased with the results of having refinished a piece of furniture, but see the doing of the task as the most enjoyable part of the process. The finished product, indeed, may only be important as it reflects or symbolizes the process.

One of the characteristics of purposeful activities is that they have a potential of being symbolic. Prior to discussions of the nature of purposeful activities, a brief digression into a description of symbolism seems in order.

SYMBOLISM

A symbol is an action, object, person, image, or word that has special complexity of meanings in addition to its conventional and obvious meaning (4,49,160,317, 386,473,492–494,565,580,660,722,723,778,790,873, 875,876). A symbol, although able to be explained in some detail after study, always has elements that are unknown or hidden. A person, for example, might be able to give a fairly good explanation of why she enjoys baking bread. However, there is something about the process and the feelings it engenders that cannot be described. That which is symbolized, the meaning of a symbol, is called the referent.

Symbols may be differentiated from a sign: an action, object, image, or word that stands for another action object, image, or word. There is no mystery to a sign; it is easily understood. There are no hidden or unknown aspects. Symbols have an emotional component, whereas feelings are rarely associated with a sign. Some examples of signs are waving one's hand to say goodbye, an advertisement in the newspaper, and a road map.

There are three interrelated aspects of symbols: representation, form, and content. Representation refers to the way in which a symbol is experienced or produced. Symbols may be represented as actions, images, words, or objects. Action symbols are expressed through the motions of the symbol producer. They are seen in purest form in dance. Action symbols are sometimes combined with and thus confused with image symbols. There is, for example, a tendency to overlook the movement aspect of dreams. More attention is given to the people in dreams than to what they are doing. Similarly in doodling, it is often the movement itself that is significant, not what is produced. Both aspects, however, usually complement each other to give a fuller notion of what is being symbolized. Image symbols, perhaps the best known way of representing a symbol, appear in dreams, fantasies, and in the visual arts. Words are often used to label symbols and, by association, the word itself may become a symbol. This is the case, for example, in the words "American flag" and "motherhood." However, words tend to be signs of symbols more often than symbols in and of themselves. Concrete object symbols are people or things that take on or are invested with symbolic meaning. Marilyn Monroe and Watergate are examples of concrete object symbols.

The two other elements of a symbol are form and content. Form refers to the manifest structure of a symbolic representation. A symbol, for example, might be represented as an image. The form of the image may be a candle, a black cat, a color, or running water. A particular symbolic form may have many referents or meanings. The content of a symbol is concerned with the referent or referents of a symbol. Symbolic content may take many forms. The following examples are by no means exhaustive but are presented to give the reader some idea of the difference between form and content.

The first example specifies forms, followed by common content symbolized by these forms.

1. Mother: place of origin; that which passively creates; substance and matter; lower body; womb; vegetative functions; unconscious; that which carries, nurtures, embraces, protects; emotional being.
2. Horse: subhuman animal side, drives, power, locomotion, beast of burden, sorcery, magic, that which heralds death (white horse).
3. Mandala forms (anything that has a circle-like form, which may include a quaternary division): oneness, unity, devotion to life (what is or that which is desired), completeness, peace.
4. Dragon or serpent: initial state of unconscious (because it "dwells in caverns and dark places"), revelation, anything frightening.
5. Metals: inner man, spiritual growth, highest illumination.
6. Tree: historical view of the developing self; passive, vegetative principle; earthbound; the body; maternal (contact with earth); life (flowers and leaves on trees); arrested growth and fear of future (stunted tree); growth; protection and shelter; nourishment; solidarity and permanence; old age; death and rebirth.
7. Snake: active, animal principle; emotionality, possession of a soul (in unison with tree); animation of the body and materialization of the soul.
8. Birds: spirits, thoughts.
9. Cross: wholeness, becoming whole, healing.
10. Helpful persons: adequate ways of dealing with unconscious content or present life situation.

The second example specifies content followed by common forms utilized to symbolize that content.

1. That which is unusually potent, particularly in relation to healing and fertility: bull, ass, pomegran-

ate, lightning, horses, hoofs, menstrual fluid, phallic-shaped objects and stones.

2. Guide to lead out of confusion: wise man, savior, redeemer.
3. Perfect being: an object rounded on all sides, unity of the two sexes, union of opposites.
4. Immortality: fruit, embryo, child, living body, stones, gems.
5. Birth-death-rebirth cycle: destruction of objects, dismemberment, cannibalism.
6. Feminine side of man (anima): anything that is characterized as having feminine qualities (e.g., mother, flower, butterfly), a beautiful young girl, an old woman, half-human object, snake, tail of fish.
7. Masculine side of woman (animus): anything that is characterized as having masculine qualities, a strong young man, a crippled man.
8. Evil or the devil: dragon, night raven, roots, body, black eagle, fire, darkness.
9. Birth: water, egg.
10. The unconscious: forest, deep water, sea, trees, fish, plants.
11. Life or soul: anything mobile, colored, or iridescent; butterfly; mind; breath; moving air; fire; shadow; blood.
12. Consciousness: light, head, angel, death of snake (overcoming of the unconscious).

Symbols may be universal, cultural, or idiosyncratic in nature. A symbol is universal to the extent that either the form or the content of the symbol has been shared by a variety of cultural groups widely different in time and place. For example, the form of a circle has been used to symbolize peace or unity in many cultural groups. The idea of evil and the life cycle are common themes in many cultural groups. These themes may be symbolized in many ways; in myths, visual arts, ceremonies, and so forth. The two examples given above to illustrate the difference between form and content made use of universal symbols. Understanding of universal symbols has been gained through a study of mythology, alchemy, fairy tales, art, and language. The form of a symbol is considered to be universal if it can be shown to exist with the same meanings in the records of numerous cultural groups who have not been closely associated in any way. The content of a symbol is described as universal if it refers to ideas or themes that have been of concern to a variety of diverse cultural groups. Universal content may not take a universal form. It may, rather, be influenced by the culture of the individual. One may find, for example, that potency is symbolized by a bull, a sports car, or a rocket. Universal content may also take a form that is idiosyncratic to the individual. The richness and vitality of universal symbols are expressed in their compounded meaning and changing form.

A symbol is considered to be cultural when it is related to the values, norms, preoccupations, and concerns of a particular cultural group. Cultural symbols are understood and shared by most members of a cultural group. Some examples of common content expressed in symbols by the predominant culture in the United States are: sex, violence, the desirability of being physically attractive, and money. Cultural forms are nonhuman objects that are relatively specific to the culture, gestures, words, and people identified as heroes or villains for one reason or another. Examples of symbols found in our culture are the computer; a raised, clenched fist; the phrase "women's liberation"; and John Wayne. Cultural symbols may endure for a long period of time or they may be transient in nature. For example, regardless of one's political orientation, the White House, for citizens of this country, has served as a cultural symbol for a considerable period of time. On the other hand, burning draft cards, a cultural symbol of the late 1960s, has lost the significance that it had at that time.

Idiosyncratic symbols are concerned with the unique experiences of the individual; his world view, life style, identity, and the people and things that are important to him. An individual's idiosyncratic symbols, for example, might deal with such content as lack of trust, financial concerns, his occupation, and worry about his son's school grades. The form of an idiosyncratic symbol varies tremendously. It may be a recurring doodle or dream, warm colors, or collecting stuffed animals. Idiosyncratic symbols may be shared among a small number of people. Many families have idiosyncratic symbols, particularly in relation to holiday celebrations or ways or expressing affection. But many idiosyncratic symbols are not shared and, indeed, the individual himself may be unaware of them.

There is considerable interrelationship between the three different types of symbols. In many cases, the content of a symbol produced by a given individual has universal, cultural, and idiosyncratic elements. Its form may also be, in part, universal, cultural, and idiosyncratic. It is important to look at the three aspects of a symbol relative to both form and content in order to gain some idea of the meaning of a symbol. In considering an owl as a symbol, for example, one may look at:

- Form: Universal—bird of prey; cultural—common decorative motif; idiosyncratic—(possible) the sound of owls heard in the woods at night as a child.

- Content: Universal—darkness, attack, to devour; cultural—wisdom, knowledge; idiosyncratic—(possible) watchful, wary.

This is, of course, an incomplete interpretation of a symbol, as are all interpretations of symbols. They can never be completely known. In addition, a description such as this also lacks the perspective of a particular individual, with his own feelings and ideas about the symbol. Although symbols can never be understood in their totality, they can only be understood superficially unless the person who has created the symbol is consulted. This description also does not express the emotional feeling, either positive or negative, attached to a symbol.

The formation of symbols is an unconscious process. It cannot be controlled by the individual nor can an individual deliberately formulate a symbol. Symbols apparently are formed through primary process organization of perceptions and come into being through the process of primary aggregation—the grouping of perceptions in some sort of a loose assemblage. This grouping process seems to be based on some similarity of the perceptions. They may be similar in time or place of perceptions, function, associated feelings, or physical properties. This grouping, based on similarity, accounts for the fact that a symbol has some common characteristics that it shares with its referent. This factor also accounts for the multiple meaning of a particular symbolic form. The form itself has many elements, each of which can become grouped with different sets of perceptions that have similar elements. It is unknown why a particular form and type of representation comes to stand for the whole aggregate.

Although the above explanation may appear to be plausible relative to cultural and idiosyncratic symbols, it still leaves a rather large question relative to universal symbols. The major issues of concern to cultural groups are, indeed, similar; all groups must deal with the common themes of birth, death, adequate food, the unknowns, love, hate, and so forth. Thus universal content is not too difficult to understand. It is the universality of some forms that causes wonder. As mentioned in Chapter 3, Jung hypothesized that universal symbols were inherited memory traces from our phylogenetic past. This seems rather questionable in terms of our current understanding of genetic inheritance. A more probable explanation is the commonality of neurological structures shared by all individuals. It is hypothesized that neurological structures predispose human beings to organize perceptions in similar ways. This is apparently true, for example, in the ways that people deal with anxiety. Although a specific defense mechanism may be more evident in one culture as opposed to another, all of the common defense mechanisms are found cross-culturally.

There is a learned quality to cultural symbols not found with universal or idiosyncratic symbols. The enculturation process, whether it takes place in childhood or as an adult, is characterized, in part, by gaining some understanding of the symbols of the culture.

Symbol formation and the interrelatedness of universal, cultural, and idiosyncratic elements in a given symbol are another example of the individual's position relative to the past and his current environment. It is an indication of the individual as a unique person, a cultural being, and a given moment in the evolution of the species. An individual's stored perceptions are a result of his uniqueness, his membership in a cultural group, and inheritance. Perceptions and their organization specific to each of these aspects of the individual cannot be separated; they are intertwined and overlapping. Symbol formation then is influenced by personal experience, the shared understandings of one's culture, and the inherent tendency to organize perceptions in a particular form.

Symbols are created by individuals and not by collective groups. Universal and cultural symbols exist as definable entities because the experiences and the perceptions of individuals have many common elements. When an individual or a collective group responds to a symbol formulated by another individual, it appears that the overt form of the symbol communicates with a gestalt of feelings and ideas (a primary aggregate) which already exists within the individual or the members of a cultural group. Emotional response to universal symbols occur in a similar manner.

The process of symbolization and symbols themselves appear to have several functions. One of the major functions is to facilitate communication between the unconscious and conscious levels of the human psyche. In many instances, unconscious ideas can initially only be expressed in symbolic form. Conversely, the unconscious can often only be reached through symbols. Symbols help to bring unconscious ideas to the level of consciousness so that they can be translated into denotative and connotative concepts: the language of consciousness. Thus previously unconscious ideas can be assimilated with conscious ideas. This allows for a widening or expansion of the self and at the same time more integration of the various parts of the self. Because universal symbols bring about awareness of ideas and concerns that are common to all people, the individual experiences his relationship to others in the past, present, and future. There is a lessening of the isolation that is an inherent part of being human—a connecting of the individual to the human experience. An individual's exploration of his own symbols helps to free energy that was utilized to maintain ideas in the unconscious. Exploration also frees some energy invested in the symbol and its referents. There is, therefore, more energy available for need satisfaction. The spontaneous production of symbols is a natural attempt to bring a balance between the conscious and unconscious.

It is believed that another function of symbols is to guide the individual by providing a more objective view of the individual's situation. Many experiences are not stored at the conscious level. Thus the conscious part of the psyche is less knowledgeable because, so to speak, it does not have all of the available information. Symbols provide information about the one-sidedness of the personality and matters to which the individual should attend. They warn of danger if the individual does not take some corrective action. Symbols may foreshadow future events. The historical precipitating factors leading to these events may be stored only on the unconscious level. A symbol that foreshadows an event is communicating information which the conscious mind has failed to perceive or grasp. Events typically foreshadowed are often transitional in nature—events that will cause a profound change in the individual's situation. Symbols may suggest a course of action that may be beneficial for the individual or give information about the consequences of a planned action.

Another function of symbols is to allow the individual to experience symbolically that which cannot be experienced in reality because of the absence of required objects or people or because of personal or cultural taboos. In this case a symbolic act or object may be utilized to allow for the need-fulfilling experience. Behavior that arises from repressed ideas or wishes is often an attempt to experience, in a symbolic manner, that which is apparently forbidden in reality. Substitute libidinal objects may be symbolic of the desired libidinal object. All substitute objects, however, are not symbolic.

Symbols are utilized by cultural groups in two ways: first, as a means of communication, and second, as a tool for dealing with the unknown. As a method of communication, symbols are a type of shorthand that facilitates the communication process. They also allow individuals to express, at least in part, that which is essentially inexpressible. As a tool for dealing with the unknown, symbols are used as a means of controlling anxiety. The unknown is often seen as a destructive force that must be bound and placated. Symbolic acts, objects, and words are used for this purpose. Man perceives himself as having some control over the unknown through the use of symbols. Symbols help to satisfy the need for safety and are usually invested with a considerable amount of feeling. The symbols that a cultural group uses for communication and control of the unknown help to consolidate the identity of the group and contribute to maintaining its cohesiveness.

There is one other area that needs to be discussed. Some relationships have been found between various aspects of the content, form, and process of art productions and unconscious ideas, feelings, use of psychic energy, need, status, and so forth. These findings were derived from a process referred to as projective techniques. This is a procedure for discovering a person's characteristic attitudes, motivations, or ideas by observing his behavior in response to a situation that does not elicit or compel a particular response, i.e., to a relatively unstructured, ambiguous, or vague situation. In studying these relationships, it is difficult to determine whether we are seeing the result of a symbolic or sign process. It is also difficult to determine whether the symbols (if they are symbols) are universal or cultural. Much remains unknown about these relationships. Some examples of these findings are presented in Table 10.1.

In conclusion, the process of forming and responding to symbols is a universal human endeavor. The understanding of another person's symbols leads to greater understanding of the person. The symbolic potential of activities and possible symbolic expression through activities is always taken into consideration in the occupational therapy process. The symbolic element of activities is, however, only one of the many important aspects of activities.

CHARACTERISTICS OF PURPOSEFUL ACTIVITIES

There are several characteristics of purposeful activities that allow them to be used as a therapeutic tool and that make them an effective tool (220,288,290,291, 309,446,535,556,731,794,801,956).

Universal

Purposeful activities are universal in the sense that they exist and prevail in all times and places. They affect, concern, and involve all aspects of the human experience. Individuals participate in purposeful activities through most of their waking hours. Even sleep in a way is a purposeful activity. All peoples, regardless of culture, are involved in the purposeful tasks of being a family member; they engage in activities of daily living, work, and play. There are differences, of course, in how people engage in these activities. The variation in detail is endless but the common element is the same: the activities are directed toward a planned or anticipated

TABLE 10-1. *Relationships between form and content found by projective techniques*

1. Symmetry
   a. Lack of = overwhelmed by unconscious content
   b. Slight lack of = no major unconscious conflicts
   c. Well balanced = self-directed, adaptive
   d. Bilaterality stressed = rigidity and compulsivity
2. Placement
   a. Centered = preoccupied with self (if extreme), self-directed (if not extreme)
   b. Off center = unmet love and acceptance needs
   c. Right of center = well-controlled psychic energy
   d. Left of center = uncontrolled psychic energy
   e. Below center = experiences the self as inadequate, preoccupied with loss, aggressive energy turned toward the self
   f. Above center = distant from people, striving for unattainable goals, seeks need satisfaction in fantasy
   g. Clinging to edge of paper = seeking support, experiences the self as inadequate
3. Size
   a. Small in relation to whole = experiences the self as inadequate, experiences self as being overwhelmed by external environment, overly dependent on others for need satisfaction
   b. Large in relation to whole = difficulty in controlling urges, compensation for experiencing the self as inadequate, overwhelmed by feelings
4. Directions of lines
   a. Horizontal = femininity, overinvolvement in fantasy, fear of external environment
   b. Vertical = masculinity, self-assertive
   c. Continual change of direction = unfulfilled safety needs
5. Pressure
   a. Heavy = psychic energy available for acting on the environment, self-assertive
   b. Light = little psychic energy available for acting on the environment, energy tied up in unconscious conflicts
   c. Variation = flexible and adaptive, unstable
6. Shape of strokes
   a. Angular or jagged = free-floating aggressive energy
   b. Long = controlled use of psychic energy
   c. Short = difficulty in controlling psychic energy
   d. Straight = assertive, avoids close interpersonal relations, deals with environment realistically
   e. Broken, sketchy = insecurity, high anxiety
   f. Thin = fear of loss of control
   g. Erasures = dissatisfaction with the self, experience of uncertainty
   h. Free and rhythmic = unrestricted
   i. Circular = femininity, tendency to withdraw, difficulty in satisfying need for love and acceptance
7. Movement
   a. Considerable = restless, seeking of need satisfaction, creativity, overwhelmed by conflicts
   b. Minimal = experience of loss, aggression turned toward self
   c. Rigidity = energy directed toward maintaining ideas at the unconscious level, attempting to control external environment
   d. Mechanical = experience of the self as nonhuman, depersonalization
   e. Even rhythm = masculine
   f. Odd rhythm = feminine
8. Color
   a. Warm = expression of satisfactory investment of libidinal drive, expression of difficulty in locating or manipulating aggressive objects, feelings are important
   b. Cool = effort to control drives, thinking important
   c. Light, watery = fear of self-revelation
   d. Bright = self-assurance
   e. Dark = experience of loss, aggressive energy turned toward self, regression to primitive levels of functioning
   f. Black and brown = conflicts related to control, constricted personality
   g. Red = self-centered, feeling and intuition important
   h. Blue = control, self-restrained
   i. Green = difficulty in controlling aggressive drives
   j. Yellow = difficulty in satisfying love and acceptance needs, feeling and intuition important
   k. Red and yellow = spontaneous in environmental interactions
   l. Orange = active adaptation to environment
   m. Purple = projection of negative affect and aggressive drive
   n. Unharmonious warm colors = difficulty in investment of libidinal energy
   o. Too much = inadequate need satisfaction, difficulty in controlling drives
   p. Too little = difficulty in forming meaningful relationships with others, self-constricted
9. Mode of handling materials
   a. Smearing = conflicts related to control
   b. Scribbling = fearful of unconscious content, conflicts related to infantile period
   c. Scrubbing, pushing, pulling, scratching, slapping, picking = difficulty in controlling aggressive drive or manipulating aggressive objects
   d. Patting, stroking = conflicts related to oral period, investment of libidinal energy in object
10. Content
    a. Inadequate = experience of loss, aggressive drive turned toward self, fear of unconscious content
    b. Excessive = attempting to keep conflicts unconscious through rigid control of the self, difficulty in entering meaningful relationships with others
    c. Organization chaotic = overwhelmed by unconscious content
    d. Flowers and fruit = feminine
    e. Boats = feminine, womb, journey

TABLE 10-1. *(contd.)*

f. Manufactured objects = masculinity, overreliance on nonhuman environment
g. Diagrams, maps, plans = projection of negative affect or aggressive drive, inadequate fulfillment of safety needs
h. Water, egg, fish = fertility, birth, renewal
i. Personification of nonhuman objects = projection of anxiety-provoking unconscious content
j. Objects in series = number of persons in family (arrangement indicative of relationships)

11. Person
    a. Head = related to thinking, intellectual aspirations, consciousness, fantasies
    b. Hair = related to libidinal investment in the self
    c. Teeth = related to aggressive drive
    d. Mouth = related to satisfaction of love and acceptance needs
    e. Eyes = related to projection of feelings and aggressive drive, feelings of shame and guilt
    f. Chin = related to strength and determination
    g. Neck = related to conscious control versus unconscious content, when pronounced, thinking more important than feeling, intellectual endeavors emphasized
    h. Arms and hands = related to mode of dealing with aggressive objects
    i. Legs and feet = related to safety needs, aggressive energy turned toward self, discouragement
    j. Sexual characteristics = depending on how treated, may indicate preoccupation with sexual matters, lack of concern, or denial
    k. Internal anatomy shown = overwhelmed by unconscious content
12. House
    a. Roof = related to conscious mental content, fantasy, intellectual operations
    b. Walls = related to individual's perceived ability to satisfy needs and deal with unconscious content
    c. Doors and windows = related to contact with environment
    d. Chimney = related to potency
    e. Smoke = conflict in home, threat of being overwhelmed by unconscious content, warmth
13. Trees
    a. Trunk = related to perceived ability to cope with internal and external environment
    b. Branches = related to ability to derive satisfaction from the environment
    c. Organization of whole = related to intrapsychic balance, integration of aspects of the self, identity
    d. Age = related to desired or perceived age of the self
    e. Roots = related to security needs, unconscious content
    f. Degree of life = related to hope, future anticipated

end result. There is also variation in when in the life cycle a particular activity is predominant. Some individuals engage in activities that other people are either unable to master or in which they are not interested in participating. Nevertheless, whatever activities people do engage in, the activities are primarily purposeful in nature.

The very universality of purposeful activities, indeed, causes some difficulty. They are so much a part of our daily life that they often go unnoticed. One tends to think little about brushing one's teeth, boarding a bus, or stopping to get one's shoes repaired. This is a part of the fabric of life that is given minimal attention. Purposeful activities tend to be given attention primarily in the negative; when something goes amiss in the usual or expected process, one may cease to perform a typical purposeful activity. A friend, for example, may repeatedly call in sick or simply not show up at work. One's first response besides general concern would be to question the individual's physical and/or emotional well-being.

Everyday purposeful activities are also usually only given attention when they must be performed with considerable thought and effort. An individual who has experienced a recent loss, for example, may find it tremendously difficult to get out of bed in the morning, to keep appointments, or even simply to make a telephone call.

Finally, we tend to take note of activities that appear to be purposeful for the individual performing the activity but the purpose cannot be deduced by the observer. One may, for example, observe a child taking all of his toy soldiers out of various drawers and boxes. There may be a very "logical" reason for this, for instance, he is in the process of selecting soldiers for the massive campaign about to be waged on the living room floor. On the other hand, the child may be engaged in this activity because he is unhappy about something and just being with his soldiers gives him a sense of comfort. In either case, the observer needs to question the child to discover the purpose of the activity.

Another way in which the universality of purposeful activities causes some difficulty is in their acceptance as a legitimate tool by others. Purposeful activities are so ordinary in nature; how can they possibly be useful in restoring or maintaining function? Therapeutic tools, it is frequently assumed, ought to be somewhat mysterious or at least not commonplace, everyday events. Occupational therapists have, at times, had some difficulty in explaining to clients and other staff members alike the use of activities in evaluation and intervention.

In a more positive vein, the universality of purposeful activities, their practicality, and their ordinariness often leads to considerable acceptance on the part of clients and other staff members. With little explanation, the obvious is often made clear. The lack of mystery and thus the relative absence of anxiety facilitates clients' involvement in intervention. The fact that purposeful activities are a cross-cultural phenomenon also facilitates involvement in evaluation and intervention, if the therapist attends to the cultural variation in detail.

Purposeful activities, then, are universal and permeate the fabric of daily life. They are a part of our life to such an extent that their significance and importance often go unnoticed. Yet without purposeful activities, there would be little to differentiate the human experience from the experience of the nonhuman world. Indeed, one could say that without purposeful activities there would be no human experience.

Fundamental to Performance Components and Occupational Performances

Purposeful activities are fundamental to optimal growth and development in a number of different ways. First, and perhaps of major importance, is that purposeful activities are the means whereby performance components are acquired. Adequate development of sensory integration; visual perception; motor, cognitive, and psychological function; and social interaction cannot occur outside the context of purposeful activities. Performance components are not acquired through random activity or mindless exercise; rather they are acquired through active goal-directed interaction with the environment. One example may suffice to illustrate this point. A typical purposeful activity of a 2-year-old child is, with pail and shovel, burying a truck in the sand area of a play yard where there are other children. Eye-hand coordination and the capacity to motor plan are being developed as the child fills and empties her pail. In walking with a full and empty pail the child is learning to make postural adjustments necessary for mature patterns of locomotion. The process of burying the truck and its eventual recovery reinforces the permanency of objects in time and place. Psychological function is being developed as the child acts on the basis of a particular interest, invests psychic and physical energy in the task at hand, and exercises a degree of self-discipline. The initial stage of social interaction with peers is beginning. No longer an observer of others, the child is learning how to engage in a task in the presence of others. Engaged in a purposeful activity, the child is developing performance components.

The above example was in relationship to a 2-year-old child. Any particular stage in the life cycle could have been used to illustrate the acquisition, maintenance, or elaboration of performance components. The point to be made is that this process takes place only through engaging in purposeful activities. It is through goal-directed interaction with the environment, through experiencing, investigating, trying out, practicing, responding, managing, controlling, and creating, that the individual acquires the basic skills for effective interaction in the environment. In using purposeful activities, then, the occupational therapist is employing a method basic to the natural developmental process.

Another way in which purposeful activities are fundamental is that they constitute occupational performances. Social roles are made up of an integrated cluster of purposeful activities. Without purposeful activities, a social role has no substance. It is what an individual does in relationship to the human and nonhuman environment that defines and delineates a social role. A woman, for example, in the role of the mother of a 13-year-old son, makes breakfast, checks to see that he has money for lunch and his keys, engages in responding to his running commentary as they watch the evening news together, reminds him it is his turn to wash the dinner dishes, quizzes him on his Spanish vocabulary, discusses the logistics of getting to the party on Friday night, and gives him a hug and a kiss as he goes off to bed. The example illustrates at least in part the purposeful activities that constitute the role of being a mother relative to an adolescent child. Without the capacity to engage in each of these activities, and many more, the role of being a mother would be impossible. Social roles are collections of activities finely tuned to needs of one's role partner. In helping an individual to engage in a variety of social roles, the occupational therapist assists the individual in becoming skilled or in regaining the skills necessary for adequate performance of the purposeful activities that constitute a required, desired, or anticipated social role.

The third way in which purposeful activities are fundamental is the extent to which they require the use of a variety of performance components. There are few if any purposeful activities, except perhaps contemplation, which do not require more than one performance component. Putting on and tying one's shoes, for example, involves knowing the right from the left, being able to bend down and maintain balance, remembering how to tie a knot, being motivated to perform the task, and selecting an appropriate pair of shoes for the social situation for which one is dressing. The multiple skills necessary for engaging in most purposeful activities provide a framework for integration of the various performance components. It is within the context of purposeful activity that performance components are not only developed but also combined to form functional units of behavior or skills. Development of one performance component without integration of that component with other components leaves the individual essentially without the means to master the environment successfully.

Conversely, the attainment of an adequate level of development of one performance component is enhanced by participating in purposeful activities in which the other required performance components have been mastered. A child, for example, who has adequate binocular vision, who is able to sit quietly and attend to a task, and who is accepting of direction from others is in a far better position to develop refined eye-hand coordination than a child who does not have these abilities. The fact that purposeful activities require the use of a variety of performance components is used by the occupational therapist both to facilitate integration of performance components and to design activities to enhance the development of one particular performance component.

Finally, purposeful activities are fundamental because it is through such activities that the individual gains knowledge about the human and nonhuman environment and about himself. Purposeful activities provide information and feedback, which is essential for further interaction with the environment and appreciation of one's assets and limitations. It is only through purposeful activities that one gains a sense of mastery and competence relative to the environment. A student, for example, may join a drama group. Assigned the responsibility of assistant stage manager, the individual must make or find appropriate props. In taking on this task, the individual learns about what materials are appropriate for the fabrication of props, how stable an imaginary throne really needs to be, and where you find dry ice in the middle of winter. The student also learns something about how people deal with anxiety as the day of performance comes closer and finally arrives. After the last performance, the student is aware that he can change scenery in the dark, that he really understands the many uses of a safety pin, and that telling an actor to count the ticket receipts while he is waiting to go on calms anxiety. The student also discovers that the cast party can be a lot of fun.

Although purposeful activities in and of themselves provide valuable feedback, recognition by others of what one has learned or accomplished is also important. The student in the above example needs the praise of his peers, a thumbs-up sign from the drama teacher, and a hug from his father. The pleasure of learning something new, the delight in mastery, is often hollow and a short-lived victory if it is not shared with and recognized by others who are significant to the individual. What was learned, discovered, or gained for the moment is often lost if it is not considered important by members of one's family and social network.

In summary, purposeful activities are fundamental to performance components and occupational performances because they are the means whereby performance components are acquired, they are the elements that constitute occupational performances, they facilitate the integration of performance components, and they are the way in which an individual gains knowledge about the human and nonhuman environment and about himself.

Made Up of Elements that Can Be Identified

Purposeful activities are formed of many parts. Each part is important and can be identified and explored in its own right. Driving a nail into a board, for example, requires coordination, some strength, and the capacity to hit an object; writing a poem requires extended concentration, creativity, and the capacity to organize abstract concepts. A person in a nurturing role relative to a child gratifies physical and emotional needs, is understanding, and permits a wide latitude of behaviors; a person in the role of a foreman makes demands for productivity, limits emotional expression, and is minimally concerned with gratifying infantile needs. When working alone, an individual may make his own decisions, indulge in daydreaming, and regulate the amount of work accomplished; in a group one is required to share decision making, meet the needs of others, and accept group norms regarding behavior.

The above examples give some idea of the elements of activities, that they are made up of many parts. Not to consider the elements of purposeful activities is to miss much of their richness and complexity. In considering a purposeful activity, an occupational therapist looks at its parts: the motions used; the procedure and process; material and equipment; the result of the process, whatever it may be; the interpersonal relations that influence the process and in turn are influenced by it; the context in which the activity occurs; its possible cultural meanings; the factor of age and gender; and the performance components required and their relationship to occupational performance.

Purposeful activities then are made up of a collection of elements that can be identified, studied, and made knowable. Because of this characteristic, purposeful activities are able to be analyzed.

Holistic

The elements of a purposeful activity are intimately related and interdependent. In working with clay, for example, the individual may be involved in wedging the clay, sculpting an object, or making a vase on a potter's wheel. Not only the nature of the clay but the process of clay manipulation must be taken into consideration in defining the activity. The type of interaction possible in a doing process that demands concentration and highly controlled motor behavior is different from the interaction possible in a doing process that requires little concentration and considerable freedom of action. In selecting a purposeful activity for evaluation or intervention, all the elements contained within the activity must be taken into consideration. The nature of specific elements may be altered or become more or less significant when combined with other elements. The holistic aspect of the activity must be understood as well as its parts.

Able To Be Manipulated

The elements of an activity may be arranged in a variety of combinations so as to arrive at a purposeful activity that is appropriate for a given client. This is the process of activity synthesis. This characteristic of purposeful activities is both an asset and a limitation. It is an asset because it allows the therapist to design an activity in a manner that he or she feels will be most beneficial for a client. It is a limitation because any participant may manipulate the elements of an activity. Lack of recognition that manipulation of elements has occurred and lack of understanding regarding the reason for the manipulation tend to impede movement toward the desired goal. The goal of a particular intervention process, for example, may be to help a client learn how to follow directions. Constructing and finishing a small wooden shelf may have been selected as an appropriate activity. However, if the client disregards the step-by-step directions provided and proceeds based on her own idea of what should be done, she has changed the intended nature of the activity. Other activity elements may need to be added to help this client reach the stated goal.

Promoting Differential Responses

An individual's response to a purposeful activity is based on the nature of the activity elements and the extent to which the individual has mastered the various performance components. The responses of an individual can often be predicted if one is aware of the nature of the activity elements and the performance components the individual has acquired. If, for example, an activity requires fine manipulation of objects in the presence of others and the individual has gained full maturation in the area of sensory integration visual perception and is able to interact in a parallel group, the individual would probably be comfortable in participating in the activity and derive pleasure from participation.

Differential responses to purposeful activity can also be looked at from another perspective. The elements of activities have inherent characteristics that strongly predispose one to particular expression of ideas and feelings and to particular types of motor behavior. Finger painting, for example, is likely to elicit ideas about being messy and early childhood experiences. One would expect rather gross movements often of a rhythmic nature and little attention to detail. When given the task of pounding in a series of nails, ideas elicited are often related to being precise or thoughts which have to do with being assertive or angry. One would expect vigorous, well-controlled gross movements. By knowing the activity elements and the typical response to various elements, one can predict an individual's response within a fairly narrow range. If an individual does not respond in the usual manner, then the therapist must identify the reason or reasons for the atypical response. It may be that the individual does not have the necessary performance components, has personal feelings and ideas that interfere with participation in the usual manner, or has culturally based beliefs that lead him to interpret the activity in a different manner than one may have anticipated.

Conversely, individuals with particular types of problems are likely to respond to various activity elements in specific kinds of ways. An individual who is anxious, for example, is likely to respond negatively to an activity that is ambiguous and lacking in an easily discernable structure. An individual who is dependent tends to respond positively to an activity that has detailed directions or one that can be shared with the therapist. By knowing the typical response of an individual with a particular problem to specific activity elements, the therapist is in a position to identify problem areas and to select appropriate activities for intervention. Differential response to activity elements also enables the therapist to design a purposeful activity that will directly address the client's particular problem area. In helping a person, for example, to identify their assets and limitations, the therapist may suggest that the client engage in an activity that has an end-product that can be judged by objective standards.

In conclusion, an individual's interest in a particular purposeful activity, lack of interest, choice of activities, and manner of engaging in an activity provide considerable information about the individual. Differential responses to the elements of purposeful activities serve as one of the guides for selecting appropriate activities for evaluation and intervention.

Able To Be Graded

Purposeful activities in their totality, and the elements of activities, are able to be graded along any number of dimensions. Some of the common dimensions used are degree of complexity, structure, stimulation provided, creativity possible, variety in procedures, and social interaction required. There are, of course, many other dimensions. A single type of activity may be graded along one dimension, e.g., number of steps, or various different activities may be placed along the same dimension. In illustration, clothes construction may be graded to involve an ever-increasing number of steps. Lacing up a pre-cut leather coin purse, making a tile ashtray, and doing a copper enameling project each require a different number of steps. The gradability of purposeful activities allows the therapist to tune activities finely to the needs of each client.

Facilitating Communication

Purposeful activities enhance communication in two ways. First, they promote nonverbal communication and thus provide a means for bringing unconscious or unshared ideas to the level that they can be conveyed to others. The action element, the doing aspect of activities, and the material and tools used provide a broad spectrum of means for nonverbal expression of ideas and feelings. This helps the therapist to understand the client in ways that are not always possible through verbal communication alone. Perhaps more important, however, purposeful activities help the client to communicate with herself. They provide an opportunity for the client to select on some level common recognizable real or symbolic ways of expressing ideas and feelings. These are often ideas and feelings that the client is unaware of or, for one reason or another, fearful of expressing directly. For those who fear recognition and/or expression of intrapsychic content on a verbal level, activities allow for communication that one does not necessarily have to "own." One can, at least initially, screen oneself from the ideas and feelings being expressed; perhaps they were inadvertent or not really meant.

Ideas and feelings that are acted out or expressed within the context of a purposeful activity are much less likely to come under conscious scrutiny and thus edited before presentation. They are also less likely to be screened out by defense mechanisms. Thus, nonverbal communication often reveals more about the self than verbal communication. This facilitates understanding of oneself and others' understanding of the individual. The actions and objects used in purposeful activities, then, serve as a catalytic agent or stimulus for eliciting unconscious or unshared ideas and feelings.

The other way in which purposeful activities facilitate communication is in relation to social interaction. When people do not know each other, when they are somewhat uncomfortable with each other, a shared purposeful activity frequently allows them to become acquainted and more relaxed. Participation in an activity allows people to have something in common to discuss and serves as a bridge for more intimate communication.

Having a Focusing, Organizing Effect

Closely related to their role in facilitating communication is the focusing aspect of activities. Purposeful activities have a converging effect, which allows feelings and ideas to become integrated in such a way that vague pieces can be organized into words. It is as if one were able to see one's ideas and feelings laid out in some way external to the self. Seen from this perspective, they are often more easily articulated in words.

Purposeful activities also have an organizing effect that can be described as both microscopic and macroscopic. Microscopic is used here in the sense that participation in a single activity helps an individual to bring his or her attention, knowledge, and skills into an integrated gestalt. It helps the individual to feel that aspects of the self are, indeed, together; it helps the individual to feel more organized. A variety of purposeful activities that occur at fairly regular intervals throughout the day or week provide macroscopic organization. The individual feels there is order and purpose in the day and week even if this order is initially externally imposed. This is one of the reasons for Meyer's and Slagle's emphases on a regular schedule of work, play, and rest. This organizing aspect of purposeful activities is particularly important for individuals who are confused, anxious, or depressed.

Purposeful activities in the context of a group provide a degree of structure and organization that is helpful to many clients. Because activity groups involve a doing process as well as discussion, an individual is given an opportunity to use presently available skills. Thus an individual who is fearful of engaging in activities has an opportunity to participate in the group on a verbal level. Conversely, individuals who are shy or who lack verbal skills may become part of the group primarily through participation in the activity. This element of activity groups facilitates initial comfort and involvement. With such involvement, the individual is then able to begin to acquire skill in deficit areas.

Another way in which purposeful activities provide structure and organization is that they have a framework which allows expression of ideas and feelings within known limits. The activity is sufficiently concrete so as to focus clients on the problems and issues that are the specific goals of intervention. Thus, for example, if the goal of an activity group is to develop work habits, group members know they are participating in the group to practice certain skills only. They are not there to acquire leisure skills nor are they there to share problems related to family interaction.

Finally, purposeful activities provide a tangible means of measuring progress. The activity is a concrete reality factor against which the individual can measure achievement and growth. Positive change can be demonstrated by the degree of movement toward completion of a particular activity or the increasing complexity of the activities the individual selects and completes. The intervention process comes to be seen as an organized, progressive endeavor.

Emphasizing Doing

The revocable world is one of language; the irrevocable world is one of action. One can say almost anything; one can promise a good deal; one can play with words and need not take them altogether seriously. But action, doing, is another thing. Actions are real; they cannot be taken back or denied. This makes actions more powerful than words and also makes them more scary.

The use of purposeful activities as a tool for intervention has become increasingly important as greater emphasis has been placed on verbal skills or language in our culture. There is a tendency to deal in the abstract rather than that which is more concrete. It is fine, for example, to know the general principle for hanging shelves or putting together a disassembled kitchen step stool. However, it is in the execution of these activities that one truly understands the principles and one's capacity to apply abstract knowledge to actual situations. When thought does not lead to some type of action, critical opportunities for learning are lost. In addition, the individual does not gain sufficient experience in understanding the consequence of action. Through participation in a wide variety of purposeful activities, the individual accumulates "a store of action experiences essential for human function; a reservoir of experiences gathered through direct engagement with the environment" (291, p. 308).

There are many individuals who, because of past experience or the lack of experience, are fearful of engaging in purposeful activity. Such individuals often have considerable verbal skill. They are most comfortable in talking about something but when there is a distinct demand to engage in a purposeful activity related to their knowledge base they become fearful. Such individuals are apprehensive that they might demonstrate incompetence. They have had little experience with the task at hand and little experience with the consequences of success or failure relative to purposeful activities. In the extreme, individuals who lack experience in engaging in a variety of activities tend to view themselves as inept or inadequate in many areas of human function. Purposeful activities facilitate collaboration in identifying difficulties in doing. The specific request to become involved in an activity minimizes denial or rationalization relative to actual proficiency in performance. Attempts to evade responsibility for task completion can easily be seen by the client and therapist alike.

It should be noted that the emphasis on doing in the occupational therapy process by no means precludes verbal communication or verbal tasks. Indeed, the development of verbal skills and the ability to engage in meaningful verbal interactions are not uncommon goals of intervention. The point to be made is that purposeful activities include a strong doing component, which is not found in traditional psychotherapy.

Frequently Involving the Nonhuman Environment

In most cases, purposeful activities involve the manipulation of the nonhuman environment. There is considerable variation in the extent to which the nonhuman environment is used. In weaving on a large floor loom, for example, the individual's major involvement may well be with the nonhuman environment. Deciding what to prepare for lunch does not entail direct manipulation of the nonhuman environment; obviously, however, a part of the nonhuman environment is being focused on in some detail. Having a conversation with a friend may not include any involvement with the nonhuman environment except perhaps drinking a cup of coffee. It should be noted that some purposeful activities do not involve any substantial manipulation or use of the nonhuman environment. All interactions with the nonhuman environment are not necessarily purposeful.

Varying on a Continuum from Conscious to Not Conscious/Unconscious

There are two dimensions of this continuum that need to be differentiated. One continuum is concerned with the difference between subcortical and cortical levels of function. Stimuli integrated at the subcortical level and the responses derived from this organization are not conscious. They cannot be recalled nor can they be articulated in language. It is usually impossible, for example, for an individual to describe in any detail how he is able to maintain his balance on a bicycle or to say how he learned except some vague statement about trial and error. The performance component of sensory integration is a subcortical process and thus is not conscious. It is acquired through purposeful activity which is, indeed, conscious, but the learning that takes place is outside conscious awareness. In helping an individual to develop a mature level of sensory integration, purposeful activity provides the needed stimuli and a structure for the organization of those stimuli. However, it is detrimental to the learning process to ask the individual to focus on the stimuli or on the way they are being organized. If attention is so directed, learning is less likely to occur. The individual might learn how to respond appropriately in a narrowly defined situation, but that is learning on a cortical level and not sensory integration. Skill acquired at a cortical level can compensate for lack of sensory integration, which may eventually be necessary, but that, initially, is usually not the focus of intervention. A mature level of sensory integration is best attained in the context of purposeful activities in which the individual's attention is drawn to the end goal or purpose, to the pleasure of the activity and the joy of mastery rather than to specific stimuli or the movements themselves. In this sense, then, purposeful activities can be said to have a not-conscious element.

The other aspect of the continuum is the conscious-unconscious dimension. This is here considered to be a cortical level of organization. In the intervention process, cognitive and psychological function and social interaction are usually learned initially at the conscious level. In the process, for example, of helping a client to increase his or her fund of knowledge, learn how to express feelings appropriately, and become skilled in group interaction, conscious awareness of what is to be learned is important. Gaining information and practicing skills are emphasized. As mastery increases, the individual needs to focus less attention on new knowledge and skills; responses become in a sense automatic. It is at this point that significant learning has taken place. The details of how to do something no longer need to be attended to; the information necessary for effective action is now at the preconscious or unconscious level. Energy is freed for other matters; the goals of intervention have been accomplished. It is important to note that this information is not subcortical in nature. It is cortical and can, if necessary, be recalled. One example may help to clarify. At the time when a child learns how to tie his shoe, great attention is, at first, devoted to this task. After several months, however, the task becomes automatic; it is accomplished quickly without any thought. When pressed, however, the individual can give a description of the step-by-step process necessary for tying a shoe.

Finally, purposeful activities have the capacity to tap the unconscious. With focus on the activity as a whole, the individual's actions are frequently influenced by unconscious or unshared intrapsychic content. This facilitates the sharing of ideas and feelings that are interfering with the individual's capacity to adapt and engage successfully in age-appropriate developmental tasks. In addition, focus on the activity as a whole facilitates working through: the process of repeatedly experiencing the effects of maladaptive, intrapyschic content on one's behavior while concurrently formulating a more adaptive way of perceiving oneself, other people, and the events of daily life. By not attending to specific skills, new intrapsychic content is more likely to be integrated Attention to specific aspects of the activity promotes the development of splinter skills, not the integration of new intrapsychic content. It should be noted that this paragraph is based on the assumptions of analytical frames of reference and does not necessarily relate to developmental or acquisitional frames of reference.

Varying on a Continuum from Real to Symbolic

All elements of a purposeful activity are real in the sense that they have tangible qualities that exist in the here and now. However, the actions and objects of a purposeful activity may be responded to or dealt with in a symbolic manner. Purposeful activities may be real, symbolic, or a combination of the two. Careful preparation of a meal for a special person is an example of an activity that has both realistic and symbolic elements. It is realistic in the sense of shopping, cooking, and setting an attractive table. It is symbolic in the sense of expressing love and wanting to give to the other individual in a nurturing kind of way.

The elements of a purposeful activity tend to be dealt with as real when the activity is designed to help the individual to develop concrete skills. A client, for example, may be involved in learning how to use a telephone, attend to the details of a task, make change, or follow the directions of the workshop supervisor. The task in these examples is clearly defined and the desired end responses are able to be described and measured by standards external to the task.

Activity elements may be or come to be symbolic in three major ways. Elements that are, for example, unstructured, ambiguous, allow for self-expression, require creativity, and nonverbal tend to promote the production and expression of symbols. Second, activity elements may be similar to a symbolic object or interaction that is used in the normal development process or part of daily life. Examples are the transitional objects of a young child, expression of feelings through artistic productions, and the giving of a gift. Some activity elements have the same characteristics as symbolic environmental elements. The process of leather lacing, trampoline play, or drilling holes is, for example, similar to the intrusive behavior used by young boys to gratify, in a symbolic manner, sexual impulses that are not able to be gratified directly. Third, activity elements may be symbolic of real environmental interactions. This is different from the relation just described in that the environmental elements as they actually exist are not symbolic. A parent interacts with a child, for example, in a nurturing manner. The care provided is real and comprehensive. It is not symbolic. A nurturing relationship may be symbolized in the occupational therapy process, for example, by an activity which involves the therapist regularly preparing and serving baking powder biscuits to a client who has never developed a trust relationship. If the client responds in such a way as to indicate that the interaction is perceived as a need-gratifying nurturing relationship, then the activity elements would be described as symbolic of an interaction typical of the normal developmental process.

In exploring or analyzing the elements of a purposeful activity, the therapist attempts to identify those aspects of an activity which contribute to its being perceived as real. The therapist also attempts to identify the potential symbolic elements of an activity. In so doing, it is instructive to look at the universal, cultural, and idiosyncratic possible symbolic meanings. The therapist also attempts to determine the elements that promote the production and expression of symbols, the elements that might be similar to symbolic environmental elements or symbolic of environmental elements. The elements of a purposeful activity can and should be explored in the abstract. It is, however, only in the evaluation and intervention situation that the therapist is able to determine whether the client is utilizing the symbolic potential of an object or interaction. Assessment is sometimes difficult because activity elements are often responded to both as symbols and as real elements. In addition, a client may respond to that which has many decidedly real qualities, in a symbolic manner.

Varying on a Continuum from Simulated to Natural

Purposeful activities as used in occupational therapy may be simulated or natural. Simulated activities are those activities that an individual engages in within the confines of a clinical setting. Such activities are simulated in the sense that they are designed to develop skills that can be used in the community. This is not meant to imply that there is anything artificial or unreal about simulated purposeful activities. They are organized, goal directed, and based on a particular theoretical system. An analogy of this type of purposeful activity can perhaps best be made with the various simulated activities that were designed to prepare the astronauts for their ventures into space. To prepare an individual for participation in the community, simulated activities ideally have several characteristics. First, they must be relevant to the development of skills the individual will need for successful participation in the community. They must arouse and sustain the individual's interest in the learning process. Finally, simulated purposeful activities are designed to resemble as closely as possible the activity patterns the individual is likely to encounter in the community. An example of the latter is helping a client to engage in personal hygiene activities shortly after waking in the morning rather than attempting to teach these activities in the middle of the afternoon. The simulated aspect of purposeful activities has led to the idea that the occupational therapy process provides a laboratory for living: a microcosm of life, learning, and work. Learning occurs through experience in an initially protected environment where the individual is able to experiment with more adaptive modes of behavior.

A natural purposeful activity is one that takes place in the community. This type of activity may occur in the company of the therapist, with fellow clients, or the client may engage in the activity independently. Some examples of natural purposeful activities are going roller skating in a local park, applying for a job, and helping one's children with their homework. Those natural activities in which the therapist is not involved are sometimes referred to as prescribed activities. Such activities are agreed on by the client and therapist for the purpose of testing and practicing new skills. In such a situation, the therapist serves as a resource person providing support and guidance relative to problem solution and reinforcement.

Typically, the intervention process begins with simulated purposeful activities and moves in the direction of natural purposeful activities. This, however, may not always be the case. Natural purposeful activities may be used initially and throughout the intervention process. An example of the latter is assisting a somewhat anxious and mildly depressed new mother to deal with infant care, becoming a parent, and the altered dynamics of the family constellation through guiding the client's direct involvement in the situation to be mastered.

SUMMARY

Purposeful activities are defined as those doing processes that require the use of thought and energy and are directed toward an intended or desired end result. They have several characteristics that allow them to be used as an effective therapeutic tool in the occupational therapy process. Purposeful activities were described as being universal, fundamental to performance components and occupational performances, made up of elements that can be identified, holistic, able to be manipulated, promoting differential responses, able to be graded, facilitating communication, having a focusing organizing effect, emphasizing doing, frequently involving the nonhuman environment, varying on a continuum from conscious to not conscious/unconscious, varying on a continuum from simulated to natural.

11 Activity Analysis and Synthesis

Purposeful activities cannot be designed for evaluation and intervention without analysis and synthesis. It is this tool that allows the occupational therapist to assess the client's need for intervention and to make a match between the interests and abilities of the client and the activities that will help to meet health needs, prevent dysfunction, maintain function, manage interfering behavior, and bring about growth or change. As previously defined activity analysis is the process of examining an activity to distinguish its component parts. Activity synthesis is the process of combining component parts of the human and nonhuman environment so as to design an activity suitable for evaluation or intervention.

Analysis and synthesis of any aspect of the human and nonhuman environment can only take place within, at least, a tentative conceptual framework or system of classification. One cannot, for example, analyze a table without having some idea of what aspect of the table is to be assessed or the purpose of that assessment. One could analyze a table, for example, relative to the uses to which it might be put, the soundness of its construction, the type of tools and materials necessary to make a table, or in terms of aesthetic design. Without a conceptual framework, analysis tends to be primarily speculative in nature. Similarly, without a conceptual framework, the process of synthesis lacks direction. For example, one may be asked to draw a map. If the individual has only a vague idea of the area to be illustrated and does not know what needs to be included in a map, it is highly unlikely that what might be drawn will constitute a useful map.

Each profession has its own conceptual framework for looking at the varied aspects of the same phenomenon. An interior decorator and an electrician will analyze a kitchen very differently. To guide his analysis, an interior decorator may make use of such concepts as sufficient storage space, height of work areas, and color scheme. An electrician is more likely to use such concepts as quality of overhead lighting, number of electrical outlets, and adequacy of wiring. Similarly, there are various ways of synthesizing information about the human and nonhuman environments. A cook, for example, synthesizes a cake and a pie in very different ways. The cook must take into consideration, among other factors, the ingredients necessary and the type of pan to be used.

Activity analysis and synthesis in occupational therapy are concerned with the study and design of purposeful activities. There are two different approaches to this task. One is the identification of the inherent components of an activity. This approach, here referred to as generic, involves analysis only, providing no guidelines for synthesis. Its primary purpose is to make activities and their elements distinct and apprehensible. The second approach, referred to as restricted, provides a conceptual framework for both analysis and synthesis. There are several types of restricted activity analysis and synthesis categorized according to purpose or use. The restricted approach builds on the generic approach.

THE GENERIC APPROACH

The conceptual framework of generic activity analysis is drawn from the domain of concern of the profession.

The full spectrum of all aspects of the domain of concern—performance components, occupational performance, age, environment—are taken into consideration. There is no universally accepted conceptual framework for generic activity analysis; the one presented below is compiled from a number of sources (220,238,290,309, 446,618,945,960). It is primarily concerned with the psychosocial aspects of occupational therapy, as this has been previously described. Thus, the motor component and visual perception will not be presented in any detail. The conceptual framework for a generic approach to activity analysis is given in Table 11-1.

The conceptual framework in Table 11-1 is essentially a guide to the study of purposeful activities. It provides one way of perceiving and considering activities in order to understand their component parts, and their potential. To facilitate use of this guide, a few suggestions may be helpful.

To analyze an activity with knowledge and skill, one must know the activity. One should know the materials, tools, and processes involved and the extent to which the activity fosters or impedes various types of human interaction. Ideally, the therapist has engaged in the activity being analyzed, or at least has studied the activity in great detail.

The activity to be analyzed should be clearly specified. One cannot study an activity in the abstract. It is almost impossible to analyze "working with clay," for example. Such a statement is far too vague; there are several ways of working with clay. It is far better to analyze "working with clay using the slab method," or "making a pinch pot." The interpersonal environment in which the activity takes place should also be clearly defined. Continuing with the example of clay, one can make a pinch pot alone, with someone else in the room available for help if needed, or sitting around a table with a small group of other people. By clearly specifying the nature of the activity, the therapist circumscribes the task of analysis within manageable limits. If this is not done, activity analysis becomes a very lengthy, somewhat unproductive project.

The activity to be analyzed should be defined as it is typically engaged in under ordinary circumstances. Although it is possible to grade and adapt many activities, this is part of restricted analysis, not generic. The purpose of generic analysis is to understand the activity as it exists—to know its inherent nature. Only with this knowledge is the therapist able to consider the potential of the activity for evaluation and intervention.

In using the guide outlined in Table 11-1, the therapist considers every point. A characteristic may or may not be relevant to the activity being studied; if relevant, it should be made clear how it is relevant. The guide is not a checklist; it is a means of helping a therapist think about an activity. Using making a pinch pot within the context of a small group, some examples of how one would use the guide follow.

- IA. Tactile and visual sensory input predominate; the clay is wet, somewhat cold and slippery, and monochromatic.
- IB. Some multiple stimulation, new responses are likely to be required, integration primarily at the cortical level.
- IIA. A fairly gross motor activity; only a moderate amount of strength, endurance, range of motion, and coordination required; client needs capacity to sit upright in a chair with little postural change required.
- IIB. Somewhat active motions at first then passive, motions are fairly rhythmic and repetitious.
- IIIA. Requires moderate degree of attention, but does not inherently command attention.
- IIIB. Some image memory required, does not require long-term memory.
- IIIC. Activity can be performed with a mild orientation deficit.
- IIID. Requires cognitive development to at least the age of six to seven years, some creativity possible.
- IIIE. Abstract thinking not required.

In studying activities, it is often useful to compare and contrast two or more activities. The differences between activities become readily apparent, as do the similarities. Comparing activities also allows the therapist to be more specific in regards to the degree to which an activity is characterized by a given component. In contrasting making a pinch pot with weaving a woolen scarf, for example, it can be easily seen that weaving is a far more structured activity than making a pinch pot.

Analysis of activities may seem like a lengthy project to the student therapist; indeed, it does take some time for the novice. However, the task goes rather quickly after some practice. Regardless of the length of time, it is really the only way to become conversant with the nature of activities and the potential that they have for evaluation and intervention.

THE RESTRICTED APPROACH

The restricted approach provides conceptual frameworks for both activity analysis and synthesis (711). This

TABLE 11-1. *Conceptual framework for the generic approach to activity analysis*

- I. Sensory integration
  - A. Sensory input
    1. Vestibular
    2. Proprioceptive
    3. Tactile
    4. Visual
    5. Auditory
    6. Olfactory
    7. Gustatory
  - B. Opportunity for integration
    1. Reflexes
    2. Multiple stimulation
    3. Sensory discrimination required
    4. Adaptive response required
    5. New response required
    6. Subcortical versus cortical response encouraged
- II. Motor function
  - A. Functional capacity required
    1. Gross motor
    2. Fine motor
    3. Strength
    4. Endurance
    5. Range of motion
    6. Coordination
    7. Basic posture required and postural changes necessary
  - B. Types of motions
    1. Passive (e.g., patting, stroking)
    2. Active
    3. Aggressive
    4. Rhythmic
    5. Repetitious
- III. Cognitive function
  - A. Attention
  - B. Memory
    1. Representation
       - a. Exocept (motor)
       - b. Image
       - c. Endocept
       - d. Concept
    2. Duration
  - C. Orientation
  - D. Thought processes
    1. Level of cognitive development required (as outlined in Chapter 5)
    2. Creativity required or possible
  - E. Need for abstract versus concrete thinking
  - F. Intelligence
    1. Complexity
    2. Number of steps
    3. Directions—demonstrated, pictorial, verbal, written
    4. New learning required
    5. Rate of learning required
    6. The ability of the task to be broken down into component parts (steps)
  - G. Factual information
    1. General knowledge required
    2. General knowledge to be gained from the activity
  - H. Problem solving required
  - I. Symbolic potential
    1. Universal
    2. Cultural
    3. Idiosyncratic
    4. Potential for facilitating the production of symbols
    5. Similarity to symbolic objects or interactions used in normal development or a part of daily life
    6. Potential for being symbolic of real environmental interactions
    7. Unconscious needs that can be expressed or gratified
- IV. Psychological function
  - A. Dynamic states
    1. Needs—expression, satisfaction
    2. Emotional expression permitted or encouraged
    3. Values inherent in activity or able to be expressed
    4. Interests that might be satisfied
    5. Motivation—intrinsic, extrinsic rewards
  - B. Intrapsychic dynamics
    1. Potential for the expression of psychodynamics
    2. Defense mechanisms—extent to which they are encourged
  - C. Reality testing
    1. External limits
    2. Readily defined way of using tools and materials
    3. Clearly defined end result—able to be measured against objective criteria
    4. Extent to which sharing of ideas and feelings is possible or encouraged
    5. Extent of feedback available
  - D. Insight
    1. Opportunity to experience the effects of one's actions on the environment
    2. Time for thinking about motives and actions
  - E. Object relations
    1. Possibility for investing libidinal or aggressive energy
    2. Suitability of objects for need satisfaction (people and things)
  - F. Self-concept
    1. Sexual identity
       - a. Traditional masculine or feminine connotation of the activity
       - b. Opportunity for symbolic expression of a sexual nature
       - c. Opportunity to interact with members of the same and opposite sex
    2. Body image—opportunity to become aware of one's body
    3. Assets and limitations
       - a. Variety of different kinds of skills required
       - b. Opportunity for feedback
    4. Self-esteem—likelihood of being enhanced
  - G. Self-discipline
    1. Volition—availability of choices
    2. Self-control—required versus external limits
    3. Self-responsibility and direction—extent to which this is possible

TABLE 11-1. *(contd.)*

4. Dealing with adversity
   a. Possibility of success or failure
   b. Degree of frustration probable
   c. Degree of anxiety probable

H. Concept of others
   1. Degree of trust required
   2. Interaction with a possible authority figure required
   3. Degree of interaction with peers

V. Social interaction
   A. Interpretation of situations—degree to which this is required
   B. Social skills
      1. Communication
         a. Amount required
         b. Degree of verbal versus nonverbal
      2. Dyadic interaction
         a. Degree of interaction with another person required or possible
         b. Degree of structure
         c. Variety of one-to-one relationships possible
      3. Group interaction
         a. Type of group—parallel, project, egocentric-cooperative, cooperative, mature
         b. Need for instrumental versus expressive roles
         c. Degree of structure
   C. Structured social interplay
      1. Cooperation
      2. Competition
      3. Compromise
      4. Negotiating
      5. Assertiveness

VI. Occupational performances
   A. Relevance to social roles
      1. Family interaction
      2. Activities of daily living
      3. School/work
         a. Work habits—task, interpersonal
         b. Preparation for vocational choice
         c. Relationship to a particular occupation
      4. Play/leisure/recreation
         a. Type of play
         b. Complexity of rules
         c. Possibility as a shared recreational activity
         d. Possibility as a hobby
         e. Possibility for the formation of friendships
   B. Temporal adaptation
      1. Past, present, or future related
      2. Related to a time-specific activity of the day, week, or season
      3. Facilitates the ordering of events in time
      4. Time imposed by the structure of the activity, participation of another person
      5. Involves the coordination of more than one social role

VII. Age
   A. Extent to which activity is age specific
   B. Relevance to age-specific developmental tasks
      1. Those that have been mastered
      2. Those for which it may facilitate mastery
   C. Adaptation to loss
      1. Facilitate mourning
      2. Promote involvement in realistic problem solving
      3. Promote engagement in old or new interests and interpersonal relationships

VIII. Cultural implications
   A. Ethnic groups
      1. Meaning
      2. Relevance
   B. Socioeconomic group
      1. Meaning
      2. Relevance
      3. Affordability in the community
      4. Educational level necessary

IX. Social implications
   A. Extent to which members of the individual's social network are or can be involved in the activity
   B. Extent to which family members are or can be involved in the activity
      1. Opportunities for family members to learn about the client's current level of function
      2. Opportunities to explore new ways of communicating and interacting
   C. Implications of the activity relative to the sick role
      1. Dependency versus independence
      2. Passive versus active
      3. Extent to which the activity will help the individual cope with chronic illness or disability
   D. Community resources—extent to which use of community resources is facilitated
      1. Actual participation
      2. Skills necessary for participation
   E. Physical environment
      1. Typical environment in which the activity takes place
      2. Extent to which the activity helps in adjustment to the demands of the physical environment

X. Other considerations
   A. Place on continuum of simulated to real
   B. Time
      1. Length of total activity
      2. Length of each stage or step
      3. Delays inherent in the process
      4. Sequential ordering of stages linked with time
   C. Extent to which activity can be broken down into parts and number of steps
   D. Equipment and materials needed
   E. Space required
   F. Noise involved
   G. Dirt—are the materials to be used dirty or do they create dirt
   H. Cost of the activity
      1. Equipment and materials
      2. Therapist's time in preparation

approach is more finely tuned with either a theoretical system, to the needs of a client, or both. There are several types.

For the Purpose of Teaching

Many activities are made up of several steps or stages and can be presented in a number of ways. Activity analysis involves determining the various subtasks and the order, if any, in which each of the tasks needs to be done. Activity synthesis involves working out the most appropriate way to present each subtask and the sequence of presentation. Analysis and synthesis are primarily based on the principles of learning, as described in Chapter 9. The client's cognitive ability is also taken into consideration, relative to synthesis.

For the Purpose of Determining Whether a Client Can Perform an Activity

This first involves analysis of an activity relative to the functional requirement of the activity. The therapist's knowledge of the performance components is used as the basis for analysis. Synthesis in this situation involves comparing the functional requirement of the activity with the client's current capacities. This approach to activity analysis and synthesis is an essential part of all types of intervention. In meeting health needs, prevention, management, and maintenance, the functional requirements of the activity are finely tuned to the client's current capacities. In the change process, on the other hand, activities are selected which have at least some functional requirements that are a step beyond the client's current abilities. This is the only way that change is likely to occur.

For the Purpose of Adaptation

In order to adapt an activity, the therapist first looks at the functional capacity of the client. With this in mind, the therapist analyzes the activity to determine what elements can be changed or altered so that the client can perform the activity. This usually requires a good deal of problem solving. Many clients, particularly those who are physically disabled, frequently enjoy participating in this process and often arrive at quite ingenious solutions. Although outside the limits of this text, analysis and synthesis, for the purpose of adaptation relative to physical disabilities, also take into consideration the possibilities inherent in various functional aids. It should be remembered that adaptation of an activity should never be such that the integrity of the activity is violated. Another activity ought to be selected.

For the Purpose of Grading

The concept of gradation is important in many aspects of occupational therapy. Many frames of reference call for the gradation of activities in order to bring about change. The concept of gradation is also important in the maintenance of function. This is particularly true in working with clients whose conditions are characterized by periods of exacerbation and remission. Activities are analyzed, then, to determine what elements are able to be graded and the degree of gradability possible. This is another time when it is useful to compare several activities. On a particular dimension, one activity may suffice for one portion of the dimension, whereas another activity may be appropriate for another part of the dimension. Activities are synthesized so that they are at the correct level on the dimension of concern.

For the Purpose of Meeting Health Needs

The therapist analyzes activities relative to the extent to which they might satisfy the various health needs. Synthesis is concerned with designing an activity that will meet the health needs of a particular client or a group of clients. Analysis and synthesis are based on the therapist's knowledge of health needs and the ways in which these might be satisfied. This information will be presented in Chapter 17.

For the Purpose of Prevention

Activities are analyzed to determine what aspect of performance components or occupational performances they might enhance. They are synthesized to include the elements believed to enhance function in a particular area. To this extent, prevention is based on frames of reference. Thus, a conceptual framework for analysis and synthesis is derived from a frame of reference. This will be discussed momentarily.

For the Purpose of Maintenance

Activity analysis and synthesis relative to maintenance are essentially similar to what was outlined above where the purposes of grading and determining whether a client can perform an activity were discussed.

For the Purpose of Management

Activities are analyzed to determine how and to what extent they inhibit interfering behavior. They are synthesized so as to take the greatest advantage of their inhibiting capacity. A conceptual framework for this type of analysis and synthesis will also be outlined in Chapter 17.

For the Purpose of Change

Activity analysis and synthesis relative to the change process are based on a conceptual framework that is drawn from a particular frame of reference. There are as many different systems of classification, then, as there are frames of reference. The frame of reference determines which elements of the activity are to be emphasized and the depth with which some of the elements are to be explored and exploited. Analysis and synthesis based on an analytical frame of reference, for example, will give particular attention to the symbolic, expressive, and interpersonal aspects of the activity. An acquisitional frame of reference concerned with occupational performances is likely to focus on the potential of the activity for providing opportunities to develop competence in and balance between social roles.

For the purpose of change, activity analysis and synthesis are separated between a particular activity's potential for evaluation and its potential for intervention. The behaviors indicative of function and dysfunction of a particular frame of reference form the bases for activity analysis and synthesis relative to evaluation. The postulates regarding change of a particular frame of reference form the basis for activity analysis and synthesis relative to intervention.

In regard to evaluation, activities are analyzed relative to their probability of eliciting behaviors indicative of function and dysfunction as enumerated in a particular frame of reference. Activities are synthesized based on knowledge of the gestalt of behaviors the therapist wishes to observe. An illustration of synthesis is selecting an activity for evaluation that is likely to elicit a number of different behaviors indicative of function and dysfunction rather than an activity that is likely to elicit only one such behavior. In synthesizing an activity for evaluation, however, two areas of function having some interdependent elements should not be evaluated simultaneously. The behavior elicited may not differentiate between the client's capacity to function in one area as opposed to the other. In evaluating task skills and group interaction skills, for example, asking the client to do a task within a group setting would not be an appropriate activity. The client's difficulty in doing the task may interfere with the ability to function in the group. Conversely, difficulty in functioning in a group situation may interfere with the client's performance of the task. The therapist, in this case, would be unable to determine if the client had difficulty in performing a task or in group interaction or both.

Postulates regarding change, ideally, state the nature, quantity, quality, and sequence of interaction with the human and nonhuman environments, which are considered to be instrumental in bringing about positive change. Thus, activities are analyzed according to whether and to what degree they embody components of the stated characteristics. For example, a postulate may state that work habits are enhanced by interacting in a situation where one is required to adhere to the directions provided. Activities would then be analyzed with respect to whether one needed to follow directions strictly in order for the activity to be successful.

Activities used in the change process are synthesized to be as consistent as possible with the entire postulate regarding change for a specific area of dysfunction. For example, a postulate might state that form perception is enhanced through visual, tactile, and proprioceptive exploration of objects. Thus, after analysis, the therapist would design an activity or a series of activities that provided the greatest opportunity for visual, tactile, and proprioceptive exploration of a variety of objects.

Conceptual frameworks for activity analysis and synthesis relative to the change process are derived from specific frames of reference. As such they are only as complete as the frame of reference on which they are based. If a frame of reference provides only vague behaviors indicative of function and dysfunction, then the conceptual framework for activity analysis and synthesis relative to activities suitable for evaluation will be vague. The same situation is true if the postulates regarding change of a frame of reference are inadequate. The conceptual framework for analysis and synthesis of activities for change will be inadequate.

CONCLUSION

Activity analysis and synthesis provide the occupational therapist with the means to understand purposeful activities and how to determine the potential of specific activities for evaluation and intervention. Activity analysis and synthesis allow the therapist to select activities that will enhance the growth and adaptation of each individual client.

12 Review of Group Dynamics

This chapter provides a brief overview of the dynamics of small groups as they exist in all aspects of the social system (102, 172, 250, 293, 336, 390, 391, 415, 442, 575, 594, 595, 633,868,915,1049). It is not an in-depth discussion of the various theories of small groups. It is presented here to outline one of the theoretical components fundamental to activity groups.

"Group dynamics" is a general term used to identify the nature of small groups and the events that typically occur in small groups. Group dynamics is sometimes subdivided into three parts: structure, process, and content. Structure refers to the totality of patterned regularities that remain largely unchanged. All groups, for example, have goals, norms, and membership roles. Process refers to regulated interchanges between different parts of the social system. Process can be related to the internal changes that occur in a group or to the interrelationship between the group and the broader social system in which it is embedded. Content refers to the substance of a particular group. All groups, for example, have goals but each group has goals that are particularly its own. The focus of this review is primarily on the structure of small groups and the interrelationship between structural parts, the process.

Research into the dynamics of small groups began, as mentioned, in the early 1940s. It has since that time been concerned with three major issues: (a) the structures common to all groups, (b) the changes that occur in groups over time, and (c) the individual in the group in terms of how the individual affects the group and is affected by it. The research that has been done can perhaps best be described as being on a continuum from "statistical" to "clinical."

Statistically oriented approaches are exemplified by various scoring or rating systems considering verbal interactions, feelings of members, task accomplishment, and so forth. This approach reduces group events to their component parts, which can be coded and treated statistically. It is based on the conviction that study of the atomistic events in groups will yield universal patterns of group life. This approach has not provided a unified theory of small groups but it has provided considerable information. One of its disadvantages is that it tends to obscure the richness, variety, subtlety, and complexity of human behavior.

Clinically oriented approaches, on the other hand, are concerned with more intuitive and theoretical processes. They do not involve explicit or systematic intervening steps in arriving at conclusions about groups. Their findings tend to be somewhat impressionistic, subjective, and ideographic. One of the disadvantages of this approach is that interpersonal behavior varies so much across situations. Findings vary, reflecting the uniqueness of the setting from which the behavior was observed rather than universal dimensions. Findings may not apply in different settings.

Both statistical and clinical approaches, therefore, have limitations. Nevertheless, in combining the findings of the two approaches a rich body of knowledge in regards to group dynamics has been developed.

DEFINITION

A group is an aggregate of people who share a common purpose and are interdependent in the achievement of that purpose. There is frequently a distinction made between primary and secondary groups. A primary group is a face-to-face organization of individuals who cooperate for certain common ends, who share many common ideas and patterns of behavior, who have confidence in and some degree of affection for each other, and who are aware of their similarities and bonds of association. Examples of primary groups are the family, the gang, some friendship groups, and some groups that are part of the informal structure found in work settings. A secondary group, in contrast, is any large group that does not allow for face-to-face contact of all members. Group members do not have close or intimate ties but they share some common interest or similarity. Within a secondary group, there may be one or more primary groups. Individuals frequently interact in a secondary group through membership in one of the primary groups that make up the secondary group. Some examples of secondary groups are the members of a church, employees in a large organization, and the faculty of a college. This chapter is concerned with primary groups.

Primary groups are usually small, being made up of three or more people but usually fewer than 20. They persist long enough so that the behavior of one member influences the behavior of other members, an informal subculture and normative system develops, and emotional attachments are engendered. There is usually a set of functionally differentiated roles even though these may be somewhat rudimentary. Members perceive themselves as being part of the group. Primary groups tend to have a memory for past experiences despite some change in membership. They are capable of learning and responding as an entity. Members are able to engage in emotional as well as instrumental behavior. Finally, a group can achieve goals well beyond the capacity of a single individual.

Primary groups are formed in three ways: spontaneously, deliberately, or through elaboration. Spontaneous groups are most frequently social in nature, not highly structured, and tend to be democratic. Deliberate groups are usually found in formal organizations, are more structured, and tend to have a fairly autocratic style of leadership. Groups formed through elaboration, exemplified by the extended family, tend to include values and norms brought from the parent group or groups. Their structure and leadership styles usually also reflect that of the parent group.

Primary groups are crucial at every stage of development: family of origin, classroom, peer groups, work groups, family of procreation. They are the major means by which socialization and enculturation take place. It is out of the associations formed in these groups that the individual fashions and has fashioned a developing and changing concept of self. Individuals learn appropriate ways of behaving in varied social situations and acquire a set of social values and attitudes that allow them to respond to the structure and pressures of the larger society. Primary groups operate as a mediating mechanism and a buffer between the individual and the wider social system. It is through them that social expectations are channeled to the individual and where these demands are softened and made manageable. Most individuals form or enter into primary groups to satisfy their needs for affection, affiliation, and security. They use such groups to control the external environment. Primary groups form the basis for reality testing and, if need be, actually create a reality. The latter is likely to occur if the wider social system is seen as threatening in some way or if it is characterized by many unknown elements and/or conflicting values and ideas.

General systems theory has frequently been used as a framework for the organization of knowledge about primary groups. As previously discussed, general systems theory, in part, is organization of phenomena in terms of a hierarchy of systems, each containing its subsystems and contained within a suprasystem. Five subsystems of primary groups have been identified:

1. the interaction system—organization of overt behavior of members;
2. the emotional system—the configurations of feelings among members and their emotional response to events that occur;
3. the normative system—a set of ideas about what is and is not appropriate behavior within the context of the group and the wider social system;
4. the technical system—a set of ideas about what the group should accomplish (goals) and how this should be accomplished (means);
5. the executive system—an interpretation of what the group is, ideas about what would be desirable for it to become, and about how it might reach that ideal.

All of these subsystems interact with each other. Individuals in a group engage in a continuous process of acting, reacting, and adapting to each other. As a consequence their interpersonal behavior becomes patterned: differential roles develop; a division of labor emerges; subgroups may form; differentiation of authority, power, and status occurs; norms and values are systematized; and a hierarchy of goals is established.

As important as the interaction of the subsystems of a group is, a group does not exist in a vacuum. A primary group is considered to be part of an open system. As such it has boundaries sufficient to maintain a certain degree of inner integrity and identity, yet its boundaries are sufficiently flexible and permeable to be able to use the environment in maintaining and perpetuating its own existence.

A group, then, exists within a suprasystem which impinges on it and on which it impinges. The goals and means of a group, for example, cannot be too divergent from those acceptable to the wider social system. If they are, the social system will attempt to alter the goals and means or, in the extreme situation, make a strong effort to disband the group. Conversely, a primary group may act as an agent of change relative to the wider social system. It may, for example, attempt to change the schools in a community or work to preserve the architectural style of a particular area. The interrelationship between primary groups and the wider social system is exemplified by the women's movement. Initiated by many primary groups which eventually coalesced into a secondary group, the women's movement substantially altered the structure of many families.

The subsystems of a group and the collection of groups that make up the suprasystem are in a constant state of assimilation and accommodation and go through repetitive cycles of disequilibrium and equilibrium. A change in one part of any system reverberates throughout the system, causing change and requiring adaptation in the other parts of the system. A system is a totality of interdependent elements, all of which exert some force on each part of the system.

The continual changes that take place in primary groups occur within the parameters of an identifiable structure. The remainder of this chapter is devoted to a brief discussion of the parts of this structure.

THE ELEMENTS OF STRUCTURE

As mentioned, structure refers to the patterned regularities of all primary groups that remain largely unchanged. Ten elements of structure will be described here.

Group Development

Primary groups have frequently been conceptualized as having a developmental cycle with specific phases. A given group may not go through all of the phases because of the particular nature of that group or because the group becomes caught in one phase and cannot move on. The phases of a group overlap, with hints of most phases found during each of the other phases. It is also not unusual for a group to regress periodically to a previous phase, particularly in a time of stress. Five, relatively discrete, phases of primary groups have been identified.

Orientation Phase

In this first stage group members tend to be eager to be a part of the group and have very positive expectations. There is, however, some anxiety regarding the unknowns: what it will be like and what will happen in the future. This is a time of getting to know other group members and of testing the boundaries of interpersonal behavior. There tends to be considerable dependency on the leader, other group members, the situation, and/or preexisting standards. A considerable amount of time is spent in defining the task, how it should be approached, and assessing the resources and skills necessary for task accomplishment. The length of time of this phase varies and is often dependent on the specificity of the task. If the group has a very specific task, this phase tends to be rather short.

Dissatisfaction Phase

This is the time of intragroup conflict and highly emotional expression; the euphoria and good feelings of the first phase are over. What group members had hoped for and the reality of the situation frequently do not coincide. Further, the state of dependency on the leader begins to be uncomfortable. Rebellion of one sort or another is seen as providing a possible solution. There is polarization around interpersonal issues, particularly in regards to the leader. There may be periods of hostile confrontation, with the leader being blamed for unmet expectations and impossible demands. This often serves to establish intermember solidarity, which may be temporary in nature. Subgroups tend to form and reform relative to their support of the leader and commitment to the task. Boundaries of acceptable behavior begin to be formed, and are severely tested. Differential roles begin to be molded. Negative feelings and negotiating for positions in the group may be so disruptive that work on the task decreases. The duration and intensity of this period is often dependent on difficulty in clearly defining what precisely constitutes the task, how difficult it is, and what skills the group members possess and can acquire to accomplish the task. The end or resolution of this phase will depend on how easy or difficult it is to resolve the sense of frustration, disillusionment, and anger. It will also depend on the extent to which group members are able to gain or organize the skills necessary for task accomplishment. The task of the group may be redefined so that it is conceptualized in a more achievable form.

Resolution Phase

This phase begins when there is a gradual decrease in dissatisfaction. Expectations are redefined to be more compatible with the situation. This leads to group members developing a more positive feeling about themselves and pleasure in task accomplishment. There is a decrease in the animosity between group members and between the members and the leader. This is accompanied by an implied or explicit agreement about what is appropriate interpersonal behavior; standards or norms evolve. Cohesiveness begins to develop with the sense of being an in-group and the expression of more intimate personal feelings. Roles come to be defined more clearly and there is a gradual increase in work on the task.

Production Phase

This stage is characterized by group members having generally positive feelings toward each other and toward being part of the experience. Members work well together with more autonomy from the leader. Less time is spent in struggling against the leader, other group members, or the task itself. Roles become flexible and functional, with more group energy channeled into the task. Structural issues have been resolved and are now supportive of task performance. The group knows very well what it is doing; it can resolve its internal conflicts, mobilize its resources, and take intelligent action. Group members are able to engage in honest interpersonal communication and have developed the means for consensually validating their experiences.

Terminal Phase

This phase is signaled by the end of the task, a time limit, some impending event that will bring an end to the group or a disintegration process (group members slowly drift away from the group). The group begins to face and be concerned about its own end, the dissolution of its boundaries, and the movement of its members into other groups. There is the sense of impending loss and anticipatory mourning. This is often a time when members assess the success or failure of their experience. If the group ends with a sense of accomplishment, positive feelings may be stronger than the negative ones of loss. Maximum productivity may come at the beginning of this period, but work on the task generally decreases toward the end.

The five phases of group development are strongly influenced by emotionally laden, or central issues.

Central Issues

In any primary group there are a number of issues inherent in the situation: dependency, hostility, hope, helplessness, freedom, individuality, competition for authority and power, assertiveness, intimacy, love, sexuality, envy, giving, and sharing. These issues can be seen as being on two continuums: unconscious to conscious; and idiosyncratic to interpersonal to collective. In other words, the group or individual may not be aware of the current central issues and a central issue may be the concern of one individual, a subgroup, or the entire group. Central issues of one type or another continually surface in group interaction and need to be identified and addressed. An issue may be reconciled but it is rarely resolved once and for all; it will likely come up again.

Sometimes central issues are neither identified nor addressed. In such a case the individual or the group acts in a variety of ways to solve the issue in devious and obscure ways, all of which tend to disrupt the work of the group. Two overlapping concepts have been used to describe this situation: hidden agenda and basic assumptions. Hidden agenda refers to a central issue that is covert and implicitly closed to direct public scrutiny and awareness. Nevertheless it emerges to influence what takes place in the group. A hidden agenda is apparent when observed behavior does not seem to be compatible with the ongoing events of the group. The concept of hidden agenda is usually applied to an individual or a subgroup who is unable to bring an issue out into the open. This may be due to unresolved personal issues that are aroused by the situation of the group, habits of public behavior characterized by indirect expression of emotions, and ideas or feelings of vulnerability.

The term "basic assumptions," on the other hand, usually is used to describe the group as a whole. A group that is currently motivated by basic assumptions functions as if its members were following some shared unconscious beliefs about their goals and why they are together. This overt behavior is not related to the realities of the situation nor designed to cope successfully with the group task. Basic assumptions, springing from emotional issues the group is unable to face, tend to obstruct and divert the group from accomplishing its task. Behavior motivated by basic assumptions serves to reduce tension and avoid immediate distress. It may take many forms: dependency, fighting over irrelevant issues, withdrawal, the formation of subgroups, and so forth. Basic assumptions do serve to enhance, at least temporarily, the cohesiveness of the group but they also act as a hindrance to the more rational problem-solving activities of the group. Primary groups are replete with basic assumptions and ritualistic activities that serve to maintain these assumptions. The periodic, critical task of a group is to look at the central issues that are affecting its capacity to function effectively. Lack of adequate attention to central issues may well render the group ineffective and ultimately lead to its disintegration.

Roles in Groups

There are a variety of roles, or patterns of behavior, that are necessary in order for a group to function adequately. These roles have been conceptualized in a number of ways, with major emphasis on either the sharing of leadership or on the role of the leader. The first approach focuses on those roles that are necessary for task accomplishment and the maintenance of the group. The second approach is concerned with the qualities and behavior of an effective leader.

The roles necessary for optimal group function have been outlined by Hare et al. (391). They are divided into two categories: instrumental and expressive. Instrumental roles are concerned with the selection, planning, and execution of the group task. The following roles are included in this category. The initiator-contributor suggests new ideas. The information seeker asks for clarification of facts. The opinion seeker asks for clarification of opinions or values. The information giver offers facts. The opinion giver states his beliefs or values. The elaborator spells out suggestions. The coordinator clarifies relationships. The orienter defines the position of the group with respect to its goals. The evaluator critic compares the accomplishment of the group to some standard. The organizer prods the group to action. The procedural technician expedites group movement by performing routine tasks.

Expressive roles are oriented to the function of the group as a whole and the gratification of members' needs. The following roles are included in this category. The encourager praises, agrees with, and accepts the contribution of others. The harmonizer mediates differences between members. The compromiser changes his own behavior so as to maintain group harmony. The gatekeeper facilitates and regulates communication. The standard setter expresses standards for the group to achieve. The group observer notes, interprets, and presents information about group process. The follower goes along with the movement of the group.

The roles outlined above are considered to be functional as they contribute to group goals. They are contrasted with dysfunctional roles, which are primarily directed toward the playing out of a hidden agenda or the unstated basic assumptions of the group. Such roles are not considered to be relevant either to the group task or to the function of the group as a group.

At any given time, the particular functional roles required for optimal group productivity depend on the nature of the task, the position of the group in relation to the accomplishment of the task, and the group's phase of development. In this approach to defining group roles, no sharp distinction is made between leader and follower roles. Those patterns of behavior, typically described as "leadership" in nature, are considered to be available to, and ideally shared by, all group members. Leadership thus becomes a multilateral responsibility. Under ideal circumstances, group members are able to identify the need for and to take a variety of roles.

Nevertheless, even in well-functioning groups, leadership does emerge. It is usually not, however, vested in one person. Rather it tends to be polarized around two individuals: the instrumental leader, who is primarily concerned with the group task, and the expressive leader, who takes responsibility for seeing to the social-emotional needs of the group. Instrumental leadership may be shared, particularly when the group has two or more distinct tasks. A department of occupational therapy, for example, may have two instrumental leaders. One instrumental leader may be concerned with the formal administration of the department and the department's relationship to the broader social system of the hospital. The other instrumental leader may be considered the clinical expert, providing guidance relative to various problems in evaluation and intervention. Regardless of the number of leaders, these specialists must cooperate in order for the work of the group to continue effectively. If this does not occur, subgroups may form around each leader, with considerable conflict ensuing. With divided loyalties, the group becomes frustrated and little work is accomplished.

The other approach to the study of group roles has focused on defining the qualities and behavior of an effective leader. Most consideration has been focused on the instrumental leader. Several characteristics have been identified. An effective instrumental leader establishes and maintains a clear definition of the group's goals and the primary task of the group. This is done through defining, and defending, the means for execution of the primary task; continually clarifying the task and the nature of the work that is required; and by helping to identify obstacles and consequences of possible decisions or choices.

An effective instrumental leader also obtains necessary information from both inside and outside the group. The leader also helps the group to be open to new and different ideas without becoming immobilized by fear or conflict. He or she assists the group in integrating the various perspectives and alternative possibilities for policy or action that emerges within the group.

The leader assesses the skills and interests of individual members and assigns tasks on the basis of this assessment. The aptitudes and preferences of individual members are recognized and protected. In doing this, the leader attempts to make use of individuals' assets and to compensate in some way for their liabilities. In other words, the leader becomes aware of the human resources of the group and determines how best these can be used.

The effective leader coordinates individuals' efforts in a productive manner. This is accomplished by planning what needs to be done, initiating each successive step, and supervising group members' work. Task performance is enhanced by evaluating what has been done, stressing proper procedures or methods, identifying deadlines, and so forth.

The leader persuades others to participate in leadership functions. This is often accomplished by delegating authority whenever possible.

Another characteristic of an effective leader is that he or she defines the group relative to the larger social system by determining the scope and permeability of the group's boundaries, regulating the flow of information into and out of the group, representing the social system to the group and representing the group to the social system, and by facilitating the group's movement toward a preferred location in the social system.

The effective leader creates and preserves for him- or herself a psychosocial position in the group which synthesizes participation and observation. Emotional immersion in the group is avoided as is extreme detachment.

Finally, the leader helps the group to address, sublimate, and/or channel central issues into the work of the group.

The characteristics outlined above are general in nature. The effectiveness of a group depends on the fit between leadership style and the particular situation of the group. Ideally the style shifts in accordance with the developmental phase of the group and the actual demands of the task over time. Flexibility in leadership style is a definite asset.

In a classic study, three types of leadership were identified: authoritarian, democratic, and laissez-faire. Authoritarian leadership is characterized by the leader determining all of the policies of the group. Each step in the task is dictated by the leader one at a time so that future steps are always uncertain to some degree. The leader usually defines the task and the work companion of each member. The leader tends to be "personal" in praise and criticism and remains aloof from active group participation except when describing or demonstrating what needs to be done.

Democratic leadership is characterized by the leader encouraging and assisting group discussion and decision making on all matters of policy. Perspective in regards to the task is gained through discussion, with general steps to the goal sketched out. When technical advice is needed the leader suggests two or more alternative procedures from which a choice can be made. Members are free to work with whomever they choose and the division of tasks is left up to the group. The leader is "objective" or "factual" in praise and criticism and tries to be a regular group member in spirit without doing too much of the work.

Laissez-faire leadership is characterized by complete freedom for individual or group decisions with a minimum of leader participation. Various materials are supplied by the leader who makes it clear he or she will provide information only when asked, taking no part in work discussion or defining the task. The leader only infrequently offers spontaneous comments on members' activities unless questioned. Essentially there is no attempt to regulate the course of events.

Another way of looking at leadership styles is based on the leader's beliefs about people or the individuals in a particular group. Two different orientations have been identified and are referred to as theory X and theory Y. An individual who is described as having a theory X orientation believes that people dislike work and avoid it if they can. People must be coerced, controlled, or threatened into working and have little ambition or interest in responsibility. Therefore people really enjoy being directed and being guided by a strong leader. On the other hand, an individual who is described as having a theory Y orientation believes that the effort expended in work is natural and pleasurable. People are capable of being self-directed and self-controlled once they feel committed to certain objectives and goals. People not only accept but actively seek areas in which they can be autonomous and responsible.

In relation to the first three styles of leadership described, people with a theory X orientation would tend to be autocratic leaders, whereas people with a theory Y orientation would tend to be democratic or laissez-faire.

No style of leadership is considered to be better than another style. It cannot be emphasized enough that effective leadership is situationally determined. What works is dependent on the people involved, what the group needs to do, and what is expected by the group members.

As mentioned there has been less study of expressive leaders. However, some specific traits have been identified. The expressive leader is concerned with preserving the social-emotional solidarity of the group—maintaining and strengthening this aspect of the group. This leader attends to the process of the group, listening to understand. The leader takes responsibility for accurate communication, being particularly sensitive to unexpressed feelings and minority points of view, and helps to keep the discussion moving along by summarizing feelings and ideas. The internal and external pressures of the group are continually assessed and kept at a manageable level if at all possible. The expressive leader gives considerable feedback to the group. Feedback takes the form of the leader: (a) describing what he or she feels or observes; (b) discussing the way in which it affects the leader and the possible effect it might have on the group; (c) checking to determine whether his or her perceptions and its effect is shared by the group; and, if this is responded to in the affirmative, (d) raising the question of what should be done about it. The leader's capacity to be supportive, to listen, and to use good judgment relative to timing are all important.

It should be noted that the traits just described may well be found, at least in part, in some instrumental leaders. Conversely, some of the characteristics of an instrumental leader may be found in an expressive leader. The difference between the two types of leaders is often more in degrees rather than in the kinds of interactions in which they engage.

Just as the style of appropriate instrumental leadership is situationally determined, whether an individual will take a leadership role is also influenced by the situation. An individual frequently takes a leadership role if (a) aware that a given function is needed in the group; (b) he or she feels able to perform it, and has enough skill to do so, or it is safe to attempt to do so; and (c) has an opportunity to do so. On the other hand, the group may select a member for leadership. If specialized skills are needed, the choice is usually fairly obvious. If no particular special skill is needed, the group usually solicits a member who seeks to organize the group, asks for and attempts to integrate contributions from others, or proposes various courses of action. The individual selected is usually a person who is able to meet the needs of the group and its expectations at that particular time.

Although a leadership role is preferred by many people, it is not a role without some limitations. The group's acceptance or rejection of a particular leader depends on the degree of compliance on the part of members, their identification with the leader, and the extent to which they internalize the values and ideas of the leader. In the beginning phases of the group, members tend to project or externalize their ideas of what a group leader should be onto the leader. This is done essentially without regard to the real qualities of the particular leader. Members usually attempt to view the leader as a strong, resourceful, and potentially nurturing figure. No matter how good the leader may be, it is nearly impossible to live up to others' idealized image of a leader. When the leader cannot meet the members' exceptionally high standards, members tend to become quite angry, and the leader frequently feels that he or she has failed the group. In addition, the high visibility makes the leader the most likely target for a variety of negative and positive feelings. Transference and countertransference are a very common occurrence in any group. Group members frequently have highly ambivalent feelings toward the leader. Individuals in a leadership position, in order to maintain their sense of identity, need to develop a high tolerance for ambivalence.

The above discussion of membership and leader roles is based on groups that are functionally task oriented. Although central issues are present, on the whole they are dealt with in a constructive kind of way that only periodically delays the work of the group. Groups that are primarily organized around basic assumptions, however, have a different way of organizing interpersonal relationships. There is no acknowledgment of or toleration for a complex view of interpersonal relationships. Basic assumptions lead to simplified constructions of reality and relatively uncomplicated membership and leader roles. This inevitably results in a loss of skill in playing a variety of roles and a constriction of role options for members and leaders. Individuals are locked into and seduced into irrational, unsatisfying, and unproductive roles. The leader is subjected to conflicting and fundamentally impossible demands: to provide unlimited nurturance, to fight and subdue imaginary enemies, to rescue the group from death and desolation. This is a thoroughly uncomfortable situation for everyone involved.

Group Goals

A group goal is the desired future state of the group that is held by a sufficient number of group members to induce movement toward that state. A group goal can also be described as a state toward which the majority of the group's effort is directed. There may be discrepancy between the "real" goal as defined above and the stated goal. A group goal may be stated, verbalized by group members; or unstated, not verbalized. Group goals may be anywhere on the conscious-to-unconscious continuum. A conscious goal is one that the group is aware of; it may be stated or unstated. An unconscious goal is outside of the awareness of group members. A group primarily motivated by basic assumptions tends to have unconscious goals.

Group goals have several functions. They provide orientation and focus for the group and set guidelines for group interaction. They constitute a source of legitimacy for the group, providing a reason for the group's existence to the group members and persons outside of the group. Goals provide a standard by which the group may judge its activities and decisions. Finally, goals provide a means by which persons outside of the group may assess and judge the group. Judgment is based on the perceived worth of the goal and the degree to which the group has attained its goal.

The goal of a group is sometimes never realized because of the nature of the goal, such as to provide adequate occupational therapy services to clients. This is an ongoing goal so to speak. When a goal is realized or perceived as unattainable, the group sets a new goal or disbands.

Some groups have more than one goal. Multiple goals may have a positive effect on the group; one goal may facilitate attainment of other goals or they may provide a greater recruitment appeal for the group. Group members may be able to gratify more needs and utilize a greater variety of their talents. However, multiple goals can also have a negative impact on the group. Various goals may be in conflict with each other either in regards to the activities necessary to reach the goal or the consequence of goal attainment. One goal may subordinate another, leading to conflict between group factions who see different goals as primary.

Group goals are not the sum of individual goals. The group goal may be different from an individual's goal; each group member may have different goals. However, a person usually joins a group because he or she believes that the group goal will facilitate the attainment of personal goals. When group members determine the group goals, the individual's relative influence in setting group goals is dependent on the degree of participation and amount of influence.

Motivation to work for attainment of group goals is heightened by participation in goal setting. Such participation leads to a better (a) fit between the goal and members' motives and goals, (b) understanding of the actions required for goal attainment, and (c) appreciation of how the behavior of the individual contributes to required group action. If the goal is not accepted by a significant portion of the group, effort is usually poorly coordinated. There tends to be a high incidence of self-oriented rather than task-oriented behavior. The factors that influence an individual's acceptance of a group goal are the personal consequences of accepting and attaining the goal and the degree to which the individual is attracted to the group. An individual usually experiences feelings of group belongingness, sympathy with group emotions, and a readiness to accept the influence of the group if he has a clear understanding of group goals and the activities necessary to reach the goal.

The best group goals are challenging rather than unrealistic—clear, and stated in operational terms. Operational goals are able to be measured. Some examples are "to make a doll house" or "to find a workable solution to a specific problem." Nonoperational goals are unable to be objectively measured; "to make a ward more liveable or to improve the group members' ability to relate to other people" are two examples. If the group's goal is by its nature nonoperational, it is usually best to break it down into operational subgoals that have some plausible linkage to the general goal. An example of operationalizing a goal is identifying "to make bedspreads for the mens' dorm" a subgoal of "to make a ward more liveable." Groups tend to function best when goals are operational because members are better able to define what activities will lead to the goal. Nonoperational goals are fairly common, however, because there is less fear of failure. There is also a tendency to avoid operational goals when the goal is primarily simply to be with other group members.

The setting of goals is a statement of the desired relationship between the group and the external environment. Group goals and activities leading to their attainment must be somewhat compatible with goals accepted by the wider social system. If there is a serious conflict, the external environment may well bring pressure on the group to change its goals or activities leading to the goal, or it may attempt to dissolve the group.

Group Norms

Group norms are patterns of behavior that are considered appropriate to the group. They govern the interaction of group members and are the means by which interaction is structured and given meaning. There is usually a range of behavior considered acceptable; any behavior that falls outside of that range is seen as deviant and usually subject to negative sanctions. Norms, which may be conscious or unconscious, develop whenever an aggregate of people interact for a period of time; this occurs because people have a need to know what others are going to do. The expectation that group members will act within the normative structure makes it possible for the individual to predict their behavior.

The norms of a group change over time, with several factors accounting for the alterations. The group may be confronted with behavior not covered by current norms: additional norms are then created to deal with the behavior. New knowledge or technology may become available to the group, which requires the development of new standards, or allows the group to disregard a particular norm. If a norm is ignored by a large portion of the group for an extended period of time, it usually ceases to be a functional norm. When a norm is perceived as being in conflict with the goals of the group, either the norm or the goal is changed.

When an individual joins an ongoing group, one of the first tasks is to learn the norms of the group and how to behave in accordance with them. This occurs through the process of socialization, which has been previously described. Full acceptance as a group member usually only occurs after the individual has learned to operate within the normative structure of the group. As a full group member, the individual is instrumental in reinforcing and in changing norms. An individual who does not follow group norms is likely to be rejected by the group. There are, however, some exceptions; individuals who are seen as having a special position in the group or who have high status may not be rejected. On the whole, the more affinity an individual has for a group, the more likely he or she is to accept the group's norms.

At times, there may be conflict between the various norms of a group. This is resolved by the group's rejecting or altering the conflicting norms or by creating another norm prohibiting recognition of the conflict. There may also be conflict between the norms of the group and norms accepted in the external environment. This may be resolved in a way similar to intragroup norm conflict, or the difference may simply be accepted by the group. When the latter is the case, group members operate on a double normative standard, behaving one way within the group and another way when interacting with and in the wider social system.

Communication

Communication is the process of transmitting, or transmitting and receiving information by means of gestures, facial expressions, words, signs, or symbols from one individual to another. Communication may be very direct or it may be quite circumspect. The degree of clarity may be deliberately planned by the transmitter or it may be regulated by essentially unconscious processes. It is, of course, ultimately the receiver who decides the clarity of a message, and indeed the meaning of the message. Communication takes many forms: repetition, monologue, collective monologue, criticism and ridicule, orders and threats, questions and answers, and adaptive give and take. The latter is probably the most fruitful form of communication; it is also probably the rarest.

Communication in a group is used for several purposes. One purpose is control. The individual or a few individuals toward whom most of the communication is directed or who direct the majority of communication toward other group members are usually the most influential members of the group. Control of the channels of communication often leads to control of the group. Communication is also used to clarify group goals. Such clarification may be related to problems in need of solution, information needed for decision making, or conflicting opinions, behavior, or group norms. Individuals who use communication for the purpose of clarification contribute significantly to the functioning of the group by helping to move the group toward its goals. Communication also allows for the sharing of feelings and ideas not directly related to the task. Such communication assists in the satisfaction of social-emotional needs and increases the solidarity of the group.

One of the major problems confronted by many groups is difficulty in open and clear communication. There are several factors that contribute to this difficulty.

If an individual does not know how his communication is going to be received or if he knows it will be received negatively, he tends to limit his communication.

Group members may be overly concerned with self-concept. Persons who perceive themselves as inadequate frequently feel they are exposing themselves to adverse criticism when they communicate with others. Conversely, individuals may limit communication to a person who they perceive as having a tenuous or poor self-concept for fear they will in some way destroy or further damage his self-concept.

There may be a lack of factual information that is pertinent to the problem or issue under consideration. The communication process ceases or is misdirected because members do not have anything to discuss.

Communication may be controlled by a one-way, hierarchical system. In this situation communication tends to be directed from the top to the bottom or from the bottom to the top. In neither case is it reciprocal.

There may be an avoidance of conflict-arousing material or a group norm that prohibits recognition of conflict. In the course of events, much information becomes directly or indirectly related to one or several of the conflict issues. Communication comes to be limited because a reservoir of conflict-arousing issues is created in the group. With an increase in taboo information, there is a decrease in information shared.

Members may lack investment and involvement in the group. Group membership or group goals or both must be significant to an individual for that individual to be motivated to communicate.

Members may have infrequent contact. There is a high positive correlation between membership contact and communication. Intervening contact with other groups and individuals frequently dilutes communication in a given group.

The communication in the group may be unclear. Communication is decreased when the receiver does not understand the information communicated by the sender. This often occurs when the sender's primary mode of communication is nonverbal and the receiver is either unaware of or unable to understand the nonverbal communication. In addition, when there is a gross discrepancy between verbal and nonverbal communication, the receiver frequently has difficulty in understanding the nature of the message being given.

Elimination of any of the above-listed factors tends to increase communication in a group. Regardless of the factors that inhibit communication, however, there are others that tend to enhance the exchange of feelings, ideas, and information.

One factor is the lack of a shared reality among group members. This usually leads to an attempt to structure and define the situation so that it is more understandable. Such an attempt is usually implemented by an increase in communication.

There may be concern over movement toward and attainment of the group goal. This factor is more related to the nature of the communication than the quantity of communication. When group members are concerned about the goal there tends to be more task-relevant communication.

A limitation in the amount of time allowed for the making of a decision is a source of external pressure that usually increases communication.

The need for communication increases when there are differences in group members' values and standards. This is especially true when there is a desire to maintain group solidarity and cohesiveness.

The possibility of and desire to enhance one's status in a group prompts an individual to communicate more. In this situation an individual tends to direct an increasing amount of communication toward high status individuals in the hopes of gaining recognition. Through recognition by and interaction with high status individuals, the individual is able to reduce the difference between his or her own status and a high status person.

Although all elements of the structure of a primary group are important, communication is perhaps the most significant. Without communication, the group becomes moribund or ceases to exist as a viable entity.

Group Cohesiveness

Group cohesiveness refers to the degree to which group members see themselves as being intimately related, connected in some way, and part of the same circumscribed unit. A high degree of cohesiveness is characterized by all members working for the common goal, a readiness of individual members to take responsibility for group tasks, individual loyalty to group members, and a willingness to defend the group from outside threat or attack. Cohesiveness arises out of two interrelated forces: individuals' affinity for a group and acceptance of each group member by the group. Individuals are attracted to a group because participation in the group is seen as a better source of need satisfaction than participation in another group. The group is accepting of an individual if that individual is seen as able to contribute to the group's goals or the satisfaction of social-emotional needs.

There are several factors that appear to contribute to cohesiveness. One such factor is a considerable amount of interaction. The nature of the interaction does not seem to matter very much. What seems to be the important factor is the amount of time people are together doing something. Closely related to this factor is propinquity: physical nearness in time and place. For example, a group of people who live together are likely to have greater cohesiveness than a group whose members live in different residences.

Similarity or complementarity of interests, personality traits, ethnic background, or some other characteristic contributes to cohesiveness. Groups that perceive many similarities between its members tend to be more cohesive than groups that do not perceive such similarity. Groups in which members complement each other in some way often have an added advantage relative to meeting the goals of the group.

General success relative to the task or goal of the group or expectation of such success is a factor exemplified in the idea that it is nice to be on the winning team.

A group whose climate is characterized by cooperation and democratic leadership tends to be more cohesive than a group not so characterized.

Competition with other groups tends to define the group in relation to an "out-group," making the group boundaries very clear. Competition tends to make goals more specific and motivates activities leading to the goal.

The status of the group in the external environment is another factor. Most individuals want a high status and tend to have affinity for a highly placed group. By membership in a high status group, the individual's overall status in the community tends to be higher. High status groups on the whole are more cohesive than low status groups.

A cohesive group has many advantages over a group that is less united. Its membership tends to be stable and the group has considerable influence over its members' behavior. This latter factor, of course, would not be considered an advantage if the group prompted behavior that was highly deviant, as defined by the broader social system. In a cohesive group members can count on each other's participation and loyalty, which leads to a greater feeling of personal security. Finally, belonging to a cohesive group tends to increase the individual's feelings of self-worth.

Decision Making

Decision making is the process of arriving at an agreed on solution to a problem. The process of decision making in a group is usually characterized by the following sequence of events: orientation, evaluation, conclusion, and implementation. In the orientation phase the problem is formulated or defined and relevant facts bearing on the decision are shared. Evaluation involves a delineation of various possible solutions. Group members share their knowledge, values, and interests, using this information as the criteria by which the facts of the situation and the proposed courses of actions are judged. There is an examination of the consequences of the different solutions and, at times, trial application of a few solutions. The group's conclusion may be arrived at through unanimous decision, consensus, majority rule, or compromise. Unanimous decision involves full agreement by all group members as to the best solution. Consensus occurs when a minority agrees to go along with the majority but reserves the right to have the decision reevaluated at a later date. Majority rule involves the larger portion of the group agreeing to one solution. The minority loses the right to have the decision reevaluated at a later time. Compromise occurs when there is a combining of two different points of view so that the ultimate decision is something quite different from either point of view. Implementation, the final phase of decision making, involves carrying out the decision.

Several assets of group decision making as opposed to individual decision making have been identified. In group decision making there is (a) a greater sum total of knowledge and information available, (b) a greater number of approaches to the problem and (c) increased acceptance and better understanding of the decision. The possible liabilities of group decision making are social pressure for a unanimous decision or consensus, domination by one individual or a small subgroup, and hidden agendas. Some examples of hidden agendas that interfere with decision making are simply wanting to win the argument, fighting for a personal cause, or not wanting the group to make any decisions.

In addition to the possible liabilities mentioned above, there are several other factors that interfere with decision making. One factor is fear of the consequence. The fear may be due to anxiety regarding the reaction of persons seen as powerful by the group, fear of added responsibility, or fear of change.

Conflicting loyalties may interfere. Individuals may have membership in two groups that have different ideas about the appropriateness of a given decision. Thus, they may have difficulty in approaching the decision-making process objectively.

Interpersonal conflict is another factor. A proposal may be rejected on the basis of dislike for the individual who made the proposal rather than on its merits. On the other hand, there may be a division of the group into two or more factions on the basis of several other issues rather than real disagreement about the decision at hand.

A methodological blunder may interfere with decision making. For example, there may be unclear formulation of the problem or issues that have a bearing on the problem. Techniques in collecting relevant information may have been poor. Group norms may limit freedom to express opinions and values. The group may rely too much on opinions rather than facts. The group may be forced to reach a conclusion before it is ready.

Another factor is inadequate group roles. Decisions are not reached because the roles necessary for decision making are not being taken by group members.

The decisions a group makes, both large and small, have a profound impact on a group. The impact may often be felt far in the future and thus influence the group for an extended period of time. It is a wise group that is able to make good decisions, and to rescind those found to be poor.

Conflict

Conflict is struggle over claims to scarce status, power, or resources in which the aim of the opponents are to neutralize, injure, or eliminate their rival. Conflict may occur between group members or between the group and the wider social system.

Conflict is a natural phenomenon; it is a response to the reality that there is a shortage of what people need and want. No group has sufficient resources to fulfill all internal needs and to meet all external demands. In a group, there is a scarcity of freedom, position, and rewards. So long as people value freedom, it is inevitable that there will be conflict between this idea and the demands for some degree of conformity, which is inherent in every group. Some people are more competent than others or more powerful. Positional conflict is unavoidable; in most groups there is some sort of a hierarchial structure with some people on the top and others on the bottom. Groups accept and reward some members more fully than others, creating another source of conflict. Although the above is described in relation to a group, a similar statement could be made in regards to the situation between the group and the broader social system.

Conflict can have a positive effect on a group. Some of the positive or functional effects of conflict are to: (a) eliminate sources of dissatisfaction, (b) revitalize existing norms in the group or alter inappropriate norms, (c) readjust the balance of power, (d) reduce an individual's social isolation, and (e) restructure the external environment by assigning different positions to the various groups which it contains.

Conflict is dysfunctional only when the group has no or insufficient toleration for or ways of dealing with conflict. It is not the conflict that is dysfunctional but rigidity of the group which permits hostilities to accumulate and to be channeled along one major path once they come out in the open. An analogy in regard to conflict is that functional conflict can be likened to putting out small brush fires, and dysfunctional conflict to having a conflagration with which to deal.

Power and Deviancy

Power is the capacity to influence others. It is an important concept in the understanding of group dynamics for two reasons: all groups have some sort of a power structure and the process of socialization into a group implies a certain type of power relation between the individual and the group.

Five basic sources of power have been identified. Briefly they are:

1. reward—the ability to give something to others that they need or desire such as money, scarce resources, attention, and affection;
2. coercive—the ability to punish in some way or to inflict a penalty such as the loss of an anticipated reward, rejection, ridicule and extra work;
3. legitimate—usually related to some official position that gives the individual the right to prescribe the behavior of others;
4. referent—comes from the person or people who are influenced, derived from their identification with or desire to be like an admired person, who then comes to have power relative to these individuals;
5. expert—derived from an individual's special knowledge or skills that are seen as important to others.

An individual's power may come from one or several of the sources outlined above. On the whole, the broader an individual's power base, the more power that person is able to wield.

Individuals without power often feel some degree of alienation from the group or, for that matter, from the broader social system in general. They may or may not be motivated to seek power. Power cannot be given; it must be taken. A person may be given power to use, temporarily, but the power is not in essence his or hers; it may be withdrawn at any time. Taking power is difficult because it is not given up easily. Those in the power structure resist because of an unwillingness to share power. When power is taken, there is frequently a feeling on the part of the one who has taken the power that those who previously had more power must be removed. This is done both to prove one's position and to ensure that the position will remain secure. Most people do not share power well, or with much style and grace.

As mentioned, the socialization process implies a certain type of power relationship between the individual and the group. The group usually, but not always, has more influence over the behavior of any given member than that member has over the behavior of the group. There are three major ways that the individual responds positively to the influence of the group. The individual may comply with the requirements of group life because the group has the power to manipulate rewards and punishment. Such an influence is usually restricted primarily to the behavior that the individual perceives as subject to the observation of the group. Second, the individual may identify with the group, accepting its influence because of wanting to establish or maintain a satisfying relationship with the group. The individual consciously takes on expected reciprocal role relationships relative to other group members. Third, the individual internalizes the norms, values, attitudes, and behavioral responses characteristic of the group and accepts the influence of the group because the ideals of the group are intrinsically rewarding.

Ideas and behavior adapted in this way tend to be integrated with the individual's existing ideas and behavior. Satisfaction is due to the affinity for the new behavior as opposed to identification, where satisfaction is due to being accepted by the group.

The socialization process does not always go smoothly or end successfully. During the process the individual may take on one or more deviant roles. Some of these individually centered rather than group-centered roles follow.

The aggressor finds ways of deflating the status of others; expressing disapproval of the values, acts, or feelings of others; and attacking the group or the problem it is working on.

The blocker tends to be negativistic and stubbornly resistant, disagreeing and opposing without reason and attempting to maintain or bring back an issue after the group has dealt with it in some way.

The recognition-seeker works in various ways to call attention to him- or herself whether through boasting, reporting on personal achievements, or acting in unusual ways.

The bon vivant makes a display of lack of involvement in the group. This may take the form of cynicism, nonchalance, horseplay, and other more or less studied forms of nonserious behavior.

The dominator tries to assert authority or superiority in manipulating the group or certain members of the group. Domination may take the form of flattery, of asserting a superior status or right to attention, giving directions authoritatively, interrupting the contributions of others, and so forth.

The help-seeker attempts to call forth sympathetic responses from other group members or from the whole group through expressions of insecurity, personal confusion, or self-depreciation.

The deviant individual is subjected to pressures to bring his or her behavior more in line with the expectations of the group. These pressures will be respected if the group is seen as valuable. If the individual insists on maintaining a deviant position, however, the group may threaten rejection. The degree to which the group is attractive to the individual will determine whether that person selects another form of behavior that will prevent exclusion by the group. A considerable amount of attention is usually given to the deviant person, with the hopes of altering behavior. If such attention is unsuccessful, the individual may be rejected from the group or leave of his or her own accord. On the other hand, the individual may rebel, rejecting all of the values and norms of the group. Or the individual may take a stance of exaggerated conformity. This is not considered to be a particularly functional group role as the individual tends not to contribute to the group; that person is essentially just there. Finally, the individual may be more creative, accepting only the pivotal values and norms of the group, and ignoring the rest.

It should be noted that groups vary considerably in regard to the amount of deviant behavior that they will tolerate. Frequently the more cohesive the group, the less it is able to tolerate deviant behavior. Nevertheless, some highly cohesive groups are able to countenance one or two highly deviant members. Toleration of deviancy is not necessarily equilateral across the group. Some members may be allowed to engage in relatively or even highly deviant behavior without much response from the group. Such nonconformists usually have considerable power relative to the group. Their degree of power places them in a privileged position not enjoyed by other group members. Occasionally an individual without any particular power base is allowed to be deviant because of a group need. The deviant individual, in this case, is permitted, or even encouraged, to engage in behavior in which other group members secretly would like to engage. The deviant acts out the fantasy of other group members.

CONCLUSION

The study of group dynamics has led some people to believe that everything should be done by and in a group. Individual responsibility is considered to be dangerous and dyadic interactions of any kind unhealthy, inexpedient, and not concerned with the welfare of any social system. It is as if such people believed that the individual is inherently evil or dangerous and thus needs to be controlled by the group. A more balanced point of view about the nature of groups would seem to be one based on the following assumptions: (a) groups are inevitable and ubiquitous; (b)groups mobilize powerful forces that produce effects of utmost importance relative to the social system; (c) groups may produce both good and bad consequences.

An understanding of group dynamics increases the possibility that desirable consequences from groups can be deliberately enhanced.

The responsible individual must determine what will be gained or lost as a result of any particular kind of group activity or as the result of solitary or dyadic interaction as opposed to a group effort.

13

Therapeutic Groups

This chapter will be devoted to a discussion of groups as a therapeutic tool. Discussion will be general in nature, applicable to verbal as well as activity groups (257,474,512,604,644,805,881,908,1013,1017,1043). The next chapter will deal more specifically with activity groups.

Groups as a therapeutic tool are based on the general assumption that psychosocial dysfunction, at least in part, is a disorder in interpersonal functioning. As such it can be more clearly understood and remedied in the context that gave rise to it in the first place. Groups play a major role in human growth and development and in the maintenance or undermining of the individual's well-being. Human beings live, work, and play in groups and thus are ill-equipped to survive without the capacity to interact effectively in groups.

There are eight other specific assumptions relative to therapeutic groups. First, groups provide all of the elements needed to promote change. They serve as a vehicle for the reduction of anxiety and a setting for reality testing. They provide feedback regarding behavior, information about alternatives that need to be considered, reinforcement of positive behavior, and nonsupport of negative behavior. The group furnishes new experiences designed to broaden the repertoire of knowledge and skills needed to cope with society.

Second, each person brings to the group idiosyncratic aims, needs, characteristic perceptions, and a sense of reality. Therefore, the acceptance of individual differences in growth and insight is vital to the atmosphere of the group.

Third, all groups move in three planes: (a) the manifest content of what is happening in the group, (b) the feelings being expressed in a variety of ways, and (c) the learning that occurs through the relationships group members establish with each other.

Fourth, to help people one needs to start with their perception of the situation. Help is more useful if it is initially directed toward the problem causing the individual and/or the group the most immediate concern.

Fifth, individuals have an innate capacity to deal with their own problems if they are provided a setting where they can feel secure enough to examine their situation.

Sixth, as an individual feels more secure, the need to shut out unwanted information decreases. This in turn enables the individual to view problems in a broader perspective, which by necessity must include the values and attitudes of society. Therefore the solution to a problem, although starting out as egocentric, must ultimately be related to the paradox that the individual can only satisfy his needs through others.

Seventh, a change in any part of an individual's life affects all other parts of his existence. Therefore the individual must investigate the ways in which he can modify his environment.

Eighth, the overall goal of group therapy is the personal development of individual members.

CONSIDERATIONS RELATIVE TO STRUCTURE

In this section each part of the structure of a group will be discussed relative to its influence on therapeutic groups. The structure of a group, if properly used, can have a positive effect on the intervention process. The therapist manipulates the structure in such a way that the group becomes a therapeutic tool.

Group Development

Every phase of a group has different characteristics. The therapist must be finely tuned to the phase a group is experiencing and regulate his behavior accordingly. It should be noted that the phases of a group overlap and that it is not unusual for a group to return periodically to an earlier phase.

Orientation Phase

An individual's reaction to any group is affected by the expectations that person has relative to the group. When expectations are not met in a group, the individual becomes less involved in the group and is less likely to gain from the situation. Thus, the therapist's first responsibility is to help group members set realistic expectations relative to the task and social-emotional aspects of the group. Here task refers to the goal or purpose of the group, e.g., evaluation, meeting health needs, prevention, maintenance, or change. Expectations relative to social-emotional aspects refers to what needs will be satisfied in the group and the degree to which the individual will be asked to express personal feelings and ideas. Preparing the client for entry into the group is very important. The client is told about the group, both the positive and negative aspects, as well as given an opportunity to express her concerns about entering and participating in the group. The better prepared the client is for the group experience, the more likely he or she is to use that experience wisely and well.

The therapist should be relatively permissive and accepting during the orientation phase, particularly in regard to group members' feelings about authority—negative or positive, realistic or unrealistic. It is also necessary for the therapist to help group members become acquainted and to facilitate adequate acceptance. Group members are encouraged to take appropriate membership roles and are given considerable assistance with beginning the task. In this phase the therapist may need to meet more of the social-emotional requirements of the group than will be necessary or even appropriate during subsequent phases. If some or all of the participants have been members of another group which they have recently left, they may need to mourn the old situation before they are able to participate in the new group. The therapist recognizes this need and helps the group members to express the sadness they are experiencing.

It is important in this phase that the therapist work out procedural matters with the group members. Ideally, this is accomplished through mutual agreement and becomes the contract between group members and between the therapist and the group. The procedures of concern are the time and length of each meeting, where the meetings will occur, when the group will end if it is time limited in nature, attendance and punctuality, holidays and vacations, type of contact outside of the group, behavior that is not acceptable within the context of the group, and what the therapist will and will not do. At this point there should be as few "rules" as possible. It is more productive for the group if the majority of procedural matters are dealt with as they arise in the course of interaction.

The above discussion is based on the assumption that the orientation phase has a positive tone. This may not be the case, particularly when membership in the group is not entirely voluntary. There may be considerable resistance and hostility and work on the task may be less than one would otherwise expect. The orientation phase in this case tends to be very short and blends almost immediately with the dissatisfaction phase. The resolution phase will also be concerned with resistance about being in the group.

Dissatisfaction and Resolution Phases

Before explicit attention is directed toward dissatisfaction, it should have been interfering with the task for some time. If attention is called to dissatisfaction too early, the group may resist acknowledging that there is any problem. Verbal acknowledgment of difficulties usually encourages members to address the problem in a fairly direct manner. The therapist assists the group by helping the members examine what they have achieved up to this point. It is helpful to discuss the goals and expectations of the group once again. It is also useful to be very specific about what the goals of the group are not. The roles that specific group members are currently taking in the group should be discussed as well as the extent to which these roles are productive relative to the task and the maintenance of group solidarity. Other aspects of the relationships between members and the relationship to the therapist should also be discussed. It is often useful to restate the nature of the task and to give increased attention to learning the skills necessary for the task and the application of these skills. Outlining the typical developmental stages of most groups sometimes gives the group hope for better times ahead. It also helps them to view their current problems from a more universal perspective rather than thinking present difficulties are a consequence of their inadequacies.

Productive Phase

Even in this most positive phase of group interaction, some difficulties may arise. The therapist must often help group members keep their skills at an appropriate level. If new goals are added, these may necessitate the learning of new skills. If subgoals are not attained in a reasonable length of time, the therapist may need to help the group from becoming discouraged. Periodic reassessment of what has been accomplished is useful. The task must not be allowed to become irrelevant; nor should social-emotional interests (unless they are part of the goal) be permitted to dominate the attention of the group. Fatigue with the task may occur and the therapist must pay appropriate attention to the periodic need for rest (e.g., a day off, doing something that is recreational in nature). The therapist encourages group members to be independent relative to his or her role as a leader and to take an increasing number of membership roles. Expectations are kept reasonable at all times.

Termination Phase

If the group is not time limited, the therapist, with the assistance of the group, must determine when optimal benefits have been realized. As the time for termination approaches, the task is completed as well as possible or brought to some kind of closure. The group evaluates what has been accomplished through a review of the overall experience. As the time for termination draws nearer, group members usually feel a sense of loss and sadness and frequently have difficulty saying goodbye. It is important for the therapist to help the group acknowledge both positive and negative feelings and the appropriateness of these mixed feelings. The therapist also helps group members to prepare for the next experience to come. The termination of a client from an ongoing group will be discussed later in the chapter.

Central Issues

Central issues predominate in therapy groups. In some groups, depending on the goal and the frame of reference being used, they serve as the vehicle for helping clients to deal with their problems in functioning. In other groups central issues are dealt with as they surface but other means are used as the primary vehicle.

It is very easy for a therapy group to become dominated by basic assumptions. This occurs because clients tend to have little skill in interpersonal relations or in openly discussing their personal feelings and ideas. The therapist, unless very watchful, can get caught up in the group's basic assumptions. When this happens, the group ceases to be a therapeutic tool and in fact can be quite detrimental. The best way to deal with groups dominated by basic assumptions is, obviously, not to let such domination develop in the first place. This is accomplished by dealing with central issues immediately once they become evident rather than putting them off, hoping they will become reconciled spontaneously. If by chance a group should become primarily motivated by basic assumptions, the best course of action usually is to suspend all supposedly goal-directed activity until the basic assumptions are brought to the surface and explored. Dealing with central issues essentially involves taking the role of an expressive leader and providing feedback. This was discussed in Chapter 12.

To the list of central issues previously outlined, therapy groups typically have a few others. These are fear of personal inadequacy, discomfort over admitting the need for help, confusion about responsibility for self or others, and uncertainty about what constitutes reality. These issues, although occurring in groups other than therapy groups, are more likely to become central issues in therapy groups.

Of all of the central issues, dependency seems to be the most prevalent. This may be due to the sick role as it is traditionally seen by the dominant culture, or it may be due to the feeling of helplessness and inadequacy which is so often a part of psychosocial dysfunction. Wanting to be dependent and concern about being dependent generate a whole set of conflicting messages directed toward the therapist: to be omnipotent, resign; to be strong, capitulate; to be nurturing and loving, remain aloof and impartial. The issue of dependency can become further colored by conflict or confusion relative to the primary task of the group. All therapy groups are designed to help clients ultimately become more independent. However, groups where the therapist teaches specific skills (e.g., work habits, activities of daily living) may appear to put group members in a dependent position vis-à-vis the therapist. In this situation the therapist must stress the ultimate goal of autonomy and design the learning experience so that clients become increasingly independent.

Although not usually identified as a central issue, the issue of a "here and now" orientation versus a "then and there" orientation is a source of concern in many therapy groups. Where a group is supposed to be on the here and now–then and there continuum varies with the goals and theoretical orientation of the group. Regardless of where the group is supposed to be, however, there tends to be difficulty in maintaining the desired place on the continuum. Therapists who wish to use the group members' present participation in the group as a means of helping them to learn new patterns of behavior may find the group focusing on past behavior and difficulties as a means of avoiding change. Conversely, therapists who wish to use present participation as a springboard to group members' understanding of their past may find the group preoccupied with the immediate situation. This too is a means of avoiding the task of the group.

The here and now of the group is always an important factor. Clients actively dealing with their here and now problems are more likely to see the relevance of the group activity. They are more likely to be able to generalize from current experiences to past ones, which may take on new meaning. To the degree to which present perceptions can be related to the past, it is possible for the person to determine if he or she wishes to continue in the same direction in the future. The therapist needs to help group members make sense of the here and now experience perhaps in terms of past behavior but most assuredly in terms of future expectations.

Roles in Groups

The therapist, concerned with optimal participation of group members and their development of functional skills, encourages role diversity. Such an orientation is tempered, of course, by the current capacity of group members. The therapist's expectations need to be well matched with what is possible and probable on the part of group members. To facilitate the taking of a variety of roles, the therapist participates in only those group membership roles that are necessary for the continuation of the group at a particular moment in time. This encourages other group members to see the necessity for various membership roles and gives them an opportunity to experiment with these roles. As a complement to this stance on the part of the therapist, there are some other methods that may be used to increase role flexibility. Some of the methods that have been found useful are: (a) discussion of the various membership roles, why they are necessary for the adequate function of a group, and the behavior that constitutes the various roles; (b) periodic assessment of the group by group members in regard to the roles currently being played and the need for additional or different roles; (c) role playing of various membership roles; and (d) members acting as observers of the group so as to see roles and role requirements from a more uninvolved position.

The therapist plays a key, if not pivotal, role in a therapy group. To be an effective therapist in a group, the individual must examine his or her own beliefs about the individual, mind and personality, what justifies the means to a goal, and where do the rights of a person end and the rights of society begin. The leader needs to identify his or her own goals and clarify values in order to develop a yardstick for evaluating performance.

The therapist is responsible for the selection and preparation of members for the group. Throughout the course of the group's existence, the therapist's superordinate task is to prevent member attrition, to deflect any forces that threaten group cohesiveness, and to create a viable social system. The therapist must form a consistent, positive relationship with the group—a relationship characterized by concern, acceptance, genuineness, and empathy. The therapist ideally fosters an environment in which the capacities of each member are protected and utilized so that each will be enabled to develop in his own way at his own pace without restricting the development of other members. The requirements of the task and the structure and composition of the group defines the kind of leadership role the therapist needs to take.

Initially, the therapist usually takes the majority of membership roles, being essentially a combined instrumental and expressive leader. As such, the therapist plays what is, at times, two conflicting roles. To be supportive while demanding attention to the task is a complex process that requires considerable skill. In order to minimize the conflict, the therapist often emphasizes one role over another in reciprocal sequence. Thus at times the therapist may take primarily an instrumental role, then primarily an expressive role, back to a more instrumental role, and so forth. In the situation where there are co-therapists, one may take an instrumental role and the other an expressive role. On the other hand, they each may take these roles in a reciprocal sequence.

As members learn to take on various group roles, the leader relinquishes these roles and reinforces their being played by group members. There are those who suggest the therapist give up the position of authority as soon as possible and seek membership status. The therapist is then in a position to interact with others on the basis of equality. This may, indeed, be the ideal, but it is certainly not the typical situation. Many members in groups, even in their collectivity, are unable to take all of the roles necessary for the accomplishment of the goals of a therapy group. As much as the therapist encourages members to take functional group roles, the therapist remains responsible for the overall direction of the group.

The dynamics of a group are much more complex than those of a client-therapist dyad. Because of the complexity, the therapist may be tempted to abandon the role of the leader of the group and retreat to the dyadic stance, relating directly to each individual group member. The leader is not as influential, not as much in control in a group as in a dyad. The leader is also the focus of much more intense and varied emotional forces. The ambiguous feelings and dissatisfaction are frequently directed at the leader because of authority, power, and personal characteristics. The leader is the individual in the group who is most likely to be idealized, castigated, and misunderstood. The therapist must be able to come to grips with the interpersonal complexities of the group in order to meet the requirements of group leadership.

The demands of therapy group leadership are such that co-leadership is fairly common. A co-therapist may be a student or beginning therapist, or the two leaders may be of equal status. The student-established leader combination allows the neophyte to learn the leadership role under the guidance of a skilled practitioner who is able to monitor the neophyte's behavior and give help and support. The drawback of this arrangement is that the difference in experiential levels may lead to tension and conflict, which the group may exploit. Co-leaders of equal status are often recommended as the ideal. They benefit from the peer involvement and are stimulated to learn from each other. Clients are able to benefit from the co-therapists' combined insight and technical skill.

Co-therapists are often recommended for those groups which are designed primarily to focus on individuals' problems as they originated in family relationships, or which focus on family-related problems. Such leadership facilitates simulation of a family-like group and provides a model for relating and communicating in that context. The equal status of the leaders is important in this situation because it portrays the possibility of the partner relationship being egalitarian in nature. There is really no need for the co-leaders to be of the opposite sex. Regardless of sex, the leaders tend to take complementary roles and attitudes.

Co-leadership, however, is not without problems. Some of the difficulties that can arise are: (a) working at cross purposes—often arising from differences relative to goals, philosophy, theoretical orientations, and training; (b) difficulty in working together because of differences in personality and interaction styles; (c) poor planning and communication, so that the co-therapists do not know who is going to do what, and when; and (d) failure to give attention to the progress of their own relationship, leading, for example, to one leader taking over, supporting clients against the other, trying to prove that one leader is nicer or better and so forth.

A good relationship between co-therapists is characterized by mutual respect, acceptance, and shared responsibility. The relationship will affect the group, with a positive relationship between co-therapists being highly correlated with the accomplishment of group goals. To maintain an adequate working relationship, co-therapists need to meet together regularly to discuss the group, to assess progress that has been made, and to plan future strategy. Co-therapists should not expect to have a problem-free relationship; differences of opinion are bound to arise. Joint supervision or consultation is useful not only when there is a problem but also as a means of increasing the effectiveness of the two leaders.

The therapist should be careful in selecting a co-leader, paying particular attention to personality and theoretical compatibility, ability, and willingness on the other's part to work as a team. Everyone should not expect to be interested in being a co-leader; some therapists prefer working as the sole leader of a group. In addition, all groups do not need co-leaders. Co-leadership is not necessarily an efficient use of therapeutic time and it is twice as expensive as sole leadership.

Group Goals

As in any primary group, therapy groups are more effective if the goals are explicit and clearly stated. It is the therapist's responsibility to define the goals of the group. Members are then selected in part on the basis of matching their needs with the goals of the group.

The goals of therapy groups vary tremendously. The different goals are not necessarily mutually exclusive; one group may have two or more goals. Goals only in part reflect a particular theoretical orientation. Two groups, for example, may have quite similar goals but the theoretical system that influences the means may be very dissimilar. A taxonomy of goals for verbal therapy groups is outlined below. A taxonomy, used to describe activity groups, will be presented in Chapter 14.

There appears to be six major categories of goals for verbal groups. The first category is the identification of the roots of the individual's problem. Through interaction in the here and now of the group, the individual is helped to view his or her problems as they originated in past relationships.

The second category is the understanding of behavior as it presently exists. The source of the individual's problems are not the chief concern but rather the group is directed toward identifying what members are currently doing that is causing them difficulty. Emphasis is on how the individual affects others and how others affect him.

Problem solving is the third category. The group's focus is on dealing with predetermined problems. Thus membership is quite homogeneous, selected on the basis of a common area of difficulty. Such problems as addiction, child abuse, retirement, adolescent adjustment, and so forth may be dealt with in this type of group. Focus is usually on how to solve or cope with the problem. Various solutions, typically, are identified and tried outside of the group.

The fourth category is the development of social interaction skills. The group is focused on encouraging interaction and communication among members. The therapist is primarily concerned with helping members to learn appropriate ways of engaging with others.

The fifth category involves being supportive. The focus of this type of group is to help members maintain as high a functional level as possible. Psychological defenses as they currently exist are reinforced and anxiety is kept at a minimum. Everyday problems of interacting in and coping with the environment are dealt with, in a fairly concrete manner, as they are raised by group members.

The sixth category involves dealing with situational stress. The problems dealt with in this type of group, in most cases, are secondary to physical illness, social dislocation, required change in life style, death, and so forth. Emphasis is placed on decreasing anxiety and frustration, providing factual knowledge about the situation, and maintaining the individual's sense of dignity and self-worth. With such assistance it is anticipated that the individual will become more integrated and able to cope with the situation at hand.

As mentioned, many groups have multiple goals. No single group may fall into only one of the categories discussed above.

Group Norms

The norms of therapeutic groups must be such that they facilitate attainment of group goals. As the above discussion indicated, the goals of therapeutic groups vary, as do appropriate norms. For example, a norm that emphasizes the importance of a high degree of self-disclosure would be appropriate in a group concerned with identifying the roots of an individual's problem. It would not be appropriate in a group concerned with the development of social interaction skills. There are, however, some norms that are necessary for all therapeutic groups regardless of goals. These are honesty, spontaneity, free interaction, nonjudgmental acceptance of others, mutual respect, dissatisfaction with present modes of behavior, and eagerness for maintenance of one's current level of function or for change. It is through a group culture characterized by such norms that the curative factors of a group are able to operate effectively.

Some of the norms of a therapeutic group may be stated explicitly by the therapist at the inception of the group. These norms tend to be procedural in nature and, as mentioned, are usually related to such matters as attendance, behavior that will not be tolerated in the group situation, and so forth. Other norms are less explicitly stated and tend to be developed through the therapist's acting as a role model and reinforcing behavior likely to lead to attainment of the defined goals.

The therapist, however, is only one member of the group. Even given the position of the therapist relative to power, therapeutic groups tend to develop and comply with norms that are compatible with their present level of function. This is a self-protective maneuver to deal with the immediate stress of the situation, a natural response. Such a response may be corrected spontaneously by the group after a short period of time; if it is not, the therapist needs to intervene. One way the therapist may change an interfering norm is to act outside of the structures of the norm. This helps group members to understand that noncompliance with the norm is acceptable, not detrimental to self-integrity or harmful to others. The therapist may also bring the dysfunctional nature of the norm to the group's attention. The way in which the norm is interfering with goal attainment is outlined as well as, perhaps, some of the reasons why the norm came into being. Bringing the incompatibility of the norm and the goals of the group to conscious awareness often helps the group to alter or eliminate the norms. The process of altering a norm is not something that happens quickly or without some distress. It is a long-term process, accompanied by some anxiety. Demands on the part of the therapist are rarely effective; gentle firmness is.

Communication

Adequate communication is central to any helping process. The majority of people who seek assistance with psychosocial problems have some difficulty in the area of communication: they may not know what other people mean; they may not know what they mean; they feel they are misunderstood. The therapist's task then is to assist group members in examining their words and behavior to see if they represent what the client wishes to communicate. There are several techniques to facilitate the process.

- Questioning: drawing the client out and asking what the client is trying to express, what the client is thinking and feeling
- Clarifying: identifying and giving labels to feelings and behavior, accenting or underscoring, emphasizing
- Reflecting: restating what it appears the client is trying to say
- Interpreting: making connections between feelings and actions, giving meaning to an experience, linking up past experiences with present behavior
- Confronting: requesting a client to look at how he or she is perceived by others in contrast with what the client would like to believe others are perceiving
- Summarizing: reviewing important points that are related and restating them in a brief form
- Informing: giving information or advice, contrasting and sharing alternatives, identifying possible consequences, using hypothetical situations and examples
- Structuring: statement of the "rules" of the helping process either verbally or by the way the therapist does or does not act in specific situations, defining and clarifying expectations, and group goals
- Silence: allowing group members time to think their own thoughts in their own way

The above techniques are designed to help group members discover what they are saying and doing relative to meaning. There are other techniques that facilitate communication in general. Some of these are: (a) reassuring, encouraging, and supporting; (b) creating and maintaining an optimal amount of tension; (c) using oneself as a role model relative to clear, concise, and meaningful communication; (d) focusing communication on the client's self-interest; (e) encouraging and allowing emotional catharsis; (f) persuasion; (g) environmental manipulation such as seating arrangement or structure of the workplace; and (h) simulated experiences such as role playing or doing exercises to illustrate a point. Most of all the therapist needs to communicate that he or she cares.

One of the most important communication processes in a therapeutic group is feedback. Feedback describing personal assets is usually received with feelings of well-being; feedback regarding deficiencies is often followed by feelings of anxiety and depression. Therefore, positive feedback is considered to be far better than negative feedback. In addition, people tend not to believe negative feedback; positive feedback thus has a higher informational value. Behavioral feedback in conjunction with verbal feedback is more effective than either type of feedback given alone. Positive feedback delivered publicly increases both the believability of the information given and feelings of self-worth. The therapist, therefore, gives as much positive public feedback as possible. In addition, the therapist provides opportunities for group members to give more feedback to each other than would usually occur spontaneously. This type of feedback also enhances group cohesiveness.

Group Cohesiveness

In order for therapeutic groups to reach their goals there must be a relatively high degree of cohesiveness. Such cohesiveness provides the security necessary for identifying and trying out new, more adaptive kinds of behavior. However, the cohesiveness of the group should not be too high. Excessive cohesiveness sometimes leads to such a feeling of togetherness and self-sufficiency that the group does not attend to what is occurring in, and the demands of, the wider social system. The group and the culture of the group become reality for group members and a haven from the ambiguities and conflicts of the broader environment. Excessive cohesiveness can also interfere with exploring alternate ways of behaving. Group members inhibit each other's growth because they fear change will decrease the feeling of togetherness of the group. Finally, excessive cohesiveness may interfere with a group member's appropriate departure from the group. A client's membership in a therapy group is usually temporary in nature. The ultimate purpose of group participation is to prepare the client to return to and function more effectively in the community. Departure from a highly cohesive group is very difficult. Thus the leader's task is to maintain cohesiveness at an optimal level: sufficiently high to provide a safe environment for change and growth, but not so high that change and growth are impeded.

Decision Making

Factors interfering with adequate decision making were discussed in the last chapter. Some ways in which decision making may be improved in a therapeutic group are: (a) open discussion of fear regarding the consequences of a decision and giving support to members who are experiencing anxiety; (b) discussion of conflicting loyalties so as to help group members to test whether the differences are basic or merely surface conflicts that can be adjusted; (c) creation of a group atmosphere in which conflict can be openly recognized and explored regardless of whether it is related to the decision to be made or personal antipathy; (d) clear formulation of the problem and related issues; (e) adequate techniques for collecting data; (f) open and free discussion of opinions and value; (g) adequate time allowed for exploration prior to arriving at a decision; and (h) helping group members to take appropriate membership roles.

The decisions to be made by the group should be carefully selected so that they are compatible with the collective knowledge and skill of the group. To ask a group to make a decision they are not capable of or ready to make is inviting unnecessary problems. A group should be asked to make only those decisions that they have the power or right to make. Going through a decision-making process to discover that one ultimately does not have the right to make the decision is demeaning at best and a thorough waste of time. If a therapist is to have veto power over a decision made by the group, this should be made quite clear initially, not after the fact. When the therapist maintains the right to veto a decision, possible reasons for disallowing the decision to stand are given before the group enters into the decision-making process. If a decision is vetoed, the therapist explains the reasons in detail. Sometimes a group does not have the right to make a decision but participation in the decision-making process is considered desirable. In this case the group is asked to serve in an advisory capacity to the therapist. When the therapist makes the subsequent decision, the process whereby the decision was made and the reason for the decision is discussed with the group. This helps the group to learn more about the decision-making process and to perceive their part in the decision that was made. The ability to participate in group decision making is an important skill for group members to acquire. Every opportunity should be made available for the practice of this skill.

Conflict

There are several common sources of conflict in therapeutic groups. There may be conflict between group norms or the norms of the group and those of the external environment. The latter usually relate to issues that are allowed to be discussed, behavior permitted, and the open expression of affection and hostility. There may be conflict between the group goals and the goals set by the external environment as appropriate for the group. Relative to activity groups, for example, the external environment may perceive accomplishment of the activity as the primary goal of the group. The activity is viewed by the group as only a vehicle for accomplishing the goals of the group. There may be conflict between group members' desire for increased growth and fear of change. Finally, there may be conflict between a group member's desire to avoid recognition of maladaptive behavior and the group's demand that such behavior be recognized and changed.

There are several ways of dealing with conflict in a therapeutic group. The therapist often needs to help the group to develop and maintain norms that permit the recognition and expression of hostility. The source of conflict needs to be identified so that in discussion the real issues may be dealt with rather than superficial or extraneous issues. The therapist usually encourages open discussion of conflict. Addressing the situation directly rather than avoidance or token discussion is recommended. The discussion should be kept to the real issues rather than allowing individuals to discuss the inadequacies of the persons involved. The therapist gives extra support to group members who have difficulty expressing hostility or dealing with conflict.

Power and Deviancy

There is considerable power latent in groups. A number of people acting in concert deliver a greater quantity of more credible information to each other than any one of the individuals would be able to deliver alone. Group members exert a tremendous amount of influence on each other. It is the therapist's responsibility to mobilize the influence of group members and to help them to use it wisely. The group leader assists individuals to motivate, reinforce, act as models, and give accurate information to each other.

The therapist also has power in his or her own right. This is derived from legitimate sources as well as from expertise and group members' identification. The therapist may also have power derived from the capacity to give rewards or to levy a penalty. The therapist too must learn to use power wisely. There are times when it may be necessary to use power vis-à-vis group members as a leverage for change. It usually is recommended, however, that the therapist use power sparingly because it places group members in a highly dependent position. Helping group members to influence each other in the direction of positive growth is usually considered the appropriate role of the therapist.

Some of the problems presented by deviant group members and ways of dealing with these problems have been discussed throughout this section. There will be further discussion in the final section of this chapter.

CURATIVE FACTORS

Irvin Yalom has identified twelve curative factors in groups (1043). He sees change in therapeutic groups occurring as through an intricate interplay of various guided human experiences. The twelve factors are considered to be interdependent, often representing different parts of the change process. Some of the factors refer to actual mechanisms of change; others are more accurately described as conditions of change. A few of these factors have been discussed previously. They are briefly stated once again so as not to interfere with the integrity of Yalom's ideas. The twelve factors are as follows.

1. Instillation of hope. This is derived from seeing that others have similar problems with which they are able to cope somewhat more effectively. It is also derived from observing improvement of others and the therapist's belief in self and the efficacy of the group. Hope not only helps to keep the client in the group but it is also therapeutic in and of itself.

2. Universality. Most individuals in a state of psychosocial dysfunction think that they are unique in their wretchedness. This is heightened by their social isolation and lack of opportunity for consensual validation. In a group situation the individual is able to perceive similarity to others. This in turn leads to the sharing of one's deepest concerns. Group members benefit from such an experience and from the ultimate acceptance by other group members. Universality can be broadened by the therapist who uses various myths, stories, and plays that speak eloquently to the human condition as it has been passed from generation to generation and across cultures. The sharing of this collective knowledge with the group often helps group members realize that their particular problems are not singular to them or other members of the group, that such problems have been faced by the human species probably since the dawn of consciousness.

3. Imparting information. Information about mental health, illness, psychodynamics, advice, suggestions, and direct guidance in regards to life problems is seen by many group members as extremely helpful. The information provided may be explicit as in didactic instruction or discussion or it may be presented in a more implicit manner. Giving information is more than its content; it implies and conveys mutual interest and caring. To be able to ask for suggestions and to give them unselfishly links individuals in a shared experience.

4. Altruism. To give to others is as important as receiving help. The intrinsic act of giving makes people feel they have something of worth to give. It makes little difference what is given: support, reassurance, suggestions, insight, sharing similar problems. Giving counteracts aloneness and marked self-absorption.

5. The corrective recapitulation of the Primary Family Group. Transference, which is likely to occur spontaneously in groups, allows the earlier experiences with parents and siblings to be reexplored. It is important that these be relived in a way that faulty perceptions are altered and new ways of interacting acquired. To do this, behavioral stereotypes must be constantly challenged; reality testing, exploration of relationships, and experimenting with new behaviors is encouraged. The group needs to avoid freezing into rigid ways of interacting, which is typical of many families.

6. Development of socialization techniques. Socialization is used here in the sense of the ability to interact comfortably with others. Groups provide an opportunity to learn basic social skills and to receive feedback in regard to social behavior.

7. Imitative behavior. Individuals benefit from observing the behavior of other group members and an opportunity to try out a variety of different modes of behavior. Imitation can be quite diffuse in that there are many models, and the individual can select from any behavior of any member of the group. Even if imitation is short lived it may help the individual to set aside stereotypical ways of interacting by experimenting with new behavior.

8. Interpersonal learning. A freely interacting group with few structural restrictions will in time develop into a microcosm of the larger social system. Group members collectively will express the values and ideas of the wider community, and will present the same demands, illogical behavior, and so forth. As in the larger social system, all types of maladaptive interpersonal behavior will be displayed. There is no need for members to describe their maladaptive behavior; they will act it out in the group. In this way a group is a laboratory where members can see their own behavior, what triggers it, and the response of others. The social microcosm created by the group also provides a realistic setting for trying out and determining the effects of new behavior.

9. Group cohesiveness. The cohesiveness of the group encourages the affectual sharing of one's inner world. In the conditions of acceptance, the individual is more inclined to express and explore ideas and feelings. In knowing and accepting parts of themselves, group members are able to relate more deeply to others and self-esteem is increased.

10. Catharsis and corrective emotional experiences. Catharsis is the process of ridding oneself of suppressed or held back feelings and ideas. It is the process of expressing strong emotional content. Although catharsis gives temporary relief, in and of itself it is not enough for change to occur. Ideally catharsis occurs within the context of a corrective emotional experience. This refers to a strong expression of emotion which is interperson-

ally directed and which represents a risk on the part of the client. An illustration of a corrective emotional experience is an individual for the first time really being able to express positive feelings toward another person. Through such an experience the individual comes to recognize the inappropriateness of avoiding certain ideas, feelings, and behavior. Ultimately this enables the individual to interact with others more honestly and more profoundly. A corrective emotional experience cannot occur unless the group is sufficiently supportive to permit the necessary risk taking. Reality testing with consensual validation must be a part of the experience as well as reflection on the experience. In addition the experience needs to include learning how to express such feelings regularly and in an appropriate manner. Emotional expression alone is not effective. The dual emotional and cognitive components of the experience are what allows it to facilitate change.

11. Existential factors. The existential factors in groups seem to consist of: (a) recognition that life is at times unfair and unjust; (b) recognition that ultimately there is no escape from some of life's pain and from death; (c) recognition that no matter how intimately one becomes involved with another person, one still faces life alone; (d) the idea of facing the basic issues of life and death and thus living one's life more honestly and being less caught up in trivialities; and (e) learning that one must take ultimate responsibility for the way that one lives one's life no matter how much guidance and support one gets from others.

This factor is derived from a melding of two elements: existential philosophy, which emphasizes choice, freedom, responsibility, and meaning in life, and a humanistic orientation, which emphasizes human potential, awareness, peak experiences, self-realization, and intimate interactions with others. The existential/humanistic orientation locates the source of support for the individual on each person's dependency on his fellow man and his willingness to help others since in the process he helps himself. The ultimate goal of intervention is seen as self-actualization or finding meaning in life. A group situation is seen as ideal for accomplishing such a goal. It is believed that self-actualization can never be attained through deliberate, self-conscious pursuit. Rather it is a derivative phenomenon that is attained only when the individual has transcended the self. Only when one has forgotten himself in an absorption in someone else can one find meaning in life. The group's focus on such issues as illness, death of others, termination, and loss is seen as one way of tapping and using existential factors in the course of intervention.

12. The desire to know. Yalom questions whether this should be considered one of the curative factors in groups. It is included here as one of the factors because there seems to be considerable evidence in the literature to support its importance.

The desire to know is described as the cognitive component of the therapeutic process. It is the need to have explanations. Such explanations decrease anxiety by removing ambiguity, by eliminating a minuscule portion of the unknown, and by inching back the darkness. Having explanations is the first step in control of any phenomenon, including the self. The desire to know is basic to the need for self-understanding. A group experience provides this understanding through the availability of information and feedback. Self-understanding promotes change because it encourages the individual to recognize, integrate, and give free expression to previously dissociated parts of the self.

Finally, Yalom briefly discusses the curative factors that exist outside of the group. He speaks of an "adaptive spiral" wherein a change in the client leads to changes in extragroup interpersonal environment, which leads to further personal change. The group experience is seen as mobilizing members to take advantage of environmental resources which in fact had long been available. The group experience removes personal obstructions that had previously interfered with the development of the client's own network of support.

The degree to which the various curative factors outlined above influence a particular therapeutic group depends on the goals of the group, the theoretical approach, and the capacity of group members. Similar to considerations relative to structure, the suggested curative factors are used selectively with more or less emphasis. Selection and emphasis is ultimately determined by the needs of a particular group.

COMPOSITION OF GROUPS AND PROCEDURAL MATTERS

There are several things that must be considered in beginning a group. The first step is to determine whether a group is necessary: what client needs are not being met, and can these needs be met most effectively in a group. There may be a variety of needs, thus the therapist sets some priorities determining which needs are most pressing. With this general survey, the therapist becomes more specific and outlines the goals of the proposed group. It is suggested that the goals be few in number and, if possible, stated operationally. Groups with few and precisely stated goals are usually far more successful than groups with numerous goals, which are vaguely stated. It is wise to remember that no group can fulfill all of the client needs that may be present in a particular setting. If the stated goals of the group do not dictate the theoretical base for the group, this is then selected by the therapist. Again, specificity is very important. Finally the therapist determines the methods to be used. Although methods are usually influenced by the theoretical base, they should nonetheless be clearly stated. Methods include the role of the therapist, communication techniques to be used, and learning experiences such as role playing. All of the above are in relationship to verbal groups. The occupational therapist would also include selection of appropriate activities.

Two other procedural issues, size and whether the group will be open or closed, need to be determined before membership selection. It has been found that groups of less than 5 and more than 10 are not conducive to attaining goals common to therapy groups. A group of less than 5 often does not have enough variety and points of views to allow the group to serve as a social microcosm. Groups larger than 10 usually present so much variation and complexity that it is difficult for therapist and group members alike to attend to and keep track of all that is going on. Seven or eight members in a group is usually an ideal size. In activity groups, the type of activity may influence the number of participants. For example, if cooking is to be used as an activity, the group should probably be no more than 5 members. A group that makes use of team sports, on the other hand, may comfortably be as large as 12 to 14 members. The extent to which the therapist is required to be directly involved in the activity may also limit group size.

Most therapy groups are closed or semi-closed. A closed group is one in which once the membership is selected and stabilized; no new members are added to the group. Closed groups usually have a defined beginning and end, with termination for all members occurring at the same time. A semi-closed group adds new members only if the group is less than the desired size or if one group member leaves. Semi-closed groups tend to be ongoing in nature, with new members being added periodically and termination taking place on an individual basis. An open group, where there is considerable movement of people in and out of the group, is usually considered undesirable because it may impede learning. Some groups are open, however, particularly those that occur in a setting where clients tend to stay for a short period of time. The goals for such groups tend to be supportive in nature or involve dealing with situational stress.

After completion of the preliminary work described above, the therapist is ready to select members for the group. The ideas outlined below are general in nature because actual selection will depend to a great extent on the goals of a particular group. The degree to which any group can represent society as a whole will affect the usefulness of that group as a testing ground for ideas and behavior. For this reason, considerable heterogeneity of group membership is suggested. On the other hand, group members must have a sufficient degree of commonality to allow for the development of cohesiveness and mutual concern. Common problem areas, but not necessarily similar diagnoses, are considered one good way of establishing some degree of homogeneity in a group. It is also considered expedient for group members to be at approximately the same level of emotional maturity, especially in regard to the immediacy of infantile needs versus more sophisticated ways of handling such needs. Another suggested homogeneous factor is similar intelligence and degree of cognitive development. This will influence the level at which ideas can be conceptualized and communicated. Heterogeneity relative to age, sex, and cultural background is frequently recommended. There are times, however, when it may be better for a group to be homogeneous in respect to these factors: groups designed to deal with specific developmental tasks, e.g., problems particular to women returning to work and family issues.

The issue of homogeneity/heterogeneity aside, it is the mix, the chemistry of the group that needs to be given attention. The therapist attempts to select a group of people who in their collectivity are motivated, able to communicate, sufficiently assertive, and capable of playing a variety of group roles. Group members then are selected or rejected in terms of the conditions under which the group is conducted, compatibility with other members, and the goals of the group. An individual may not be appropriate for a particular group but that does not mean he or she is inappropriate for all groups.

The above-mentioned factors—group goals, theoretical base, method, size, whether the group is open or closed, and criteria for membership—are usually outlined in what is referred to as a group protocol. This document is essentially a plan for the group which the therapist intends to follow. It serves both as a guide for the therapist and as a means of communicating to others about the nature of the group. This latter function of a protocol helps other staff members to understand the group and to refer clients appropriately.

In a semi-closed group, new members are periodically added. One, of course, may only be able to reject those candidates that are grossly inappropriate. On the other hand, the therapist may have more choice. The potential member should be ready to join a group. With the exception of a group designed to deal with situational stress, it is not a good idea to place a person in a group at the time of a specific crisis in his or her life. At this time the individual tends to be self-preoccupied, concerned with maintaining some semblance of integration, and totally disinterested in the problems of others. Most clients when first admitted to a mental health facility are in such a state. Clients in crisis usually benefit more from a one-to-one relationship with the therapist.

In addition to the prospective member, the therapist also needs to look at the group. In adding members, the therapist is concerned with what is missing rather than only with what is present. There is an attempt to maximize the range of member characteristics while at the same time maintaining compatibility of membership. The therapist avoids placing an individual in the group who would be likely to become a psychological isolate in that particular group.

Preparation of a new member for joining an ongoing group is similar in most respects to preparing members for the beginning of a group. Some additional areas, however, need to be covered. The client is helped to realize that initially he or she may well feel excluded from the group. The client is also prepared for the unusual culture of the group. The culture may be difficult to understand because he or she did not participate in its development. Fears about the high level of sophistication of group members, the openness with which feelings are expressed, or concern about seeing the "sicker" side of other members may be expressed. The therapist encourages the client to enter and participate at his or her own rate, not feeling any pressure to become a "good" group member immediately. Finally, it is useful for the therapist to describe the major events of the past few meetings to the new member.

The therapist also must be concerned about the group that is admitting a new member. This is a difficult, emotional time for the group; it is also a time that offers great potential for growth. Group members may see the newcomer along several dimensions. The new member may be viewed as an interloper; an untrustworthy stranger who may destroy or take over the place that an established member has won for himself in the group. Conversely, the newcomer may be seen as someone at odds with the group who will never be accepted. Depending on the issues currently being dealt with in the group, the new member may be seen as an ally; a savior or a new victim to become the scapegoat of the group. The group essentially has two alternatives: it can indoctrinate the new member into the culture of the group in such a way that the status quo does not change; or it can allow the newcomer to examine the present traditions and norms and make recommendations that will increase his or her security in the group. The more functional, mature, and secure group usually takes the latter course of action.

It is the therapist's responsibility to prepare the group for the addition of a new member. When a new person is being considered for membership, the current members are given an opportunity to discuss this imminent event. It is often useful to explore some of the fantasies members may have about the newcomer and the effect that the inclusion will have on the group. Plans for welcoming and orienting the anticipated member should be made by the group. If circumstances permit, it is sometimes helpful to have group members assess the suitability of a potential member by inviting him or her to a group meeting. This should not be done, however, if the group does not have any real part in the decision. Group members should be reminded that in the process of assessment there is no need to do a replay of the Inquisition. If at all possible, a new member is added to the group only if the group is prepared to welcome the person or at least willing to be accepting.

Termination of a single group member is a common event in most groups, except in those situations where the group terminates as a whole. Termination may occur if the client's behavior is such that it is seriously impeding the progress of the group. This course of action is only taken after every effort has been made to make the group situation comfortable for the client. A group member who is evidently experiencing severe difficulty in the group should be seen individually by the therapist. A one-to-one discussion is recommended because interaction within the group setting has obviously not been helpful. In meeting with the client, the therapist attempts to identify the source or sources of stress. If the source of stress is such that leaving the group is seen as the only alternative, the therapist makes the experience as constructive as possible. It is not the client who has failed but the form of intervention. The therapist helps the client to identify other forms of intervention that may be of assistance or accepts the client's position that now is not the optimal time for intervention. The door for further assistance is always left open. At some point the client should bring formal closure to being a group member within the context of the group. Again the therapist makes this experience as positive as possible for both the individual and the other group members. At later meetings the group should be encouraged to deal more directly with their feelings about the individual leaving the group: whether these feelings be relief, anger, a sense of failure, or a combination of these. The therapist as an individual must also deal with the same feelings.

Termination for a successful group member is, at least ultimately, a more positive experience. Ideally termination is seen as one stage in the individual's growth—growth that will continue after the individual leaves the group. Some problems may, however, arise in the termination process. The group may not want the individual to leave the group because he or she is such an effective and valued group member. The therapist may have the same feelings. The individual may delay departure from the group because of the security it provides, and the scariness of the tasks ahead. As the time for departure nears, the group becomes less important for the individual as affinity is withdrawn from the group and invested in other people and other groups. The therapist helps the group and the individual to deal with separation and loss and to engage in mourning. The therapist also gently redirects the group to focus on the tasks which they have not yet completed.

CONCLUSION

The structure and dynamics of a primary group can be used to benefit individuals who are experiencing problems in functioning. The curative potential or factors of a group situation can be used selectively to facilitate growth and adaptations. Primary groups, the original matrix in which socialization occurs, are effective in promoting continued growth.

14 Activity Groups

The last two chapters, I hope, have provided some background information useful for the understanding of activity groups. It should be noted before proceeding that occupational therapists do not use verbal groups; they are not one of the legitimate tools of occupational therapy. Verbal groups are the legitimate tool of several other professions. Members of these professions are educated to use verbal groups effectively; occupational therapists are not. An understanding of the structure and dynamics of groups and the therapeutic aspects of groups are fundamental to both verbal and activity groups. However, these phenomena combined with purposeful activities makes activity groups far different from verbal groups.

Activity groups, as previously defined, are primary groups made up of and designed to assist individuals who share common concerns or problems related to the acquisition or maintenance of performance components, and occupational performances. They are also used as a means of satisfying health needs. Activities are an integral part of the groups' here-and-now interaction within the context of the group; or else a specific gestalt of activities, engaged in by group members outside the group, become the focus for group discussion. Activity groups are used in both the evaluation and intervention processes. As a means of evaluation, activity groups assist the client and therapist in identifying difficulties in functioning. As a means of intervention, activity groups are used in meeting health needs, prevention, management, maintenance, and the change process. Relative to intervention, activity groups may be concerned with acquiring group interaction skills or learning how to cook, for example. The activity in such a situation occurs within the context of the group and is used as the vehicle for acquisition of the identified skills. Conversely, an activity group may be concerned with such skills as how to apply for a job or how to organize various tasks inherent in being a homemaker. In this type of an activity group participants are involved in attempts to engage in the above-mentioned activities outside the structure of the group. The experiences of each individual are brought into the group for discussion and exploration. Group interaction may involve sharing of experiences, giving information, role playing, providing support, and suggesting solutions to identified problems.

The addition of activities to a therapeutic group alters the nature of the group. It becomes something different than a verbal group. Thus it is necessary to consider the components of activity groups in their own right.

Prior to proceeding, it should be noted that little formal research has been conducted relative to activity groups (781). The ideas presented in this chapter are speculative in nature and are derived from fairly unsystematized observation.

CONSIDERATIONS RELATIVE TO STRUCTURE

This section is concerned with a discussion of the structural elements of groups as they are affected by the addition of activities to therapeutic groups.

Group Development

The nature of the activity selected by group members and/or the way in which the activity is carried out may symbolically mark the stage of development of an activity group. In the orientation phase, for example, members tend to want to work on an activity together, being most cooperative about sharing and helping each other. The group's high expectations may be evident in their selection of a complex task that may well be beyond the collective skill of the group. The dissatisfaction stage is often symbolized by the group electing to do individual projects or by working on a shared project in a very disjointed and physically distant manner. The productivity phase usually is marked by a return to more cooperative activities now more realistically defined relative to the skills of the group. The terminal phase may be characterized by an activity that symbolizes unity or closure or in some way describes the process of the group and the growth which members have experienced.

Another way in which the developmental phases of the group may be evident is along the continuum of simulated-to-natural activities. Depending on the type of activity group, initial activities may be entirely simulated. As the group progresses through the various phases, activities are likely to become more natural. A group of upper-extremity amputees, for example, may initially practice dressing, using hand tools, opening doors, manipulating a billfold, and the like. Later they may go out and eat at a restaurant together.

In regard to specific phases, activities often facilitate adjustment of the group. In the orientation phase, group members who have difficulty with interpersonal relations often find that the activity provides a focus for interaction. The responses of others can be tested by observing how they interact with the nonhuman environment and in the context of an activity. The activity provides some degree of interpersonal distance, which may be initially more comfortable for some group members. During the orientation phase the group may need considerable assistance with the activity. The skills necessary to engage in the activity may have to be taught by the therapist.

During the dissatisfaction phase work on the activity may be extremely slow or it may stop altogether. One of the major decisions the therapist must make in dealing with factors that interfere with reaching the stated goals is whether to interrupt the activity and involve the group in a verbal discussion of a problem or to make alterations in the group more indirectly through feedback and reinforcement. The course of action taken by the therapist will depend on the type of activity group and the capacity of group members to use discussion as a means of modifying behavior.

To enhance the productive phase, it is often helpful to use a wide variety of activities. This assists group members to maintain interest in the goals of the group and minimizes the fatigue factor. Engaging in an occasional activity that has little to do with the goals of the group is also helpful. The complexity of the activities used in the group are likely to increase in this phase. Care does need to be taken so that this increase is neither too slow nor too rapid.

During the termination phase the group completes their final activity. The activity may be specifically selected to deal with the issues of this period. The activity then can be used as a focus for assessing what has been accomplished and as a means of saying goodbye.

Central Issues

Basic assumptions that are interfering with the goals of the group are frequently evident in the way in which group members engage in activities. Group members may manipulate the activity in such a way that it no longer has any relationship to the goals of the group. Group members may also collectively respond to an activity in a highly unusual manner. This is often a sure sign that one or more basic assumptions are influencing the group. The symbolic potential of many activities may be used by the therapist to promote expression of basic assumptions. The assumption is often almost literally acted out in the doing of the activity. This kind of symbolic illustration helps the group to focus on the assumption in a fairly direct manner. It also allows for some distance from the assumption, which often makes recognition and exploration easier. It is almost like talking about a picture of one's self as the first step in being able to talk about oneself.

The relationship between basic assumptions and activities can, in part, be illustrated in regard to dependency. The responsibility, sharing, and mutual help involved in doing an activity often lead to a decrease in dependency. On the other hand, dependency may be increased in those activity groups involving the teaching of a specific skill by the therapist. This can be minimized in part by using the discovery method of teaching and, if possible, by having group members teach each other. Mastery in the performance of a variety of activities decreases dependency.

Activity groups on the whole are primarily concerned with the here and now. The activity of the group facilitates this orientation by emphasis on doing. Doing is an immediate, concrete event that exists in the present. The focusing, organizing effect of activities also serves to maintain the attention of the group on the task at hand.

Roles in Groups

Purposeful activities form a natural nucleus for the development of instrumental roles relative to participation in an activity. These functional membership roles are usually the first ones taken by group members. Instrumental roles relative to the social-emotional goals of the group and expressive roles are usually learned somewhat later.

The number of roles the therapist continues to play in an activity group varies with the type of group. In a group, for example, where interaction is primarily parallel in nature, the therapist takes the majority of membership roles. In other activity groups where the interaction is on a more mature level, the therapist eventually may need to take very few membership roles.

Activity groups may or may not have co-therapists. If there are co-therapists, their responsibility may split along somewhat different lines than those in a verbal group. One therapist may become the activity specialist, being particularly concerned with helping group members to participate in the activity. The other therapist may become the goal specialist, being primarily concerned with helping group members to relate the activity to the goals of the group. The goal specialist, for example, may help the group to look at what they learned about their capacity to be assertive through participation in the task. The goal specialist may also be in a better position to observe the dynamics of the group. This division in role responsibilities by no means occurs in all activity groups with co-therapists; the division, if any, may be along entirely different lines. The taking of differential roles by co-therapists in any group is often more dependent on the personalities of the co-therapists than on the type of group.

Group Goals

The fact that purposeful activities are made up of a number of elements that are able to be manipulated enhances the attainment of group goals. Activities can be selected and finely tuned to meet the needs of a group at any particular time.

The goals of activity groups tend to be more concrete than those evident in verbal groups. It appears that making the link between the activity and the goal helps to clarify the goal for both the therapist and the group members. The close link between purposeful activities and the performance components and occupational performance seems to form a bridge which facilitates goal clarification.

As mentioned, the activity, on the other hand, can be a source of confusion in regard to the goal of an activity group. The difference between the activity as a vehicle and as a project which is to be completed is sometimes difficult for group members to understand. If this should be the case, the therapist must be very explicit in explaining and demonstrating the difference.

Group Norms

The norms of an activity group tend to be more numerous than those of a verbal group. Not only are they concerned with acceptable content for group discussion and interpersonal behavior, but also behavior relative to participation in the activity of the group. When the activity of the group has external criteria for evaluation, the group needs to set standards for adequate performance. Because of the greater number of norms in an activity group, conflict between norms is more likely.

Communication

The ways in which purposeful activities enhance communication has been outlined in Chapter 10. It is suggested that the reader review this section.

Group Cohesiveness

Purposeful activities by their very concreteness provide a tangible way of identifying with the group. They are something all of the group members share in common. Participation in the activity of the group brings members together in close proximity and provides evidence that they are working together. Cohesiveness is also increased when the activity is such that it can be shared with group members outside the group. In addition, the sense of "we have produced" enhances the feeling of being an integrated group.

In centers where there are several activities groups, mild competition between groups relative to some activity or series of activities facilitates cohesiveness. Who can win or do the best is a strong incentive for a group to work cooperatively. The therapist, of course, must guard against letting the competition get out of hand. It should be regulated in such a way as to enhance cohesiveness but should not be allowed to interfere with the goals of the group.

Decision Making

The ultimate responsibility for selecting an appropriate activity belongs to the therapist. The process of deciding on an activity, however, can often be utilized as one means of attaining the goals of the group. Group members, therefore, may take a major portion of the responsibility for activity selection. The therapist retains veto power, but this is rarely used if the group is given the responsibility only when it is ready. A group is ready to engage in selecting an activity when it: (a) understands and accepts the goals of the group; (b) possesses a sufficient degree of cognitive skill to select an appropriate activity; and (c) is able to arrive at a decision.

Regardless of the type of group, the therapist may have to help with activity selection in the beginning phases of the group. One useful way to help the group select an activity as well as to learn how to select an activity is for the therapist to present three or four alternatives. The group then discusses the pros and cons of each and is helped to arrive at a decision. This method limits the amount of stimuli with which the group must deal and helps the group understand the nature of an appropriate activity. The process the group went through to arrive at the decision may be reviewed by the therapist in order to facilitate future decision making. After this initial phase, members in several types of activity groups are given primary responsibility for activity selection. It is through selection and carrying out an activity that group members are enabled to attain the goals of many types of activity groups.

Conflict

The possibility of conflict between the goals of an activity group and completion of the activity has been discussed. In addition, conflict may arise in conjunction with selection of the activity and how that activity should be carried out. Some of this conflict is real in the sense that it is directly related to the issue being contended. At other times the conflict may simply be the overt expression of underlying conflict that has nothing to do with the activity issue. At still other times it may be a combination of the two. The therapist and group members must locate the source of real conflict and deal with it appropriately.

Power and Deviancy

Purposeful activities are extremely powerful. This is particularly true when they take place in the context of a group. The powerfulness of activities in this case comes from two sources: the irrevocability of action and the fact that action tends to be less censored than words. An individual's actions and the collective actions of the group are clearly available for everyone to see; they are there in the public arena, open for examination. They cannot be taken back or easily denied. Second, purposeful activities tap the unconscious, presenting ideas and feelings that are likely to be relatively unmonitored by the individual or the group. Purposeful activities provide a fertile source of information that can be used by group members for self-understanding and as the basis for altering maladaptive ideas and feelings.

Purposeful activities also can have an effect on the power structure of a group. Expert power can be derived from knowing how to do the activity being used as the vehicle for intervention. A group member who has the necessary knowledge and skill to be considered somewhat of an expert in the activity is in an advantageous position in the power structure of the group. This is particularly true if the group member has more knowledge and skill than the therapist relative to the activity. One means the therapist can use to equalize the power difference between herself and other group members is not to have expertise in the selected activity. The learning of the activity together often helps the group to perceive the therapist from a far different perspective. The process of shared learning is also often a fruitful means for helping group members to attain the group goals.

In conclusion, the structural elements of activity groups are influenced by the inclusion of a doing process. At times activities add another dimension to a structural element; at other times they enhance an element.

CONSIDERATIONS RELATIVE TO CURATIVE ASPECTS

The combining of purposeful activities and the curative aspects of groups may affect either the purposeful activity or a curative aspect. The effect may be to make one element more complex or the effect may be synergistic. Synergy here refers to the combining of elements that work together cooperatively to increase the effectiveness of both. In other words, the combined action of purposeful activities and the curative aspects of groups may be more potent than either of these elements acting alone.

Some of the major relationships between purposeful activities and the curative factors of groups are as follows.

1. Instillation of hope. One of the elements of hope is the experience of seeing oneself able to do, to be able

to perform in a functional manner. Engagement in a purposeful activity, regardless of how simple, fosters hope. The individual may be slow to perceive change relative to feelings about himself or interpersonal relations. Increasing capacity to engage successfully in ever more complex and demanding activities is frequently more readily observable. Such a change is also more easily seen in others. Thus purposeful activities may help to maintain a feeling of hope in the ultimate outcome of the intervention process.

2. Universality. Universality is an inherent characteristic of purposeful activities. The timelessness and the pervasive nature of purposeful activities enhance the factor of universality in groups; the converse is also true. Here again is an obvious synergistic relationship between a curative factor of groups and purposeful activities.

3. Imparting information. Purposeful activities provide information in three major ways. Through engagement in purposeful activities, the individual is quite clearly able to observe what he or she is and is not able to do. Second, in a properly designed situation, the individual is able to identify the relationship between feelings, thoughts, and action—the influence of emotions and ideas on interaction in the environment. Third, learning how to engage in a variety of different activities contributes to the individual's fund of knowledge about how to do, how to manipulate the human and nonhuman environment effectively.

4. Altruism. Sharing an activity with another person or helping someone to engage in an activity provides an opportunity to give to others. This type of giving is initially often much easier than giving on a more personal level. In addition, purposeful activities provide a structure for giving that is not as readily available in a verbal group. The individual is able to see more clearly how he can be of help to another person, and is able to see the effect of that help.

5. The corrective recapitulation of the primary family group. Typical family interaction takes place in the context of doing, particularly in relationship to activities of daily living and leisure time pursuits. Purposeful activities can be used, in part, to simulate the familial environment where initial learning took place. Through shared participation in these types of activities, the individual is also able to explore new, more adaptive ways of engaging in intimate interpersonal interactions. The variety of activities available, if used effectively, mitigates against the development of stereotyped interactions.

6. Development of socialization techniques. Purposeful activities provide a vehicle for shared interaction with others. An activity, initially, can be used as an aid to interaction and as a springboard to more personal interaction. It should be noted, however, that the capacity to participate in an activity with one or more persons is a valuable skill in and of itself.

7. Imitative behavior. Observation of other group members engaging in purposeful activities provides another source for imitation. The individual is able to see how other people engage in doing processes and how they relate to others in the context of that doing. Again, the structure provided by purposeful activities serves to organize imitated behavior into a meaningful gestalt; it serves to integrate pieces of behavior into wholes.

8. Interpersonal learning. Purposeful activities provide another, very significant, element to the group as a social microcosm. They make the microcosm more reflective of the larger social system in that they present the demand for doing, for performing. The inclusion of purposeful activities provides a more accurate perspective of the relationship between interpersonal behavior and engaging in a doing process—a perspective not always apparent in verbal groups.

9. Group cohesiveness. This factor was discussed in the last section relative to purposeful activities.

10. Catharsis and corrective emotional experiences. Catharsis and corrective emotional experiences can be promoted by selecting activities that are likely to elicit and allow for the expression of specific feelings not being addressed by a group member or the group as a whole. Activities can also be designed to facilitate reflection on the experience, consensual validation, and appropriate expression of emotions.

11. Existential factors. The universal element and the symbolic potential of activities may promote recognition of the existential position regarding the human experience. Sharing and helping others may assist the individual in transcending the self and, therefore, ultimately reach the point of self-actualization. Finding meaning in life may also be facilitated by engaging in a variety of purposeful activities with the intention of identifying what experiences lead to expression of one's own idiosyncratic uniqueness.

12. The desire to know. Purposeful activities provide information about the self, other people, and the nonhuman environment. They assist the individual to see the various relationships between these interacting elements. The integrative aspect of purposeful activities helps the individual to use disparate parts of the self in a unified, holistic manner.

In conclusion, this section has described some of the ways that the curative aspects of groups are related to and interact with purposeful activities. The first two sections of this chapter were an illustration of the interrelationship of the three theoretical systems that support activity groups: the structure and dynamics of primary groups, the curative factors of groups, and purposeful activities. With this as a foundation, the following section is devoted to an outline of the various types of activity groups.

TYPES OF ACTIVITY GROUPS

Traditionally, activity groups have not been subdivided into various types. They were discussed in general terms as if all activity groups were alike. If more specificity was needed, a particular group was usually identified by its goal (e.g., a prevocational group or a socialization group) or by the activity used (e.g., gym group or cooking group). This way of labeling groups, however, is rather imprecise; it tells the listener very little about the group. A group identified by its goals gives no clue about the activities used or about the process; a group identified by its activity implies no specific goal. A cooking group, for example, may be oriented to (a) teaching clients how to cook, (b) helping clients to be more effective in group interaction, (c) satisfying oral needs or the need to be nurtured, or (d) helping clients to understand their ideas, feelings, and values related to food and eating. Any of these goals may be quite appropriate for a "cooking group," but the label does not give sufficient information. Neither groups identified by a goal or an activity provide any indication of the theoretical system on which the group is based. Descriptions of various activity groups can be found elsewhere (33,53,78,80,121,133,241,280,283,287,290, 364,411,517,526,528,564,571,613,639–641,675,706, 708,791,929,953,982,997).

It appeared thus, that there was a need for a common vocabulary relative to activity groups which more clearly describes their nature. It was out of this apparent need that a taxonomy for activity groups was developed (711). This classification is based on some similarity in the general goal of the group, the types of frame of reference that may be used as the basis for a particular type of group, clients who may benefit from participation, the role of the therapist, and suitable activities. These elements will be used to describe the various types of groups in the following discussion.

There are six major categories of activity groups, with some of these categories being further subdivided. Each will be described as a discrete entity. In actual clinical practice, however, a given activity group may be a blend of two or more of the described categories. They are presented as discrete entities here because it is felt that one should know what one is blending before proceeding.

Evaluative Groups

Evaluative groups are designed to assess an individual's capacity to function within a group. It provides information, for both client and therapist, in regard to the client's capacities and limitations in regard to group interaction. The rationale for evaluative groups is similar to that of any other evaluative situation: in order to assess a particular skill one must observe an individual in a setting that provides an opportunity for the individual to demonstrate the skill in question. It is true that a therapist may observe clients' interactions with others in various settings, e.g., in the day room, during a general meeting of all of the clients, or in the coffee shop. In such situations, however, the client is often unaware he or she is being observed and thus may feel no particular reason to demonstrate the ability to function in a group situation. It is far better, therefore, to provide a structured situation for the observation of interpersonal skills. The client is aware that she now has an opportunity to demonstrate skills. The therapist is able to observe in a situation that has known demands and limitations.

An evaluative group may be based on either an acquisitional or developmental frame of reference. Although the setting used is similar, the conclusions drawn will vary depending on the frame of reference being used. In other words, each frame of reference categorizes function and dysfunction relative to the ability to interact in a group somewhat differently. In illustration, a therapist using an acquisitional frame of reference is likely to focus on the appropriateness of the client's behavior, on the client's ability to relate to others, and on the various membership roles the client is able to take. A therapist using a developmental frame of reference would attempt to determine where the client is in relationship to the development of group interaction skills. (The stages of development in this area were outlined in Chapter 5.)

Participation in an evaluative group is appropriate for any clients who, in their past interactions, have demonstrated some difficulty in interpersonal relations. Participation is also appropriate for any client who is likely to be involved in an activity group during the intervention process. Intervention for the latter category of clients may not be concerned with developing the capacity to engage more effectively in groups. Nevertheless some aspect of intervention may take place in the context of a group. An activity group may, for example, be used to meet health needs or to help an individual adjust to the loss of a social role. Participation in an evaluative group gives the client and therapist some idea about the client's capacity to engage with others in a group setting and the type of group that may be best for that particular client.

An evaluative group usually meets only once and lasts for about 45 minutes to an hour. Granted, this is a relatively short period of time, but it is usually sufficient for initial evaluation. More refined assessment takes place during the continued evaluation, which is always a part of intervention. Typically four to six clients are included in an evaluative group. In groups of less than four, interaction tends to be more dyadic than group oriented. A maximum of six clients is suggested because it is very difficult for the therapist to observe more than six people adequately. The participants for a given evaluative group are usually selected in a rather pragmatic manner. Those clients who have come into the facility in a given period of time and who need to participate in an evaluative group are usually included in one group. If there are more than six clients, then two evaluative groups are used or discrete evaluative groups are formed at shorter intervals.

Prior to the meeting of the evaluative group, the therapist meets individually with each client to explain the purpose of the group. When all the participants are assembled, the therapist introduces the members of the group to each other and once again briefly explains the purpose of the group. It is the therapist's responsibility to select the activity. Group members are responsible for planning how they will organize the activity and its implementation. The therapist defines the parameters of the activity and provides the necessary tools and materials or makes them readily available. The therapist does not participate in the group; the therapist's role is to observe the interaction among group members. When the group members are engaged in the activity, only questions that are specifically directed toward the therapist are answered. The therapist tries, however, to keep such questions at a minimum. The therapist's role, as described above, is explained to the group members.

After the group has completed the activity or when the designated time for the group meeting has come to an end, the therapist brings closure to the meeting by making some positive comments about the group's interaction and thanks each member for participating. After the meeting, the therapist meets with each of the clients. This is not done in the context of the group meeting because the clients do not know each other well enough for discussion that deals with personal issues. In these individual meetings the therapist shares observations with the client and encourages the client to share ideas about interactions in the evaluative group. The client is encouraged to describe whether interactions in the evaluative group are typical of participation in other group situations. Discrepancies between the therapist's observations and those of the client are also identified and discussed. Ideally, the client and therapist come to some agreement about the client's assets and limitations relative to the capacity to interact comfortably and effectively in a group.

An activity suitable for an evaluation group is one that (a) requires group planning and collaborative interaction for implementation and (b) can reasonably be completed in the allotted time period. The selected activity should also be one that is compatible with the general characteristics of the population served by the facility. The therapist thus takes into consideration the age, educational level, cultural background, and so forth of the population being served. Table games, construction projects such as making a space station out of "Lego" blocks, and making a mural are some activities used in evaluative groups. In selecting an activity for an evaluative group, th therapist is somewhat less concerned with whether the activity is of particular interest to group members. However, it certainly does help if the members can become easily engaged in the activity.

It is important to remember that an evaluative group does not include any kind of planned intervention. By not participating in the group, the therapist allows the interaction to proceed in whatever way it unfolds. The only time the therapist intervenes is if one client is disrupting the group so severely that the group becomes immobilized. In such a case the therapist briefly tries to correct the situation by defining the broad limits of socially acceptable behavior in a group situation. If this is not effective, the therapist removes the offending client from the group. This whole situation may be avoided if the therapist is somewhat selective about who is to be included in an evaluative group. Through general observation, the therapist is usually able to identify clients who are likely to be extremely disruptive to a group. Such individuals should not be included in an evaluative group. They may, however, be included at a later time when their behavior is under somewhat better control.

Task-Oriented Groups

Task-oriented groups are designed to help members to become aware of their needs, values, ideas, and feelings as they influence action, and to test the validity of this intrapsychic content (287). Task-oriented groups are not designed to develop skill in group interaction per se; however, this may occur spontaneously through participation in the group. The goals of this type of group are primarily concerned with developing self-awareness or self-understanding. Task-oriented groups are based on analytical frames of reference.

The process of selecting, planning, and carrying out group activities is the means through which members become aware of the relationship between thoughts, feelings, and actions. The activities elicit behavior, which is explored relative to the thoughts and feelings that prompted the behavior. These thoughts and feelings are then examined to determine if they are appropriate to the objective situation at hand. Members are helped through feedback to look at the environment in a more realistic manner and to act on the basis of that reality. Through experimenting with and practicing more effective patterns of interacting, more adaptive ideas and feelings replace those that are less adaptive. Effective interaction on the basis of the new ideas and feelings serves to make them more permanent.

An example may be useful at this point. A woman in the group may engage in an activity in a very submissive kind of way, always accepting those parts of the activity that are not very interesting, such as mixing paint or cleaning up at the end of the work period. The therapist and other members help the individual to become aware of her behavior; discussion may lead to the fact that the individual believes she is not worthy enough to engage in any of the more interesting or enjoyable aspects of the activity. The individual is helped to test her belief about being unworthy against the perceptions of other group members. They in turn help the individual to see that this idea about herself is not based on the objective reality of her considerable, previously demonstrated, capacities; it is a belief that has no basis in reality. The group then helps the individual to be more assertive and to insist that she take on more interesting components of the activity. Through doing this repeatedly, the individual begins to believe, hopefully, that indeed she is a worthy person.

Clients suitable for a task-oriented group are those individuals who possess the capacity to function at a fairly high level but have values, ideas, and feelings that are inhibiting use of that capacity. Individuals who have experienced a change in social roles and individuals who are experiencing difficulty in adapting to chronic disability are particularly appropriate for a task-oriented group. Candidates for a task-oriented group should have a fair amount of verbal skill and ability to interact with others in a group setting.

Activities suitable for a task-oriented group are those directed toward creating an end-product or a demonstrable service for the group as a whole and/or for persons outside the group. The concreteness of this type of activity elicits and structures the expression of feelings and ideas. It also provides a measure of the individual's and group's progress. In a task-oriented group the task is selected by group members. They are responsible for the preliminary planning, the procurement of the necessary tools and materials, and the accomplishment of the activity. The activity then becomes the focal point around which interaction develops; it becomes a problem that the group must solve. The activity helps each group member to organize and use those aspects of function which are healthy and assists clients in becoming aware of and dealing with deficiencies in functioning.

Appropriate types of activities for a task-oriented group may be described in a variety of ways. Activities may be short term, such as going bowling, or long term, such as planting a vegetable garden. Activities may be self-gratifying, such as making and eating a meal together, or altruistic, such as constructing toys for a nearby children's shelter. The type of activity chosen by the group frequently indicates what the group is concerned with at a given point in time. A group preoccupied with gratification of dependency needs, for example, may concentrate on activities that are related to food or making something for themselves. A group concerned about status and self-identity may select and initiate complex tasks, such as silk screening original greeting cards or setting up a darkroom for the development of film. Groups concerned about discharge or termination may plan activities that will take them out into the community, such as exhibiting art work at a community center or doing volunteer work with delinquent youths.

The issues that are discussed in the group are primarily initiated by group members, with encouragement from the therapist when this is necessary. During the initial stages of the group, most discussion centers around the activity itself. Such discussion is appropriate in that group members are still exploring the new situation and getting acquainted with each other. Discussion of the activity gives the group an opportunity for reality testing. Various suggestions, fantasies, and wishful thinking may be expressed and contrasted with the reality of the concrete situation. Through mutual feedback, the group learns to discriminate between those activity suggestions that are feasible and those that are inappropriate or too complex for the group to handle at the present time. Selecting and planning a task also help group members to experiment with their ability to solve concrete problems.

As the group becomes more cohesive and a trusting relationship develops among group members, the group usually begins to discuss problems relative to interpersonal relations. There is an awakening interest in each other as individuals and a beginning desire to understand and know other group members on a more intimate level. Slowly the group develops the ability to discuss feelings about themselves relative to sharing and participating with each other in accomplishing an activity. Group members become aware of how the image they have of themselves is reflected in their behavior. The ability to express negative as well as positive feelings is slowly acquired.

During the productive phase, the task-oriented group provides an experience in which the client is readily able to see the influence of his values, thoughts, and feelings on actions, on relationships with others, and on the completion of the task. The client is also able to see how others perceive his behavior. The discussions that take place in the group encourage awareness of behavior, insight into why one is behaving in a particular manner, and ways in which inappropriate or inaccurate ideas and feelings may be altered. With the support of the group and the therapist, group members are encouraged to try out ways of behaving that are more congruent with the ways in which the individual would like to perceive himself and other people.

It should be noted that the activities that take place in a task-oriented group are not the focus of the group. Rather attention is given to how group members individually and collectively carry out the activities. The effectiveness of the group is not measured by task accomplishment but by the degree to which the group affords a client the opportunity to develop new ideas and feelings about self and others that are constructive and rewarding.

The role of the therapist in a task-oriented group is of primary importance. In the initial phase of group development, the therapist often needs to play a fairly active leadership role. It is frequently necessary to help the group to define its goals and reason for being. The group may need some definite, imposed structure in order to come to some agreement on an appropriate task. The therapist not only states the criteria for an appropriate activity but may also need to suggest activities and to guide discussion. In this way the group is assisted in learning how to engage in problem solving and decision making. Later the therapist may need to be fairly active in helping members to become aware of their thoughts, feelings, and actions, to focus on interpersonal relationships and task accomplishment, and to deal with group conflict. This is usually accomplished by use of the several techniques outlined in Chapter 13. In addition, the therapist often suggests ways in which an individual may explore and practice new patterns of behavior. As the group develops, the therapist plays a less active role in these areas when group members become able to take on these responsibilities.

Perhaps the most difficult part of being a therapist in a task-oriented group is to know when to move in and help the group and when to let the group struggle on its own. Typically, the therapist will find him- or herself moving back and forth between a relatively active and relatively passive role as the focus of the group changes from time to time. The therapist encourages group members to accept the responsibility of co-therapist relative to other members of the group. This assists group members to understand that they are able to play an effective part in helping each other.

Developmental Groups

Developmental groups are simulations of the various types of nonfamilial, primary groups usually encountered in the normal developmental process (706). There are five subtypes of developmental groups that are reflective of the various groups encountered in the developmental process as outlined in the play/leisure/recreation component of the life cycle. It is suggested that the reader review the appropriate sections in Chapter 5.

In the first subtype, parallel groups, individuals work or play in the presence of others, engaging in some degree of mutual stimulation but with minimal sharing of activities. In the second, project groups, individuals are involved in short-term activities that require some shared interaction, cooperation, and competition. The activity is seen as paramount, with little interaction outside the context of the activity. In the third, egocentric-cooperative groups, group members select and implement relatively long-term activities through joint interaction. The individual's manner of interacting is based on enlightened self-interest. The individual recognizes that his rights and needs will be respected only if he respects the rights and needs of other group members. In the fourth, cooperative groups, group interaction is primarily concerned with mutual need satisfaction and the sharing of ideas and feelings. The activity is considered to be secondary to need fulfillment. In the fifth subtype, mature groups, group members are able to take a variety of membership roles selectively to maintain a balance between task accomplishment and the satisfaction of group members' needs.

Developmental groups, in their pure form, are designed to assist clients in acquiring group interaction skill in a stage-by-stage manner. Each of the subtypes of developmental groups is structured to teach one level of group interaction skill, and nothing else. Clients thus are placed in a group that is one stage beyond the level of group interaction skill the client appears to have mastered at the time of initial evaluation. If the client, for example, has the ability to interact in a parallel group, he or she is placed in a group at the project level. Group members collectively are engaged in learning one level of group interaction skill. Once that level is acquired, the group as a whole may advance to the next level. This occurs when all group members learn at about the same rate. If this is not the case, after mastering the stage of group interaction skill the group is designed to teach, a client moves into another group that is functioning at the next stage.

Pure developmental groups (i.e., groups specially designed to teach one level of group interaction skill) are practical only in a large treatment facility. There needs to be a sufficient number of clients at various levels to support the formation of the various subtypes of developmental groups. In a smaller treatment facility it may be possible to have only one group concerned with the development of group interaction skill. Such a group, here referred to as "middle range," is designed to teach most levels of group interaction skill. It is structured like an egocentric-cooperative group, a type of developmental group that will be discussed shortly. Middle-range groups are not conducive to teaching the extreme ends of group interaction skill; other arrangements for learning are sometimes necessary.

Developmental groups are based on developmental frames of reference. Thus it is assumed that in order for an individual to attain the most advanced level of group interaction skill, that person must master each stage in an orderly sequence. To master each stage, a certain structure and type of interaction must be available. In addition, basic principles of learning are used. Regardless of the level of group interaction skill the therapist is attempting to develop, the therapist designs the learning situation so that the client (a) is both aware of and helped to engage in appropriate behavior and (b) receives reinforcement of, or feedback about, behavior, or both. The therapist tells the client what behavior is expected prior to entering into the group and periodically reminds group members of what is and is not appropriate behavior in the group.

Before a client can receive reinforcement for desired behavior, the behavior must occur. The therapist may simply wait for an approximation of desirable behavior and then reinforce that behavior selectively. This is the process of shaping. Just waiting for behavior to happen can take a long time. There are, however, several methods the therapist may use to elicit the desired behavior. One method is to encourage a client to imitate another group member who is functioning fairly well in the group. Or a therapist may suggest to a client that he try to act in a particular way, giving him ideas about what he might say and do. A way of acting that is ineffective or inappropriate for the group may be pointed out to the client. The client in this situation is then encouraged to interact in a different manner without any specific suggestions given. Trial and error learning is encouraged, with the client receiving feedback about the appropriateness of experimental behavior. Or the group may pause periodically in their activity to examine what behavior has been useful to the group and the individual and what behavior has been harmful or of minimal use to the group or the individual. This process both reinforces the learning of appropriate behavior and gives group members clues as to the kinds of behavior they might try. A discussion of this kind is kept as nonpersonal as possible. Group members are not singled out and told they did something right or wrong. Although using immediate examples of what occurred in the group, the discussion is oriented to talking about what kind of behavior is useful in this type of group and what behavior is not useful. Discussion is focused on practical issues of group interaction, not personal issues. Finally, the group may temporarily discontinue its current activity and experiment with various ways of acting through role playing. Role playing may center around a situation that has just occurred in the group or on a general problem within the group.

The use of reinforcement and feedback is very important in developmental groups. The therapist may take responsibility for this aspect of learning, but ideally enlists the help of all group members. This is accomplished by assisting group members not only to understand what is appropriate behavior for a particular group but also assisting them to learn how to give and withhold reinforcement and to provide feedback.

With the above as background information, developmental groups are appropriate for any client who has difficulty in the area of group interaction. The type of developmental group suitable for a given client would depend on the client's level of group interaction skill.

The following discussion describes each type of developmental group in its pure form. The ways in which group interaction skill may be learned in a middle-range group is also described.

A Parallel Group

Some clients are not initially ready to learn how to participate in a parallel group. They are either so mistrustful of others or so self-preoccupied that they have little interest in or capacity to interact in a group. When the policies of a facility do not require that a client immediately participate in a group, it is usually better for a client who is not ready to start learning group interaction skill to be seen individually by the therapist. Intervention would then be devoted to development of basic trust between client and therapist.

When a client who is not ready to learn group interaction skill must be placed in a middle-range group as soon as entering the treatment facility, few demands for participation are made initially. Ideally, the client is welcomed by group members and is given an appropriate amount of attention and support. The client may be excused from participation in the group activity, only at this point required to be with the group. When the client indicates readiness for some participation, considerable assistance is given by the therapist. Assistance is focused on the development of trust between the client and therapist. It is only after such trust is established that the client will be able to participate in the group on a parallel level.

In teaching a client how to participate at the parallel level in a middle-range group, the therapist and other group members encourage and reinforce behavior that is appropriate for interaction in a parallel group. They are concerned with helping the client to work at a task in the presence of other group members, to be aware of other group members, and to have some sort of minimal interaction with others. Additional demands for more advanced group interaction are kept to a minimum. When it is impossible for the client to have an individual task, the person who is the client's partner should be aware that the client has little idea about how to share. The other person will have to take major responsibility for organizing the task in such a way that the client can participate. The other person may end up doing most of the work, or none at all. Group members must be helped to be aware that a person who does not have the ability to participate in a parallel group often does not know how to ask for or give need satisfaction without assistance from others. Need satisfaction and help must be provided by group members. The client is only required to engage in only the most basic types of interpersonal relationships. Basic here refers to recognizing the presence of other group members and not being disruptive to group interaction.

When a client is ready to begin learning how to participate in a parallel group and the learning is to take place in a pure group, that client is adequately prepared for the new situation. The therapist tells the client what the group will be like, what kinds of activities the group members are involved in, and what will be expected of him by the group. The group leader is introduced if the client does not know this person already.

The therapist plays a very active leadership role in a parallel group. This is because individuals at this level are able to play very few group membership roles. Group members' needs for safety, love, acceptance, and esteem are met by the therapist. The therapist reinforces any behavior appropriate for a parallel group—engaging in an individual task; observing a group member or looking at the activity in which the member is engaged; making eye contact; recognition of other group members by smiling, nodding, or greeting; sitting next to someone; asking a question; answering a question; engaging in a simple, casual conversation; and so forth. The process of shaping and differential reinforcement is often used. Usually the therapist ignores inappropriate behavior. When behavior is actually disruptive to the group, however, the therapist asks the client either to stop or to leave the room. Clients who are continually disruptive in parallel groups are probably not yet ready to be in a group.

The therapist helps clients select individual activities and gives assistance in carrying them out. The activities suggested to each client are kept well within the client's ability. When an activity is fairly easy for a client to accomplish, it will not require full attention. Thus, the client is more likely to show some interest in other group members. Activities suggested to clients are ones that increase the possibility of interaction. Activities that must be done in a special area or at an individual table are discouraged, as are activities that take up a large area. A copper enamel kiln, for example, is often kept in a special area. Looms are frequently set on individual tables. Because of the nature of the activity, the client tends to work alone, having little contact with other group members. When a client is engaged in an activity that requires a large work area, other group members tend to move away from the table or not to join the client. Two or more group members doing the same type of activity is encouraged because this often increases interaction. Group members share something in common and therefore have something to talk about.

A Project Group

The therapist continues to be a definite leader in a pure project group and takes major responsibility for selecting appropriate activities and satisfying group members' needs. Behavior appropriate for a project group is reinforced by the therapist and other group members if they are able to do so. Examples of behaviors that are reinforced are two or more group members doing an activity together, cooperating and sharing, mild competition, giving and seeking assistance, and simple interaction beyond the requirement of the activities.

The therapist helps group members select short-term tasks that either allow for or require the participation of two or more persons. A "short-term" activity is one that requires interaction for less than half an hour. This is, however, an arbitrary period of time. The point being made is that clients at this level are frequently not able to sustain interaction with the same individuals for a long period of time. For an activity that takes longer than a half an hour, the therapist usually breaks up the activity so that part of it is done one day and another part is done the next time the group meets. A client is often involved in a number of shared activities in one group meeting, working in various dyads and triads. Group meetings are kept fluid, with a number of small subgroups participating in a variety of activities. Only occasionally are all group members involved in working together in a shared task. The skills required to engage successfully in an activity with more than two or three people are usually not available to individuals at this level of interaction. It is also important that activities be shareable. For example, three or four people making a cake together borders on the ridiculous. Simple team sports and games are appropriate activities for project groups. Some examples are relay races, volleyball, badminton, croquet, red rover, pool, card games, and the like. Other activities that might be used are preparing for a short skit, a rhythm band, group singing, making holiday decorations, a shared woodworking project, and making a meal.

The goal of a project group, it should be noted, is to help clients learn how to participate in a shared activity. Finishing the activity in a given period of time or creating a perfect end-product is not emphasized. The therapist gives group members plenty of opportunities to experiment with ways of sharing. Trial-and-error behavior is encouraged. The therapist stresses the idea that if a task does not get done or the results of the task leave something to be desired, there will always be a chance to try again.

When a client is to learn how to participate in a project group in the context of a middle-range group, the therapist and other group members encourage and reinforce behavior that is appropriate for interacting in a project group. Doing short-term activities with others is emphasized. Above and beyond the task, the client is helped to remain aware of other group members, to ask and to respond to questions, and to follow along with what the group is doing. More complex interpersonal behavior, however, is not required. Group members continue to attempt to identify and meet the needs of the client without asking the client to be very explicit in stating his needs. If possible, the client is involved in shared tasks that are not pressured by time or need for perfection.

An Egocentric-Cooperative Group

In a pure group designed to teach skill necessary for interaction in an egocentric-cooperative group, the therapist takes much less of a leadership role; the roles the therapist takes are finely tuned to what group members are able or almost able to do. The therapist ceases to take a particular membership role or takes on a specific membership role according to the learning needs of the group. The strategy here is to allow the group to function as independently of the therapist's direction as possible without letting it flounder to the point of disruption. Group members are not given immediate assistance, but neither are they left totally without help.

The therapist and group members reinforce any behavior that leads to successful selection, planning, and carrying out a relatively long-term activity. Group members take primary responsibility for organizing activities, although initially they may need considerable assistance. The therapist may make several suggestions and ask the group to select an activity from the suggested list, or just two activities may be suggested. On the other hand, group members may be asked to present any ideas that come to mind without any prejudgment as to whether it is a good or bad suggestion. The group then looks at the appropriateness and feasibility of the various suggested activities. The group may need information from the therapist about how to arrive at a decision and the various types of decisions. In planning the activity, group members may require help in considering all aspects of the activity—what tools and materials will be needed and how to get them, in what order the activity should be carried out, how long will it take, and so forth. While group members are engaged in implementing the activity, the therapist may need to give encouragement when the going gets rough or interest wanes, guide the group in problem solving, give individual help to one member who is experiencing difficulty, and so on. As group members learn to select, plan, and implement a long-term task, the therapist's assistance decreases. Eventually the therapist serves more as a resource person, relative to the activity, than as a group leader.

Almost any activity that allows or requires five to nine people to work together is suitable for learning egocentric-cooperative group skills. There are, however, some things to be avoided. Repetition of similar types of activities limits the opportunity for group problem solving. Too many activities that involve each group member making something for him- or herself tend to minimize interaction. Spectator kinds of activities decrease the sense of mutual self-involvement and responsibility. During the initial stages of the group, it is often better for the group to select activities that can be completed in two or three meetings of the group. Long, involved activities that take several days are better left until the group has become more stable and cohesive.

In addition to helping group members to learn to work together in planning and implementing an activity, the therapist is concerned with helping group members to meet each other's esteem needs. Members are assisted in learning how to express their own needs for recognition of achievement, and to identify and meet the esteem needs of other group members. The therapist may act as a role model, expressing his or her own need for recognition and fulfilling the esteem needs of other group members. Reinforcement and feedback relative to expressing and gratifying esteem needs is provided by the therapist, who also encourages a similar response from group members. The group as a whole may discuss: "How do you indicate that you want someone to give you praise and recognition?" "How does someone act when he wants his esteem needs met?" or "How do you let someone know he is doing a good job?"

Learning about group norms and group members' rights and responsibilities is also an important part of being able to interact in an egocentric-cooperative group. Reinforcement is given for identifying and following group norms, for demanding one's rights be respected, and for taking responsibility for respecting the rights of others. In parallel and project groups, these behaviors are reinforced by the therapist. In an egocentric-cooperative group, however, more conscious attention is given to these matters. The group may take time to talk about the norms of their group, to identify what their group's norms are, to discuss whether and how a norm helps the group to function, or to compare the norms of their group with other groups to which they belong. It is helpful if the group has an opportunity to establish group norms consciously. Rights and responsibilities of group members may also be discussed.

Group members are encouraged to accept each individual in the group and to give assistance in showing acceptance. However, at this level of group interaction skill development, the therapist continues to meet group members' needs for love and safety. The capacity to engage in satisfaction of these needs in the context of a group is not learned until the next stage. With so much emphasis on the development of group task skills, individual members need to know they are appreciated for themselves regardless of their capacity in the area of doing. The therapist's responsibility for meeting safety needs is important for an egocentric-cooperative group. In order to feel free to experiment with group task skills, the group must have a sense that there is someone who will not let them go too far or get into serious trouble. The therapist asks the group to consider the various consequences of their decisions. Beyond that, the therapist indicates that, if at all possible, he or she will identify any harmful consequences the group may not have considered. It is in knowing that the therapist will ultimately protect them that the group is able to engage in the risk behavior necessary for learning at this level of development.

Learning how to participate in an egocentric-cooperative group in a middle-range group is fairly simple. A middle-range group functions approximately at this level. The individual is being asked to participate in a type of group that is only one level above the group interaction skill he or she already has. Few precautions need to be taken. The individual is simply helped to learn how to participate in the life of the group.

A Cooperative Group

In a group designed solely for the development of the ability to participate in a cooperative group, the therapist may take the role of a participant, an advisor, or a combination of these two roles. As a participant, the therapist expresses feelings and ideas with relative freedom and avoids an authoritarian position. The therapist and group members take mutual responsibility for reinforcing and providing feedback relative to the behavior to be learned in this type of group. Some examples of the behaviors that are reinforced are: any expression of positive or negative emotion and ideas, appropriate expression, identifying and meeting another person's needs, identifying and expressing one's own needs, and sharing ideas and feelings about oneself. Development of a fairly high degree of cohesiveness is important for this type of group. Individuals need a strong sense of trust and of liking for fellow group members to enable them to experiment freely with the expression of very personal aspects of the self. Thus the therapist helps the group to develop a strong sense of identity and specialness.

Suitable activities for this type of group allow for and encourage the expression of ideas and feelings. Since the activity is secondary to need fulfillment in a cooperative group, activities often have no significant end-product. Examples of useful activities are listening to music, writing and reading poetry, reading plays, doing individual art work, making a group mural, free movement to music, or modern dance. The format for this type of group usually alternates between doing an activity and talking about the feelings and ideas that were aroused by the activity.

The purpose of this type of group is to develop cooperative group interaction skill. The purpose is not awareness and alteration of the many different values, feelings, and ideas that may be interfering with need satisfaction. That is the purpose of a task-oriented group, as was previously discussed. In a group designed for learning cooperative group skill, group members are helped to enjoy the experience of being with each other on an emotional level and how to interact at this level of interpersonal relations in a group situation. There is no attempt to develop in-depth self-understanding or to alter feelings and ideas. The purpose of the group is simply to be able to share on an emotional level.

In the other type of group designed to teach cooperative group interaction skill, the therapist serves primarily as an advisor. The therapist may initially play a relatively active role in the formative period of the group, later withdrawing to a more peripheral position. In this position the therapist is available to the group for consultation, support, and assistance, but does not participate in their day-to-day, ongoing interactions. The formation of the group may be formal or informal. In a formal formation, the therapist brings together a number of clients who are ready to begin learning cooperative group interaction skill and who share some common interests or characteristics. They may, for example, be interested in growing plants or be of approximately the same age. The common interest should not, however, be so important that group members spend most of their time seriously involved in that interest. For example, in a group formed around an interest in photography, members may spend so much of their time together taking, developing, and printing pictures that they never attend to the intimate, personal aspects of the self. Ideally, the interest is sufficiently general so that it does not become the dominant component of the group.

In a group brought together in a formal manner, the therapist introduces the participants and emphasizes that the purpose of their being together is to have fun, to enjoy each other, to share. The idea is to go off together and do whatever they want. After helping the group get started, the therapist, in essence, stays home. Group members know that the therapist-advisor is available if the group as a whole wants to talk about something that is happening in the group or if individual members want to talk. After providing some individual support, the therapist tries to bring the problem of a single member back to the group, helping the group to find ways of solving problems of interaction together.

When a cooperative group is formed in an informal manner, a number of clients spontaneously begin to interact as a group. They break off from a larger group, form a clique, and literally or figuratively go off together to enjoy each other's company. They spend considerable time together, often in the wider community. The therapist, so to speak, adopts the group, aiding them in their desire to be together and letting them know he or she is available to help with any problems that may arise. The formation of these spontaneous groups occasionally is a cause for concern to other staff members, particularly in a psychiatric setting. They feel that the formation of cliques or splinter groups weakens the sense of community of the larger group, making it less effective as a learning situation. They may feel that any clique is automatically going to be detrimental to its members, and that participants will have a negative effect on each other. Although splinter groups detrimental to group members do occasionally develop, this should not be the therapist's first assumption. Rather, the therapist should look at each individual and what the group members seem to be doing together to determine how and why the group formed. When most of the group members are ready to learn or have begun to learn cooperative group interaction skills and if the atmosphere of the group is such that it contributes to a positive learning, the therapist encourages and protects the formation of the group. The spontaneous development of a group skill is, in a sense, more "natural" than the formal formation described above. It is quite similar to what occurs in the normal developmental process. Group members tend to be less conscious of their learning about how to express feelings and satisfy needs. However, this in no way seems to interfere with the learning process.

Groups devoted to the development of cooperative group interaction skill tend to be time-limited and closed. The group is formed, and there may be some initial movement of people in and out of the group, but from that time on the group remains fairly stable. Continual movement of people in and out of this type of group is not conducive to learning. Group members must have a strong feeling of togetherness in order to share intimate feelings. Continual change in group membership limits the possibility of the group developing this sense of group identity. The group ceases to exist when most members have developed the ability to participate in a cooperative group, or have found community-based groups in which they are able to continue to learn this skill. The group tends to dissolve in a rather spontaneous manner; members move out of the group as they no longer feel a need for the group. The few group members left are usually helped to move into another cooperative group that is just being formed.

Another way a therapist may help a client learn how to participate in a cooperative group is to assist the client in locating an appropriate group outside the treatment center. This may be somewhat difficult because the majority of community groups tend to be primarily concerned with task accomplishment. However, some places such as groups sponsored by religious organizations, community centers, senior citizen clubs, and the like may have groups formed primarily for bringing people together. These groups often give only secondary emphasis to accomplishing a particular task. Thus, they may be suitable for learning cooperative group interaction skill. Involvement in almost any community program may give the individual an opportunity to join an informal group. This would be similar to the formation of a spontaneous group described above. The therapist gives the client encouragement, support, and advice while moving into a community-based group. The client knows the therapist is available for any type of assistance needed while becoming part of the group.

There are some problems in teaching cooperative group interaction skill in a middle-range group. The client may be encouraged to identify and meet the safety and love and belonging needs of other group members. Similarly, the client may be helped to identify and express his or her own needs. There may be people in the group, however, who are unable to meet the client's expressed needs. Therefore the client must learn to be selective in terms of whom to turn to for need satisfaction. This makes learning somewhat more difficult. Reinforcement may be given for expressing emotions and sharing personal feelings. Some group members may not be ready for learning in these areas; there tends, thus, to be a lack of reciprocation. Middle-range groups usually focus on task accomplishment, are open ended, and are only fairly cohesive. All of these factors impede the development of a strong feeling of liking and trust, which is necessary for the sharing of personal aspects of the self. It is usually far better for the individual to learn cooperative group interaction skill in the context of a spontaneous group or a group based in the community.

A Mature Group

In a group primarily concerned with learning how to participate in a mature group, the therapist acts as much as possible as a group member rather than a leader. The therapist takes only those group membership roles that are necessary for the continuation of the group at a particular moment in time. This encourages other group members to see the necessity for various membership roles and gives them an opportunity to experiment with these roles. The therapist and group members provide reinforcement for any appropriate behavior leading to task completion or need satisfaction. Emphasis is placed on maintaining an adequate balance between the tasks and need fulfillment, between instrumental and expressive roles. A group designed to teach mature group interaction skill helps group members to integrate the capacity to select, plan, and carry out a group activity and the capacity to satisfy one's own needs and the needs of others in a group situation. The other new skill learned in this type of group is how to satisfy the needs of group members with whom the individual shares little in common. Thus, in selecting group members, the therapist tries to choose people for the group who have a variety of interests and backgrounds and people who are different in age and gender.

Any activity that allows for or requires a number of people to work together is appropriate for this type of group. The activity usually demands a relatively perfect end-product or has an inherent time limit for its successful completion. These characteristics of the activity help group members engage in mutual need satisfaction even when there is a strong demand to attend to the task. In the initial period of learning, however, it is probably best to avoid this added pressure if possible.

A group designed for the learning of mature group interaction skill tends to be self-conscious. The group periodically stops its ongoing activity to examine what is occurring in the group. Group members attempt to determine if necessary instrumental and expressive roles are being taken and, if not, what roles need to be taken. Group members may take turns being an observer rather than a participant. This allows the individual to see how various roles are played. In addition, the group is able to get feedback from someone who is relatively uninvolved in the group's present interactions. The group may take time out to talk about various group membership roles or to experiment with taking roles in role-playing situations.

One area of concern for both clients and therapist is the therapist's position as peer in the group. The therapist must act like a peer, taking no more responsibility or authority than would be expected of other group members. Conversely, group members must learn to accept the therapist as a peer, not asking the therapist to take more responsibility or deferring to the therapist because of the authority position in other settings. Sometimes group members are too dependent on the therapist or request, in subtle ways, that the therapist take more of a leadership role. Sometimes the therapist inadvertently allows group members to become dependent or takes a leadership role. A group observer, whether it be one of the group members or an outsider, can often give the group feedback about the role of the therapist. When necessary, group members and the therapist work together to alter the role of the therapist to become more of a peer.

It is preferable, however, for a client to learn mature group interaction skill through participation in a group in the wider community. Groups that are functioning at the level of a mature group usually have little difficulty in accepting a person who is ready to learn to interact in a mature group. They are usually able to give the reinforcement and feedback necessary for learning. The therapist helps the client to find an appropriate community-based group. The therapist offers support, advice, and encouragement as the client begins to participate in the new group. The therapist may meet periodically with a group of clients who are involved in learning mature group interaction skill in various community-based groups. This group would be structured as a "concurrent topical" group: a type of group that will be discussed later in this section.

Isolated aspects of mature group interaction skill can be learned in a middle-range group. However, participation in such a group does not give the client the true experience of being in a mature group, which is really the best situation for learning. When there is no opportunity to participate in a mature group or a group designed to develop mature group interaction skills in the treatment center, the therapist and client usually try to locate an appropriate group in the wider community.

In conclusion, developmental groups are designed specifically to help clients to acquire group interaction skills in a stage-by-stage sequential manner. It is assumed that an individual learns how to interact in a variety of groups by participating in groups that require increasingly complex ways of interacting. Developmental groups may be differentiated from task-oriented groups in that they are not designed to focus on self-understanding or the alteration of values, thoughts, and feelings.

The idea behind developmental groups, that the group is structured to be compatible with a particular level of group interaction skill, is used in other types of activity groups. In this case, a particular level of developmental group (e.g., parallel or project) serves as the structure for teaching skills other than group interaction skill. Such groups are based on an acquisitional frame of reference and are usually "thematic" groups. However, not all thematic groups make use of a developmental group structure. Conversely, a thematic group that is structured to be at a particular developmental level is not considered to be a developmental group.

Thematic Groups

The fourth type of activity group to be discussed is a thematic group: a group that focuses on gaining knowledge, skill, and attitudes necessary for mastery of performance components and occupational performances. It is concerned with learning how to participate in a circumscribed, clearly defined set of activities. The activities of concern to a particular group are practiced and learned within the context of the group. The goal of a thematic group is to acquire sufficient facility in a set of activities so that group members are able to engage in these activities, independently, eventually within the community. A thematic group takes place primarily within the sheltered environment of the treatment center, although the resources of the surrounding community may be used in the process of practicing various activities. Acquisitional frames of reference are used as the basis for thematic groups.

The goals of a thematic group are such that attention is only given to the process and dynamics of the group when deficits in the process are so severe that they are interfering with attainment of group goals. The group is not designed to teach or deal with those areas of function identified in the discussion of task-oriented groups and developmental groups. Thematic groups are not concerned directly with intrapsychic content; their concern is more on a behavioral level.

The capacity to interact in a group is not dealt with in thematic groups unless the acquisition of skill in group interaction is described as nonstate specific. Group interaction in this case would be described in the context of an acquisitional frame of reference. A thematic group concerned with this orientation to the capacity to function in a group would have goals such as acquiring the ability to share tools and materials, ask for help, carry out a task in a cooperative manner, make appropriate suggestions, and converse in a casual manner with others. These skills would be taught all at the same time with no consideration of sequence. In thematic groups attention is usually given to the interpersonal relationships that the individual will need to have for participation in a specific set of activities.

Common areas of focus in thematic groups are activities of daily living, work, and play/recreation. A thematic group concerned with activities of daily living, for example, may be a grooming group, which is oriented toward such things as how to maintain one's hair in an attractive manner, how to select and care for clothing, how to care for finger and toe nails, and maintenance of a reasonable level of neatness and cleanliness. A cooking group may focus on what is an appropriate and balanced diet, meal preparation, and how to shop in an economical manner. A community orientation group for physically handicapped clients may go out into the surrounding neighborhood to explore the use of public transportation, eating in a restaurant, dealing with the reactions of strangers to one's physical disability, and locating various stores, banks, and recreational facilities accessible to the handicapped.

A thematic group that focuses on the area of work may be a prevocational group. Such a group is concerned with helping clients to learn the kind of behavior that is expected in a work setting, to develop basic work habits, or to practice work skills that may have been affected by disease or injury. The activities used in a prevocational group include assembling or packaging products on subcontract, making small wooden toys using an assembly-line format, making the noon meal, or taking care of the patient library. Regardless of the activity, the atmosphere is business-like and work oriented. Group members are expected to come on time, stay for the entire period that the group meets, complete assigned tasks, dress appropriately, and enter into casual conversation with fellow workers in such a way that conversation does not interfere with the job at hand.

Problems in the area of recreation may also be dealt with in a thematic group. In such a group, members may try various recreational activities together, such as playing computer games, participating in a touch football game, going to a concert, or visiting a local street fair. The purpose of this is to help group members to learn recreational skills and to discover what type of recreational activities they enjoy. It must be remembered that the above descriptions of thematic groups are only examples. There are thematic groups that are concerned with a good number of other, different goals.

It is essentially impossible to describe the types of activities suitable for a thematic group. The activities used are dependent on the knowledge, skills, and attitudes to be taught. The characteristics of appropriate activities are outlined in the frame of reference which is used as the basis for the group.

Selection of clients for a particular thematic group is determined by the goals of the group. Clients are placed in a given group when their learning needs match the objectives of the group. Thematic groups are appropriate for individuals in a wide range of diagnostic categories and age groups. The only really limiting criterion is that a potential member be able to function at least at the parallel group level.

The role of the therapist in a thematic group varies, depending on the specific goals of the group and the degree of sophistication of group members. The therapist's interaction will be somewhere along the continuum of highly supportive and didactic to being a knowledgeable guide. Using the examples of thematic groups provided above, the therapist might give a brief lecture/discussion on unit pricing, play the role of a somewhat sympathetic foreman, or suggest various sources of information regarding current recreational activities in the community. As in developmental groups, giving feedback, providing reinforcement, and acting as a model are very important relative to accomplishing the goals of thematic groups.

Topical Groups

A topical group is primarily a discussion group that focuses on participation in a circumscribed set of activities that take place outside the context of the group. There are two types of topical groups: anticipatory and concurrent. An anticipatory topical group involves discussion of some activities in which group members will be participating in the near future. A concurrent topical group involves discussion of some activity in which group members are presently involved. The two types of topical groups, although separated here, often blend together. For example, a group may begin as anticipatory, eventually becoming concurrent. The areas of concern in topical groups are very similar to those of thematic groups except that topical groups deal with these areas on a more advanced level. For example, a thematic group might be concerned with the development of work habits; a topical group would be concerned with learning how to find a job. The other major difference between thematic and topical groups is that topical groups are more concerned with direct interaction in the community. Activities tend to be natural, whereas in thematic groups activities are likely to be simulated. The majority of topical groups are based on acquisitional frames of reference.

Topical groups focus on engaging in activities in the community that are relatively new for the client or on engaging in activities in a manner different from the way the client participated in these activities in the past. Some examples may be useful at this point. An almost classic illustration of an anticipatory topical group is a discharge group. Members in such a group are often concerned with such things as arranging for future required treatment or intervention, reestablishing relationships with family and friends, finding a job, using leisure time, locating suitable housing, and securing supplementary funds for continued, medically related problems. Thinking through possible areas of difficulty and planning ahead often help the individual make more appropriate and satisfying arrangements for at least the immediate future. Knowing that others feel hesitant about leaving a protective environment and at least some awareness of the problems that may be encountered provide support in the knowledge one is not alone and the security inherent in anticipating problems.

Some examples of concurrent topical groups follow. A home adaptation group may be concerned with discussing physical alteration of the home environment in order to make it more comfortable, efficient, and safe given the group member's particular physical limitations. Such things as the feasibility of kitchen alterations, the need for a different type of telephone equipment, how to secure funds for financing needed alterations, and the best way to get the local grocery store to select and deliver requested merchandise might be discussed. A homemaker's group may be concerned with exploring how to establish priorities in household tasks, the efficient and effective use of time, sharing tasks with other members of the household, and gaining appreciation for tasks accomplished. A parent group is often concerned with the practical aspects of providing a nurturing environment for their children. Some issues that may be discussed are: what do you do when a child refuses to eat properly, should siblings fight out their own battles without parental interference, when should a child be able to use the family car, and what does a parent do knowing that a daughter has broken the conditions of her probation.

The process of a topical group involves discussion in the area of particular concern to the group. Problems or anticipated problems are identified and explored. Possible reasons for a problem and solutions are outlined. In a concurrent group the individual is encouraged to try a likely solution. At the following meeting that person reports back to the group the results of applying that solution. Success is properly commended; lack of success is further explored. After attempting to discover the reason for temporary failure, other solutions are suggested. Once again the individual is urged to try out a likely solution. The process continues until the problem appears to have been satisfactorily resolved. The therapist and group members offer clarification, support, feedback, reinforcement, encouragement, and advice as is needed by the individual. Role playing may also be used.

The therapist as much as possible shares leadership with other group members. Essentially, the therapist acts as a role model so that group members can learn how they can help each other. The general, overall orientation of the group is that "we are all here together to solve some particular problems relative to living and working with others." One of the responsibilities of the therapist, if not taken by other group members, is to keep the group focused on the circumscribed set of activities with which the group was designed to deal. The group may occasionally wander away from the task at hand. This is particularly likely to happen when a group member is experiencing serious difficulty in another area or when the individual is experiencing a generalized state of disorganization and decrease in function. Digressions are often necessary and helpful if they do not occur too frequently. With appropriate timing, the therapist refocuses the group back to the set of topics germane to the goals of the group.

As mentioned, the activities pertinent to a topical group take place outside the context of the group. Suitable activities are primarily determined by the goals of the group. Prescribed activities are a frequent element of topical groups. These activities, suggested by the therapist or at times other group members, are designed to help a client deal with a particular problem. Some examples of prescribed activities are playing with one's child for one-half hour per day without allowing any other interactions to impinge on that time, making a list of all tasks that must be completed by the time one's parents come to visit, going to a department store and buying one piece of clothing, calling an acquaintance on the phone, and so forth. Prescribed activities are often suggested to help a client to begin to engage in a set of activities that in their totality seem formidable to the client. The above examples also illustrate the process of breaking down or reducing an activity to manageable units. This is often a significant means of facilitating goal attainment in a topical group.

A topical group is made up of individuals who share a similar cluster of anticipated or current problems in functioning. The cluster of problems forms the nucleus of the group and is the basis for group identity and cohesiveness.

Differences in age, gender, cultural background, and so forth are usually not of particular importance. Group members ideally should be at the egocentric cooperative level of group interaction or above. Group members should also have sufficient verbal and cognitive skills to engage in discussion and problem solving.

Instrumental Groups

An instrumental group is an activity group designed to meet health needs or to maintain function. Instrumental groups—as opposed to task-oriented, developmental, thematic, and topical groups—are not concerned with change. They are concerned with helping an individual satisfy current needs or to continue to function at the highest level possible for as long as possible.

The difference between meeting health needs and maintenance of function in an instrumental group is sometimes blurred or occurs at the same time in a given group. These aspects of intervention will be discussed more completely in Part 4. For now the differences may be described as one of emphasis. Meeting health needs is concerned with enhancing the individual's sense of physical, psychological, and social well-being. As such, in a general way, it does promote the preservation of function. Maintenance, on the other hand, is more narrowly focused, being concerned with a specific aspect of function. Maintenance usually involves one or more of the performance components. Two examples may help to illustrate instrumental groups.

One health need is group association—the need for regular interaction with an aggregate of others who share common interests and are accepting of the individual. Another health need is pleasure—the need to engage in activities that the individual perceives as enjoyable. An ongoing instrumental group that involves participation in various arts and crafts is suitable for meeting the above-described health needs. The structure of such a group is regular meetings in an attractive, comfortable environment where group members feel secure. Although attendance at group meetings is not required, the atmosphere created by the therapist is sufficiently congenial that attendance by the majority of group members is regular and viewed as an important aspect of the day. Within such an atmosphere, the client is able to find a level of group interaction that is comfortable. The degree of interaction is left up to the individual. No particular pressure is applied to interact with group members beyond that currently comfortable for the individual. Within the context of the group the individual is encouraged to engage in any activity available in the setting. Assistance with any aspect of the activity is provided by the therapist. In such a setting the individual has an opportunity to experience the degree of group association with which he or she is comfortable and to be involved in activities that provide pleasure. The therapist is not concerned with bringing about change in the individual's behavior. The purpose of the group is to be with people, to have fun, to enjoy.

An example of an instrumental group concerned with maintenance of cognitive function and social interaction is a current events group. Members meet regularly to discuss, for example, local, state, and national politics, international events, and the price index, and maybe to gossip a little. The therapist makes the group comfortable for each member, encourages interaction, and helps group members to think through and present their ideas in an organized and logical manner. The goal of the group is not to bring about change but rather to provide an optimal environment in which an individual is able to perform at his highest potential. As such, the group also provides a sense of satisfaction and enjoyment.

Individuals suitable for an instrumental group are those who cannot independently meet their health needs or those who need encouragement and assistance in the maintenance of function. Appropriate activities are determined by the needs which are to be met and the type of function to be sustained. It is the therapist's responsibility to design activity experiences that will meet each client's various health needs, given his present level of function, and to design activities that will maintain function. Instrumental groups similar to all types of activity groups involve a collaborative relationship between client and therapist. It is through this collaboration effort that a satisfying program of action and interaction is established for the time, place, and capacities of the client.

In summary, activity groups are made up of and designed to assist individuals who share common concerns or problems related to the acquisition or maintenance of performance components or occupational performances and to the meeting of health needs. Various activities may be an integral part of the group here-and-now interaction or a specific gestalt of activities external to the group may be the focus of discussion.

DIFFERENCES BETWEEN ACTIVITY GROUPS AND VERBAL GROUPS

The essence of activity groups might be further clarified by comparison to verbal therapy groups. There is no sharp, definitive contrast between activity groups and verbal groups. There are degrees of variation along three different continuums. These continuums are centrality of activity, immediacy of events, and circumscribed focus.

Centrality of activities refers to the degree to which group members are involved in a shared, purposeful activity. Activity groups tend to cluster at the high or positive end of this continuum. Activity groups are concerned with a doing, action-oriented process as opposed to talking about such a process in a relatively abstract manner. Manipulation of and interaction with the nonhuman environment is an important component of activity groups. In contrast, verbal groups tend to be concerned with discussion about intrapersonal and interpersonal interactions. The individual's involvement in everyday activities is usually of far less concern. Interaction with the nonhuman environment tends to be of minor concern.

Immediacy of events refers to the degree to which a group focuses its attention on here-and-now events or events that are likely to occur in the immediate future as opposed to then-and-there or past events. Activity groups tend to focus on here-and-now and near future events. Verbal groups tend to give far more attention to then-and-there events.

The third continuum relates to the degree of circumscribed focus. Circumscribed focus refers to the specificity of group goals and legitimate areas of discussion. Activity groups tend to have fairly delimited goals and legitimate areas of discussion. For example, an activity group may be primarily concerned with how to use and budget one's time or how to find suitable housing. Verbal groups tend to have more general goals and legitimate areas of discussion. For example, a verbal group may have as its goal to increase self-awareness. In such a case there would be few if any areas of human experience that would not be suitable for discussion.

It is essentially a combination of the three continuums mentioned above—centrality of activity, immediacy of events, and circumscribed focus—which differentiates activity groups from verbal groups. Figure 14-1 illustrates the continuums.

The combination of the three continuums is an important consideration. Any given activity group or verbal group may be at any point on each of the three continuums. Collectively, activity groups tend to be more to the right side of the continuum as diagramed in Fig. 14-1, whereas verbal groups tend to be toward the left side of the continuum. There are variations on three dimensions, not one arbitrary factor that distinguishes activity groups from verbal groups.

CONCLUSION

Part 3 of this text has described the legitimate tools of occupational therapy as they relate to the psychosocial components of the profession. It is through the use of these tools that the therapist participates in the evaluation and intervention process—the focus of the remainder of this text.

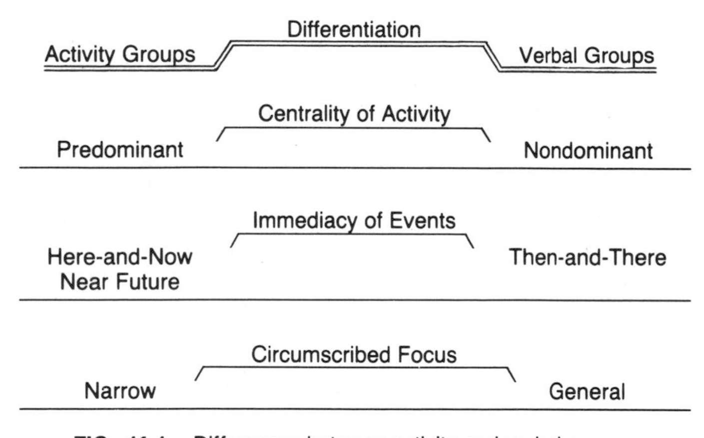

FIG. 14-1. Differences between activity and verbal groups.

Part 4

Evaluation and Intervention: An Overview

Parts 1–3 have set the stage for this and the subsequent parts of the text. They have provided the background information necessary for evaluation and intervention, the essence of the occupational therapy process. Part 4 is addressed to the sequence of events that leads up to the identification of the client's problem areas and continues to the ultimate point of their most expedient resolution. Expectant here refers to the most feasible or best possible solution given the nature of the problem and the current circumstances that impinge on the problem. This sequence of events is shown in Fig. P4-1: evaluation, the setting of goals and priorities, formulating a plan for intervention, the intervention process, reevaluation to determine progress, termination, and communication (129,190,960). As the diagram indicates, the events of evaluation and intervention take place in an orderly fashion, with one event naturally leading to the next. The communication process; keeping records and making verbal and oral reports, is an ongoing process that takes place throughout the sequence.

The various processes outlined above will be discussed in Chapters 15 through 19. The change process will be discussed separately in Part 5.

One point to be emphasized here is that evaluation and intervention are a collaborative process. It occurs *with* the client, a cooperative venture. Therapist-client collaboration is a highly significant determinant of the success of evaluation and intervention. Cooperative interaction with other members of the health team and with individuals significant to the client is also important. It is always good for the therapist to remember that he or she is only one element in a total matrix of interactions that will either facilitate or impede evaluation and intervention. Although only one element, the therapist is respon-

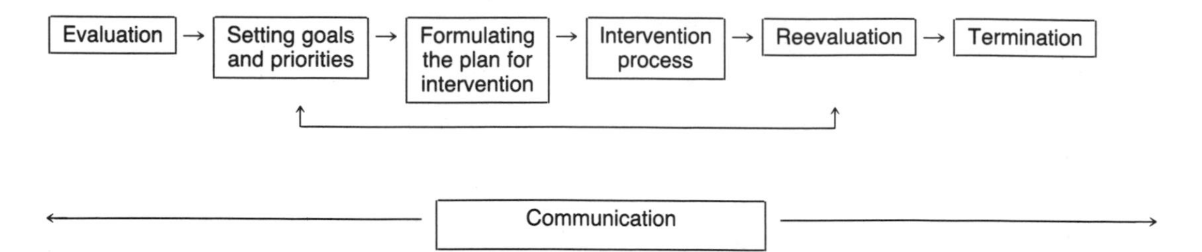

FIG. P4-1. The evaluation and intervention process. (Adapted from Trombley and Scott, ref. 960.)

sible for contributing to the matrix in such a manner that it, as a totality, works for the client's benefit.

15 Evaluation

Evaluation, as previously defined, is the process of assessing whether an individual requires assistance in meeting health needs in his or her current environment, is in need of intervention directed toward prevention, is able to benefit from involvement in the change process, or is in need of a program of maintenance or management. Evaluation takes place prior to and periodically during the course of intervention. It is concerned with the current status of the individual as opposed to intervention, which involves some process modification of current status.

Evaluation has the following purposes (3,916,956,960).

- To identify whether an individual has a problem in functioning and if that problem can be modified by the occupational therapy process.
- To understand the nature of the individual's problems and the effect they may have on his or her life.
- To learn something about the individual relative to social roles, social and cultural background, available support system, values, skills, and interests.
- To understand the individual's functional capacities and strengths as well as deficits.
- To gain some idea of the individual's potential for change.
- To determine appropriate objectives for intervention.
- To facilitate the selection of relevant frames of reference.
- To devise an expedient plan for intervention.
- To enlist the individual's cooperation and interest in the occupational therapy process.
- To begin the process of establishing rapport.
- As an ongoing process, to determine at what point intervention is to be altered or discontinued.

The purposes outlined above are listed roughly in the order of the questions addressed in the evaluative process. The order, however, does not indicate that any one purpose is more important than another.

Evaluation as a collaborative process involves the client and therapist working together to identify the client's assets and limitations. Thus the client should be aware that he or she is being evaluated, what he or she is being evaluated for, and what is expected during the evaluation process. Evaluative findings are shared with the client. Ideally, the evaluative process is designed to help the client identify his or her own problems in living. Self-discovery of problem areas is often more meaningful to a client than having someone else tell that person what the problems are.

Evaluation should take place as soon as possible after the client is admitted to the treatment center. The only exceptions are when the client is so seriously physically ill that he or she is unable to engage in any meaningful interaction or when the client has severe psychiatric symptoms that are being treated with drugs. In the latter situation it is sometimes better to wait a few days until medication has had at least some effect. By waiting, the therapist is likely to get a more accurate picture of the patient's problem areas. In addition, the client is usually much more able to cooperate in the evaluative process.

The period set aside for initial evaluation is relatively short, a few days perhaps but definitely not more than a week. Intervention can thus be initiated without undue delay. A short initial evaluation period may mean that some desired information is not available. However, no matter the length of time set aside for evaluation, additional information is almost always desired. Initial evaluative findings are always considered tentative and thus subject to change. This is one of the reasons reevaluation is part of the occupational therapy process.

Evaluation should be as efficient as possible. When several team members are to be involved in evaluation of the same client, evaluation is planned so that there is minimal overlap in the information each person requests of the client. This is most easily accomplished if each person on the evaluation team knows what information each other team member usually requests of a client. It is a waste of both staff and client time for many staff members to investigate the same area. Thus, for example, if the nurse usually assesses activities of daily living relative to hygiene and grooming there is no reason for the occupational therapist to evaluate this area as well.

With these introductory remarks, this chapter is divided into four sections: sampling of behavior, sequence and process, sources of data, and emotional aspects.

SAMPLING OF BEHAVIOR

Evaluation in occupational therapy is based on behavior—what an individual says or does. Obviously the therapist cannot observe all of the individual's behavior and thus, similar to evaluation in most areas of human function, evaluation in occupational therapy involves a sampling of behavior (402,577). It is from this sample of behavior that one, at some risk, makes a statement about the individual's capacity in that area of human function. Classroom tests are an example of the sampling aspect of evaluation. From the student's response on the test, the teacher makes some judgment about the degree to which the student has mastered the subject matter the test was designed to assess.

Another aspect of evaluation, also illustrated in the example given above, is that the evaluation process must provide an opportunity for the individual to exhibit specific behaviors. Opportunity is important in the above statement, for the absence of usual or expected behavior is as significant in evaluation as the presence of such behavior. To design an appropriate evaluative situation, then, the therapist must know what aspect of the domain of concern he or she wishes to assess, the behavior that best provides information about that area, and the situational stimuli that are most likely to elicit the desired behavior.

An evaluative situation is only useful if it provides an accurate measure of the area of human function it is designed to assess. Two important concepts concerned with the issue of accuracy are reliability and validity (13,359,402,516,877,901,988). Reliability is the extent to which it is possible to obtain similar results upon repetition of the evaluative situation. It is an estimate of the degree to which an individual will exhibit the same type of behavior in the evaluative situation if it should be repeated a number of times. Obviously, an evaluative situation that allows for a considerable variation in behavior provides less accurate information than an evaluative situation that does not. There are several types of reliability, most of which have been studied in relationship to paper-and-pencil tests. The major types are (a) Test-retest: If the same test is given again, after a suitable interval to minimize differential practice effects, will comparable information be obtained? (b) Parallel forms: If comparable forms of the test (i.e., duplicate, equivalent, or alternative forms) are given at essentially the same time, will comparable results be obtained? (c) Internal consistency: Do the several parts of the test (each half, every other question, etc.) yield the same information?

The therapist, using evaluative tools such as a check list, questionnaire, or some other type of inventory completed by the client, should assess the reliability of the tool. In this case, the test-retest method of determining reliability is probably the most expedient. Interview schedules (the series of questions to be asked in an interview) and evaluative situations that involve the use of a purposeful activity should also be subjected to a study of their reliability. Although different than a paper-and-pencil situation, the test-retest method is probably also appropriate.

Finally, any evaluative situation that involves observation and the completion of some kind of a check sheet should be evaluated relative to its "inter-rater" reliability. This type of reliability is a measure of the degree to which several different therapists arrive at the same conclusions when they observe a specific interaction using the same check sheet. Reliability in this case is often increased by good definitions of behavioral categories and by practice on the part of the therapists. An evaluative situation used by many therapists should, as much as possible, yield comparable information.

The other concept concerned with the accuracy of an evaluative situation is validity. Validity is the degree to which an evaluative situation measures what it purports to measure. There are three major types of validity: content, criterion-related, and construct.

1. Content validity is established through a rational analysis of the content or substance of the evaluative situation. Its determination is based on the individual's

subjective judgement. There are two subtypes of content validity: face and logical. Face validity involves a person examining the evaluative situation and concluding that it measures what it is supposed to measure. Logical validity (also known as sampling validity) involves a careful definition of the domain of behavior to be measured by an evaluative situation and the logical design of the situation to cover all the important areas of the domain. Logical validity is somewhat more sophisticated than face validity and it is recommended that it be made part of the process of developing an evaluative situation.

2. Criterion-related validity involves the comparison of evaluative findings to some standard outside the evaluative situation. There are two types of criterion-related validity: predictive and concurrent. Predictive validity involves the comparison of evaluative findings to some predicted future behavior. This is accomplished by gaining information from the evaluative situation for a given group of individuals. Later information is collected relative to the specified criterion. Findings from the two sources of information are then compared to determine the extent to which the evaluative situation predicted future performance. A good example of tests that have been found to have fairly good predictive validity are the Scholastical Aptitude Test and the Graduate Record Examination. Concurrent validity involves the comparison of information derived from the evaluative situation and the criterion situation with both measures being obtained at the same time. An example of establishing concurrent validity for an evaluation situation designed to assess work habits would be to (a) evaluate a sample of employees of a given company using the evaluative situation, (b) obtain the annual worker evaluation report for each worker in the sample from the personnel office, (c) compare the findings of the evaluative situation with the company report. Predictive validity is not usually used to assess the accuracy of occupational therapy evaluative tools. There are two reasons for this: it is usually not necessary and it is extremely expensive. Concurrent validity, although also somewhat expensive, could and should be used to assess many of the evaluative tools used by occupational therapists.

3. Construct validity is the degree to which an evaluative situation measures the theoretical construct it is designed to measure. Based on a current theory regarding the aspect of human behavior being measured, the developer of the evaluative tool makes predictions about findings when the tool is used to assess specific population. These predictions are then tested. In illustration, there is an evaluative tool used by occupational therapists to assess the extent to which clients have mastered the various developmental levels of group interaction skill (see p. 708). One way in which the construct validity of this tool could be assessed is to use the tool to evaluate children and adolescents at various age levels. The prior prediction would be that individuals at a given age level, for example 6 years, would have mastered the ability to participate in an egocentric-cooperative group but would not have mastered the ability to participate in a cooperative group.

Establishing the validity of an evaluative situation is no easy task. It is rarely if ever attempted until a relatively high degree of reliability has been demonstrated. It is essentially a waste of time and energy to validate an evaluative situation when the situation is not able to elicit similar kinds of behavior consistently from the same individual.

Many evaluative situations or tools have almost built-in potential for error. Thus, reliability and validity tend to be somewhat low. Briefly, some of the problems found in the use of common evaluative situations follow.

Analogous Situations

This refers to evaluations that take place in an environment designed to simulate the natural environment in those areas that are considered important relative to the purpose of the evaluation. One of the major problems with analogous situations is that behavior is extremely variable and environmentally dependent. Cross-situational stability for many kinds of behavior is not particularly high. There is always some question about whether the type and frequency of behavior seen in an analogous situation are similar to the individual's behavior in the natural environment. Thus, for example, an individual in an evaluative group may be quite dependent and demanding. This behavior may not be at all evident in the individual's usual environment. Another major problem with analogous situations is the dearth of normative data, i.e., the usual performance of a given group. Thus, the therapist must rely on subjective inferences and subjective norms in interpreting the information derived from assessment utilizing analogous situations.

Questionnaires

One problem with questionnaires is response bias. The individual becomes "set" for whatever reason to respond in a particular kind of way. Everything, for example, may be viewed in a very positive light, or negatively. Social desirability is another factor that may cause a problem. The individual essentially responds to the questionnaire in a way that he or she thinks would be a socially acceptable way to respond. The response thus has little relationship to the individual's own ideas or feelings. The situation in which the individual completes the questionnaire may influence the kinds of responses given. Immediate events have a strong influence on response and the flavor of the response. Another important factor is the length and complexity of the questionnaire. If too complex or lengthy, the individual may lose interest in the whole process and answer in a superficial and/or haphazard manner.

Interview

There are many subjects that people are hesitant to discuss with another person, particularly a relative stranger. Some of these subjects are deficits in function, behavior that deviates from social norms, sexual interactions, money, and religion. The interviewer also influences the response of the individual. The individual is likely to tell the interviewer what he or she thinks the interviewer wants to hear. For example, if the individual thinks the interviewer is only interested in the individual's problems in functioning, this is all that the individual will talk about. The interviewer will hear nothing about those areas in which the individual is managing his or her affairs quite nicely. Another factor that influences the responses in an interview is its structure, i.e., questions requiring a short answer versus questions allowing for considerable elaboration and so forth. People tend to say different things, depending on the kinds of questions that are asked.

The evaluative situations or tools commonly used by occupational therapists in assessing psychosocial components have, on the whole, not been subjected to rigorous study. Thus, there is little information about their reliability or validity. This is not to say that they are not reliable or valid. They may well be; we simply do not know at this time. This is an area that needs considerable work. As the profession grows and matures, hopefully, it will study and thus gain more confidence in the efficacy of its evaluative procedures.

SEQUENCE AND PROCESS

The sequence and process of evaluation are intimately connected. They are separated here for ease in presentation. In actual clinical practice, however, these two elements are intertwined. Sequence of evaluation refers to the various steps of the evaluation phase, whereas process refers to the kinds of decisions the therapist makes throughout the evaluation phase.

The Sequence of Evaluation

The sequence of evaluation begins when the therapist is requested to evaluate a client or the therapist initiates the process independently (29,74,129,189,190,220,705, 916,956,960). The first step in the sequence is screening, sometimes referred to as informal evaluation. Screening is the process of ascertaining whether or not an individual is a potential client for occupational therapy and, if that is the case, of determining what type of formal evaluation is necessary. Screening may involve one or more of the following: review of medical or other records, an interview with the individual and/or a family member, discussion with other professionals who are familiar with the individual, informal observation of the individual interacting with others and/or while engaged in manipulation of nonhuman objects, and the administration of a formal screening tool. All of these are not necessarily required for adequate screening. The therapist simply must gather sufficient data to determine whether the individual might benefit from occupational therapy and if so what areas of function need to be assessed in detail.

An individual is considered able to benefit from occupational therapy if he is currently unable to meet his health needs, is at risk relative to becoming dysfunctional in performance components or occupational performances, shows evidence of dysfunction in these areas, or is having difficulty maintaining function, given the nature of his disability. Screening involves a general assessment of these four areas. Behavior that might need to be managed is usually considered after it is determined that an individual could benefit from occupational therapy.

During the screening process, the therapist, using criteria that will be outlined in the next chapter, assesses whether the individual's health needs are being met. The performance components as described in Chapter 3 are used as the basis for screening in these areas. The information provided in Chapters 4 and 5 is used as the basis for screening occupational performances. Age and environment are always taken into consideration in screening as they are for formal evaluation.

Through screening, then, the therapist is able to make some determination about the type(s) of evaluation which will be necessary. If the client is a potential candidate for the change process, the therapist decides what frame of reference would be appropriate to use. This is determined before formal evaluation, because the kinds of information sought and the evaluative tools used will be influenced by the selected frame of reference. Through screening, for example, the therapist may discover that a 65-year-old client's thinking is quite concrete and not particularly logical and that he has some serious difficulty in manipulating the nonhuman environment. An analytic frame of reference probably would be inappropriate for this individual because of cognitive deficits. The individual's age may preclude the use of a developmental frame of reference. Thus, an acquisitional frame of reference may be the most expedient. There are many factors that are taken into consideration in selecting a frame of reference; this example was only used in illustration. Criteria for selecting a frame of reference will be discussed in more detail in Part 5.

Screening usually, but not always, involves a meeting between the potential client and the therapist. The purpose of the meeting varies, depending on the method of screening used by the therapist. It may, for example, be used simply to meet the client and to introduce oneself as a preliminary step to further interactions. It may be used to informally observe the client's behavior and to gain some preliminary information about the client's assessment of his situation. It may involve a formal interview or the administration of a specific screening tool. The purpose of the meeting should be clear to the therapist and communicated to the client.

Regardless of the specific purpose, the first meeting between client and therapist is very important (91, 98,266,567, 786,790,887). Initial impressions are formed quickly and are often difficult to change, particularly when they are negative. To make this first meeting as successful as possible, the therapist attempts to find a place to talk that is relatively free from distractions. The therapist introduces him- or herself and encourages the client to do likewise. The therapist then briefly explains the occupational therapy process, defining both the therapist's role and that of the client in evaluation and intervention. The purpose of this first meeting is also made clear. Explanations are given at a level that the client seems able to understand. (It is sometimes difficult to determine whether the client understands what the therapist is saying; two indicators are whether the client asks questions relevant to the information presented and whether she is able to respond to questions.) Also, one does not overwhelm the client with information or questions. This can be confusing, with the result that the client remembers little of what was said. The client is encouraged to ask questions and express immediate concerns. Answers to questions are as honest and forthright as possible. The therapist should never be afraid to say, "I don't know." Reassurance is given realistically in a genuine manner. Time is always left for casual conversation if the client is able to tolerate this type of interaction. The therapist indicates concern for the client as an individual with unique qualities. The client is never made to feel that evaluation is an impersonal, assembly-line procedure. It is, rather, presented as a personal assessment in which the client is intimately involved. When it appears that the client is a potential candidate for occupational therapy, the initial meeting is ended by the therapist indicating the next step in the evaluative process. This may commence promptly or an appointment may be made for meeting together in the immediate future.

Formal evaluation, if indicated, occurs subsequent to screening. The purpose of formal evaluation is to verify the existence of the problem found in screening, to further define the problem, or to dismiss the results of screening as spurious. In addition to assessment of health needs, performance components, and occupational performances, the therapist is concerned with identifying the client's expected environment. Expected environment refers to the anticipated life situation of the client. It includes the social roles that will be required of the client in that environment and the knowledge, skills, and attitude that must be integrated for successful participation in these roles. As a general rule, the therapist uses 6 months or 1 year as a time guide, depending on the severity of the client's condition. Thus, in determining the expected environment, the therapist asks the general question, Where is the client likely to be and what will he or she be doing 6 months (a year) from now?

The environment in which the client may eventually live might be a total institution, a sheltered environment, the preintervention environment, a new unsheltered environment, or any combination of these. A total institution is a place of residence, work, and recreation where a large number of like-situated individuals, separated from the wider society, lead an enclosed, formally administered round of life. Examples of total institutions are a state mental hospital, an institution for the mentally retarded, and some extended-care facilities. A sheltered environment is one in which the individual is protected from many of the usual demands of the social system. A half-way house, a group home, sheltered workshop, or a boarding house in which many of the individual's needs are provided for by salaried employees are examples of a sheltered environment. The preintervention environment is the environment in which the client lived prior to hospitalization or is living during the intervention process. A new, unsheltered environment is one in which the individual must meet the usual demands of the social system, but in a setting that is different from the preintervention environment.

In determining the expected environment, the client and therapist are concerned with such questions as: Where will the client be living? With whom? What will the client's responsibilities be in his or her home? Will the client be going to school or working? What kind of job will he or she probably have? What kind of avocational pursuits will be available for the client? Identifying the expected environment helps both client and therapist set intervention goals and priorities. The expected environment may change during the intervention process; thus it is always discussed during each reevaluation.

There are several factors to consider in preparation for formal evaluation. One previously mentioned is the frame of reference to be used. This, in turn, determines to some extent the evaluative tools or situations to be used. When there are choices, the therapist must decide which evaluative tool would be more acceptable to the client, or the client may be given a choice if that seems appropriate.

The sequence of evaluative interactions also must be considered. For example, when an evaluation is based on a developmental frame of reference, the therapist usually begins with a task that is likely to be well within the individual's capacity and then moves on to more developmentally advanced tasks. The individual's age will also influence sequencing. Children and adolescents often are more cooperative when sedentary evaluation procedures are presented first and followed by procedures that involve more physical activity. Evaluation with an elderly individual may be more effective if the opposite sequence is used. The sequence should be sufficiently varied to maintain the client's interest but also have some logic that is reasonably discernible to the client.

Whether and what aspect of evaluation should take place individually or in a group setting is another factor to take into consideration. Evaluation procedures that require a good deal of interaction between client and therapist should take place in a dyad. The same is true for procedures requiring very close observation of refined aspects of behavior. Evaluation in a group setting is appropriate for assessing an individual's capacity to engage with others either in dyadic interactions or in the context of a group task. A group setting may also be used if the end result of the evaluation task is more important than observing the process. Thus, the completion of an inventory or questionnaire may be accomplished more economically in a group setting followed by individual discussion with each client. In this case evaluative findings are concerned only in a tangential way with the interaction of the individual with the aggregate of others.

The therapist must decide whether the initial evaluation is to be a complete survey or if it would be more appropriate for evaluation to take place in a limited number of areas only. A partial evaluation, for example, may include assessment of a client's ability to engage in simple tasks and to function in a group. At a later time, during the reevaluation session, difficulties in activities of daily living might be explored. All of these areas (and others) would be assessed at the same time in a complete or total initial evaluation survey. Partial evaluations are probably best for clients who appear to have deficits in almost all areas of function and for clients who are in an acute state of distress. Clients who appear to have less difficulty in functioning are usually able to participate in a total initial evaluation.

Evaluation should take place in an environment that is physically safe, pleasant, and free from extraneous distractions. Physical safety is particularly important for clients who have physical or sensory impairment. The ambience of the evaluation environment should be such that it is acceptable to the majority of clients. It ought to be clean, neat, and well-lighted, without being sterile in appearance. In general, it should simply be a comfortable place in which to be. Extraneous distractions such as noise, many objects that are likely to arouse interest, people moving in and out of the environment, and so forth can be detrimental to the evaluation process. This is particularly true for clients who are somewhat confused, hyperactive, or who have a short attention span. Finally, evaluation should be planned in such a way that it engages the individual's interest in the process and leaves the individual with a sense of satisfaction and completion. The latter is important. Evaluation, as will be discussed at the end of this chapter, is often a trying experience for the client. Thus, the client should leave the situation feeling that he or she has done a commendable job and has successfully completed an important piece of work.

With adequate preparation and planning the *process of formal evaluation* should go fairly smoothly. However, it is important to note that even the best laid plans may occasionally not meet the immediate needs of the client. Thus during formal evaluation, the therapist should always remain flexible, adapting his or her behavior as much as possible to assist the client in being comfortable and able to cooperate.

Prior to the beginning of evaluation, the procedure is explained, including what is expected of the client. Explanations should be honest, age appropriate, and congruent with the individual's current capacity to understand. Anxiety, confusion, preoccupation with other matters, and depression may limit comprehension, at least initially.

The therapist's behavior during evaluation should be relaxed and attentive to the client. Feedback and encouragement are given freely and honestly as they are called for in the situation. The only time this may be inappropriate is during the administration of a standardized test. Directions for giving the test may specify the behavior of the examiner. In this case the therapist may be required to maintain a sense of distance to avoid giving the individual clues that may affect performance. Generally the therapist does not intrude upon the evaluative tasks until it is quite evident that the individual cannot perform the task independently. The therapist may then suggest the client discontinue the task or the therapist may help the client complete the task. This is done to alleviate, in part, the client's possible feeling of failure. It is, of course, taken into consideration in interpreting the data.

Although the therapist's behavior is relaxed during the evaluative procedure, the therapist remains in control of the situation. Limits are set in regard to what behavior will and will not be tolerated. These may be presented nonverbally simply by the therapist's behavior or they may need to be stated verbally and at times rather firmly. Even though the individual may know what the limits of the situation are, there are times when these may be tested. This is particularly truc in thc case of children and adolescents. The therapist restates the limits and if necessary uses physical contact to control the deviant behavior. Behavior that interferes with evaluation should be noted. It may well be that such behavior will need to be managed as part of the intervention process.

Time is an important factor in the evaluation procedure. The therapist should meet the client at the appointed time. Delays tend to increase the client's anxiety and, perhaps more importantly, show a marked disrespect for the client. During the evaluation procedure the therapist does not permit interruptions either from visitors or the telephone. The only exception is when there is a real emergency. Interruptions break the continuity of the evaluation, may interfere with concentration, and, again, they indicate disrespect for the client. The client should be aware of the length of the evaluation meeting and this time limit should be adhered to. Young children and individuals who have difficulty conceptualizing time are warned 5 or 10 minutes before the end of the evaluation meeting so that the close of the meeting does not appear to be too abrupt. These comments regarding time are also applicable to the intervention process.

The individual's right to refuse to participate in an evaluative task is always respected. There are three major reasons for refusal. The individual (a) may be afraid to risk failure, (b) may think that he or she knows how to perform the task but lacks the self-confidence to experiment, or (c) may choose to refuse as a way of demonstrating independence and self-sufficiency. If refusal is treated in a matter-of-fact manner, the individual will often attempt the task if it is suggested by the therapist at a later time in the evaluation process. Risk-taking and cooperation usually increase as the client begins to trust the therapist. For some people trust comes neither easily nor quickly.

Evaluation should be terminated at the first indication of real fatigue. Individuals who are tired are unable to perform at their highest level. Discontinuation because of fatigue also indicates concern and caring on the part of the therapist. Fatigue is indicated by such behavior as rubbing or closing the eyes, decreased motor and/or verbal behavior, and careless mistakes that were not previously evident. Fatigue is most likely to be evident in small children (particularly if the evaluation does not coincide with their typical active periods of the day), individuals who are physically ill, the elderly, and individuals who are on high doses of medication.

Real fatigue should, however, be differentiated from feigned fatigue or boredom. Feigned fatigue is often an attempt to avoid the evaluation situation. Rather than terminating the meeting, the therapist helps the client to look at possible reasons for avoidance. Good preplanning of the evaluative meeting so that there are a variety of tasks that are likely to be stimulating and interesting to the client usually minimizes the probability of boredom. However, if boredom does occur, a change in the task often quickly relieves the feeling.

Note-taking during evaluation is common and usually an accepted procedure. It is often quite necessary if the therapist is to recall the individual's performance accurately. Although it may seem clumsy at first, with a little practice note-taking can be accomplished quickly and unobtrusively. However, close interaction with the client and detailed observation of the client's behavior may preclude note-taking. If this is the case the therapist should record observations immediately after the evaluative meeting. Specific time should be set aside for this in the therapist's schedule. The end of the day is not a good time to write down observations. The therapist is usually tired and the immediacy of the evaluative meeting is often lost because of the number of intervening events. If the client questions the therapist about taking notes, a simple explanation is given. Some clients ask if they may see the notes. There is no reason why they should not; evaluation is a collaborative experience. It is often more meaningful, however, for the therapist to share the evaluative findings with the client after the therapist has had time to organize the data and make some interpretations. Raw data, hastily written, often give the client little information, if the client can read the notes at all.

The last step in the sequence of evaluation is reevaluation. This is the periodic assessment of the client's progress or lack of progress during the course of intervention. It is a formal, regular part of the intervention process. It is *formal* in the sense that time is specifically set aside to look at what improvements the client may or may not have experienced. All problem areas are reassessed, the data are interpreted and compared with prior evaluative data to note changes. Reevaluation is *regular* in the sense that it takes place at specific predetermined times during intervention. The timing of periodic evaluation will depend on the nature of the individual's problem and on the changes informally observed in the client's performance during intervention. Although timing varies, once a month is probably the longest time that should elapse between periodic evaluations.

When reevaluation indicates that the long-term goals of intervention have been reached, intervention is terminated. When the immediate or short-term goals have been reached, more advanced goals are set. A new plan is written and intervention continues. This is the ideal sequence of events. However, it is sometimes discovered that the client has made no progress since the initial evaluation or last reevaluation. It may also appear that the client has more problem areas than those originally identified.

If intervention is not progressing in the anticipated manner, the client and therapist need to look at the following.

1. The type and amount of medication the client is receiving. It is possible that the client might receive more benefit from another kind of medication. On the other hand, the client may be taking too much or not enough medication. The responsible physician is consulted.

2. The immediate goal(s). The immediate goal for intervention may have been set too high. That is, the goal may have been too advanced for the client to reach at the present time. When this is the case, simpler or more basic goals are set, a new plan is written, and intervention continues. At other times it may be found that the immediate goal is not truly compatible with the client's wishes. He may have thought he wanted to reach the stated goal but he may not really want to do so. Another goal more compatible with the client's wishes is selected, at least for the present time.

3. The intervention situation. To discover factors that might be interfering with intervention it is often helpful to compare the intervention situation to the principles that underlie meeting health needs and management and to the postulates regarding change of the frame of reference being utilized. Perhaps crucial principles are not being used or are not being followed properly. Similarly, if intervention is taking place in the context of a group, the structure and dynamics of the group are considered. For example, there may be group norms that are inhibiting change or the communication process may be faulty. When factors in the intervention process are found to be interfering with the goals, the therapist and client attempt to make the necessary changes.

4. Elements outside the intervention situation. Some elements that may be interfering are the following:

a. There may be divergent ideas, within the setting, about the effectiveness of various types of intervention. This may occur, for example, when some of the staff believe that the use of psychoactive drugs is the only type of treatment that is effective, or that only in-depth verbal psychotherapy will alter behavior. When some staff members hold either of these beliefs, they tend to see occupational therapy as only keeping clients busy and out of trouble while the "real" treatment is taking effect. When this attitude is communicated to clients, even on a nonverbal level, clients may experience conflict, hesitating to devote time and energy to the occupational therapy process.

b. The atmosphere of the treatment facility or the current life situation of the client may not be conducive to intervention. Decisions about a client's privileges or discharge date may be made in a highly arbitrary manner, for example, or there may be an excessive number of rules and regulation. Clients cannot participate in intervention when their basic human rights and needs are not being respected, or if they are preoccupied with personal emergency. Examples of the latter would be concern about a severely ill parent or imminent loss of usual income.

c. People important to the client may be indicating in some way that they do not wish the client to change. A mother, for example, may become frightened when her dependent, passive daughter begins to assert herself. The mother does not know how to cope with this new behavior and indicates to the daughter that she is more comfortable with the daughter's former behavior.

When the client and therapist find factors outside the intervention situation interfering with intervention, they work together to bring about the necessary changes. Identification of these factors alone may be sufficient to allow intervention to continue in a more positive manner. These disruptive factors, however, cannot always be altered, or at least not at the present time. It may be necessary for intervention to be discontinued. Sometimes the situation is such that a therapist is not able to help a client: this is an unhappy fact of life that a therapist must learn to accept.

Reevaluation may also include assessment of areas of function not included in the initial evaluation. The therapist, for example, may feel that the client is now ready to examine his ability to work or to explore ways in which he has used his leisure time.

Periodic evaluation also offers an opportunity to reassess the client's expected environment. The essential question is whether the expected environment should be the same as the one identified at the time of initial evaluation or of the last periodic evaluation. The client or therapist may feel that the previously agreed upon expected environment will not provide sufficient support for the client. Or the proposed expected environment may be seen as too sheltered; the client might be more comfortable in an environment that allows for more independence and decision-making. Finally the client's interests, values, and ideas about himself may have changed. One client, for example, may decide she does not want to return to college, another may feel that he would now like to try living in a senior citizens' residence rather than living alone. When the expected environment is to be different from the one originally planned, the client's assets and limitations must be reassessed relative to the new expected environment. Does the client, for example, need less, more, or different skills for this new environment? It may be necessary to set different long-term goals.

Reevaluation is the last phase in the evaluation process. Little has been said, however, about how the therapist arrives at the various conclusions that ultimately lead to defining a client's areas of function and dysfunction. This aspect of evaluation is here referred to as process.

The Process of Evaluation

In the process of evaluation, the major responsibility of the therapist is to decide what data to collect, to collect data that are as accurate as possible, and to decide what the data mean. Evaluation is a special kind of decision-making (35,567,624,786,960). The therapist is confronted by an array of data: searching and shifting through the array, rejecting some aspects of the available data, and seeking more data to supplement the existing information. The solution to the problem consists of identifying the client's assets and limitations and specifying the kind of intervention that is likely to be most helpful. At the beginning of the evaluation process, the therapist uses a pattern recognition procedure to focus quickly on a group of possible problems. This is the screening process that gives the therapist a rough idea of what the problem may be. The addition of further data and personal experience allows the therapist to reach a conclusion with a relative degree of confidence.

The therapist as a decision maker must, however, come to grips with uncertainty. Variability is the law of life. No two bodies are alike, no two psyches are alike, and no two individuals react alike or behave alike under conditions of psychological stress, trauma, or disease. Thus, the degrees of error in clinical practice are fairly large and universal. Evaluation is best conceptualized as a matter of probability. The therapist, therefore, must learn to accept ambiguity, uncertainty, and open choice. There are no assurances that one is right, nor is there certitude that one is wrong. Evaluation is not an exact science, nor will it ever be as long as there is individuality and uniqueness.

With these brief introductory remarks, the process of evaluation consists of three phases—data collection, interpretation, and validation—which are continually repeated (74,220,290,705,916,956,960).

The first concern of the therapist is data collection, the major question being what data to collect. In some situations there is superabundance, in other situations data are negligible at best. In gathering data the therapist must focus on that information which reflects both adaptive behavior and functional limitations relative to the occupational therapy domain of concern. There is likely to be a good deal of extraneous information which, although interesting, is not pertinent to the occupational therapy process. What is and is not pertinent is difficult to define and will depend to some extent on the frame of reference being used as the basis for evaluation. In using an acquisitional frame of reference, for example, the therapist may not be interested in the information derived from some type of projective technique, whereas a therapist using an analytical frame of reference may be interested in such information.

Although the therapist seeks specific data, the focus should not be so narrow that other potentially significant data are ignored. In evaluating a client's capacity to engage in a task, for example, the therapist may note that the client completed the assigned task with no difficulty. However, in the process of doing the task, the client spoke extensively about a summer she had spent in Vermont when she was a teenager. This may or may not be useful information. It is, nonetheless, noted by the therapist, for it might prove to be useful in the future. Vision may be a useful illustration of the data collection process: Central vision then is analagous to the gathering of specific information, whereas peripheral vision refers to awareness of seemingly extraneous information that may or may not be significant. As in vision, what is central and what is peripheral at any moment in time often shifts while collecting data.

This phase of the evaluation process includes the selection of tools and methods by which information is to be obtained, as well as the use of these tools and methods. The selection of evaluative procedures is not particularly well structured in occupational therapy. There is, for example, no agreed on method for screening. Selection thus is dependent on many factors, including the nature of the presented problem, the characteristics of the client, the setting, the frame of reference being used, and the therapist's personal preference. There is within the profession a relatively strongly expressed desire for more specific guidelines in regard to the selection and use of evaluative tools. This need does have some merit. To some extent, however, the need grows out of a fear of ambiguity and lack of certitude, elements that are inherent in any evaluative process no matter how highly structured. In a more positive light, the lack of specific guidelines gives the therapist considerable latitude in selection, which may ultimately be more useful in identifying the unique set of problems presented by each client.

The process of gathering information involves the notation of "raw data," i.e., the recording of facts, behavior, and events. It is the process of taking note of something as opposed to ascribing meaning. For example, recording that a client continually requests assistance and often asks the therapist if he or she is doing a task correctly is data collection. Saying that this client is dependent is not data collection; it is interpretation. The information gathered during the evaluation process is always initially recorded as raw data. In this way no information is lost. It may be referred to repeatedly without the loss of information, which always occurs in any type of categorization. The initial recording of only interpretations does not allow the therapist to return to the data in the future for reassessment. In addition, first interpretations are often not particularly accurate. Without recourse to raw data the therapist is ill-prepared to alter initial interpretations.

The next phase of the evaluation process is interpretation. This is the process of assigning meaning to raw data, of reformulating the data in such a way that they become useful for planning intervention. It is the process of responding to the question, "What does it mean?" The first step in the process involves organization of the data. It involves analysis of the data and placing pieces of data into specific categories. These categories, in a broad sense, are assets and limitations relative to health needs, performance components, and occupational performances. An additional category is possible interfering behavior that may need to be managed. To make matters a bit more complicated, a datum may fit into one or more categories. Organization of data can be likened to putting together a giant jigsaw puzzle, with only a rather hazy idea of what the final picture will be. And in this jigsaw puzzle some of the pieces are interchangeable, appropriately placed in more than one position. Lest the novice therapist be put off, the process of organizing data becomes considerably easier with experience. It is a challenge, figuratively a puzzle to be solved; and considerable gratification is derived from its apparently successful solution.

Organization of data is followed by assessing the data for the purpose of problem identification. Assessment involves clinical judgement. Clinical, here, refers to clients. Judgment is the forming of an opinion, estimate, notion, or conclusion from available data. It has the connotation of relative objectivity, knowledge, and wisdom that is applied to matters affecting action, good sense, and discretion. Clinical judgment is only "relatively objective"; it really exists on a continuum from the objective to the subjective. Objective judgment is a decision free from personal and emotional bias and based on criteria that are comprehensible to any competent observer. A judgment is considered to be most objective if it is derived from data collected by instruments that are not dependent on the opinion or accuracy of the individual observer. Subjective judgment, on the other hand, is based on criteria that are not described or discernible. It often refers to decisions derived from data collected without the aid of instruments. There is an assumption in these definitions, of course, that only instrumental observation is verifiable—which is not necessarily the case. Clinical judgment then is a process that is frequently not totally objective, but then neither is it entirely subjective. The recent activity related to the development of a standardized test in occupational therapy is evidence of the profession's concern about more objective ways of identifying clients' problems. This is commendable, but it also should be remembered that no evaluative tool can ever be totally objective and reliable; clinical judgment will always entail a considerable amount of subjectivity. Clinical judgment is learned. It is not inherent, a gift someone is born with, nor is it bestowed at graduation; it is an important skill that must be acquired. Good clinical judgment is based on knowledge and experience and learned through participation in the process under good supervision.

Through clinical judgment, the therapist arrives at a statement of the client's assets and problem areas. Problem areas will be conceptualized and stated somewhat differently, depending on the frame of reference being used. Using an analytical frame of reference, for example, a client may be described as having difficulty in dealing with loss. The same client might be described as being dysfunctional in the area of temporal adaptation using an acquisitional frame of reference. It should be noted that a statement of the client's problem areas is not the same as the goals for intervention. Goals are determined on the basis of the client's expected environment and in consultation with the client. Goal setting will be discussed in detail in Chapter 17.

Interpretation can only be made on the basis of available information. When a considerable amount of information is lacking, the therapist has two choices. The therapist may simply say there is not sufficient evidence to determine the client's assets and limitation in a particular area. Or the therapist may make a tentative statement, identifying it as such and indicating that further investigation will take place during intervention.

The third step in evaluation, validation, is the process of seeking confirmation regarding the accuracy of one's interpretations. The best source for confirmation is the client. This is one of the reasons it is suggested that the therapist share evaluative findings with the client. Occasionally, however, a client is not ready to acknowledge difficulty in a particular area. In addition, some clients are not able to provide validation, particularly young children, the severely retarded, those who do not seem to be in good contact with reality, and clients who are diagnosed as having a chronic organic mental disorder. Thus, at times confirmation may be sought from family members, fellow therapists, or other staff members. Observation of the client in a situation different from that of the evaluative procedure is also useful. Validation is not "finding out whether one's interpretations are right or wrong"—it is rather a shared learning process with no final, arbitrary expert. The therapist may observe behaviors indicative of function or dysfunction which are not observed by other staff members. The behavior of any individual often varies from situation to situation; what is observed, therefore, may also differ.

The evaluation process—data collection, interpretation, and validation—is, as mentioned, a process that is continually repeated. It does not happen just once, but rather it is a continuing cycle that recurs throughout the occupational therapy process.

Evaluation up to this point has been discussed pretty much in the abstract. Little has been mentioned specifically about the means for collecting data. It is to this area that the next section is addressed.

SOURCES OF DATA

This section provides an overview of the different sources of information used by the occupational therapist (74,220,618,916,956,960). Some of these sources or methods of obtaining information are used alone. Others are combined and used together at the same time. An interview, for example, also includes observation. This section does not deal with specific evaluative tools commonly used to assess psychosocial components of occupational therapy. These will be outlined in the following chapter. Eight general sources of information are discussed here.

Observation

Observation means to regard with attention, to watch and listen carefully, with alertness, taking particular note of detail. Observation is used as part of almost all evaluative procedures and is critical in the gathering of useful data. During observation obvious behaviors are noted but the less tangible feelings and ideas are also of great importance. The significance of nonverbal behavior was discussed previously. By way of review, in observing, the therapist is attentive to such things as the client's posture, body movements, gestures, facial expression, changes in physical attitude relative to various people and events, clothes (style and color), grooming, jewelry, perfume, and so forth. In observing verbal communication, the therapist not only listens to what is being said but also makes note of the choice of words, their organization into phrases and sentences, tone of voice, accent, and inflection. Interaction between the client and the nonhuman environment is also an important source of data. The client's choice of an activity, ways of handling tools and materials, typical motions, orderliness, amount of care taken, and so forth provide useful information.

Observation outside the context of a formal evaluation procedure frequently provides another dimension to evaluate findings. Where it is possible, the therapist ought to observe clients interacting in different situations. The client is likely to be more informal and spontaneous when involved in different role relationships. An additional perspective of the client's values, interests, assets, and limitations can be gained, for example, in observing the client in the dining room, day room, at ward meetings, and during participation in recreational activities.

As an observer, the therapist should be as unobtrusive as possible, attempting not to influence the client and the client's interactions. This stance may be attained to some degree if the therapist is present only in the role of an observer. It is much less possible when the therapist is interacting with the client. Still the therapist must attempt not to intrude any more than is necessary. This is one place where self-knowledge is particularly important. The therapist who knows the kind of impact he or she has on people and the way that people typically react to him or her is in a better position to interpret the client's behavior. As an observer the therapist must also observe him- or herself in the situation. Note should be made of possible ways one may have influenced the client: for example, interest shown to specific topics, reactions to irritating behavior, response to the client's ideas, and so forth. It is also important to remember that the client is likely to influence the therapist. The client's behavior, for example, may make the therapist more or less attentive. Even when the therapist takes a rather distant position relative to the client, there is always some degree of interaction and thus mutual influence.

Regardless of what occurs within the observation situation, the therapist brings a number of predetermined ideas and feelings to it (3). Some examples of these "sets" are:

- What the therapist knows about the client.
- The expectations the therapist has relative to how the client will and/or ought to behave.
- Knowledge regarding the evaluative procedure.
- Feelings about oneself as a person and as a therapist.
- Internal states such as anxiety, preoccupation with other matters, fatigue, and so forth.
- Personal biases and cultural values.

It is important for the therapist to be aware of these cognitive sets and to work toward eliminating them as much as possible. Sets cannot, however, be totally eliminated; no one can make himself into a pure sponge. The therapist's awareness of his or her sets makes it possible to look at the data gathered in a somewhat more objective manner.

Observation is facilitated and made more objective by the therapist knowing beforehand what kinds of data to look for and what behavior is likely to occur in the observation situation. Although the therapist is looking for specific information, other data may be available in the situation. The analogy of central vision and peripheral vision relative to the data-gathering process is particularly applicable to observation. Even with a clear idea of the information desired, the therapist should never be so focused in intent that he or she forgets to give attention to supposedly extraneous data.

Some people are apparently naturally better observers than others. However, like clinical judgment, it is a skill that can be learned. It is best acquired through practice and good supervision.

Records and Meetings

The information gathered from records and meetings with other staff members or professionals involved with a client can provide valuable information. These sources of data are almost always used in initial screening, but they are also used in formal evaluation and planning intervention.

Medical records, ideally, provide information about the client's past medical history and current medical problems. They provide the client's diagnoses or tentative diagnoses, prognoses, precautions if any and a listing of medications being taken by the client as well as other treatment being provided, and the client's response. Daily nursing notes are of particular importance in that they often provide information about the client's adjustment to the institutional setting, skill in self-care, interactions with others, and behavioral problems. If the client is a child, a developmental history is usually available or at least the medical records may provide an enumeration of the child's major developmental milestones.

Medical records and records from other institutions may also provide information from a variety of specialists. Some of the data pertinent to the occupational therapy process that may be available are:

- Speech therapy—Information about the client's capacity to communicate effectively.
- Recreational therapy—Information about the client's ability to engage in cooperative and competitive situations, social skills, leisure time interests.
- Physical therapy—Information about the client's physical capacities and limitations.
- Rehabilitation counseling—Information about the client's work history, current limitations relative to work, vocational skill and interests, and future plans relative to work.
- Dietary—Information about the client's special dietary needs and restrictions.
- Social service—Information about the client's home, family, social network, socioeconomic status, and cultural background.
- School—Information about the child's academic achievements, adjustment to the school situation, and any special problems in learning.

- Psychology—Information about the client's intelligence, unconscious processes, personality structure, interests, and evidence of organic mental disorders.
- Psychiatry—Information about the client's unconscious processes, defenses, degree of control, capacity to deal with stress, concept of self, current issues of concern, deviant behavior, and precautions.

Although a potential source of considerable information, reading records is not necessarily an easy task. It takes some experience to find and sort through the material. There is frequently considerable information, such as lab reports, that is not relevant to the occupational therapy process. Abbreviations are frequently used. There are standard abbreviations that may be found in any good medical dictionary. Nevertheless, records are often filled with personal abbreviations or those particular to a specific setting. These must be learned or somehow deciphered. Handwritten notes may also present some problems. Parts of the report may be out of date, and thus it is important to check when a particular report was written. Finally, because something is written in a report, it does not mean that it is accurate. Everyone is liable to be in error at times, and personal biases, insufficient information, lack of understanding of the client's cultural background, language barriers, and being under time pressures often lead to inaccurate reporting. Reports that contain raw data are likely to be more accurate than those that present interpretations.

Another source of information is meetings with other personnel who have been or are involved with the client. These may be group meetings such as rounds, team meetings, admission conferences, and the like. Or meetings may be on a one-to-one basis with the various specialists outlined above. Meetings often provide information that is not available in the client's records. Although such information may be more in the nature of personal impressions, it sometimes gives an added dimension to written reports and fills in some of the inevitable gaps.

Meetings are particularly important when the client's records are sparse. This is likely to occur when the client has had no previous medical or psychosocial problems or when the client is new to a given facility. In the latter case, it is often a good idea for the therapist to contact appropriate specialists at the last agency with which the client had contact. Securing permission from the client or the client's family is, of course, necessary. The therapist should be sure to find out if the client has previously been involved in occupational therapy.

The therapist sometimes questions whether or not to read reports or discuss the client with other specialists before or after his or her own evaluation with the client. The advantage of gathering data before one meets the client is that the therapist has some clues about the client's difficulties. This provides information that may be useful in planning evaluation and forewarns the therapist of difficulties that may be encountered. The disadvantage of prior information is the possibility of paying more attention to written reports and the comments of specialists than to what the client is actually saying and doing during the evaluation procedure. The therapist may look for reported behavior, disregarding other critical behavior. The advantage of reading reports and talking to other specialists only after evaluating the client is that the therapist is not biased by previous information. Thus the therapist's interpretations provide an independent point of view about the client. Other reports can then be used as a means of validation. The disadvantage, of course, is that the therapist knows nothing about the client prior to the initial interview. It is probably best for the beginning therapist to try both methods before deciding which is best.

Interview

An interview is a planned conversation usually conducted for the purpose of giving and receiving information. Interviewing, as a source of data, will be discussed only briefly here. It will be described in considerably more detail in Chapter 16. An interview with a client is probably the most valuable source of information available to the therapist, with some exceptions. Nevertheless, the client, on the whole, knows more about him- or herself than anyone else. It is unfortunate that the client's statements are sometimes overlooked—what he or she says about the nature of the difficulties is at times ignored or considered to be the statements of an individual who is sick or who lacks the psychological sophistication of the therapist. In addition, some novice therapists are hesitant to ask the client direct questions. Contrary to some popular opinion, clients are truly human beings and not some ill-defined subspecies; also they do not break. The hurt that they experience is much better relieved by a confident, direct approach. The need to speak indirectly is more related to the therapist's insecurities and lack of confidence than to the client's objective state.

An interview is usually successful if the therapist is clear about the purpose of the interview and the kinds of information desired. A solid knowledge base is important, for this serves as the foundation for planning the interview, i.e., the areas to be covered and the questions to be asked. Good observation is also necessary if an interview is to be successful.

There are two major types of interviews—general and focused. A general interview is concerned with obtaining a broad spectrum of information about the client's past and current circumstances. It usually covers all aspects of the occupational therapy domain of concern. The initial interview with the client and/or with the family is usually general.

A focused interview is concerned with one particular area that has been previously defined. Focused interviews may occur any time during the occupational therapy process and may or may not be conducted in conjunction with the use of other evaluative tools. Some examples of focused interviews are obtaining a detailed work history, review of progress up to a given point in intervention, an object history (a review of the nonhuman objects that have been important to the client), and a terminal interview. The latter takes place before the client leaves intervention and is designed to assist in bringing closure to the occupational therapy process.

Regardless of the type of interview, most therapists find it useful to use an interview schedule. This is an outline or a list of planned questions relative to the areas to be covered in the interview. An interview schedule is a way of making certain that as much information as possible is gained from the interview and that no important aspects are forgotten. The schedule, it should be noted, is used as a guide and not as a questionnaire.

Standardized Tests

A standardized test is composed of empirically selected materials. It has definite directions for use, adequately determined norms, and data on reliability and validity (13,74,359,516). Empirical here refers to the selection of test items through experimental means. Directions for use outline very specifically how the test is to be given, including materials to be used, directions to be given to the testee, time limitations, if any, and the behavior of the test administrator. Directions are also given for scoring and interpretation. Norms are a single value or a range of values constituting the usual performance of a given group. They are established on the basis of testing a large sample of individuals who have known relevant characteristics (e.g., age, sex, cultural background, geographic area, etc.). A standardized test is usually useful only if it has a relatively high degree of reliability and validity. Standards vary for stating whether a test has sufficient reliability and validity to be useful, depending on what the test purports to measure. In general, it can be said that a test that has a test-retest reliability of more than 0.70 and criterion-related validity of more than 0.50 is a fairly good test. (Reliability and validity are stated here as correlation coefficients.)

The results of a standardized test can be considered accurate or trustworthy only if the test is administered strictly according to the directions given and if the individual being tested has the same characteristics as the sample used as the basis for establishing norms. It is unethical for a therapist to report the score of a standardized test as such if the above criteria were not met. A therapist may modify a standardized test or administer it to an individual who is not part of the normative group. Useful information might be gained from such an endeavor but the therapist is no longer using a standardized test.

In addition to the considerations outlined above, Banus (74) outlines a list of questions that may serve as a guide in deciding whether to use a standardized test and/or what standardized test to use. Some of these questions are:

- What is the purpose of the test?
- Does it screen for the presence of a problem or probe the depths of a known problem?
- Do I need to survey a wide range of behavior or zero in on a few related behaviors?
- Are there omissions in the test development that might bias the standardization because all relevant factors were not taken into consideration?
- Have the reliability and validity of the test been researched by persons other than its authors?
- How can I get the time and money to learn how to use or obtain the credentials for the test I want to use?
- Is an alternative but equivalent method of testing available that fits my time and budget?
- How much time is needed to administer, score, interpret, and report the findings?

The majority of the standardized tests used in occupational therapy are related to the developmental assessment of children.

Activity Evaluation

Activity evaluation is a specially designed evaluative situation that involves the client's participation in one or more purposeful activities. Aside from interviews, it is probably the most common type of evaluation used in assessing psychosocial components in occupational therapy (112,412). In order for an activity to be effective as an evaluative tool, the therapist must be very specific about (a) the area being assessed, (b) the behavior indicative of function and dysfunction in that area, and

(c) the behavior that is usually elicited by the activity. In selecting an appropriate activity, the therapist "matches" the behavior he or she wishes to observe with an activity that usually elicits such behavior. This process, previously discussed, requires considerable knowledge of activities and skill in activity analysis and synthesis.

One advantage of the use of activities as a source of data is that the number of areas that can be assessed in this way is fairly large. Activities are sufficiently varied that the selection of a particular activity can, in part, be determined by the age, cultural background, education, interests, and so forth of the client. The third advantage is that the client is readily able to see assets and limitations which, in turn, facilitate collaboration in the evaluative process.

There are several different types of activity evaluations. They may take place in a dyad of client and therapist or a group. They may be used to assess performance components as well as aspects of occupational performances. They may be structured in that one task with specific directions is given or they may be unstructured; the client may do anything he or she wished with the tools and materials provided, or the client may be asked to select an activity from several that are available. Activity evaluations usually take place in conjunction with a focused interview and/or the use of a check sheet.

Inventories and Questionnaires

An inventory has the connotation of an enumeration of various items whereas a questionnaire provides an opportunity for a more in-depth exploration of a specific area. As a means of data collection, inventories and questionnaires tend to blend together. They are usually completed by the client at leisure to be returned to the therapist at some specified time. At the time when an inventory or questionnaire is given to a client, the therapist explains its purpose, gives any necessary directions, allows the client to look it over and ask any questions. After the therapist has had an opportunity to study the completed inventory or questionnaire, it is usually discussed with the client in a focused interview.

There are, of course, some clients who will not be able to complete an inventory or questionnaire independently. This may be due to lack of the necessary cognitive ability, poor reading and writing skills, poor command of the language, or inability to concentrate on such a task at the present time. The therapist may assist the client in completing the inventory or questionnaire or decide that another method of data collection is more appropriate, given the client's present situation.

One of the advantages of inventories and questionnaires is that they give clients an opportunity to think about themselves and what information they want to share with the therapist. This is far different from an interview where the client is required to be more spontaneous in response. Many clients after an interview, in retrospect, wish they "had said something more about this," or they "forgot to tell the therapist about that." Although the client may share this information later with the therapist, there is sometimes a feeling that the moment is lost or the client may be hesitant to bring up the subject. Thus, inventories and questionnaires help the client to organize thoughts and integrate them in a manner that facilitates communication.

An example of an inventory is an activities of daily living check list where the client is asked to identify those activities that he or she is able to perform or would like to be able to perform. A work history is often obtained through a questionnaire. An example of a combined inventory and questionnaire is an evaluative tool known as an Activity Configuration. This tool is designed to provide information about how the client uses his or her time and the extent to which this temporal arrangement is need satisfying.

Check Sheet

This evaluative tool is used by the therapist in conjunction with other means of collecting data, in particular, observation and activity evaluations. They are used as a guide for the therapist during actual evaluation or later as a way of summarizing data. As a guide, check sheets are very similar to interview schedules in that they provide assistance in remembering what data need to be collected relative to various areas. As a means of summarizing data, check sheets serve to describe the frequency of given behaviors according to a key. For example:

1. = Almost never
2. = Seldom
3. = Occasionally
4. = Frequently
5. = Most of the time
6. = Almost always

Another way that check sheets are used to summarize data is to specify the skills the client has currently mastered and those that it will be necessary to master for successful participation in the expected environment. This method helps identify problem areas and provides a graphic means of communicating with the client.

Projective Techniques

Projection is a term used to describe the process whereby the individual reveals a good deal about thoughts and feelings through words and/or actions. This is a very ordinary phenomenon that one observes daily in family members, friends, and associates. As a means of collecting data, projective techniques refer to the presentation of unstructured ambiguous stimuli that allow the client to respond more on the basis of thoughts and feelings rather than on the external reality of the situation. Projective techniques provide, in a sense, a window into an individual's intrapsychic processes. Not a clear window, rather one covered with mist and sometimes considerable frost, but a window nonetheless.

Projective techniques as used by occupational therapists are a part of or a subtype of activity evaluations. Unstructured activities are used as a means of facilitating projection or of making it a more prominent part of the client's response (90,290,416,584,614,749). If the therapist wishes to use the projective dimension of behavior as part of evaluation, the therapist must seek considerable feedback and validation from the client. In other words, the therapist discusses with the client what his actions and what he has created mean to him. Collaboration between client and therapist is of great importance in order for the therapist to make accurate interpretations. The therapist also needs considerable knowledge of symbolism, psychodynamics, psychoanalytic theory, and of self. Projection, as a natural phenomenon, should not be treated as if it were something particularly scary, but it should be treated with respect.

Projective techniques ought not to be used as a means of collecting data unless the information is to be used directly in discovering the client's assets and limitations and in planning intervention. The misuse of projective techniques in the early 1960s as outlined in Chapter 2 need not be repeated in the 1980s; we did that already.

Resource Material

It may be necessary for the therapist to go back to the textbook when confronted with an unfamiliar diagnosis. An understanding of the client's condition relative to classical symptoms, course, prognosis, and counter-indications for various types of interventions is critical information. It may also be necessary for the therapist to review the therapeutic and possible side effects of the client's medication and any precautions before planning either evaluation or intervention.

In conclusion, the occupational therapist has many excellent sources of information to use as the foundation for client evaluation. All should be used with full recognition of their potential and deficits, and with care. No means of collecting data is any better than the clinical judgments used by the interpreter.

EMOTIONAL ASPECTS

Initial evaluation is frequently quite difficult for the client. The idea of "being evaluated" has many connotations (91,98,266,567,786,790,887)—most of them negative, giving rise to feelings of vulnerability and fear. Some of the thoughts clients may have are:

- The therapist will find out my secrets, she can read my mind;
- The therapist will judge me and find me deficient, inadequate, or bad;
- The therapist will tell other people, particularly those who are close to me;
- The therapist will laugh at me;
- The therapist is far superior to me in every possible way;
- All of the problems I have are my fault.

With the above-mentioned ideas and feelings, the client's initial response to evaluation may not be very positive. There are several responses that are quite common. The client may experience pain-anxiety, making cooperation very difficult and/or performance anywhere near usual capacity. The client may be suspicious, engage in denial, be hostile or indifferent. The client may not be particularly truthful. The client may be condescending toward the therapist, questioning the therapist's right to evaluate and, in general, try to make the therapist feel inferior or angry. On the other hand, the client may be overeager to please and act in a highly infantile manner.

The client may respond in one of the ways mentioned above or various responses may be combined in an idiosyncratic pattern. It is useful to remember that these responses are normal and, if not taken to an extreme, are healthy defenses. Understanding these responses is facilitated by the therapist figuratively putting him- or herself in the place of the client and considering how one might feel and react.

There are several things the therapist can do to minimize the possibility of negative feelings and responses during initial evaluation. First, the therapist tries to develop some degree of trust on the part of the client. This is usually accomplished by being warm and accepting and by acting like a real, caring individual. It is often helpful to articulate some of the possible negative ideas and fears that the client may have about the evaluation process. The collaborative nature of the evaluation process should be emphasized as well as the fact that the therapist will be sharing the data gathered and interpretations with the client. The therapist tries to create the sense that "we are in this together." Above all, the therapist should be gentle.

The picture outlined above regarding possible client responses admittedly is somewhat negative. Not all clients are fearful of initial evaluation. Many clients who are fearful do not respond in an adverse manner and manage their concerns about evaluation in a positive and adaptive manner. It is also good to note that emotional response to periodic reevaluation tends to be far less severe. By that time a sufficient degree of rapport has usually been established between client and therapist so that the client, if experiencing anxiety, is much better able to share such anxiety with the therapist.

The beginning therapist also frequently has some difficulty with initial evaluations. It may be a frightening experience regardless of prior preparation. There are many thoughts that come to mind or hover close to consciousness. Some of these thoughts and ideas are likely to be as follows: One feels stupid, lacking in adequate knowledge and skill for the task that lies ahead. The responsibility is too much. One individual has no right to evaluate another; such an undertaking is morally offensive. The client will think I am inept and so will my supervisor and other staff members. The client will be difficult and probably not like me. Evaluation means that one really has to set goals and engage in intervention.

Fidler (660) has perhaps best articulated the fear that surrounds evaluation and intervention. She has described this experience as:

> The scariness involved in identifying one's self as an agent of change. The assumption of such a role is frightening, of course, because intervention, treatment planning, requires not only evaluative statements but also a statement of expectations. You are called upon to say this is where I feel another individual is, this is where I feel to the best of my knowledge he should go, and this is how such movement can best be accomplished.

The initial fears surrounding evaluation diminish in time, but they may never entirely disappear. The best course of action in dealing with these fears is to recognize them and accept the fact that they exist. It is also useful to share one's anxiety with knowledgeable others who can understand and provide support and to remember that others have and do share your trepidations.

In conclusion, Abrew (3) has conceived of evaluation as a feedback loop or the constant interaction between the client, the therapist, and the tools used in the evaluation process. The client brings himself as an individual with his fears and anxieties, his pain, his assets and limitations, his beliefs. The therapist brings him- or herself as an individual, with evaluative skills, judgment and experience, and beliefs. Evaluative tools may be more or less reliable and valid; they may be biased relative to age, culture, educational level, and language; they make specific demands on client and therapist alike. Each of these parts of the loop—client, therapist, and evaluative tools—impinges on each other to facilitate or impede the evaluative process . . . or both.

16

Evaluative Tools

Evaluative tools are aids to facilitate the gathering of information that will be used to identify the client's assets and limitations. The purpose of this chapter is to describe some of the major evaluative tools used to assess psychosocial function and dysfunction (412). It is divided into three parts: interviewing, tools used for assessing performance components, and tools used for assessing occupational performances.

INTERVIEWING

Interviewing is probably the most powerful, sensitive, and versatile evaluative instrument available to the occupational therapist. The type of interview discussed here is general in nature (91,98,266,567,631,786,887, 916,956). Interviews that focus on one particular area will be described later in this chapter. Discussion of a general interview will include a description of purpose, process, content, assessment of cultural background, interviewing family members, and special circumstances.

Purpose

A general interview has several purposes or functions:

1. It serves as a medium through which a good working relationship between client and therapist is initiated, developed, and, hopefully, sustained.
2. It assists in identifying what is required by both parties to communicate effectively with each other.
3. It defines respective roles and obligations.
4. It provides a means for collecting data about the client that is sufficient for the formulation of a good case history and ultimately for identification of areas of strengths and weaknesses.
5. It allows the therapist to test various hypotheses about the client's possible areas of difficulty.
6. It guides the therapist as to how to best communicate recommendations to the client and family and to engage their cooperation.
7. It establishes mutually acceptable conditions for continuing collaborative involvement.

Verbal and nonverbal communication of information between client and therapist is the essential element of a good interview. The therapist is concerned with demonstrating interest in understanding the client and his or her point of view and in communicating that understanding to the client. Conducting an adequate interview, thus, is more than the client responding to a list of stereotyped questions. Each item of information frequently requires clarification and amplification. All information must be carefully weighed as to its clinical significance and its possible relationship to the client's strengths and weaknesses. To obtain the necessary information, the therapist must selectively guide the client through the entire process. Each item of information requires interpretation that in turn may necessitate a further intelligently guided search for additional information.

Throughout the interview, the therapist attempts to order and assign meaning to the information obtained. This involves a process of analysis and synthesis of information in the course of which the therapist repeatedly constructs and tests hypotheses through further and direct inquiry—until corroborating or refuting information emerges. In the attempt to order information and assign meaning, the therapist continually scans his or her own clinical and personal experience and knowledge for points of familiarity and congruence.

The intellectual processes that occur during and/or subsequent to a general interview have been outlined by Prior and Silberstein (786). With some modification these are as follows:

Acquiring unedited factual information provided by the client, which may or may not be accurate or precise. This information provides the foundation for other, more complex thought processes.

Understanding the facts as related by the client through further questioning and discussion.

Organizing the facts as related by the client and not as interpreted by the therapist.

Sorting out or analyzing the obtained data into related categories. This usually includes differentiating minutiae from significant information and classification of information relative to whether it is an asset or a liability.

Reassembling or synthesizing the data into patterns of recognizable areas of function and dysfunction. This, of course, requires knowledge of what is normal and atypical relative to the client's age, culture, and social environment.

Evaluating the synthesized data by asking the client questions to confirm or refute the therapist's tentative assessment.

This intellectual process is frequently not linear but rather reoccurs in a cyclical manner. However, without this process the purpose of an interview is lost. It cannot provide adequate information for an accurate assessment, and it provides no guidelines for determining what other evaluative tools would be appropriately utilized in the future.

Process

A therapist's primary task in carrying out an interview is to provide the right atmosphere, to be a good listener, and to ask only those questions that help the client tell his own story. In a good interview the client is able to talk freely about things that are important to him, such as his fears, problems, and conflicts.

The setting of the interview should be one in which the client feels that there is an adequate amount of privacy and that nothing will be overheard by others. Interruptions are kept to a minimum with the atmosphere being calm and unhurried. The client may be more comfortable if the therapist does not sit behind a desk but rather places the chairs in a conversational arrangement. On the other hand, the psychological distance of a desk may make the client feel more secure. The therapist thus may give the client the option of where to sit. A reasonable amount of time should be set aside for the interview, and the client should know the length of the interview. Forty-five minutes is usually adequate for the completion of an interview. If all of the necessary information is not gained in the alotted time, the therapist arranges to meet with the client in the near future. The therapist need not feel that he or she must or should learn everything about the client or understand the client completely in one interview.

The beginning of the interview is frequently the most difficult and awkward time for the client. On the other hand, the client may welcome the opportunity to have someone with whom to talk. At the start the therapist takes the initiative by introducing him- or herself. The therapist asks the client to identify him- or herself and provide basic information such as age, marital status, type of employment, and so forth. There may be a brief period of informal talk after which the therapist initiates discussion of the client's situation. It is usually best to start with how the client views the situation or problem at this point in time rather than request a detailed account of the beginning and the course of the problem. The latter is valuable information but it is usually better to guide the client in this direction after he or she has had an opportunity to state immediate concerns.

In conducting an interview it is essential to follow some routine pattern of questioning to ensure coverage of all aspects of the client's problem and life situation. An interview is not, however, carried out through use of a questionnaire or through a bombardment of questions. The client is gently and understandingly led to relate his story in his own words and way. The method of questioning should be brief and simple and in language that is understandable to the client; the therapist may use the client's own terminology, at least until there is mutual agreement as to what the terminology means. Only one question is asked at a time. Questions may be open-ended—so phrased that the client must respond with phrases or sentences; or direct—only a "yes" or "no" response is required. Best results are usually achieved by initiating inquiry into each new area with open-ended questions followed by progressively more specific (direct) questions until the subject is fully clarified. The therapist tries to formulate each successive question on the basis of what the client has just said. Leading questions or questions that suggest answers are avoided. It is perfectly acceptable to let the client digress a little. However, the therapist must keep in mind what information the client has not yet given or clarified so that he or she can return later to ask the necessary questions at an appropriate time. Questioning should be unobtrusive so that unnecessary interruptions are avoided. The therapist's task, it should be remembered, is to listen attentively and quietly and to extract meaning from what the client is saying. Although points are clarified through discrete questioning, overstructuring is avoided. The client should in no way be prevented from telling his own story or be influenced to relate what he feels the interviewer wants him to say. If the client is permitted to talk freely he will often volunteer essential information that the therapist may not be able to elicit through direct questioning.

As mentioned, the client may be anxious about evaluation and deal with that anxiety in a variety of different ways. The therapist needs to remain self-assured, calm, and unhurried, providing guidance and reassurance. Respect and understanding for the client's difficulty in talking about painful or embarrassing topics should always be maintained. The client should not in any way be pushed but, rather, ample time should be given along with some encouragement. It is often wise to create a balance between talking and silence. Too much silence may create anxiety on the part of the client. On the other hand, some silence is good, for it allows the client to reflect, gather his thoughts, and consider how he would like to proceed. If a client becomes upset, begins to cry, or responds with an angry outburst, the therapist remains quiet, gives a word of reassurance, and indicates that such an emotional display is understandable and quite acceptable. In every interview there are bound to be distortions, omissions, memory lapses, or exaggerations. The therapist should be slow to point these out and tactful if and when he or she does. As the client becomes more comfortable, he often corrects these himself.

Finally, the therapist is concerned about bringing an interview to an end. If the client demonstrates fatigue or serious discomfort, the interview is terminated early. The reason for early termination is given to the client and an appointment is made for another meeting. Aside from the above circumstances, an interview is terminated on time even if all desired information has not been acquired. The client is told the interview is about to end and is asked if there is anything else he would like to add at this point. Just as the interview is coming to a close, the client may introduce a new piece of information as if it were a mere afterthought. Such information is dealt with briefly, and the client is reassured that it will be discussed in more depth at the next meeting. The client may feel that he has exposed embarrassing aspects about himself. Concern may be expressed about the therapist's opinion of him and matters of confidentiality. Again, reassurance is given. In bringing the interview to a close, the therapist summarizes the essential features of the client's story. This is done both to verify that the therapist has understood what the client has said and to bring an appropriate closure to the interview. In most cases arrangements are made for another meeting, or the therapist describes the next step in the evaluation process. If the client seems unduly upset at the end of the interview and is confined to a clinical setting, it is often a good idea to stop by and see the client very briefly later in the day or the next morning. At this time additional support and reassurance are given.

Content

The content of an interview refers to the type of information the therapist seeks to gain from the client. What information the therapist needs will vary with the client's presenting problems and the circumstances of the interview. As mentioned, the therapist need not explore areas in the interview that have been adequately covered by other members of the team. The therapist in this case conducts the interview so as to build on what is known; to add to the understanding of the client's situation. A general interview will also vary depending on whether it is part of a screening process or a formal evaluation. A screening interview tends to be of lesser depth than an interview that is part of a formal evaluation. The areas covered are, however, fairly similar.

The content areas outlined below are concerned with the psychosocial aspects of the individual's life situation. When the interview is also to be concerned with physical dysfunction, additional areas would be addressed.

In general, then, the occupational therapist is concerned with gaining information relative to the following:

1. Biographical data: the client's full name, sex, age, place of residence (address and telephone number), date and place of birth, ethnic group, religion, primary spoken language, marital status, educational level, and current occupation;
2. Presenting problem: the client's current problems, whether the onset of the problem is sudden or of a chronic nature, the cause ascribed to the origin of the problem or to its exacerbation (all of this as described by the client);
3. Current health status: the client's present assessment of physical and mental health and concerns relative to these areas, in particular fears and anxieties;

4. Past health history: the client's medical history, both physical and psychological, past illnesses or injuries, type of treatment or intervention, way in which the client has adapted to past life tasks, developmental history (particularly important for a child or adolescent);
5. Family: the client's family of origin; what home life was like, kinds of interpersonal relations; brief characterization of parents, siblings; feelings toward them; what the client believes they felt toward him; family attitudes toward social interactions, education, work, sexuality; the family's economic status and group identification (ethnic, religious); family experiences of note (separation, divorce, chronic illness, quarreling, abuse, etc.). The client's current familial interactions: composition; interpersonal relationship with partner and children, sexual relationships; relationships among family members; health status of family members; major sources of stress (money, in-laws, etc.); types of interaction with family of origin;
6. Activities of daily living: the client's patterns of eating, exercise, and sleep; activities of daily living responsibilities; who takes care of other responsibilities; sense of adequacy; areas of particular difficulty;
7. School/work: the client's grades in school, how he or she gets along with teachers and classmates, any particular area of difficulty; nature of job, past employment history, relationship with co-workers and supervisors, effectiveness at job, conditions of work, physical and psychological pressures; job or school satisfaction;
8. Play/leisure/recreation: client's usual play or leisure activities (what activities and with whom), friendships, involvement in community organizations, use of alcohol and drugs, general satisfaction;
9. Environment: the client's living conditions, type of community, degree of safety, support system available, degree of comfort in environment.

The above listing may seem quite lengthy, particularly to the novice therapist. However, most clients can provide this information in a relatively short period of time. But it should again be remembered that all this information need not be acquired in one interview. In an initial interview it is better to gain less information than to rush through at the expense of not establishing adequate rapport with the client.

Cultural Factors

Cultural differences are an important factor in evaluation and intervention (395). The first set of questions that needs to be addressed is the extent to which the individual's behavior is influenced by the shared understandings of culture, by his or her idiosyncratic world view and personality, or is a manifestation of difficulties in psychosocial function. The second set of questions has to do with whether the individual behavior is primarily influenced by the shared understandings of his or her culture and whether these understandings are quite different from those of the therapist, in which case then what does one do. All of these questions will not be addressed here. Those related to intervention will be discussed in Chapter 17.

During initial evaluation, discussion with the individual regarding involvement with and dependency on parents, other relatives, and friends within his or her ethnic group often serves to indicate the individual's degree of adherence to the shared understandings of the ethnic group. This will provide some information about the individual's orientation to health and health care and will likely give some clues to the individual's probable behavior as well. The following is a list of questions that can be instrumental in gaining additional information regarding the individual's ideas about his or her condition:

1. What do you think has caused your problem?
2. Why do you think it started when it did?
3. What do you think your condition does to or for you? How does it work?
4. How severe do you think your condition is? Do you think it will last a long time or will it soon improve?
5. What kind of help would you like to have?
6. What are the most important results you would like to get from this help?
7. What are the chief problems your condition has caused you?
8. What do you fear most about your condition?

These questions, of course, may be phrased in a number of different ways. The important point is to gain information about how the individual perceives the nature of the condition.

There are several factors that contribute to variations in health beliefs and behavior of members of a given ethnic group. It is good to remember that although the individual may be fairly well enculturated to the dominant social group (in the United States, white, Anglo-Saxon, Protestant), he or she may return to ethnically derived ideas in the stressful situation of illness or disability. One of the factors that contributes to variation is the extent to which the individual has been exposed to the ideas of modern medicine and popular standards of health care. This is likely to be dependent on level of formal education, generation, relationships with ethnic group and family, experience with "good" medical services for self or for family members, and urban as opposed to rural residence. The individual's income may influence ability to carry through on long-term expensive health regimens and the support systems available for long-term care. The individual's occupation may determine his or her willingness to discontinue work and take the sick role. This could be an asset or a liability in the intervention process. Compliance with activity, diet, and other dictates of a regimen may also be related to occupation. Attitudes toward work, whether the individual's work is of a migrant or fixed nature, whether it is manual or sedentary, and regularity of employment are all important factors influencing beliefs about health care.

When the client and therapist do not speak a common language, the interview must take place through a translator. The translator is asked to use the client's own words rather than an interpretation of what the client is saying. To ensure accuracy of translation, the translator is asked to request clarification from the client or therapist if he or she does not understand what either is saying. It is always difficult to use a translator when sensitive matters or matters that might cause the client embarrassment need to be discussed. The possibility that the client may not be totally open should be kept in mind.

Interviewing Family Members

There are several advantages to interviewing one or more members of the client's family. They are a valuable source of additional information, particularly when the client is unable to give a clear account of present and past situations. They may serve as a check on the reliability of the client's report if there should be any question that it is not entirely accurate. Through an interview with family members, the therapist is able to gain some understanding of the dynamics of the family and the client's relationship with other family members. There is likely to be evidence about the effect of the client's situation on the family; and the effect of the family on the client's situation. Finally, through a general interview, the therapist begins to learn how to relate to family members. In this way the therapist may be in a position to help the family as well as to enlist their help in assisting the client.

The issues of openness and confidentiality are always important. When the client is an adult, it is wisest to gain the client's consent to interview a family member. If a family member was interviewed prior to meeting the client, the client is told this when the client and therapist first meet. In most cases it should be made clear to both client and family that the therapist holds conversations with either in strict confidence. Thus, the therapist does not tell the family about what was discussed with the client and conversely does not tell the client what was discussed with the family. Moreover, the therapist never acts as a conveyer of messages between client and family. Rather, the therapist encourages direct communication between client and family.

The principles relative to a general interview outlined above are equally applicable to an interview with family members. The same process takes place and the same content is covered. Thus, essentially the same procedure is used as was used in conjunction with the client. However, the therapist must demonstrate understanding of family concerns, fears, and anxieties. Time must be given to listening to their problems, which may or may not be directly related to the client's situation. An interview with a family should be such that the family feels the therapist has the best interests of the family as well as the client in the forefront.

Special Circumstances

In general, by being attentive to the client and concerned about the client's comfort, the therapist will ultimately succeed in obtaining adequate information. There are, nevertheless, some clients who have special kinds of problems. The following are some suggestions that may facilitate an interview with such clients:

The client who is severely physically ill or debilitated. A lengthy interview is not recommended under these circumstances. Several brief 10- to 15-min interviews distributed over a period of time are usually the wisest course of action.

The client with degenerative dementia. The therapist must judge the extent of the client's problem as well as evaluate the reliability of the client's report. Defects in attention, memory, and abstract thinking often lead to difficulty in obtaining an accurate history. If the client is capable of providing some information, interviewing techniques are adopted to make the effort as productive as possible. Questions are worded simply with the client being given an ample period of time to respond. Questions may be repeated to check the consistency of responses. Interview sessions are kept brief. A family member or friend may be able to provide additional information.

The client who has a schizophrenic disorder. Although usually oriented to person, time, and place and having an intact memory, the client may have considerable difficulty communicating in a direct manner. The client may be preoccupied with fantasies and hallucinations; thinking may be disorganized and behavior bizarre or marked by extreme withdrawal. It is important to remember that almost all individuals with this disorder have difficulty in relating to others. The therapist needs to be very patient and repeatedly draw the client back to the subject under discussion. Silently sitting with the client for a period of time may lead to some increase in communication. The information provided by the client, though fragmentary and incomplete, is usually very valuable. In interpreting the data, the therapist should always consider the possible symbolic meaning of the information provided by the client.

The client who is severely depressed. The client may complain of being unable to remember or think clearly. There is considerable preoccupation with pessimistic thoughts. The client is not likely to volunteer information or to elaborate on any information provided; responses are likely to be brief. The therapist needs to be gentle but fairly persistent. Open-ended questions are usually not recommended, at least not in an initial interview. Questions that can be answered by yes or no or a short sentence usually lead to the best results.

The client who is mentally retarded. Questions are kept at a level commensurate with the client's capacity to understand. Open-ended questions are usually inappropriate as are those that require abstract thinking or speculation. Inquiry should be addressed to concrete information that will be viewed as relevant by the client.

The client with expressive aphasia. Such an individual may be extremely frustrated because of an inability to communicate clearly. However, the client is frequently able to communicate through gestural signs for yes and no. Thus, questions must be carefully phrased so they can be answered by the client.

The client with a hearing defect. If the client has a hearing aid, strongly recommend that it be brought to the interview and turned on. The therapist should always speak clearly, directly face the client at all times, and keep hands away from his or her face. At times it may be effective to conduct the interview through an exchange of written messages. If so, it is extremely important to attend to one's own and the client's nonverbal communication. Some deaf clients rely on sign language as means of communication. When this is the case an interpreter should be used during the interview.

The above outline of special circumstances is admittedly brief. The number of special circumstances is probably infinite. This aspect of the interviewing process was discussed to alert the reader to the need for being adaptive in conducting a general interview. Each client and each family member will have their own idiosyncratic needs. It is important that the therapist be able to identify these needs and to modify the interview accordingly.

ASSESSMENT OF PERFORMANCE COMPONENTS

The evaluative procedures to be described here and in the next section do not necessarily fall into orderly categories. Some tools assess one performance component; others may assess more than one performance component. The same is true relative to tools used in the evaluation of occupational performances. To make matters a bit more complicated, some tools were developed within the context of a particular frame of reference; others were not. The evaluative tools used in the assessment of psychosocial function in occupational therapy are not well organized or highly refined.

The tools that are discussed here are those that appear to be most commonly used in the profession (413). The author has taken the liberty of making some modifications in several of the tools which have not been standardized. This was done in the interest of clarity and completeness and not with the intention of modifying the nature of the tool.

Evaluation of Sensory Integration

Evaluation of sensory integration relative to children has been studied much more thoroughly than any other of the psychosocial components. The test battery used is the Southern California Sensory Integrating Tests (SCSIT) in conjunction with the Southern California Postrotary Nystagmus Test (SCPNT) and suggested behavioral observations (58,59,64). The SCSIT consists of the following 17 subtests:

- Space visualization
- Figure-ground perception
- Position in space
- Design copying
- Motor accuracy
- Kinesthesia
- Manual form perception
- Finger identification
- Graphesthesia
- Localization of tactile stimuli
- Double tactile stimuli perception
- Imitation of postures
- Crossing midline of body
- Bilateral motor coordination
- Right-left discrimination
- Standing balance—eyes open
- Standing balance—eyes closed

The test has been standardized using a group of children with average intelligence and no apparent motor difficulties. It provides normative data for children from about 4 to 9 years of age, depending on the particular subtest. The test-retest reliability is between 0.89 and 0.12, depending on the subtest and age level. Validity has primarily been discussed relative to content. Criterion-related validity has not been studied, or at least not reported.

Through factor analysis, scores of the subtest seem to cluster into four syndromes or types of disorders. These are

1. Tactile defensiveness (lack of integration of the tactile subsystem);
2. Postural and bilateral integration;
3. Praxia;
4. Form and space perception.

(It should be noted that the author has taken form and space perception out of sensory integration and placed it in a separate category. See Chapter 3 for a discussion of this. The inclusion of form and space perception here as a syndrome related to sensory integrative deficit is for the purpose of accurately describing the Southern California Test Battery.)

Of the syndromes listed above, one is rarely seen in a child exclusive of all others (59, p. 5).

> Dysfunction is operationally defined as a meaningful cluster of test scores that fall a standard deviation or more below age expectations or below other meaningful test score clusters in the same child. "Meaningful" is obtained from the tendency toward covariance among test scores of children with learning disorders as shown in the factor analyses.

The SCPNT measures an aspect of vestibular function. Nystagmus is an involuntary, rapid, back-and-forth movement of the eyes usually arising from a fairly high degree of stimulation of the semicircular canals. Children with learning disabilities may have a hyperactive or hypoactive postrotary nystagmus response.

A group of behavioral observations is the last part of the sensory integrative test battery developed by Ayres. The behavior to be observed is concerned with postural-ocular reactions and other neurological signs such as abnormal reflexes.

The SCSIT Battery is primarily suitable for administration to children who are of normal intelligence but demonstrate problems in the academic subjects of reading, writing, and mathematics. The Battery should be used only as a nonstandardized tool with individuals who have characteristics different from those of the normative group. One cannot make the assumption, for example, that a 13-year-old child should be able to get a perfect score on all of the subtests. It is not known, in fact, whether this is the case. The test should be used cautiously with children who are mentally retarded, who have a diagnosis of cerebral palsy, or who are severely emotionally disturbed. If used, the results are interpreted with due consideration of the other multiple factors, which may well be affecting performance. Because the Battery is being used in a nonstandardized manner, test scores are not formally reported.

The administration and interpretation of the SCSIT Battery are very complex, and considerable study and practice are required to attain mastery. To become qualified, Ayres suggests that the therapist be knowledgeable in the construction and interpretation of psychological tests, statistics, and the nature of sensory integrative dysfunction. The therapist should also have considerable perceptual-motor skill, for smooth administration requires a high degree of manual dexterity. A thorough acquaintance with the SCSIT manual is essential. It is also suggested that a potential examiner administer the Battery at least 20 times in a clinical situation and interpret the findings under the supervision of a person who is proficient in the use of the Battery. The Center for the Study of Sensory Integrative Dysfunction provides a course of study leading to the development of proficiency in the use of the Battery. Another means of gaining proficiency is through graduate study in sensory integrative function and dysfunction, which is offered at a few universities. The latter provides more in-depth study and focuses on intervention as well as evaluation. The Center's course of study to date is concerned only with evaluation.

The SCSIT is, as mentioned, only suitable for evaluating children. It has, however, been suggested in the literature that some adults diagnosed as schizophrenic have sensory integrative deficits. This is a tentative hypothesis and should be viewed as such. There are no standardized tests to determine levels of sensory integration function of adults. King believes that examination of an individual's usual posture and movement patterns is a suitable means of determining sensory integration problems (533). She feels that specific postures and movements are a result of chronic difficulty in vestibular processing. This, in turn, leads the individual to take a position that is a spontaneous reaction to the fear of falling. It also inhibits movement, for self-initiated motion may lead to the possibility of falling.

The postural and movement patterns that King believes are indicative of sensory integrative dysfunction are:

1. A pronounced head-to-toe S-shaped posture with head and abdomen protruding forward;
2. A shuffling gait with difficulty in walking in a normal heel to toe fashion;
3. An inability to raise the arms above the head to anything approaching a vertical line;

4. An immobility of the head and shoulder girdle with difficulty rotating the head on the vertical axis or to roll the head to the side, forward, or back;
5. A tendency to hold the arms and legs in a flexed, adducted, and internally rotated position both when sitting and standing;
6. The thumb held in adduction, atrophy of the thinar eminence, ulnar deviation of the wrist, and a weakness of grip.

These postures and movements can be assessed by observation and by asking the client to attempt to engage in the above indicated movements.

Evaluation of Cognitive Function

There are two ways to assess cognitive skill: an addendum to a general interview and Task Skill Assessment. The addendum provides information about cognitive function as it is demonstrated through communication. Task Skill Assessment gives data regarding cognitive function as it is demonstrated in action.

As an addendum to a general interview, cognitive skill is assessed through observation of particular kinds of behaviors and through asking rather specific questions (567,786). In the interview, the therapist takes special note of the following:

1. General responsiveness. Is the client alert, accessible, appropriate? What is the rate of response?
2. Grooming. Is the client neatly groomed and appropriately dressed? What kind of statement is the client attempting to make relative to appearance?
3. Manner. How does the client present him- or herself—friendly, cooperative, negative, fearful, suspicious, etc.? Does the client have any nervous habits or mannerisms? What are the client's typical posture and facial expression? What is the client's overall motor pattern—tense, restless, retarded, relaxed, and so forth?
4. Speech. How does the client speak and express him- or herself, i.e., tone of voice, rate of speech, verbal production slow or apparently blocked, vocabulary used? Is the client's speech coherent and easy to follow or is it rambling, circumstantial, and disconnected?
5. Mood. Is the client depressed, elated, high? Does the client appear anxious, apprehensive, or fearful?
6. Emotions. Are the client's feelings appropriate and congruent with the ideas expressed and/or overall life situation? Is there a general stability in feelings or emotional lability?

In addition to observation, specific questions often facilitate evaluation of various cognitive components.

1. Orientation. Question the client regarding the date, time of day, and where and who he or she is.
2. Memory. Does the client know what he ate for breakfast, or when her first child was born, for example? The questions asked to assess short- and long-term memory should be such that the therapist is able to check on the accuracy of response.
3. Concentration. Is the client able to accurately repeat a series of five numbers?
4. Insight. When questioned about present problems is the client able to give an accurate account of the situation that is compatible with the beliefs of his or her cultural group?
5. Judgment and problem solving. Given the present situation, what are the client's plans for the future? Are they realistic and well thought out?
6. Thought processes. Is the client able to define the difference between two related concepts such as laziness and idleness? Is the client able to give an abstract interpretation of a proverb such as "people in glass houses should not throw stones"? When the therapist presents a different point of view or interpretation in regard to something the client has said, is the client able to understand and consider the new formulation? Are the client's thoughts logically related to each other and coherently expressed?
7. Mental content. When questioned, what does the client describe as major concerns and preoccupations? The therapist attempts to determine whether the client has delusions, phobias, obsessions, or hallucinations and the nature of these. However, the therapist is also interested in the client's dominant ideas, attitudes, and beliefs; the client's feelings about herself, guilt, and worries.
8. Knowledge. When questioned does the client know anything about current events, i.e., how to return merchandise to a department store, the local police emergency number, for example? The questions asked should be such that most individuals of the client's age and life situation would be able to respond readily.

In the above outline of an addendum to a general interview, intelligence can only be estimated. Perhaps the best clue is the client's vocabulary, given the educational and cultural background.

Task skill assessment is an evaluative tool designed to evaluate an individual's cognitive function as it relates to doing (708,915,956). Task skill is the ability to carry out activities requiring the use of various tools and materials and the completion of several steps. It is concerned primarily with manipulation and use of the nonhuman environment. Task skill, although primarily cognitive in nature, also involves the use and integration of some visual perception, psychological, sensory integrative, and motor components. This is, of course, true of any doing process.

Task skill assessment involves requesting a client to complete a specific activity independent of any assistance. Adequate directions and tools and materials necessary to complete the activity are made readily available. The evaluation ideally takes place in a one-to-one situation. When it is necessary to evaluate more than one client at a time, the therapist does not encourage interaction between the clients. Such encouragement may interfere with a client's ability to complete the activity.

In selecting an appropriate task, the therapist analyzes a variety of activities, asking him- or herself whether a given activity could be completed successfully by a fully functioning individual who is similar to the client in age and intelligence. The client's gender and cultural background are also taken into consideration in selecting an activity. Two suggested activities are projects made from interlocking blocks such as Legos or from an erector set. The advantages of these two types of activities are (a) they can be graded in complexity, (b) they can be disassembled and used repeatedly, (c) they have a quality of play. The latter is often important for it takes some of the anxiety out of the evaluative situation.

The form presented as Table 16-1 may be used by the therapist as an aid to observation. A scoring of 1 through 4 is suggested. A rating of 1 is given if the client experiences considerable difficulty in a specific aspect of the activity whereas a rating of 4 indicates no difficulty. The numbers 1 to 4 should be considered as being on a continuum. In using the form a number is entered into the "Present" column. The "Comments" column is used to record specific things the client did or said that led the therapist to assign the number. Entries in this column are as specific as possible. This is the place for the "raw behavior" mentioned earlier. The "Future" column is tentatively completed at the time of initial evaluation. A rating of 1 to 4 is assigned based on the client's expected environment. The guiding question is what degree of cognitive function, or task skill, the client will need to manage in his or her expected environment. As mentioned, expected environment is always tentative at the beginning of intervention. Its usefulness here is to determine whether the client needs help in this area. For example, the client who is planning on returning to a job where told exactly what to do and

TABLE 16-1. *Summary of task skill*

Behavior	Comments	Present (1–4)[a]	Future (1–4)[a]
Willingness to engage in doing task			
Adequate posture for task			
Sufficient physical strength and endurance			
Demonstrates adequate gross and fine motor coordination			
Sustained interest in task			
Normal rate of performance			
Ability to follow oral, demonstrated, pictorial, and written directions			
Appropriate use of tools and materials			
Acceptable level of neatness			
Appropriate attention to detail			
Ability to solve problems that arise in performing task			
Ability to organize task in a logical manner			
Tolerates frustration			
Self-directed			

[a] 1, Considerable difficulty; 4, no difficulty.

how to do it is going to need less skill in problem solving than the client who is self-employed.

After the client has completed the evaluative activity or has completed as much as he or she can, the therapist discusses the activity with the client. The Survey of Task Skill may be used as the basis for discussion. The client and therapist sometimes fill out the form together, with differences in points of view being discussed. The form may also be used as a concrete aid in talking about the client's expected environment.

Evaluation of Psychological Function

Two evaluative tools will be discussed relative to psychological function: the Fidler Battery and the Free Choice of Selected Activities. Each of these, to some extent, involves the use of projective techniques. This was briefly discussed in the last chapter. It is suggested that the reader review that section and the section on symbolism in Chapter 10.

The Fidler Battery, originally developed by the Azimas, was later revised by Gail Fidler (67,749). It is derived from a psychoanalytic orientation and is designed to identify intrapsychic content through the production and exploration of symbols. The Battery is made up of three activities. Administration of the Battery involves:

1. Giving the client a box of colored pencils and drawing paper and asking the client to draw whatever he or she wishes;
2. Giving the client a variety of different colored fingerpaints, water, and paper suggesting that they be used in any way the client wishes;
3. Giving the client a ball of moist clay and telling him or her to make anything the client wishes.

After the client has completed each activity, the therapist asks the client to talk about the method of proceeding, organization, color, content, feelings, ideas, and associations that he or she has relative to the production. When all three activities have been completed and discussed, the therapist asks the client to describe the various relationships he may have perceived between the three activities and the products produced.

It is suggested that the Battery be given in a quiet room where the client and therapist are alone and undisturbed. The therapist sits at the work table with the client in such a position that he or she is able to observe the client's facial expressions and work. Directions are repeated if necessary but no suggestions are made. During discussion of each activity, the therapist attempts to gain as much information as possible but does not lead the client or attempt to elicit information that the client is not able or willing to express. The therapist does not make any interpretation to the client during administration of the Battery but rather guides the discussion so that all aspects of each activity are explored.

Data gained through the administration of the Battery and the discussion are interpreted in conjunction with information acquired in a general interview and any other available data. It is best not to "read" too much into the data gained from the Battery. Rather, it is important to really listen to the client. The therapist should never think that he or she knows more about the client than the client knows about him- or herself. It is, however, useful to try to enter into the subjective experience of the client.

The Fidler Battery is used most appropriately and successfully with clients of average or above intelligence who have some degree of verbal skill. Its use is inappropriate with clients who are diagnosed as paranoid, aphasic, who have visual perception problems or a predominance of primary process thinking, or with individuals who are mentally retarded.

Free choice of selected activities is an evaluative tool that can be used with any type of frame of reference, i.e., analytical, developmental, or acquisitional. The discussion following the activity would most likely deal with the symbolic meaning of the client's choice of activity, the materials used, motions, and product produced when an analytic frame of reference is being utilized. This may also be true to some extent if a developmental frame of reference is being used. The discussion would be more oriented to everyday affairs when an acquisitional frame of reference is being used as the basis for evaluation and change process.

When using free choice of selected activities as an evaluative tool, the client and therapist meet alone for approximately an hour. The therapist offers the client a choice of approximately five activities. The client selects one. The therapist provides whatever directions are needed, and the client is asked to carry the activity through to completion. The therapist offers assistance only if it is evident that the client cannot finish the activity. The therapist observes the client without initiating any conversation. If the client attempts to engage the therapist in conversation of a casual nature, the therapist participates. This is not a time for the client to discuss the nature of his or her problems. If the conversation drifts in this direction too seriously, the therapist tells the client that the problems can and will be discussed later and gently changes the subject. What the client says during the doing process is important but

TABLE 16-2. *Interpersonal Skill Survey*

Behavior	Comments	Present	Future
Demonstrates ability to initiate, respond to, and sustain verbal interaction			
Expresses ideas and feelings appropriately			
Aware of others' needs and feelings			
Participates appropriately in cooperative and competitive situations			
Able to compromise and negotiate			
Able to be assertive			
Takes appropriate group roles			

more information can often be gained if the conversation is not directly related to the client's current difficulties in functioning.

Following completion of the activity, discussion is focused on the client's selection of a particular activity, how it was performed, the client's feelings and ideas about the process and end product, and what the client thinks the activity says about his- or herself as a person. It is sometimes useful to ask the client what would be the next activity selected if there was sufficient time for its completion. The reason for this choice is then discussed.

The five activities available for selection should be short term (20 min to a half hour) and require little direction on the part of the therapist. Each of the activities should have very different characteristics with variation along the dimensions of structured-unstructured, simple-complex, gross-to-fine motions, soft-to-resistant material, destructive-constructive, facilitating-to-inhibiting symbolic expression, and color. The activities selected should, of course, be appropriate to the client's age, gender, and cultural background.

Evaluation of Social Interaction

There are two evaluative tools available for the assessment of social interaction: Interpersonal Skill Survey and Group Interaction Skill Survey. Both make use of an evaluation group as outlined in Chapter 14. It is recommended that the reader review this section.

The Interpersonal Skills Survey is derived from an acquisitional frame of reference. Presented as Table 16-2, it is used as a guide for observing a client's behavior in an evaluation group. A rating of 1 to 4 is used in a manner similar to that outlined in the discussion of Survey of Task Skills. It also may be used as a point of departure for discussion between client and therapist after the meeting of the evaluation group (956). It is often helpful to show the client the survey already completed, with the therapist explaining why certain ratings were given. The client is then encouraged to express opinions about his or her behavior in the group and whether this behavior is typical of participation in other group situations. Discrepancies between the therapist's observations and those of the client are then discussed. Hopefully some agreement can be reached. During this interview, the client and therapist may also discuss the client's expected environment. If possible, they decide the type of interpersonal skills the client is going to need for successful participation in this environment.

The Group Interaction Skill Survey is derived from a developmental frame of reference (708). The reader is referred to Chaper 5 and the sections on play/recreation/leisure for ages 1 through 18 years for a description of the development of group interaction skills. The Group Interaction Skills Survey presented as Table 16-3 is used as a guide for observing a client in an evaluative group. The purpose of the guide is to help determine a client's level of development relative to group interaction. In the left-hand column the therapist checks the behavior that is most indicative of the client's interaction in the group. If a client exhibits all of the behavior listed under a particular type of group, it is fairly safe to say that the client would be able to participate in that type of group in a variety of situations. However, all behaviors may not be checked under a particular type of group because the client has moved beyond that kind of interaction. For example, one behavior listed under project group is "occasionally engages in group activity. . . ." The client may participate consistently in the group activity, indicating that the individual has moved beyond

TABLE 16-3. *Group-Interaction Skill Survey*

Type of group	Notation
Parallel group	
Engages in some activity, but acts as if this is an individual task as opposed to a group activity	
Aware of others in the group	
Some verbal or nonverbal interaction with others	
Appears to be relatively comfortable in this situation	
Project group	
Occasionally engages in the group activity, moving in and out according to his or her own whim	
Seeks some assistance from others	
Gives some assistance when directly asked to do so	
Egocentric-cooperative group	
Aware of group's goal relative to the task	
Aware of group norms	
Acts as if he or she belongs in the group	
Willing to participate	
Meets esteem needs of others	
Able to get others to meet his or her esteem needs	
Recognizes rights of others	
Not overly competitive	
Cooperative group	
Makes own wishes, desires, and needs known	
Participates in group activity but seems concerned primarily with his or her own needs and needs of others	
Able to meet needs other than esteem needs	
Tends to be most responsive to group members who are similar to him or her in some way	
Mature group	
Responsive to all group members	
Takes a variety of instrumental roles	
Takes a variety of expressive roles	
Able to share leadership	
Promotes a good balance between task accomplishment and satisfaction of group members' needs	

the project group level of interaction. With this type of exception in mind, when a client does not exhibit all of the behaviors listed under a particular kind of group, it is likely that the client has not mastered interaction in that type of group. The survey form again is useful for structuring the interview after the end of the evaluative group meeting. The focused interview is conducted in a manner similar to that outlined for assessment of interpersonal skills.

The types of evaluative tools described in this section are appropriate for the evaluation of performance components. There are other tools used for assessment of occupational performances. These are described in the following section.

TABLE 16-4. *Activities of Daily Living Survey*

Activity	Present	Future
Personal hygiene		
Elimination		
Bathing		
Grooming		
Dressing		
Dressing appropriately		
Washing, ironing, and mending clothes		
Eating		
Feeding one's self		
Knowledge of nutritional needs		
Meal planning		
Using kitchen appliances		
Using measuring and cooking utensils		
Cooking for self		
Cooking for household members		
Cleaning up		
Maintaining some order in kitchen		
Food storage		
Communication		
Use of telephone		
Use of telephone directories		
Writing personal and business letters		
Filling out forms		
Home		
Locating and securing housing		
Furnishing and decorating home		
Routine cleaning		
Major cleaning		
Minor household repairs		
Maintenance of household appliances		
Care of yard and lawn		
Utilities conservation		
Home safety and security		

ASSESSMENT OF OCCUPATIONAL PERFORMANCES

There is somewhat less overlapping in the evaluative tools used for assessment of occupational performances. However, similar to the assessment tools for performance components, they are not as complete and well designed as, hopefully, they will be in the future.

Evaluation of Family Interaction

The majority of information regarding familial roles is usually obtained from a general interview with the

TABLE 16-4. *(contd.)*

Activity	Present	Future
Community resources for household repairs and maintenance		
Travel		
Walking		
Using public transportation		
Using a map		
Buying, maintaining, and driving a car		
Securing a taxi or other forms of private transportation		
Traveling outside one's immediate neighborhood		
Traveling outside the city		
Safety precautions in travel		
Health care		
Appropriate use of medication		
Making and keeping necessary medical appointments		
Taking care of minor illnesses		
Simple first aid		
Management of weight		
Engaging in excercise		
Adequate time for sleep		
Knowledge of contraceptives and venereal disease		
Wise use of potentially addictive substances		
Shopping		
Making lists for required items to be bought		
Shopping for Personal items		
Clothes		
Household goods		
Shopping for quality and best prices		
Keeping receipts, instructions, and warranties		
Money management		
Daily money transactions		
Banking interactions		
Budgeting		
Paying bills		

client and with other family members. Observation of the client with family members is also useful. There are so many familial roles that vary with age, culture, and life circumstances that only one role, that of being a parent, is described below. Essentially, in regard to all familial roles, the therapist and client attempt to identify whether the client is participating in various required roles in a way that is satisfying to him and to his role partners. The question of concern is, "Is this individual participating in familial roles in a manner congruent with his or her age, cultural group expectations, and life situation?"

In regard to being a parent, some facets of this familial role that the client and therapist need to consider are the client's capacity to (708):

- Care for the child's physical needs (food, clothing, safety, etc.);
- Care for the child's emotional needs (aware of age-appropriate needs, able to demonstrate affection);
- Engage in play/recreational activities with child;
- Communicate in a forthright manner with child (does not give double messages, gives child an opportunity to discuss matters of concern, encourages expression of thoughts and feelings);
- Discipline the child in a consistent manner (sets limits, adequate balance between freedom and control, maintains self-control when child does not meet behavioral expectations);
- Show concern for and promote child's formal and informal education;
- Give the child appropriate responsibilities;
- Relinquish the nurturing relationship in a manner that promotes the child's continued development.

These areas need to be discussed particularly if there is concern on the part of the client or other family members about the client's ability to be an adequate parent.

Evaluation of Activities of Daily Living

As mentioned in Chapter 4, activities of daily living cover a broad area of human behavior. Thus the Activities of Daily Living Survey (Table 16-4) is probably not complete, nor is it likely to be suitable for every client population. It is thus presented as only a sample of a type of evaluative tool to assess function relative to activities of daily living (488,708,956). The "Present" column is checked if the client is able to perform the activity listed in the "Activity" column. The "Future" column is checked if the client will need to be able to perform the activity in the expected environment. It is also checked if the client indicates that he or she would like to be able to perform this activity in the future.

One way of assessing activities of daily living is to discuss the Survey with the client. This may be sufficient if the therapist is fairly sure the client is able to honestly assess his or her capacity to function in this area. Many clients, however, are not able to do this. In addition, some people are hesitant to admit to difficulty in such "ordinary" activities. Thus, a specially designed activity evaluation is sometimes required. This involves asking the client to demonstrate competence in various activities of daily living. Only those activities the client is likely to need to do are evaluated. Ideally this is done in the client's expected environment. If this is not possible, a simulated situation in the clinical setting may be used. Specific means for evaluation are so dependent on what is available in the clinical setting that it would be impossible to delineate them in any realistic way. Designing appropriate evaluative situations is, then, left up to the knowledge and creativity of the therapist. The therapist often must be rather ingenious in devising situations that will allow both therapist and client to gain sufficient information for adequate assessment. If various doing experiences are used, the therapist discusses the data gained from the experience with the client using the Activity of Daily Living Survey as a guide.

TABLE 16-5. *School Survey*

Do you attend school regularly? Do you arrive on time? Do you usually go to all of your classes?
What do you like about school?
What do you dislike about school?
What subjects are you studying now and what were your latest grades in these subjects?
What subjects do you like the best and why?
What subjects do you like the least and why?
(In answering the two above questions consider all subjects you have taken, not just what you are taking now.)
What qualities do you like best in a teacher? What qualities do you like least?
How well do you get along with your teachers?
What kind of interactions do you have with your teachers outside class?
What is your typical behavior in the classroom? Do you participate in class discussions or activities? Are you able to pay attention? Do you take notes?
What do you do if you are having a problem with a particular subject?
How do you feel about your classmates?
How would your classmates describe you?
What do you do during free periods and at lunch time?
Does anyone help you with your homework?
How do you prepare for a test?
What type of tests do you like best?
Does taking a test make you feel excessively anxious? If so, how do you deal with this anxiety?
What are your future educational plans?
(Consider the elective subjects you would like to take, whether you would like to go to a different school, plans for college, what your major might be.)
How do your parents feel about your education and how are you doing in school?

Evaluation of School/Work

Although many of the basic skills necessary for successful participation in school and work are the same, the two areas will be discussed separately here.

TABLE 16-6. *Work Survey*

Behavior	Comments	Present	Future
Comes to work on time			
Stays at work for required period of time			
Appears able to work a normal work day			
Sustains attention to work tasks			
Performs tasks in a normal amount of time			
Plans work period so that a required amount of work is accomplished			
Organizes tasks relative to realistic priorities			
Works at increased speed when required			
Carries on appropriate conversation when working			
Returns to work when interrupted			
Takes direction from a work supervisor			
Alters behavior appropriately on the basis of constructive criticism			
Seeks direction from work supervisor when necessary			
Requests only an appropriate amount of need satisfaction from supervisor			
Evokes a pleasant response from others			
Socializes with others during work breaks			
Gives assistance willingly			
Follows the norms of the work setting			

When there is evidence that a child or adolescent is experiencing difficulty in *school*, the therapist's major task is to determine the source of the problem. The therapist and client must attempt to identify what is the primary source of difficulty and what are the secondary sources which are a consequence of the primary difficulty. This is no easy task as many times there is a cumulative effect, i.e., the interaction of multiple difficulties. Problem areas to consider are (a) a learning disability, (b) lack of interpersonal skills relative to authority or peers, (c) preoccupation with concerns that are unrelated to school, (d) an educational situation that is not responsive to the client's needs, (e) parental lack of interest in the client's school experience.

Information about the client's capacity to function in school can be gained from an interview with the client, parents, and the client's teacher or advisor. School records, if available, are a valuable source of information. Observation of the client in the school setting is also a good source of data. When direct observation in the school is not possible, some information about a client's capacity to interact with classmates may be obtained from observation of the client in an evaluation group. Involving the client in a situation in which he is required to follow the directions of a person in authority may provide information about the client's relationship to her teachers.

The School Survey (Table 16-5) may also be used as a source of information (106,290,306,772). As a questionnaire, it is suitable for many clients 12 years of age or older. When used in such a manner, it is given to the client to complete by him- or herself. After completion and after the therapist has had an opportunity to read it, the client and therapist discuss it together. The survey may also be used as a guide for a focused interview with a younger client, parents, or teachers.

Assessment relative to *work* is first concerned with where the individual is in the work cycle (698). The following outline may be used as a guide (see Chapter 5 for further clarification): Fantasy choices. Tentative occupational choice (interest, capacity, value, transition). Realistic choice (exploration, crystallization, specification). Established in an occupation (selected area of specialization, clear career goals). Reassessment

TABLE 16-7. *Leisure/Recreation Survey*

Activity	With whom	Present[a]	Future
Swimming			
Table games (cards, chess, Scrabble, etc.)			
Photography			
Drama groups			
Discussion groups			
Choral groups			
Woodworking			
Reading			
Playing a musical instrument			
Listening to music			
Social dancing			
Pool			
Needle work (sewing, knitting, etc.)			
Running			
Bicycling			
Movies			
Going to parties			
Visiting (neighbors, friends, family)			
Entertaining			
Union activities			
Bowling			
Lectures			
Attending classes			
Gardening			
Shopping			
Religious services and organizations			
Poetry			

[a]F, frequently engaged; O, occasionally engaged; *, enjoyable. See text.

of career goals. Adjustment to final years of employment. Adjustment to retirement.

As mentioned, the work cycle of some women may be different from that of the male norm. Thus, superimposed on the work cycle just outlined, for women the therapist should consider whether the client is in the phases of: Discontinuation of employment for the purpose of child rearing; contemplating/preparing for return to employment; adjusting to return to employment.

With the client's place in the work cycle identified, assessment, where appropriate, focuses on the client's past work history, present assets and limitations in the area of work, and future work plans. Information may be gathered through a questionnaire or an interview. How the information is gathered depends on the client's educational level and ability to complete a questionnaire (290,518,635,698,708,727). Regardless of the method used to gain information, the necessary data include: Approximate dates of beginning and leaving each job; job title and specific tasks the client was expected to perform: approximate salary; reason for leaving each job; attendance record; relationship with work supervisors; kind of supervision with which the client is most comfortable; relationship with co-workers in the client's var-

TABLE 16-7. *(contd.)*

Activity	With whom	Present[a]	Future
Going to a restaurant or bar			
Hanging out			
Political organizations			
Modern dancing			
Sketching			
Painting			
Gymnastics			
Boxing			
Wrestling			
Cooking			
Baseball			
Basketball			
Football			
Tennis			
Racketball			
Golf			
Skiing			
Sculpture, pottery			
Building models			
Computer games			
Calisthenics			
Television			
Casual conversation			
Fixing things			
PTA			
Volunteer work			
Community action groups			
Other			

ious jobs; which of the jobs the client liked best and why; what three jobs the client feels would be most interesting at this time; what specific work skills the client has (e.g., typing, operating a special kind of machine, skills in selling, managerial skills, computer programming, etc.); attitude toward work.

If the client has a job to which he or she wants to return or had a job in the not too distant past and wishes to get a similar job, evaluation is specific to that type of work (708). In other words, assessment is concerned with the client's ability to perform in a given kind of work situation. The client and therapist discuss the job in order to determine what types of interpersonal relations and task skills are necessary to perform the job successfully. It is often helpful for the client and therapist to prepare a written list of the necessary behaviors. This is then used as a check sheet on which the client's ability to perform the job is recorded. Data for completing the assessment may be gained from an interview, the client's participation in an evaluation group, and in an evaluation designed to assess task skills.

Another and perhaps more realistic way to assess the client's capacity to engage in a specific type of job is for the client to participate in a work situation. Such a

TABLE 16-8. *Activity configuration*

Part I

Time	Monday	Tuesday	Wednesday	Thursday	Friday	Saturday	Sunday
Morning							
7–9							
9–11							
11–1							
Afternoon							
1–3							
3–5							
5–7							
Evening							
7–9							
9–11							

Part II

A. What needs does the activity satisfy? What needs are not satisfied during this activity or not satisfied because of engaging in the activity?
B. I have to do this activity. I want to do this activity. Or both?
C. I want to do this activity, and I think this is good. I want to do this activity, and I think this is not good. Others make me do this and I am glad they do. Or others make me do this and I wish they did not.
D. I do this activity very well. I do this activity well enough. Or I do not do this well enough.
E. I feel joy, liking, love, fear or anxiety, dislike, hatred, anger, depression, guilt, or some other emotion while engaging in this activity, I feel ______ and ______.

situation may be available in the treatment center, in the community, or in a sheltered workshop. For evaluation to be valid, the client should participate in a work experience that is as similar as possible to the type of job for which the client is being evaluated. The client works in the job situation for approximately a week. The client is observed by the therapist periodically as well as by her supervisor on the job. At the end of this period the client, therapist, and, if appropriate, the supervisor go over the previously prepared list of required behavior. Each of the behaviors is discussed to determine whether or not the client is able to perform in that area.

The evaluation procedure outlined above is primarily oriented to assessment of an individual who has a fairly good work history and a realistic idea of the type of work in which he or she would like to engage. When a client has not worked recently, has not worked for an extended period of time, or has never worked, a different kind of work evaluation is required. This evaluation focuses on the client's capacity to function in a general work situation, not in a specific job. The Work Survey, appearing as Table 16-6, may be used as a guide for evaluation. Participation in a sheltered workshop program or in an ongoing work group is the best situation for evaluating general behavior needed for successful participation in a work setting. A work group is a thematic activity group designed to teach adequate work habits. Three to five days is usually sufficient time for evaluation. After this period the client, therapist, or work group leader discusses the Work Survey together. A rating of 1 to 4, as previously described, is used to identify the client's assets and limitations relative to work.

Evaluation of Play/Leisure/Recreation

Assessment of a child's play usually includes an interview with a parent and with the child and observation of the child playing (74,462,463,552,884,944,946). The latter should take place in a room where there is a variety of available toys, games, and equipment suitable for gross movement. After acquainting the child with what is available, the therapist allows the child to select any available activity. Free play is encouraged with no prohibition against moving spontaneously from one activity to another. If invited to participate in any play activity by the child, the therapist becomes a willing participant. As a participant, however, the therapist allows the child to take the lead in determining what will be done and how it is to be done. If the child is hesitant in engaging in any type of play, the therapist initiates a play activity with the child. The activity selected should be one that the child is likely to enjoy. It should be interesting and appropriate to the estimated developmental age of the child. Once engaged, the child is given the leadership position. If possible, the therapist also observes the child playing with other children. This may be in an informal situation or in some type of a structured play group.

Through the interviews and observation the therapist attempts to gain the following information:

1. The extent to which the child engages in:
    a. playing with toys;
    b. imaginative/innovative play, alone and with others;
    c. rough and tumble play;
    d. arts and crafts, construction of objects;
    e. spontaneous games with rules negotiated;
    f. organized games with formal rules;
    g. active and quiet play;
    h. play that involves cooperation and competition;
    i. being read to, looking at picture books, reading;
    j. watching television, alone and with others;
    k. playing games of strategy and chance.
2. What the child plays with;
3. How the child plays with toys and other materials;
4. What type of play is liked best, what is avoided or liked least;
5. With whom the child plays;
6. How the child plays with other children and adults;
7. What body postures the child uses during play;
8. How long the child plays with objects, with people;
9. Where the child plays;
10. When the child plays.

The Leisure/Recreation Survey (Table 16-7) may be used as a guide for evaluating this area of occupational performance (651,708,884). The activities listed should be considered an enumeration of possible leisure/recreational activities. A more precise and typical survey may need to be developed for a particular client population. The client may be given the Survey to complete alone or the client and therapist may complete it together. A suggested code for filling in the "Present" column is: F = frequently engage in the activity; O = occasionally engage in the activity; * = an activity that the client enjoys rather than participates in because it is expected or there is nothing else to do.

In discussing the survey, the client and therapist consider whether the client's use of leisure time is adequate relative to variety, active and sedentary activities, time spent alone and time spent with others, being interesting, providing need satisfaction. As mentioned, there is considerable variation in the way people spend their leisure time. Thus, the therapist must be cautious in interpretation. The "Future" column is checked if the client would like to engage in a particular activity in the future. The "With whom" column can be used by the client and therapist to assess the balance between solitary and shared activities.

Friendships can be considered to be on a continuum from casual to intimate, with chum relationships usually occurring once or twice during adolescence. Evaluation of friendships usually takes place in the context of a general interview, but it may also be the basis for a focused interview (708). The outline below may be used as a guide to assist the therapist in formulating appropriate questions:

Casual friendships. Sees some people occasionally perhaps once or twice a month. Engages in a regular activity with some people such as members of a softball team but rarely sees them outside this context. Sees some people regularly such as neighbors or co-workers and occasionally spends some leisure time with them.

Good friendships. States that these are friends regularly seen, expresses a liking for these friends, and experiences pleasure in being with them; enjoys doing things with friends as well as just sitting and talking.

Intimate friendships. The client thinks of a few other people as being particularly important, although not necessarily using the word love to describe the relationship. The client talks, however, very much as if he or she loved these people. The client accepts their limitations as well as their assets and is willing to make sacrifices for them. He or she turns to these people for help with personal problems. The individual feels very close to these friends but does not feel a loss of personal autonomy. There is no jealous possessiveness, and the client readily accepts the fact these friends may have intimate relationships with other people.

Chum relationships. The client currently has or had in the past one or two friends with whom he or she spent considerable time almost every day; if unable to be with the friend, he or she called the friend for lengthy conversations on the phone. The individual trusted this friend and shared very personal information. The individual experienced feelings of jealousy when he or she thought the friend was giving too much time and attention to someone else.

Evaluation of Temporal Adaptation

In addition to the client's general statements about use of her time, the Activity Configuration is a useful tool for assessment of temporal adaptation (164,708,994). The Configuration, outlined as Table 16-8, is made up of two parts. Part I, a detailed listing of all activities that are part of the client's typical week, is usually filled out by the client alone. Then using Part II as a guide, the client and therapist discuss each activity mentioned. In general, the client and therapist attempt to determine how the client is using his or her time and the extent to which this use of time is satisfying for the client.

SUMMARY

This chapter has outlined various evaluative tools used by occupational therapists for assessment of psychosocial function and dysfunction. Attention was given to interviewing and to the tools used to assess performance components and occupational performances.

17

Types of Intervention

Intervention has been defined as a collaborative effort on the part of the client and therapist directed toward goals they have previously established. For the sake of clarity and specificity, intervention has been subdivided into five types: prevention, meeting health needs, the change process, maintenance, and management. This chapter addresses all types of intervention except the change process, which is discussed in Part 5. The last section of the chapter concerns the process of goal setting and implementation.

PREVENTION

Prior to discussing prevention in occupational therapy, some background information relative to prevention in the area of health might be useful.

Background Information (152,186,827,975,987)

The human race has more than once been threatened by extinction because of plague and pestilence. Although there were periods of massive decrease in population, the human race has managed to survive. Nevertheless, disease has had a great impact on history. It has been the cause of mass migration, virtual elimination of cultural groups, altered national customs, and has influenced religious development and determined the outcome of wars. On the whole, disease and epidemics were considered to be an act of God. Civilization for the most part was content to take action to protect itself only when disease actually occurred. Although some attempts were centered on curative medicine, resorting to prayer and/or fleeing in terror were much more prevalent. Prevention was, in general, not considered particularly important.

Nevertheless, action to prevent ill-health and its consequence has been taken in one form or another in even some of the earliest of cultures. The actions taken have varied, depending on the nature, organization, and circumstances of the particular group and on the values, knowledge, and technical means available to it. Even many very primitive groups kept their surroundings clean and appeared to recognize that certain diseases were contagious. The ancient Jews practiced a variety of preventative measures. They were concerned about cleanliness of the body, disinfection of dwellings after illness, sanitation of camp sites, disposal of excreta and refuse, protection of the water and food supply, and hygiene relative to sexual intercourse and maternity. The Greeks made a decisive change from magical-religious practices to a more rational naturalistic method of dealing with illness. They believed that good health could be maintained by living moderately, regulating diet and exercise, and minimizing stress.

Prevention as we know it today could perhaps be said to have begun in the seventeenth century with Leeuwenhoek's development of the microscope. Although other people had previously formulated the theory that infections were the result of minute organisms that invaded the body, this theory did not gain any real recognition until it could be demonstrated scientifically. In the latter part of the eighteenth century, the idea that governments were responsible for the health of their people began to receive some recognition. In England, Jeremy Bentham urged that legislation relative to environmental sanitation, communicable disease, and the administration of medical care be enacted (92). Preventative medicine as a true scientific discipline, however, did not really come into being until after Pasteur's discoveries in the nineteenth century.

Preventative medicine is a branch of applied biology that seeks to reduce or eradicate disease by removing or altering the responsible etiological factors. The application of preventative medicine is assisted by epidemiology. This scientific discipline is concerned with the occurrence, distribution, and the types of diseases of mankind in time and in various places. Second, it is concerned with the relationship between disease and the life-style of any particular group. Understanding the nature of a disease and the causal elements involved in its occurrence provides, to a greater or lesser degree, a basis for prevention. There is frequently adequate knowledge to justify classification of a certain disease as preventable. Its continued presence is chiefly due to the lack of methods for placing effective control measures in operation. Certain controls would limit personal freedom to a level intolerable for many people. Particularly in Western society, where social values are such that individuals prefer a fairly high degree of personal freedom to the adequate prevention of some diseases. The degree of successful prevention depends to some extent on the urgency and dimensions of the health problems, but it is also dependent on political, economic, cultural, and ideological factors as well. Some areas where preventative measures are possible but have been only marginally successful are improved nutrition, air and water pollution, and the protection of workers in a wide variety of occupations. There continue to be outbreaks of such diseases as diphtheria and poliomyelitis despite the availability of preventative measures. Historically, prevention has involved a combination of government policies and programs, private group undertakings, and family and individual actions relative to health. It is only in the coordination of all of these that prevention can succeed.

Over the course of time preventative medicine has had many successes. It has found the means for controlling, if not eradicating, such diseases as smallpox, cholera, typhoid, malaria, yellow fever, tuberculosis, deficiency diseases, rubella, erythroblastosis (RH incompatibility), and phenylketonuria (PKU). Preventative medicine has been far less successful in dealing with the chronic diseases that are so endemic in the population today. Little has been accomplished in the prevention or control of cancer, cardiovascular and renal conditions, diabetes mellitus, arthritis, musculoskeletal conditions, and the changes associated with aging. Rosen (827) has commented that the situation with respect to noncommunicable chronic diseases is analagous to the state of affairs around 1870 in terms of understanding and preventing communicable diseases.

It should also be noted that medical education and training is oriented to the diagnosis of disease and its treatment—not to prevention. The exceptions are in the area of immunization and deficiency diseases. In addition, the system of payment for medical services does not encourage the involvement of physicians in prevention except in those systems where there is prepayment. Many recent advances in prevention have been led by groups other than medicine. Some examples of preventative measures fostered by nonmedical groups are identification of individuals who are carriers of dysfunctional recessive genes and genetic counseling, birth control, amniocentesis, induced abortion, screening for defects at birth, and intensive enrichment programs in early childhood.

Traditionally, in discussing prevention three levels or types of prevention are identified: primary, secondary, and tertiary. Primary prevention is concerned with reducing the incidence of disease and disability in a given population. It involves counteracting the factors responsible for the occurrence of illness. Efforts are directed toward changing attitudes, values, and actions in regard to conditions and behaviors that foster disease and disability. This is usually accomplished through education, direct service, and political action addressed to current and anticipated problems.

Secondary prevention involves reduction of the severity and duration of the disorders through early identification and prompt treatment or intervention. It also involves efforts to prevent any secondary difficulties that may arise out of the immediate problems of coping with the effects of an existing disease or disability.

Tertiary prevention involves reducing the rate of dysfunctional performance among disabled individuals within the community.

One final concept that needs to be defined is community medicine (152,165,166,759,827). Community medicine involves both prevention and curative procedures. It differs from traditional medicine in that its approach is to families and other groups in the population, primarily those who are not being adequately served by other available agencies. Of particular concern are social and occupational situations that affect health. Community medicine in the United States was essentially initiated by the passage of the Barton-Hill Act, legislation briefly discussed in Chapter 2. This was the first step toward effective health planning and resource development on a national scale. There was an effort to not only increase the number of hospital beds, but also to elimate maldistribution of facilities. Among the number of criteria that needed to be met to qualify for funds were preventative programs that included health maintenance, disease prevention, and health education.

Prevention in Psychiatry

The above discussion focused primarily on prevention relative to physical medicine. Prevention in the area of psychosocial dysfunction presents some issues that are not so apparent in the prevention of physical disease and disability (85,135,165,166,202,607,717,759,958).

The ultimate goal of prevention relative to mental health is a more satisfying and effective life for people, with a reduction in the stresses and strains that appear to contribute to psychosocial dysfunction. The difficulty in reaching this goal is due to a lack of knowledge regarding etiology and prognostic or therapeutic factors that might provide a useful basis for classification. Medical diagnosis implies a theory of etiology or pathology and treatment, and by inference, possible methods of prevention. This is not the case in psychiatry. Diagnostic categories are ever changing; there is no agreement on etiology or pathology or on preferred treatment. Proposals for prevention, then, are not and cannot be based on the same scientific foundation traditional to programs of prevention in physical medicine. To make the situation more complex, there is no agreement on the aims and purpose of human life against which an illness-health continuum might be evaluated. This lack of agreement leads to the absence of a good, accepted definition of mental health.

Psychiatry in the 1960s promised a marked reduction in the incidence of mental illness and received massive amounts of federal and state money to fulfill that promise. With all of the effort and expenditure of monies, there is no evidence that there has been a reduction in mental illness. Some of the disillusionment with psychiatry experienced by many people today arises from a promise made but never fulfilled.

Another problem with prevention relative to mental health is that psychosocial dysfunction appears to arise from complicated interrelated factors. Genetic factors, molded by biological and psychological factors, influence the developing infant from the moment of conception through intrauterine, familial, and ultimately extended social experiences. The vicissitudes of later sociocultural pressures are also a factor. The capacity to cope with internal and external stress seems to be related to the ability to maintain a steady or homeostatic state that facilitates adaptation without excessive anxiety. The problem is that we have little idea of how that desired homeostasis is attained.

Given the present state of knowledge, prevention can only be directed to factors *believed* to be pathogenic in the hopes that they will lead to a reduction in psychosocial dysfunction. Prevention is, then, based more on social and ethical values rather than on any scientific foundation that specific factors cause mental illness.

Some of the current areas of concern in psychiatric prevention are (202):

Paranatal factors

1. Deficits in nutrition and physical health of the mother; drugs, alcohol, and specific viral infections which lead to congenital anomalies and mental retardation;

2. Chronic psychological distress of mothers during pregnancy leading to a significant increase in postpartum vulnerability to physical and psychological disorders.

It is important to note that sophisticated medical technology has resulted in the survival of many premature and low birth weight babies who exhibit a high level of chronically handicapping conditions and increased incidence of behavioral and psychological disorders later in life. Prevention in this area and the ethical issues involved are just beginning to be addressed.

Family issues

1. The large increase in single-parent families where there may be a conflict between the economic needs of the family and the nurturing needs of young children;

2. Changes in ideas about gender roles may lead mothers to feel that there is little meaning or worth in what they are doing and that there is minimal community support for their role as a parent;

3. The lack of adequate training for individuals who are providing day care for young children;

4. The lack of family structure characterized by adequate organization, flexibility, a large number of adaptive strategies for conflict resolution, and a clearly defined hierarchical structure with at least two generations discernible;

5. Inadequate support given to parents during the early years of child-rearing which will allay their fears, correct distortions, and, in general, increase parental effectiveness;

6. Transitional states of dysfunction seemingly related to attempts to master particular developmental tasks that are not adequately differentiated from more fixed psychopathological patterns.

The school system

1. Lack of a sufficient number of trained personnel to engage in early case finding relative to physical, emotional, and learning problems;

2. Inadequate provisions for the learning-disabled child leading to secondary emotional and behavioral problems;

3. The demand that teachers give considerable attention to the mental health of students without recognizing that there are limitations in what educators can do while at the same time instructing students in basic academic skills;

4. Public law 94-142 requiring schools to provide for the education of handicapped children even though school systems often have neither the personnel nor the skills to manage the problems of some of these children;

5. The chaotic state of many schools may require students to engage in deviant behavior in order to survive in this pathological environment.

Delivery of psychiatric services

1. Lack of adequate differential diagnoses relative to physical versus psychological disorders—particularly in the elderly;

2. The care of the chronically disturbed individual who does not meet the current criteria for continued hospitalization (represents a danger to him/herself or others) nor is provided with adequate facilities and support in the community.

The above list of areas of concern, it should be noted, is by no means complete. Only some of the major areas were mentioned.

There are three main approaches to prevention used by psychiatry: education, administrative action, and direct service.

Public education has taken two forms—within the school system and through the media, with the latter probably being more effective. It is evident that some change in attitude has taken place, particularly concerning the relationship of mental health to crime, delinquency, addiction, suicide, and so forth. People are more aware of the stresses caused by urban industrial life and the effects of these on both physical and mental health. There is also greater awareness of the relationship between physical and mental health. The apparent biochemical nature of some mental illness and the effectiveness of some psychotherapeutic drugs have resulted in a somewhat more positive and accepting attitude toward mental illness.

Administrative action involves prevention by influencing laws, statutes, regulations, and customs. The goal is to reduce preventable stress or to provide services to assist people facing stress to engage in appropriate problem solving. Administrative action may be fostered by an individual practitioner or by local, state, and national groups. A word of caution is appropriate here relative to attempting to alter customs. A culture, as previously discussed, is made up of a system of interdependent elements. One must be aware of those dynamic elements and take care not to make matters worse.

Direct service in prevention involves interaction with an individual or the people immediately around that individual. The goal is to attempt to change the emotional forces in a person's environment. Such interactions are based on the theory that mental health is related to the quality of interpersonal relationships—family, friends, work group, and so forth—and to the degree to which needs are being met. Therefore, the practitioner is concerned with improving interpersonal relationships or remedying disordered ones. Most efforts have been directed toward dealing with key people in the community or institutions, the rationale being that they influence a considerable number of other people because of their position in the structure. Therefore, by helping them to improve their interpersonal relations, other people in the structure will be helped indirectly.

In conclusion, psychiatry has been and remains concerned about prevention. As a profession it has not been particularly successful. This rather poor showing is related, at least in part, to the multiple factors that influence mental health and the limited knowledge about these factors.

Prevention in Occupational Therapy

Prevention, as one type of intervention, is relatively new to occupational therapy (24,176,184,259,261,298, 299,333,357, 371,372,483,583, 617,830,831,989,1008, 1009,1024). The idea only began to be accepted in the early 1970s when the concept of community medicine gained considerable popularity. Although now an accepted part of occupational therapy, it is not an area in which many therapists work exclusively. There are therapists, however, who engage in preventative activities as a small part of their practice or as members of professional associations. There are several reasons why occupational therapists have not been more active in prevention. Some of the major ones are:

1. Traditionally occupational therapists have been concerned with assisting the chronically disabled individual, not individuals who are healthy or, at least, relatively healthy;
2. The base of operation for occupational therapists has by and large been a hospital or clinical setting, not the community. Occupational therapists have, indeed, used the community to facilitate intervention but more as an extension of the clinic than a primary setting;

3. There are far fewer job openings or opportunities in prevention than there are in dealing with the other aspects of intervention;
4. A good theoretical basis, a functional, satisfactory rationale and guide for services to the healthy community has not yet been developed;
5. There is no research that demonstrates the effectiveness of occupational therapy preventative programs.

The above-listed restraining factors may disappear gradually as the profession gains more knowledge and skill relative to prevention.

One area where conflict may continue, however, is the chronic versus the well population. That occupational therapists have always been concerned with those who are chronically disabled is not the point being discussed here. Rather, with the increase in the age of the population and the survival of many individuals who are developmentally disabled or who have acquired disabilities, the number of people needing occupational therapy services is on the increase. The question then is can occupational therapy as a profession afford to turn any major portion of its efforts toward prevention. This question is simply raised here for your consideration. There is no easy answer when a profession is faced with a dilemma about where to allocate its resources.

One more point needs to be raised before continuing. As mentioned, the idea of prevention in occupational therapy is relatively new. The other types of intervention—meeting health needs, maintenance, management, and the change process—have been a part of occupational therapy from its inception. Prevention does not always fit nicely into this traditional scheme. This is particularly true in the case of maintenance and prevention. There is some overlap, for example, in the case of instruction in work simplification; is this maintenance or prevention? This is also true relative to the change process. A life skills development program for psychiatric clients, for example, is considered by some to be prevention. Others consider it a part of the change process. This author would take the latter stance. Confusion in the literature about what is and is not prevention is mentioned here for two reasons. First, so that the reader in reviewing the literature is aware that discrepancies will be found. Second, this type of confusion can lead to a misunderstanding about the theoretical base that supports a particular type of intervention.

The theoretical foundation and rationale for prevention, as mentioned, have not been well articulated in occupational therapy. The following ideas relative to prevention have, however, been mentioned:

Occupational therapists have always been concerned about the quality of life of all age groups, regardless of an individual's degree of illness or wellness;

Active, purposeful interaction with the environment not only is indicative of health, but serves to develop the characteristics that define health;

Successful participation in occupational performances facilitates the development of performance components. In turn, adequate and continued development of performance components enables the individual to participate in more complex and refined occupational performances;

Dysfunctional or maladaptive behavior is frequently caused by disorders in the environment with which the individual interacts. Thus, rather than seeking deficiencies within the individual, it would seem wiser to deal with the environmental disorders.

On the basis of the above premises, somewhat more philosophical than theoretical, occupational therapists have engaged in a variety of preventative programs. The lack of a good theoretical foundation for prevention *is* of concern to the profession. One way that professions do evolve is to engage in a new set of activities, forming a theoretical foundation as they study the effects of their endeavors. This should, of course, be done with caution and serious study, guided by experience and wisdom.

Some of the preventative programs in the area of psychosocial function that occupational therapists are involved in are:

- Intensive care neonatal units to provide education, consultation, and direct service relative to the stimulation needed for adequate development in particular of the tactile and vestibular systems;
- Well-baby clinics with emphasis on screening for developmental delays and parent education;
- Nursery and day care programs as consultants to the staff in respect to creating an adequate environment for optimal development and for the purpose of identifying developmental delays;
- Workshops for parents and for parents and children together to facilitate the parent-child relationship as it changes and develops over time;
- Programs for teenage mothers and other expectant parents to facilitate understanding of child development, the ever changing needs of the child, and parenting skills;
- Involvement in school systems to screen for physical, emotional, or learning problems and to facilitate the mainstreaming of handicapped children;
- Industrial and home design programs for making recommendations to prevent accidents, promote safety, and minimize architectural barriers;

- Community planning groups to provide consultation concerning comprehensive health programs, architectural planning, housing that promotes an optimal mix of the various age groups, and recreational facilities and programs;
- State agencies to assist in the setting of standards and in the translation of federal guidelines for application in the state;
- Working with the military to improve the quality of life for single personnel and families by constructing a network of services which stress prevention;
- Retirement planning programs designed to help individuals to develop new interests and skills, to understand the relationship between life style and maintenance of health, and to emphasize the importance of regular and stimulating interaction with others;
- Programs for the elderly which provide for involvement in different settings and the availability of counseling services in regard to health, financial matters, dealing with loss, family relationships, and so forth.

The above list of preventative programs in which occupational therapists are involved was drawn from a survey of the literature. Therapists may be involved in other programs that have not yet been reported.

One other aspect of prevention that is of concern to occupational therapists is crisis intervention (165,166, 759,830,831). As used here, crisis refers to a situation in which a person faces serious obstacles to important life goals. At least for a time, the obstacles seem insurmountable. It is a period of disorganization during which many different, unsuccessful attempts at solution are made. Associated with or as a consequence of crisis there is likely to be one or more of the following: problems in communication; disruption of occupational performances; confusion of values; loss of usual coping mechanisms; and the sense of being overwhelmed by feelings such as anxiety, grief, anger, and impotence. Crisis frequently occurs at the time of developmental passages, divorce, serious illness or disability, death, disasters such as fire or floods, and other conditions that lead to a severe disruption of one's usual environment or living situation.

The cultural context in which the individual lives influences perception of the situation. First it defines the severity of the situation. Second, there is considerable variation in the degree to which a particular situation has been taken into account by the individual's culture. If it has been seriously considered, there are frequently very clear-cut prescriptions of what one should do in the particular circumstances. These expectations, at least, provide some guidelines for the individual. It is important to note that cultural expectations may, however, hamper a realistic solution to the problem. When the culture offers no prescriptions of how one ought to respond and behave, the individual is left without the collective wisdom of his or her culture. This can be a devastating state of affairs, compounding efforts to effectively deal with the crisis. An example of this is the birth of a severely impaired child.

An individual cannot exist in a state of crisis for any extended period of time. Eventually some kind of adaptation is achieved which may or may not be in the best interests of the individual, or others with whom the individual is involved. Solutions based on projection or displacement, for example, may be at the emotional expense of others. Poor solutions may lead to regression or a precarious state of mental health.

On the other hand, when the crisis comes to a successful resolution, the individual arrives at a new state of equilibrium. This is usually accomplished through both external and internal adaptation. In other words, the individual alters the environment in such a way as to make it more comfortable and need-fulfilling, and redefines ideas, values, and goals in such a way as to facilitate adjustment. The capacity to deal effectively with a particular crisis situation is believed to have a positive influence on the individual's capacity to handle future crisis situations and on his or her general state of mental health.

Crisis intervention is designed to help individuals arrive at a more viable solution to the serious problem at hand. This is not to say that many people are not able to resolve a crisis in an adaptive manner alone or with the aid of family members and friends. However, there are times when an individual needs assistance from someone who is less emotionally involved and who has experience in assisting individuals in crisis.

The goals of crisis intervention are (a) to alleviate the impact of immediate or anticipated disruptive stressful events and (b) to help mobilize the manifest and latent psychosocial capacities and social resources of those directly affected for coping adaptively with the effects of stress. In general, this is done through enabling the individual or individuals to reaffirm or further clarify values, reopen or improve communication, reestablish or make constructive role adjustments, and to engage in reality-based problem solving.

Crisis intervention is centered on the problem, not on the individual. Thus, it is not considered necessary to analyze the personality or past experiences of the individual which may be making it difficult for the person to deal with the crisis in an effective manner. Rather the therapist makes a direct effort to assist the individual with the problems at hand. One of the therapist's functions is to help the individual personalize information. This is done because there is often a difference between knowing what is "good" or "right" and acting on that knowledge. The therapist acts as an enabler, letting the individual or the system do the work. The therapist avoids inflicting additional pain, reduces guilt, and above all treats the individual with respect. An effort is made to increase the individual's hope and the possibility of success. The therapist essentially offers him- or herself as a supporting and helping person. Because of the support offered by a small group, crisis intervention is often more effective if it takes place in a topical group.

Caplan (165) emphasizes the importance of what he refers to as "worry work." He feels that when an individual is faced with a crisis it is necessary to worry; that worry is purposeful. The work related to worry is that of the internal adjustment that is stimulated by signal anxiety. There are several factors that may influence worry work. One factor is the revival of old memories, of old fantasies of loss due to previously unresolved problems of a similar nature. These become symbolically linked to the current crisis. Another factor is the actual, real environmental threat that is impinging on the individual. The temporal nature of the crisis also is important. It may start and get worse, start and finish, or start and get slowly better. The first situation interferes with worry work the most. Finally, worry work is influenced by the individual's state of physical health, constitutional toughness, repertoire of coping responses, ability to withstand frustration, and degree of success in dealing with crisis in the past. Individuals who do not worry usually are not stimulated to do the necessary work of adjustment and adaptation. The result is often disordered behavior, psychosomatic reactions, or poor solutions.

The above discussion has primarily focused on helping an individual deal with a current crisis. Crisis intervention is also used to help an individual deal with an anticipated problem. Adequate anticipation of a problem relieves at least some of the burden and thus keeps the difficulty in a more controlled range. Evidence suggests that if certain positive types of inner attitudes are formed before the danger materializes, the chances of becoming traumatized or of developing disorganized behavior are reduced. When events take place as an individual anticipates, the occurrence of unpleasant episodes does not come as a surprise. The individual feels reassured that events will proceed in the expected fashion. Worry is also considered to be important in anticipated crisis. In worrying, the individual is likely to fantasize or mentally rehearse various unpleasant occurrences. That person is thus motivated to seek out and heed realistic information about the painful and distressing experiences he or she will probably encounter.

Anticipatory worry should take place in the presence of support and in an atmosphere of hope. In this way worry can be kept at a level compatible with the reality of the situation—not too much and not too little. Through receiving support of others in advance, the individual has increased confidence that he or she can handle the problem.

In helping an individual anticipate a problem, the therapist describes in detail what the individual is likely to perceive, hear, feel, smell, and so forth. The therapist does not do the individual any service by telling a nice story. The painful realities need to be presented. At the same time, the therapist helps the individual identify ways of dealing with the problems. The support and help that are likely to be available are described. At times it is possible to help the individual foresee some of the potential problem areas and take steps to prevent them rather than solve them. The hope of successful outcome within the range of predictable reality is offered.

Apathy is fairly common in the anticipation of crisis. Apathy may arise from two sources: (a) the individual does not realize there will be a danger or (b) the individual realizes only too well that there is a danger but feels that he or she just cannot cope with its consideration. In the first case, stimulation in regard to the danger will increase the individual's effectiveness in adequate preparation. In the second case stimulation often only increases apathy. General support is about all the therapist can offer; intervention relative to anticipated crisis would not be effective at this time.

In conclusion, prevention, one aspect of intervention, is fairly new in the practice of occupational therapy. It is beginning to be developed as the profession gains knowledge and skill in this area. Crisis intervention has the strongest theoretical foundation and demonstrated effectiveness. It fits well into the domain of concern of the profession with its strong emphasis on problem solving. It is also an orientation that is well suited to topical activity groups, both concurrent and anticipatory.

MEETING HEALTH NEEDS

Meeting health needs (137,290,403,646,709) has been defined as the process of satisfying or fulfilling inherent human needs so that an individual may experience a sense of physical, psychological, and social well-being. These needs are considered to be universal in that they are shared by all people, regardless of their current state of health. Health needs may be differentiated from those needs that arise from the consequence of physical or psychosocial dysfunction. A need for prosthetic training or the infantile dependency of an adult, for example, are not considered to be health needs. They are not shared by everyone and they are the result of trauma, deficit, or stress. These needs would be of concern in the change process.

For the purpose of this text, health needs are described as:

Psychophysical: The need for adequate and attractive food, clothing, and shelter and an optimal amount of sensory stimuli, gross motor activity, and rest. Of concern here are the individual's physical surroundings, i.e., the nonhuman environment. It includes the kind and variety of available food, how it is prepared and served, the opportunity to be well-groomed and dressed, and a place to live that is warm, in both the physical and the psychological sense, and safe. The lack of optimal sensory stimuli is of particular concern if an individual is confined to bed or if the individual lives in an environment that is drab and unchanging. Sufficient gross motor activity is considered necessary for optimal function in all areas. Adequate rest refers to both the need for sleep and the need for solitude. When at least the minimal essentials for meeting psychophysical needs are not available, the individual's attention is almost exclusively focused on seeking satisfaction. Other needs are considered relatively unimportant.

Temporal balance and regularity: The need for an adequate balance between work, play, and rest; a consistent ordering of events; and the opportunity to have some options in how one uses time and orders events in time. This need was discussed quite extensively in Chapter 4 in the section on temporal adaptation.

Safety: The need to interact in an environment that is experienced as relatively free from harmful situations. Such an environment is characterized by (a) general agreement about what is right and wrong, (b) predictable responses from others, (c) knowledge regarding what behavior is expected of each individual, (d) recognition of the individual's right to need satisfaction, (e) lack of arbitrary decision-making, (f) some degree of change as a consequence of the individual's action, (g) a limited number of things the individual cannot understand or influence, (h) security for one's possessions, and (i) freedom from physical harm. This need includes the right to have sufficient information so that the individual can make informed decisions about the type of treatment and intervention in which he or she wishes to engage. Typically people avoid situations that are perceived as unsafe. When most situations are so viewed, the individual tends to restrict interaction. This, in turn, limits the opportunity to gain satisfaction of other needs.

Love and acceptance: The need to be accepted by others as being a unique and very special person. The individual must be accepted for him- or herself rather than for something he or she has accomplished in the past, is doing now, or will do in the future.

Group association: The need for regular interaction with an aggregate of others who share common interests and goals. It is the need to have a sense of kinship with others.

Mastery: The desire to understand and to some extent control oneself, other people, and the nonhuman environment. It is the desire to figure out how things work, to do something skillfully, to test one's abilities, to match wits with another person. When motivated by this need, an individual engages in an activity because it is interesting and challenging.

Esteem: The need to receive recognition from others. It is the need to secure respect for doing, for being productive or creative. Esteem needs can only be satisfied if an individual has an opportunity to do something that is perceived by others as worthwhile. The activities engaged in to satisfy this need are not necessarily pleasurable in and of themselves.

Sexual: The need for recognition of one's sexual nature, for association with both sexes, and for release or sublimation of sexually induced tensions.

Pleasure: The need to engage in activities that the individual perceives as enjoyable in and of themselves. It differs from mastery in that activities that satisfy this need may not be particularly challenging to the individual. They are activities engaged in just for fun.

Self-actualization: The need to be oneself, to do something that is of particular importance to oneself. Activities engaged in to satisfy this need are self-oriented in that recognition or acknowledgment from others is not required for satisfaction. The need for self-actualization differs from the need for mastery in that mastery involves some kind of struggle or contest. In satisfying the need for self-actualization, there may be a struggle but that is not the point of the activity. The poet, for example, may work very hard to write a poem just exactly the way he wants it to be. But that is not why he writes poetry. He writes to satisfy a desire to express his ideas. It is his way of attaining self-actualization.

This is, of course, only one way health needs can be categorized. Other systems may be preferred, depending on one's work setting, theoretical orientation, and world view. A specific way of categorizing health needs is not as important as grasping their nature and differentiating them from needs that arise from trauma, deficit, or stress.

Although the above outline of needs is an elaboration of the work of Marlow, a strict hierarchy is not implied. However, satisfaction of psychophysical safety and love and acceptance needs is considered to be more basic than the other needs. In other words, only after these two needs are fulfilled, at least to some degree, is the individual able to focus attention on the satisfaction of other needs. The importance or priority of the less basic needs will vary depending on the individual. Some people, for example, are more concerned about gratification of sexual needs than are other people.

People meet their needs in a number of different ways. A particular activity may satisfy one need for one person and another need for another person. For example, some people cook because they are hungry (psychophysical need), others cook because they like the praise they receive from family and friends (esteem needs), and still others cook simply because they like to cook (pleasure). It should also be remembered that one activity may satisfy a number of different needs for an individual.

A therapist is concerned about meeting health needs when clients are deficient in occupational performances or performance components to the extent that they are unable to seek need satisfaction independently or to interact effectively in various environments that will provide need satisfaction. This may be a result of a client's deficit or environmental limitations. Many institutions, for example, do not provide environments that are conducive to satisfying health needs or even impede interaction in available satisfying environments. Many communities do not readily provide for the satisfaction of health needs for those who are disabled.

The responsibility of meeting health needs is shared by other members of the health team, clients, and the community. This process neither can nor should be perceived as the responsibility of the occupational therapist alone. However, the occupational therapist must often take a prominent position in creating need-satisfying environments. The therapist's understanding of human growth and development, the need-satisfying potential of purposeful activities, and the importance of meeting health needs facilitate the taking of this leadership role.

In order to clarify the process of meeting health needs, three different levels may be considered. The first level is direct satisfaction of the client's health needs by the therapist. The therapist does this by organizing individual and group activities within the occupational therapy department. Such activities are oriented to satisfying health needs and helping clients locate and make use of need-satisfying environments in the institution or the community. At the second level the therapist works with clients and various members of the health team to create structures and practices within the institution that are conducive to the satisfaction of health needs. At the third level the therapist is involved in working with clients and community members to develop structures and practices in community institutions so that these institutions are responsive to the need satisfaction of the disabled.

These three levels are by no means mutually exclusive. In working with clients to bring about change in various need-inhibiting practices within an institution, for example, interactions may be so structured that clients are also receiving direct gratification of some of their health needs. In helping clients make use of community facilities that provide an opportunity for need satisfaction, the therapist may enhance the potential of such facilities for providing need satisfaction for the disabled. A note regarding the first level: some occupational therapists feel that they have fulfilled their responsibility regarding health needs when they operate only in the confines of the first level. It is unlikely that interaction on this level alone will be sufficient for the satisfaction of clients' health needs.

The process of meeting health needs at the first level, similar to all types of intervention, involves evaluation, goal setting, implementation of a program, continuous reevaluation, and program alteration when appropriate. Initial evaluation is oriented to assessment of the client and to the immediate environment. The major question addressed is what needs, if any, are not being satisfied in the client's present environment? General signs of lack of need satisfaction are restlessness, anxiety, complaining, statements about being bored, and getting into mischief. In an interview with the client, the extent to which the client is experiencing need satisfaction or frustration is discussed. After a brief explanation of health needs, if necessary, each of the needs outlined above is reviewed. Observation and discussion of the client's typical day may provide further information. In addition to age and sex, the therapist is also concerned about the client's cultural background, interests, and general level of function relative to the performance components. This information will facilitate collaborative program planning with the client. The therapist assesses the environment by questioning, "Does this environment appear to offer the type of need satisfaction required by this client?"

With the above information, the therapist and client are in a good position to decide what needs are and are not being met. Before developing a plan, it is useful to ask the client how these needs were met in the past and how he or she thinks these needs could be met under the present circumstances. The therapist may suggest various activities, being as creative and inventive as possible. It is important for the therapist not to let his or her own values interfere with the client's fantasies about various activities or the client's choice. Need satisfaction is by definition a pleasurable experience and it is only the client who can define his or her own pleasure. At times, of course, the therapist must bring some reality into the discussion. The therapist and client then plan a program that will satisfy at least some of the client's health needs. This may involve individual and group activities within the institution or activities in the community. Help in selection and encouragement during initial involvement may be necessary. This is particularly important for the client who perceives little possibility of need satisfaction. As the client gains a higher level of function in the performance components, some alteration in the program may be required. As the client moves toward discharge from the institution, every attempt should be made to help locate situations within the community that are likely to contribute to satisfaction of his or her health needs.

The first step in meeting health needs on the second and third level is assessment of the institution and community environment (home and the wider community) in regard to the extent to which they readily provide for satisfaction of health needs. The process of altering structures and practices in any social system is usually difficult and time-consuming. Planning and implementation of actions to meet health needs on these two levels should be done in conjunction with the involved clients if at all possible.

To alter structures and practices in any social system, the therapist must have knowledge about the formal and informal structures of organizations and group dynamics. The former was discussed in Chapter 4 in the section on work; the latter in Chapter 12. In addition, the therapist must have knowledge of how social change is brought about. The process, frequently referred to as innovation, will only be discussed briefly here.

Bringing about change to the point where it is fully accepted as opposed to a passing alteration in the usual course of events is not an easy task (215,243,381,388, 422,702,867,893,894,1048). The ability to innovate, like any other skill, is learned through practice. Prior to actually engaging in innovative behavior, the therapist must have a sincere belief in the occupational therapy process and a commitment to the profession. The therapist must be convinced of the worth of the services the profession provides and accept the profession as a reference group. The therapist must recognize that being an occupational therapist is more than an 8-hour-a-day job; that it often takes time away from leisure pursuits. To be an innovator the therapist must be knowledgeable, articulate about and skilled in the practice of occupational therapy. Finally, the therapist must be able to establish and maintain a comfortable working relationship with a variety of different types of people and occupational groups. The therapist should be in the habit of being concerned about and meeting the needs of others within the context of both formal and informal organizational structures.

In considering an innovation, the therapist selects a situation that is amenable to change. It is a waste of time to attempt to alter a situation that the therapist is fairly sure is currently unchangeable. It is best to start out small. The capacity to set limited goals is definitely an asset. As the informal structure is often more flexible, change initiated in this area tends to meet with more success. In planning how to alter a situation that is detrimental to meeting health needs, problem-solving techniques are used. These are outlined in Chapter 3 in the discussion of cognitive function.

The situation is studied with the idea of identifying elements that will facilitate change. Some aspects to consider are: the people the therapist should talk with, what one will say to sell the idea, possible objections and how these may be dealt with, what to do after everyone agrees with the general idea, and how the innovation can actually be implemented. The assistance of one's immediate supervisor ought to be sought. It is also very useful to gain help and support from people who have a high status in the organization. In approaching these people, the therapist should be self-assured, able to explain the nature of the innovation, and most important, why the innovation ought to be accepted. The why of the innovation should be described in such a way that it is compatible with the goals of the organization.

In implementation of an innovation, the most appropriate solution is identified and initiated. The therapist must persevere in the face of obstacles. And there are very likely to be obstacles. Initial failure in acceptance of an innovation should not impede further action. It appears that lack of perseverance is the major reason innovations are not fully accepted. The therapist essentially needs to keep faith in the idea that organizational change which will enhance the capacity of others to function effectively is both desirable and possible. Knowledgeable consideration of the problems and well thought out selection of appropriate strategies tend to minimize any anxiety the therapist may have as well as enhance the probability of success.

The above digression was concerned with the process of how to ensure the satisfaction of health needs on the second and third levels. It should, as mentioned, be initiated in conjunction with clients and, where appropriate, other staff members, the client's family, and representative from the community.

The factors or situations that will satisfy a particular health need for a given person are subject to much individual variation. Table 17-1, then, gives only suggestions to prompt the reader's own imagination and creativity.

The suggestions give only some clues of how to meet health needs. That is all that can really be provided in any text. The final important point in understanding the concept of meeting health needs is to differentiate that aspect of intervention from the change process.

When a client and therapist are involved in the change process, they are concerned with bringing about some predetermined, planned alteration in the client's typical repertoire of behavior. In the process of meeting health needs, the client's typical repertoire of behavior *may* change but the nature of the change is not predetermined or planned. The purpose of meeting health needs is to allow the client to be more comfortable, not to alter behavior in any permanent fashion. The change process deals with the consequence of physical or psychosocial pathology or deficits. Meeting health needs involves helping a client to gain satisfaction despite current physical or psychosocial dysfunction. Two examples may help to clarify. Suggesting that a client participate in an instrumental group which does not require independent problem solving is intervention directed toward meeting health needs. Helping a client develop the ability to problem solve independently would be described as the change process. Identifying activities that will allow a client to satisfy esteem needs given his or her present capacities and limitations is part of the process of meeting health needs. Helping a client to acquire additional skills so that he or she may participate in activities that are more highly prized by the client's social system is part of the change process.

Other differences between meeting health needs and the change process are time orientation, degree of immediate pleasure, and the therapist's role. Meeting health needs is oriented to the present, the here and now; it concerns the immediate felt needs of the client. The change process, on the other hand, is oriented to the acquisition of knowledge, skills, and attitudes that will be required for future interaction in the community or in some type of more sheltered environment. During intervention designed to bring about change, current needs may be momentarily ignored. An adolescent girl, for example, might prefer chatting with her friends rather than spending time learning how to shop for and prepare food.

The process of meeting health needs is designed to provide immediate pleasure for the client. The change process may be pleasurable in the sense that the client is aware that it will contribute to his or her future well-being. However, the change process often does not provide immediate pleasure. Participation in altering dysfunction is frequently tedious, time-consuming, painful, and fatiguing.

The difference in the therapist's role in meeting health needs as opposed to the change process is in the degree of demand and overt assistance provided. Two examples may be useful to clarify. A therapist may arrange for a young girl to pursue her solitary hobby of reading as a way of helping her meet her current health needs. At other times, the therapist may insist that the girl participate in an activity group designed to develop group interaction skills. A therapist may give a client considerable help in making a toy box for his grandson but insist that he work toward independence in dressing.

The change process and meeting health needs may occur simultaneously. However, the differences outlined above suggest difficulty in combining the two processes. A clear distinction in time for engaging in the change process and meeting health needs tends to facilitate goal setting, planning, and implementation. Such a distinction often clarifies for both client and therapist the reason for engaging in particular activities.

Meeting health needs is considered to be complementary to the change process. It appears that change on the part of the client is less likely to occur in an environment that does not provide need gratification. If an individual must expend the majority of his energy seeking need satisfaction, there is likely to be little energy or interest available for learning new patterns of behavior.

MAINTENANCE

Maintenance (50,53,283,589,956,1025), as one aspect of intervention, has been previously defined as the process of preserving and supporting an individual's current level of function. Types of maintenance can be subdivided relative to time and focus of concern. In regard to time, maintenance may occur concurrent with the change process or subsequent to the change process. Focus of concern may be performance components or developmental task. Figure 17-1 may be useful in understanding the relationship between these various subtypes of maintenance.

In other words, maintenance may be concerned with performance components and/or developmental tasks regardless of whether it takes place concurrent with the change process or subsequent to it. Although Fig. 17-1

TABLE 17-1. *Suggestions for satisfying health needs*

Psychophysical needs
Remember the importance of ethnic food
Many people like junk food, it is relatively inexpensive, can be delivered, and is likely to be a welcome relief from institutional cooking
There is very little reason why hospitalized clients cannot wear their own clothes
Hospital gowns and clothes do not have to be inherently unattractive and ill-fitting
Within reason, clients should be surrounded by personal objects that have particular meaning to them, e.g., photographs, stuffed animals, some toys, figurines, a quilt
Living quarters can be colorful, interesting, and well kept
A good haircut does wonders for feelings about oneself; a hair stylist should be readily available;
Walking is good exercise, even if inside, although far better out in the fresh air
Active games and sports should be encouraged; a gym is invaluable but even a corridor can be used creatively
Electronic games, television, visits from other patients, and simple craft activities are a good source of stimulation for patients who are bedridden
A quiet place for reading or contemplation is a primary requisite for some people
Temporal balance and regularity
A variety of activities should be available
Remember that treatment, the change process, and maintenance are work
Play and relaxation are a necessary part of the human experience
The pace of daily activities should be designed to accommodate the client's energy level
A regular routine or order to major daily events should be evident
Individual divergence from a regular routine set by others should be accepted and within some limits encouraged
There is no reason for most adults to have to go to bed at any particular time
Safety
The rules and customs of the setting should be explicitly stated
Rules should be kept to a minimum and should be simple, reasonable, and within the capacity of individuals to follow
The physical environment should be known to the client either through a tour or a detailed map with fire exits and routes clearly indicated
People are not afraid of fire drills; inconvenienced, yes, but not afraid
Arbitrary responses from others are a detriment to good mental health
The individual should be told that it is perfectly acceptable to get angry (with some limits on the *expression* of anger), be scared, cry, ask questions, and express affection
Information in regard to the nature of the individual's illness or disability, diet, medication, medical procedures, expected course of events, and so forth should be provided directly. Waiting for the client to ask is a way that the team protects itself; it rarely has anything to do with the client's needs
The individual's right to say no and make demands should be explicitly stated and honored
It should be demonstrated to the individual that his or her possessions are secure even if this means a padlock for a personal cabinet or key to the room
Physical safety from being attacked by others, from falling, or from being injured in some other way should be paramount in helping the client to organize his human and nonhuman environment
Love and acceptance
The question always is how can you as a therapist demonstrate love and affection
Treat the client as unique, not a diagnostic category, not an age group, not as a member of a particular culture, but as a singular human being
Give special privileges, bend the rules
Touch with care
Be prompt for appointments and always attentive
Share your self, your ideas and feelings, something about yourself
Give gifts such as a joke, poem, piece of news or gossip, the plot of the current book you are reading
Find environments where the client will be accepted for him- or herself, or help to create such an environment
Group association
Arranging situations so that people who have interests and ideas in common can get together
Include all clients in group interactions even if they are unable to get out of bed
Create a place where people can get together for conversation and shared activities
Initiate interaction through introducing activities that can be shared
Encourage group participation but only with full awareness of each client's capacity for group interaction
Initially clients may not be interested in group participation; respect this need for more solitary activity or for simply observing
Organizing a party a couple of times a month in and of itself has little if any relationship to satisfying needs for group association
Mastery
Arts and crafts that require manual and cognitive skill
Puzzles, computer games, games of strategy
Activities that require gross motor skill: skate board, swimming, volley ball, badminton, tennis, softball, canoeing, and so forth
Debate, discussion of current events, writing short stories
Puppetry, song writing, performing
Photography (an excellent activity for those confined to bed)
Esteem
Volunteer work in an institution or in the community
Visiting people, calling them on the telephone, or being a pen pal
Display and/or sale of arts and craft objects made by clients
Fixing things, making things to give to others, or providing some kind of service
Earning money
Demonstrating some particular talent for the pleasure of others
Sexual
Remember that sexual needs are essentially unrelated to age and are important throughout the life cycle
Treat the client as a sexual being according to the individual's own definition of appropriate interaction between the sexes
Flirting is on the whole enjoyable and harmless
Provide means whereby the client has an opportunity to interact with both sexes
Masturbation is a healthy need-satisfying activity
Oral and manual sex are also very enjoyable
Provide sexual information
Home visits present opportunities for satisfaction of sexual needs; encourage them on a regular basis
Privacy, for most people, is a prerequisite for satisfaction of sexual needs; arrange this, if possible, whether the individual is at home or in an institution
Pleasure
This is a very idiosyncratic need which is satisfied in a number of different ways
It may be satisfied by reading Shakespeare, watching a horror movie, or gambling
Although the therapist may suggest a variety of activities, it is the client who decides what is pleasurable, not the therapist
Self-actualization
Like pleasure, this need is satisfied in a very individualistic kind of way
Various creative activities are often found to be need satisfying, e.g., gardening, or meditation, or taking care of one's home

Time	Focus	
	Concurrent Performance components	**Concurrent** Developmental tasks
	Subsequent Performance components	**Subsequent** Developmental tasks

FIG. 17-1. The relationship between time and focus of maintenance.

presents performance components and developmental tasks as separate entities, in actuality this is not necessarily the case. Social interaction, for example, is a performance component, but the acquisition of increasingly more sophisticated and differentiated social skills is a developmental task. The distinction is made here primarily for ease in presentation.

The time aspect of maintenance will be discussed first within the context of performance components. Concurrent maintenance is the process of conserving function in one or more areas while attempting to alter dysfunction in other selected areas. Concurrent maintenance may be illustrated relative to intervention with a client who has recently suffered a cerebral vascular accident. An area that may need to be maintained is the individual's accurate self-concept. The change process is likely to be concerned with the enhancement of motor function and visual perception. In evaluation relative to the need for concurrent maintenance, the therapist asks the following question, "Aside from those areas where there is evidence of dysfunction, are there other areas in which it appears that the individual will need assistance in preserving function during the change process?" The key phrase here is "need assistance." There are many individuals who are well able to maintain function independently without any help from the therapist. Thus, using the example just given, some clients will be quite able to maintain an adequate self-concept without assistance; others will not be able to do so.

The need for concurrent maintenance is dependent on several factors. The major ones seem to be the individual's living situation during the period of the change process, the degree of support from family and friends, and the individual's general state of physical and mental health. The way in which the client elects to play the sick role is also an important factor. The more independent stance the individual takes, the more likely he or she is able to maintain function in unaffected areas without the assistance of the therapist.

In the process of maintenance, nothing new is to be attained, nothing is altered, no change is planned. This is what makes this aspect of intervention maintenance and not the change process. Nevertheless, frames of reference are used as the theoretical basis for planning a maintenance program. They are used, however, somewhat differently than they are used in the change process. As a guide for planning maintenance, the therapist first selects a frame of reference that is addressed to the appropriate area of function. Second, the therapist, from the information provided in the frame of reference, attempts to answer two questions: (a) What factors in the environment are important in maintenance of the given area of function? (b) What behavior on the part of the individual is necessary for the maintenance of the given area of function?

Planning a maintenance program based on a frame of reference can be illustrated by continuing with the example relative to self-concept. One important aspect of an adequate self-concept is perceiving the self as being self-directed. This aspect of self-concept is addressed in the frame of reference known as Recapitulation of Ontogenesis (see Chapter 24). The pertinent postulate regarding change is: Self-direction is acquired through practice in being self-directed, communication by significant others that one is capable of being independent and reinforcement of such behavior. The postulate, it should be remembered, is concerned with how to help a client to *become* self-directed. When maintenance is the issue, however, the client has the particular skill in question. Using the example, the client is able to be self-directed, therefore the therapist must extrapolate from the postulate regarding change in order to answer the two questions presented above. The plan for maintenance deduced from this postulate might be as follows:

1. Provide as many alternatives as possible;
2. Allow and encourage the client to make choices;
3. Encourage decision-making and independent behavior;
4. Reinforce all self-directed behavior regardless of what the therapist thinks about the wisdom of a particular choice.

Such a program of intervention will, hopefully, maintain the client's capacity to be self-directed throughout the course of the change process.

Subsequent maintenance is the process of conserving the degree of function that has been attained during the change process. It takes place after termination of the change process. Subsequent maintenance typically occurs in the chronic phase of disability and is initiated in the individual's home or in a sheltered environment of one type or another. The theoretical basis for planning subsequent maintenance is similar to that outlined above for concurrent maintenance. There are, however, some other factors to consider.

It is important to remember that the chronic phase of disability is not a continuous plateau. There are times that the individual may need to reengage in a change process. This should not be confused with maintenance. In other words, because of alterations in the client's age or life circumstances, for example, the client may need direct assistance in gaining increased knowledge, skills, and attitudes. The individual, for example, may need assistance with temporal adaptation or in gaining the capacity to become a worker.

Moreover, there are some chronic conditions that are characterized by periods of remission and exacerbation or by a downward course. In such a situation a maintenance program must be periodically altered relative to the client's current condition. Often very finely tuned adjustments need to be made in order for the recommended program to be effective.

It is occasionally forgotten that many clients with a psychiatric diagnosis have a chronic condition. The capacity to function in the community is often dependent not only on the regular ingestion of appropriate medication but also on adequate support for the maintenance of performance components and developmental tasks. In addition, such individuals often need assistance in organizing their daily life in such a manner that it supports adequate function. A general program of maintenance for individuals with a chronic psychiatric condition should be designed to help the client:

1. Maintain a state of good physical health;
2. Avoid excessive amounts of stress;
3. Arrange for sufficient amounts of work, rest, and relaxation;
4. Identify events or situations that are likely to be difficult;
5. Deal with such events and situations one at a time;
6. Be aware of signs that indicate an exacerbation of one's condition;
7. Become one's own caretaker.

Although the above program of maintenance is probably suitable for individuals with any chronic condition (if not for the general population), it is particularly important for individuals with a chronic psychiatric condition.

Of primary importance in subsequent maintenance is the implementation of the program by the client and continued participation in the program for a long period of time or through the remaining life-span. A high level of success seems to be dependent on several factors (155,935):

1. A well-established trusting relationship with the individual who recommends the plan;
2. Presentation of the plan in such a way that it includes prior discussion with the client; an explanation of why the plan is necessary; clear instructions presented verbally and in writing; definite specifications as to time, amount, degree, and so forth; and an opportunity to learn the various procedures involved under the guidance of the therapist;
3. A plan that does not take too much time, energy, or effort, or cause too much discomfort;
4. A plan that is relatively compatible with the important daily activities of the client and family members;
5. Relatively immediate evidence that the maintenance program is effective concerning its purpose and that the perceived good effects are not outweighed by a negative impact on the client's sense of identity or life-style;
6. A client who is sufficiently lucid to follow the plan and not in such a state of anxiety that he or she needs to deny the seriousness of the condition or the need for a maintenance program;
7. The financial resources of the client are not excessively strained by adherence to the plan;
8. There is regular follow-up by the therapist, including an opportunity for the client to call the therapist by telephone whenever he or she has any questions or concerns.

The above factors, which are believed to contribute to the success of a maintenance program, can be used as a guide by the therapist in designing and presenting a maintenance program. Although all of the above factors are important, follow-up is probably the most significant. Support, reinforcement, and knowing that someone really cares and is concerned are essential in order for anyone to follow a long-term maintenance program.

The above discussion of concurrent and subsequent maintenance was primarily concerned with performance components. The following discussion of maintenance will focus on developmental tasks. What was previously said regarding maintenance in general should be kept in mind as it is also applicable to maintenance relative to developmental tasks.

Developmental tasks, as used here, refer to those skills and patterns of interactions which are required and/or expected in various phases of the life cycle. They include, or perhaps more accurately are best described by, the acquisition and elaboration of occupational performances through the course of life cycle. The major developmental tasks were outlined in Chapter 5. Maintenance relative to developmental tasks involves providing an environment that enables an individual to preserve those developmental tasks that have been mastered, to consolidate those developmental tasks that the individual is currently involved in mastering, and to prepare for those developmental tasks that need to be mastered in the immediate future. The theoretical base for planning a program of maintenance relative to developmental tasks is derived from the therapist's knowledge of human growth and development. A summary of such a knowledge base is outlined in Chapter 5. The question the therapist uses as a guide is "What are the environmental factors necessary for the maintenance of a particular individual's current life tasks?"

The idea of maintenance relative to developmental tasks may be clarified by differentiation from meeting health needs and the change process. Maintenance relative to developmental tasks is somewhat like meeting health needs in that it allows individuals to function at their optimal level while engaging in the change process. Both processes are essentially need-satisfying. The difference is that maintenance relative to developmental tasks is age-specific. Most adolescents, for example, are very concerned with perceiving themselves as being like their peers. One way that the mutual sense of identity is consolidated is through a common liking for certain types of music and clothes. Thus, the therapist might attempt to maintain an adolescent's sense of common identity by providing appropriate music and by encouraging the wearing of some articles of clothing that are currently in fashion. The music on the adolescent ward for orthopedic patients may be somewhat disconcerting to an adult visitor and the costumes a bit bizarre, but such an atmosphere is good evidence that attention is being given to the developmental tasks of these adolescents.

The distinction between the change process and maintenance relative to developmental tasks is somewhat more pronounced. A therapist is involved in the change process when interactions with a client are directed toward enhancing the learning of skills that are usually acquired prior to the client's current chronological age. The goal of the change process is essentially remedial in nature. A therapist is involved in maintenance relative to developmental tasks when he or she assists in providing an environment that is conducive to the preservation, consolidation, and preparation for developmental tasks that are typical for the individual's chronological age. For example, helping a 9-year-old child learn how to engage in parallel play is the change process, whereas organizing a play group for pre-kindergarten hospitalized children is maintenance.

A similar distinction can be made concerning subsequent maintenance. Intervention is directed toward the change process when a client is, for whatever reason, unable to master developmental tasks even when the optimal environment for such development is readily available. Intervention is directed toward maintenance when the therapist assists the client in finding a typical environment for mastery of an emerging developmental task. Aside from this, the client needs no other assistance in continuing with developmental tasks.

Although the maintenance of all developmental tasks is important, the one area sometimes forgotten is in relationship to familial roles (405,982). It is important that the therapist assist clients in preserving their familial roles both while hospitalized and after discharge. Preservation is far more likely to be successful if it begins immediately after dysfunction occurs rather than waiting until the client "feels better." It is very easy for the client and family members to alter interactions so that the client is allowed only to play the sick role. Transferring from the sick role back into family roles can be difficult, particularly when the client's condition becomes chronic in nature. The therapist, thus, should encourage the client to participate actively in the ongoing affairs of the family, performing what tasks and interpersonal elements of his or her roles are possible. If the client is hospitalized, beyond regular visits by family members, the client should be encouraged to have frequent contact with family members by telephone.

One final remark about maintenance. This aspect of intervention has for many years been viewed, at best, as the least desirable type of intervention. It is often seen as too simple, unexciting, and lacking any challenge. It is certainly seen as less prestigious than prevention or the change process. This is an unfortunate state of affairs because maintenance, particularly subsequent maintenance, contributes a great deal to the well-being of clients. Good programs of maintenance retard regression and allow those who are chronically disabled to be active participants in the community of others.

MANAGEMENT

Management (74,290,956,981), as previously defined, is the process of minimizing undesirable or disruptive behavior so that the therapist and client can deal more directly and effectively with areas of dysfunction. Undesirable or disruptive behavior may be behavior that is indicative of dysfunction. As such, it is not of direct concern in the change process. The change process is addressed to the dysfunction per se, however that may be defined. It is not addressed to the manifestation of dysfunction. In some frames of reference, for example, minimal attention to personal hygiene and grooming is considered indicative of perception of the self as an unacceptable human being. The change process based on such a frame of reference would be directed toward developing a better sense of self-worth. The client's hygiene and grooming would not be of concern because of the expectation that this area would improve as soon as the individual developed a greater sense of self-worth. If, however, the client's hygiene was so poor that it was detrimental to his or her general health or excessively offensive to others, this would be dealt with through management. Management is only concerned with minimizing or controlling undesirable or disruptive behavior. If the change process is successful, such behavior will gradually disappear as the individual acquires more functional skills in dealing with himself and the environment.

Undesirable and disruptive behavior may not be related to any particular area of dysfunction but rather be more general in nature. Recognizing dysfunction, electing to engage in a change process, or perhaps being in a strange environment is likely to cause anxiety, which may be manifested in a variety of ways. For example, an 18-year-old girl who has recently become paraplegic may exhibit a facade of indifference to her severe disability and take a sexually provocative stance, both of these behavioral patterns being unrelated to her real feelings and detrimental to engaging in the change process. A 5-year-old child in a state of acute panic is unable to participate in any kind of formal evaluation. The therapist then must be concerned with these behaviors that arise out of anxiety. In dealing with such behaviors, the therapist not only decreases anxiety but also increases the individual's capacity to participate in the change process.

Perhaps of gravest concern in the area of management is the client who is potentially suicidal. Following are some guidelines the therapist may use to plan interaction with a suicidal client (504):

1. The belief that a person who talks about suicide will not actually take his own life is a myth;
2. Take the client's ideas about committing suicide seriously;
3. Do not issue a provocation to suicide by, for example, telling the client that he would never do such a thing;
4. Go easy in making any value judgment;
5. Do not get carried away by the "good reasons" a person has for suicide;
6. Know what resources are available in the institution or community;
7. Know your own attitude toward life, death, and suicide;
8. Listen. This allows the client to discharge at least some of the tensions that have brought him to the point of self-destruction. The opportunity to talk with another person will help the client sort out other possibilities for himself. This is a time for just listening; interpretation, in-depth questioning, and advice-giving are not appropriate;
9. For a depressed individual, one of the most crucial times is when his mood begins to elevate. The client feels better and is able to think more clearly. It is at this point that the individual, seemingly out of the horror that he has just experienced, becomes even more bent on suicide in order never to have to experience that type of mental torture again;
10. Although ordinary precautions should be taken, people who seriously want to commit suicide will do so.

When a client is successful in ending his or her life, it is natural for the therapist to experience anger, guilt, and sorrow. These feelings should not be hidden or considered aberrant. Rather, they should be experienced openly and discussed with others. Through successfully dealing with one's own feelings, the therapist is in a far better position to help other clients who are potentially suicidal.

Management of other undesirable and disruptive behavior, although not necessarily life-threatening, is nevertheless a task that takes some thought and planning. There are a considerable number of behaviors that need to be managed. Not all of them can be discussed here. Thus, the following is presented as more of an introduction to the subject rather than an in-depth study.

One of the primary principles used as the basis for managing undesirable and disruptive behavior is derived from the learning theory of operant conditioning. This principle, which has to do with the effect of reinforcement, was described in Chapter 9. Briefly, behavior that is not reinforced tends to drop out of a person's repertoire of usual behavior. Combined with differential reinforcement, this has been found to be an effective way of managing behavior. Differential reinforcement is the process of giving reinforcement for one kind of behavior and not giving reinforcement for another type of behavior. When used in management, differential reinforcement involves not reinforcing undesirable or disruptive behavior through attention or some other kind of need satisfaction. While doing this, the therapist reinforces behavior that is necessary for active involvement in the other aspects of intervention. It should be remembered that use of reinforcement in management is not designed to develop a new repertoire of behavior on the part of the client; that is the change process. Reinforcement in management is designed to temporarily control behavior until the client is able to deal more effectively with the demands of the environment.

The following are some additional suggestions regarding the management of more specific kinds of deviant behavior. These suggestions are based on a theory regarding how people typically respond to various types of activities and on the past experience of many therapists as to what seems to be effective in the management of some behavior.

Confusion. Massive amounts of structure seem to be most effective. This includes the general environment as well as specific activities. The client's daily routine should be well organized with little free time. The client should be required to make few if any decisions. Reassuring devices such as giving the client a schedule of daily activities and a floor map of the treatment facility are sometimes useful. General reassurance is also important.

Anxiety. Because anxiety may arise from a number of sources, there are a variety of ways of managing this disruptive response. One or a combination of the suggested methods may be effective with a particular client. Sincere reassurance is almost always effective. Some clients respond best to an undemanding environment where a wide latitude of behavior is permitted. Other clients are more comfortable in a structured environment where there is little time to think and few decisions to be made. One of the major antidotes for anxiety is purposeful activity. It distracts, has an organizing effect, and demonstrates to the individual that he or she can accomplish something even while in a state of anxiety. The therapist thus encourages participation in any activity in which the client shows the least bit of interest. At times the therapist must be somewhat directive in order to get the client to initially become involved in the doing process.

Hostile and/or critical behavior. The best course of action seems to be dealing with the client's behavior in a matter-of-fact way, in a commonplace or prosaic manner. It is important to try not to provoke anger, not to argue or show anger toward the client, regardless of one's own feelings.

Infantile or childish behavior. It is often wise to accept some of this behavior. In the face of considerable stress, temporary regression is not uncommon and, indeed, is probably healthy. There are many people who believe that temporary regression ultimately leads to more adaptive responses. While giving some support to regressive behavior, it is often also necessary to indicate fairly strongly that more "adult" or mature behavior will be expected in the near future.

Suspiciousness. Be as open as possible and explain everything in a simple and straightforward manner. Answer all questions in great detail, and be comfortable with that. It is not, however, useful to repeat explanations when it is quite evident that the client already understands. Do not be taken into the client's web of suspiciousness and begin to be as distrustful of events and people surrounding the client as the client is.

Denial. The best course of action seems to be to work around the client's denial. If the client is not yet ready to deal with major issues or difficulties start with something minor. Focus on something the client wants to do, learn, or accomplish. Direct confrontation is rarely useful and could be harmful to the client's capacity to deal with the present situation.

Intellectualization. Any kind of lengthy discussion about the client's difficulties should be avoided. Get to the point of doing, not talking, as soon as possible. Initially, participate with the client in an activity. For a client who uses intellectualization as a way of avoiding involvement in any kind of active doing, management is concerned with getting the client to engage in purposeful activities. The issues that surround the client's fear of doing are dealt with in the change process.

Withdrawal, depression, hypoactivity, or motor retardation. Hypoactivity or motor retardation may be the consequence of medication. If this is the case, avoid suggesting strenuous activity and provide for regular rest periods. When the behavior of concern here is a direct manifestation of dysfunction it is important to be with the client, to sit with him, making few demands. Very slowly engage the client in some kind of activity. Initial activities should be very simple such as walking down the corridor, watching television together, or the therapist playing solitaire and inviting the client to watch and advise. Avoid any demand for lengthy conversation. Gentle humor may be useful.

Aggressive, unreasonable behavior. The therapist should define limits relative to what will and will not be permitted. The purpose for the limits should be clearly stated. Keep limits consistent, clear, and reasonable. Restate and enforce limits as often as necessary. Inconsistent reinforcement of limits is confusing to the client and may result in aggressive behavior simply to test the therapist's capacity to enforce them, and the therapist's patience.

Difficulty in controlling behavior. Planned ignoring of deviant behavior is sometimes useful. On the other hand, extra attention and affection when the client appears to be losing control are frequently effective in assisting the individual to monitor his own behavior. Extra help in a situation that is likely to be difficult is also useful. In a group situation the therapist may appeal to the client's sense of fairness and responsibility to the group; or, after a reasonable warning, the client may be removed from the group. A change in the client's current activity or restructuring the activity may be useful, as is tension release through gross motor activity. The therapist may openly state the problem of lack of control and ask the client how he thinks this problem can be solved. Behavior often becomes more reasonable when the client is allowed greater participation in decision-making. This can be facilitated by listening to the client and providing feedback relative to the client's reality testing. Finally, physical contact often reassures the client that he can control his own behavior.

The above suggestions regarding management should be taken as just that—recommendations only. They are not meant to be recipes. What will work for one therapist may not work for another; what will work for one client may not work for another. A plan for effective management may only be determined after an initial period of trial and error. This is a very pragmatic aspect of intervention.

In conclusion, there is considerable variation in the amount of deviant behavior that therapists are able to tolerate. Some therapists do not seem the least bit bothered by considerable deviancy whereas others find this difficult or almost impossible to countenance. A therapist who has difficulty tolerating excessive deviancy should not consider him- or herself to be too rigid, controlling, or unsympathetic. There is, within some limits, no reason why the therapist should be fearful of stating expectations for client behavior. If a particular behavior is bothersome to the therapist, he or she has a right to demand different, more socially acceptable behavior. It is important to remember that a therapist cannot be effective if uncomfortable in the intervention process.

GOAL SETTING AND IMPLEMENTATION

The first part of this chapter described four aspects of intervention in some detail. It is now time to return to a discussion of the sequence of events relative to evaluation and intervention outlined in the introduction to Part 5 (290,705,956,960). The sequence was discussed in Chapter 15 through the point of problem identification. This section will continue the discussion of the sequence up to the point of termination. It will be divided into four parts: setting goals and priorities, formulating a plan for intervention, implementation, and cultural differences.

Setting Goals and Priorities

Problem identification, as mentioned, is a statement of the client's limitations in all areas; possible areas of potential deficit (prevention); health needs that are not being met; areas that require maintenance; behavior that needs to be managed; and limitations relative to performance components and/or occupational performances. Problem areas, however, are not necessarily the goals of intervention (629,661,705,960). For any number of reasons, all problem areas may not be addressed in intervention.

In general, a goal is a conscious end result toward which behavior is directed. In the occupational therapy process, goals are usually identified as long-term and short-term. Long-term goals specify the end result of intervention, i.e., the expected level of functioning the client will achieve by the time of termination of intervention. They are frequently stated in relationship to occupational performances.

Short-term goals are sub-goals or the building blocks that ultimately lead to one or more of the long-term goals. In setting short-term goals the sequence and priorities of intervention are established. Sequencing refers to what will be done first, second, and so forth. Sequencing implies priorities or what is the most important at any particular time in the intervention process. Typically, prevention and meeting health needs receive first priority, concurrent maintenance and management are second, the change process is third, and subsequent maintenance fourth or the last priority.

Goals are set relative to only those aspects of intervention which are to be of concern. In other words, when there is no need for management, for example, no goals are set relative to this aspect. Each area of concern may have a number of goals. Several health needs, for example, may need to be met; the change process may be concerned with sensory integration and social interaction. Thus many short-term goals may be dealt with at the same time.

The designation of short-term and long-term goals is traditional in occupational therapy. It was derived from viewing the change process as a sequence of events which leads to a specified end point. Such a designation may or may not be appropriate for all aspects of intervention. Rather than thinking in terms of long- and short-term goals, it may, at times, be more accurate to think of serial or singular goals. A serial goal is one in which discernible sub-goals are easily identified, e.g., long- and short-term goals. A singular goal is one in which sub-goals are nonexistent or not easily identified. In prevention, for example, serial goals would be appropriate for describing the steps whereby adolescent mothers are helped to learn about child care and the parenting process. In describing crisis intervention another aspect of prevention, the concept of a singular goal, may be more useful. A statement of a singular goal would also seem more appropriate when specifying the objectives of meeting health needs, maintenance (both types), and management.

Regardless of whether one is formulating serial or singular goals, they should be stated in the most specific or concrete manner that is possible. Ideally, they are stated in behavioral terms—a specification of what the client is going to be able to do or what he is not going to do any longer. An example of a poorly stated goal relative to the change process would be "improved self-concept." If deficit in this area was identified, in part, by the client's sloppy appearance and subservient manner, a more appropriate statement of the goal would be that the client wear clothes appropriate for his weight and height and compatible with the norms of his cultural group and the absence of subservient behavior in interaction with others. Concrete goals stated in behavioral terms help the client and therapist to determine whether or not the goal has been attained. Goals stated in a vague manner are very difficult to assess.

Finally, short-term goals should be limited both in terms of number and, relative to the change process, in terms of the amount of change expected. A limited number of goals helps to focus the intervention process. If there are too many goals, both client and therapist may become confused and lose sight of the objectives of intervention. The amount of change expected is limited so that neither the client nor therapist becomes discouraged. If short-term goals are too ambitious it is quite possible that the client will become unmotivated and/or feel he or she is not making adequate progress. It is far better to set a series of short-term goals that can easily be attained in a short period of time.

There are several factors that are taken into consideration in setting goals:

1. The client: Goals are set in collaboration with the client. Ideally the client and therapist sit down together and decide what the goals of intervention will be. This is done by reviewing the information gained in the initial evaluation. Areas of difficulty are identified and priorities are set. Goals are written and become part of the client's file. There are, however, times when this ideal course of events does not come to pass.

During discussion of the goals, the client and therapist may have the same goal in mind but use different words to define that goal. Such difficulties in communication can be corrected through discussion and through careful attention to the meaning of the client's words.

When, however, it is evident that the client's ideas about goals are disparate from those of the therapist, certain steps may be taken to minimize the differences. The first thing the therapist might do, after eliciting the individual's ideas about the condition, is to explain his or her own views in a manner understandable to the individual. Discrepancies in points of view are likely to become apparent and should be discussed openly. One way of dealing with discrepancies is essentially to educate the individual with the intention of changing some ideas. This tends to be a relatively long-term process, so immediate results should not be expected. It may or may not be successful. On the other hand the therapist may attempt to work within the client's orientation. In this case goals are formulated that are considered to be reasonable by the therapist and which do not violate or at least respect the individual's conceptual system. Another method that might be used is to negotiate a compromise. The client and therapist agree to a group of goals that accommodates each of their views of the situation to some degree but does not require either one to accept the other's ideas of the situation.

The goals selected must be meaningful to the client. If they are not, it is unlikely that the client will actively engage in intervention. In such a case everyone is wasting his time. As intervention progresses, the client may be more willing to look at other problem areas and to set more realistic goals.

Occasionally a client is not able to enter into discussion regarding goals. This, for example, may be the case with a client who is profoundly mentally retarded, depressed, psychotic, or confused. In this situation the therapist formulates a few short-term goals and begins intervention. The client is told what the immediate goals are even if it does not appear that the client will understand them. Goal setting is discussed later with the client when, hopefully, he or she is more able to enter into such a discussion.

2. The team: Goals are formulated in collaboration with those fellow staff members who are to be involved in assisting the client. Through discussion between staff members and the client, general common goals for the client are agreed on. Each member of the team is then able to formulate more clearly specific goals with the client. Sharing in this manner ensures that the staff goals are in harmony with and complementary to each other. This is important because incompatible goals will lead

to confusion on the part of the staff and the client and inhibit the client's movement toward a more adequate state of function.

3. Knowledge about the disease process or deficit and the client's prognosis: Such information allows the therapist to formulate goals that are realistic in light of the client's condition.

4. The client's expected environment: This factor was discussed in some detail in Chapter 15 in the section on the sequence and process of evaluation.

5. Realistic external constraints: In formulating goals there must be a realistic possibility for implementing a plan to achieve the objectives. The setting of impractical or idealistic goals is bound to lead to disappointment on the part of both client and therapist. Some of the external constraints to be taken into consideration are the client's financial resources; the customs and policies of the institution concerning the length of time each week the therapist may be involved in intervention with one client and the length of time the client is expected to stay in the institution; the setting in which intervention will take place, including space, facilities, equipment, and materials; and the resources that are available in the immediate community.

It is within the context of evaluative findings, both assets and limitations, and the factors outlined above that goals for intervention are formulated. The next step in the occupational therapy process is to formulate a plan designed to meet the specified goals.

The Plan for Intervention

A plan for intervention (287,705,956,960) is a written statement of what the client and therapist intend to do to attain the goals that have been set. It describes the activities that will be used, the nature of the therapist's interaction with the client, the setting(s) in which intervention will take place, and if applicable, the type of activity group(s) that will be used. The plan includes each area of intervention that will be addressed, not just the change process. It is stated specifically in reference to each immediate short-term and singular goal with a more general statement about how each of the subsequent short-term goals and thus the long-term goals will be attained. The latter is stated in a more detailed manner prior to the initiation of intervention relative to a new short-term goal.

A plan for intervention is developed in collaboration with the client. However, collaboration in this instance is of a somewhat different nature than in the case of formulating goals. The process is less mutual in that the therapist here is definitely the expert. Clients, with some assistance, usually are quite capable of formulating goals that are meaningful to them. If the client knew how to reach those goals, there would probably be very little need for intervention. The therapist as the expert has the responsibility of developing a plan whereby the client is enabled to reach the desired goals. This is not to say that the client is not involved in developing a plan for intervention. The plan is discussed with the client. The client is helped to see the relationship between the goals he or she helped set and the activities and interpersonal relationships he or she and the therapist will be engaged in to reach these goals. The various groups that the client may participate in are described and the role in each group is outlined. The client may suggest changes in the plan, and these changes are made if at all possible.

There are several factors to be taken into consideration in developing a plan for intervention.

Selecting Suitable Activities

Selecting suitable activities involves the analysis and synthesis of activities. Essentially, the therapist identified those elements believed to be responsible for the implementation of the stated goals. These elements are drawn from the information provided in the first part of this chapter, the therapist's knowledge of human growth and development, and the postulates regarding change of pertinent frames of reference. Activities are analyzed to determine if and the extent to which these elements are present. Activities are synthesized or in some cases merely selected so that all the necessary elements are present in the intervention situation. In synthesizing an activity the therapist is careful to maintain the integrity of the activity. In other words, the essential nature of the activity remains intact. An example of an activity that has lost its integrity is a client sanding the wood for a bird house and the therapist doing all other parts of the activity. An activity may be synthesized in such a manner that it is suitable for achieving more than one goal; in fact, this is recommended. However, more than one activity is often necessary in order that all the appropriate elements are present in the intervention situation.

The Therapist's Behavior

The therapist's behavior should be clearly specified. This area is sometimes overlooked in formulating a plan for intervention. The therapist's behavior relative to management is of particular importance but it is also important in the other aspects of intervention. Postulates regarding change frequently provide guidelines for the therapist's behavior. Chapter 8 also provides some principles relative to the therapist's interactions with clients.

The Client

Activities should be selected so that they are congruent with the client's current level of function relative to all performance components. This principle should be operant in all aspects of intervention except the change process. In the attempt to improve function, an activity may be synthesized so that one element of the activity is somewhat beyond the client's typical repertoire of behavior relative to a given performance component. This is what makes the activity effective as a means of change. The other elements of the activity should be compatible with the client's current level of function. This allows the client to make use of his or her assets in other areas to enhance function in an area of deficit. An example of synthesizing an activity in this manner is in the development of skill at the project level of group interaction. The various activities used in such a group are selected to be well within group members' present capacity, thus allowing them to give their attention to learning how to function in a group.

The client's age, sex, cultural background, and interests are also taken into consideration when developing a plan for intervention. This compatibility is very important, for without it the client may well reject the plan and refuse to participate in intervention. Obviously this is not a desirable situation. With some creativity on the part of the therapist and the therapist giving close attention, particularly to the interests of the client, compatible activities can almost always be synthesized.

Some clients have particular problems such as perceptual, sensory, or motor deficits that must be taken into consideration in developing a plan for intervention. This may require some adaptations of activities. In making such alterations the therapist must keep in mind two points: (a) the integrity of the activity as defined above and (b) the maintenance of the essential elements of the activity. The latter refers to making quite sure that in the process of adaptation those elements considered necessary for successful intervention are not lost. For example, the satisfaction of esteem needs is unlikely to occur if the client requires considerable assistance in watering the plants in the lounge area. The client knows he has not accomplished the task independently. If adaptation is such that the essential elements of an activity are compromised, it is far better to select a different activity.

The plan for intervention should be designed so that there is a high probability of success. The vast majority of individuals who have psychosocial problems do not need to experience failure. For many it is the last thing in the world that they need. At times, particularly in the initial stages of intervention, activities are synthesized so that success is assured. Later, in the intervention process when it is necessary for the client to deal realistically with identifying his or her assets and limitations and the issue of success and failure, activities are synthesized to facilitate learning in these areas.

Finally, the meaning of the activities to the client must be taken into consideration. As discussed in Chapter 9, any activity has a symbolic potential whether it be universal, cultural, or idiosyncratic. A client's response to an activity may be negative or positive, depending on the meaning the individual assigns to the activity. In the process of discussing the plan for intervention with the client, the therapist should attempt to assess the meaning of the suggested activities to the client. An immediate negative or positive response is important to note but beyond that it may be important to understand the why of such a response. This is particularly true in relationship to the change process when an analytical frame of reference is used. Regardless of the why, in the initial phase of intervention the client's negative reaction to a particular activity should be respected. Another, more acceptable activity is arrived at through discussion with the client.

It is essential to remember that planning intervention is often characterized by negotiation and compromise on the part of the therapist and the client. A therapist who has mastered these two skills is in an excellent position to gain the cooperation of clients.

In conclusion, the overall plan for intervention should be suitable for facilitating progress toward meeting the stated goals; it should be clearly related to the objectives. The plan should be realistic, taking into consideration the limitations of time, space, and availability of staff.

With completion of an adequate plan for intervention, the client and therapist are ready to proceed with the task ahead.

Implementation

The process of implementation can be divided into three parts: orientation, productive, and termination. In the orientation phase the therapist reviews the goals and the plan for intervention with the client and describes in detail the way that the program will be carried out. If all or part of intervention is to include the involvement in a group, the client is introduced to the other group members and given some time to adjust to the group before specific demands are made. The reader is referred to Chapter 13 for a detailed discussion of this process. The client is also introduced to other staff members, such as the supervisor of a work group, if they will be participating in the intervention process. The orientation phase is the first test of the plan for intervention. Through observation, the therapist assesses whether the activities outlined in the plan are too easy or too hard. The client should just be able to do the activity with some facility, but nevertheless find it challenging. When this is not the case, appropriate adjustments are made in the plan and the activity. If the client is not participating in the plan—not attending assigned groups, for example, or being physically present but not engaging in activities—the therapist investigates the situation. An attempt is made to identify the reasons for nonparticipation. The client's comments about reasons for noninvolvement are listened to with great care. Disregarding this information frequently interferes with movement into the productive phase. When necessary, the plan for intervention is altered so as to be more compatible with the client's wishes. Often, however, the client simply needs additional encouragement. This is particularly true in the orientation phase, when the client is entering a new situation and is being asked to learn things that are very difficult for him or her to do.

The productive phase begins when any necessary initial adjustments are made in the plan and the client settles down to the work of intervention. The therapist should always be aware of the possibility of fatigue and provide adequate rest periods if necessary. Active participation in intervention requires considerable energy on the part of the client. What seems like a fairly simple activity to the therapist may be quite tiring for the client. The therapist also monitors the client's use of tools and other equipment. The client's safety should always be of paramount concern. The therapist, therefore, makes sure that the client is using tools correctly and that they are put in a safe place when not in use. The integrity of the plan for intervention is carefully maintained until the first reevaluation or until such time that there is evidence of a need for change. The therapist observes the intervention process to ensure that the interaction is compatible with the plan and, in particular, the frame of reference(s) being used. Reevaluation takes place periodically during the productive phase as outlined in Chapter 15. At that time it may be found that the client is able to move on to more advanced short-term goals. The plan for intervention is then expanded to include a specific outline of how these goals are to be achieved. Other adjustments in the plan relative to singular goals may also need to be made at this time.

Throughout the intervention process there should be a sense that the client and therapist are participating in a mutual interaction. They are partners in a joint venture—their roles are different but their responsibility is mutual. It is helpful if the therapist always remembers the individual's inherent capacity to judge what is harmful or beneficial to the self. This capacity may be stunted by dysfunction but it remains viable in most people. Thus, attention should be given to the client's expressed opinion regarding the progress of the intervention process, for the information the client provides is tremendously important. Disregarding this information all too often is responsible for lack of movement toward function.

In the productive phase, particularly if it is lengthy, the client may periodically lose interest or become less willing to work at the task of intervention. It is often a tedious task, time-consuming, not always rewarding, and may indeed be painful. Thus, the therapist must maintain the client's interest and investment in the process. This may be accomplished through setting reasonable short-term goals, an occasional one or two days off, ample opportunity for recreation and being with family and friends, and a lot of encouragement. It is also vital that the therapist maintain his or her own consistent interest and involvement in the intervention process and the client's progress.

The final part of intervention, the termination phase, signals the ending of the intervention process. Because of the many factors involved, this phase will be discussed in some detail in the next chapter.

As a part of most intervention processes, the therapist is concerned with instructing individual clients or groups of clients in how to do a specific activity. The way this is accomplished and the extent to which it is appropriate will depend on the nature of the client's dysfunction, the frame of reference being used, and the plan for intervention as a whole. Nevertheless, it is important that the therapist have some knowledge of the process of teaching an activity. The occupational therapist must know how to teach an activity so that the client understands clearly how the activity should be done or the various ways that it can be done. Good instructions minimize the time needed for correcting mistakes and for direct supervision of the client. Good instruction also enhances the possibility of successfully completing the activity.

The guidelines for instruction are derived from the Principles of Learning outlined in Chapter 9 and from the methods of instruction suggested by Hopkins (444). They, however, are more specific and addressed only to the teaching of an activity. The Principles of Learning are more general and apply to the acquisition of many types of behavior and not simply to how to do an activity. There are five steps involved in instruction: preparation for instruction, preparation of the client, presentation of the activity, try-out performance, and follow-up.

Step 1. Preparation for instruction

a. The activity is analyzed to identify the component parts and the significant steps. This process was discussed in Chapter 11 in some detail;
b. Consideration should be given to how much of the activity can be taught at one time, given the nature of the activity and the functional level of the client;
c. The proper tools, necessary materials and equipment should be ready for use;
d. The work area should be arranged so that it is free of unnecessary objects, safe, and comfortable.

Step 2. Preparation of the client

a. Establish some degree of rapport with the client if this has not already been accomplished, allay any evident fears, and encourage participation;
b. Determine how much the client knows about the activity so that instruction may be given at an appropriate level;
c. Be sure the individual understands the purpose for learning the activity;
d. Ask the client to take or assist him or her in taking a comfortable and correct position for performance of the activity.

Step 3. Presentation of the activity

a. Give verbal directions as well as demonstration of the process. Written and pictorial directions may be useful, depending on the nature of the activity and the learning ability and preference of the client. Providing an example of the finished product or of steps in the process is also sometimes useful;
b. When demonstrating, work at the side of the client so that the process can be easily seen. Demonstrating while opposite the client may be confusing;
c. For individuals with deficits in the area of cognitive function, the activity may need to be simplified. Directions should be given one step at a time in a clear, concise, consistent, and concrete manner;
d. Present instructions slowly and periodically ask if there are any questions;
e. Teach the process step by step, stressing key points and areas where common errors are made;
f. Teach no more than can be mastered at one time.

Step 4. Try-out performance

a. Ask the client to perform the activity step by step with the therapist or immediately after the activity has been demonstrated;
b. Anticipate errors or, if necessary, correct them as they occur;
c. If appropriate, have the client repeat the activity several times so that the client is sure he or she can perform it correctly.

Step 5. Follow-up

a. Allow the client to work independent of the therapist if that is compatible with the plan for change. The therapist should not hover over the client;
b. Tell the client whom to ask for help if difficulties arise;
c. Check progress at appropriate intervals to identify any problems and to give encouragement. Less frequent follow-up is necessary as the client's competence and confidence increase.

As mentioned, the above outline is provided as a guide only. Modifications may be required to meet the specific needs of particular clients. In addition, the way in which instructions are given must be compatible with the plan for intervention.

The previous discussion concerning implementation assumed the therapist's direct involvement with the client. However, this may not always be the situation. Depending on the setting and the plan for intervention, other therapists or staff members may assume the major daily responsibility for carrying out the plan or the plan may be carried out by personnel in another community agency. In the former situation, the therapist who collaborated with the client in evaluation, goal setting, and developing a plan for intervention may now assume the role of supervisor of the therapist responsible for implementation of the plan. Thus, the therapist's relationship with the client is indirect. It is, however, often appropriate for the therapist to periodically stop by, say hello to the client, and inquire after his or her general well-being and progress. In the situation where intervention takes place in another community agency, a grammar school, for example, the therapist may act as a consultant. This consulting relationship may be established with the agency, the client, or one or more family members. In many situations the use of resources away from the primary treatment center is recommended for at least part of the intervention process. Such a course of action facilitates the client's reinvolvement in being a participating member of the community.

Formulating goals and developing a plan for intervention and implementation may seem rather complex and time-consuming to the neophyte therapist. It is that. But with some practice, the process becomes relatively easy and simple in most instances. It just takes some experience and good supervision.

Cultural Differences

There are several issues that may be encountered in the intervention process which are related to differences in cultural background of the client and therapist (395,672,940). Language is one area where difficulties may arise. A therapist who regularly interacts with members of an ethnic group who speak a language different from that of the therapist should attempt to gain a working knowledge of that language with emphasis on words and phrases that are commonly used in the intervention process. Bilingual cards with simple requests and information are sometimes a useful device for communication at those times when a translator is not immediately available. Relatively free visiting with relatives and friends is often arranged for clients who do not speak the common language of the facility.

Interactional norms vary from one culture to another. A young therapist may have some difficulty gaining respect and trust from an individual who comes from a culture where knowledge and wisdom are equated with age. Also, such an individual, if elderly, may expect to be shown considerable deference and what the therapist may feel is an unusual amount of consideration. The client may have rather high standards of modesty, particularly relative to cross-gender interactions. These feelings should be respected by the therapist. The therapist's ethnic background, social class, gender, or professional occupation may make the client reticent to talk openly. This can usually be overcome by encouragement, listening intently, and not hurrying. Clients vary relative to the degree of personalness which they consider appropriate in interacting with a therapist. They may want a quite formal relationship or on the other hand prefer that it be much more casual and friendly. Degree of personalness is also related to the client's preference for being addressed by his first or last name and the extent to which the client accepts "touching" as one way of communicating. Some clients respond well to a directive approach whereas others are comfortable with a more equalitarian approach. Some clients are very uncomfortable when there are disagreements with the therapist. Other clients do not mind differences of opinion, and, in fact, might even enjoy such encounters.

In many cultures the family plays a very important role. Thus the degree to which the client is free to decide on a course of interaction independent of family may depend on ethnic group membership. The most influential member of the family varies from one ethnic group to another. There are also differences regarding with whom the therapist is expected to discuss health issues and problems. Some ethnic groups believe that the family should be with an ill or disabled member at all times. Visiting, the physical care of the client, preparing special foods, and so forth are seen as the proper role of the family. Most cultures have various rituals surrounding terminal illness and death. These, of course, are respected under almost all circumstances and are treated with deference and thoughtful consideration.

Although the above suggestions are outlined relative to cultural variations, many are applicable to interaction with all clients, regardless of whether there is evidence of cultural differences between client and therapist.

CONCLUSION

Intervention is often best thought of as a cyclical process involving setting goals, planning how to achieve these goals, implementation of the plan, reevaluation, setting new goals, and so forth. The process, however, usually does come to an end. It is to this aspect of the occupational therapy process, termination, that the next chapter is addressed.

18 Termination

Termination is the last phase of the intervention process. It is frequently a time of turmoil for the client because of doubts regarding his or her capacity to manage in the community. For ease in presentation, this chapter is divided into two parts—process and emotional issues.

THE PROCESS

Although termination of intervention is usually described in the singular, there are really two types of termination—final and partial. Final termination refers to the separation between therapist and client which is considered to be the endpoint in their relationship (916,956,960). The client and therapist bid each other goodbye with the expectation that they will not meet again. Partial termination, on the other hand, refers to a separation that is temporary in nature but that marks the end of one kind of a relationship and the beginning of a new relationship (74,155,935). The best example of partial termination is when a client has gained all possible benefit from the change process and is ready to return to the community with a regular program of maintenance. Termination would be partial in this situation if the therapist was responsible for follow-up of the maintenance program. The client and therapist would have continued contact through, for example, the client's bimonthly visits to the clinic, home visits by the therapist, or discussions by telephone. The client and therapist relationship changes from the relatively intimate daily contact of the treatment facility to a relationship that is less intimate and more distant in time and place. Another example of partial termination is a developmentally disabled child who leaves a treatment facility or a course of outpatient intervention with the full knowledge that he will return again some time in the future for additional involvement in the change process. The difference between final and partial termination is primarily a matter of degree. Final termination is more anxiety-provoking for the client and is concerned more directly with the issue of separation. In the remainder of this chapter a distinction between final and partial termination will be made only when there is a marked difference between the two relative to process or emotional issues. It is suggested, however, that the reader remain aware of the two types in the discussion that follows.

Termination is identified as the last stage of intervention. This is accurate in the sense that it is the major focus during the last few days or weeks of intervention. It is inaccurate in that termination should be of concern and addressed throughout the intervention process. Termination actually begins during evaluation when the client's anticipated expected environment is identified. With at least some idea where the client is going to be and what he or she is going to be doing, intervention is at least, in part, oriented to the time of termination. The expected environment is discussed during each reevaluation and, if necessary, altered as circumstances require. The periodic discussion of the expected environment facilitates consideration of and realistic planning for the future. This diminishes denial and fantasy and ultimately makes termination a less anxiety-provoking process.

In conjunction with tentatively identifying and discussing the expected environment, the therapist is concerned with the resources of the client; those immediately available and those potentially available. It is often useful for the client and therapist together to identify the client's immediate resources. Many times clients are surprised at how many resources they have. On the other hand, some clients are somewhat taken aback to discover how few resources they have. Such a situation may be anxiety-provoking, with the therapist needing to provide considerable support. Timing of initiating discussion of resources, thus, is important. Although becoming aware of one's limited immediate resources can be difficult, it ultimately, with some guidance, helps the client to look at the future realistically and make appropriate plans. In reviewing immediate resources, the major areas of concern are the client's financial status, housing, and the support system available, including family, friends, and neighbors.

Potential resources are people, situations, organizations, and institutions available in the community which may provide care and/or support for individuals who are unable to live a healthy and satisfying life independently. Some examples of potential resources are federal, state, and private sources of financial support for the disabled, special housing, group homes, day programs, visiting homemaker and nursing services, sheltered workshops, state-sponsored vocational rehabilitation programs, recreational programs for the disabled, special schools, organizations concerned with a specific disability such as United Cerebral Palsy and the Arthritis Foundation, extended care facilities, and so forth. Potential resources are available in all communities although admittedly, some communities have a far greater number than others.

It is the responsibility of the therapist to be knowledgeable of potential community resources that may be useful to the type of client population with which he or she is concerned. Knowledgeable refers to knowing what resources are available, how to gain access to these resources (people to call, procedures required, etc.), eligibility, and limitations.

In identifying resources and in connecting the client with available resources, the occupational therapist often works in close cooperation with a social worker. To this cooperative effort, the therapist brings a well-defined understanding of the client's assets and limitations. This is often crucial in determining what resources are most appropriate for a particular client. The social worker may take primary responsibility for helping the client to consider and select appropriate resources. However, there are situations in which a social worker is not available, or this aspect of client care is not part of the job description of the social worker. The occupational therapist, then, must take on this responsibility.

In providing an orientation to potential resources, the therapist must consider the client's capacity to comprehend, make decisions, and initiate contact. These factors will influence the therapist's approach and the extent to which the client will need direct assistance in gaining access to appropriate resources. When a client is functioning at a fairly high level, the therapist's major responsibility is to provide information and to tell the client how to get further information. The therapist and client may discuss the pros and cons of various resources, but the choice of which resources to use is up to the client. The therapist encourages decision-making and the taking of relevant action. The therapist does not make decisions for the client or act on behalf of the client. This attitude is adopted out of respect for the client's right to make his or her own decisions and to encourage the client to take responsibility for planning his or her own life.

When a client is in a far less functional state, the therapist's discussion of potential resources involves considerably more than providing information. Direct assistance is given in the selection of resources and in making specific contacts. The therapist may help the client complete the necessary forms and accompany the client to required interviews. Visits may be made with the client to peruse various organizations or facilities.

The orientation to potential resources often involves family members. Ideally they are always involved regardless of the age or functional capacity of the client. There are times, however, when the client does not want the family to be involved in decisions regarding the use of potential resources. These wishes should be respected. When family members are involved, discussions in regard to community resources should include the client. The therapist's major role is to provide information and to encourage mutual decision-making between the family and client. When a family is disorganized or, for some other reason, unable to make decisions and take relevant action, the therapist must take a more active part in helping the family to make adequate use of potential resources.

The process of termination is influenced by the factor of time. The period of time in which the client is involved in intervention may be limited by financial considerations, the policies of the facility, or law. When time is limited, it is often easier to assist the client in remaining conscious of and in planning for final or partial termination. Consideration of the future becomes almost automatically a natural part of the intervention process. The drawback of time-limited intervention is that the long-term goals that were set may not have been met. This could be a result of the setting of too ambitious goals. However, even when very realistic goals are set, there are occasions when these goals are not achieved. The client may have to move to another facility rather than return to the community, or intervention is discontinued with the hope that the client will attain a higher level of function through her own efforts in the community. Neither of these two situations enhances the termination process. It makes it more difficult for both client and therapist to bring a comfortable closure to the intervention process.

Time for intervention, on the other hand, may be unrestricted. In this situation, decision-making regarding the client's readiness for termination of intervention becomes a collaborative effort involving the client, the therapist, and other members of the team. The criteria used to determine readiness for termination are (a) if the client's problem areas have been sufficiently altered so that the client is able to function effectively in the expected environment, (b) if the client's remaining areas of dysfunction can be best dealt with through participation in a different kind of treatment or intervention process, and/or (c) if no additional progress can be expected, at least at the present time. When time is unrestricted, the idea of termination frequently becomes a less conscious part of intervention. Because of the lack of time pressure, intervention may be more lengthy than is really necessary. Termination itself, however, may be more comfortable as the decision was arrived at through a mutual process rather than by fiat. There is often a sense of completeness to the experience which may not be present in time-limited intervention.

Regardless of the element of time, it is helpful during the termination phase for the client to separate from involvement in intervention gradually. This may take several forms: the hospitalized client may be encouraged to spend an increasingly greater time in the community, e.g., during the day, overnight, or for a weekend. There may be a decrease in the number of regularly scheduled sessions for intervention. The client may be involved with a decreasing number of team members. Gradual withdrawal from intervention tends to decrease the client's dependency and assists the client in realizing that he or she has attained at least a fairly adequate amount of functional capacity.

If the plan for intervention includes subsequent maintenance, there is preparation for this during the termination phase. The maintenance program is described to the client with full explanation as to its purpose. Adjustments are made to make it as compatible as possible with the client's anticipated living situation and lifestyle. Any necessary new skills required for adequate participation in the program are taught and practiced to the point that the client feels comfortable. The termination phase may also include the teaching of energy conservation techniques and, for the physically disabled client, making structural adaptations in the home environment. The latter, of course, should be carried out in consultation with the client and other family members. Factors that influence the success of subsequent maintenance were outlined in more detail in Chapter 17.

Some clients' expected environment is not their preintervention environment. It may be, as mentioned, a total institution, some type of sheltered environment, or an unprotected environment which is new for the client. Although all of intervention is directed toward preparing the individual for participation in a particular environment, special effort may be directed toward this goal during the termination phase. Anticipatory or concurrent topical groups are particularly useful in this phase of intervention. This type of activity group was described in Chapter 14. In such groups, the client has an opportunity to identify possible problem areas, problem solve relative to various solutions, engage in trial interactions, and discuss difficulties encountered. The role playing of typical situations that might occur or have occurred is a particularly useful technique.

For clients who are somewhat hesitant about moving into a new environment, the therapist may need to take a more active stance. For example, if a client is going to live in a sheltered environment, it is often helpful for the client and therapist to visit the facility, meet the staff members who will be primarily responsible for the client, talk to some of the residents or participants in the program, and, in general, get a feel for the environment. The degree to which the therapist becomes directly involved in a client's transition to a new environment is dependent primarily on the functional capacity of the client. The therapist should be sufficiently self-aware to provide only the degree of assistance that is actually needed by the client and not assistance that is primarily motivated by the therapist's own needs. This will be discussed further in the next section.

In the termination phase the client and therapist give themselves ample time to review together what took place during intervention, e.g., what has been gained through the process, the dark moments, the times of great success, and their own relationship. Plans for the future, of course, are discussed. Even with all of the sharing, there needs to be a specified time for saying goodbye. Ideally, this is not a time when the intervention process is reviewed or specific problems are considered. It is a time to share the last moments of a significant relationship.

There are two issues that are often raised regarding termination, the giving of a gift and whether there should be contact between client and therapist after final termination. There are no generally accepted guidelines for dealing with these two issues. Thus, the suggestions provided are those of the author. Accepting a gift from a client which is given as a token of appreciation is well within the bounds of typical human relations. Any kind of extravagant gift, however, should not be accepted. Rejection of such a gift should be accomplished with a full explanation of why the gift cannot be accepted. A gift given to express appreciation and well within the financial capacity of the client should be accepted graciously and without embarrassment. The therapist may also be inclined to give a token of affection and expression of best wishes to the client. If the inclination is there, the therapist, if comfortable, should act on it. The gift should be simple and something that the therapist knows will be significant to the client. For the client, a gift from the therapist may have a tremendous long-term significance. There may be times when the client will feel insecure, inadequate, and long for the protection that he or she felt during the intervention process. The therapist's gift may well become a symbolic statement that someone cares, understands, and knows. In the dark of the night, the gift may remind the client that he or she can make it.

After final termination, some clients feel the need to occasionally talk with the therapist. They may telephone or stop by to say hello. The need for such contact is not unusual and should be accepted as part of the separation process. The therapist, first of all, should not see such a need as pathological or evidence of excessive dependency. Interaction is best kept at the casual level but with evidence of concern for how the client is faring and what is happening in daily life. In the usual course of events, the client becomes more secure in his or her life situation and contact with the therapist gradually diminishes to the point of no contact or an annual Christmas card. If contact continues for an unusually long time and/or is characterized by excessive dependency, the therapist should firmly state the parameters of the relationship and reinforce the client's capacity to go about living without assistance from the therapist. If the goals of intervention have been met, the latter situation is a relatively rare occurrence.

There are two major variations in the process of termination as outlined above. The client, for any number of reasons, may be suddenly transferred or discharged before the goals of intervention have been met and without any opportunity to participate in the termination phase of intervention. This is certainly not an ideal situation but nevertheless it does occur. If possible the therapist should contact the client to inquire about his or her situation and to provide reassurance. It is the therapist's responsibility to consider and hopefully find an effective means of ensuring that the client will have continuity in the intervention process.

The other variation is standard operating procedure for some short-term inpatient psychiatric programs. The client's period of hospitalization is likely to be only a few days or, at the most, a couple of weeks. In this type of setting, the therapist's major responsibilities are meeting health needs, helping the client reintegrate, and evaluation. On the basis of evaluative findings, the therapist makes recommendations concerning the type of intervention the client appears to need in order to function at an optimal level. A complete evaluation summary is sent to whoever will be responsible for the further care of the client. In a short-term treatment facility, the therapist-client relationship is less intense. Termination is primarily focused on preparing the client for the kind of treatment/intervention that lies ahead. Preparation involves giving information about what will be happening and the probable emotions the client will experience. In many ways, this type of termination is similar to anticipatory crisis intervention as was outlined in the last chapter in the section on prevention. A considerable amount of support is also important. The therapist's role in a short-term inpatient psychiatric facility will be discussed in greater detail in Chapter 27.

The process of termination as outlined above has only alluded to the emotional element, a very significant factor in successful terminations. The remaining portion of this chapter is devoted to the discussion of this element of the termination process.

EMOTIONAL ISSUES

Termination, a time of change in roles and relationships, is frequently surrounded by a number of emotional issues (81,99,290,705,956,981). Particular feelings may be experienced by the client, family members, and by the therapist.

For the client, termination of intervention, regardless of the circumstances, is frequently a traumatic experience. The client's major question, although it may take several forms, is "Can I make it?" The client may experience fear or anxiety and anger. The latter feeling may be derived from two sources. The client may perceive termination as rejection and/or the client may believe that the therapist and other team members did not do enough and that with more effort on their part, the client would be able to function at a higher level. These beliefs of the client are often not based on reality but are a way of dealing with separation. On the other hand, these beliefs may have some basis in reality. Clients sometimes are rejected by staff members and not all clients receive optimal care. Whatever the reason for the client's negative feelings, it is important to realize that they are very real for the client. Ignoring them, thinking they will go away, is not an effective means of helping the client deal with separation. These feelings must be addressed by the client and therapist together.

Clients respond to the feelings associated with separation in a number of ways: feigned independence, angry outbursts, denial of any benefit from intervention, contrary behavior, complaints, excessive demands, and regressions, to name just a few. Regression is probably the most common reaction. The client suddenly decides, usually on an unconscious level, that he or she is really not able to function. The client's behavior often begins to be very similar to behavior at the beginning of intervention.

There are several ways in which the therapist may help the client through the termination phase:

- Discuss the history of the intervention process—what was and was not accomplished, what was most and least effective;
- Help the client identify current assets and limitations;
- Encourage the client to function at his or her highest level, make demands. The client's observation of his or her own capacity to function is frequently far more effective than anything the therapist could possibly say;
- Recognize the client's fear and indicate that this is a usual and normal reaction to termination;
- Accept and absorb the client's anger. A logical and reasonable discussion is rarely effective. Retaliation on the part of the therapist is inappropriate and should be avoided at all costs;
- Let the client regress to a degree and temporarily. This may help the client to feel better, and it will in no way interfere with the client's ultimate capacity to function effectively;
- Give honest support and reassurance while still recognizing some of the difficulties that are ahead;
- In the case of partial termination, the therapist defines his or her new role relative to the client and expectations in regard to the client's behavior;
- Accept the client's gratitude gracefully.

Any one or all of the above methods may be helpful to the client. Most of them are used with the intention of facilitating the client's capacity to discuss feelings and ideas about termination and what the future is likely to bring. In discussion, the client may repeatedly return to the traumatic events, if any, that surrounded the initial need for intervention. Talking about these events frequently helps the client place them in some reasonable perspective and accept them as part of a total life experience.

The client's family may have their own set of emotional issues. They are likely to have fears regarding the client's return home and/or concern about how the client will fare without regular contact with the therapist. They often have fantasies and expectations that are not grounded in reality. This may be true regardless of how closely the therapist has worked with the family during the course of intervention. The closer the therapist has worked with the family, however, the more likely that their expectations will be compatible with the client's objective state of function. The therapist may help the family during termination by giving accurate information concerning the client's assets and limitations; providing a detailed description of the home maintenance program, if any; reviewing the resources that are available to the client and family; and outlining the type of behavior on the part of the family that will be most beneficial to the client. It is also useful if the therapist suggests various recreational or leisure activities that the client and family may enjoy together. Such activities frequently help the transitional period go more smoothly and the client to reassume appropriate family roles and responsibilities. As with the client, the therapist should help family members talk about their fears and fantasies. The sharing of ideas, with adequate feedback, is probably the best way for anyone to sort out the real from the unreal.

Finally, termination may give rise to several emotional issues for the therapist. This is particularly true for the beginning therapist but, regardless of experience, it may still be a time of conflicting feelings. Some of the feelings the therapist may have are:

Guilt and feelings of inadequacy. These feelings often come from the wish or belief that one could or should have done more in helping the client to function more adequately. There may be a tendency to engage in the fantasy of "if only . . .".

Anger. This feeling often is a response to the client's anger. The therapist may feel that the client is profoundly ungrateful in face of the belief that one did more than anyone else would have done to assist the client. There is a feeling of not being respected or appreciated and that the client has no right to be angry.

Relief. The client was difficult to work with, perhaps unmotivated, or even obnoxious. Recognition of this feeling, no matter how well founded, can also lead to feelings of guilt. The idea that one is more than delighted to have a client leave intervention leads some therapists to question their basic concern for other human beings and their capacity to be a good therapist. This, of course, is rubbish; there are some clients who are very difficult to work with and not particularly nice people.

Protectiveness. This feeling tends to be aroused when the therapist has legitimate concern about the future well-being of a client. It may also occur, however, when the therapist feels that he or she is the only one who can assist in nurturing the client's further development. This idea is likely to have little basis in reality.

Sadness and concern. This is a usual feeling that comes with any separation. It should be accepted as such, with the recognition that such feelings are indicative of caring about and liking another individual.

In dealing with the above feelings, it is best for the therapist to recognize them and accept them for what they are. It is important also for the therapist to discuss these feelings with other staff members and a supervisor.

Although the above discussion has focused on some of the negative factors relative to termination, the experience can be and should be positive. When well-handled, the termination phase of intervention can be a good growth experience for all parties involved. When approached by the therapist with such an orientation, the transition from intervention to greater or full participation in the community can serve as a firm foundation for further development.

19 Communication

Communication, the giving and receiving of information, is a significant part of the occupational therapy process. Communication with the client and family members has been discussed throughout this text. This chapter, however, is devoted primarily to communication between the therapist, other members of the treatment/intervention team, and appropriate administrative personnel. More specifically, it is concerned with the following topics: the importance and purpose of communication, interdepartmental communication, written communication, and oral communication.

IMPORTANCE AND PURPOSE OF COMMUNICATION

A profession serves and is responsible to a particular society or social system. One of a profession's obligations is to be accountable, to provide evidence in regard to the nature of the services provided and the effectiveness of such service (111,185,249,366,385,596,676, 921,1028). Without adequate accountability, the society has every right to raise questions about the nature and efficacy of what they are paying for. Vague statements and the assumption that the society should believe or have faith in the profession are hardly sufficient. Society wants and has a right to adequate documentation: a clear statement of the goals of intervention, the means used to attain these goals, and the extent to which goals are achieved.

The occupational therapy process usually takes place within the context of a team of other professionals. For intervention to be effective, team members must communicate with each other in a somewhat structured and organized manner (27,381,388,894). Without such organization, team members would be working in isolation, each essentially going off and doing whatever he or she thinks is best. There would be no coordination and more than likely this would lead to less than optimal, if not inadequate, client care. At best, the care is unlikely to be well coordinated.

The therapist needs good records to determine the nature of the client's assets and limitations and to plan adequate ongoing intervention for individual clients. Adequate records also provide some of the raw data that the therapist may use in developing hypotheses to formulate or test a particular theory, or to determine the efficacy of a given method of intervention. It is in this way that the profession remains viable and effective in serving society.

More specifically, the purpose of good communication is to (74,170,327,619,916,956,960,1000):

- Provide clear, concise, objective data about the client in order to define problem areas, formulate goals, plan intervention, and to document changes in behavior;
- Permit good articulation between the client's involvement in occupational therapy and the other services concerned with the client's care;
- Share and problem solve with other team members so that the client receives optimal care;
- Provide the necessary justification for the cost of evaluation and intervention;
- Document the occupational therapy process so as to meet the requirements of Professional Standards Re-

view Organization (PSRO) and other forms of utilization review such as the accreditation of a facility;
- Facilitate the continued study and development of the occupational therapy process.

Because of the importance of communication, it is imperative that accurate records and reports are made and kept current. It is also imperative that sound systems of communication with other staff members are worked out and used on a regular and consistent basis.

Engagement in adequate communication is a time-consuming process. There are meetings to prepare for and attend, and there is a considerable amount of written work to do. The latter is often seen as particularly difficult by the neophyte therapist. The therapist may be tempted to give insufficient attention to communication in the press of many other responsibilities. Such an inclination should be resisted as communication is essential to adequate practice. The therapist who does not take the time and effort to communicate probably is being professionally irresponsible.

INTERDEPARTMENTAL COMMUNICATION

The cornerstone of effective client intervention/treatment is good interdepartmental communication (175,216, 245, 257, 290, 348, 367, 373, 702, 926). Both formal and informal channels of communication are extremely important and lack of use of either impedes client care. The channels used at any particular time will depend on the structure and traditions of the facility and on the type of information to be communicated. Interdepartmental communication has been found to be defective in many institutions. The reason for this deficit varies from institution to institution, but there seem to be several common underlying factors:

1. Communication in institutions may be nonreciprocal. The information communicated by one individual may have little bearing on the communication directed toward her by another individual. One of the reasons for nonreciprocity is the hierarchical structure of most institutions. Those high in the hierarchy are dependent on those below for information. The information given by lower status persons, however, tends to be highly selective, presented in a stereotyped manner, and often does not contain relevant facts. The communication from high status persons tends to be in the form of orders, or at least is perceived in that manner. Because of an inadequate exchange of information, communication from high status persons is frequently not relevant to the situation or not seen as reasonable.

2. Institutions are characterized by a paucity of meaningful information. In many institutions, staff members lack specific information that will allow them to function in an effective manner. When attempts are made to initiate reciprocal communication, it is often found that the individuals involved are unable to understand each other. Intraprofessional jargon may be the only language available to the individuals. This jargon is frequently not understood by those who are not members of the profession. Moreover, staff members may be so used to using stereotyped language that they themselves do not realize that they do not know the meaning of the words.

3. There is a tendency in institutions to rely on informal communication. Occupational therapists are often very proud of the breadth of their informal communication system in relation to members of other departments. Although there is nothing inherently wrong with informal communication, one could raise the question of why so much of it is necessary. The occupational therapist may avoid formal channels of communication out of fear that the information given regarding clients is mediocre or lacking in sophistication. There is also often a complaint that information given through formal channels is ignored. If this is the case, one might question the relevancy of the information or the form in which it is presented.

4. Frequently members of one department are completely ignorant of the role and function of members of another department. Thus they see no reason for communication. Closely related to this factor is ignorance regarding the particular problems and concerns of another department. Without this knowledge communication may be irrelevant and meaningless. The communication between departments may simply not be understood. Through empathetic understanding of others, an individual is far more able to regulate the content and timing of communication accurately and to interpret the latent message of the response.

5. The members of many professions suffer from feelings of inferiority, particularly those directly concerned with client care. These feelings are frequently related to the recognition that there is much that is unknown about psychosocial dysfunction. One is often powerless to help a client regain function. Feelings of inferiority, and the fear that lack of knowledge and skill will be recognized by others, limits communication. The individual thus comes to operate on the principle that the less said, the less others will know what one is doing. This principle is also utilized when an individual feels that he or she is engaging in evaluation or intervention procedures that might be seen as illicit by members of other departments. A therapist may be involved in experimental or very creative work with clients, but fear

of misunderstanding and disapproval inhibits any communication about this work.

6. Feelings of inferiority also lead departmental members to jealously guard the domain they have carved out for themselves (44,247). This domain is usually defined in terms of some process relative to client care. One's sense of worth comes to be tied to the process as opposed to the underlying function of the process, which may or may not be known. Movement of others into this domain or territory is perceived as threatening. One means of assuring that encroachment does not occur is to limit communication.

7. Feelings of inferiority may give rise to marked status consciousness. When a person perceives her status as low or when she is uncertain whether she can maintain her position, she tends to become preoccupied with status. In such a situation it has been found that individuals tend not to communicate to others of equal or lower status. They direct communication to persons of higher status or to no one. If an individual is unable to change status level, communication directed to high status persons tends to be irrelevant. Neither of these patterns of communication facilitates client care.

8. Another factor that interferes with interdepartmental communication is lack of concern for meeting the social-emotional needs of persons in other departments. This is often due to ignorance regarding the importance of this component of communication. Although it takes some extra time and effort, communication that occurs concomitant with satisfying social-emotional needs tends to be better understood and more effective. As in any group endeavor, concern only with task impedes the accomplishment of the task.

9. Much of the interaction that takes place between institutional personnel tends to be ritualistic. Rituals are highly stylized and carefully prescribed sets of gestures and words performed by socially designated persons. Rituals tend to come into being when individuals attempt to deal with the unknown. For this reason they are common in hospitals and other health facilities. Rituals do have many positive functions; however, they tend to impede communication. What goes on during a ritual is often erroneously perceived as communication. People then feel that no additional communication is needed. Communication does not take place in ritualistic interactions; other settings or situations must be utilized.

Although the above-mentioned factors which impede interdepartmental communication may seem overwhelming, they are amenable to change. Through individual and joint action, effective interdepartmental communication can be initiated and sustained. The following suggestions are offered as a guide:

1. There is an intimate relationship between reciprocal communication and meaningful information. If the participants in a communication process are giving and receiving meaningful information, the process is far more likely to be reciprocal. The therapist can make the content of communication more meaningful by identifying what information others want. Often this is accomplished by helping others to understand what information the therapist has. Similarly, the therapist must identify what information others have that would be useful. Such information is then requested from these persons.

2. Jargon should be avoided as much as possible. It serves a useful purpose at times but it is also used to hide lack of knowledge. If an individual is unable to translate jargon into common everyday language, he probably does not understand the meaning of the jargon. People may very convincingly use such terms as "reality testing," "thought disorder," "ego function," etc., without really being able to define their meaning. Elimination of jargon and stereotyped language is best begun by translating all written and oral communication about client care into common language. Subsequent to this step, the therapist can help persons in other departments to do likewise.

3. The administrator and staff of an occupational therapy department must insist on their right to use formal channels of communication for giving and receiving the information needed for adequate client care. Chance meetings in the hall or quick conferences in the coffee shop, although important, do not allow for an adequate exchange of information. If one feels respect for and competence in the job being performed, then one must seek and demand similar respect from others. One of the ways of accomplishing this is through the use of formal channels of communication. Implicit in this statement is the assumption that one is communicating relevant information in an intelligent manner.

4. By showing interest and concern and asking appropriate questions, the therapist is able to gain considerable information about the role and function of another professional group or department. It is best to approach this exploration with an open mind. Prior concepts about what a department does or is "supposed to do" may be misleading. One wishes to gain information about department members' perception of their role and function. Further information may be gained by actually observing department members in action. Their behavior may give a more accurate idea about what they do than a verbal interchange. Both sources of information are, however, important. One is able to understand the present role and function of department members as well as

gain information about the ideal for which members strive.

5. Listening and observing also assist one in identifying the problems and concerns of another department. It is sometimes bothersome to listen to others complain. However, the information gained and the opportunity provided for the other person to express feelings greatly facilitate the communication process. Information regarding the problems of another department should never be used as a weapon against the department or as a source of gossip. This is unkind and at times destructive. Such information should only be used in a constructive manner.

6. One's feelings of inferiority can be minimized by accurate recognition of the knowledge and skills one currently possesses. Feelings of inferiority are appropriate only when the therapist ceases to attempt to gain further knowledge and skill. The therapist must not only recognize limitations in him- or herself, but also the fact that there is much still unknown about psychosocial dysfunction. Such recognition allows all institutional personnel to look at problems realistically and to approach them in an open and experimental manner. Pretending that one has answers or that the client is not improving through some fault of his or her own only covers up problems and does nothing to solve them.

7. In approaching others, the therapist should be aware of the possibility that the other person may feel inferior. The person may act in a superior manner, but underlying inferiority feelings may be present. The other person should not be approached as if he or she is all-knowing. If so approached, that person may feel compelled to take on this role. This causes added discomfort, which will further impede communication. In communicating with others, the therapist presents known information in a matter of fact manner and freely admits to lack of knowledge or skill in the area under consideration. Answers to questions are not demanded. Rather the therapist approaches the situation as an opportunity to share information and opinions. Ideally, collaborative problem solving takes place. An attitude of willingness to try the ideas of other people, to experiment, and to honestly evaluate an attempted solution is particularly helpful.

8. Communication with others is improved if the therapist does not fear disapproval from others. This assumes, of course, the therapist has honestly explored his or her actions, evaluated the purpose and rationale for them, and acted within the limits of his or her knowledge and skill. These are questions the therapist must answer for him- or herself or with the help of a supervisor. If the therapist has acted appropriately, he or she need not fear disapproval. Some people may still disapprove; it is rare when one's actions meet with universal acceptance. However, without unnecessary fear, the therapist feels free to communicate, regardless of some negative responses. This, in turn, helps others to communicate more readily.

9. Although a special domain of action may interfere with expedient communication, it must be recognized and respected if it exists. Attempts to eliminate the domain of another person or department are usually not effective. Rather they tend to make the parameters of the domain more rigid. One must move with caution into another person's territory. Attempting to take over or indicating in any way that the other person has not done an adequate job should be avoided. The only way that adequate communication can take place when territoriality is in question is to seek cooperation and to make the other feel that he is gaining far more than he is losing. The latter should be based on an honest appraisal of the situation, not an empty promise. Communication cannot take place if people are not dealt with honestly at all times.

10. Concern about status is a part of human nature. However, normal concern does not necessarily blind one to the need for communication with persons of equal or lower status. Channels of communication with these persons should be diligently cultivated as are the channels between oneself and high status persons. This is not done simply to be "nice." People of equal or lower status are often able to give far more help in attaining goals than persons in higher status positions.

11. Social-emotional needs must be fulfilled as a part of the communication process. Concern for others as human beings, in addition to recognition of their roles in the institution, is very important. Reflection on past situations where one was treated as some sort of a nonhuman object without needs will help the reader to understand the necessity for meeting social-emotional needs.

12. Recognition and acceptance of rituals indirectly help communication by making people more comfortable. Although individuals can be helped to see that rituals are not a particularly useful form of communication, direct confrontation usually provokes extreme anxiety. Confrontation should be slow and regulated by the participants' capacity to use this information. In the meantime the therapist must use other settings and situations for the purpose of communication.

13. Finally, openness in communicating tends to be contagious. If the therapist is comfortable in communicating with others, others will feel more comfortable in turn. Interdepartmental communication will be greatly enhanced.

WRITTEN COMMUNICATION

There are several records and reports that therapists are expected to write. These will be discussed momentarily. However, the initial focus of this section is on some basic principles about written communication.

The hallmarks of good written communication are as follows (91,98,266,786,1000):

Knowledge of the reader. It is important that the therapist knows with whom he or she is communicating, what they want to know, and what they do not want to know.

Clarity. The words used should be specific. Indefinite terms (good, large, etc.) are subject to individual definition and should either be avoided or further explained. The terminology used should be understandable to all members of the health team. Uncommon terminology, abbreviations, and symbols should be avoided. If it is necessary to use a word that is not likely to be known, it should be defined. Jargon that is particular to one's own profession should be avoided. Grammar, spelling, and punctuation are important. All written work should be edited to correct mistakes in English. If reports are handwritten, they should be legible. It is a waste of time to write something that no one else can read. Whether handwritten or typed, all reports should be neat.

Completeness. There should be complete descriptions of the types, frequency, and extent of activities of concern, those of the client and those to be used in intervention. The reader should not have to make assumptions about what data have and have not been collected. When a particular aspect of function has not been assessed, for example, this should be stated in the report. Similarly, adequate function in a particular area should be stated, not just those areas in which there are problems. Completeness is also concerned with the use of whole sentences—not just phrases and words. Contractions should be avoided.

Consecutiveness. Data should be presented in a logical manner. Each part should follow in an orderly fashion that is discernible to the reader. If client fatigue or time precluded the collection of all data at once or in order, for example, the information should be recorded in sequence with notations concerning the omissions so that ultimately the record will be consecutive and complete. When notes are written in paragraph form, the first sentence of each paragraph states the major idea to be discussed in the paragraph. The idea is then elaborated or explained in subsequent sentences. Reports may be written in outline form if it is acceptable to the facility and the therapist finds this method successful in recording and communicating the pertinent information.

Finally, all written communication is dated and signed, including designation of therapist's title. In some facilities, reports made by student therapists must be cosigned by the responsible supervisor.

Types of Written Reports

There are six major types of written reports: client history, evaluation summary, plan for intervention, periodic notes, final discharge summary, and special reports. Each of these will be discussed briefly (84,89, 107,290,327,619,631,705,786,871,956,960,1000).

Client History

Some facilities do not require the occupational therapist to write a formal client history. The major portion of the client's history is taken and reported by one or more other members of the health team. Additional pertinent history gathered in the course of occupational therapy evaluation is included in the evaluation summary.

In the event that the therapist is responsible for writing all or a portion of the client's history, it should be presented as the client's own story. Whenever possible, the client's own words are used. This ultimately provides the most information to the reader, for it conveys the client's understanding of him- or herself and of his or her current life situation. It also gives the reader some idea of the client's ability to recall events, organize thoughts, and to communicate this information to others. Thus, the therapist should avoid translating the client's statements into what the therapist believes is better English or language that is commonly used by the health team. Any interpretations are out of place in a history. The purpose of a written history is to present raw data, not to identify the client's problem areas. Information is presented as accurately as possible so that the therapist and other members of the health team can draw their own conclusions. The client's untranslated perceptions and expressions provide the most objective data from which later interpretations and conclusions can be made. In order to facilitate this type of presentation, the client's responses, if direct quotes, are placed in quotation marks. If the client's statements are paraphrased, the statement is preceded by "the client says," "the client desires," etc. The informants should be identified whether it be the client, his wife, or mother, and so forth. When there is more than one informant, it should be evident what information was provided by each informant. The format of written histories should all follow the same order. This not only allows for logical presentation, but also facilitates the later retrieval of a specific piece of information. A suggested order of presentation is:

- Biographical information
- Presenting problem(s)
- Current health status
- Past health history
- Family
- Activities of daily living
- School/work
- Play/leisure/recreation
- Environment

These various categories are outlined in detail in Chapter 16 in the section on interviewing.

Evaluation Summary

An evaluation summary is a presentation of the conclusions drawn from the initial assessment. The form in which evaluative findings are presented varies from facility to facility. Thus, the following outline is general in nature, describing the information that ought to be included. The evaluation summary is so titled and states the client's name, sex, age, and the date. Other biographical data are usually not necessary, as these are available in the client's history. The introductory remarks usually include a listing of the evaluative tools used as a means for gathering data. The client's general status, i.e., degree of confusion, cooperation, etc., is described as well as any extenuating circumstances such as a less than optimal situation for evaluation. This provides the reader with some idea of the accuracy of the evaluative findings.

Statements about each of the aspects of intervention are then made. These statements include areas in which there may be potential problems (prevention), the extent to which the client is able to meet his or her health needs independently, areas of function that will need to be maintained, any behavior that will require management, and the client's areas of function and dysfunction as specified in the frame of reference(s) being utilized (change process).

In summarizing information relative to the change process, each function-dysfunction continuum included in the frame of reference is mentioned. Areas of function are usually stated first, followed by those areas in which there is dysfunction. All statements include supporting evidence. The following two sample statements may be useful: "The client is able to meet all health needs independently as evidenced by his relaxed manner, involvement in a number of activities which he states are satisfying, and his capacity to ask questions about his condition and the care that he is receiving"; "The client has difficulty in concentrating on a task as evidenced by wandering around the room and engaging in considerable extraneous conversation when requested to engage in task-oriented behavior." In providing evidence for a statement, only a sample of the behavior used as the basis for the interpretive statement needs to be provided. For ease in reading, the statement is presented first, followed by the evidence. The reverse format, presenting the evidence first, followed by an interpretive statement, often requires the reader to go back and review the evidence again. This should not be necessary and is essentially a waste of time. When the initial evaluation was not complete, areas not assessed are mentioned with the reason for their exclusion at this time.

The evaluation summary is placed in the client's institutional or facility chart with the evaluative summaries from other members of the team. A copy of the summary is kept in the occupational therapy files with the notes taken by the therapist during evaluation and any of the Surveys, Check-Lists, or completed questionnaires used in the evaluation process.

Plan for Intervention

This a report of the goals of intervention and a description of the means that will be used to attain these goals. Singular goals relative to meeting health needs, maintenance, and management are usually presented first, followed by serial goals. Each long-term goal is stated with the short-term goals for each listed. Goals, as mentioned, are stated in behavioral terms if at all possible. It is often useful to mention the client's expected environment, as this gives more meaning to the goals and places them in a recognizable context. The sequence in which various goals will be addressed is described.

The activities, including the therapist's interaction with the client, which will be used to reach the singular goals, are outlined. In regard to serial goals, the activities and therapist's interactions are described for the immediate short-term goals. Tentative activities and interactions that will be used to attain the long-term goals are briefly outlined. Further elaboration will be included in periodic notes. In describing the activities that will be used to reach singular and immediate short-term goals, the therapist needs to be quite specific. It is not enough to say what activities will be used; a description of how they will be used is important. For example, if a short-term goal is the ability to solve problems where the solution is readily available, the activity described in the plan for intervention may be, "The client will be involved in small woodworking projects that have very explicit step-by-step directions and a list of suggestions as to how to deal with various problems that may arise." Similarly, if the client is to be involved in a group, the major emphasis of the group is explained. Thus, a client with difficulty in the area of recreation may be involved in a "group that is actively exploring recreational facilities in the community." Or a client who is somewhat confused or deficient in the area of reality testing might be placed in "a cooking group in which the therapist and clients devote considerable time talking about what is going on in the immediate situation." Finally, if applicable, any precautions that will be observed during intervention are noted.

In some centers, the evaluation summary and plan for intervention are combined in one report. One method for doing this is the SOAP report (97,223,956). SOAP is an acronym for the organization of data in the following manner:

Subjective—the client's view of his problem(s);
Objective—the clinical findings in regard to the problem, directly observable behavior;
Assessment—the findings derived from formal evaluation;
Plan—a statement of the goals of intervention and the activities and interpersonal interactions that will be used to reach the goals.

The advantage of a structure such as a SOAP report is that the same organization is used by all members of the team. This allows for ease in sharing information. Inconsistencies or conflicts in goals or methods are readily apparent.

Periodic Note

A periodic note is written after each reevaluation. It includes a summary of the changes that have taken place since the initial evaluation or the last reevaluation. Focus is on the client's position relative to goals and other significant changes in behavior. If areas of function not included in the initial evaluation are assessed at the time of reevaluation, the findings are noted. Any alteration in the client's expected environment is also indicated. Changes in goals, singular, long-term, or short-term, are specified with the reasons for the change given. The therapist states whether the current activities and interactions will be continued, whether one of the tentative activities outlined in the original plan will be initiated, or whether a new activity will be used. The tentative or new activity is then described. When there is no observable change in the client's behavior or no change is anticipated in goals or activities, this is so stated. Collectively, periodic notes should give an accurate overview of a given intervention process and the client's progression through that process.

Final Discharge Summary

This is usually written at the point of termination of intervention or at the time the client leaves the facility. In the latter case, the client may still be involved in subsequent maintenance. The summary includes a brief statement of the initial evaluative findings, the goals for intervention, the activities and interactions utilized in intervention, and the client's status relative to the goals at the time of discharge. Any discharge plans such as the client's intention to join Alcoholics Anonymous or to participate in a recreational program for physically disabled teenagers are noted. When a client is to be involved in a subsequent maintenance program, the plan for the program is briefly described. The final discharge summary, where appropriate, is used as the base line to determine whether the subsequent maintenance is being effective in conserving function.

Special Report

A special report describes a significant, unusual event that is essentially extraneous to the intervention process. Some special reports such as those dealing with accidents are often made on a form provided by the facility. Other special reports are written directly in the client's chart. Most facilities have a list of incidents that must be reported. Some common incidents requiring a special report are (a) a client's attempt to physically injure himself or another person; (b) physical abuse of a client by a staff member; (c) accidents involving a client or a staff member; (d) a rapid mood swing; (e) a marked change in behavior or appearance; (f) a suicide threat, either covert or overt; (g) information regarding drugs or alcohol; (h) a threat or attempt to leave the institution without the required permission; (i) loss of tools or equipment that could be used in a harmful manner; and (j) nonattendance at a required activity if the client is considered harmful to himself or others. In writing a special report, the therapist describes the incident and provides all supplementary data that are relevant. The context in which the incident occurred or in which the information was gained is clarified. There is, however, some information about the client that should be communicated immediately. This will be discussed in the following section.

ORAL COMMUNICATION

The basic principles outlined for writing records and reports are applicable to oral communication as well. In addition, there are a few other principles to keep in mind:

1. Be prepared for oral presentations so that evaluative findings, goals, plans for intervention, and the theoretical knowledge that serves as their foundation can be clearly articulated.
2. Keep presentations short and to the point. Rambling on should be avoided at all costs.
3. Do not give people more information than they are able to hear and consider at one time.
4. Listen to what other people say.
5. Encourage questions and, in turn, do not be hesitant in asking questions.
6. Try to create a dialogue.
7. Speak clearly and sufficiently loud so as to be heard by all concerned parties.

There are three major situations where oral communication is required: staff meetings or conferences, informal situations, and special reports. Although there is some overlapping, each of these will be discussed separately.

The major purposes of a staff meeting or conference are the sharing of information, ideas, and opinions; problem solving; and decision-making by members of the health team. These meetings are usually held regularly so that participants are essentially members of an ongoing small group. The dynamics of groups as discussed in Chapter 12 are therefore applicable for understanding the interactions that occur in these meetings. It is suggested that the therapist be continually aware of the dynamics. In so doing, the therapist is better able to regulate communication so that information is presented at a time that it is likely to be heard and understood. The therapist will also be a more effective communicator if comfortable in taking a variety of group roles. Although staff meetings and conferences are primarily task oriented, they also are a situation in which staff members are able to satisfy many of their social-emotional needs. Thus, to the casual observer, some staff meetings may appear to be excessively devoted to the strong expression of feelings and opinions, joking, fooling around, gossiping, and the like. It is important for the therapist to be comfortable and participate in this aspect of meetings. Ultimately such participation will facilitate the therapist's communication with other team members and the satisfaction of some needs.

There are many times when a therapist meets in an informal situation with other members of the health team. These meetings may be spontaneous, in which case the therapist has little time for preparation. It is important that the therapist be able to say that he or she does not have a particular piece of information. Trying to fabricate something is inappropriate. It is far better for the therapist to say that he does not know and will get the information shortly and follow up on this promise. The therapist, of course, must be well prepared for preplanned informal meetings. Confidentiality should always be kept in mind. The informal situation should provide sufficient privacy so that the conversation is not overheard by others, in particular, clients and family members. Thus, quick conferences in the hallway or the coffee shop should be avoided unless a sufficient degree of privacy can be assured. Finally, as mentioned, informal communication should not be viewed as a substitute for the use of formal channels of communication.

Special reports, as discussed in the last section, involve communication about significant, unusual events. Incidents requiring such reports were outlined. When the situation is serious, this "emergency information" is given verbally to one's supervisor, the ward personnel responsible for the client, the client's physician, or anyone else who is authorized to take some kind of definitive action. The setting in which the therapist works usually dictates the most appropriate person to which this information should be given. If the therapist is in doubt, the information is communicated to all of the above-mentioned people. Information of this nature, which is given verbally, is also put in writing so that it becomes part of the formal record.

CONCLUSION

Communication is a tremendously important part of the evaluation and intervention process. Without adequate communication, the therapist is essentially working in a vacuum. This is an uncomfortable and sometimes dangerous situation to be in. Initially, for the neophyte therapist, the process of communication may seem cumbersome and time-consuming. With practice, effective communication does become easier and even pleasurable. Attention to this facet of professional responsibility early in one's clinical work is recommended.

Part 5

The Change Process

The change process, the development or restoration of function to the highest possible level, is the focus of Part 5. Being placed in a separate section does not in any way mean that the change process is of lesser or greater importance than the other aspects of evaluation and intervention. It is presented separately only because the subject is rather complex and the description therefore somewhat lengthy. In the following discussion of the change process, the reader is asked to keep in mind how it fits with the other aspects of the occupational therapy process. It cannot be considered alone, for in so doing the therapist's orientation to the totality of client care would be lost.

Frames of reference serve as the foundation for the change process. Thus, the first chapter in this part describes the purpose and structure of frames of reference in general. Chapters 21, 23, and 25, respectively, describe the three major types of frames of reference—analytical, developmental, and acquisitional. This includes a discussion of the major current frames of reference used in occupational therapy which fit into each of these categories. The latter discussion will be brief and critical in nature. The reason these frames of reference are not presented in detail is that most of them have not been formulated in such a way that they provide an adequate guide for the change process.

Chapters 22, 24, and 26 describe an example of a frame of reference that is representative of each of the three categories. The three frames of reference presented here in their entirety represent the author's attempt to take the best from the current frames of reference included in each category. These parts, with some additions, *hopefully* have been synthesized in such a manner that the three frames of reference provide an adequate blueprint for evaluation and intervention. The word hopefully is italicized to indicate that no frames of reference in occupational therapy are formulated in such a way that they meet the criteria for a perfect frame of reference. More specific frames of reference are likely to be formulated in the future as the theories constituting the profession's body of knowledge become more refined and are further varified.

With these introductory comments, the reader is invited to study the nature of the change process in occupational therapy.

20

Frames of Reference

Frames of reference, intimately related to the model of the profession, form the link between theory and change process. Their structure and content provide a guide for evaluation and intervention. It is to these characteristics of frames of reference that this chapter is addressed.

THE LINK BETWEEN THEORY AND THE CHANGE PROCESS

Theoretical systems are descriptive. The function is to predict relationships between a circumscribed set of events or phenomena. No action is implied or recommended. They are not designed to deal with practical situations. By way of illustration, theories of group dynamics describe the various stages of group development, group roles, systems of communication, and so forth. They say nothing about how to use a group for various purposes; they provide no guidelines for fostering the effectiveness of a group. They simply delineate what happens in small groups and on the basis of that characterization make predictions, given certain circumstances, about what will happen in a group. Ways of manipulating and using groups have been deduced from theories of group dynamics, but the theories per se are not concerned with such matters (75,119,140,174,307, 346,427,550,627,646,720,777,780,917). Theories do not answer the questions of how, when, relative to whom, and so forth.

There is no direct link between descriptive science and professional work. Two occupational groups in which this is well illustrated are architecture and medicine. In architecture there is an interrelationship between physical scientists, architects, and the practical worker in the field; in medicine there is an interrelationship between biological scientists, medical researchers, and practicing physicians. The architect, using knowledge derived from the physical sciences, designs buildings that, among other things, are structurally sound. The medical researcher, using knowledge from the biological sciences, in part, is responsible for testing chemical compounds to determine their effectiveness as medication and to provide guidelines for their use. Architects and medical researchers then provide the connection between theory and the application of knowledge. They provide the means whereby abstract theories are restructured into a form that makes them usable for dealing with practical situations.

In some occupational groups such as those identified above, there are specified categories of people who are responsible for making the link between theory and application. In other occupational groups no such specified categories of people exist. This is true for occupational therapy and for most of the other health-related professions. The forming of necessary links has been primarily left to those in the professions who are particularly interested in the process.

Without the connection or link between theory and application, either the scientist or the practitioner may begin to engage in essentially irresponsible behavior. The scientist may develop and act upon sporadic flashes of interest in application. Such an individual is not a member of a profession and thus acts outside the context of any cohesive set of philosophical assumptions, ethical code, body of knowledge, or domain of concern. More importantly, this individual acts outside his or her area of expertise and without any discernable legitimatization by society. An example is a chemist who, identifying a new compound, decides to sell it to the public to cure any number of human ills. This is practicing medicine without a license; something that is frowned on in our society. Other examples are the use of programmed instruction to teach elementary school subjects by scientists who are not educators and the use of biofeedback in rehabilitation by scientists who are not members of any of the health professions.

The profession that does not understand the relationship between theory and application may do one of two things. First, practitioners may not see any connection between the body of knowledge of their profession and the tools and techniques used in daily practice. Over time, practice becomes separated from the theories on which it was founded. Interaction with clients becomes stylized and carried out by rote. Practitioners who are unaware of the theoretical foundation of their work engage in the application of technology only.

Second, without adequate links between theory and practice a profession may become primarily oriented to a set of philosophical assumptions. Philosophical assumptions, as mentioned, are a statement of the values, purpose, and reason for the profession's existence; they define the ends or goals of the profession. The profession's body of knowledge, on the other hand, provides the information used as the basis for reaching the goals of the profession. It provides the means. When a profession bases practice on an aggregate of beliefs, a grounding in empirical theory becomes irrelevant and unnecessary. Faith has its place in the human experience and is extremely important. It cannot, however, serve as the sole foundation for a profession. One would, for example, be foolish to walk into a building that was constructed out of a set of philosophical assumptions. Similarly, in an attempt to overcome deficits in function, one would not seek assistance from a profession whose practice did not rest upon a specified body of knowledge.

The essence of the problem then is how to connect the two extremes of theory and practice. It is for this reason that linking structures have been developed. Two professional groups that have given considerable attention to their linking structures are education and psychiatry. These are, respectively, referred to as "theories of instruction" and "theories of practice." The concept and composition of frames of reference was derived from a study of these two types of linking structures. Characteristics were distilled and combined to create a structure particularly suitable for occupational therapy.

The label given to the linking structure for occupational therapy—frame of reference—does not make use of the term "theory." This term was not included in order to eliminate any confusion regarding theory and linking structures. Theories, as mentioned, are descriptive, with no action implied or recommended. Linking structures, on the other hand, although based on theory, are normative. They provide a schema for the practitioner and their function is to provide a guide for action.

A linking structure for a profession is considered to be very important. Only after such a structure evolves is it possible for (a) an occupation to become a profession, (b) a profession to grow, and (c) individuals within a profession to engage in scholarly activities relative to the profession itself.

With these introductory remarks a detailed description of frames of reference follows.

DEFINITION

A frame of reference is a set of interrelated, internally consistent concepts, definitions, and postulates derived from or compatible with empirical data that provide a systematic description of or prescription for particular designs of the environment for the purpose of facilitating evaluation and effecting change relative to a specified part of the profession's domain of concern (705,711).

Some clarification of this definition seems in order. "A set of interrelated internally consistent . . ." refers to the idea that all concepts, definitions, and postulates within a given frame of reference must be congruent. The theoretical base of a given frame of reference is often formulated by using elements from a number of different theoretical systems. Parts of a theory sometimes do not mesh easily with parts taken from other theories. In a good frame of reference, then, all the components of the various theories utilized fit together in a logical and concise manner; they have internal consistency.

"Derived from or compatible with empirical data . . ." refers to the idea that frames of reference must rest on a firm theoretical foundation. Frames of reference ideally are based on theories that have been verified by considerable research. In actuality, this is not always the case. Frames of reference in occupational therapy are sometimes based on theories that have been subjected to little empirical testing. Such frames of reference are utilized for two reasons. Without them, practitioners' interactions with clients would be guided only by intuition or a compassionate desire to serve mankind. On the other hand, if therapists just used frames of reference based on verified theory, only a very few clients would be accepted for intervention. Many clients would be deprived of at least some opportunity to develop skills necessary for community living. Obviously, neither of the above courses of action is desirable. A therapist, then, evaluates and plans intervention on the basis of currently available knowledge, fully recognizing the tremendous number of unknowns inherent in the process.

"Provides a systematic description of or prescription for a practitioner's interaction . . ." refers to two functions of frames of reference. The first function is descriptive in that it describes what a practitioner using a given frame of reference does. A frame of reference in this sense is essentially a "word picture" of the practitioner's interaction in the evaluation and intervention process. The second function of a frame of reference is prescriptive: it provides directions as to how a practitioner may interact in the evaluation and intervention process. Thus, frames of reference provide information for the neophyte therapist relative to how to assist a client. These same directions are, of course, also provided for experienced therapists who wish to use a new frame of reference. Frames of reference are prescriptive but they are not recipes; they provide guidelines for practice only.

"Particular designs of the environment . . ." refers to statements about the conditions that foster learning and the development of competence. Frames of reference describe activities and interactions—the nature of the optimal environment—in which learning or change is most likely to occur.

"A specified part of the profession's domain of concern . . ." refers to the limited nature of any given frame of reference. A particular frame of reference defines in detail and amplifies one or more aspects of the profession's domain of concern. A frame of reference may be addressed to only one performance component, as exemplified in Ayres' frame of reference regarding the sensory integration; it may on the other hand be concerned with all of the performance component. This is evident in some developmental frames of reference. Finally, frames of reference may be concerned with one or more of the occupational performances. The parameters of any particular frame of reference tend to be narrow and addressed to a circumscribed area of function and dysfunction.

In addition to the criteria outlined above, a good frame of reference has four other characteristics. It provides:

1. An explicit statement of its boundaries, the limitations under which it is proposed, for whom it is applicable;
2. A statement of goals and/or a description of competent performance;
3. An outline of the ways in which the initial level of performance is assessed and the competent level of performance;
4. Sufficient information so that it is possible to collect data to study the short- and long-term effects of its implementation.

In the process of intervention, more than one frame of reference may be used as a guide in the change process. This is particularly true when a client has multiple problems or areas of dysfunction. For example, a therapist will use a variety of frames of reference simultaneously or in sequence to deal with the physical, psychological, and social sequelae of a client who has experienced a cerebral vascular accident. No frame of reference in occupational therapy provides guidelines for helping an individual re-learn activities of daily living, adjust to alterations of physical appearance, cope with becoming somewhat dependent, and dealing with family members' reaction to the client's disability.

Occupational therapy has many different frames of reference that are addressed to the various aspects of the profession's domain of concern. In addition, there is sometimes more than one frame of reference concerned with the same aspect of the profession's domain of concern. For example, one might use an analytical frame of reference as the basis for change in the area of psychological function. Or one might use a frame of reference based on the Skinnerian theory of operant conditioning as the basis for intervention in the same area. Different frames of reference addressed to the same element of occupational therapy's domain of concern may cause conflict within the profession. However, this should not be viewed as detrimental to the profession or a sign of hopeless confusion. Such conflict enhances the vitality of the profession and assists in the clarification of ideas.

Because of the variety of frames of reference applicable to the psychosocial components of occupational therapy, the therapist fortunately has an opportunity to make a selection. In selection, the setting of intervention and the nature of the client population are significant factors. Moreover, the therapist's area of expertise, life view, and inclinations are also of great importance in selecting a frame of reference.

STRUCTURE

Frames of reference have a particular structure that facilitates the connection between theory and application (705,711). The focus of this section is structure; the content of particular frames of reference is described in subsequent chapters. In outline form then, the structure of a frame of reference is made up of:

1. A statement of the theoretical base,
2. Delineation of function-dysfunction continuums,
3. A listing of behaviors indicative of function and dysfunction,
4. Postulates regarding change.

Theoretical Base

The theoretical base of a frame of reference delineates the concepts, definitions, and postulates necessary for an adequate description of and rationale for the type of change suggested by the frame of reference in its totality. It is referred to as the *base* because it identifies the parameters of the frame of reference and serves as the matrix from which all other parts of the frame of reference are deduced. What is included in a theoretical base varies somewhat, depending on the parts of the domain of concern to which the frame of reference is addressed or on the types of evaluation and change process for which it is to serve as a guide.

In general, the theoretical base describes the nature of the area of human function(s) of concern in the frame of reference and the effects of interaction with people and things on that area of human function. More specifically, normal development and developmental deviations are described, factors that influence normal and deviant development are delineated, and interactions with the human and nonhuman environments that are believed to alter deficits in the direction of function are defined. When a deficit is unalterable, the theoretical base describes the means by which substitute functions are developed.

A theoretical base may be formulated out of one theoretical system, or concepts, definitions, and postulates may be drawn from several different theoretical systems. The latter is more often the case because many theories important to the practice of occupational therapy are primarily static. A static theory describes some types of relationship between various phenomena but does not account for change or alteration. Examples of static theory are neuroanatomy, which describes the structures of the nervous system and their spatial relationship one to another, and Freud's theory of psychosexual development. Neuroanatomy describes the potential for movement of the body, but it does not describe how nerve impulses are transmitted to ensure the coordinated movement of body parts. Freud's theory of psychosexual development delineates stages of sexual development but it does not say how individuals move from one stage of development to another. In contrast, dynamic theories deal with the issue of change, movement, alteration, and so forth. Examples of dynamic theories are neurophysiology, which is the study of how nerve impulses are transmitted, and learning theories, which attempt to account for relatively permanent changes in behavior.

If a static theory is used as part of a frame of reference, a dynamic theory of one sort or another must be used. The theoretical base of a frame of reference concerned with neuromotor function, for example, would most likely include concepts, definitions, and postulates from neuroanatomy and neurophysiology. The theoretical base of a frame of reference concerned with sexual development may use Freud's theory of stages of sexual development but would also need to include some aspects of a dynamic theory to describe how movement from one stage to the next takes place (317). On the other hand, Talcott Parsons' theory of social development, for example, describes both stages of social development and the environmental factors that facilitate movement from one stage of development to another (766). Thus the theoretical base of a frame of reference concerned with social development may be drawn entirely from Parsons' theory.

A theoretical base may or may not deal with "cause" or antecedent events believed to be related to dysfunction. Causal or antecedent events are only included if they contribute to an understanding of evaluation or change. When antecedent events are irrelevant to evaluation and intervention, it is unnecessary, and at times confusing, to describe these events in the theoretical base. Dysfunction or deficit may arise from and be maintained by any number of known or unknown factors that have influenced the individual. If the factors considered to be antecedent to dysfunction are located in the individual's past history, they are not amenable to change. If the factors leading to dysfunction are considered to be currently operating in the individual's present environment, then dysfunction is located in the environment and not the individual. For example, a woman may be depressed because her husband and children do not express any appreciation of her role as a mother and homemaker. Although, indeed, the woman may need some assistance, the frame of reference that deals with this issue most directly is addressed to the dysfunction of the husband and children, not to that of the woman.

A theoretical base is adequate only if its conceptual system and postulates are well defined (516,750,877, 901,988). Three important criteria for judging any conceptual system are economy, exclusivity, and measurability.

Economy refers to judicious or sparing use of concepts. Only concepts absolutely necessary for comprehensiveness ought to be included.

Exclusivity refers to a sharp differentiation of one concept from another. Such a differentiation should be made though a very specific definition of each concept. A good definition describes a concept in such a way that it becomes a singular phenomenon, a specific category. A good definition of a concept identifies the higher order abstraction from which the concept originates and delineates that concept from all other concepts included under the higher order concept. For example, the definition of a turtle begins with "a reptile of the order Chelonia . . ." and continues with a description of the unique characteristics that differentiate that turtle from any other chelonians. A concept can be understood and shared only if it is well defined. Ideally, the definition of a concept is so clear that anyone can categorize phenomena in a fashion similar to the originator of the concept.

The concepts of a theoretical system must ultimately be measurable. Abstract concepts are important, but if they can not be reduced to metric definition they ultimately serve no useful purpose. Measurability is important for two reasons. First, in order to verify a theory it must be tested through research. Research can only occur if the concepts of a theory can be described in such a way that they can be measured. Second, the phenomena of concern in a theoretical base is function and dysfunction; unless these elements can somehow be observed and measured it is impossible to evaluate or to determine if any change has occurred. A concept that can be measured is referred to as a variable, a concept that has been operationally defined. Admittedly, it is sometimes difficult to reduce a concept to the level of a variable. This is particularly true in the case of intrapsychic phenomena.

Postulates, the third structural component of a theoretical system, state the relationship between two or more concepts. In a well-organized theory each of the concepts are clearly related to all other concepts. This is illustrated in the first diagram (left) of Fig. 20-1. Concepts that are defined are in some way related to each other. The second diagram (right) is an illustration of a poorly structured theory; all of the concepts are not connected to all other concepts by a relationship statement, a postulate.

In summary, the theoretical base of a frame of reference describes the area(s) of human function of concern in the frame of reference and interactions with the human and nonhuman environment believed to alter deficits in the direction of function. Antecedent events or current factors that influence dysfunction are included in the theoretical base of a frame of reference only to the extent to which they facilitate an understanding of the evaluation and intervention process. The conceptual system and postulates of a theoretical must be well defined.

Function-Dysfunction Continuums

Collectively, function-dysfunction continuums are a definition of the element that constitutes the area of human function(s) addressed in the frame of reference. A gradation is implied from total inability to engage in a particular function to complete mastery of that function. An example of a function-dysfunction continuum is:

Group interaction skill:

Inability to participate in a parallel group → Ability to participate in a mature group

The term "continuum" is important in understanding this part of the structure of a frame of reference. It was chosen to indicate that there is essentially no break or line of demarcation between that which is considered function and that which is considered dysfunction. Function is considered to be relative to age, cultural background, and present life circumstances. For example, an adolescent in our society is not expected to have a full-time job; an individual of 25 years of age is expected, in most cases, to be able to work successfully in a full-time job. The individual who is unable to manage money is not considered to be in a state of dysfunction in activities of daily living if there is someone in the environment who is willing and able to look after the financial affairs of the individual. Function and dysfunction, then, is viewed as an uninterrupted line and relative to the life situation of a particular individual. It is this lack of a clear demarcation of function or dysfunction that makes the idea of "expected environment" important in the evaluation process and in setting goals.

The function-dysfunction continuums outlined in a frame of reference are deduced from the theoretical base of a frame of reference. In the theoretical base an aspect of human function is described, with deficit and mastery being discussed in general terms. The nature of function and dysfunction is made more specific in this part of a frame of reference. For example, in the theoretical base, "interpersonal skills" may be defined as an aggregate of abilities that an individual must have in order to interact successfully with others. In the section devoted to delineation of function-dysfunction continuums, the general category of interpersonal skills is broken down into its component parts. The function-dysfunction continuums

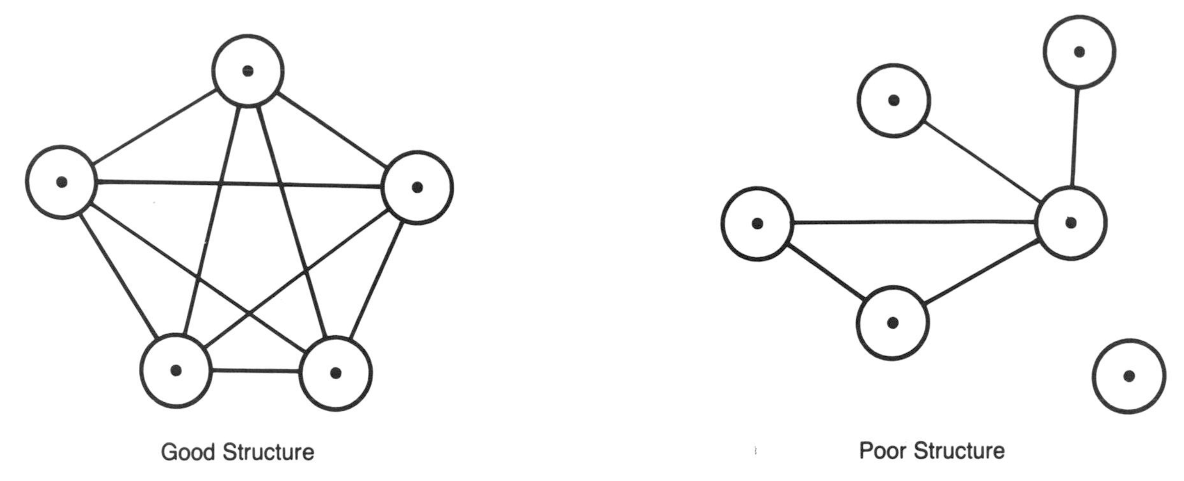

FIG. 20-1. The structure of theory. ●, Concepts; ○, definitions; —, postulates.

might then be awareness of others' needs and feelings, cooperation with others, ability to express ideas and feelings appropriately, taking appropriate group roles, and so forth.

A frame of reference may have one or several function-dysfunction continuums. Most frames of reference have more than one continuum, but no particular number is appropriate. The criterion for judging numerical adequacy is whether the continuums identify all of the component parts of the human function(s) to which the frame of reference is addressed.

When there is more than one continuum in a frame of reference, they should be relatively mutually exclusive and stated on the same conceptual level. The word relatively is emphasized here. An individual is a holistic entity. Although areas of human function are subdivided, this is done with full recognition that at the daily interaction level, each function influences the adequacy or inadequacy of all other functions. Relatively mutually exclusive refers to the definition of continuums in such a way that they have few characteristics in common. A negative example is activity neatness and attention to detail; these areas have many similar elements. A positive example is ability to cross the midline and eye-hand coordination.

All of the function-dysfunction continuums of a given frame of reference should be on the same conceptual level. For example, it is better to identify dimensions such as work habits, activities of daily living, and interpersonal skills as function-dysfunction continuums in a given frame of reference than to identify dimensions such as reality testing, ego strength, and impulse control. Work habits, activities of daily living, and interpersonal skills are fairly equal relative to conceptual level. Reality testing, ego strength, and impulse control are not on the same conceptual level: reality testing and impulse control are considered to be two of the several ego functions. They are thus subsumed under ego functions. Function-dysfunction continuums that are relatively mutually exclusive and stated on the same conceptual level greatly facilitate the process of evaluation and intervention.

Behavior Indicative of Function and Dysfunction

Behaviors indicative of function and dysfunction are essentially a listing of behaviors that serve to identify function and dysfunction relative to the continuums of a particular frame of reference. Collectively, they provide an operational definition of each continuum and serve as the basis for evaluation. To facilitate evaluation, behaviors indicative of function and dysfunction are stated in the most specific way possible. Ideally they are stated in such a way that they are at the level of direct observation. For example, "poor body schema" is not as specific as "unable to identify positions of body parts with vision occluded." The degree of specificity possible often depends on the continuums under consideration. Behaviors indicative of function and dysfunction tend to be closer to the level of observation in those frames of reference, for example, which deals with occupational performance than those addressed to psychological function.

Some frames of reference provide a listing of both behaviors indicative of function and behaviors indicative of dysfunction. Other frames of reference provide a listing of behaviors only relative to function or to dysfunction. In such a case the absence of behaviors indicative of function in an individual's repertoire is a sign of dysfunction. And conversely, the absence of behaviors indicative of dysfunction in an individual's repertoire is a sign of function in that particular area.

In most frames of reference one behavior alone is not sufficient to identify function or dysfunction. The presence or absence of a gestalt of behaviors provides the best basis for evaluation of dysfunction. In that function-dysfunction continuums are rarely entirely mutually exclusive, a particular behavior indicative of function or dysfunction may be listed under two or more continuums. For example, "minimal attention to personal hygiene" may be stated as being indicative of negative feelings about one's self or indicative of lack of skill in the area of self-care. Usually only by awareness of the gestalt of behaviors indicative of function and dysfunction is the therapist able to engage in accurate evaluation. Too much overlapping of behaviors indicative of function or dysfunction is, however, a sign that the continuums in the frame of reference are not sufficiently mutually exclusive and/or are not on the same conceptual level.

What is identified as dysfunction in one frame of reference may be described as behavior indicative of dysfunction in another frame of reference. For example, in one frame of reference anxiety regarding travel may be identified as a behavior indicative of unmet security needs. In another frame of reference anxiety regarding travel may be identified simply as an area of dysfunction. The goal of intervention in the aforementioned frame of reference may be to assist the client in identifying unconscious ideas relative to feelings of insecurity. The goal of intervention relative to the latter frame of reference would be to assist the client in learning how to travel without experiencing anxiety. Thus, what is dysfunction as opposed to behavior indicative of dysfunction varies from one frame of reference to another. The change process is directed toward minimizing dysfunction with the assumption that behavior indicative of dysfunction will gradually cease to be a part of the client's repertoire of behavior as the individual moves toward a state of function. In the interim, some behavior indicative of dysfunction, such as acute anxiety, may need to be managed. Behavior indicative of dysfunction is never directly dealt with in the change process.

Behavior indicative of function and dysfunction forms the conceptual framework for activity analysis and synthesis relative to designing evaluative situations. This process was outlined in some detail in Chapter 11. The evaluation process was discussed in Chapter 15. Therefore, neither of these topics will be discussed here. In some frames of reference, however, specific evaluative techniques are suggested. Ideally these techniques are described in such a manner that they can be duplicated by any therapist to elicit the desired behavior. The way in which the elicited behavior or findings are to be interpreted should also be provided. This, it must be emphasized, is the ideal. Most of the evaluation procedures one finds in frames of reference have some broad criterion for interpretation; however, it is also necessary to use a good deal of clinical judgment.

Postulates Regarding Change

Postulates regarding change are descriptive or prescriptive statements, deduced from the theoretical base, which state the principles by which an individual is assisted in moving from a state of dysfunction to a state of function. They state the nature, quality, quantity, and sequence of interactions with the human and nonhuman environments which are believed to facilitate change. Postulates regarding change also state principles that guide the therapist in selecting the short- and long-term goals, the step-by-step progression of intervention in each area of dysfunction, and the postulates applicable during each stage of intervention. The last information is usually included in one general postulate.

Postulates regarding change, then, serve as a guide to the therapist in designing an environment to promote change. They state the characteristics of appropriate activities, not specific activities. The role of postulates regarding change in relationship to activity analyses and syntheses was discussed in Chapter 11. Suffice it to say at this point that postulates regarding change are concerned with interactions relative to the human and nonhuman environment. Thus, in designing activities, the occupational therapist considers his or her interpersonal interactions with the client and interaction process relative to the nonhuman environment and the interplay between the two. The therapist never considers interpersonal relationships outside the context of the nonhuman environment or the nonhuman environment outside the context of interpersonal relationships. All activities then have an interpersonal component and a component of interaction with the nonhuman environment.

By convention, postulates regarding change are stated in a specific form. The beginning phrase or stem of a postulate states the area of function with which the postulate is concerned. The remaining portion of the postulate describes environmental interactions. Thus, a postulate such as "purposeful motor activity enhances the integration of sensory stimuli" is not acceptable because the area of function is stated at the end of the postulate. A more appropriately arranged postulate is "the ability to trust another human being is acquired through extensive interaction between two persons in which one individual receives consistent and relatively immediate need satisfaction, is not required to give any reciprocal satisfaction, and is free to engage in any behavior that is not destructive to the self or others." This convention was developed simply because a statement of function at the beginning of a postulate makes it easier for the reader to comprehend.

In a postulate regarding change, the area of function-dysfunction is usually stated in the positive. For example, a postulate beginning with the phrase "secondary process thinking is increased by . . ." is more acceptable than "primary process thinking is decreased by . . ." This convention is probably based on the belief of most practitioners that the development of adaptive behavior is far more important than simply diminishing maladaptive or dysfunctional behavior.

In addition, and perhaps far more important, a postulate regarding change is addressed to the nature of the external environment and not to what the client will somehow accomplish in an undefined manner. An example of a postulate that describes the external environment is "A more accurate self-concept is acquired through feedback from others regarding the individual's capacity to engage in a variety of different kinds of activities." An example of a postulate addressed to what the client will do is "A more accurate self-concept is acquired through understanding of one's assets and limitations." The point to be made is that postulates regarding change are articulated to guide the therapist in synthesizing or designing activities that will facilitate the development of function. The second postulate stated above does not provide such guidance.

Postulates regarding change may be general or specific. A general postulate applies to a number of or all the continuums identified in a particular frame of reference. A specific postulate applies to one continuum. The following examples illustrate these two types of postulates:

1. A general postulate. Perception in a given sensory system is enhanced by general sensory stimulation which is sufficiently intense to be received by the central nervous system yet does not cause overarousal.

2. A specific postulate. Development of occular control is facilitated by encouraging the client to focus on stationary and moving objects both within the central field of vision and peripheral to the central field of vision.

The first postulate relates to the integration of sensory stimuli regardless of the particular sensory system under consideration. The second postulate is concerned with ocular control, which is only one aspect of sensory integration.

Some frames of reference have only general postulates regarding change, others have only specific postulates, and still others may have both types. The types of postulates contained within a given frame of reference are relatively unimportant. What is important is that the postulates are deduced from the theoretical base and adequately describe or prescribe the process of change relative to the continuums to which the frame of reference is addressed.

In summary, the structure of a frame of reference consists of a theoretical base, function-dysfunction continuums, behaviors indicative of function and dysfunction, and postulates regarding change. There are a variety of different frames of reference in occupational therapy. This variety provides for professional viability and choice on the part of practitioners. The common structure of frames of reference facilitates communication. Even in the midst of disagreement there is at least a shared language.

RELATIONSHIP TO THE OCCUPATIONAL THERAPY MODEL

In general, frames of reference are deduced from the model of the profession (75,341,457,572,666,716,780, 828,861,892,1036). In other words, the theoretical base of a frame of reference draws on various systems that are part of the body of knowledge of the profession. The function-dysfunction continuums are an elaboration of one or more aspects of the profession's domain of concern. The tools suggested in a frame of reference consist of one or more of the tools considered legitimate by the profession. Frames of reference that are not deduced from the profession's model are considered to be, at best, irregular or eccentric. Individuals who use frames of reference that deviate significantly from the parameters of the profession's model are usually subject to formal or informal sanctions by the profession.

As indicated, the above statement is generally true, but not always. Frames of reference sometimes begin to be used in occupational therapy prior to their theoretical base being a part of the recognized body of knowledge of the profession or their continuums part of the domain of concern. They often are developed out of practice, with the theoretical system on which they are based being either taken from a discipline or another profession or formulated at the same time. The only real relationship they have to the model of the profession is that they are, in a very broad sense, compatible with the philosophical assumptions and parameters of the profession. These tentative frames of reference, ideally, are subjected to evaluation through well-planned research. The two major research questions addressed are "Does intervention based on this frame of reference result in positive change on the part of the client?" and "In what setting and/or with what group of clients is application of this frame of reference most effective?" It should be noted that this type of research is not directly concerned with testing the theoretical system on which the frame of reference is based. Only the effectiveness of the frame of reference is being assessed. When the effectiveness of a frame of reference has been documented at least to some extent, the theoretical system on which it is based usually becomes part of the body of knowledge of the profession and the continuums part of its domain of concern. The frame of reference is added to the profession's collection of recognized frames of reference. This, as mentioned, is the ideal. Frames of reference have been accepted by the profession based on intuitive feelings that a given frame of reference is good and works and/or simply through widespread use. In other words, acceptance is based on belief rather than empirical testing. Acceptance of a frame of reference on the basis of shared belief only is primarily due to the embryonic state of the professions' collective knowledge about and skill in research methodology. This deficit is now in the process of being remedied as more and more occupational therapists are completing advanced professional programs of study.

Frames of reference, then, in actuality become part of the profession in two different ways. They are derived from the model of the profession, or they are developed almost in a peripheral manner, ultimately being accepted by the profession.

The differences between frames of reference and the model of the profession, perhaps, at this point need some clarification. They differ in three ways: magnitude, universality of acceptance, and degree of guidance.

In relationship to magnitude, a model defines and gives boundaries to a profession in its totality. A particular frame of reference, on the other hand, gives boundaries to a small aspect of the profession's body of knowledge and domain of concern. Models are broad in focus whereas frames of references are limited and narrow in focus.

A model, as mentioned in Chapter 1, is accepted almost universally by the profession and by the society to which the profession is responsible. A given frame of reference is often only accepted by a limited number of practitioners within a profession. For example, in occupational therapy, only some practitioners accept King's frame of reference regarding sensory integration as an appropriate guide for intervention relative to clients diagnosed as schizophrenic. A model, because it is more generally stated, tends to engender far less disharmony. Frames of reference, being more specific and transient, often tend to become the focus for considerable professional disagreement. However, such conflict also may lead to clarification of concepts and productive research. This in turn, enhances the model of a profession.

Third, a model defines the profession. A frame of reference guides the practitioner in the immediacy of day-to-day interaction with clients. A model offers no principles that describe or prescribe evaluation and the change process in any specific kind of way. A model is, essentially, simply a reservoir of the collective beliefs, knowledge, and skills of the profession. A frame of reference tells the practitioner how to use or apply a portion of that knowledge and skill to enhance the function of clients.

Finally, the concept of frame of reference, the idea that we need a linking structure between theory and practice, is by no means universally accepted by the profession. There are three major reasons for lack of acceptance:

1. There are those who do not like the constraints of a frame of reference. They prefer a less structured, often referred to as an eclectic, approach to the change process. The need to define the process and to be able to articulate a theoretical rationale for that process is seen as unnecessary. Working within the constraints of a frame of reference is viewed as diminishing the client's individuality and the therapist's spontaneous, intuitive response.
2. There are those who feel that frames of reference, as they presently exist in the profession, are too narrow and application too complex. Frames of reference are considered to be narrow in the sense that they are often applicable to only one aspect of the client's deficit in functioning and not to the multiple problems presented by many clients. Thus, one must often use more than one frame of reference simultaneously or sequentially. This is seen as a highly complex enterprise. These individuals would prefer frames of reference to be far broader in scope.
3. On a more philosophical level, there are those who object to the diversity that is exemplified in the idea of frames of reference. These are individuals who seek a comprehensive theory of occupational therapy. Their assumption is that once we have a comprehensive theory that covers all aspects of client care, a variety of frames of reference will be unnecessary. Another assumption

seems to be that a comprehensive theory will be so stated and that it will be immediately applicable as a guide to practice. Thus, there will be no need for a linking structure between theory and practice.

With all of the objections to the concept and idea of frames of reference, there is no evidence that frames of reference will become a permanent part of the configuration of occupational therapy. However, until redefined, replaced, or rendered obsolete, it appears that frames of reference are part of the profession for the time being.

With this orientation to the nature, structure, and function of frames of reference, the various types of frames of reference and specific frames of reference will be discussed in the following chapters.

21 Analytical Frames of Reference

DESCRIPTION

Analytical frames of reference provide a structure for linking psychoanalytic theories, the symbolic potential and reality aspects of activities, and the process of altering intrapsychic content in the direction of providing a more adaptive basis for interaction with the environment (290,307,317,427,492,646,705,711,969). The assumptions fundamental to analytical frames of reference are:

1. Intrapsychic content is the major factor which influences behavior;
2. Intrapsychic content can best be altered by bringing it to a point where it can be examined and evaluated in the context of a shared reality;
3. Repeated interactions in situations that elicit intrapsychic conflicts, with adequate guidance, facilitate conflict resolution and the addition of new, more adaptive intrapsychic content.

The above, rather lengthy definition, more than likely needs some elaboration. Psychoanalytic theories constitute a body of knowledge formulated by Freud, with elaboration and modifications by many of his followers. Central to this body of knowledge are the concepts of unconscious motivation, conflict, and symbolism. The theories are concerned with many aspects of the human experience. The three major areas of concern are psychodynamics, states of psychosexual and psychosocial development, and the process whereby intrapsychic content is altered. It is important to note here that psychoanalytic theories of development are used as a means of understanding needs and characteristic ways of achieving need satisfaction in various stages of development. They are not used as the basis for assisting a client to experience the stages of development sequentially. This process may be part of a developmental frame of reference. Finally, there are many shades and varieties of psychoanalytic theories. Thus, a frame of reference based, for example, on Sullivanian theory will be somewhat different than that based on Jungian theory.

In analytical frames of reference purposeful activities are viewed as being concerned with action, its role in communicating intrapsychic content, and the use of such nonverbal communication for the benefit of the client. The symbolic potential of activities—the actions, the objects used in the action process as well as those that result from the action, and the interpersonal relations that influence the action and are in turn influenced by it—is emphasized. Activities are considered to (a) have inherent characteristics that elicit expression of specific intrapsychic content, (b) serve as the basis for a shared reality, and (c) provide an experiential laboratory that facilitates the intrajection of new intrapsychic content.

Relative to the occupational therapy domain of concern, analytic frames of reference are addressed to psychological function. (Some aspects of social interaction are occasionally included). Frames of reference other than analytical are also addressed to this performance component considered in analytical frames of reference.

Intrapsychic content refers to ideas, feelings, needs, and values. The content of most concern in analytical frames of reference is, first, that which is unconscious, preconscious, and that which is conscious but not readily, if ever, shared with other people. Second, analytical frames of reference deal with aspects of intrapsychic content that are in conflict—the simultaneous activation of opposing or mutually exclusive impulses, desires, or tendencies. An example would be a felt need and a particular set of values which prohibits satisfaction of the need.

It is assumed that intrapsychic content is the major factor influencing behavior. In other words, how one thinks and feels, i.e., one's internal experiences, are far more consequential than environmental factors or specific learned responses in selecting a course of action or engaging in particular kinds of behaviors. This is in contrast to developmental and acquisitional frames of reference in which environmental influences and/or one's repertoire of behavior is seen as far more influential than internal experience. The totality of an individual's intrapsychic content is, however, considered to be strongly influenced by life experiences. How a person thinks and feels about himself and others is believed to be a result of past interactions with others. This belief or assumption, however, is only in part used as the basis for the change process.

In regard to the change process, analytical frames of reference describe (a) how intrapsychic content is brought to the point where the client is able to share it on the verbal level and (b) the process whereby intrapsychic content is altered in some way so that the client is able to reject it or deal with it more effectively. The latter, often referred to as "working through" is the process of having the client experience the same intrapsychic conflicts over and over again, with the help of the therapist, until the client can independently face and master the conflicts in ordinary life. It is the process of repeatedly experiencing the effects of maladaptive intrapsychic content on one's behavior while concurrently formulating a more adaptive way of perceiving one's self, other people, and the events of daily life.

The two parts of the change process—the sharing of intrapsychic content and working through—are considered to be a necessary sequence of events. One part of the sequence without the other is not believed to be conducive to permanent change. In other words, the sharing or communication of intrapsychic content is not considered to be sufficient. An individual can often rather easily talk about ideas, feelings, values, and needs and not make any attempt to alter those that are in conflict or are maladaptive. This is an example of the familiar colloquialism "all talk and no action." On the other hand, trying to face and master conflicts in ordinary life without understanding the nature of the conflict is usually either unsuccessful or leads to the development of a splinter skill. The latter refers to the learning of a pattern of behavior by rote. A pattern so learned tends to be divorced from the individual's feelings and sense of identity and often has a hollow, unnatural quality. It also demands considerable thought and effort. Intrapsychic conflicts that have been adequately shared and worked through eventually lead to patterns of behavior that are spontaneous, require little conscious effort, and are felt to be very much a part of the self.

Analytical frames of reference are concerned with intrapsychic content. Lack of skill in various areas of human function is considered to be a sign of maladaptive or conflicting intrapsychic content; it is considered to be behavior indicative of dysfunction. The change process is directed toward alteration of intrapsychic content. It is assumed that skills needed for productive interaction in the community will spontaneously be learned or relearned after the resolution of conflict or the introjection of more adaptive intrapsychic content. This is quite a different orientation than one finds in developmental or acquisitional frames of reference. In both of these types of frames of reference, lack of skill development in various areas of human function is the primary area of concern. Intrapsychic conflict or maladaptive content, if mentioned at all, is identified as a result of lack of skill in one or more areas; it is behavior indicative of dysfunction. The change process in developmental and acquisitional frames of reference is directed toward acquiring skills in various aspects of human function. It is assumed that problems relative to intrapsychic content will disappear spontaneously with the acquisition of skills.

It has been found, however, that the assumptions just outlined are not compatible with the behavior of all clients. Alteration of interpsychic content does not always lead to the spontaneous learning or relearning of skills, and the development of particular skills for living does not always spontaneously lead to alteration of intrapsychic content. Thus, in the change process an analytical frame of reference may be combined with a developmental or acquisitional frame of reference, the latter being more typical. Usually an analytical frame of reference is used as the basis for the change process initially followed by the use of an acquisitional frame of reference. However, they may also be used simultaneously. When used either sequentially or simultaneously, it is important for the therapist to be aware of which is being used when. The postulates regarding change for these two frames of reference are very different. Thus the activities used, the way they are used, and the therapist's interactions with the client are all very different.

The theoretical base of an analytical frame of reference, in general, describes the individual as continually striving for need fulfillment, expression of primitive impulses, and control of inherent drives. In the usual course of events, the individual acquires a value system that allows him or her to meet needs, express impulses, and control drives in a manner that is both satisfying to the self and acceptable within the norms of the individual's cultural group. This process occurs because through acceptance of the norms of one's cultural group, the individual is accepted as a full-fledged member of the group and thus receives all the rewards commensurate with such membership. At the same time this process is occurring, the individual selectively internalizes a relatively accurate set of ideas about him- or herself, other people, and the world in general.

This process, however, does not always occur in the manner outlined above. There are many reasons for this, the primary one being a less than optimal environment for growth. For whatever reason, the individual may experience needs, drives, and impulses as being in conflict with each other, with the reality of the environment, or with the value system. Such conflictual experiences tend to arouse anxiety, which in turn leads to repression of the conflict. The individual either pushes these conflicts out of consciousness, or remains aware of the conflict but does not share it with others. However the individual deals with conflict, it still tends to influence behavior. Likewise, the individual may selectively internalize a set of ideas about him- or herself, other people, or the world in general which are woefully inaccurate and maladaptive. These ideas tend to be dealt with in the same manner as conflicts and also tend to influence behavior.

The theoretical base of an analytical frame of reference also describes the symbolic potential of activities, their capacity for facilitating the communication or sharing of intrapsychic content, and the way in which they can be used in the process of working through. The theoretical base also describes how change is brought about. In addition, such processes as exploration of intrapsychic content, testing the validity of intrapsychic content, insight, free or guided associations, interpretations, and transference are also usually described.

Function-dysfunction continuums are sometimes not well defined in analytical frames of reference, and they are frequently not mutually exclusive. The reason for this is that intrapsychic content rarely comes in neat little packages. It tends to be interrelated, lacking in any apparent order, and without firm boundaries. This is the nature of intrapsychic content, especially that which is unconscious and has nothing to do with dysfunction per se. When specified, function-dysfunction continuums may focus on:

1. Conflicts believed to be typical of various states of development, e.g., oral, anal, genital, latency, phallic;
2. Conflict areas unrelated to developmental states such as love, hate, aggression, sexuality, autonomy, trust, and death and loss;
3. Maladaptive intrapsychic content such as inaccurate ideas about oneself and other people.

Behavior indicative of dysfunction, in general, is any behavior that cannot be explained, given the realities of the situation, and/or any behavior that is causing the individual to be uncomfortable with the self or with other people. The link between disordered behavior and the nature of the individual's dysfunctional intrapsychic content is made through the use of a system of psychodynamics. As previously defined, psychodynamics is any of several systematic means of explaining the relationship between the individual's past and present environment, intrapsychic content, and behavior. This process is discussed in some detail in Chapter 3 in the section on psychological function. More specifically, the nature of the client's intrapsychic content is evaluated through study and understanding of past history, current behavior, and symbolic communication.

Postulates regarding change in an analytical frame of reference tend to be less specific than in the other two types of frames of reference. One of the major reasons for this is that the change process tends to be cyclical in nature, with much repetition of sharing, making association, interpretations, the development of insight and working through. This is in contrast to developmental frames of reference where the process is far more likely to be linear. The other major reason for nonspecificity is that there is considerable variation in what may occur in a given intervention session with a client. At times, for example, when the focus of a session is to be working through, events may transpire so that it would be far more appropriate to focus on sharing intrapsychic content or on reality testing.

Postulates regarding change in analytical frames of reference also tend to be vague in regard to the setting of goals. No guidelines for sequential goals are usually provided. The change process usually begins, then, in an area in which the client and therapist agree is causing difficulty. From there the change process usually evolves and is addressed to contingent or very different areas. This lack of well-defined goals does present some difficulty in periodic reassessment and for determining an appropriate point of termination. Identifying progress and a time for the end of the change process tends to be somewhat subjective. It is frequently based on how the client feels about him- or herself and on the degree of comfort in environmental interactions.

The use of an analytic frame of reference is appropriate with clients who show evidence of intrapsychic conflict or maladaptive intrapsychic content because of past faulty experiences in interactions in the environment or with clients who have experienced a marked alteration in their life situation. The latter may occur, for example, when an individual suddenly becomes disabled, when there is a serious loss, such as the death of a spouse, or when an individual moves into a very different culture. Individuals who have experienced a great change in their life situation may well have had no difficulty in the past situation; their intrapsychic content was quite adaptive. It is adjustment to the new situation that is causing them difficulty. Thus the individual may need to acquire a more appropriate set of ideas about him- or herself and perhaps about other people and the world in general. A marked alteration in life situation may also bring to the fore some past unresolved conflicts such as those related to independence or loss. Analytical frames of reference are particularly applicable for helping the individual deal with such conflicts.

Finally, participation in a change process based on an analytic frame of reference requires a fairly high degree of cognitive function, verbal skill, and psychological sophistication. Regarding cognitive function, the individual needs to have at least an average intelligence quotient and be able to use secondary process thinking. The capacity to engage in a moderate amount of problem solving is also necessary. Although analytical frames of reference make use of a considerable amount of nonveral communication, the content of such communication must, at some point, be verbalized. In other words, the content must be brought to the level wherein it becomes sharable, i.e., the level at which it can be discussed, explored, and subjected to validation in a shared reality. This requires verbal skills as it is only on this plane of discourse that the necessary type of sharing can take place. In the initial phase of the change process, the client need not be particularly verbal. However, in attempting to use an analytical frame of reference, the therapist should have some sense that the client possesses the capacity to engage in a meaningful verbal exchange. Psychological sophistication refers to the client's ability to recognize that one's ideas, feelings, values, and needs, to some degree at least, influence behavior. Without this recognition, the client is unlikely to be interested or engage in a change process that is based on an analytical frame of reference. The client is likely to feel that the therapist has taken leave of his senses, or at best, is insensitive to the client's needs and cultural background. The therapist is likely to be very frustrated. A change process based on an analytical frame of reference is not, therefore, suitable to all clients. When used as a guide for change with a client who is able to participate and when it is used by a knowledgeable and skilled therapist, an analytical frame of reference is a very powerful tool.

With this general description of analytical frames of reference, the remaining portion of the chapter is devoted to a discussion of the two analytic frames of reference currently used in occupational therapy: The Fidlers' and Object Relations Analysis.

REVIEW OF THE ANALYTICAL ORIENTATION

The Fidlers

This discussion of the Fidlers' orientation to the occupational therapy process is derived from their book, *Occupational Therapy: A Communication Process in Psychiatry* (290). Although they have elaborated on some of the ideas in this book, they have not presented, in writing, any complete revision of their orientation. In this discussion emphasis is placed on that part of their text which is primarily concerned with the change process and which is based on psychoanalytic theory.

The Fidlers' orientation is the first frame of reference formulated after the sterile period of the symptomatic approach (outlined in Chapter 2). As such it still has some of the flavor of that approach. The Fidlers write from a period when the medical model was still used as the basis for describing the occupational therapy process. In addition, the three types of frames of reference now used in occupational therapy had not been clearly defined nor had the five types of intervention been identified and differentiated. Finally, the Fidlers do not use the structure of a frame of reference to describe their orientation. This is understandable as the need for a link between theory and application had not yet been recognized. Because of the factors outlined above, the Fidlers' orientation is somewhat difficult to describe in the more current language of the occupational therapy model. As in any translation and in one that, by necessity, is greatly abridged, a considerable amount of the content will not be discussed and much of the richness and subtlety of their orientation will be lost. It is therefore suggested that the reader study *Occupational Therapy: A Communication Process in Psychiatry*. In the interim, the following is a summary and discussion of their orientation.

The Fidlers' work is primarily based on the psychoanalytical approach of Henry Stack Sullivan. Concerning a dynamic theory of change, Sullivan, although using somewhat different terminology, is fairly closely related to the traditional psychoanalytical school. There is, however, one major exception. Sullivan felt that, at times, the gratification of infantile needs could be necessary in order for an individual, chronologically beyond the infantile stages, to advance to more mature stages of interaction. Gratification of needs, as used by Sullivan, does not fall within the parameters of an analytical frame of reference. Rather it is one of the hallmarks of a developmental approach. Sullivan, thus, was in part psychoanalytically oriented and in part developmentally oriented—a combination of approaches which are compatible only when clearly distinguished from each other and their interrelationship specifically defined. Sullivan does not do this well and neither do the Fidlers. Lack of clarification concerning the differences between analytical and developmental approaches has led to considerable confusion in occupational therapy.

The Fidlers' approach differentiates between treatment, mental health processes, and rehabilitation. Treatment is considered to be concerned with the "elimination of pathology and as such is concerned with the illness of the patient" (287, p. 24). The Fidlers' reliance on the medical model is quite evident here in the terminology used. Treatment is divided into three categories:

1. "The psychoanalytic approach places primary emphasis on the unconscious, exploring the unconscious needs, drives and conflicts of the patient and resolving these by means of awareness and understanding within the therapeutic relationship" (287, p.24). This approach is the traditional psychoanalytic orientation.
2. "The supportive approach recognizes the significance of the unconscious phenomenon and helps the patient to gratify his needs by sublimation. It deals with conflicts by establishing constructive defenses rather than by exploring and uncovering" (287, p.25). This approach is primarily concerned with need gratification whether it be direct, in a symbolic manner, or through sublimation.
3. "The directive or repressive approach uses the patient's existing ego integration to repress unacceptable feelings and behavior... through structures and a relationship which is supportive and which requires appropriate behavior" (287, p. 25). This approach is really quite close if not the same as management as described in Chapter 17.

Although a distinction is made between these three types of treatment in the beginning of the text, they are not differentiated either in the discussion of evaluation or of intervention. They are blended together in some combination apparently relative to the needs of a particular client and/or the emphasis of the clinical facility. Guidelines for this blending are not specified. The psychoanalytic approach as described by the Fidlers is similar in many respects to the change process as defined in this chapter. It will, thus, be the primary focus of this section.

Before proceeding, however, the Fidlers identify two other aspects to their approach: mental health processes and rehabilitation.

> Mental health processes may be defined as those methodologies that are directed towards developing and sustaining an environment and culture based on the inherent worth and integrity of the human being. Such concepts recognize man's need for love, acceptance and a sense of belonging and his need to share with others and to perceive himself as a productive contributing member of society (287, p.25).

As described, "mental health processes" are essentially identical to "meeting health needs" as that aspect of intervention was discussed in Chapter 17.

> Rehabilitation may be defined as those efforts and procedures that are directed towards helping the patient to learn to use more effectively his existing integrative capacities and his assets and abilities towards developing and refining skills that will enable him to assume appropriate economic and social responsibilities outside of the hospital (287, p.27).

This definition of rehabilitation and its placement outside of treatment is derived from the medical model. In that model, treatment is considered to be the elimination of pathology whereas rehabilitation involves dealing with sequelae or the residual effects of a pathological process. The occupational therapy model makes no such distinction; it does not make use of the concepts of either pathology or sequelae. Second, as used by the Fidlers, rehabilitation is based on an acquisitional not an analytic orientation, although this is not clearly stated in their book. Third, no frame of reference is provided for rehabilitation, it is only discussed in the most general of terms. In that rehabilitation appears to be acquisitional in orientation and no frame of reference is provided, it is not discussed further here.

To return to the Fidlers' description of the psychoanalytic orientation, the following discussion summarizes their ideas using the structure of a frame of reference. As mentioned, this is not the structure used by the Fidlers.

The Fidlers emphasize the following concepts in their *theoretical base*:

1. Communication is seen as the essence of the occupational therapy process—the process and end product of activities allowing the individual to communicate thoughts and feelings they cannot communicate on a verbal level. Inability to communicate effectively, to put subjective thoughts and feelings into words, is seen as the core problem from which other difficulties in psychosocial functions arise.

2. The role of the unconscious is seen as very important, particularly in relationship to how it influences behavior. Knowledge of psychodynamics is considered necessary for understanding both behavior and activities. The formation of symbols, a process that takes place unconsciously, is also considered important.

3. Object relations, particularly how it relates to the nonhuman environment, is emphasized. Only positive or libidinal object relationships are discussed. Negative or aggressive object relationships are implied but not specifically identified as such.

4. The importance of interpersonal relationships in the change process is noted. This includes both the dyadic relationship between client and therapist and the client's interactions in groups. Although many aspects of interpersonal relationships are discussed, particular mention is made relative to the role of reality testing and consensual validation in the change process.

5. Activities are described in much detail. Particular attention is given to the symbolic potential of activities and their capacity to (a) allow for the expression of feelings, ideas and thoughts that cannot be expressed verbally; (b) provide an opportunity for reality testing; and (c) allow the individual to work through previously unconscious conflicts.

Finally, the Fidlers describe two interrelated sequences regarding the change process. One is that doing, or appropriate activities, leads to thinking, which leads to verbalization, which leads to awareness, which in turn leads to the integration of previously unshared or unconscious content with conscious content. The other sequence is described as follows: "As particular needs and problems are worked through various aspects of the occupational therapy experience will assume varying degrees of importance, i.e., gratification of infantile needs, vs. reality testing vs. re-establishment of defenses" (287, p.119).

The major problems with the Fidlers' theoretical base are that concepts are not well defined and occasionally different labels or terms are used for the same concept. Concepts tend to be loosely connected rather than interrelated in clearly stated postulates. The boundaries of the frame of reference are not well delineated; there is little said about for whom it is applicable or the limitations under which it is proposed. The goals of the change process are not specifically stated.

About *function-dysfunction continuums* the Fidlers speak of five areas of concern:

> 1. Concept of Self: To assess how the patient perceives himself and how he functions within this concept. The nature of his body image, identification, self-esteems, etc.
>
> 2. Concept of Other: How he perceives others and how he may expect to relate to others. What expectations he has concerning relationships, how he views authority and peers; what interpersonal distortions exist; and how he behaves in relationship to these.
>
> 3. Ego Organization: The nature and extent of his capacity for reality testing, the validity of his perceptions and the nature and degree of his capacity to organize, control, predict, follow through, etc. The extent of his recognition of the real-unreal of the me-not me and the quality of his defenses.
>
> 4. Unconscious Conflicts: A delineation of areas of unconscious conflict, of frustrated basic needs and drives, of conflicting impulses and needs and areas of functioning that generate anxiety, elicit defenses, etc.
>
> 5. Communication: The nature and manner of communicating feelings and thoughts, the nature and extent of verbal and nonverbal communication, his use of symbols, effectiveness of communication, areas of difficulty, etc. (287, p.103).

The continuums are deduced from the theoretical base, are mutually exclusive, and stated on the same conceptual level. The five areas are quite broad with several subareas mentioned. The latter should perhaps be considered the continuums rather than the five labeled areas. The use of etcetera following the stated subarea implies that there are other subareas. It is unclear as to what these might be.

The Fidlers do not give any specific listing of behaviors indicative of function and dysfunction. An "Outline for Evaluation" is provided. It consists of three major categories: relationship to the therapist, relationship to the group, and relationship to the activity. In each category a series of questions are listed. Under relationship to the activity, for example, the following questions are presented: "What are the characteristics of the activity the patient selects?;" "How does the patient respond to and deal with the realistic and/or symbolic characteristics of the activity?;" "What feelings are expressed in the content and in the way he handles the material, the process?" At the conclusion of the questions there are two lists of terms. One of behavioral characteristics such as aggressive, infantile, rigid, and so forth. The other delineates defense mechanisms such as denial, projection, and intellectualization. No evaluative tools are described, although obviously some type of activity is used in the evaluation process.

The relationship between the "Outline for Evaluation" and the continuums is not clearly stated. The Fidlers simply say that the therapist makes interpretations to arrive at some evaluative statements concerning each of the continuums. The need for knowledge about oneself and an understanding of psychodynamics are emphasized in order to make accurate interpretations. No other guidelines for evaluation are provided.

The Fidlers do not present any *postulates regarding change*. They do provide three case examples of how occupational therapy may be used in the change process. The examples are compatible with the theoretical base and the continuums.

The Fidlers do discuss activities in general and provide an "Outline for Activity Analysis." This is divided into 17 categories, with several questions being listed in each category. The categories are motion, procedures, materials, and equipment, creativity and originality, symbols, hostility and aggressiveness, destructiveness, control, predictability, narcissism, sexual identification, independence, and group relatedness. The Outline is not specific to the continuums and there are no guidelines for activity synthesis. In another chapter, the Fidlers discuss the utilization of activities. They describe some characteristics of activities which they believe are helpful for dealing with specific areas. The areas discussed are (a) self-concept and identity, (b) sexual identification, (c) infantile oral and anal needs, (d) dependency, (e) hostility, (f) reality testing, and (g) communication. These areas are only in part similar to the function-dysfunction continuums as described above.

This is the weakest part of the Fidlers' frame of reference; there are no real guidelines for planning or implementing a change process. Without additional information and good supervision, it would be very difficult to apply this frame of reference.

Object Relation Analysis

Object relations (705) as used in this frame of reference identify the process wherein the individual becomes attached to or invests in objects—people, things, and ideas—that satisfy needs. Through exploration of the satisfaction of needs and factors interfering with that satisfaction, the individual comes to know himself more completely and is therefore better able to satisfy his own needs and those of others. The frame of reference is described as being applicable to those individuals who are experiencing serious difficulties in living and also as one means of enhancing the function of any individual.

The theoretical base of object relations analysis is formulated out of various theories. Those used most extensively are Maslow, Freud, Jung, the Azimas, Arieti, and Naumberg. Jung's ideas are perhaps most influential, particularly, in terms of the frames of reference's general tone or mood. The major concepts used in the theoretical base are:

1. Needs, drives, and objects—These concepts are defined separately and their interrelationship is described in terms of object relations as outlined in Chapter 3.

2. Affect—An inner, subjective experience that may or may not be expressed. It is the feeling or emotion one experiences relative to objects.

3. Will—The will is defined as the individual's capacity to select a specific course of action. The individual is seen not as driven by internal forces but as a being that has the capacity to make choices. Needs are described as providing motivation for action. The will accounts for the selection and investment of libidinal and aggressive energy in appropriate objects.

4. Attending and the formation of complexes—Attending is the term used to identify the whole spectrum of consciousness: conscious, preconscious, personal unconscious, and collective unconscious. A complex is a gestalt of repressed affect, energy, and intrapsychic content associated with some type of conflict. The process leading to the formation of complexes is described.

5. Cognition—This is similar to the description of cognition as discussed in Chapter 3.

6. Symbolism—As used in this frame of reference, symbolism is similar to the definition and discussion in Chapter 10.

The interrelationships of the concepts outlined above are identified as:

> 1. The behavior of man is described in terms of a dynamic balance between needs, drives, affect, cognitive processes and the will;
>
> 2. Through the interrelationship of these inherent elements, man relates to objects in such a way as to realize his unique potential;
>
> 3. This relationship, however, is rarely perfectly tuned, and imbalance leads to inattention to aspects of the self and the environment. Some of these aspects or complexes are actively relegated to the unconscious; other complexes are not allowed to emerge from the unconscious. It is these unconscious complexes which interfere with self actualization;
>
> 4. Man has also acquired the capacity to make contact with these split-off, unknown parts of the self and to integrate them with the conscious self. Phylogenesis has endowed man with the cognitive processes of symbol formation and conceptual thinking. Through the use of these processes, in conjunction with his other inherent elements, man is able to correct the imbalance between that which is conscious and that which is unconscious and thus continue towards self-actualization" (705, p.37).

The major problem with the theoretical base of this frame of reference is the lack of a dynamic theory. The change process is only alluded to and not really discussed in any detail. In addition, the goal of the frame of reference, self-actualization, is not well-described; it is most certainly not operationally defined.

Dysfunction is described as the presence of one or more complexes that are interfering with the individual's ability to seek and obtain need gratification. Twenty-five complexes, each constituting a continuum, are listed. They are as follows:

1. Feelings of inferiority
2. Differentiation from the nonhuman environment
3. Trust in one's fellow man
4. Control of sexual impulses
5. Emotional separation from one's parents
6. Establishing mature love relationships
7. Finding one's place as a contributing member of a social system
8. Selecting a guiding system of values
9. Physiological and psychological changes
10. Inevitability of death
11. Perception of the self as an unacceptable object
12. Lack of gratification of safety needs
13. Lack of gratification of love and acceptance needs
14. Lack of gratification of esteem needs
15. Investment of aggressive energy in the self
16. Free-floating libidinal energy
17. Free-floating aggressive energy
18. Threatened emergence of unconscious content
19. Acceptance of the shadow side (unacceptable aspects of the self)
20. Animus and anima (the opposite sex characteristics of the self)
21. Relatedness to the nonhuman environment
22. Thinking function superior (concerned with logic and objectivity)
23. Feeling function superior (adjustment is based on the value placed on or judgments made about people and events)
24. Sensation function superior (adjustment is primarily through sensory processes and sensual experiences)
25. Intuition function superior (adjustment through identification of possibilities, acts on the basis of premonitions)

Aside from the fact that there seems to be an extraordinary number of continuums, there is little gradation implied. Some of the continuums are not mutually exclusive, such as "feelings of inferiority" and "perception of the self as an unacceptable object." The continuums may not appear to be on the same conceptual level, nevertheless they are if one remembers that the labels used designate a gestalt of unconscious affect, energy, and ideas that are associated with a conflict.

Each of the continuums are followed by a list of behaviors indicative of functions and dysfunction. In the interest of space, two examples will have to suffice:

"Thinking Function Superior
a. analyzes the situation and arrives at specific conclusions
b. able to bring order out of confusion
c. emphasis upon objectivity, logical thought processes
d. comfortable with theoretical material, abstract ideas
e. minimal evidence of other functions
f. symbols which refer to consciousness
g. difficulty in expressing feelings regarding productions
h. cool colors
i. emphasis on head of reproduced human figure

Feeling Function Superior
a. feelings finely differentiated and given close attention
b. able to evaluate objects relative to their positive and negative aspects and acceptance of both aspects
c. avoids negative thoughts
d. relates well to people
e. sees the value or importance of what should be done and goes ahead and does it
f. sets standards
g. minimal evidence of other functions
h. symbols which refer to emotionality
i. verbalizes about productions primarily in terms of feelings
j. warm colors (red, yellow)" (705, p. 68).

Suggested tools for evaluation are an interview and the Fidler Battery. The latter is described in Chapter 16. The interview suggested is similar to the general interview outlined in this text, again in Chapter 16.

The behaviors indicative of function and dysfunction are somewhat overlapping but not so extensively that differentiation between most of the continuums can be made. The behaviors to be used for assessment are compatible with the suggested evaluative tools. The behaviors are sufficiently specific that they provide guidelines for interpretation and for identifying the various complexes that are apparently disturbing the client. The therapist, obviously, must be fairly facile in the interpretation of symbols.

Postulates Regarding Change

The following postulates are given:

1. Complexes are identified and brought to consciousness through affectual-cognitive exploration of symbols produced by the individual relative to his past, current and future situation.
2. They are integrated into consciousness through conceptual representation and secondary process organization of the complex content.
3. With integration into consciousness, psychic energy previously invested in the complex is freed and available for use in need satisfaction.
4. The information gained through integration of unconscious content therefore becomes available to guide willful selection of appropriate or substitute objects for need satisfaction.
5. Exploration and integration of complexes is facilitated by reproduction of symbols originally produced in dreams

> and wakeful fantasy, the production of exocept, motoric and image symbols in the use of art media and the companionship of a knowledgable and empathetic guide (705, p.70).

Postulates 2, 3, and 4 are deduced from the theoretical base, but they do not provide guidelines as to how to design an environment that will facilitate change. Rather, they describe what happens relative to the individual. Thus, these are really not postulates regarding change. Postulates 1 and 5 are concerned with the change process. They are, however, extremely vague and alone do not provide sufficient guidance for planning or implementing a change process. There is an additional section of the frame of reference which discusses the change process in somewhat more detail. Although not presented as postulates regarding change, the following areas are discussed:

- Factors that need to be taken into consideration in the exploration of symbols;
- The role of cognition in the integration of the content of symbols with conscious content;
- Types of suitable activities (primarily art media) and how these may be used;
- The role of the therapist as a knowledgeable companion and guide in the change process;
- Suggestions in regard to giving interpretations to the client.

None of these areas except for cognition are discussed in the theoretical base. Notably lacking in the frame of reference is any reference to the process of working through. It is occasionally alluded to but never discussed. Although Object Relation Analysis provides somewhat better guidelines for implementing the change process than the Fidler's frame of reference, neither is adequate as a blueprint for action.

In the next chapter an analytical frame of reference will be outlined which draws on these frames of reference but which is, hopefully, more clearly described.

22 Reconciliation of Universal Issues: An Analytical Frame of Reference

The title of this frame of reference essentially describes its area of focus. Universal issues are those themes, concerns, or matters of substance that are an intrinsic part of being human. They are here identified as reality, trust, intimacy, adequacy, dependence/independence, sexuality, aggression, and loss (see Chapters 3 and 5 for appropriate references). Universal issues are a recurrent phenomena. Each of them is apparent at every stage of the life cycle, although they may be manifested in different ways at various times in the course of the life cycle. The issue of intimacy, for example, is often raised when one begins to form close friendships, contemplate marriage, become a parent, enter into a mentor-neophyte relationship, and so forth. A review of Chapter 5 will further illustrate the recurrence of the various universal issues.

Universal issues are only reconciled, never resolved once and for all. Here reconciled is used in the sense of bringing into agreement or harmony; making compatible or consistent. What is reconciled is the individual's thoughts and feelings relative to the various universal issues and the objective situation of the environment. Any marked change in the individual's life situation, whether it be internal or external in nature, is likely to bring one or more universal issues to the forefront of the person's attention. In such a position, these issues must somehow be addressed or dealt with. Some accommodation must be made to reconcile the issues, to temporarily lay them to rest.

The goal of intervention, based on this frame of reference, is to assist the individual in reconciling those universal issues currently of concern. This is not only done to help the individual manage his or her present life situation but it is also done with the belief that successful reconciliation of universal issues at one point in the life cycle will foster adequate reconciliation in the future. For example, at the time of retirement from remunerative employment, the issue of one's adequacy may become a predominant concern. If the individual is able to reconcile the issue at this time, it may be easier to deal with the issue as it once again may be raised when the individual is faced with diminished motor function and sensory acuity.

This frame of reference is concerned with psychological function. Its use is appropriate for individuals who are unable to reconcile universal issues because of maladaptive intrapsychic content that has resulted from faulty life experiences. Its use is also suitable for individuals whose life situation has been markedly altered so that the way in which they have reconciled universal issues in the past is no longer appropriate given their current circumstances.

The major limitations of this frame of reference is that it is only applicable with individuals who have normal or above intelligence, facility with secondary process thinking, some verbal skills, and the capacity to relate, at least to a moderate degree, to another person.

THEORETICAL BASE

To a great extent, the theoretical base of reconciliation of universal issues is made up of theoretical systems that have been previously described in the text. These systems thus, in the interest of economy, are only briefly summarized. The reader is referred to a more complete discussion in the previous parts of the text. The theoretical base consists of four parts: universal issues, aspects of psychological function, activities, and the change process.

Universal Issues

As mentioned, universal issues are those themes, concerns, or matters of substance that are an intrinsic part of being human. They are here defined as:

Reality: An awareness of the physical and interpersonal factors, including the attitudes and emotions of others, that exists in the environment, as well as the collective beliefs and values of a particular social system.

Trust: Confidence in the integrity of another person or persons.

Intimacy: A willingness to form long-term relationships of friendship, love, and/or nurture, and a willingness to abide by the commitments of such relationships.

Adequacy: Concerns about whether one is managing one's daily affairs and responsibilities in a competent manner.

Dependence/Independence: The degree of comfort one has in seeking and accepting the assistance of others, as well as acting without assistance.

Sexuality: The way in which an individual feels about and deals with sexual urges and tendencies.

Aggression: The way the individual feels about and acts on the urge to overcome obstacles to gain need satisfaction, to push forward his or her own interests or ideas, and to seek dominance in social situations.

Loss: The way in which the individual responds to being deprived of something of importance for which there is no hope of recovery; death and other types of personal losses.

The reconciliation of universal issues involves an alteration of intrapsychic content primarily. Subsequent to such an alteration, the individual is likely to change behavior, as well as attempt to manipulate the environment. Ideally, the reconciliation is such that it is viewed as positive by the individual. Adequate reconciliation results in a general feeling of well-being and places the individual in an optimal position for reconciling universal issues in the future. Poorly reconciled or unreconciled universal issues tend to lead to maladaptive behavior and/or the experience of rather severe discomfort. When an individual has had difficulty dealing with a particular issue in the past he or she is likely to have problems coping with that issue the next time it needs to be dealt with.

Aspects of Psychological Function

Universal issues form a nucleus around which intrapsychic content is organized. More specifically, they each serve as a core for a gestalt of needs, emotions, values, interests, and motivations (dynamic states); elements of self-concept; and ideas about other people.

Intrapsychic dynamics are a part of the theoretical base of the frame of reference. They provide the means for explaining the relationship between intrapsychic content and behavior which, in turn, facilitates the evaluation process and an understanding of the client.

Reality testing is considered from two perspectives in this frame of reference. First, processing and organizing intrapsychic content so that it is congruent with a shared reality is one of the universal issues. Second, the process of reality testing is used as one part of the process of helping an individual reconcile universal issues.

The development of insight in relationship to how one's thoughts and feelings concerning various universal issues may impede reconciliation is part of the change process. Insight and the role of reality testing will be discussed further momentarily.

Object relations per se are not the focus of this frame of reference. Some of the same phenomena is being addressed but the conceptual system used is not the same.

Finally, self-discipline is not dealt with in this frame of reference. As an aspect of psychological function it is, however, fairly closely related to the universal issues of adequacy.

Activities

All of the characteristics of purposeful activities, as described in Chapter 10, are part of the theoretical base of reconciliation of universal issues. There are five, however, that are of particular importance: promoting differential responses; facilitating communication; having a focusing, organizing effect; varying on a continuum from conscious to not conscious/unconscious; and varying on a continuum from real to symbolic. These characteristics are described as follows:

Promoting differential responses. This characteristic refers to the idea that the elements of purposeful activities strongly predispose one to particular expressions of ideas and feelings and to particular types of behavior. When an individual does not respond in the usual manner, this alerts the therapist to intrapsychic content that may account for a divergent response to the activity. Conversely, individuals with universal issues that have not been adequately dealt with are likely to respond to various activity elements in specific kinds of ways. This knowledge facilitates evaluation and allows the therapist to synthesize a purposeful activity that will either enhance communication and/or working through.

Facilitating communication. The action elements, the doing aspect of activities, and the materials and tools used provide a broad spectrum of means for nonverbal expression of ideas and feelings.

Having a focusing organizing effect. Purposeful activities have a converging effect which allows feelings and ideas to become integrated in such a way that vague pieces can be organized into words.

Varying on a continuum from conscious to not conscious/unconscious. Purposeful activities have the capacity to tap the unconscious. With focus on the activity as a whole, the individual's actions are frequently influenced by unconscious or unshared intrapsychic content. This facilitates communication. In addition, focus on the activity as a whole facilitates working through. By not attending to specific skills, new intrapsychic content is more likely to be integrated. Attention to specific aspects of the activity promotes the development of splinter skills, not the integration of new intrapsychic content.

Varying on a continuum from real to symbolic. The symbolic potential of activities is emphasized in the communication aspect of the change process, the production of symbols being an excellent means of tapping unconscious or unshared intrapsychic content. It is suggested that the section on symbolism in Chapter 10 be reviewed at this point. The real component of activities is emphasized, to some extent, in the working-through aspect of the change process. This is done to provide an opportunity for the individual to integrate new intrapsychic content. With attention focused on the reality of the activity, the individual is not immediately aware of personal thoughts and feelings. Thus, integration, which must take place out of awareness, is facilitated.

The Change Process

Figure 22-1 diagrams the change process (9,290,307, 317,368,386,427,492,646,705) in reconciliation of universal issues. It is presented in the hope that it will assist the reader in finding a way through all the terminology presented below. The middle of the diagram—Communication, Insight, Assessment, and Working through—presents the usual sequence of the change process. The larger arrowheads going toward the right indicate that the change process, in general, moves in that direction. The smaller arrowheads indicate that the process is rarely linear, often moving back and forth between the major phases. Communication is subdivided to indicate that more than one process occurs in this phase. Activities and transference, at the top of the diagram, are the two major tools used in the change process. The arrows are so placed to indicate their use throughout the change process but with major emphasis in the first and last phases. Associations and Interpretations, at the bottom of the diagram, are two types of verbal interaction which, again, take place throughout the change process. The arrows are so placed for the same reason as outlined above. Each aspect of the change process will now be discussed in some detail.

Communication

As part of the change process of an analytic frame of reference, communication has been discussed in Chapter 21. Essentially it is the process of transforming inner private subjective ideas, emotions, and experiences (whether they be conscious or unconscious) into an external public form and the examination and evaluation of this intrapsychic content. An external public form refers to words, to language. Stated somewhat differently, private ideas, emotions, and experiences must be brought to the verbal level. It is only at this level, in this form, that they can be examined and evaluated.

The process of bringing unconscious or unshared intrapsychic content to the point of sharing frequently involves the organization and presentation of this intrapsychic content in a symbolic manner initially. This apparently happens automatically once the individual is given an opportunity to engage in activities that involve a variety of tools and materials and that allow for some degree of freedom in using these tools and materials. The variety and freedom allow the individual to express intrapsychic content more openly than is usually possible in activities that have little variation and strict limits. In addition, they allow for expression on a nonverbal level through the veil of symbols. From the level of symbolic expression, intrapsychic content must then be brought

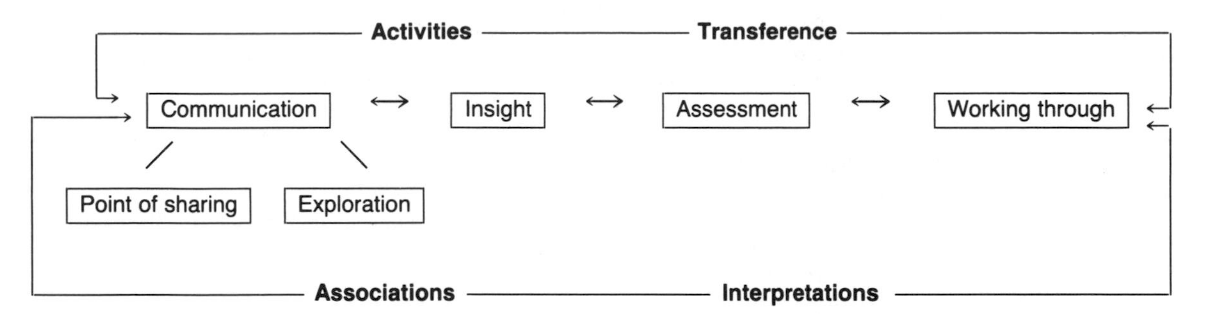

FIG. 22-1. The change process in reconciliation of universal issues.

to the verbal level. This is accomplished primarily through associations and interpretations, processes that will be discussed shortly.

The second component of communication is exploration, the examination and evaluation of intrapsychic content that is at a verbal level. Exploration involves first disclosing ideas, emotions, and experiences to test their validity in a shared real world. Sometimes referred to as reality testing, this process essentially involves the client and therapist working together to answer the question "Are the client's ideas, emotions, and meaning the client has assigned to different experiences compatible with the client's current life situation and the nature of the external environment in which the client presently exists?" A considerable amount of feedback from the therapist (and, if exploration takes place in a group, from other group members) is necessary for the client to answer this major question.

Exploration involves examining the relationship between now verbalized intrapsychic content and the conduct of daily affairs. It is the process of making the link between ideas and emotions and the way in which one behaves. To make this connection, interpretations are again used. This in turn leads to insight.

Insight

As used in this frame of reference, insight refers to the conscious understanding of the meaning and purpose of one's behavior. The development of insight may be a slow process with small increments of understanding occurring over a period of time. On the other hand, insight may occur quite suddenly and all at once. In this case it is often accompanied by the idea "Why didn't I understand the relationship before? It is so simple and obvious!" Some degree of insight is a necessary part of the change process. Without making the link between intrapsychic content and behavior, the individual perceives his or her behavior as unlawful or capricious and ideas and emotions as singularly unimportant relative to environmental interactions. Some degree of insight is prerequisite to the next two phases of the change process—assessment and working through.

Assessment

Assessment refers to the choice to maintain or alter some aspect of one's intrapsychic content. This choice ideally is conscious and made with forethought. There are aspects of the choice, however, that are often less than conscious. Although the individual may say that he or she would like to make changes, there may be unconscious resistance to this course of action. Change is difficult and in this case means giving up some parts of the self which have been significant for a long period of time. Conflicts regarding modification of intrapsychic content are likely to be aroused periodically throughout the change process. If the individual decides, after due consideration, that no modification of intrapsychic content is necessary or desirable, the change process ends at this point. The individual has gained insight into the relationship between intrapsychic content and behavior; an important discovery. However, such a discovery alone usually leads to neither alteration of intrapsychic content nor behavior. When an individual choice is to alter some aspect of intrapsychic content, it is often accompanied by a decision to begin to address one or more of the universal issues that has been previously avoided, poorly reconciled, or reconciled in a way that is now incompatible with the individual's current life situation. The individual essentially decides to engage in the process of working through.

Working Through

This is the process of the client experiencing the effects of maladaptive intrapsychic content over and over again until able to deal with such content in an effective manner. Concurrently it involves formulating a more adaptive way of perceiving oneself, other people, and the events of daily life and of reconciling one or more universal issues. This is accomplished with the assistance of the therapist and, when it occurs in the context of a group, fellow group members. Help is provided by the therapist through the design of activities that are likely to elicit the ideas and emotions that are maladaptive for the client. This allows the client to deal with the content over and over again in a variety of situations. The purpose of this kind of interaction is to help the client sort out the gestalts of intrapsychic content, rejecting that which is invalid or not congruent with reality and integrating that which is valid or reality based.

Some maladaptive intrapsychic content may never actually be rejected. It remains, but the individual becomes so familiar with it that it evolves into something less scary, less powerful, and thus less influential in the conduct of daily affairs. Another way of describing this process is that through repeated interaction in situations that elicit maladaptive intrapsychic content, the individual acquires new intrapsychic content that allows him or her to handle or deal with the old maladaptive content. New intrapsychic content also allows the individual to reconcile universal issues in a way that is satisfying to the self and others. Through repeated behavior that is influenced by new intrapsychic content, the content loses its sense of being foreign or alien and eventually becomes a comfortable part of the self.

Nevertheless, in the process of repeatedly interacting in situations that have been difficult for the client in the past, "old" maladaptive intrapsychic content often intrudes. The client then returns to the former way of dealing with other people and events and coping with universal issues. These setbacks, if adequately interpreted, are not considered detrimental to the change process. As a matter of fact they enhance the change process, for they provide the matrix out of which new intrapsychic content is integrated. It is important to remember that the process of working through takes considerable time and energy, hence the name for this process. It is also a process that may arouse considerable anxiety in that the client frequently is engaging in new behavior and behavior that was previously forbidden by his or her former way of perceiving self and the world.

Activities and Transference

Activities as part of this frame of reference have been previously discussed. Transference was also discussed in Chapter 8 in the section on conscious use of self. It was defined there as an unconscious psychological process characterized by a response to a person in a manner similar to the way in which one responded to a significant individual in one's past life. Transference on the part of the client is encouraged in this frame of reference. It is used to help the therapist understand the client's intrapsychic content and thus typical modes of interaction. By assessing the client's responses, the therapist is usually able to determine whether the client has formed a transference relationship. To be able to make such a determination, the therapist needs considerable self-awareness and an understanding of how clients typically react to him or her. When a client's behavior toward the therapist is atypical, it is very likely that the client has formed a transference relationship. In such a case further study is needed to determine the client's perception of the therapist, e.g., as an authority figure, a nurturing individual, a peer, someone who is inadequate, and so forth. The client's response to the therapist based on transference gives the therapist information on how the client feels about him- or herself in relation to whatever kind of person the client perceives the therapist to be. This information is used, at appropriate times, to assist the client in communicating thoughts and feelings more directly, in making connections between intrapsychic content and behavior, and in the process of working through. This is accomplished through making appropriate interpretations.

When intervention takes place in the context of a task-oriented group, the client may form a variety of transference relationships with other group members. The meaning and the understanding of these relationships are also used in the change process.

The therapist facilitates the development of transference relationships by acting in a fairly neutral manner, by trying not to represent oneself as a unique individual with a particular life style, a special set of interests, and a specific value system. Admittedly, this is somewhat difficult to accomplish. Nevertheless, by presenting oneself as a "blank screen," the therapist enables the client to engage in transference relationships and thus facilitates the change process.

It is important to note that the client may form a variety of transference relationships with the therapist during the course of the change process. At one time, for example, the client may perceive the therapist as similar to a grandson, at other times as a forbidding uncle, and so on. The therapist must keep account of the client's various and varying perceptions, for many times the therapist is being cast simultaneously in a number of roles. This is important, for accurate interpretations can only be made when the therapist is aware of the client's immediate perception.

Association and Interpretations

Association

The process of making associations facilitates the communication of intrapsychic content. It involves relating whatever comes to mind while or subsequent to engaging in an activity. The external events and phenomena act as a stimuli for the verbalization of a variety of ideas, emotions, and needs. What is said is believed to be determined by and an expression of the individual's intrapsychic content. In using purposeful activities as stimuli for associations, the client is encouraged to talk about all elements of the activity—the real and symbolic motions, material, process, end product, and interpersonal elements.

Free or controlled associations may be used. In free association, the client is asked to report anything that comes to mind. This may lead, through a chaining process, to almost anywhere. In controlled associations, certain limits are placed on the client's responses, although a range of choice is always available. The limits placed are those of the activity. In other words, the client is asked to keep primarily focused on the elements of the activity under consideration. Controlled associations are preferred for two reasons. First, this method helps the client organize thoughts and feelings around an immediate "here and now" experience. It provides a structure that is often helpful to clients. Second, there is some reason why the client engaged in a specific activity in a particular way at a given time. Moving away from the activity, which often happens in free association, may not permit the client and therapist to discover that reason. Jung suggested that controlled associations were most useful in understanding symbols (492). He believed that the production of a symbol is the expression of something very definite the individual is trying to communicate. Ignoring this fact does a great disservice to the potential of the unconscious for providing useful information. Free association nevertheless, is used at times, as, for instance, when the client is unable to make any controlled associations.

To assist the client to learn how to engage in this process of controlled or free associations the therapist explains the process and, at times, may demonstrate the process by sharing his or her own associations to the activity. The information gained through associations, in addition to other observations, are used to formulate interpretations.

Interpretation

As used in this frame of reference, interpretation refers to giving meaning to experiences. It involves identifying relationships between experiences; between intrapsychic content and behavior; between past, present, and, perhaps, future life situations. The purpose of interpretations is, in a sense, to bring order out of chaos.

Two kinds of interpretations have been identified, horizontal and vertical. Horizontal interpretations refer to the identification of common elements in the client's present life situation. A client, for example, may act in a very superior manner relative to other members in her task-oriented group and later comment that the house plants she is tending are stunted and unhealthy looking. Connecting these two events is horizontal interpretation. Vertical interpretation refers to the identification of common elements in the client's past, present, and, perhaps, future life situation. For example, a client may draw a house surrounded by scaffolding. Through making associations, the client mentions that she was always frightened when her mother was not home when she returned from school. At the termination of intervention the client will be living alone, in an apartment for the first time. Identification of the common elements in these three events is vertical interpretation.

Formulating accurate and meaningful interpretations and presenting them at an opportune time is no easy task. It must be learned from practice and in conjunction with skilled supervision. There are, however, some guidelines that have proved helpful over time. These are outlined below.

To be useful and meaningful to a client, interpretations must touch the client's being. When it does, the client's response will be emotional, experiential, and cognitive. The therapist never tries to convince the client of the correctness of the therapist's interpretations. This limits the client's independence and makes him or her a subordinate partner in the change process. Therefore, any interpretation that does not win the true assent of the client is considered invalid for the present. The therapist and client either leave elements unconnected for that time or search for another interpretation. The client will experience a sense of fit when an interpretation is accurate. It is only then that the interpretation is right in the sense of being meaningful to the client.

An interpretation is useless if the client is not ready to hear or comprehend the relationship being suggested. Thus, the therapist must be truly with the client in order for him to experience the client's readiness. Interpretations are usually most successful when they are focused on a relationship that is near to the point of being recognized by the client.

Interpretations dealing with the client's concerns in the here and now of the immediate situation are most useful. The client, for example, may complain of a headache, a fairly regular occurrence for him, and a few minutes later tell the therapist that he has lost a tool borrowed from the occupational therapy department. The interpretation that might be made is that the client's headache may be due to fear of being criticized for carelessness. This interpretation is likely to be more easily accepted by and useful to the client because he has experienced the headache and the possibility of criticism at the same time and in the immediate situation. Interpretations made when the client is not experiencing anything relative to the interpretation tend to be meaningless and, if at all, registered only on the cognitive level. The necessary emotional-experiencing aspects are missing.

Interpretations should be used sparingly. Too many interpretations confuse and often overwhelm the client to the point that he or she no longer listens. Even if attentive, it is usually only on the cognitive level. The process becomes intellectualized and without feeling. Excessive interpretations by the therapist tends to place the client in a passive position; spontaneity and self-direction are limited.

Collaboration, as always, is important. It is often facilitated by stating interpretations in a tentative or questioning manner. This helps both client and therapist to view the therapist's role as a guiding participant, as opposed to an all-knowing, superordinate being. The client is usually, then, more comfortable when disagreeing with the therapist. The client will also feel more free to alter a part of the interpretation, to accept only some part of the interpretation, or to reject it. The words the therapist uses also enhance collaboration and integration. Each client has a unique manner of speaking. Thus, it is often useful for the therapist to use the client's terms or expressions when suggesting an interpretation. This tends to establish contact with the client's most intimate ideas and feelings. However, this way of stating interpretations should not be used all the time. The therapist's own typical vocabulary or way of speaking offers another dimension for the client's consideration. It would be unreasonable to deny this additional perspective to the client.

It is suggested that the therapist use direct terms to discuss human experiences as opposed to euphemisms. This indicates to the client that intimate experiences can be spoken about in a simple and matter-of-fact manner. The therapist must exercise caution, however, for what is a euphemism to one person may be a specially meaningful word to another. Therefore, the identifying labels a client uses should be explored to discover their exact meaning. For example, some people use the expressions "intercourse" and "making love" to speak of very different kinds of sexual experiences. Substituting one for the other may make very little difference, but on the other hand, it may be a way of distinguishing between two very different interactions.

It is best for both client and therapist to not use technical terms or psychological jargon. When a client uses such terms it is sometimes a way of not speaking directly, making the experience into an intellectual exercise, or of speaking negatively about oneself or others. When this occurs the therapist suggests that the client try to select other words for the discussion. By so doing, the true meaning of what the client is saying is likely to become more evident both to the client and to the therapist. The therapist's use of technical terms may be misunderstood by the client or taken as a derogatory comment. Such words as "compulsive," "controlling," and "infantile," etc., have a negative meaning to much of the lay population. Moreover, the use of technical terms often makes the client feel as if he or she were something out of a textbook, a "case" rather than a person.

Gaining self-knowledge is a painful experience but in all growth there is some pain. The therapist helps regulate the pain of growth, not eliminate it. Thus, false reassurance and withholding painful interpretations are not helpful to the client. Both interfere with the client's growth and demean intelligence and courage. The destructive pain of therapy emanates more from interpretations that carry a derogatory, critical evaluative theme than from an honest articulation of the therapist's perceptions. Interpretations that demonstrate a sincere interest in the client and a nonjudgmental understanding attitude toward behavior, emotions, needs, and ideas go a long way in regulating the hurt of growth. It is also good to remember that interpretations are not always threatening to a client. Often they are experienced with a good deal of relief. A bit of the confusion is taken away; more about the self comes to be understood.

Gaining self-knowledge can be a lonely experience even when accompanied by a perceptive therapist. In discovering the uniqueness of oneself, the sense of commonality with others may be lost. Conversely, lack of self-knowledge can also generate a feeling of aloneness. The individual perceives him- or herself as so unique that it is difficult to relate to others. For these reasons, it is suggested that the therapist help the client to view problems, at least in part, as the essence of the human condition. Interpretations dealing with universal symbols and/or are presented in the form of fables, proverbs, or well-known quotations are often useful for this purpose. The client in this way is helped to experience membership in the human group.

As mentioned, the nature of the client's transference relationship with the therapist provides a valuable source of information. Exploration and interpretation of the transference relationship is helpful in that it involves dealing with what the client is experiencing. It therefore has an immediacy that is rare in any discussion of the past. Before the client's transference relationship is interpreted it should be at the point where it is relatively well established, but not to the point where it is so intense that the client is blind to the real client-therapist relationship. At an opportune moment, the client is likely to focus on the transference relationship, either directly or through formulated symbols. If this does not occur, the therapist introduces this significant aspect of the change process by inquiring what the client thinks or experiences relative to the therapist. The exploration that follows is often extremely fruitful in revealing intrapsychic content that has heretofore been unconscious and/or never shared.

During the change process, clients sometimes engage in various behaviors directed toward maintaining content in the unconscious. This is referred to as resistance. When it occurs, interpretations regarding unconscious content are not useful to the client and tend to be ignored. It is necessary to help the client to recognize his or her resistance prior to engaging in exploring that which his or her behavior is keeping out of consciousness. This is done by focusing on the resistance itself and frequently on the transference relationship. It is important to remember that that resistance is not consciously willed; the client is not deliberately attempting to impede the change process. The client's behavior is as unknown to the client as the unconscious content which it is directed to ward off.

As intervention progresses, the therapist encourages the client to make his or her own interpretations. In a way this could be considered one of the subgoals of the change process—to develop the client's capacity to understand the relationship between thoughts and feelings and behavior independent of the therapist. This can be accomplished through the client's active engagement in interpretations. The therapist helps the client to make interpretations independently by (a) enumerating several possible connections; (b) pointing out aspects of the client's symbols, past life, or current situation unnoticed by the client; (c) articulating basic themes that seem to be evident; and (d) reminding the client of past statements, omissions and apparent contradictions. Most importantly, the therapist does not make an interpretation when it is apparent that the client will be able to articulate a relationship in a very short time. In waiting, the therapist allows the client adequate time for thinking through and organizing the various significant connections.

By helping the client learn to make interpretations and in suggesting interpretations, the therapist creates an atmosphere of encouragement and quiet sharing.

The importance of symbols in the communication and working through phases of the change process has been discussed. Understanding the meaning of a symbol involves a combination of making associations and formulating interpretations. There are several factors to keep in mind when elucidating the meaning of symbols.

Symbols are and can only be produced by an individual. They cannot be separated from that individual: past, current, and future life situation; philosophical, religious, and moral convictions; place in the life cycle and cultural background. Symbols should be explored with an attitude and orientation of innocence, that is, no fixed meaning is assumed regarding any symbol. They should be explored with a sense of discovery and with the individual who has produced the symbols. Most symbols have common referrents which provide some landmarks in understanding intrapsychic content. Yet, a symbol produced by an individual also has idiosyncratic aspects. To assign a fixed meaning to a symbol is to inhibit discovery of how the symbol relates to that individual. The common referrents of a symbol are utilized in evaluation to assist in identifying a client's problem areas. In the change process itself, however, no predetermined meaning can be assigned to a symbol.

The meanings of symbols are discovered through exploration of their various aspects: form and content; personal, cultural, and universal elements. The whole becomes known through its parts. The meaning of a symbol may also be discovered through exploration of the context in which it occurs, through other symbols that occur at the same time, through other symbols that have been formulated in the past, or through symbols that will be produced in the future. The meaning of a symbol is often obscure until it is related to other symbols. Symbolic content that takes the same or a different form repeatedly often provides more information than a symbol that occurs only once. This is, however, not a hard and fast rule. Looking for similarities in symbols is sometimes a fruitful undertaking, for comprehension of the relationship between two symbols occurring together may provide a clue to the meaning of both. It is also helpful to address the question "For what purpose was the symbol produced?" Why now, why in this time and place?

Symbols are invested with energy and emotions. Without these components a symbol is lifeless, an empty shell. Such symbols cannot serve as a guide to an individual for they are without dynamic force. When a symbol is not consciously connected to needs or emotions, it has no meaning to the person. Some symbols are produced without conscious awareness of their emotional component. The individual may feel neutral toward the symbol, or, at best, somewhat curious. Such symbols may come to life only through exploration of their meaning to the individual. Awareness of the feeling component may be miniscule and allusive at first. This may be due to the feelings being foreign or disagreeable to the individual. In such a case expression of the feelings requires patient nurturing. At other times emotions may come with a mighty rush, even to the point of almost overwhelming the individual. When this occurs it is the individual's sense of being in control of the self which needs support. Just as symbols without emotions are lifeless, symbols whose content remains unknown are also without life. They cannot be a dynamic factor in the growth of the individual. The energy, emotional, and content components of a symbol must be brought together and integrated for symbols to have real meaning.

Symbols can never be completely understood. In exploring symbolic communication, one is, at best, able to comprehend only those aspects currently relevant to the client. Although one may intellectually explore all aspects of a symbol, it is usually only those aspects associated with feeling or connected with feeling through exploration that are of current significance. The process of abstracting currently significant content helps the client focus on and therefore make some use of symbols in the present. Other aspects of the symbol may become known only at a future time. A symbol once produced may remain a part of the individual for some time. It may periodically become reactivated, reexplored by the individual and, in turn, yield new information. A symbol contains a set of information at the time it is produced. But the various aspects may have meaning only as the individual continues to grow and develop.

Exploration of a symbol is a very personal matter. Only the symbol producer can judge if the content of a given symbol is applicable to him- or herself. There is a feeling of fit or rightness when the individual comes upon the pertinent meaning of a symbol. The therapist may discover the meaning of a symbol and, indeed, may have much data to support the discovery, but if this does not feel right to the client, the identified content is not currently applicable. The client may not be ready to accept the content on a conscious level; acceptance may only occur much later. On the other hand, the therapist's interpretation may not have been accurate; the connection made is meaningless and therefore useless to the client. One, however, need not be overly concerned with the accuracy of the interpretation. A client may feel good about a particular interpretation only to discover later that another interpretation is more accurate. "Sooner or later the psyche rejects the mistake, much as an organism does a foreign body" (493, p. 65).

Symbols can be explored by an individual in isolation, but exploration shared with a knowledgeable and empathetic participant facilitates the process. The other, in essence, accompanies the individual on a journey of self-discovery. This is the role of the therapist. All individuals are unaware of or blind to parts of themselves. Thus there may be aspects of symbols which they produce that they do not perceive. The therapist may well be able to point out these aspects for the individual's consideration. The therapist's controlled associations to the symbol may open up areas that are unknown to the client. Individuals tend to have a relatively stereotyped view of themselves. The therapist may suggest a new view or a wider perspective. Similarly, the therapist may see relationships between the client's current situation and symbols, aspects of symbols, or a given symbol which are not perceived by the client. The therapist is able to nurture feelings and give support when feelings are overwhelming.

Discussion about a symbol requires the use of words. This, in turn, places ideas, emotions, and needs in a public arena where they can be subjected to validation. It is important to emphasize that the therapist never imposes him- or herself on the client; rather leads, guides, supports, provides companionship with empathy.

In summary, the theoretical base of Reconciliation of Universal Issues describes the interrelationship between universal issues, intrapsychic content, aspects of psychological function, activities, and the change process. The change process was described as having four recurrent phases: communication, insight, assessment, and working through. Throughout these phases, activities, transference, associations, and interpretations are used as the basis for modifying intrapsychic content so as to allow the individual to adequately reconcile one or more universal issues.

THE CONTINUUMS AND BEHAVIOR INDICATIVE OF FUNCTION AND DYSFUNCTION

The listing in Table 22-1 gives the titles of the function-dysfunction continuums and some behaviors indicative of dysfunction relative to each of the continuums. Behavior indicative of function is not provided for, in most cases it is simply the absence of behavior indicative

TABLE 22-1. *Function-dysfunction continuums and associated behaviors*

Reality

Confusion
Distorted perception of one's body
Identity diffusion
Considerable ambivalence
No internalized value system
Preoccupation with philosophy or religion
Seeks a number of opinions from others regarding how to deal with a particular problem
Difficulty making decisions regarding a course of action
Confusion regarding appropriate behavior
Lacking basic information regarding the environment
Behavior erratic without any apparent motive or theme
Emphasis on objectivity and logical thought processes
Fear of the undefined
Mandula or geometric shapes
Symbols that refer to reaching upward for guidance or downward for a base of support
A circumscribed border
Emphasis on head of reproduced human figure

Trust

Expresses fear of others
Acts shy and fearful of the therapist
Difficulty communicating ideas and feelings because of concern about the response of others
Perceives most other people as unworthy or unacceptable
Sees others as critical, hostile, competitive, and/or seductive
Ambivalent toward others
Always questioning, suspicious of others' intentions, secretive
Difficulty in getting along with others, has few friends
Avoids unstructured activities, prefers activities over which he/she has control
Prefers not to share an activity
Wants to know rules
Productions show isolated objects; human figures are absent, vague, or threatening
Symbols have destructive or controlling aspect

Intimacy

No evidence of mature love relationships relative to friends, spouse, or children
Preoccupied with self
Relationships with others are cold, mechanical, and lacking in feeling
Complains about difficulty in getting close to other people
Experiences isolation from others
Speaks of loneliness
Fears rejection
Lack of empathy toward others
Highly controlled in expression of emotions
Much concern about nonhuman objects
Warm intense colors or very cool colors
Takes great care in drawing one human figure
Preoccupied with stroking and patting

Adequacy

Functions inadequately
Poor vocational history or school performance
Minimal attention to personal hygiene and dress
Many statements regarding personal inadequacies
Restricted interaction in the environment
Lack of self-direction
Dissatisfaction with the self
Negative feelings about one's body
Other people considered better than the self in an indiscriminate or nondifferential way
Glorification of parents or persons in authority
Preoccupied with what others think about the self
Much expression of guilt and shame
Difficulty in excepting limitations of the self, sees any limitation as total relative to the entire self
Productions that depict others as larger or more powerful than the self
Size of production small relative to space and materials available
Human images very vague and/or appear to be inadequate
Trees young and appear to be weak
Light sketchy lines

Dependence/Independence

Preoccupied with independence, sees even legitimate dependency as bad
Independence is equated with aloneness and loneliness
Excessively dependent
Accepts even abuse to maintain dependent relationship
Makes little effort to be independent
Vague fears and restricted interaction relative to the environment
Difficulty in taking responsibility for the self
Looks to others for guidance and decision-making
Dependent on parents beyond age where it is considered usual in one's cultural group
Evidence of need to be in control of all situations
Productions contain many father and mother symbols
Self portrayed as infantile
Productions have passive or overly active quality
Dominant figure in production is above or set apart
Prefers structured activities

Sexuality

Does not mention sexual matters or talks excessively about them
Promiscuous or inhibited in sexual interactions
Excessively sexually provocative or acts in an asexual manner
Extreme in orientation to own gender (ultramasculinity, feminine little doll)
Rejection of opposite sex, endowing them with negative, stereotyped characteristics
Rejection of opposite sex characteristics in self or others
Rigid differentiation of sex roles
Symbols expressing sexual intercourse to the exclusion of other content
Sexual aspects of human figures emphasized or absent
Highly disguised or predominant masculine or feminine symbols
Opposite sex symbols have unattractive characteristics

Aggression

Perception of the self as the primary obstacle to need satisfaction
Anxiety or guilt regarding identification, investment in, or manipulation of aggressive objects
Self-destructive behavior
Anti- or asocial acts
Verbally abusive with others for no apparent reason
Preoccupied with power and control
Dark colors and symbols referring to destruction or evil
Deformed, threatening-appearing human figures; ominous tone
Scrubbing, pushing, pulling, scratching, slapping modes of handling materials
Angular, jagged strokes; heavy pressure
Intense warm colors

Loss

Negative feelings toward the body as a whole or affected part
Denial, avoidance, or overprotection of affected part
Treats affected part as not an element of the self and/or as a nonhuman object
Resistance to or disinterest in rehabilitation efforts
Depressed
Denies disability
Cannot express feelings relative to loss or loss is central to thinking for an excessive period of time
Activity is excessive but not purposeful except as defense against loss
Attempts to act as if aging process is not taking place
Preoccupation with self-care
Human figures young and well formed
Productions contain objects having an eternal quality
Symbols of birth-death-rebirth cycle or immortality
Fear of death, which may or may not be based on factual information
Mandula forms
Dark colors
Old or withered trees
Symbols referring to the soul
Symbols of transition

of dysfunction (A review of the section on symbolism may be useful at this point.)

The major purpose of evaluation is to determine the status of the client's universal issues. The client and therapist need to identify whether universal issues have been adequately and appropriately reconciled for the present time or whether they are unreconciled. It is also necessary to determine the client's cognitive function in the areas of thought process and levels of conceptualization. Although not directly addressed in Reconciliation of Universal Issues, adequate capacities in these aspects of cognition are necessary for participation in a change process based on this frame of reference.

A general interview and the addendum to a general interview are used in the evaluative process. One of the following tools should also be used: Fidler Battery, Free Choice of Selected Activities, or Activity Configuration. The Fidler Battery is probably the most appropriate of these three tools. However, some clients object to participation in this type of evaluative procedure owing to negative ideas about a psychoanalytical orientation. Free Choice of Selected Activities is the next most appropriate tool. It, however, may not be an effective tool for clients who need considerable structure or who have serious difficulty making any kind of a decision. The Activity Configuration is probably the least appropriate of the three tools, but it may well be the only activity-oriented evaluative procedure acceptable to some clients. This is particularly true for clients who are not especially psychologically sophisticated. In using the Activity Configuration relative to this frame of reference, the therapist gives the greatest attention to Part II of this tool. The evaluative tools mentioned above are described fully in Chapter 16.

POSTULATES REGARDING CHANGE

Short- and long-term goals, the areas of initial focus and the desired end results of the change process are determined jointly by the client and therapist, with major emphasis on the client's choice of where to begin.

The change process may take place in a dyad of client and therapist or in activity groups. Groups are probably a more effective environment for change because of the various curative factors. The most commonly used activity group is a task-oriented group. However, topical and thematic groups may be used in the process of working through.

Change is brought about most effectively by interaction in a supportive, accepting, and empathetic environment.

Communication as it relates to bringing unconscious or unshared intrapsychic content to the point of sharing is facilitated by engaging in activities that offer a variety of tools, materials, processes, and interpersonal relationships and in activities having a high symbolic potential.

More focused communication may be facilitated by engaging in activities that embody, highlight, call forth, or symbolize the universal issues that appear to be of concern to the client. The following activity characteristics are suggested:

1. Concerns about the nature of reality can best be identified by activities that are unstructured yet with a demand for evaluation; by unfamiliar tools, materials, and actions; by involvement in situations that are ambiguous and elicit a number of ideas as to how one might respond; and by activities that involve questioning of oneself.
2. Concerns related to trust are best identified through participation in activities that require sharing and where success or failure depends in part on the actions of one's partner(s).
3. Concerns related to intimacy are best identified through participation in activities that require extensive interaction with others, particularly in dyads, such as the sharing of personal information directly or in a symbolic form, and activities that require physical contact.
4. Concerns related to adequacy are best identified by participation in activities that require manual dexterity, multiple processes and steps, new learning, that require material that needs to be controlled, chance for failure, and end products that can be judged by objective standards.
5. Concerns about dependence/independence can best be identified by participating in activities that require either reliance on another person for task accomplishment, the need to adhere to a step-by-step procedure, and minimal independent thinking or activities that require independent action, responsibility, and that are somewhat ambiguous.
6. Concerns about sexuality are best identified through participation in activities that involve interaction with members of both sexes, in traditionally sex-specific activities, and in activities that focus on the human body.
7. Concerns about aggression are best identified through participation in activities requiring gross and aggressive motions, material that is resistive and/or difficult to control, and few external controls.
8. Concerns about loss can best be identified by participation in activities that focus on the human body; on the creative, expressive, unstructured media; that are moderate in scope; that make use of dark colors; the nature of the activity or the end product is oriented either to the past or the future. (In helping an individual

in this area, what the therapist wants to do is very gently tap the grief, to assist the client to get some idea of its content and dimension, and to focus on the loss.)

The characteristics of the activities described above are designed to elicit unconscious and unshared intrapsychic content. They are designed to force the issue into the open or to a more conscious level. As described, such activities may be too threatening for some clients. If that is the case, the therapist makes the activity less intense or demanding without allowing it to become so benign that little or no meaningful intrapsychic content or universal issues are elicited. Now to return to the postulates regarding change.

Communication as it relates to exploration is facilitated by

- Indicating the extent to which particular universal issues have been appropriately reconciled relative to the client's age, cultural group, and life situation;
- Pointing out the relationship between intrapsychic content and unreconciled universal issues and the effect these have on the doing process and interpersonal relationships;
- Giving the same information or feedback repeatedly in a variety of situations;
- Receiving feedback from the nonhuman environment as to the effects of one's behavior as it is influenced by intrapsychic content and universal issues.

Insight occurs spontaneously as a consequence of adequate exploration and interaction in an accepting and supportive environment.

Assessment is facilitated by an environment that outlines the consequences of various available courses of action, encourages and supports risk-taking behavior, provides reassurance as to the availability of assistance in the task ahead, and allows for free choice and respects the choice that is made.

Working through is facilitated by activities that:

- Elicit maladaptive intrapsychic content and unreconciled universal issues;
- Provide an opportunity for the client to engage in behavior that is more in line with the intrapsychic content and reconciliation of universal issues which are now desired by the client;
- Are graded to allow the client to experience increasingly more complex interaction without undue stress;
- Provide for a variety of settings and sufficient time so that new intrapsychic content and strategies for reconciliation of universal issues may be adequately integrated;
- Allow for participation in activities sufficiently interesting to the client that they are engaged in as a total entity without the client giving attention to the learning of specific skills.

The following activity characteristics are suggested as a means of facilitating working through in specific areas:

Reconciliation of the issue of reality is facilitated by participation in activities that require judgment of what is real or accepted in the particular situation; activities that require action based on judgment; activities that demonstrate variation in people's values and beliefs; and activities that require action based on one's own values and beliefs regardless of whether they are shared by others in the immediate environment.

Reconciliation of the issue of trust is facilitated initially by participation in activities that require little trust but are moving slowly in the direction of activities that require considerable trust; interactions should begin with people who are similar in many ways to the client followed by interaction with less similar people.

Reconciliation of the issue of intimacy is facilitated by initially engaging in activities that require little sharing on an interpersonal level; involvement in the care of nonhuman objects (plants, animals) is often useful; in moving toward more interpersonal sharing, the doing aspect of the activity should be undemanding relative to skill and energy required.

Selection of activities for reconciliation of the issue of adequacy is determined to some extent by the areas in which the client feels more inadequate; by gradation of activities from simple to those that require increasingly greater competence; by a variety of activities so that the client is able to experience assets and limitations; and by feedback from other individuals as well as the activity.

Reconciliation of the issue of dependence/independence is facilitated by participation in activities that are graded either relative to increasing independence or increasing dependence (the direction of the gradation will be determined by the client's present capacities and current life situation) and by activities that encourage sharing with others regardless of whether the client is moving toward greater dependence or independence.

Reconciliation of the issue of sexuality is facilitated by interaction in an environment where the client's sexuality is accepted; by participation in single and mixed sex groups where the client is encouraged to engage in a variety of activities that traditionally have been identified as masculine and feminine (engagement in both types of activities); and by participation in situations where there is increasingly frank discussions of and information about sex-related issues, including attitudes of others, the safety of having sexual intercourse, one's likely capacity to engage in sexual intercourse, contraceptives, and alternative means of sexual gratification.

Reconciliation of the issue of aggression is facilitated by participation in activities that initially provide few obstacles to need satisfaction with gradation toward activities that present more impediments relative to immediate satisfaction; toward activities that are graded relative to the need for gross and assertive motions and the degree to which external limits are set by the nature of the activity or by other individuals; and toward activities that are increasingly challenging to the client relative to their complexity and the extent to which they require mastery.

Activities suitable for dealing with the issue of loss will be described in two different categories—the individual confronting his or her own death and the individual who has sustained a loss.

Reconciliation of the issue of confronting one's own death is facilitated by participation in an environment that accepts death as part of the life cycle, that encourages the open discussion of death, and that provides adequate support for the individual, encouraging as much independent activity as possible; by participation in activities that provide an opportunity to express and share ideas and feelings about illness and death with others who are able listeners; by reality testing to correct misconceptions if this is in the best interest of the client; by activities that can be shared with family members and friends; activities that involve treasured objects; and activities that prompt a life review such as going through the family photo album and reading old newspapers and letters.

The latter activities allow the client to identify ideas about the self and other people and test them in the reality of death (the idea of laying ghosts to rest, of cleaning house). The process frequently causes the arousal of the full spectrum of human emotions which can be experienced in contrast to each other. It also encourages the individual to identify values and to separate those that are enduring.

Reconciliation of the issue of a recently sustained loss is facilitated by participation in rhythmic repetitive activities that may provide some comfort; activities that encourage expressing grief; shared activities that prompt the client to talk about the past, present, and future, about what the client would like to do, and why he or she can or cannot; by listening and reality testing on the part of the therapist, including providing honest and factual information; by helping the client engage in any kind of activity in which he or she shows the slightest interest (encourage the client, do not push; self-selected activities are more beneficial to the client); by participation in activities that allow for experimentation with ways of filling the void of loss; by assisting in the formulation of realistic plans for the future when the client has acknowledged, at least to some degree, that the loss has been sustained; and by accepting the level of function that the client wants and thinks is realistically possible.

Remember that as the client tries new activities and judges competence, he or she may again identify more loss and repeat the earlier steps of grieving, sadness, and negative feelings about self. As each new activity is encountered, the client may have to face many new realities about abilities and situations.

This completes the postulates relative to the four phases of the change process. The following three postulates are addressed to those processes that occur throughout the four phases.

1. Transference is facilitated by the therapist acting in a fairly neutral manner, which involves *not* presenting oneself as a unique person with a particular life-style, set of values, and specific set of interests.
2. Associations are facilitated by encouraging the client to talk about all elements of an activity: the real and symbolic, motions, materials, process, end product, and interpersonal elements.
3. Interpretations facilitate the change process by identifying relationships between intrapsychic content and behavior and between past, present, and, at times, future life situations. By following the guidelines presented in the theoretical base, interpretations are likely to be both meaningful and useful to the client.

SUMMARY

Reconciliation of Universal Issues is concerned with the modification of intrapsychic content in such a manner that the individual is able to reconcile universal issues in a more adaptive manner. Eight universal issues are identified as being of major importance. They are reality, trust, intimacy, adequacy, dependence/independence, sexuality, aggression, and loss. The change process is described as having four phases: communication, insight, assessment, and working through. Activities, transference, associations, and interpretations are used throughout in order to facilitate the integration of more adaptive intrapsychic content.

The application of this frame of reference with a variety of client populations is discussed in Part VI.

23 Developmental Frames of Reference

Developmental frames of reference provide a structure for linking theories of human development, the age-specific nature of many activities, and the process of acquiring the basic skills necessary for successful interaction in the environment (58,64,67,74,339,616,618, 711,801,938,960). The assumptions fundamental to developmental frames of reference are:

1. Behavior is primarily influenced by the extent to which the individual has mastered previous stages of development.
2. In the typical maturation process the individual progresses through specific stages of development in various areas of human function. In each stage the individual's behavior or skill is qualitatively different than it is relative to a past or future stage in that area.
3. Interaction in an environment that simulates the usual optimal environment for the mastery of a particular stage of development in a given area will allow the individual to acquire the necessary behavior in an integrated manner. The individual must pass through all stages of development in a particular area to acquire maturation in that area.

The first section of the chapter is devoted to an elaboration of the above definition. The remaining portion of the chapter provides a review of the developmental orientation in occupational therapy.

Theories of human development constitute a body of knowledge devoted to describing various stages of human growth and how an individual moves from one stage to another. There is no one general theory of human development covering all areas of human function. Rather there are many theories, each dealing with a circumscribed aspect of human function. Thus, there are respective theories, for example, regarding the maturation of reflexes, psychosexual development, and the development of cognition. There are also several, often conflicting theories, about the same aspect of human development. This is particularly true in the areas of psychological and social function. A developmental frame of reference may be addressed to the application of one theory of development or the application of several theories.

In developmental frames of reference, purposeful activities are primarily viewed as embodying characteristics that are essential for the mastery of a particular stage of development in a given area of human function. The symbolic potential of activities is sometimes taken into consideration. This is true in the application of developmental frames of reference which are based on psychoanalytically oriented theories of psychosexual development. In such a case, activities are analyzed to determine the extent to which they might, in a symbolic way, satisfy various infantile needs. For example, in considering gratification of oral needs, one would analyze activities to ascertain whether they involved eating, sucking, blowing, encourage dependency, and so forth.

It is important to note that in developmental frames of reference, the symbolic potential of activities is not used to facilitate communication. Communication as described in the discussion of analytical frames of reference is not a part of developmental frames of reference. In other words, bringing unconscious or unshared intrapsychic content to the point where it can be shared is not considered important. The client need not be consciously aware that an infantile need is being gratified. The potential of activities to satisfy infantile needs in a symbolic or disguised way enables the client to receive satisfaction without having to recognize directly that he or she is at such a primitive state of development. Such recognition is extremely uncomfortable for many people as is the direct gratification of infantile needs.

In developmental frames of reference that are not based on psychoanalytically oriented theories, the reality of activities irrespective of their latent or covert symbolic potential is usually given priority. Activities are analyzed to determine the extent to which they might contribute to the age-specific development of performance components or occupational performances in a realistic manner. For example, one stage of cognitive development is characterized by the capacity to use simple tools. In the typical developmental process it appears that this skill is acquired through participation in tasks requiring the use of readily available tools. Thus activities would be analyzed to determine if the use of simple tools is necessary for successful completion of the activity.

Finally, in developmental frames of reference, activities are viewed primarily as a vehicle for acquiring stage-specific behavior rather than as entities to be mastered in and of themselves. By way of illustration, a group of clients may be involved in designing and making greeting cards to sell. The purpose of their involvement in this activity is to learn how to take appropriate roles in group situations. It is not to learn how to make greeting cards; this would be mastery of the activity. Designing and making greeting cards for the purpose of developing one stage of group interaction skill is the use of activities as a vehicle. It should be noted, however, that activities are occasionally considered as entities to be mastered in developmental frames of reference.

The first assumption of a developmental frame of reference is concerned with the belief that how an individual functions in the here and now is determined by whether that individual has successfully completed or passed through age-appropriate stages of development. The nature of the individual's present environment is not considered to be of great importance in influencing current behavior. Thus, for example, if a person is not ready to master participation in a cooperative group, he or she will either avoid such a group or interact in the group as if it was some other, less advanced type of group.

The second assumption addresses the belief that the area(s) of human function of concern in the frame of reference develops in a stage-specific manner. Stage specific refers to a series of steps, phases, or periods in the process of development. At each stage something new is added to the individual's repertoire; there is something qualitatively different in the way an individual is able to interact in the environment. This is exemplified in the child learning to sit, crawl, stand, walk, and so forth, sequentially. This may be contrasted to quantitative change such as the refinement or elaboration of behavior. Examples of quantitative change are increase in vocabulary or the acquisition of better eye-hand coordination. Quantitative development may take place during a particular stage or after the stage has been completed. Thus, in the development of language, at one stage the child acquires the ability to form a declarative sentence. This is an example of a qualitative change. As the child continues to mature, he or she will learn to form more complex declarative sentences; this is quantitative development. Developmental frames of reference are primarily concerned with qualitative changes in various areas of human function. It is assumed that once a basic skill or ability is acquired, refinement and elaboration will follow in the usual course of environmental interactions. In distinguishing the difference between qualitative and quantitative development, it is often useful to visualize qualitative development as a stairway with each step representing a specific stage of development in a given area of human function. Qualitative development may be visualized as a smooth ascending diagonal line, an ascending curve that plateaus or that plateaus for a period of time and then begins to descend. The appropriate visual representation of quantitative development would depend on the area of human function being illustrated.

Development in a particular area of human function is considered to be cumulative. That is, behavior acquired at a previous stage is not lost but rather integrated with the behavior acquired at the next stage of development. Thus, when an individual has reached a mature level of function in a particular area, behavior is the result of the accumulation or addition of successive parts or elements.

The third assumption fundamental to developmental frames of reference refers to the belief that mastery of a particular stage of development can occur in an environment that has characteristics similar to those elements believed to be essential for the mastery of that stage in the normal developmental process. Activity experiences are thus designed to be like situations that are thought to be influential in the acquisition of the stage-specific behavior in the typical course of development.

The third assumption also refers to the belief that each stage of development in a particular area needs to be mastered in order for an individual to be fully functional in that area. It is believed that no stage can be skipped or by-passed; stage-by-stage learning must take place. Lack of mastery of one or more stages frequently leads to the acquisition of splinter skills. This is stage-specific behavior that has been learned by rote, in a mechanical or nonintegrated manner. As mentioned, behavior so learned takes considerable energy to maintain and is the first behavior to be lost from the individual's repertoire in times of stress. Thus, when a developmental frame of reference is being used, the teaching of splinter skills is avoided and stage-by-stage learning is emphasized. However, when an individual, for whatever reason, cannot advance beyond a specific state of development, it may well be necessary to assist the individual in developing splinter or, perhaps more accurately, compensatory skills. This is only done after every effort has been made to help the individual master stages in a sequential manner. When splinter or compensatory skills are being taught, the change process involves the application of an acquisitional frame of reference, not a developmental frame of reference.

Relative to the occupational therapy domain of concern, developmental frames of reference currently in use in the profession are addressed to one or more of the performance components, activities of daily living, and to play as preparation for work. The other occupational performances have not been addressed. There is, however, no reason why they could not be dealt with through a developmental approach. That is, there is nothing inherent in developmental frames of reference prohibiting their use as the bases for change relative to family interaction, school/work, recreation/leisure, and temporal adaptation. Such frames of reference simply have not been formulated.

Developmental frames of reference in occupational therapy tend to focus on the first years of the life cycle and early adolescence. There are probably several reasons for this but the following seem to be significant:

1. Many developmental frames of reference grow out of occupational therapists' experiences in working with children and young adolescents. Frames of reference were formulated specifically to serve as the foundation for working with this population.

2. Occupational therapists tend to be more knowledgeable about child and early adolescent development. The understanding of adult development and development of aged individuals has only recently been of concern to them and included in basic professional education.

3. There is considerable evidence to indicate that stage-specific development of the performance components are, by and large, completed by mid- or late adolescence. This is not to say that it is thus assumed that development ceases at the end of adolescence. Rather, after this age development tends to be quantitative in nature. That is, basic behavioral patterns are elaborated and refined in order that individuals may adequately cope with the demands and responsibilities of adult life.

Whether a particular developmental frame of reference is concerned with the entire life cycle or with only a part of the life cycle is not important. All that is necessary is that the parameters of the frame of reference are clearly defined and the reason for limited parameters specified.

The major goal in the application of a developmental frame of reference is to help an individual master all stages of development in the areas addressed in the frame of reference that are appropriate, given the client's age and expected environment. A client is assisted in reaching those stages of development which are compatible with chronological age. When a client's age is such, for example, that he or she should only have mastered three of five stages in a particular area, then the change process is terminated when the last of these three stages has been attained. When a client's age is such that all five stages should have been mastered then the change process is usually not terminated until the final stage has been mastered. There are some exceptions to this. The client may be able to master the more advanced stages in a particular area without assistance from the therapist. Continued learning, then, would take place in the context of daily interaction in the community rather than in or under the auspices of the protective environment of a clinical setting. On the other hand, a client may not need to acquire complete competence in a particular area because such a degree of competence is not required in the expected environment. For example, an individual who is not obligated to engage in a nurturing relationship in his expected environment and has no interest in doing so need not master this advanced level of dyadic interaction.

The theoretical base of developmental frames of reference provides a description of the sequential stages of development of those areas of function addressed in the frame of reference. In addition, the theoretical base describes those factors in the environment, both human and nonhuman, which are believed to be responsible for movement from one stage of development to the next stage of development. When static developmental theories—those that only describe stages—are used, the theoretical base must also include a dynamic theory—one that describes how change occurs. One or a combination of learning theories may be used for this purpose. It is important to note that the inclusion of learning theory does not make a frame of reference acquisitional. The requirement that stage-by-stage mastery is essential is not negated by the inclusion of learning theory.

Developmental delays or deficits may be caused by any number of factors: neurological impairment, a less than optimal environment for growth, and so forth. Development may be retarded from very early in the life cycle, or lack of age-appropriate mastery in a particular area may be caused by traumatic injury or extreme and extraordinary environmental stress. However, discussion of the various reasons for developmental delay or deficit is usually not included in the theoretical base of developmental frames of reference. Causal factors are not considered important; the individual's current status is. The therapist essentially is only concerned with where the individual is, developmentally, at the time of initial evaluation. The etiology of developmental delay or deficit is, however, important in identifying the individual's expected environment and in setting realistic goals for the change process.

Function-dysfunction continuums in a developmental frame of reference consist of specific areas of human function. Each continuum is divided into stages; the number of stages varies depending on the area being addressed. Also, each stage may consist of several components or skills which are acquired in that area of human function at approximately the same time. In the description of the continuums, the approximate chronological age for the normal acquisition of each stage is usually given.

Some developmental frames of reference consist of only one continuum in that they deal with only one area of human function. Others consist of several continuums as they are concerned with a broader spectrum of human function. In illustration, a frame of reference based on Erikson's "eight stages of man" or Freud's outline of psychosexual stages would have only one continuum (271,317). Whereas, frames of reference that include continuums concerned with cognition, sensory integration, interpersonal relations, and so forth would have several continuums. In multicontinuum developmental frames of reference, each area of function is considered to be interdependent, with the other areas of function specified in the frame of reference. Thus, it is assumed that deficit or lack of age-appropriate development in one area of function will inhibit appropriate growth in other areas. Normal development across various areas of function tends to be uneven for any given individual. This is a natural and typical phenomena. If, however, development in one or more areas lags too far behind that of other areas, the individual is likely to have problems in the total developmental process. It is as if serious deficit in one area acted as a drift anchor, slowing down development in other areas.

Behavior indicative of function and dysfunction consists of a listing of specific behaviors an individual usually exhibits if he or she has or has not mastered a given stage of development. It should be noted that behaviors indicative of function and dysfunction are usually given for each stage, not for the continuum as a whole. One difficulty in delineating behavior indicative of function and dysfunction in a developmental frame of reference is related to the apparent difference between an adult who has not completed a relatively primitive stage of development and a child just prior to acquisition of the stage-specific behavior. This, of course, needs to be taken into consideration in interpreting evaluative findings.

The evaluation process involves determining whether an individual has mastered age-appropriate stages of development. Because development is a continuous process, mastery of a particular stage is not necessarily easy to identify. Frequently one sees some degrees of mastery across contiguous stages. In illustration, take a continuum that is made up of five stages. After evaluation with a particular client the therapist may see the following pattern:

Stage A—Complete mastery
Stage B—Almost complete mastery
Stage C—A fair amount of mastery
Stage D—Some mastery
Stage E—No mastery

In this case, it is fairly safe to say that the client is "at" stage C, with some components of stage B not yet mastered, and beginning the acquisition of some components of stage D.

In evaluation based on a developmental frame of reference, there are two factors that may cause some confusion for the neophyte therapist. The first is related to the client's past history. There is a tendency to equate what appears to be a growth-inhibiting environment at the usual time of mastery of a given stage with unsuccessful completion of that stage on the part of the client. The client, however, may have completed that stage even without an optimal environment or may have completed the stage later in a different, more growth-facilitating environment. The therapist is only concerned with the client's degree of mastery at the time of evaluation. The attainment of mastery of a particular stage may have been delayed or difficult to acquire. But this information is not relevant to the evaluation process.

The other factor is related to the tendency of people to compensate for lack of mastery, to acquire splinter skills, or to learn by rote. Because of this the individual may appear to have mastered the final stage of a particular area of human function at the time of evaluation. For example, because a client has attended college one should not assume that he or she has acquired the final state of cognitive development. Thus, the therapist must evaluate very carefully and not arrive at a conclusion about mastery without sufficient data.

Postulates regarding change in developmental frames of reference may be general or specific. General postulates may be addressed to all of the continuums in the frame of reference or to only one or two continuums. General postulates are often deduced from the learning theory(s) described in the theoretical base. The presentation of such postulates is based on the assumption that although the behaviors learned at each stage of development of various areas of function vary, the crucial factors that allow for the learning of the behavior are similar. Specific postulates state the characteristics of the environment that are believed to allow for movement from one given stage of development to the next stage of development. When specific postulates are used, there is a postulate regarding change for each stage of every continuum included in the frame of reference. Moreover, if one stage of development includes more than one component, there may be a different postulate regarding change for each of the components. Many developmental frames of reference have both general and specific postulates regarding change.

Postulates for setting short- and long-term goals are the same for all developmental frames of reference. In general, these postulates are the following:

1. The change process is initiated in that area of human function in which stage-specific learning is the most primitive. Most primitive refers to when the stage should have been mastered in the normal course of development. It does not refer to the sequential number of the stage, i.e., first, second, etc.

2. The change process is initiated at the stage immediately subsequent to the last stage that has been completely mastered. Using Fig. 23-1, the change process would begin with stage B.

3. The change process continues in that area of function through each sequentially more advanced stage until mastery in that area is equal to learning in the area in which stage-specific mastery is the next most primitive.

4. Change in this second area is then initiated.

5. The sequence continues until the client has (a) attained an age-appropriate level of mastery in all areas, (b) attained sufficient mastery for adequate function in the expected environment, or (c) reached what appears to be the highest level of mastery possible for him or her at this time.

Figure 23-1 provides an illustration of how these postulates relative to goal setting are applied.

Such a detailed outline is, of course, not needed in uni-continuum frames of reference. The change process begins at the stage immediately subsequent to the last stage that has been completely mastered.

The use of developmental frames of reference is appropriate for a broad spectrum of clients: individuals who are diagnosed as having psychiatric problems, individuals who are mentally retarded, individuals who have developmental delays in the psychosocial area due to restricted experiences because of physical illness or disability, and for individuals who are experiencing difficulty mastering an age-appropriate developmental task. The particular developmental frame of reference used must, of course, be addressed to those areas of human function which are problem areas for the client and include stages of development which the individual has not mastered.

It should be noted that developmental frames of reference are not just applicable to children or young adults. Although a particular developmental frame of reference may only deal with stages of development that are usually mastered by the end of adolescence, this does not mean that the frame of reference is not applicable for individuals who are beyond that age. Many clients will not have mastered these stages of development in various areas of function regardless of where they are in the life cycle. However, a developmental frame of reference that is addressed only to child and adolescent development should probably not be used for clients over about fifty years of age, even if they have not mastered the stages outlined in the frame of reference. The use of an acquisitional frame of reference is likely to be more appropriate. This recommendation concerning age and developmental level should be taken as only a suggestion. There are many exceptions when the use of a developmental frame of reference may be appropriate.

In contrast to analytical frames of reference, participation in a change process based on a developmental frame of reference does not require any particular level of cognitive function or verbal skill. As a matter of fact, some developmental frames of reference are ideally suited for clients who are markedly deficient in these areas.

The application of developmental frames of reference, similar to analytical frames of reference, requires a somewhat lengthy period of time. Thus both these types of frames of reference are inappropriate for short-term intervention. As a general rule, neither type of frame of reference should be used in situations where the client

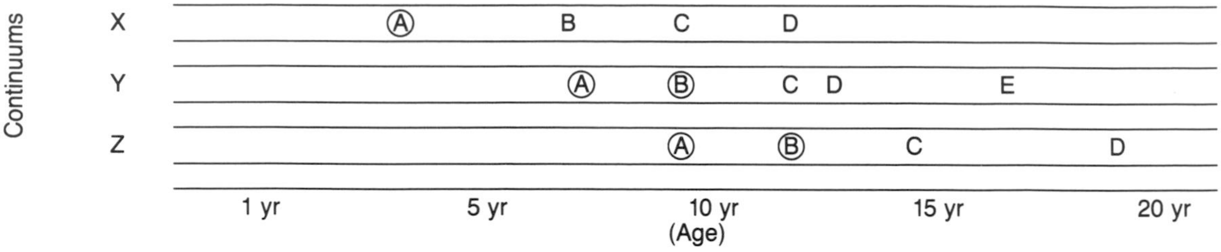

Continuums	
X	Ⓐ B C D
Y	Ⓐ Ⓑ C D E
Z	Ⓐ Ⓑ C D
	1 yr 5 yr 10 yr (Age) 15 yr 20 yr

The client is 15 years of age.
○ = Mastery of that stage of development at the time of initial assessment.
Long-term goal = mastery of Z–C
Short-term goal in sequence: Goal 1 = mastery of X–B; Goal 2 = mastery of X–C; goal 3 = mastery of X–D and Y–C; (Stages from different areas of function usually mastered at the same time in the normal developmental process may be dealt with simultaneously in the change process.); goal 4 = mastery of Y–D; goal 5 = mastery of Z–C

FIG. 23-1. The sequence of goal setting in developmental frames of reference.

will be involved in intervention for less than a month. The use of an acquisitional frame of reference is usually more appropriate in such situations.

With this general description of developmental frames of reference, the remaining portion of this chapter is devoted to a brief discussion of those major developmental frames of reference primarily concerned with psychosocial components and currently used in occupational therapy.

REVIEW OF THE DEVELOPMENTAL ORIENTATION

Ayres

The first major developmental frame of reference was proposed by A. J. Ayres and is concerned with sensory integration (58,64). Through her work, primarily with learning disabled children, Ayres identified four major syndromes related to deficits in sensory integration. These are:

1. Tactile defensiveness: Characterized by adversive responses to certain types of tactile stimuli, particularly light touch instituted by others; by diminished tactile discrimination; and frequently by hyperactivity and distractibility.
2. Postural and bilateral integration: Deficit is characterized by poorly integrated primitive postural reflexes, immature equilibrium reactions, poor ocular control, and lack of integration of the two sides of the body.
3. Praxia: Deficit is characterized by difficulty in planning skilled or nonhabitual motor tasks.
4. Form and space perception: Deficit is characterized by difficulty with eye-hand coordination, form consistency, figure-ground perception, position in space, and spatial relations.

Each of these syndromes is considered to arise from faulty development of some aspect of subcortical processing. Function in these areas is described as being acquired by stages through the normal maturation of the nervous system and adequate interaction with the environment. Deficits in development are determined through the use of SCSIT, SCPNT, or some nonstandardized modification of these tests. Remediation in general, involves "providing planned and controlled sensory input with usually—but not invariably—the eliciting of a related adaptive response . . ." (58, p. 114). Adaptive responses are purposeful, goal-directed actions that are more mature and complex than the individual has emitted before. Repeating already learned responses is not considered effective in bringing about change. However, repetition is felt to be important for consolidation of the changes that have occurred.

Ayres provides a detailed theoretical base for her frame of reference and clearly identifies continuums and behavior indicative of function and dysfunction. The continuums or syndromes are not necessarily mutually exclusive, a factor in the frame of reference which Ayres readily identifies. The relationship between data gathered from the use of SCSIT and SCPNT and the identification of function and dysfunction is fairly clearly stated. Nevertheless, the interpretation of the data is a relatively complex matter. Both general and specific postulates regarding change are provided, with many examples of various techniques deduced from these postulates described. Ayres' frame of reference is one of the most complete available in occupational therapy.

The following are some of the issues that have been raised relative to this frame of reference and to sensory integration as a performance component.

There is some question regarding the degree to which the neurological structures and their functions, stated as being basic to the sensory integrative process and used as support for the frame of reference, are an accurate description of the way in which the brain processes information. There is, however, so much unknown about the brain that the question cannot really be answered at this time.

The literature often either states or implies that sensory integration is basic to most other areas of function. This is especially true in the area of cognitive function. The capacity to read, write, and deal with mathematical problems are to some extent cognitive in nature but they are only a small component of cognitive function. Individuals with learning disabilities are often of above average intelligence, and there is no evidence to indicate that their cognitive development, as described by Piget, is deficient (774). It is thus more accurate to view sensory integration as one area of human function equal but not superordinate to all other areas. Deficits in sensory integration may cause delayed or inadequate development of the other performance components, but the converse is also true. All performance components are interrelated but that relationship is not hierarchial.

There is some question regarding just what type of change is occurring in intervention directed toward improving sensory integration. Ayres states that

> new anatomical pathways are not developed but already existing neuronal connections which are lying more or less dormant are used with greater ease and frequency. . . . Therapy is believed to use potentially existing synapses or mechanisms although the possibility of establishing new synapses, especially in the young child is not overlooked (58, p. 128).

Whether this is the case or not is unknown. It may well be that the individual is simply acquiring skills without any alteration of the nervous system.

Many proponents of intervention based on Ayres' frame of reference seem to identify deficits in sensory integration in individuals with a very wide variety of disabilities. Some of the literature seems to suggest that almost all individuals screened by occupational therapists have deficits in this area. Proponents of a particular frame of reference do, at times, become somewhat carried away and imprudent in their claims. This is mentioned by way of a reminder to the neophyte therapist.

Finally, as mentioned in Chapter 16, the reliability of the evaluation techniques developed by Ayres is not very high nor has validity been established. In addition, the efficacy of the application of Ayres' frame of reference is only just beginning to be studied. There is further discussion of this frame of reference in Chapter 31.

Ayres' concern about sensory integration and her frame of reference influenced the developmental frames of reference formulated by Llorens and Mosey. These frames of reference will be discussed momentarily. Ayres, however, probably had the greatest influence on King.

King

The frame of reference formulated by L. J. King is described by her as being specific to adults diagnosed as having process or reactive schizophrenia (533). She describes these reactions as nonparanoid in nature with process schizophrenia being characterized by schizophrenic-like behavior evident in childhood which gradually becomes more pronounced, with the individual slowly slipping into psychoses. Reactive schizophrenia is characterized by at least marginally adequate function until encountering a severe stress situation.

Although based on Ayres' work, King's frame of reference is primarily concerned with the integration of vestibular stimuli. This aspect of sensory integration is seen as basic to the integration of all other types of stimuli. King does not, however, describe the integration of vestibular stimuli as stage specific. Thus, her frame of reference is actually not developmental. It is being discussed here only because it is frequently categorized as developmental by members of the profession.

King's theoretical base is primarily devoted to presenting an argument for deficit in the integration of vestibular stimuli being a causal factor of nonparanoid schizophrenic disorders.

The function dysfunction continuum in this frame of reference, as mentioned, is the integration of vestibular stimuli. Behaviors indicative of dysfunction were outlined in Chapter 16.

Postulates regarding change emphasize the importance of gross motor activities which:

1. Encourage motions that are the opposite of protective primitive reflex patterns (i.e., extension, abduction, and external rotation);
2. Emphasize attention to the active doing or the accomplishment of some goal rather than on the motor processes involved;

3. Are experienced as comfortable and pleasurable by the individual.

King's frame of reference has only been formulated relatively recently and may well be revised and amplified in the future. At this point it has been presented in a rather sketchy manner, with the assumption that the reader is familiar with Ayres' frame of reference. Although narrow in the population to which it is addressed, King's frame of reference has stimulated considerable interest. Evaluation of the effectiveness of its use is just beginning. Hopefully these efforts will continue.

There are many critical issues raised by this frame of reference. These are best understood in the context of a review of research relative to schizophrenic disorders. Such a discussion is presented in Chapter 31.

Llorens

Also drawing upon the work of Ayres, L. A. Llorens' orientation is, however, broader, taking into consideration more areas of human function and the entire life cycle (618). By way of introduction, Llorens' developmental approach comes out of the late 1960s and early 1970s when a variety of frames of reference were being formulated as well as efforts being made to articulate a comprehensive theory of occupational therapy. The distinction between these two entities was not clearly defined at that time. This is reflected in Llorens' work, which can best be described as a cross between a frame of reference and a comprehensive theory. Her work will be discussed here as a frame of reference for two reasons: It more closely resembles a frame of reference than a comprehensive theory, and it is generally treated as a frame of reference by the profession.

In formulating her frame of reference, Llorens used the developmental theories of Ayres, Erikson, Freud, Gesell, Hovighurst, Pierce and Newton, and Piaget. Seven basic areas of human function are identified: neurophysiological, psysical-motor, psychosocial, psychodynamics, social-language, sociocultural, and activities of daily living. The satisfactory integration and assimilation of these seven basic areas is referred to as "Behavioral Expectations and Adaptive Skills" and is divided into three subcategories: developmental tasks, ego adaptive skills, and intellectual development. Finally, the concept of occupational performance is also included in the theoretical base. It is described as including "work, education, play, self-care, and leisure." Although not specifically stated, it appears that occupational performance is a third order of human function. This level is apparently dependent on adequate mastery of age-specific behaviors or skills at the two lower levels. Schematically it seems best to visualize Llorens' way of organizing the various dimensions of human development as a pyramid: the seven basic areas of human function as the foundation of the pyramid, the three subcategories of behavioral expectations and adaptive skills as the middle portion, and occupational performances as the top of the pyramid.

Llorens outlines human development by providing an overview of the life cycle which is divided into eight phases. Possible deficits in development are described through the presentation of 15 brief case studies.

Purposeful activities are discussed in two different ways. The first is through a guide for activity analysis, which includes six major dimensions for the examination of activities: sensory, physical, psychodynamic, social, practical, and attention and skill aspects. The second way that purposeful activities are described is through the categorization of types of activities: sensory, developmental, symbolic, and daily life tasks. Interpersonal relationships are described but treated separately from activities. The four types of activities and interpersonal relationships are further subdivided into those that are typical in each of the eight phases of the life cycle.

Llorens suggests various evaluative procedures: personal interview, behavioral observation, sensorimotor tests, projective techniques, and intellectual assessment.

In regard to the change process, Llorens states that

> It is through the skilled application of activities and relationships that the occupational therapist provides growth experiences to assist in closing the existing developmental gaps and preventing potential developmental maladaptation in. . . . [various] spheres of development both across developmental areas and throughout the life cycle (618, p. 37).

Llorens continues by stating that

> Sensorimotor activities, developmental activities, symbolic activities, daily life tasks and interpersonal relationships specifically significant to particular age ranges in the growth process are the tools used by occupational therapists in . . . intervention.

Intervention is primarily described through the presentation of plans for intervention relative to the 15 case studies previously mentioned.

Llorens has formulated a developmental frame of reference which seems to cover the majority of areas of human function of concern to occupational therapists plus the entire life cycle. Its strong points are the overview which it presents of the life cycle and the emphasis it places on considering the possibility of developmental deficits or lags in clients with a wide variety of diagnoses and from various age groups. However, as a frame of reference, Llorens' presentation lacks specificity, which makes it a somewhat less than adequate guide for formulating plans for change. Some of the major problem areas are briefly identified below.

The theoretical base does not provide a dynamic theory. There is no description of how an individual moves from one stage to the next in the normal developmental process. There seems to be an assumption that the reader knows a good deal about the dynamics of human development in the areas addressed and that therefore no detailed explanation is necessary.

Second, the presentation of three levels of human function is confusing. Admittedly it is extremely difficult to categorize the multiplicity of human functions in any sort of meaningful way. There is much overlapping of areas and combining of areas to form more complex gestalts of behaviors. However, Llorens' three levels seem excessively redundant. For example, activities of daily living are placed on both the first and the third level; cognitive function, to some extent included in the neurophysiological area, is also a part of intellectual development, one of the three subcategories of the second level. As a consequence of this redundancy the function-dysfunction continuums are neither mutually exclusive nor on the same conceptual level. This, in turn, leads to difficulty in evaluation.

The third problem area is related to the description of purposeful activities. The two methods of description—a conceptual framework for activity analysis and categorization of activities by types—tend to confuse rather than clarify. No reason is given for the two different presentations nor is there any discussion of how they relate one to the other.

The fourth problem is concerned with the interpretation of evaluative data. Behaviors indicative of function, as presented, are not particularly detailed nor are they specifically tailored to what one might observe using the suggested evaluative procedures or tools. Llorens does emphasize the importance of knowledge and skill in evaluation in the area of human development and clinical judgement. However, more specific guidelines concerning evaluation would be useful.

Finally, Llorens does not provide any postulates regarding change. The information presented is not sufficiently specific to provide guidelines for goal setting and planning intervention.

Llorens' frame of reference has been widely used as a structure for organizing strategies for evaluation and intervention. However, direct application is only possible through drawing on additional information regarding human growth and development and purposeful activities.

The last major developmental frame of reference in occupational therapy is "Recapitulation of Ontogenesis," which was formulated by Mosey in the late 1960s. This will not be discussed here since a revision of that frame of reference is presented in its entirety in the following chapter. The major revisions made are in the interest of simplification and greater clarity.

24 Recapitulation of Ontogenesis: A Developmental Frame of Reference

Recapitulation of ontogenesis was selected as the label for this developmental frame of reference because it seems to describe what happens in the change process (705). More specifically, the term recapitulation means to repeat or to do over again. Ontogenesis is the term used to identify the stage-by-stage development characteristic of a particular species. The change process in a developmental frame of reference, then, gives the individual an opportunity to progress sequentially through those stages of development which had not been attempted or were never completely mastered.

This frame of reference is addressed to all of the psychosocial performance components. It is appropriate for individuals who have, for whatever reason, not mastered all the stages of development outlined in the frame of reference. There are no particular restrictions on the applicability of this frame of reference other than those described in Chapter 23 relative to all developmental frames of reference.

AN OVERVIEW

Recapitulation of ontogenesis is addressed to the development of "adaptive skills"—essential, learned patterns of behavior. As outlined below, adaptive skills are not concerned with all aspects of development but only with those that are considered crucial for successful participation in the various occupational performance. Occupational performances are not, however, addressed in this frame of reference. The term "adaptive" is used here in the sense of being able to negotiate within the environment in such a way as to be able to satisfy one's own needs as well as those of others. It is used in the sense of creative use of the environment—not in the sense of conformity.

Six major adaptive skills have been identified as well as the subskills, which sequentially form the foundation for each mature skill (see Chapter 5 for references). The subskills delineate the developmental stages of each skill; when all of the subskills have been acquired, the individual is said to have reached full maturity in a particular adaptive skill. The following outline gives a brief definition of each of the adaptive skills. The subskills or stages that constitute each skill are listed in the sequence in which they are usually learned. Some of the subskills consist of more than one part which henceforth will be referred to as components. The components of a subskill are not considered to be sequential except in a few instances which will be identified later in the discussion of each subskill. The six adaptive skills are as follows:

Sensory integration skill. The ability to receive, select, combine, and coordinate vestibular, proprioceptive, and tactile information for functional use.

1. The ability to integrate the tactile subsystems (0–3 months).
2. The ability to integrate primitive postural reflexes (3–9 months).

3. Maturation of mature righting and equilibrium reactions (9–12 months).
4. The ability to integrate the two sides of the body, to be aware of body parts and their relationship, and to plan gross motor movements (1–2 yr)
5. The ability to plan fine motor movements (2–3 yr).

Cognitive skill. The ability to perceive, represent, and organize sensory information for the purpose of thinking and problem solving.

1. The ability to use inherent behavioral patterns for environmental interaction (0–1 month).
2. The ability to interrelate visual, manual, auditory, and oral responses (1–4 months).
3. The ability to attend to the environmental consequence of actions with interest, to represent objects in an exoceptual manner, to experience objects, to act on the bases of egocentric causality, and to seriate events in which the self is involved (4–9 months).
4. The ability to establish a goal and intentionally carry out means, to recognize the independent existence of objects, to interpret signs, to imitate new behavior, to apprehend the influence of space, and to perceive other objects as partially causal (9–12 months).
5. The ability to use trial-and-error problem solving, to use tools, to perceive variability in spacial positions, to seriate events in which the self is not involved, and to perceive the causality of other objects (12–18 months).
6. The ability to represent objects in an image manner, to make believe, to infer a cause given its effect, to act on the bases of combined spatial relations, to attribute omnipotence to others, and to perceive objects as permanent in time and place (18 months–2 yr).
7. The ability to represent objects in a endoceptual manner, to differentiate between thought and action, and to recognize the need for causal sources (2–5 yr).
8. The ability to represent objects in a denotative manner, to perceive the viewpoint of others, and to decenter (6–7 yr).
9. The ability to represent objects in a connotative manner, to use formal logic, and to work in the realm of the hypothetical (11–13 yr).

Dyadic interaction skill. The ability to participate in a variety of dyadic relationships.

1. The ability to enter into trusting familial relationships (8–10 months).
2. The ability to enter into association relationships (3–5 yr).
3. The ability to interact in an authority relationship (5–7 yr).
4. The ability to interact in a chum relationship (10–14 yr).
5. The ability to enter into a peer, authority relationship (15–17 yr).
6. The ability to enter into an intimate relationship (18–25 yr).
7. The ability to engage in a nurturing relationship (20–30 yr).

Group interaction skill. The ability to engage in a variety of primary groups.

1. The ability to participate in a parallel group (18 months–2 yr).
2. The ability to participate in a project group (2–4 yr).
3. The ability to participate in an egocentric group (9–12 yr).
4. The ability to participate in a cooperative group (9–12 yr).
5. The ability to participate in a mature group (15–18 yr).

Self-identity skill. The ability to perceive the self as a relatively autonomous, holistic, and acceptable person who has permanence and continuity over time.

1. The ability to perceive the self as a worthy person (9–12 months).
2. The ability to perceive the assets and limitations of the self (11–15 yr).
3. The ability to perceive the self as self-directed (20–25 yr).
4. The ability to perceive the self as a productive, contributing member of a social system (30–35 yr).
5. The ability to perceive the self as having an autonomous identity (35–50 yr).
6. The ability to perceive the aging process of oneself and ultimate death as part of the life cycle. (45–60 yr).

Sexual identity skill. The ability to perceive one's sexual nature as good and to participate in a relatively long-term sexual relationship that is oriented to the mutual satisfaction of sexual needs.

1. The ability to accept and act on the basis of one's pregenital sexual nature (4–5 yr).
2. The ability to accept sexual maturation as a positive growth experience (12–16 yr).
3. The ability to give and receive sexual gratification (18–25 yr).

4. The ability to enter into a sustained sexual relationship characterized by the mutual satisfaction of sexual needs (20–30 yr).
5. The ability to accept the sex-related physiological changes that occur as a natural part of the aging process (40–60 yr).

The Adaptive Skills Developmental Chart, Fig. 24-1, is an attempt to illustrate the sequential, interdependent nature of adaptive skills. The shaded areas relative to each adaptive skill indicates the age range in which each subskill is usually mastered. It should, of course, be remembered that there is much individual variation in the age of mastering which is still well within the normal range.

The theoretical base of recapitulation of ontogenesis is made up of much that has been previously discussed in this text. More specifically, it consists of the psychosocial performance components (Chapter 3), socialization (Chapter 4), the life cycle (Chapter 5), and all of the tools of occupational therapy (Part 3). In the discussion of each adaptive skill, emphasis is placed on identifying those elements within the environment that are believed to be responsible for the mastery of each developmental stage of the six adaptive skills.

The function-dysfunction continuums of recapitulation of ontogenesis are, of course, the six adaptive skills. An individual is considered to be in a state of function when there is evidence of integrated learning of those subskills appropriate to chronological age and/or are needed for successful participation in the expected environment. The individual is said to be in a state of dysfunction when there is evidence of a lack of integrated learning of these subskills. Behavior indicative of function and dysfunction as well as appropriate evaluative tools is outlined in the discussion of each of the adaptive skills.

Some therapists have found that the Adaptive Skills Developmental Chart is useful for summarizing evaluative findings. A perpendicular red line is drawn to the right of the most advanced subskill the client has mastered in each adaptive skill; a perpendicular blue line is drawn to the right of the most advanced subskill of each of the adaptive skills which ought to have been mastered given the client's age or which the client needs for successful participation in the expected environment. This is a graphic way of delineating the client's current status as well as the long-term goals of the change process. Intervention is then directed toward the sequential mastery of all subskills falling between the red and blue lines.

There are three general postulates regarding change in recapitulation of ontogenesis. The first two were discussed in Chapter 23. They are, first, that adaptive skills are acquired through participation in growth-facilitating environments. On the basis of this postulate, the therapist designs activities that simulate the specific growth-facilitating environment believed to be necessary for the mastery of a given subskill. The environmental elements required for the mastery of each subskill and the significant activity characteristics is outlined later in this chapter.

The second general postulate is concerned with the sequence of the change process. The initial goal of the change process is mastery of the most primitive subskill that the client has not learned in an integrated manner. The change process is addressed to this adaptive skill until the subskill level is equal to the subskill level of the next least-developed adaptive skill. Change is then initiated in this area. This sequence continues until the client has mastered all subskills that are appropriate for his or her age or that are needed for successful participation in the expected environment. More than one subskill may be dealt with at the same time in the change process if these subskills are mastered at approximately the same time in the life cycle. Reference to the Adaptive Skills Developmental Chart may be useful for determining the appropriate sequence of the change process.

The third general postulate regarding change is that the need for mastery serves as a motivational and regulatory force in the development of adaptive skills. This need allows the individual to experience what is good and right for him or her at any given time. In other words, if appropriate environmental elements are available, an individual will make use of them for the continued acquisition of adaptive skills. In essence, the change process involves tuning into and tapping this need for mastery. The therapist's knowledge of human development and clinical judgment is, of course, important. It is the therapist's responsibility to select appropriate learning experiences; to provide activities that will facilitate mastery; to determine when the client is ready to move on to the learning of more advanced subskills; and to provide support, encouragement, and reinforcement. However, if the client shows evidence of more than the usual degree of anxiety, resistance, or frustration, it is recommended that the therapist reassess the client's current level of development and the environment that has been planned for learning. The activities made available to the client may not be appropriate at this particular time. Intervention designed to facilitate the mastery of adaptive skills must be a collaborative experience if it is to nurture growth.

The remaining portion of the chapter is devoted to the discussion of each of the adaptive skills.

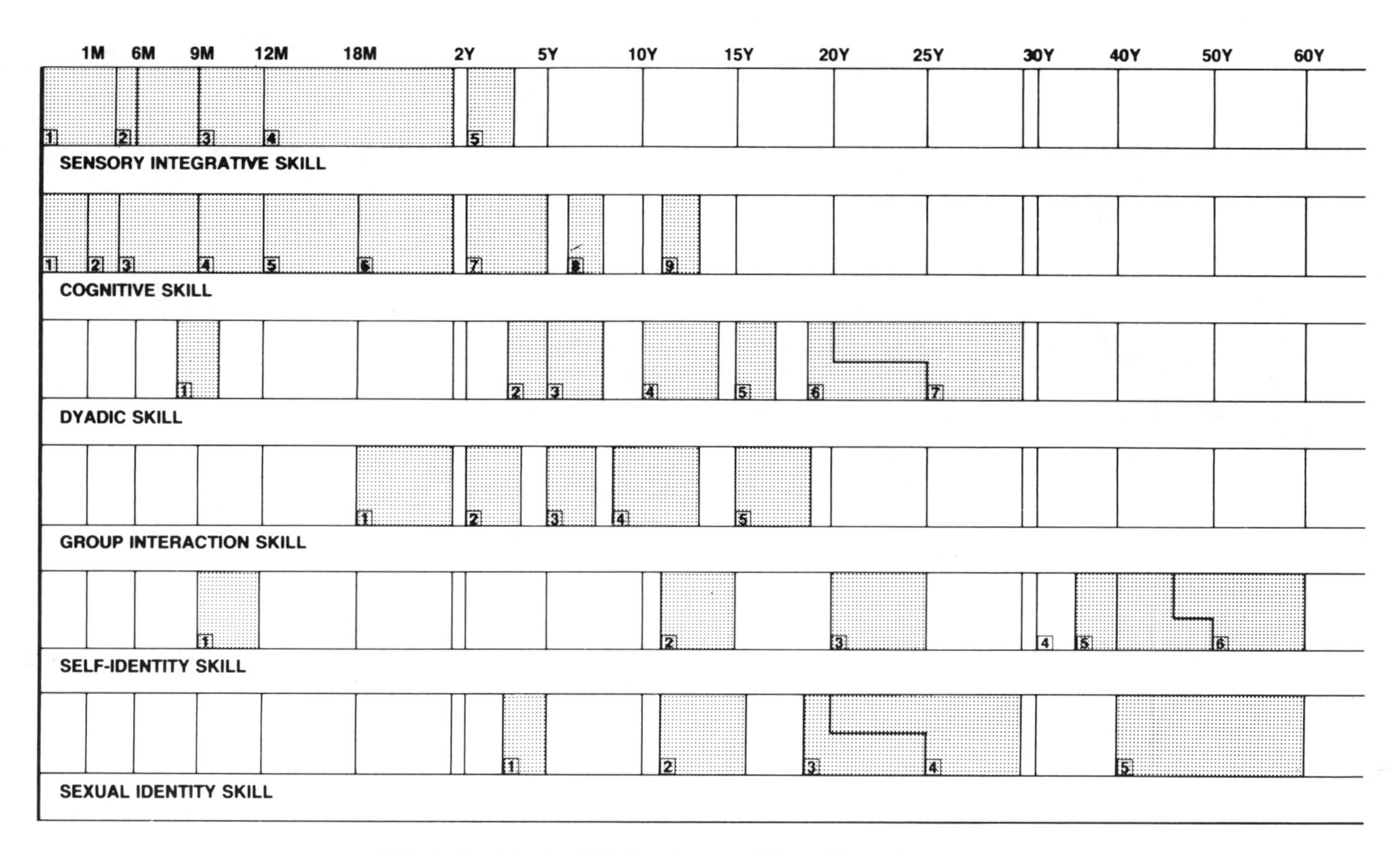

FIG. 24-1. Adaptive Skills Developmental Chart. M, month(s); Y, years.

EVALUATION AND THE CHANGE PROCESS

Sensory Integration Skill

The following description of sensory integration skill is based on Ayres. However, rather than a delineation of syndromes, this presentation outlines the sequential development of sensory integration as presented in Chapter 5. Admittedly, this is a simplification of Ayres's work, a factor that should be kept in mind when using this part of recapitulation of ontogenesis.

Evaluation of this adaptive skill is based on the data gathered through the SCSIT outlined in Chapter 16. However, this should only be done if the client is a member of the normative population and if the therapist is skilled in the administration of these tests. When either of the criteria is not able to be met, it is recommended that the therapist use the behaviors indicative of function and dysfunction (outlined below) as the bases for designing appropriate evaluative situations.

The following general postulates regarding change apply to the mastery of all stages of sensory integrative skill.

First, sensory integration is enhanced by providing planned and controlled sensory input that elicits a related adaptive response. (There are times, however, when an adaptive response is not considered important. This is particularly true in the initial phases of the change process when the provision of appropriate sensory stimuli is more important than eliciting an adaptive response.)

Second, sensory integration is enhanced by sensory stimulation which is sufficiently intense to be received at the subcortical level but not so intense that it causes overarousal.

Third, adaptive responses are enhanced by increased tactile and proprioceptive stimulation associated with the involved muscle groups.

Fourth, more refined and discriminate adaptive responses are facilitated by grading stimuli events from gross to fine.

Fifth, sensory integration is facilitated by providing an opportunity for the individual to engage in motor activities that are not a part of his or her usual repertoire of behavior. However, repetition of newly learned adaptive responses helps to consolidate and maintain those subskills that are in the process of being mastered.

Sixth and finally, the most appropriate activities for facilitating sensory integration are those that arouse the client's interests and are experienced as pleasurable.

With these introductory remarks, the five stages of sensory integrative skill are described as follows:

The Ability to Integrate the Tactile Subsystems (0–3 months)

An adequate balance between the protective and discriminatory tactile subsystems allows the individual to differentiate between injurious and noninjurious tactile stimuli and to inhibit the appropriate system on the bases of this information.

Behaviors indicative of mastery of this subskill are the ability to tolerate stimulation of light touch receptors, accept tactile stimulation initiated by others, locate a point of tactile stimulation fairly accurately, perceive double tactile stimulation, identify simple geometric shapes drawn on the back of the hand (graphesthesia), and identify shapes through manual manipulation.

An individual has not mastered this subskill if the behaviors listed above are not present. Other indications of lack of mastery are the feeling of discomfort and the desire to escape when the individual is uncertain about or not in control of the tactile stimuli that he or she may receive; hypersensitivity to pain, cold, sounds, and odors; unreasonable anger or belligerence when inadvertently touched by another person; and the avoidance of activities that involve physical contact. Lack of mastery may also be indicated by a seemingly uncontrollable urge to touch everything in the environment.

A balance between the tactile subsystems is acquired through stimulation of those tactile receptors that respond to pressure, as opposed to light touch. This tends to inhibit the protective system. In addition, the individual must have an opportunity to experience many different kinds of noninjurious tactile stimuli. Stimulation of the hands, forearms, and face promotes perception because of the rich supply of tactile receptors located in these areas.

The change process relative to mastery of this subskill involves massive stimulation of the tactile receptors, especially those receptors responding to pressure. A rough cloth or brush of appropriate stiffness is usually used to stimulate receptors on the face, forearms, and hands. This may be done by the therapist but the preferred method is for the individual to give tactile stimulation to him- or herself. This method is recommended for two reasons: (a) the individual is less likely to respond in a negative manner to self stimulation, and (b) stimulation can be initiated several times a day. Many individuals who lack a balance between the protective and discriminatory tactile subsystems find that self-stimulation has a soothing, organizing effect at those times when they are feeling anxious, upset, or jumpy. Other areas of the body may also be stimulated by rubbing or brushing. Additional stimuli are provided by using various textured carpets and rugs during floor activities. Rolling inside a barrel lined with a rug is also a useful activity. When facilities are available, water play, swimming, water hose activities, hot and cold showers, and covering the body or body parts with sand provide additional tactile stimulation. Such stimulation occurs concomitant with purposeful motor activity that should be perceived as safe and predictable by the individual. Tactile stimulation is not utilized if there is evidence of hypertonicity. If stimulation gives rise to pallor and increase in heart or respiratory rates, or a strong negative reaction, it is discontinued or altered in such a manner that the above-listed responses do not occur.

The Ability to Integrate Primitive Postural Reflexes (3–9 months)

The primitive postural reflexes of concern here are the tonic-labyrinth reflexes (flexion of arms and legs in the prone position and extension in the supine position) and the tonic neck reflexes (extension of the arm toward which the head is turned, flexion of the other arm, and a similar or opposite reaction in the lower extremities).

These reflexes are believed to be integrated when the individual does not exhibit any difficulty in maintaining a pivot prone position (extension of neck and extremities when in the prone position), or there is evidence of the tonic neck reflex or trunk rotation when the head is passively turned or vertical movement of arms when asked to hold arms out in front of body with eyes closed. These reflexes are considered not be to integrated if the individual exhibits the above-mentioned behaviors.

Primitive postural reflexes are integrated through taking positions that are directly opposite from the reflex position. The ability to take the opposite position is facilitated by vestibular stimulation. It also appears that stimulation of the pressure receptors of the chest and stomach when an individual is in a prone position leads to assumption of the pivot prone position. Flexion of the neck in a supine position tends to cause flexion of the extremeties. These reactions themselves appear to be reflexive in nature.

One method that has been found to be effective involves the use of a scooter board (thorax-sized board on wheels). Maintaining a prone position on a scooter necessitates extension of neck and extremities. This position may be further facilitated by rolling down an inclined plane (increases vestibular stimulation) and pressure stimulation of the back extensors. The supine tonic labyrinth reflex may be inhibited by taking a supine position on the scooter board or on a swing. The tonic neck reflexes are integrated through eliciting the reflex and then taking a standing or kneeling position with the arm opposite from the way in which the head is turned and in an extended position supporting the body. The arm on the side of the body toward which the head is turned is maintained in a flexed position. The position taken by the legs depends on their reflex reaction. There should be extension of the leg that is receiving increased flexer tone from the tonic neck reflex. The turned-head position is facilitated by holding a towel between chin and shoulder, which also provides increased tactile stimulation. The need for equilibrium reactions in maintaining these positions enhances integration of the reflexes. The individual should engage in activities that promote inhibition of the postural reflexes several times a day. It is recommended that they be preceded by or take place concurrent with vestibular stimulation. Such stimulation can be gained from swinging, spinning, twirling, rolling, etc. The activities described below for developing equilibrium reactions are also useful for integration of postural reflexes.

Maturation of Mature Righting and Equilibrium Reactions (9–12 months)

Mastery of this subskill leads to the development of balance or adequate equilirium reactions.

An individual reacts appropriately to vestibular stimuli when able to maintain one- and two-leg standing balance with eyes open and closed, easily retain balance when the body's center of gravity is shifted, and stabilize trunk and proximal parts when using distal parts to carry out an activity. Absence of these reactions indicates lack of mastery in this area.

The development of appropriate reactions to vestibular stimuli is enhanced through vestibular stimulation and repeated attempts at making bodily adjustments in response to alteration in vestibular stimulation.

Some methods that have been used for alteration of dysfunction in this area are passive swinging or spinning in a net hammock in the initial phase of the change process to assist in subcortical reception of vestibular stimuli. Some individuals with deficit in this area appear to have a very high threshold for vestibular stimuli; there is need for massive input. Self-initiated spinning or swinging is used later in the change process as this both arises from adaptive behavior and promotes adaptive response. Other methods are activities that involve rolling in a barrel (lined with a rug in order to increase tactile stimulation); maintaining balance on a large beach ball while in a prone, supine, sitting, and kneeling position (the therapist holds on to the client's hands or feet until he or she has gained sufficient skill to safely engage in this activity without resistance); scooter activities (independently or with another person pulling the scooter at an increasingly greater speed); balancing on a rocking board in sitting, kneeling, and standing positions; sliding down an inclined plane sitting or kneeling on pieces of slick paper; balancing on a T-stool; walking on different types of stilts; and walking on a rail. Activities selected to increase equilibrium reactions are structured so that the individual's attention is distracted from the act of balancing itself. This enhances integration at a subcortical rather than at a cortical level. Activities requiring co-contraction of postural muscles while distal parts are involved in the performance of a task are particularly helpful in enhancing integration.

Integration of Two Sides of the Body (1–2 years)

Through mastery of this component, sometimes referred to as bilateral motor coordination, the individual becomes aware of and learns to coordinate the two sides of the body.

Mastery is indicated by the ability to cross the midline visually and manually without hesitation and perform bilateral activities with ease. Lack of learning is the absence of these types of behaviors and a seeming disregard for one-half of space or one side of the body.

Integration of the two sides of the body is acquired through reciprocal movement of the extremities, bilateral activities, and activities that require manual and visual crossing of the midline of the body.

Change in this area begins with such gross reciprocal activities as creeping, crawling, clapping, bicycling, playing with hulahoops, jumping with two feet, and swimming. Bilateral activities requiring the joint use of two hands are used next (e.g., moving large objects, hitting a suspended ball with a cardboard tube held at either end, and batting a ball). Complementary bilateral activities and unilateral activities are initiated as the individual's skill increases. Concurrent with use of the above activities, the individual is involved in tasks involving movement away from, toward, and across the midline of the body. Blackboard activities and calisthenics, which require these types of movement, are suggested. Special attention should be given to increasing tactile and proprioceptive stimulation (for instance, rubbing body parts and use of weighted cuffs). When there is evidence of marked perceptual and motor deficit on one side of the body, emphasis is placed on this neglected side. If there is evidence of poor motor planning on one side of the body, the methods outlined below for the development of motor planning are utilized.

Awareness of Body Parts and Their Relationships (1–2 years)

This aspect of sensory integrative skill is sometimes referred to as body scheme. It involves knowledge of the various body parts, their static relationship to each other, and the relationship of parts during movement and in different postural positions.

An individual who has mastered this component is aware of body parts and their relationship to each other, is able to identify various fingers when they have been touched by an examiner (vision occluded), name the various body parts, state the relationship between parts, and identify the position of his or her body parts without aid of vision. Dysfunction in this area is indicated by the inability to engage in these behaviors.

Awareness of body parts and their relationships is acquired through purposeful movement; observation of the body of self and others, and activities that involve integration of tactile, proprioceptive, and visual information.

Some activities for change deduced from the above postulates are movement of body parts through their full range of motion with assistance from the therapist, without assistance, and against resistance; imitation of the therapist's movements; visual inspection of the self, another person, or a representation of the human body accompanied by identification of body parts and discussion regarding the relationship of one part to another; drawing around body parts; sculpting and drawing the human body and putting together a representation of the human body; identifying various objects and textures with vision occluded, sand play, and finger painting (primarily for adequate finger identification).

Planned Gross Motor Movements (1–2 years)

Gross motor planning is the ability to plan and carry out large movements in a skilled and coordinated manner.

Adequate gross motor planning is indicated by the ability to engage successfully in activities that require gross motor actions, to carry out nonstereotyped gross motor activities skillfully, and to imitate postures taken by an examiner accurately. Deficit is indicated by the inability to successfully engage in these activities.

The individual acquires the ability to plan gross motor movements through participation in gross activities that require increasingly more precise and complex planning for their proper execution.

There are several suggested methods for increasing gross motor planning. Activities are graded from "simple" to "complex." Initially, the therapist may take the individual passively through the required motions, which will increase sensory input and thus facilitate planning. Proprioceptive input is further increased by co-contraction of postural muscles and weighted cuffs. The motions required in the activities should be nonstereotyped or actions that the individual does not ordinarily perform. The therapist, for instance, would not have the individual walk up a flight of stairs—the therapist may request, however, that the individual go up the stairs backwards. Once a particular motor activity is learned or does not require the individual's attention, it is no longer useful for treatment and a new activity or some modification must be introduced. The therapist initially suggests various gross motor activities; later, the individual is asked to make up his or her own motor tasks, describe the task to the therapist, and then execute the task.

Self-initiated activities require planning prior to action and thus facilitate the development of this aspect of sensory integrative skill. Some activities useful for the development of gross motor planning are modified rolling, crawling, walking, and scooter board activities; obstacle courses involving hopping, jumping, walking, crawling, and climbing, rhythm bands, circle games, body stunts, ball games, gymnastics, "Simon says," postural imitation, and pantomimes of common tasks. Although subcortical levels are involved in the learning of motor planning, the motor cortex is of particular importance. In change directed toward enhancing motor planning, therefore, the individual is engaged in activities that require his or her full attention. The therapist may need to remind the patient to focus on what he or she is doing.

The Ability to Plan Fine Motor Movements (2–3 years)

Fine motor planning is the ability to carry out highly refined and integrated movements in a skilled and coordinated manner.

Adequate fine motor planning is indicated by the ability to successfully engage in activities that require fine motor responses, imitate intricate and refined postures taken by the examiner, and return a hand to a position previously assumed with the help of the examiner (without the aid of vision). Deficit is indicated by the inability to successfully complete such activities.

The individual acquires the ability to plan fine motor movements by engaging in refined activities that require increasingly more precise and complex planning for their proper execution.

The principles and methods outlined above for enhancing gross motor planning apply as well to the development of fine motor planning. Some appropriate nonstereotyped activities are hand puppets, tracing, jacks, paper folding, ring toss, peg boards, sewing cards, and various crafts.

Cognitive Skill

Cognitive function was discussed in general terms in Chapter 3 and its development in Chapter 5. Mature cognitive skill has been defined as the ability to perceive, represent, and organize objects, events, and their relationship in a manner that is considered appropriate by one's cultural group. Although there are some cultural differences, mature cognitive skill is usually considered to be the use of denotative and connotative concept representations and secondary process organization for conscious thought and shared communication.

Exocept, image, and endocept representation are acquired in the process of developing mature cognitive skill. These types of representation remain available to the individual; some perceptions continue to be stored as exocepts, images, and endocepts. Even after the development of mature cognitive skill many persons prefer to use a lower level type of representation. Thus, an individual may use image representation more frequently than connotative representation. This in no way indicates that the individual has a lesser degree of cognitive skill, for he or she is able to use connotative representation when necessary. The reason for preferring one type of representation over another is unknown. However, it does appear that effectiveness and efficiency influence the type of representation selected for solving a particular problem. In learning to ski, for example, most persons find that use of exocept representation is more effective than image representation. It may be possible to use connotative representation to think about redecorating a room, but most persons find it easier and more efficient to use image representation.

Movement from primary process organization to secondary process is not completed until the individual has acquired all of the cognitive subskills. The various aspects of secondary process organization are acquired at different times. For example, the ability to distinguish what is internal and external to the self is learned before deterministic causality. Tertiary process organization will not be considered in the discussion of cognitive skill because it is not felt to be necessary for adequate environmental interaction. It is a relatively rare ability acquired by only a small percent of the population. It is, however, considered to be a learned ability which can only be acquired after the individual has developed all of the cognitive subskills. Secondary process organization must be completely integrated before it is possible to engage in tertiary process organization.

Concerning evaluation of cognitive skill, the best available tools are the addendum to a general interview and the Task Skill Survey outlined in Chapter 16. The description of behavior indicative of subskill mastery and lack of mastery provided below may assist the therpist in developing other evaluative procedures for assessment in this area.

There are no general postulates regarding change for this adaptive skill. Evaluation and intervention relative to nine stages of cognitive skill development are as follows.

The Ability to Use Inherent Behavioral Patterns for Environmental Interaction (0–1 months)

The inherent behavioral patterns of concern here are sucking, grasping, crying, gross bodily movements, and recognition of and attention to visual and auditory stimuli. We cannot be certain whether or not this is an acquired or an inherent subskill. Lack of inherent behavioral patterns is more likely owing to neurological deficit rather than to inadequate learning. The first of the two reasons for describing the subskill here is that it provides a base for considering the other subskills. This is particularly true in regard to causality and acquisition of new responses. At this stage of development temporal contingency between two events appears to be interpreted as one event causing the other, and the individual's own actions are perceived as responsible for all external happenings. As will be discussed later, inherent behavior patterns that lead to pleasurable consequences tend to be repeated and consolidated into new behavioral patterns. The second reason for describing this subskill is that it does appear to be developed further through environmental interaction.

This subskill is considered integrated when the infant is able to locate the nipple with some facility, has a strong grasp and sucking response, cries and is stimulated to cry when hearing another baby cry, is able to move body parts in a gross and vigorous manner, and appears to attend to visual and auditory stimuli. Non-integration is indicated by the absence of these behaviors.

Inherent behavior patterns are believed to be enhanced through the availability of objects and events which permit, elicit, and sustain the behavioral patterns.

In the change process, poor sucking and grasp responses may be facilitated by providing objects that are suitable for sucking and grasping. Stimulation of the tactile receptors located around the mouth and in the palm of the hand also increases sucking and grasp responses. Looking and listening responses may be increased by the presence of a variety of pleasurable stimuli. Unrestrictive clothing and the tactile and vestibular stimuli that are a part of playful interaction with another individual enhance gross and vigorous movements of body parts. Although it seems somewhat strange to speak of increased crying response, consistent response to the needs that generate the crying relates crying to environmental interaction. It appears that an infant sometimes cries simply for the sake of crying rather than in response to an experience of need deprivation: allowing such crying—within reason—may indeed be a way of enhancing the crying response.

The Ability to Interrelate Visual, Manual, Auditory, and Oral Responses (1–4 months)

In this stage of development some of the inherent behaviors mentioned in the first stage are organized into patterns. The following behaviors indicate that the subskill has been learned: anticipating sucking in response to visual, positional, and auditory cues; more active looking and the ability to follow objects in motion; more active listening and seeking the source of auditory stimuli; smiling responses to the human face; vocal responses when alone and in the presence of others; evidence of intentionality in thumb sucking; anything placed in the hand is usually inspected visually and brought to the mouth; anything placed in the mouth is grasped; attempts to grasp any objects in close visual field; and imitation of actions that are a part of current behavioral repertoire (does not imitate new actions). Lack of several of the above behaviors indicates that the subskill has not been learned.

The patterns of behavior that are a part of this subskill appear to be learned because they are need-satisfying. The environmental elements required are objects that provide visual, auditory, and tactile stimulation; objects that can be manipulated, grasped, and sucked; and playful interaction with a limited number of others who experience such playing as pleasurable.

Alteration of deficiency in this subskill essentially involves supplying the above-listed environmental elements during the majority of the time an infant is awake.

Attending to the Environmental Consequence of Actions with Interest (4–9 months)

This component of the third cognitive subskill refers to the repetition of certain motor acts that influence the surrounding environment—the first active exploration of the world. Prior to this time, attention has been directed primarily toward the individual's own body or the very near environment. Learning of this component is indicated by intense study, manipulation, and rotation of objects; experimental actions directed toward objects; attention-getting behavior; deliberate and systematic imitations of behaviors already in the individual's repertoire; and repetition of imitated actions in order to reproduce it in others. The absence of these behaviors indicate lack of learning.

This component is acquired through the opportunity to explore and interact in an environment that is interesting, consistent in response, influenced by the actions of the individual, and one that stimulates mutual imitation.

For change to occur the environment must contain objects that are interesting to the individual. The therapist must sometimes be quite ingenious to find such objects, particularly in the treatment of an adult. Exploratory and manipulative behavior often needs to be encouraged if it does not occur spontaneously. Objects must be such that they can be manipulated in a number of ways without damage to them. There should be no set rules for manipulation—this must be a free experience. The best activities to use are those that allow the client to observe readily his or her effects on the objects involved. This is particularly important relative to the therapist's response. The client must be able to observe his or her impact on the therapist; and the response of the therapist should be as consistent as possible.

Representing Objects in an Exoceptual Manner (4–9 months)

Exoceptual representation is the memory of stimuli in terms of the action response to the stimuli or action directed toward the stimuli. Integration of this component has taken place when the individual initiates an appropriate motor response to unfamiliar objects that are similar to objects in the usual environment and when there is evidence that the individual recognizes that the intensity of a given act will influence the intensity of the result. Lack of learning is indicated by the absence of these responses.

This component is learned through interaction with many objects belonging to the same class and with objects responding to variation in the intensity of action directed toward them.

The change process essentially involves providing the types of objects mentioned in the postulate and encouraging the client's interaction with these objects.

Experiencing Objects (4–9 months)

This component refers to the individual's ability to recognize that objects have some permanence. (However, it is not until the next stage that the individual recognizes that objects exist in their own right, independent from the individual's actions.) Learning of this component is indicated by anticipation of the ultimate position of a moving object from observation of its trajectory; searching for lost objects (the individual, however, will act as if an object no longer exists if it is covered while he or she watches); and anticipation of the whole object when only a part is seen. The individual has not learned this component if these behaviors are not present.

It seems that this component is acquired through the opportunity to manipulate and become familiar with a number of objects.

In the change process there should be emphasis on manipulation. Although vision is important, information received through proprioceptive and tactile receptors are particularly important in acquiring the ability to experience objects.

Acting on the Bases of Egocentric Causality (4–9 months)

Egocentric causality is the belief that one's own actions are completely responsible for object response. There is a quasimagical quality about this type of causality. Behavior that indicates learning this component is the use of gestures to influence the environment, the gestures being essentially unrelated to the response desired.

This component is learned through playful interaction in which various magical gestures frequently lead to specific responses that are experienced as pleasurable by the individual.

The therapist applies this postulate by repeatedly making responses that may be experienced as pleasurable by the client when the client initiates a given behavior. There is no attempt to teach reality-oriented cause and effect in this aspect of the change process. The magical, playful quality of this component must be kept in mind.

Seriate Events in Which the Self Is Involved (4–9 months)

This component refers to a primitive idea of before and after, relative to events in which the individual's own actions are a part of the sequence. Learning this component is evident when the individual exhibits awareness of a specific order of events in which he or she has been repeatedly involved. Lack of awareness indicates dysfunction in this area.

This component is learned through interaction in an environment that involves a regular sequence of activities.

When teaching this component there must be a recognizable routine of events in which the client participates. A consistent sequence must be maintained.

Establishing a Goal and Intentionally Carrying Out Means (9–12 months)

This component refers to the ability to establish a goal prior to action and to select and initiate actions deliberately that will lead to the goal. The goals of concern here are simple in nature, as are the means. An observer of this action receives an impression of unequivocal intentionality. Integration of this component is indicated by removal of objects in order to reach some desired object and by the impression of deliberate selection of goals and means. (It is difficult, however, to describe specific behavior that causes an observer to attribute deliberateness to an act.) Nonintegration of this component will be seen by actions that seem to be inadvertent and unplanned.

This component is acquired through repeated opportunities to independently establish goals and select and carry out means.

In teaching this component, the therapist makes activities available in which the client may engage without assistance. The client should be allowed to manipulate objects any way he or she chooses. Intervention by the therapist is liable to hamper learning.

Recognizing the Independent Existence of Objects (9–12 months)

Independent existence refers to an understanding that objects have permanence, that their existence is not dependent on the individual's manipulation or visual perception. Some writers describe acquisition of this component as "differentiation between the self and other objects." The independent existence of the self as well as other objects is recognized. A behavior that indicates learning of this component, for example, is removal of an object that covers or hides a desired object. Lack of learning is evident when an individual acts as if an object no longer exists even though it is covered while he or she watches.

An individual learns to recognize the independent existence of objects by experimenting with momentary loss of contact with objects. An example of momentary loss is the mother and child playing peek-a-boo.

Some suitable activities deduced from this postulate are putting objects in a covered box and taking them out again, client and therapist hiding objects under a towel or behind a screen, very simple hide-and-seek, and the therapist and client hiding separately under a blanket.

Interpreting Signs (9–12 months)

Interpretation of signs refers to anticipation of future events on the basis of a current event. Acquisition of this component is indicated by sign recognition relative to familiar events in the environment and ease in identifying signs in a new situation. Lack of learning is indicated by lack of overt response to signs.

Sign interpretation is acquired through interaction in an environment where there is a regular sequence of events.

Activities based on this postulate are similar to those suggested for alteration of deficit in the ability to seriate events in which the self is involved. The intervention situation is arranged so that the therapist and client engage in a consistent series of activities. The pattern of events that take place are similar from one session to the next.

Imitate New Behavior (9–12 months)

With acquisition of this component, the individual is able to observe simple behavior which is not a part of his or her usual repertoire and imitate the isolated behavior or initiate behavior that is structurally analogous. Learning this component is indicated by the ability to imitate simple new behaviors.

This component appears to be learned through interaction with people who engage in simple behaviors that are imitable, given the individual's current motor capacity, and through encouragement of this imitation.

Apprehending the Influence of Space (9–12 months)

This component is more exploratory than an integrated ability. The knowledge acquired during this stage is consolidated and actively used in the next stage of cognitive development. Adequate participation in this stage is indicated by the active study of differences in size, shape, perspective, and change in objects resulting from different positions of the head. Lack of participation is indicated by the absence of this exploratory behavior.

This component is learned through interaction in an environment that encourages exploration of objects in space (the self as well as nonhuman objects) and the availability of a variety of object-space relations.

Some techniques deduced from this postulate are activities that involve placing the body and body parts into various size spaces and around various size objects, encouraging the client to move objects in space to study apparent size change, and activities that involve viewing objects from different positions.

Perceiving Other Objects as Partially Causal (9–12 months)

With learning this component, the individual realizes that the other objects are causal, but believes that the cause-effect relationship is set in motion by his or her actions; the true volition of other people is not recognized. Acquisition of this component is indicated by the use of physical contact in an attempt to bring about desired events. Nonintegration of this component is indicated by the use of magical gestures in the effort to initiate pleasurable events.

This component is acquired through interacting in an environment in which physical contact is more effective in bringing about desired events than magical gestures.

Using this postulate in the change process, the therapist provides reinforcement for nonmagical gestures and withholds reinforcement for magical gestures. Shaping is often utilized in teaching this component.

Using Trial-and-Error Problem Solving (12–18 months)

Trial-and-error problem solving is the active manipulation of objects to bring about a desired result. Goals are reached by new and unfamiliar means. Learning is indicated by the ability to solve simple problems through active manipulation of objects. The objects required for solution must be available in the immediate environment. Lack of learning is indicated by disinterest in any activity requiring trial-and-error problem solving.

This component is learned through interaction in situations requiring the use of trial-and-error problem solving.

In applying this postulate, the therapist provides interesting nonhuman objects that present problems that can be solved through active manipulation of objects and object parts.

Using Tools (12–18 months)

Tool use involves the manipulation of one object by application of another object rather than the hand. Component learning is indicated by the use of objects in a tool-like manner when the desired result cannot be attained by use of the hand. Lack of component learning is indicated by disinterest in tasks requiring the use of tools.

Tool use is learned through interaction in tasks that require the use of readily available tools and reinforcement of such activity.

Perceive Variability in Spatial Position (12–18 months)

This component refers to the realization that spacial positions are not fixed. It also refers to the ability to reach a desired destination by various routes. If the most direct or obvious route is blocked, the individual is able to utilize an alternative route. Learning is indicated by the ability to retrieve an object by a route that is different from the trajectory of the object.

Perception of variability in spatial positions is acquired through exploration of the relationships between objects, space, and movement.

Seriate Events in Which the Self Is Not Involved (12–18 months)

This component refers to memory of the order of a simple sequence of events through observation of these events rather than through participation. Learning is indicated by the ability to repeat a simple sequence of acts after observing another person perform these acts. Lack of learning is indicated by the inability to repeat a sequence of demonstrated acts or confusion regarding the proper sequence.

This component is acquired through interaction in an environment where there is an opportunity to practice sequential ordering.

Perceive the Causality of Objects (12–18 months)

With learning this component the individual loses the sense of omnipotence and recognizes that others are causal. The effect of gravity is also recognized. The individual perceives him- or herself as a recipient of the causal activities of others. Learning is indicated by evidence that the individual understands that he or she as well as others have a causal effect on the environment. Lack of learning is indicated by a feeling of omnipotence relative to other people, throwing down rather than dropping objects, and waiting for nonhuman objects to move spontaneously.

The individual acquires the ability to perceive the causality of objects through interaction in an environment where there is opportunity to observe the causal effects of others.

Representing Objects in an Image Manner (18 months–2 years)

Image representation is memory of stimuli in terms of an internal, pictorial, quasi-reproduction. Learning of this component is indicated by the ability to engage in covert trial-and-error problem solving, to imitate an absent model, and to recognize that pictures of objects and real objects are related.

The interactions responsible for the learning of this component are unknown. However, reinforcement of covert problem solving may facilitate learning and identifying objects from pictures.

Make-Believe (18 months–2 years)

This component refers to the capacity to reenact familar events by using inadequate objects and treating them as if they were adequate. There is differentiation of the "let us pretend" orientation from the real event. This ability to distinguish between the real and not real becomes more highly refined with continued maturation and learning. However, it is at this point that the basic ability is acquired. Learning this component is indicated by the ability to engage in make-believe and to understand that it is make-believe. Dysfunction in this area is indicated by the inability to differentiate between real and make-believe, disinterest in make-believe activities, or excessive engagement in such activities.

This component is acquired through an opportunity to engage in make-believe activities alone and with others and through interaction with another who enjoys make-believe but who also reinforces recognition of the difference between make-believe and real events.

In teaching this component, the therapist must provide inadequate objects that are similar in some respects to adequate objects; these must be specific to events that are familiar to the client. It is particularly important to be aware of cultural differences. The client should be allowed to go through the entire process of make-believe without interruption by the therapist. For example, destructive (within reason) behavior must be as readily accepted as more constructive behavior. Limiting any aspect of make-believe interferes with the client's learning the distinction between what is real and not real.

Infer a Cause Given Its Effect (18 months–2 years)

This component refers to the ability to recognize that familiar inanimate objects do not act spontaneously. When apparently spontaneous movement does occur, the individual is either able to identify the cause or engage in activities that are likely to lead to identification of the cause. Learning this component is indicated by interest in locating causal sources; lack of learning is indicated by the acceptance of the spontaneous movement of inanimate objects or actually attributing spontaneous movement to inanimate objects.

This component is acquired through interaction in an environment where cause and effect is readily apparent and where exploration of cause and effect leads to reinforcement.

Acting on the Basis of Combined Spatial Relations (18 months–2 years)

With the learning of this component the individual is able to estimate roughly whether of not one object will fit into another and to manipulate objects so that they will fit into a given space. Acquisition is indicated by minimal overt trial-and-error behavior in activities involving placement of objects of various sizes within matching spaces.

Combined spatial relations are learned through manipulation of objects in space.

On the basis of this postulate, the therapist provides objects that allow the client to study the position-filling and displacement properties of objects.

Attributing Omnipotence to Others (18 months–2 years)

Acquisition of this component appears to be necessary in helping the individual to understand clearly that he or she is not omnipotent. A beginning understanding of the causal effects of others is acquired in the last stage of cognitive development. However, some belief in self-omnipotence continues to be present. Learning this skill is indicated by the belief that others control natural phenomena (for instance, rain or the growth of flowers) and that others know the thought processes of the self; dysfunction is indicated by continued belief in the omnipotence of the self.

This component is probably acquired through interaction in an environment where others are perceived as trustworthy and effective in manipulating the environment in a manner that is pleasurable to the individual.

Perceiving Objects as Permanent in Time and Place (18 months–2 years)

This component seems to be an integration of the other, more primitive components that are concerned with learning about the independent existence of objects and time and space relations. It is considered learned when an individual's conscious thought processes appear to be characterized by recognition of temporal and spatial relationships and the relative absence of condensation and displacement. Lack of learning is indicated by confused temporal and spatial relations and frequent condensation and displacement.

This component appears to be learned through positive reinforcement of verbal and nonverbal behavior based on culturally accepted temporal and spatial relations and nonreinforcement of condensation and displacement.

Representing Objects in an Endoceptual Manner (2–5 years)

Endocept representation is memory of stimuli in terms of a felt experience. The nature and method of learning of this type of representation is not well understood. The only reason it is believed to be learned at this age is from reports of experiences that have occurred during this part of the life cycle. The experiences are represented in an endocept manner; therefore, this type of representation must be available. Behavior indicative of endocept representation is primarily seen in the adult who is able to discuss the difference between an endocept representation and that which is communicated relative to the representation; a child at this stage of development does not usually have the verbal capacity to describe these differences. However, many persons are not aware of or able to communicate their own endocept representation. At this point in our understanding we do not know how to evaluate the presence or absence of this component, nor do we know how this component is learned. In fact, there is some question of whether the learning of this subskill component is necessary for full maturation of cognitive skill.

Differentiating Between Thought and Action (2–5 years)

This component refers to the ability to recognize that ideas and overt behavior lead to different consequences. Although unsubstantial phenomena (dreams, thoughts, fantasies) are still perceived as quasi-tangible reality, they are seen as differing from action in the environment. In learning this component, part of the omnipotence ascribed to others is lost; the individual recognizes that others cannot read his or her thoughts. Learning is indicated by recognition that thoughts cannot directly influence the environment unless they are translated into action, and by awareness of the unreality of dreams and fantasies. Lack of learning is demonstrated by the continued belief that others are aware of one's thoughts, by fear of fantasizing about actions that would be harmful to others, and by a belief that thoughts influence others.

This component appears to be learned through interaction in an environment in which response to verbalized thoughts is different from response to action, and in an environment in which response is based on the action of the individual rather than on the basis of assumed thoughts, desires, or needs.

In planning activities deduced from this postulate, the therapist must remember that verbalized thoughts are very different from actions even when these thoughts are concerned with injury to self or others. It is typical for many therapists to respond to clients on the basis of the deduced needs or desires of the client. These deductions are often quite accurate and facilitating to the intervention process. In teaching this component, however, the therapist must take care to respond to the obvious meaning of verbal and nonverbal behavior only.

Recognizing the Need for Causal Sources (2–5 years)

Through learning of this component, the individual comes to believe that there must be an identifiable cause for every effect. The cause ascribed to an effect, however, may be idiosyncratic and not related to cause and effect relationships considered usual by one's cultural group. Learning is indicated by the ability to identify a causal source for any suggested effect and by the apparent need for such identification. Lack of learning is indicated by the absence of these behaviors.

The learning of this component seems to be motivated by safety needs, in particular the need to have a limited number of unknowns in the environment. The component seems to be acquired through interaction in an environment where requested causal relationships are given in language and detail that is comprehensible to the individual and in an environment where some idiosyncratic causality is accepted by others.

Representing Objects in a Denotative Manner (6–7 years)

Denotative representation is memory of stimuli in terms of words that stand for or name objects—the word is perceived as part of the object or equivalent to it. Learning of this component is indicated by relatively accurate use of language; age-level reading; action-oriented, pictorial, and concrete definitions of words; awareness of higher and lower level classification; the ability to form classes on the basis of similarities; and to add ar subtract classes to form supraordinate or subordinate classes.

This component appears to be learned through interaction in an environment where rich and extensive verbal behavior is emphasized as a means of communication.

In teaching this component it is important for the therapist to use extensive verbal communication and to reinforce the client's use of accurate verbal communication; interactions that emphasize manipulation of the nonhuman environment may interfere with learning. Meaningful conversation is of prime importance. In the initial phase of teaching, it may be necessary for the therapist to select a topic for discussion. The therapist uses his or her knowledge of what might be interesting and stimulating to the client(s) as the basis for selecting appropriate topics.

Perceiving the Viewpoint of Others (6–7 years)

This component refers to the ability to coordinate one's own perceptions with those of others. Learning is indicated by the ability to take the role of others (but not through imitation, as is typical in the play of young children), to perceive one's own point of view as only one of many possible points of view, and to be comfortable in considering various ways in which an object or event might be considered. Lack of learning is indicated by egocentric, inflexible points of view.

The ability to perceive the viewpoints of others is acquired through interaction in which the individual receives positive reinforcement for taking others' viewpoints into consideration.

Interactions in which argument and disagreement are nondestructive but frequent are useful for development of this component. It is suggested that argument and disagreement take place primarily with peers and that there be minimal interference or direction from the therapist. The opinion of an authority figure is often accepted without question or accepted only overtly. Neither process is conducive to the learning of this component.

Decentering (6–7 years)

Decentration is the process of distinguishing several features or characteristics of an object. Learning is indicated by a balanced view of all characteristics of an object and by use of this information in thinking and making judgments. Lack of learning is indicated by perception of a single outstanding characteristic of an object, concern with surface phenomena only, and stereotyped attitude and action toward a considerable number of people and things.

Decentration is learned through interaction in an environment in which the individual receives reinforcement for recognizing and using many characteristics of objects.

Appropriate activities for teaching this component are ones in which the individual must consider several factors if he or she is to be successful in that activity. These activities should involve interaction with both the human and nonhuman environment.

Representing Objects in a Connotative Manner (11–13 years)

Connotative representation is memory of stimuli in terms of words consciously perceived as labels for a classification of some common characteristics. Learning is indicated by flexibility in thinking, the ability to recognize that different labels may be assigned to the same phenomena, and by facility in formulating connotative concepts. Dysfunction in this area is indicated by difficulty in recognizing phenomena when there is contextual change, conscious thought that moves from particular to particular, the belief that concepts are unique to a given phenomena, and the inability to form connotative concepts.

Learning this component appears to be implemented through demand for, practice in, and reinforcement of connotative representation. In teaching this component it is suggested that the therapist provide problems that demonstrate the limitations of the other types of representation but in particular of denotative representation. Guidance in solving these problems and specification of the thinking process involved helps the individual in perceiving words as labels. Consideration of different theoretical systems dealing with the same phenomena is also useful.

Using Formal Logic (11–13 years)

Formal logic is here defined as the ability to maintain one premise during a reasoning sequence, and to base conscious thought and action on deterministic causality. The premise taken as the point of departure may vary from culture to culture, but it must be compatible with at least some of the ideas of the individual's culture group. Learning is indicated by the behavior listed above. Lack of learning is indicated by the inability to return to the original point of departure in a reasoning sequence, contradictions during the sequence, selecting an original premise that is not accepted by one's culture group, inability to perceive or correct contradictions in logic, and continued use of phenomenalistic causality.

This component appears to be learned through interaction in an environment where the use of formal logic is followed by positive reinforcement.

In translating this postulate into a change process, it is suggested that the therapist provide opportunity for practice in keeping one premise during a reasoning sequence. Debate is particularly helpful in this area. Requesting that the client review his of her correction of errors in the sequence (given the initial premise), and practice in going through the sequence again are also suggested. Finally, differential reinforcement of various premises considered acceptable by the client's cultural group is also a useful device for facilitating the development of this component.

Working in the Realm of the Hypothetical (11–13 years)

"Hypothetical" here refers to that which is future, unknown, conjecture, or open to speculation. Learning of this component is indicated by the ability to engage in thinking that goes beyond the immediate here and now of current object interaction; to imagine "what might be," perceiving both the obvious and the subtle; to deal with chance or probability; and to solve problems by isolating all of the possible variables and relationships and, through experimentation and logical analysis, to determine which of these possiblities is validated by the present data.

This component appears to be learned through an opportunity to deal with the hypothetical and reinforcement of behaviors indicative of component learning

Dyadic Interaction Skill

Dyadic interaction skill is the ability to engage in meaningful interactions with another individual; in its mature form it is the ability to participate in a variety of dyadic relationships. It focuses on those one-to-one relationships usually referred to as friendship, intimacy, nurturing, and interaction with authority. In developing this skill, the individual learns to perceive others as unique and different from the self. Unless there is strong evidence to the contrary, one learns to act on the assumption that other persons are worthy of respect, nonthreatening to self-integrity, and regard that person as an acceptable person.

Evaluation of this adaptive skill is usually accomplished through the use of the Interpersonal Skill Survey and an interview. The interview should focus on general feelings regarding others; the nature of the client's superficial and more intimate friendships; interactions with parents, spouse or partner, and children; any caretaking or mentor-neophyte relationships the client may have had; and typical patterns of behavior relative to persons in authority positions. Some information may also be acquired through interpretation of symbols produced by the client.

There are no general postulates for dyadic interaction skill. The subskills are as follows:

The Ability to Enter into Trusting Familial Relationships

This subskill, beginning at 8–10 months, is the development of confidence in other family members, experiencing them as need fulfilling and highly pleasurable to be with. Learning of this subskill is indicated by recognition of and a pleasant response to individuals who offer need satisfaction, perception of others as basically need-satisfying, and the ability to distinguish one need from another (but in a relatively gross manner). In addition to the absence of the behaviors listed above, lack of learning is indicated by profound self-preoccupation, seeking need satisfaction in fantasy, marked dependency, suspiciousness of others, and withdrawal. It is also indicated by symbols that refer to birth, womb, that which nurtures and protects, orality, and free-floating libidinal energy.

This subskill is learned through experiencing a nurturing relationship. A nurturing relationship is here defined as an extensive interaction between two persons in which one individual receives consistent and relatively immediate need satisfaction, is not required to give any reciprocal satisfaction, and is free to engage in any behavior that is not destructive to self or others. The individual who gives nurturance must be accepting, permissive, delight in giving nurture and experience strong positive feelings toward the individual who is receiving nurturance.

In a change process based on this postulate, the therapist attemps in every way possible to meet whatever needs are presently being experienced by the client. These may be needs that are verbalized by the client or ones that are carefully deduced from his or her behavior. Individuals who have not learned this subskill often experience the need to be fed and physically held. When this is the case and the client is able to accept direct gratification of these needs, the therapist offers direct satisfaction. However, many clients are unable to accept direct gratification. In this situation the client may be able to accept symbolic gratification. The need to be fed, for example, may be satisfied symbolically by such things as offering cigarettes, candy, chewing gum, soda, and coffee; preparing a meal or snack together (the client participating only to the extent that he or she wishes); and activities that make use of the mouth (blowing, sucking, singing, talking, etc.). The need to be held may be satisfied symbolically by such things as touching the client's hand or shoulder, assisting the client with self-care activities, and involvement in activities that allow for some physical contact within the context of the activity.

There are some clients who have not learned this subskill, who do not experience the need to be fed and physically held. (It should never be assumed therefore that these needs are being experienced.) With this type of client the therapist is essentially concerned with gratifying any need (except sexual) that the individual is experiencing. For example, the client may want to engage in some activity that is familiar, learn a new activity, go to a movie or out for a walk, complain, talk about problems, play cards, etc. If at all possible, given the ingenuity of the therapist, the client is assisted in doing whatever he or she wants to do. A commitment to engage in the activity for any period of time is never required. As a general rule of thumb the therapist never asks the client to clean up, finish a task, be neat, do something for the therapist, work without assistance, do anything he or she doesn't feel like doing, thank the therapist, or even respond in a pleasant manner.

Permissiveness was mentioned as one of the characteristics of a nurturing relationship. However, this is subordinate to the client's needs. If the client is not comfortable in a permissive environment, the environment is altered—many clients feel more secure in a structured environment. The therapist offers suggestions, makes decisions, provides directions, and limits hostile expression to the extent that the client indicates need for these types of responses.

Providing a nurturing relationship is not an attempt to encourage a client to regress to a more primitive stage of development. The client who needs a nurturing relationship is at a primitive stage of development already; although he or she may not act in an infantile or regressed manner. During the change process the client's behavior may become more infantile. This is permitted if it does occur, but it need not occur for change to take place. There is no attempt to make the client dependent. Individuals who lack this subskill are dependent even though this may not be manifest in overt behavior. If the client acts in a dependent manner, his or her dependency needs are met directly. If the client indicates that he or she has a need to maintain an independent stance, however, this need is also met.

The question of whether of not other staff members on the clinical setting must also enter into a nurturing relationship with the client is sometimes raised. This is not necessary for successful intervention. The client is responded to in a manner similar to the way in which the staff responds to other clients. This is, of course, assuming that staff members respond to clients in a humane manner—with profound recognition of individual needs. The client is required to adhere to the rules of the treatment facility, engage in self-care activities to the extent that he or she is able, and participate in assigned tasks and required activities.

Another question often raised is whether the client will ever move beyond a nurturing relationship. Phrased a different way: "If most of the client's needs are gratified, will the client ever move in the direction of independence and self-sufficiency?" The answer is "yes"—just as a child demands autonomy and begins to want to do things for him- or herself, so will the client. It is only those individuals who have not had adequate gratification of psychological, security, love, and acceptance needs who continue to demand and require dependent and caring-for relationships with others.

Entering into a nurturing relationship with a client is no easy task; it is very demanding of the therapist, who is often required to give far more than is required in any other type of client-therapist interaction. The therapist must be in a position where the majority of the therapist's needs are being met through interactions outside the change process and must have considerable energy to invest in the client. In addition, the therapist must feel affection and liking for the client and be comfortable in making no demands. A therapist should probably not attempt to engage in a nurturing relationship if the above-listed factors are not present.

The Ability to Enter into Association Relationships (3–5 years)

An association relationship is a type of interaction between two persons which is relatively casual, easily disrupted, minimally concerned with need gratification, and usually involves engagement in a shared task. Learning of the subskill is indicated by the ability to form casual relationships to interact with a peer comfortably and for a relatively long period, and to engage in simple competitive and cooperative interactions. Lack of learning is indicated by absence of these behaviors as well as withdrawal, lack of self-assertion, and a predominant use of symbols that refer to the environment as overwhelming.

This subskill is learned through interaction in an environment where association relationships are available and reinforced. The individual needs for safety and love and acceptance must be met outside association relationships.

In teaching this subskill, the therapist encourages the client to share a task with another person; the task must, of course, be compatible with the individual's capacity and interest. The shaping process is often used in teaching this subskill. The client should have an opportunity to engage in several association relationships if at all possible. It is not necessary for the therapist to be present during the client's interaction with others unless there is a need for immediate and continuous external reinforcement. The client's safety and love needs are met by the therapist.

The Ability to Interact in an Authority Relationship (5–7 years)

In learning this subskill, the individual begins to perceive authority figures as different from parents. They are seen as relatively powerful but not as powerful as parents. Acceptance of direction from an authority figure in a positive and cooperative manner indicates learning of the subskill; lack of learning is indicated by overcompliance, refusal to accept direction, and marked fear of authority figures. Predominant use of symbols that refer to potency and self-inadequacy may also indicate lack of learning.

This subskill is acquired through interaction with nonfamilial authority figures who make reasonable demands and provide at least some reinforcement for meeting demands.

In teaching this subskill, the therapist must first establish a close relationship with the client. It may be necessary to use shaping to establish that behavior which has been described as being indicative of skill learning. When the client is able to meet the demands made by the therapist, the therapist provides situations in which the client has an opportunity to interact with other authority figures. Appropriate behavior relative to the new authority figures is reinforced by the authority figures and the therapist for as long as necessary.

The Ability to Interact in a Chum Relationship (10–14 years)

A chum relationship is one in which another person is experienced as being extremely important to the self and the needs of the other are felt as equal to the needs of the self. This is an emotionally charged relationship characterized by mutual trust, sharing of confidences, and minimal competitive interaction.

An individual has engaged in chum relationships when he or she is able to perceive and meet the needs of others, experience his or her own humanness, and feel compassion for and empathy with another person. Lack of learning is indicated by the absence of these behaviors and the frequent use of symbols that refer to distance from people and by experience of the self as nonhuman.

This component is learned through interaction with peers who are developmentally ready to engage in a chum relationship. The environment must allow for privacy and provide an opportunity for separateness.

The therapist is not directly involved in teaching this subskill. The therapist has advanced, hopefully, beyond this stage of development and is not, therefore, a suitable person for this shared learning experience. The therapist facilitates learning by helping the client to locate other individuals who are ready to engage in a chum relationship and by allowing that relationship to develop. Approval of the relationship is communicated to the client. The therapist does not question the client about the relationship unless the client indicates a wish to discuss it. In this way, the therapist respects the privacy that is needed for development of this subskill. The intensity and secrecy of the chum relationship has a tendency to arouse anxiety in some therapists, particularly when there is evidence of shared deviant behavior. If there is grossly deviant behavior, the therapist must help the pair to alter their behavior or in extreme cases interrupt the relationship; if the deviant behavior is mild it is recommended that the therapist ignore it. In making a judgment in this matter, the therapist must weigh the harmful effect of the deviant behavior against the importance of learning this subskill. The significance of this subskill is frequently not given sufficient consideration. We often err on the side of interrupting chum relationships that could ultimately lead to the development of very important human abilities.

The Ability to Enter into a Peer Authority Relationship (15–17 years)

Peer authority refers to a superior-subordinate relationship in which the individual perceives the authority figure as similar to the self except for their relative positions in a given situation. Learning of this subskill is indicated by realistic perception of the authority figures power, comfortable interaction with authority figures, recognition that there is a distinction between appropriate behavior relative to an authority figure when he or she is acting in an authority role and appropriate behavior in all other interactions with the individual, and the ability to judge the competence of orders issued by the authority figure and to act on the basis of that judgment. As in the case of the second dyadic interaction subskill, the predominant use of symbols refering to potency and self-inadequacy may be indicative of lack of learning.

This subskill is acquired through interaction in an environment where there is an opportunity to take superior and subordinate roles and to observe others taking those roles. Additional learning of this subskill takes place through interaction with authority figures who provide reinforcement of those behaviors that are indicative of acquisition of this subskill.

One of the common techniques developed from the first postulate is formation of an activity group concerned with publishing a newspaper of newsletter. The role of editor is rotated, thus giving each group member an opportunity to take subordinate and superior roles. Involvement in one committee as chair and in other committees as a member is also a useful device for teaching this subskill. In application of the second postulate, the authority figure (whoever this may be) must clearly delineate power relative to the client; avoid unreasonable demands and arbitrary behavior; interact with the client outside of authority situations, specifically indicating the difference in the behavior expected; and encourage questioning of the authority figure's competence and directions. The authority figure must be comfortable in the authority position and be capable of seeing the client as a peer.

The Ability to Enter into an Intimate Relationship (18–25 years)

An intimate relationship is mutually need-satisfying and characterized by a firm commitment to one's partner which is maintained regardless of normal demands for sacrifice on the part of self. With development of this subskill the individual has acquired the true capacity for love of another person. Intimate involvement over a sustained period of time is possible and pleasurable, for there is a comfortable sharing of responsibility, with both individuals able to give and receive from the other.

Learning of this subskill is indicated by the ability to experience love, maintain sustained relationships, mutual need satisfaction and sharing, but nevertheless a continued sense of autonomy when participating in intimate relationships. Lack of learning is indicated by absence of those behaviors, perception of ordinary demands by others as excessive and grounds for severing a relationship, and dyadic interactions characterized by jealous possessiveness and preoccupation with the relationship.

This subskill is acquired through interaction in an environment where there are people available who are capable of establishing intimate relationships and living with others in a situation in which one is required to share responsibilities for tasks and need satisfaction.

As was the case in the third dyadic interaction skill, the therapist does not teach this skill directly. Instead, he or she helps the client locate appropriate persons and situations for learning—providing support, advice if requested, and validation of the client's capacity to engage in an intimate relationship. To teach this subskill, the therapist must experience delight in the client's movement into intimate relationships, which, in a very essential way, exclude the therapist. Communal living of one type or another often provides an excellent environment for learning this subskill; living with others outside a familial situation initiates demands and provides reinforcements that facilitate learning.

The Ability to Engage in Nurturing Relationships (20–30 years)

A nurturing relationship is characterized by satisfying the needs of another person without demanding reciprocal satisfaction. Learning is indicated by unselfish giving of one's time and energy to other people, the giving of an unconditional love that respects the rights of the other for growth and uniqueness, and the ability to withdraw libidinal energy when the other person is able to function independently. Engagement in or the desire and ability to engage in a nurturing relationship is often indicated by predominant use of symbols that refer to the birth-death-rebirth cycle, perfect being, that which nurtures and protects, femininity, and oneness or unity. Lack of learning is indicated by the absence of these behaviors or symbols, avoidance of nurturing relationships, ambivalence toward persons in need of nuturance, no enjoyment in the growth of others, premature withdrawal of interest in the nurtured person (or a tenacious holding on), anxiety and excessive feeling of loss when the nurtured person moves out of the relationship, difficulty in investing libidinal energy in created objects or difficulty withdrawing energy once investment has occurred, and anxiety and feelings of loss when sharing created objects with another.

Preliminary development of this subskill arises from caretaking activities relative to plants and animals and from taking partial responsibility of young children. Full development is dependent on interaction with another person who requires nurturing. The environment in which this relationship occurs must be seen as safe by the nurturing partner with sufficient and consistent need gratification and reinforcement of nurturing interactions. This allows for adequate time and energy to devote to nurturing. The ability to terminate the relationship depends on environmental opportunity for reinvestment of energy in other people and things which allows for continued gratification of those needs that are satisfied in the nurturing process.

Group Interaction Skill

Group interaction is the ability to be a productive member of a variety of primary groups. Through acquisition of the various group interaction subskills, the individual learns to take appropriate group menbership roles, engage in decision-making, communicate effectively, recognize group norms and interact in accordance with these norms, contribute to goal attainment, work toward group cohesiveness and assist in resolving group conflict.

The best way to evaluate for the extent of group interaction skill learning is to observe the client interacting in a small group. Evaluative groups as discussed in Chapter 14 are ideal, particularly in conjunction with the Group Interaction Skill Survey (Chapter 16).

The discussion of group interaction skill will be brief in that it essentially involves the use of developmental groups. These types of activity groups were discussed in some detail in Chapter 14.

The subskills of group interaction skill are as follows:

The Ability to Participate in a Parallel Group (18 months–2 years)

A parallel group is perhaps more an aggregate of individuals that a group in the strict sense of the word. It is a group characterized by individuals working or playing in the presence of others, by minimal sharing of tasks, and by some mutual stimulation. Learning of this skill is indicated by the ability to work or play in the presence of others, awareness of others in the group, and some verbal or nonverbal interaction with fellow group members. Lack of learning is indicated by absence of these behaviors, in addition to discomfort in the presence of others and interaction with others as if they were nonhuman objects.

This subskill is acquired through interaction in an environment where there is opportunity to work or play in the presence of others who are nonthreatening to the self. Need satisfaction and reinforcement of behavior necessary for adequate parallel group interaction must be available from a person who is important to the individual. The work or play tasks with which the individual is involved must be compatible with current capacities.

A therapist who is engaged in a group designed on the basis of the above postulates is often tempted to demand a type of sharing which is beyond the capacity of anyone who is in the process of learning this subskill. This is detrimental to learning. There should be sufficient tools, materials, or toys for all group members. The therapist is primarily concerned with providing task assistance, meeting the needs of each group member (in particular the needs for safety, love, and esteem), and giving reinforcement for behavior necessary for sucessful parallel group interaction.

The Ability to Participate in a Project Group (2–4 years)

A project group is characterized by membership involvement in short-term tasks requiring some shared interaction, cooperation, and competition; perception of the task as paramount with minimal interaction outside of the task. Learning is indicated by the ability to engage in short-term shared tasks, seek assistance from other group members, give assistance willingly and adequately, and evidence that the individual understands that one must help others to receive help from others. Dysfunction in this area is indicated by absence of these behaviors, the tendency to work alone, avoidance of contact with others, and fear that others will interfere with task completion.

This subskill is acquired through interaction in an environment in which there are sharable short-term tasks that are interesting to the individual as well as other persons who are compatible and willing to seek and give task assistance. Need satisfaction and reinforcement of behavior necessary for adequate project group interaction must be available from a person significant to the individual.

In teaching this subskill the therapist continues to meet the needs of the various group members. He or she also provides or helps the group select tasks that require interaction of two or more persons for completion. The intervention situation must be such that clients feel free to engage in trial-and-error behavior. Abortive attempts at task completion should be accepted. Tasks that must be completed by a specific time or tasks requiring creation of a perfect end product interfere with the learning of this subskill.

The Ability to Participate in an Egocentric-Cooperative Group (5–7 years)

Egocentric-cooperative groups are characterized by group members selecting, implementing, and executing relatively long-term tasks through joint interaction and individual response based on enlightened self-interest; the individual recognizes that his or her rights will be respected only through respect for the rights of others. Similarly, the individual realizes that his or her needs (particularly esteem needs) will be met only through meeting the needs of others.

Acquisition of this subskill is indicated by the ability to identify group norms and goals, use of this knowledge as a guide for action, some experimentation with various group membership roles, perception of self as a group participant with a right to belong to groups, respect for the rights of others, the ability to meet the esteem needs of others and to gain satisfaction of esteem needs. Lack of learning is indicated by absence of the above behavior, avoidance of competition (or preoccupation with competition), hesitant movement from one group to another, and a feeling that one does not belong to any group and will never be accepted regardless of behavior.

This subskill is learned through interaction in an environment where there is an opportunity to practice selecting, planning, and implementing shared, long-term tasks; cooperative and competitive behavior; various group membership roles; and seeking gratification of and gratifying esteem needs. Behavior that is indicative of adequate subskill learning must be reinforced by group members and a significant other. Security, love, and some esteem needs must be met by someone else significant to the individual.

The above postulates do not appear to require elaboration. The only further comment is that the group is encouraged to select, plan, and execute their tasks with minimal assistance from the therapist. The therapist serves primarily as a resource person.

The Ability to Participate in a Cooperative Group (9–12 years)

A cooperative group is characterized by homogeneous membership and mutual need satisfaction. The task is often considered to be secondary to need fulfillment. Learning of this subskill is indicated by the ability to express both positive and negative feelings in a group, to perceive the needs of others, and to meet the needs of fellow group members.

This subskill is acquired through interaction in an environment where there are others who are compatible and similar to the individual as well as developmentally ready to engage in a cooperative group. If group members have these characteristics, it is believed that they will provide all the reinforcement necessary to learn to perceive and satisfy the needs of others accurately; the presence of an authority figure is detrimental to the development of this subskill.

The therapist is not directly involved in teaching this subskill; instead, he or she assists the client in finding people with whom this subskill may be learned. These persons might be located in a setting outside the treatment facility. The therapist offers the client support and some need satisfaction until able to acquire this from the outside group. To facilitate learning of this subskill within a clinical setting, the therapist may form a group of compatible individuals and then may continue to interact with the group until the members become comfortable with each other and the group develops some sense of cohesiveness. The therapist then withdraws from the group and relates to them in the role of an advisor.

The Ability to Participate in a Mature Group (15–18 years)

A mature group is charaterized by heterogeneous membership, participant flexibility in taking a variety of membership roles, and a balance between task accomplishment and the satisfaction of group member needs. No sharp distinction is made between leader and follower roles—leadership functions are shared by all group members. (A description of group membership roles is provided in Chapter 12.) In a mature group, participants take those instrumental and expressive roles required for adequate group functioning at any particular time.

Learning of this subskill is indicated by comfort in heterogeneous groups and the ability to take a variety of membership roles. Lack of learning is indicated by preference for a same sex or other types of homogeneous groups and excessive preoccupation with task acomplishment or satisfaction of social-emotional needs.

This subskill is acquired through interaction in heterogeneous groups which maintains an adequate balance between task accomplishment and need satisfaction and which provides an opportunity for exploration, practice, and reinforcement of a variety of membership roles.

In teaching this component, the therapist interacts as a co-equal group member. The therapist takes a minimal number of membership roles as a way of encouraging other group members to take these roles. Some suggested techniques for increasing learning of membership roles and role flexibility are verbal exploration of the various membership roles and behavior necessary to fulfill these roles; periodic examination of the group by group members in regard to membership roles currently being played and the need for additional or different ones; role playing of membership roles currently being played; and members acting as observers of the group to see roles and role requirements from a less involved position.

Self-Identity Skill

The *self* includes the individual's physical body; a given space surrounding the body; and ideas, feelings, needs, abilities, limitations, past experience, and future potential. *Identity* is the individual's perception of self and includes knowledge and judgments about and feelings toward the self. Mature self-identity is the ability to perceive oneself as an autonomous, holistic, and acceptable person who has permanence and continuity over time.

Ideally, assessment of self-identity subskill learning involves observation of the client interacting with people and objects, discussion regarding the client's judgment and feelings about him- or herself, and interpretations of symbols produced by the client. This is an adaptive skill that is particularly difficult to assess when a client seeks assistance. The stresses that have led to a need for help tend to cover or impede manifestation of learning in this area. Because of an inability to cope with stress, the individual often verbalizes highly negative judgments about and feelings toward him- or herself. This behavior frequently reflects current anger toward the self more than self-identity subskill learning. For this reason, evaluation in this area may be delayed. When this is not feasible, interpretations should be made with caution.

The subskills of self-identity skill are given in the following.

The Ability to See the Self as a Worthy Person (9–12 months)

The term worthy is defined here as the perception of oneself as deserving of need satisfaction. The individual who has learned this subskill will seek need gratification with the expectations that this will be a successful endeavor. Lack of learning is indicated by withdrawal; no expectations of need gratification; extended periods of depersonalization of all or parts of the self; self-destructive behavior; and percepton of the self as harmful to others, evil, or dirty. Lack of learning is also indicated by the predominant use of symbols that refer to the self as evil, the womb, unity (in the sense of that which is desired), and the birth-death-rebirth cycle.

This subskill is acquired through participating in a nurturing relationship. The reader is referred to the discussion of the first dyadic interaction skill for a description of this therapeutic relationship.

The Ability to Perceive Assets and Limitations of the Self (11–15 years)

In learning this subskill the individual comes to an understanding of what he or she is able and not able to do. Limitations are accepted—with perhaps some desire to alter these limitations and attempts to do so. The individual recognizes at the same time that some limitations do not reflect total ineptness; there is a dawning recognition that everyone has deficits that must be accepted. The individual's assessment of assets and limitations is relative to skill in using the body in both a gross and fine manner, attractiveness, intellectual achievements, social skills, and interests.

Learning of this subskill is indicated by a realistic assessment of assets and limitations, acceptance of limitations, and the ability to perceive one's body as a positive object regardless of athletic skills or the lack of attributes that are currently fashionable. The tone and effect of the client's symbols referring to aspects of the self also give information about accurate assessment of capacities and limitations.

This subskill is learned through interaction in an environment that provides the individual with an opportunity to observe his or her assets and limitations, to alter limitations to the extent which he or she is able, and to receive feedback regarding assets and limitations.

To learn this subskill, the client must have an opportunity to engage in a wide variety of activities. Feedback from the therapist should be accurate and freely given. The client's sensitivities are taken into consideration, but this does not prohibit the therapist from giving an honest response regarding what the client is and is not able to do. Activities having clearly established standards, prescribed modes of action, and predictable results are also useful in providing accurate feedback to the client.

The Ability to Perceive the Self as Self-Directed (20–25 years)

This subskill refers to the individual's recognition of the self as capable of and responsible for satisfying his or her own needs, establishing personal goals, and selecting a preferred life-style. Learning is indicated by recognition that needs are satisfied only through the efforts of the self; by feelings and actions indicative of beginning independence from parents; by the ability to articulate current and future personal goals and to experience these goals as established by the self; by the individual living in a manner that is comfortable for him- or herself and not necessarily one that is valued by the cultural group; and by perception of the self as competent in dealing with ordinary life problems. Predominant use of symbols that refer to the unconscious, to that which nurtures and protects, stunted growth, self-inadequacy, experiencing the self as being overwhelmed by the external environment, overinvolvement in fantasy, insecurity, and experience of uncertainty indicate lack of learning in this area.

This subskill is acquired through practice in being self-directed, through communication by significant others that one is capable of being independent, and through reinforcement of such behavior.

In applying this postulate, the therapist is primarily concerned with the client's behavior outside the treatment facility. Although initial attempts at being self-directed may occur in the treatment facility, the client is encouraged to turn outward toward the external environment as soon as possible. This is suggested for two reasons: (a) the client cannot learn this subskill until he or she has acted effectively in the external environment, and (b) it is often very difficult to order one's behavior independently in a treatment facility. The therapist indicates to the client that he or she is able to establish personal goals, determine a life-style, and deal with ordinary life problems (for example, find an apartment, make travel plans, buy clothes, etc.). This support for the client helps to sustain efforts if there should be an initial failure. The therapist's occasional temptation to offer more than support and occasional advice is never actualized, for this would interfere with subskill learning. As far as possible, reinforcement should be the client's pleasure in successfully engaging in self-determining behavior. This is most likely to occur if the client is truly free to make his or her own choices.

The Ability to Perceive the Self as a Productive, Contributing Member of a Social System (30–35 years)

This subskill refers to the individual's awareness of being a part of a community or social system and an understanding of how the roles he or she plays assist in maintaining or constructively altering that social system. The roles that the individual perceives as productive and of a contributory nature may be relative to the family, the church, the political system, the economic system, education, or the arts and sciences.

Learning is indicated by the ability to identify roles that are important to the self, the ability to articulate in a positive manner how these roles contribute to the social system, a sense of knowing "what I am," and recognition of one's place in a social system as well as a feeling of participation in that system. Lack of learning is indicated by the absence of these behaviors, an egocentric concept of self which is totally divorced from a productive role in the community, continued preoccupation with "what I am," perception of one's roles as worthless or degrading to the self, a feeling that one's talents or abilities are not being utilized and lack of effort to seek utilization, and no evidence of productivity outside the economic system. The tone and feelings associated with symbols that refer to the individual's and others' roles in a social system also provide useful information in assessing learning in this area.

This subskill is acquired through interaction in an environment that provides an opportunity for exploring roles relative to the social system; training necessary for gaining the knowledge, skills, and attitudes required for preferred roles; and through acknowledgment by the social system that these roles are significant.

In teaching this subskill the therapist provides opportunities for the client to explore roles relative to the social system and supports the client while the exploration is taking place. The client's age, cultural background, abilities, and interests are utilized in helping the client select particular areas for exploration. An apprentice relationship with others who are engaged in roles which the client finds meaningful is useful in teaching this subskill; in such an apprentice relationship the individual interacts as a participant-learner. The training necessary for selected roles may be offered by the therapist or some other person in the treatment facility. It may also be possible for the client to acquire such training wholly through an apprentice relationship—or formal training may be necessary. Whatever the situation, the therapist assists the client in acquiring whatever type of training is necessary. Perhaps the most difficult part of the teaching process is helping the client locate others who will provide acknowledgment that the roles he or she has selected are significant to a social system. Many social systems give such recognition only for roles that are fairly complex and overtly contributory. The therapist, then, must be resourceful in locating and helping the client relate to others who are able to provide this necessary acknowledgment and reinforcement.

The Ability to Perceive the Self as Having an Autonomous Identity (35–50 years)

This subskill consists of the development of a profound knowledge of self. It goes far beyond the second self-identity skill, which is concerned with perception of one's assets and limitations. It refers to the individual's recognition of his or her essential being and, by extension, a willingness to act on the bases of that knowledge. With acquisition of the ability to perceive the self, the individual is in a position where he or she can begin to meet self-actualization needs.

Learning this subskill is indicated by evidence that the individual has continued satisfaction of all needs subordinate to the self-actualization need; by disregard for some of the nonessential norms of one's cultural group if necessary in order to accomplish something that is perceived as special, unique, and highly significant to the self; by a profound and sympathetic understanding that it is only through the support of those willing others that one is able to do a very special something; by knowledge that this is the only course of action one can take and continue to be; and by a special feeling of self-fulfillment when the individual is engaged in actions that are consistent with who he or she is. The symbol that tells us most about the learning of this subskill is the mandala. When an individual produces this symbol without any sense of longing but with joy and the experience that "this is me," he or she is well on the way to developing the subskill.

Unfortunately, we do not have a clear understanding of how this subskill is developed. We do know that all needs (using Maslow's hierarchy) subordinate to the self-actualization need must be met, and it also appears that it is very helpful when there are some persons in the environment who are capable of recognizing the individual's potential for and appreciating the result of self-actualization.

There is some question concerning whether or not this subskill is prerequisite for learning the most advanced subskill. With the recognition of our limited knowledge in this area, it may not be necessary for the therapist to be concerned about this subskill when mastery of the final subskill seems to be more imperative.

The Ability to Perceive the Aging Process of Oneself and Ultimate Death as Part of the Life Cycle (45–60 years)

An individual may perceive the aging process as enhancing the capacity to deal with self and others, but it is the rare person who perceives it as a joyful, anticipated experience. The aging process diminishes capacities, severs relationships with loved ones, and presents practical problems. Learning this subskill is indicated by resigned acceptance of the aging process and death, perception of one's life as useful and productive, engagement in activities that are compatible with actual physical and psychological capacities, and continued perception of the self as a contributing member of the social system. Lack of learning is indicated by the absence of these behaviors; excessive preoccupation with physical enhancement, religion, or making provisions for distribution of accumulated objects; denial of chronological age; and feelings that one is rejected by others. The tone and affect of symbols referring to death, the birth-death-rebirth cycle, need satisfaction, potency, life or the soul, oneness or unity, spiritual growth, historical view of the developing self, and old age also provide information regarding learning.

This subskill is learned through interaction in an environment in which the individual's capacities are recognized; there is an opportunity to continue to be a productive member of a social system; there are people who are capable of giving and receiving love; the degenerative process and death are accepted by others as part of the life cycle; the profoundly unknown aspect of death and the state of being after death are seen as legitimate concerns and acceptable topics of conversation; and support is provided for the mourning of loss.

In teaching this subskill the therapist attempts to locate or provides an environment suitable for learning.

Sexual Identity Skill

"Identity," as used in regard to this adaptive skill, refers to awareness of, feelings about, and judgments regarding one's sexual nature; and interactions with others as a sexual being. Mature sexual identity skill is the ability to perceive one's sexual nature as good and to participate in sexual relationships that are oriented to the mutual satisfaction of sexual needs. An individual who has attained full maturation of sexual identity experiences delight relative to the sexual aspects of the body and the body of others. He or she perceives the genitalia and secondary sexual characteristics as a source of pleasure for the self and the means of providing pleasure for others. The individual is aware of his or her own periodic need for the release of sexual tensions and the needs of others with whom he or she is sexually involved. The needs of both partners are taken into consideration and regulate the extent and nature of sexual interactions.

There are many ways to evaluate sexual identity subskill learning: observation of the patient relative to same-sex and opposite-sex interactions; discussion with the client regarding past and current sexual relationships, feelings regarding his or her own sexuality, and whatever fantasies he or she may have regarding sexuality; and interpretation of symbols produced by the client. All three areas provide valuable information.

The stages of sexual identity development are as follows:

The Ability to Accept and Act on the Bases of One's Pregenital Sexual Nature (4–5 years)

In learning this subskill the individual perceives sexuality as good, acceptable to others, and a source of pleasure. He or she also perceives that direct genital behavior is unaccepted in this period of his or her lifespan and that overt expression must be held in abeyance until a more appropriate time.

Learning of this subskill is indicated by knowledge regarding the sex of self and others, comfort in interacting with same-sex or opposite-sex individuals, and flexible definition of appropriate sexual roles. Lack of learning is indicated by the absence of these behaviors; perception of the self as an asexual being; promiscuous homosexual or heterosexual behavior, which has a flavor of confused sexual identity or a search for sexual identity; denial of sexuality; avoidance of people or interactions that are perceived as sexual in nature; perception of all aspects of sexuality as dirty, bad, or harmful to self and others; continued genital attachment to the parent or parental figure of the opposite sex; and a search for persons similar to the same-sex parent with avoidance of persons similar to the opposite-sex parent. The manner in which the individual uses symbols that refer to sex and the obvious absence or predominant use of sexual symbols also provide useful information regarding the learning of this subskill.

This subskill is learned through interaction in an environment where there is recognition of the individual's sexual nature, where there are individuals of both sexes who are comfortable with their sexuality, suitable individuals of the same sex who encourage emulation of appropriate sex-specific behavior as defined by the cultural group and education that is compatible with the individual's age. Interaction in a same-sex peer group facilitates inhibition of genital sexuality and consolidates pregenital sex-specific role learning. Some interaction in heterosexual groups helps the individual to learn about relating to the opposite sex. Finally, learning of this subskill is enhanced through interaction with a variety of nonhuman objects which provide an opportunity for experimenting with sex-specific modes of behavior and through symbolic expression of genital-sexuality. Denial of or negative reactions to sexually motivated behavior, the sexual aspects of the body, or private autoerotic behavior are detrimental to the learning of this subskill.

The Ability to Accept Sexual Maturation as a Positive Growth Experience (12–16 years)

Sexual maturation refers to the development of primary and secondary sexual characteristics, resurgence of sexual impulses, and cultural requirements regarding appropriate nongenital behavior for genitally mature individuals. Learning is indicated by perception of the self as a genitally mature individual, control of sexual impulses without excessive effort, experiencing the self as sexually desirable, a positive attitude toward one's primary and secondary sexual characteristics and integration of these characteristics with the other aspects of one's body schema, and the ability to engage in what is currently accepted as appropriate nongenital behavior for genitally mature individuals. In addition, an individual who has learned this component is able to engage in courting behavior with a relative degree of discretion regarding sexual activity. Lack of learning is indicated by the absence of these behaviors, denial of sexual impulses or perception of them as threatening to the integrity of the self, promiscuous sexual activity, perception of the self as only a sexual object with little recognition of other aspects of the self, preoccupation with primary and secondary sexual characteristics and a feeling that they are inadequate or excessive, a negativistic attitude toward the opposite sex (women perceived as inferior, silly, or stupid; men perceived as mean, dirty, or ill-mannered). Lack of learning is also indicated by predominant use of symbols that refer to negative feelings regarding the sexual asects of the body, being overwhelmed by sexual urges, and symbols referring to the opposite sex.

This subskill is learned through interaction in an environment where there is reinforcement for giving attention to and caring for the body, interaction with same-sex and opposite-sex peers who provide validation of one's sexuality, guidelines for acceptable sexual activity, and appropriate sex education. In addition, the environment must recognize differing opinions regarding appropriate sex-specific roles. The individual must have an opportunity to explore a variety of behavior patterns and be free to take those roles most compatible with his or her goals and life-style.

In teaching this subskill the therapist must be comfortable in discussing all aspects of sex but in particular the sexual aspects of the body of both sexes, the functions and responses of the sex organs, and various norms that govern sexual behavior. One suggested technique for enhancing attention to the body is to engage the patient in drawing or sculpturing the nude body of both sexes with concurrent comfortable discussion regarding the body. The therapist helps the client locate some same- and opposite-sex peers who are capable of providing validation of the client's sexuality. The therapist provides support, encouragement, and guidance to assist the client in interacting comfortably with these individuals. Although the therapist may provide an opportunity for one-to-one discussion of norms that may be used to guide sexual activity and information regarding sex, it is suggested that this take place in group. The consequences of selecting various norms to guide one's sexual activities should be explored. Sex education should be comprehensive, detailed, and specific, and should cover the physiological, psychological, and sociological aspects of sexuality. If there is likely to be a lengthy period before the group members will be able to engage in genital sexual activity, discussion should also focus on various ways of dealing with sexual impulses.

The Ability to Give and Receive Sexual Gratification (18–25 years)

Learning of this subskill is indicated by the individual's awareness of sexual needs, the quality and quantity of sexual responses, and the stimuli that maximize his or her ability to respond. The sexual needs of others are recognized and there is appreciation of the variation in sexual responses. Techniques for satisfying self and others are available to the individual, and he or she is able to vary responses according to the needs of others. Sexual intercourse is seen as a way of expressing affection and satisfying physiological needs. Lack of learning is indicated by the absence of these behaviors. The way in which the individual deals with symbols refering to sexual intercourse also provides useful information in the assessment of this subskill.

This component is learned through interaction in an environment where there is an opportunity to engage in autoerotic activities without guilt and an opportunity to participate in sex play and sexual intercourse with others (or another) who perceive such activity as good, beautiful, rewarding, and fun.

In most cultural groups in the United States, autoerotic activities and sex play prior to a marital relationship are considered acceptable. Sexual intercourse prior to marriage, however, is still not acceptable to many cultural groups. The advantages of autoerotic activities, sex play and premarital intercourse are the opportunities to explore the sexual responses of self and other without the additional complication of initial adjustment to marriage. It is important to remember, however, that intercourse outside of the marital relationship which generates anxiety or guilt is not conducive to learning this subskill.

In helping a client learn to give and receive sexual gratification, the therapist assists him in locating suitable persons for such learning. The therapist provides support and advice, clarifies values, and offers encouragement as needed.

The Ability to Enter into a Sustained Sexual Relationship Characterized by the Mutual Satisfaction of Sexual Needs (20–30 years)

Acquisition of this skill does not necessarily occur at the time of marriage or within the confines of a marital contract, nor does occasional and transient sexual activity outside of a sustained relationship necessarily indicate the absence of this subskill. Learning is indicated by conscious awareness of one's commitment to a sustained sexual relationship, knowledge of the implications of such a commitment, and an intimate relationship with one's sexual partner. Typical relationships with other people are nongenital in nature, but appreciation of the sexuality of the other remains an important part of the relationship. Lack of learning is indicated by the absence of these behaviors, a relatively rapid sequential change in sex partners, or a number of simultaneous partners, perception of one's self or sexual partner as sexually inadequate, primary concern with the sexual satisfaction of the self or one's partner, and perception of marriage as primarily a limitation of one's sexual freedom. There do not seem to be any specific symbols that provide information relative to learning in this area.

This subskill is acquired through interaction in an environment where there are suitable others who have the capacity to learn this subskill and a desire to do so, a general sense of security, and sufficient time to focus upon the sexual needs of the self and one's partner.

The therapist assists a client in learning this subskill in a manner similar to the one outlined for teaching the third sexual-identity skill.

The Ability to Accept the Sex-Related Physiological Changes That Occur as a Natural Part of the Aging Process (40–60 years)

Learning of this subskill is indicated by acceptance of menopause for a woman and altered sexual responses for a man, with continued perception of the self as a sexual being and enjoyment of sexual interactions. Lack of learning is indicated by prolonged mourning over the perceived loss of sexuality; feelings of worthlessness; no attempt to participate in genital sexual activities or interest in such activities; disregard for the appearance of the self, personal hygiene, appropriate clothes, or maintenance of normal weight; excessive preoccupation with appearance, extreme attempts to maintain a youthfulness that is incompatible with chronological age; and the need for continued reassurance that one is a desirable sexual being. Lack of learning is also indicated by predominant use of symbols referring to potency, fertility, life-death-rebirth cycle, unmet needs, and loss.

This subskill is learned through interaction in an environment where the individual's sexual nature is recognized and accepted; there is opportunity to participate in nongenital sexual roles that are particularly meaningful to the individual and opportunity to find another sexual partner if there has been loss of the usual partner.

In teaching this subskill the therapist assists the client in locating and using an environment with the above-listed characteristics. The therapist provides support, encouragement, and guidance as needed; the client's sexual nature and needs are taken into consideration by the therapist at all times.

SUMMARY

Recapitulation of ontogenesis is a developmental frame of reference addressed to those aspects of development considered to be crucial for adequate and satisfying participation in a variety of social roles. Identified as adaptive skills, these essential elements were described as sensory integrative skill, cognitive skill, dyadic interaction skill, group interaction skill, self-identity skill, and sexual identity skill. In discussions of the stages or stage components of each of the adaptive skills, behavior indicative of mastery and lack of mastery was described as well as the elements within the environment believed to be responsible for the mastery of each stage of development. Finally, the way in which these environmental elements are used as the basis for designing appropriate learning experiences were outlined.

25 Acquisitional Frames of Reference

Acquisitional frames of reference provide a structure for linking learning theories, the reality aspect of purposeful activities, and the process of acquiring specific skills needed for successful interaction in the environment (307,427,646,705,960,969). The assumptions fundamental to acquisitional frames of reference are as follows:

1. Behavior is primarily influenced by interactions in one's current environment.
2. Areas of human function are considered to be relatively independent, quantitative, and non-stage-specific.
3. Adaptive behavior is acquired by direct interaction in an environment designed for learning a particular skill.

The first section of the chapter is devoted to an elaboration of this definition of acquisitional frames of reference. A review of the acquisitional orientation in occupational therapy is presented in the final section.

Learning theories constitute a body of knowledge that describes the way in which individuals acquire a repertoire of behavior. Learning, as previously defined, is a process wherein there is a

> change in a subject's behavior in a given situation brought about by his repeated experience in that situation, providing the behavior cannot be explained on the basis of native response tendencies, maturation or temporary states of the organism (e.g. fatigue, drugs, etc.) (427, p. 17).

There are several theories of learning, none of which adequately account for all types of learned behavior. The most common theory of learning used as the foundation of acquisitional frames of reference in occupational therapy is operant conditioning; or at least that was so in the 1970s. The next most common foundation for acquisitional frames of reference are the "principles of learning" as described in Chapter 9.

In acquisitional frames of reference, purposeful activities are primarily viewed in relationship to their reality component. The symbolic potential of activities is rarely if ever taken into consideration. Rather, activities are considered relative to their potential for facilitating the learning of particular skills. To some extent activities are viewed as vehicles, but they are far more likely to be viewed as entities to be mastered. In illustration, if a client needs to learn how to cook, he or she may well be presented with a variety of graded cooking tasks. Through participation in these tasks the client, hopefully, learns the basics of meal preparation. This is what the tasks were designed to do. This is not to say that the client may not gain increased skill, for example, in problem solving and general coordination. But that was not the major purpose of engaging in the tasks; they were designed as entities to be mastered, not vehicles for learning something else. Finally, in acquisitional frames of reference, the age-specific nature of activities are only of general concern. Age is a factor in activity analysis and synthesis, but it is not given as close attention as in developmental frames of reference.

The first assumption of acquisitional frames of reference is concerned with the belief that the way people act is primarily influenced by the current environment in which they exist. Behavior is not, as in analytical frames of reference, considered to be the result of internal states of the person. Intrapsychic content, on the whole, is not given much attention in acquisitional frames of reference. It is not necessarily denied as being an identifiable phenomena but it is just not considered of particular importance. If addressed at all, intrapsychic content is described as the consequence of behavior. Thus if behavior is altered, intrapsychic content will be altered. There is no need for intrapsychic content to be shared or subjected to reality testing. For example, if an individual learns to act in an independent manner, that person will eventually come to view him- or herself as someone who is able to function independently. The converse assumption, if you will remember, is basic to analytical frames of reference.

In some acquisitional frames of reference, the dynamic states of the individual are given some attention. These frames of reference may, for example, postulate an inherent need to explore and master the environment, or they may assume that each individual has a particular set of interests and/or goals. These dynamic states are usually described as the source of motivation and/or as the reason for preferring certain types of interactions in the environment. It should be noted that altering interests and goals, per se, is not the major focus of these acquisitional frames of reference.

Finally, regarding the first assumption, the individual's current environment is thought to be far more influential than the repertoire of behavior the individual has acquired in the past. It is the present environment that is believed to support behavior—be it adaptive or maladaptive—not learning or the lack of learning in the distant past.

The second assumption identifies one of the major differences between acquisitional and developmental frames of reference. In acquisitional frames of reference, areas of human function, on the whole, are not considered to be closely interrelated. Thus, for example, if an individual has difficulty in interpersonal relations, this need not interfere with his or her capacity to manipulate the nonhuman environment. This is not to say that areas of human function are considered to be completely independent one from the other. However, the relationship is seen as less interrelated as that described relative to the developmental frames of reference.

In addition, areas of human function are seen as quantitative and nonstage-specific. The acquisition of a repertoire of behavior is conceptualized as the refinement and elaborations of skill without any demarcation of stages. An example of this point of view is seen in Guilford's theory of cognitive development; he views it as a quantitative increment of a collection of closely related skills. In contrast, Piaget conceptualized the development of cognition as having clearly differentiated stages. One of the assumptions of developmental frames of reference, as previously discussed, is that the development of most areas of human function is stage-specific.

The third assumption fundamental to acquisitional frames of reference refers to the belief that on the whole, the necessary skill for interacting in the environment can be learned directly without any need to go back and experience various stages of development. For example, when an individual has not developed culturally acceptable work habits it is not considered necessary to follow the ontogenetic development of work habits. Rather it is assumed that work habits can be taught without recourse to deficits in earlier phases of the life cycle.

This, it should be remembered, is a general assumption and should not be taken too literally. There are some acquisitional frames of reference that give some attention to the typical sequence of development of complex skills. Others suggest that some areas of human function be mastered before attention be given to other areas. In identifying the difference between developmental and acquisitional frames of reference, it may be useful to visualize typical ontogenetic development as center stage in development frames of reference. In contrast, ontogenetic development serves as the backdrop for acquisitional frames of reference.

The concepts of splinter skills and learning by rote are not used in acquisitional frames of reference. A particular skill either has or has not been learned; it is either part of the individual's repertoire of behavior or it is not. The concept of "frequency of behavior," is, however, used in some acquisitional frames of reference. This refers to the extent to which an individual uses a particular skill or gestalt of behavior. The change process, then, may be directed not only to teaching new skills but to increasing the frequency of use of a particular skill that is already a part of the individual's repertoire. Conversely, the change process may be concerned with decreasing the frequency of certain maladaptive behaviors.

Relative to the occupational therapy domain of concern, acquisitional frames of reference may be addressed to any one or several of the performance components or of the occupational performances. They tend, however, to be concerned with cognitive function, social interaction, and occupational performances. They seemingly are concerned with these areas of human function because behavior in these areas is more concrete or readily able to be observed.

The general goal of an acquisitional frame of reference is to help the individual acquire an adequate repertoire of behavior relative to his or her current life situation or expected environment. Acquisitional frames of reference are, in a way, rather pragmatic and in essence are applied in response to the question, "What does this client need to learn in order to manage her daily affairs?" The concept of expected environment plays a major role in determining the goals of the change process for a specific client.

The theoretical base of an acquisitional frame of reference usually provides a detailed description of one or a combination of learning theories. The areas of human function addressed in the frame of reference are also described. These may be discussed in general terms as was the case in Chapters 3 and 4, which outlined the performance components and occupational performances, respectively. On the other hand, the ontogenetic development of the areas addressed may also be described. The purpose of the latter would be to assist the therapist in identifying what specific skills the client should have in his or her repertoire, given the client's age. However, this is only used as a general guide and not in the strict way that it is utilized in a developmental frame of reference. The inclusion of stages of development in the theoretical base of an acquisitional frame of reference may, at times, be a source of some confusion. There is, admittedly, some overlapping of acquisitional and developmental frames of reference. One must often look at a frame of reference in its entirety to determine whether it is an acquisitional or developmental frame of reference.

Causal factors are usually not discussed in the theoretical base of an acquisitional frame of reference. If they are discussed, attention is usually given to general environmental factors that interfere with the development of an adequate repertoire of behavior. These usually include (a) lack of an opportunity to learn because of the individual being confined, for whatever reason, to a restricted environment and/or (b) existence in an environment in which adaptive behavior did not receive adequate reinforcement. In either case, causal factors are not considered of particular importance.

Function-dysfunction continuums in acquisitional frames of reference tend to be numerous and fairly specific. In acquisitional frames of reference that are broad in scope, the continuums identify a wide spectrum of behaviors considered to be necessary for satisfactory interaction in the environment. In more circumspect frames of reference, for example, one that was concerned only with the area of work, there would, of course, be fewer continuums outlined.

Behaviors indicative of function and dysfunction tend to be described at the level of direct observation in acquisitional frames of reference. This is far more true than in either analytical or developmental frames of reference. In addition to using only the presence and absence of particular behaviors to determine whether an individual is in a state of function or dysfunction on a given continuum, the frequency of the client's use of a particular skill (as delineated by a continuum) is also taken into consideration. Some acquisitional frames of reference, however, do not include behaviors indicative of function and dysfunction. This is particularly true in frames of reference based on a strict interpretation of operant conditioning. In this orientation there is no distinction made between a skill or the entity to which the change process is addressed and the behavior that indicates whether an individual does or does not have that skill. There is just behavior; nothing more and nothing less.

An example might be useful in illustrating this point. In frame of reference A there is a continuum identified as "sustained interest in a task." The behaviors indicative of dysfunction are that rather than working at a task, the individual wanders around the room, gazes out the window, talks to other people, talks to herself, never completes a task, leaves the room, etc. In frame of reference B, one that is based on a strict interpretation of operant conditioning, there would be no continuum such as "sustained interest in a task." Rather, the entities of concern in the change process would be what is identified above as behavior indicative of dysfunction. Thus, the therapist is likely to be concerned with eliminating the above behaviors directly and probably through nonreinforcement of such behaviors. Ideally, differential reinforcement would be used wherein the therapist reinforces task-oriented behaviors and does not reinforce the types of behaviors listed for A. The difference between the actual change process utilized in type A and type B acquisitional frames of reference may not be all that great. However, there is a difference in orientation and in how the frames of reference are presented.

Evaluation in acquisitional frames of reference tends to be focused more on the client's present interaction in the environment than on past history. The client and therapist are primarily concerned with what the client is able and not able to do in the here and now. Evaluation usually involves discussion regarding current interactions in the environment and the client's participation in evaluative situations that involve engaging in tasks alone and/or with others. Interview content and activity-oriented evaluation situations are designed to focus on environmental interactions requiring the use of the various human capacities of concern in the frame of reference being utilized. Evaluation may also include assessment of the individual's current environment to identify factors that may be responsible for maintenance of particular maladaptive behaviors.

Almost all acquisitional frames of reference have general postulates, i.e., postulates that are addressed to all of the continuums included in a particular frame of reference. These postulates are deduced from the learning theory or theories included in the theoretical base. Some acquisitional frames of reference also have specific postulates that are concerned with each of the separate continuums. These continuums usually describe characteristics of the environment that are believed to facilitate learning in a particular area. The characteristics identified are not necessarily similar to the environmental characteristics that are believed to be responsible for typical development in the usual course of the life cycle. For example, an acquisitional frame of reference concerned with the development of work habits might contain a postulate regarding change that describes the essential characteristics of a sheltered workshop. In the usual course of the life cycle, work habits are not acquired through participation in a sheltered workshop. This difference in the content of specific postulates is one of the factors that distinguishes acquisitional frames of reference from developmental frames of reference.

The criteria for goal setting are usually far less specifically stated in acquisitional than in developmental frames of reference. The criteria also vary from one acquisitional frame of reference to another. However, in most acquisitional frames of reference, the client's expected environment is used as the basis for establishing long-term goals. Concerning short-term goals and the sequence of the change process, the frame of reference may provide some suggested guidelines or leave that part of planning to the client and therapist's discretion. Pragmatically, intervention usually begins in that area considered to be the most important or useful for the client to acquire at that time. This is ideally determined by the therapist and the client together.

The use of acquisitional frames of reference is appropriate for a wide variety of clients. More specifically it is suitable for any client who has not developed an adequate repertoire of behavior or who, because of alteration in life situation, needs to develop new skills for managing daily affairs. Acquisitional frames of reference are suitable for any age group and no particular level of cognitive or verbal skill is required. They are particularly suited for short-term intervention. Acquisitional frames of reference are probably the most frequently used in helping the families of clients cope with the problems of adjusting to and living with a disabled family member. The continuums in such a frame of reference would, of course, be somewhat different than those in a frame of reference designed for clients. But the essence of the frames of reference would be the same—the learning of more adaptive behavior.

With this general description of acquisitional frames of reference, the remaining portion of this chapter is devoted to a brief discussion of those acquisitional frames of reference primarily concerned with psychosocial components and currently used in occupational therapy.

REVIEW OF THE ACQUISITIONAL ORIENTATION

The first acquisitional frame of reference was "habit training" as formulated by Slagle. This was discussed briefly in Chapter 2 and will not be described further here for it is no longer used in occupational therapy. It is only mentioned to put the acquisitional orientation into some perspective. As is discussed later in this section, in part, habit training was used as the basis of formulating the occupational behavior frames of reference.

Action-Consequence

In more recent times the first acquisitional frames of reference were based on operant conditioning. Most of them were rather narrow in scope, dealing with a few areas of human behavior and/or a specific diagnostic category (236,335,438,482,606,641,740,896,948,990, 998). Perhaps the most general is Action-Consequence, which is concerned with a much broader spectrum of behavior (705). The areas of concern are activities of daily living, avocational pursuits, and work. Each of these areas is described as being made up of tasks or manipulation of the nonhuman environment and of interpersonal interactions. Suggested evaluation procedures include an interview that focuses on the client's general capacities in the areas of daily living activities, avocational pursuits, and work; and performance assessments that are concerned with task skills and interpersonal relations. The postulates regarding change are general in nature and are, of course, deduced from operant conditioning. No specific postulate is provided, but there is a brief description of the change process in each area of concern. There is also a section on the application of the postulates regarding change which is presented in a general way and is not specific to each of the areas of concern.

There are three major difficulties with the Action-Consequence frame of reference:

1. The theoretical base does not account for everything that is contained in the rest of the frame of refer-

ence. For example, daily living activities, avocational pursuits, and work are not discussed; the use of groups is discussed in describing the change process, but groups are never mentioned in the theoretical base.

2. Behavior indicative of function and dysfunction are not clearly delineated. There are, however, many examples of functional and dysfunctional behavior throughout the presentation which provide some guidelines for interpretation of evaluative data.

3. The description of the change process is fairly brief and would probably be more useful if presented in more detail.

Perhaps the most important consequence of the formulation and application of frames of reference based on operant conditioning is that it made occupational therapists aware of the potential of learning theories as a theoretical foundation for the change process. In addition, the frames of reference provided an alternative to the analytical and developmental orientation, which are not suitable for all clients.

Activities Therapy

The next major acquisitional frame of reference formulated was Activities Therapy (708). This frame of reference not only has a broader theoretical base but it deals with more areas of human function than Action-Consequence. The theoretical base consists of principles of learning, group dynamics, and a description of the areas addressed in the frame of reference. These areas, which also form the continuums, are divided into three categories. These categories and the areas of human function which they include are (a) basic skills—task skills and group interaction skills; (b) the public self—activities of daily living, work, recreation, and intimacy; (c) the private self—cognitive system (concept of self and others and basic knowledge about the world) needs, emotions and values.

Behavior indicative of function and dysfunction is delineated by example rather than by enumeration. Evaluative procedures are outlined with some guidelines for interpreting data gathered through these procedures. Postulates regarding change are not specifically stated. There is, however, a fairly extensive description of the change process which discusses each of the continuums, with emphasis on how they are interrelated.

The major difficulty with activities therapy is that it is not entirely acquisitional in orientation. It is really a combination of all three types of frames of reference. Combining types of frames of reference is, of course, perfectly acceptable, but only if the theoretical base includes systems that support more than one orientation; activities therapy does not. For example, the areas of group interaction skill and intimacy (somewhat like dyadic interaction skill) are treated as stage-specific. The change process relative to all areas included in the category of the private self is described essentially with an analytical orientation. The theoretical base of activities therapy does not provide sufficient support for either a developmental or an analytical orientation. The one advantage of activities therapy is that for the most part it does provide fairly adequate guidelines for intervention, even though these are not presented as postulates regarding change. It would, however, be a much stronger frame of reference if its theoretical base was more complete.

Occupational Behavior

The last part of this section is addressed to a collection of frames of reference that has come to be categorized as Occupational Behavior. As mentioned in Chapter 2, these frames of reference were primarily formulated by therapists associated with the Southern California group. This orientation can perhaps be best understood by first reviewing some of the major ideas of Reilly, the founder of this group (798,799,800).

Reilly felt that occupational therapy had become too preoccupied with kinesiology, neurology, and psychoanalytic theory. Essentially she was saying that the profession was devoting most of its attention to performance components. As an alternative, Reilly strongly urged the profession to return to the ideas about occupational therapy that were promoted by Mayer and Slagle—i.e., work, play, and rest—and the balance between these areas of life experience. In other words, occupational therapy should turn its attention to the occupational performances of school/work, play/leisure/recreation, and temporal adaptation. Reilly did not include family interaction as one of the roles that should be of concern to occupational therapists. Mayer and Slagle never mentioned this area of human experience; nor, for that matter, were they concerned about any types of close interpersonal relationships (678,904,905,906,907). Similarly, Mayer and Slagle gave little if any attention to activities of daily living. Thus, this area is rarely dealt with by Reilly except in the context of the child learning how to participate in household chores.

Reilly was particularly interested in play (801). She viewed the play of a child as being the major means whereby individuals learn the basic skills necessary for becoming a worker and participating in adult recreational/leisure activities. Reilly describes preparation for these two social roles through play as follows:

- *Individual play*. An opportunity to explore the environment and what one is and is not able to do, with minimal outside constraints; an adventure in examining, investigating, questioning, and searching.
- *Arts and crafts*. A means for evaluating one's competence relating to the understanding of and having some control over the nonhuman environment; judgment is based on the end product produced.
- *Games played with other people*. An opportunity to learn the idea of rules and principles that govern acceptable behavior in particular social situations. The individual also learns how to relate to, share, and cooperate with peers.
- *Chores or tasks imposed by another person*. A means for learning how to relate to authority.

Reilly has a distinct view of human beings. An oft-quoted statement of hers is, "That man through the use of his hands as they are energized by mind and will, can influence the state of his health." (798 p. 2). This statement has been interpreted in a variety of ways, the most common being (a) that doing and engaging in purposeful activities is essential in the maintenance of health and in remediation in problems that interfere with a state of health and (b) that the individual has an inherent need to explore and master the environment and to be competent.

The first part of the interpretation emphasizes the importance of purposeful activities, the only tool that Reilly felt was legitimate for occupational therapy. The last part of the interpretation speaks to the importance of intrinsic motivation, both in human development and in the change process. Extrinsic motivation, or the demand for growth and change by others, was considered by Reilly as neither appropriate nor very effective.

Finally, Reilly emphasizes the importance of viewing the individual as being an open system. That is, individuals are strongly influenced by the environments in which they participate. Behavior is considered to be learned and regulated by the stimuli or requirements of the environment which prompt action and by the feedback which one receives as the result of that action. (See Chapters 2 and 12 for a discussion of open systems.)

On the bases of these major ideas the occupational behavior orientation evolved and led to the formulation of a number of frames of reference. Space does not permit a description of all of them; there are approximately 28. The following outline categorizes these frames of references according to the major focus and gives some idea of the various elements addressed.

1. *Play*: Theories regarding play, various types of play, stage-specific development of play, effects on the individual of lack of participation in play, skills needed in order to play, various skills that can be acquired through play, what is essential in environment for play to occur, Facilitating play (232,303,462,526, 552,680,681,813,945,946,977).
2. *Play-work*: Role theory, socialization, role transitions; play as preparation for work; transition from play to work; transition from the work role to spending the majority of one's time in leisure/recreational activities; maintenance of play/work skills and habits during hospitalization; use of activity groups in facilitating role transitions (306,365,405,653,883, 884,892).
3. *Work*: Nature of work; socialization, role theory; theories of occupational choice and gender differences in that process; work habits, remediating deficits in occupational choice process (69,106,107,652,769, 772,999).
4. *Temporal adaptation*: The nature of time; balance between work, play, and rest; development of a sense of external time; adapting to the temporal expectations of one's culture; differing perspectives of time; deficits in temporal adaptation; remediating temporal adaptation deficits (519,520,734).

There is considerable overlapping between the occupational behavior frames of reference, and they are all essentially compatible with each other. The majority are focused on intervention relative to specific populations of children and adolescents, with a few addressed to mentally retarded individuals and adults in the process of role transition owing to retirement or to an acquired physical disability.

The theoretical base of the occupational behavior frames of reference are usually complete, containing both a description of the area of concern and a dynamic theory.

Function-dysfunction continuums and behaviors indicative of function and dysfunction are only occasionally enumerated. The majority of the frames of reference, however, provide rather lengthy scales, inventories, interview protocols, and/or questionnaires. The writers of these frames of reference seem to assume that the description of an evaluative tool negates the need for continuums and behaviors indicative of function and dysfunction. This is a questionable assumption.

Postulates regarding change are provided in only two or three of the frames of reference. This seems somewhat extraordinary in that most of the frames of reference have a dynamic theory from which postulates regarding change could be fairly easily deduced. Following Reilly's idea that the best way to consider the individual is through the case method approach, case studies are often included in occupational behavior frames of reference.

These case studies, which describe evaluation and intervention, are apparently presented in lieu of postulates regarding change. Although case studies are useful in illustrating how a frame of reference might be applied, they cannot take the place of general principles designed to guide the change process. No two clients are alike. Thus there is rarely, if ever, an exact fit between a case study and the needs of a particular client. If case studies were a suitable guide for the change process, there would be no need for theory or frames of reference.

Nevertheless, it is from reading the case studies that one gets the impression that these frames of reference are, on the whole, acquisitional in nature. Although development in the area addressed is often included in the theoretical base, it appears to serve as a backdrop for evaluation and intervention. Intervention is rarely described as a stage-by-stage process. Rather, change seems to be directed toward the acquisition of specific skills.

One final comment. As mentioned, the various occupational behavior frames of reference tend to be narrow in focus relative to the population for which they are formulated, and there is considerable overlap. The narrowness of focus limits the applicability of a specific frame of reference. A few broader based frames of reference would probably be more useful to the profession. It hardly seems that we need 28 frames of reference to provide guidelines for dealing with three parts of our domain of concern.

Irrespective of the above comments, the occupational behavior orientation and the frames of reference which it has generated has made a significant contribution to the profession. Play, work, and temporal adaptation, although part of the domain of concern of occupational therapy from its inception, had, at least during the 1940s through the 1960s, not received the attention they deserved. Occupational behavior has given the profession a more balanced view of its domain of concern.

The following chapter describes an acquisitional frame of reference that draws on the various frames of reference summarized in this section.

26 Role Acquisition: An Acquisitional Frame of Reference

The label "role acquisition" was chosen for this frame of reference because its application is primarily concerned with the learning of those social roles required of the individual in the expected environment. It is essentially a combination of the frames of reference outlined in Chapter 25: Action-Consequence, Activities Therapy, and the Occupational Behavior frames of reference. Hopefully it is stated in such a way that some of the deficits noted in these frames of reference are eliminated.

This frame of reference is addressed to some aspects of motor and cognitive function, in particular those aspects enabling the individual to complete a variety of tasks successfully; to social interaction; and to all of the occupational performances. It is appropriate for individuals who have not learned how to participate in required social roles or who wish to participate in these roles in a more effective manner. It is particularly applicable for individuals who are experiencing difficulty with role transitions (becoming a parent, retirement, etc.) or individuals who, because of their current life situations, must learn how to participate in their social roles in a somewhat different manner. The major limitation of this frame of reference is that it should probably not be used as the initial frame of reference for individuals who have severe deficit in motor function, sensory integration, and perhaps psychological function. It is often the frame of reference of choice after the initial use of or in conjunction with an analytical frame of reference. It is also frequently used as the basis for intervention after an individual, for whatever reason, is no longer able to advance further through the application of a developmental frame of reference.

THEORETICAL BASE

Similar to the other two frames of reference described in their entirety, the theoretical base of role acquisition is made up of theoretical systems that have been previously described in the text. These systems, thus, are only briefly summarized. It is suggested that the reader review the detailed description of these areas in previous parts of the text. The theoretical base is discussed in five parts: the nature of the individual, what needs to be learned, how learning takes place, typical and atypical development, and appropriate tools.

The nature of the individual. The individual has an inherent need to explore the environment. Out of this exploration arises a desire to be competent, which, in turn, leads to a desire to master various aspects of the human and nonhuman environment (1014,1015,1016). The desire to master is selective in that it is primarily related to those areas that reflect the interests of the individual. When an interest is predominant, it can best be described as a goal: an end toward which the individual is willing to expend considerable time and energy. Interests and goals are developed through exploration of the environment and are influenced by the individual's generic endowment, success in particular areas, and the worth placed on certain interests and goals by the individual's family and cultural group.

What needs to be learned. To a great extent, what an individual must learn is specified by the society and cultural group in which he or she lives. These societal requirements can best be conceptualized as a number of role categories (see references, Chapter 5). Within these categories specific roles taken and how one participates in these roles are influenced by the individual's interests and goals. An individual who is considered to have adapted to and to have become a contributing member of society is skilled in participating in a variety of roles and manages these roles in a relatively organized fashion. In so doing, the individual is able to take care of basic needs and fulfill expectations for the self and that others have for him or her.

Basic to all social roles are task skills (competence in manipulating the nonhuman environment) and interpersonal skills. These basic skills form the elements out of which all role performances are built. They are elaborated and adjusted according to the requirements of specific roles. It should be noted that in typical ontogenetic development, basic skills are learned and refined within the context of participation in social roles. The relationship between basic skills and social roles can perhaps best be thought of as a spiral. Starting with primitive basic skills present at birth, the individual enters the role of family member and caretaker of the self (activities of daily living), wherein more basic skills are learned; the child then takes on the role of a player, which accounts for the development of more basic skills and so on, with more refined basic skills being learned as well as the addition of more social roles. This spiral-like development continues throughout the life cycle.

Four categories of social roles are considered to constitute the major roles required by an individual. There are, of course, variations in each of these categories, depending on the individual's age, cultural group membership, inherent capacities, and particular interests and goals. These four categories of roles are family interaction, activities of daily living, play/recreation/leisure, and work.

In order for an individual to fulfill all social roles in a manner satisfying to self and others, these roles must be organized in some relationship to time. In other words, sufficient time must be made available for participation in each required social role. This aspect of human experience, referred to as temporal adaptation, is also elaborated and refined as the individual takes on more and increasingly complex social roles. Returning to the illustration of the relationship between basic skills and social roles, temporal adaptation could also be added to that spiral.

The nature and development of social roles is a part of the theoretical base of this frame of reference. These areas are discussed in detail in Chapters 4 and 5.

How learning takes place. Learning relative to basic skills, social roles, and temporal adaptation can best be discussed from two different perspectives: the socialization process, a sociological perspective, and theories of learning, a psychological perspective. Although these will be summarized separately, they are interrelated both in the context of typical ontogenetic development and in intervention.

Socialization is the process of acquiring a particular social role. In addition to the person learning the role, two important elements of the socialization process are the agent(s) and the setting. The agent(s) is responsible for defining the expectations of what is to be learned, manipulating rewards, and providing feedback. The relationship between the agent and individual learning the role is all-important. With a relationship of respect and affection, extra weight or meaning is added to the rewards given and feedback offered. The agent(s) of socialization may be a participant in the role to which the individual aspires. In such a case the agent may be an instructor in appropriate behavior, a role model, or both. In other situations the agent may be a role partner. In this situation there is frequently considerable mutual role learning taking place. The setting for adequate socialization, ideally, is one in which the relevant behavior is elicited, evoked, required, and permitted. Practice should be possible and encouraged. Feedback should be available from other individuals and from the outcome or consequence of one's behavior. The setting should also be such that it arouses interest in exploring and the desire for mastery.

For the purpose of this frame of reference, the principles of learning as described in Chapter 9 will serve as the psychological dimension of the learning process. By way of summary, these principles are the following:

1. Learning is influenced by the individual's inherent capacities, current assets and limitations, age, sex, interests, and past and present cultural group membership.
2. Attention and perception influence learning.
3. The learner's motivation is important.
4. Learning goals set by the individual are more likely to be attained than goals set by someone else.
5. Learning is enhanced when the individual understands what is to be learned and the reason for learning.
6. Learning is increased when it begins at the individual's current level and proceeds at a rate that is comfortable for the individual.
7. Active participation in the learning process facilitates learning.
8. Reinforcement and feedback as the consequence of action are important parts of a learning experience.

9. Learning can be enhanced through trial and error, shaping, and imitation of models.
10. Frequent repetition or practice facilitates learning.
11. Planned movement from simplified wholes to more complex wholes facilitates integration of what is to be learned.
12. Inventive solution to problems should be encouraged as well as more usual and typical solutions.
13. The environment in which learning takes place is an important factor.
14. There are individual differences in the ways anxiety affects learning.
15. Conflicts and frustrations, inevitable in the learning situation, must be recognized and provision made for their resolution or accommodation;
16. There needs to be continuity between the learning situation and the experience for which the learning constitutes preparation.

It is within the framework of the sociological and psychological perspective of learning that the acquisition of basic skills, social roles, and temporal adaptation take place in this frame of reference.

Typical and atypical development. In the typical developmental process, the individual interacts in an environment where he or she is relatively free to explore and to acquire interests, goals, and competencies. The environment, ideally, also provides adequate agents and settings for the learning of required and desired social roles. Learning occurs because the individual wants to master and receive the rewards that are contingent on full participation in various roles. In the process of acquiring a variety of roles, the individual, in addition, has the opportunity to learn how to manage these roles relative to time so that they are experienced as adequately paced and satisfying.

Atypical development occurs when the environment is not conducive to learning, either in the past or at the present time. Role patterns may also be disrupted by illness, loss of a role partner, and other types of major alterations in the individual's life situation. In this case, it may be necessary for the individual to (a) reorganize role priorities and the amount of time allotted to various roles; (b) learn new skills so that she is able to participate in usual or new roles; (c) redefine one or more roles in a way that is more compatible with present abilities; and, (d) give up a particular role.

Some individuals are able to manage a disruption in role patterns independently or with the assistance of people within their social network. Other individuals need outside assistance in reestablishing a satisfactory pattern of role participation.

Appropriate tools. All of the legitimate tools of occupational therapy are used in the application of this frame of reference. There are, however, aspects of purposeful activities underscored here. Of particular importance are the following characteristics:

1. Emphasize doing. The principles of learning, a fundamental element of this frame of reference, in part, stress the importance of active participation of the learner in the learning process. Although knowledge may be gained through verbal interaction, skill is rarely acquired in this manner. Skill is usually developed through an active engagement in a doing process.
2. Vary on a continuum from conscious to not conscious/unconscious. The conscious level of learning is stressed initially in application of Role Acquisition. In other words, conscious awareness of what is to be learned is important. The individual needs to give careful attention to environmental stimuli, to responses of the self, and to the effect of those responses on the environment. As competency is gained, the individual needs to focus less attention on the particulars of a given interaction, and this is a sign of mastery. But initially, conscious attention to the nuances of what is to be learned is important.
3. Vary on a continuum from real to symbolic. The reality of purposeful activities is emphasized in this frame of reference. The tangible here and now qualities of activities serve as the basis for learning. Some clients may, on occasion, respond more to the symbolic component of an activity. When this is evident, it is noted by the therapist; it may well assist in a better understanding of the client. However, during intervention, the therapist gently draws the client away from symbolic response to one that is more appropriate to the realistic dimensions of the activity.
4. Vary on a continuum from simulated to natural. In application of role acquisition, intervention is often initiated through the use of simulated activities. However, as soon as possible, there is a shift to natural activities. Natural activities, on the whole are better suited to the learning of social roles. However, natural activities should not be used until it is fairly evident that the client is able to engage in such activities with at least some degree of comfort.

The other legitimate tool that needs to be emphasized relative to this frame of reference is activity groups. The types of activity groups appropriate to this orientation are evaluative, thematic, and topical. Task-oriented groups are not appropriate because they are designed to help individuals become aware of intrapsychic content, a goal that is not a part of role acquisition. This frame of reference is designed to alter behavior with the assumption that in so doing, ideas about oneself and other people and feelings will be altered. Developmental groups per se are not used in this frame of reference. That is, they are not used for the purpose of learning group interaction skills in a stage-by-stage sequential manner. Nevertheless, it is often appropriate to structure some groups in the application of this frame of reference along development lines. Some thematic groups, for example, may be structured like an egocentric-cooperative group; some topical groups may essentially be mature groups. The point to be made here is that the groups used in the application of this frame of reference may be structured in a manner similar to developmental groups. The way in which a group is structured is dependent on what is to be learned and the capacity for group interaction of the clients involved.

This, briefly and in very summary form, is the theoretical base of role acquisition.

THE CONTINUUMS AND BEHAVIORS INDICATIVE OF FUNCTION AND DYSFUNCTION

There are seven major categories of function/dysfunction continuums in Role Acquisition. Within each of these categories there are one or more continuums. In the outline below, most of the continuums are described in relationship to behavior indicative of dysfunction. Unless otherwise indicated, the absence of these behaviors indicates function. The categories and continuums are as follows:

Task Skills

1. *Willingness to engage in doing tasks.* Avoids engaging in tasks, talks more than engages in productive activity, remarks on his or her ineptness in performing tasks, seems fearful when engaging in a task.

2. *Adequate posture for tasks.* Sits in a slouched manner, acts as if a table or some other piece of furniture is needed for support, takes a posture that is inappropriate for the task, slow in making necessary changes in posture.

3. *Physical strength and endurance.* Tires very easily, asks for or takes an inordinate number of rest periods, complains of being tired, avoids activities requiring vigorous gross movements, complains of being too weak to engage in some activities.

4. *Gross and fine motor coordination.* Clumsy carrying out tasks, avoids tasks requiring a fair amount of coordination, performs tasks very slowly because of need to concentrate on coordinated movements. (When difficulty in this area appears to be due to sensory integrative deficit, this frame of reference is not used to deal with this area.)

5. *Interest in task.* Short attention span, spends most of the time engaged in nontask-oriented behavior (walking around, daydreaming, etc.), wants to or frequently does change tasks, leaves most tasks uncompleted.

6. *Rate of performance.* Is excessively slow in performing a task, accomplishes little in comparison to others, spends considerable time on task-oriented but nonproductive activity.

7. *Ability to follow oral, demonstrated, pictorial, and written directions.* Not able to follow directions given in one or more of the stated ways, does not bother to follow directions, repeatedly asks for oral directions when these have been given and/or when pictorial or written directions are available, does not return to directions to check whether the task is being done correctly.

8. *Use of tools and material.* Does not know how to use many tools and materials; uses tools and materials in ways that are markedly atypical; careless with tools, disregarding the safety of self and others; does not care for tools properly; is wasteful of material.

9. *Acceptable level of neatness.* Is excessively sloppy during task performance, end product appears slipshod or slovenly, does not clean up after completing a task.

10. *Attention to detail.* Excessive attention to detail, perfectionistic, is not certain what aspects of a task are more or less important; conversely there may be excessive disregard of details, hurries through tasks with little attention to details.

11. *Ability to solve problems that arise in performing tasks.* Gives up when problems are encountered or immediately asks for help, makes little attempt to solve problems, solves problems in an inappropriate manner.

12. *Ability to organize task in a logical manner.* Appears not to think about task prior to beginning; does not have all the items needed for task completion close at hand; does not consider what should be done first, second, and so forth; wastes considerable time because of lack of organization.

13. *Tolerates frustration.* Becomes upset when confronted with a problem, has difficulty in accepting delays, becomes agitated when he or she makes a mistake, has difficulty in accepting any kind of negative feedback, does not like to have to repeat steps or do something over again.

14. *Self-directed.* Follows other's choice of activity rather than selecting an activity independently; avoids beginning a new or different activity; when selecting an

activity, has difficulty carrying through on the decision made.

Evaluation of task skill is usually accomplished through data gathered from a general interview and the Survey of Task Skills. It should be remembered that task skills refer to all doing processes that involve the manipulation of the nonhuman environment. It does not refer only to the ability to engage in arts-and-craft activities.

Interpersonal Skills

1. *Ability to initiate, respond to, and sustain verbal interactions.* Ignores others, is shy to the point of having extreme difficulty in initiating engagement with another person, does not respond when others attempt to initiate a conversation, can not make small talk, sustains verbal interaction for only a short period of time, does not seem able to follow a conversation.

2. *Express ideas and feelings.* Does not express own ideas, expresses ideas as if they were not one's own, expresses ideas at a time or in a setting that is inappropriate, expresses ideas in a circumspect or tangential manner, overly controlled in the expression of feelings, overly expressive in the display of emotions, expression of emotion is atypical relative to the individual's cultural group. Can only express a limited range of emotions (i.e., negative or positive), has difficulty in asking for and/or accepting help.

3. *Aware of others' needs and feelings.* Acts as if others do not have needs and feelings or acts as if his or her own needs and feelings are always of paramount importance, is unaware of how behavior affects others, uses knowledge of others' needs and feelings for selfish ends or to injure others, shows disrespect for others' needs and feelings.

4. *Participates in cooperative and competitive situations.* Deals with situations where cooperation is required as if one were a free agent and did not need others to accomplish the task at hand, treats cooperative situations as if they were competitive, avoids competition, is excessively competitive, in a cooperative or competitive situation cannot follow the "rules" of the situation, has difficulty in dealing with being the winner or being the loser in a competitive situation.

5. *Compromise and negotiation.* Unable to see the merit of others' point of view, is adamant in seeing one's own point of view as good and right, perceives compromise as demeaning, is belligerent in negotiations, will not accept the assistance of a third party in a negotiation process, undermines any type of negotiations, views compromise and negotiation as a sign of weakness.

6. *Assertiveness.* Is unable to state own opinions comfortably, intimidated by those in an authority position or by individuals on which one is, to some extent, dependent, acts as if one's own self-interests were unimportant, makes unnecessary concessions, acts as if being assertive is unacceptable behavior, is overly assertive.

7. *Takes appropriate group roles.* Is not aware of the needs of a group relative to task accomplishment and the need satisfaction of members, does not take differential roles as required, avoids recognizing role change in others, responds in a stereotyped way in group situations, avoids interacting in groups.

Evaluation of interpersonal skills is typically accomplished through use of an interview, an evaluation group, and the Interpersonal Skill Survey.

Family Interaction

There are four major areas identified in this category. The first three—child, adolescent, and parent—are specific in that the behaviors necessary to fulfill these roles are fairly common in most cultures. "Child" and "adolescent" each consist of one continuum whereas "parent" consists of eight continuums. The fourth area, consisting of one continuum, is "general family interaction." It consists of such roles as courtship interactions, partner relationships, in-law relationships, the adult roles of being a daughter or son, adult sibling relationships, being a grandparent or grandchild, and so forth. It is described as "general" for two reasons. There is considerable variation in familial roles, given the individual's age, family, constellation, current life situation, and cultural group membership. Second, required behavior can best be conceptualized as the adequate elaboration of task and interpersonal skills to meet the demands and expectations of a particular familial role within a given family. The continuums, then, are as follows:

1. *Child.* Does not follow family expectations regarding acceptable behavior, does not obey parents on a regular basis, is not able to get along with siblings, does not participate in family activities, does not assist with household chores (as requested or as regular responsibility), is overcompliant, is too demanding and/or dependent, does not respect the rights of other family members.

2. *Adolescent.* In addition to those behaviors indicative of dysfunction outlined immediately above, the adolescent is not able to identify the needs of other family members, is unable to provide support for parents and siblings, does not assist in the care of younger siblings, spends an inordinate amount of time away from the home, asks for more than the family is able to afford

financially, does not assist family financially if needed, gives little attention to the dynamics of the family, acts within the community in such a way as to represent the family in a bad light, does not respect family values in the process of defining own values.

3. *Parenting.*

Child's physical needs: Does not provide adequate food, clothing, and shelter; does not secure periodic physical, dental, and eye examinations; does not maintain a safe home; does not secure adequate child-care assistance (baby sitter, child care centers, etc.).

Child's emotional needs: Is not able to demonstrate affection, is apparently unaware of child's emotional needs, avoids interaction with child, expresses strong negative feelings toward the child.

Play/recreational activities with child: Does not provide appropriate toys, is unconcerned about child's recreational activities, interacts in only a few stereotyped activities with child, does not see play/recreation as part of parental role.

Communication: Does not communicate in a forthright manner, gives double messages to child, denies child opportunity to discuss matters of concern, communication is not geared to the child's level of understanding and interests, unnecessarily limits expression of own thoughts and feelings.

Discipline: Does not set forth specific behavioral expectations, is not consistent in disciplining the child relative to expectations, does not maintain adequate balance between giving the child freedom and imposing limits, is not able to maintain self-control when child does not meet behavioral expectations, abuses child.

Education: Does not demonstrate concern for child's education, knows little or nothing about the child's academic performance or behavior in school, does not assist in or provide guidelines for the child's completion of homework assignments, has no contact with the school, does not encourage the child to attend school on a regular basis.

Responsibilities: Does not give the child appropriate self-care and household responsibilities, allows the child to be excessively dependent, gives the child responsibilities beyond his or her capacity, does not adequately reward the child for taking appropriate responsibilities.

Relinquish the nurturing relationship: Does not encourage adolescent's independence, rewards dependent behavior, makes demands on the adolescent for need satisfaction which are inappropriate to a parent-child relationship, uses guilt to maintain the relationship, demands independence of the adolescent before he/she is ready for such independence.

4. *General family interaction.* Is unable to communicate ideas and feelings in an appropriate manner; is not able to give emotional support; is not able to take on acceptable degree of responsibility for the relationship; is overly dependent and/or demanding; treats role partner in a demeaning fashion; is physically, sexually, or psychologically abusive; is not able to engage in activities of daily living that are appropriate to the relationship; is unable to engage in the mutual satisfaction of sexual needs. (All of the above should be viewed in terms of the various familial roles being considered.)

Appropriate evaluative tools relative to family interaction are a general interview and observation of family members together.

Activities of Daily Living

A list of the various activities of daily living is provided in the Activities of Daily Living Survey, Chapter 16. The reader is referred back to that Chapter for a description of this area and suggested evaluation procedures.

School

1. *Class attendance.* Frequently does not go to school, does not attend all classes, is late for classes and/or leaves class early.

2. *Classroom behavior.* Does not pay attention, disturbs other pupils, does not do assignments in class, does not take notes, does not participate in class discussions.

3. *Relationship with teachers.* Does not do what the teacher asks, ignores or is insolent to teachers, does not ask for guidelines or assistance when needed, is overly dependent on teachers, only manages to get along with certain teachers, cannot adapt to the style of some teachers.

4. *Relationship with classmates.* States that he or she has no friends in school, is excessively shy with classmates, is a loner, does not spend time with classmates between classes or at lunch time, teases or bullies classmates, frequently gets into fights, acts as if superior to other classmates, is not liked by classmates.

5. *Academic performance.* Grades are below what one would expect given the individual's apparent abilities, grades are markedly uneven across subjects and/or grading periods, does well in only those subjects that he or she likes, does not seem to put forth much effort, blames poor academic performance on others.

6. *Preparation for classes.* Does homework infrequently, homework is done without sufficient attention

to detail, homework is not turned in on time, needs excessive assistance from family members in doing assignments or in organizing time so that homework is completed, has difficulty with particular kinds of homework assignments.

7. *Participation in academic evaluations.* Does not study adequately for tests, hurries through examinations without giving appropriate attention to each item, becomes excessively anxious prior to or during tests, is overly preoccupied with grades.

Work

1. *Age-appropriate.* Concerns and interests in the work world are not age appropriate (see Chapter 5 for more specific behaviors indicative of function in this area).

2. *Attendance.* Attendance at work is irregular, frequently late to work, leaves work early, has difficulty tolerating a full day of work.

3. *Knowledge and interests regarding work.* Does not know what kind of job is appropriate given his or her assets and limitations, does not know what kind of work he or she would like, applies for inappropriate jobs.

4. *Find work.* Does not know how to look for a job, does not know how to use community resources to find work, does not know how to apply for a job, unable to fill out application forms, does not know how to participate in an interview.

5. *General attitude.* Does not feel the role of being a worker is an important social role, does not see self as a worker, is happier when not working, makes little effort to find a job if unemployed, can only take the worker role in a deviant subculture.

6. *Performance.* Manifests fear or anxiety as a response to the demand to be productive, acts impulsively, is apathetic and/or withdrawn, does not organize tasks relative to priority, does not work at increased speeds when required, cannot tolerate interruptions, does not easily return to work after interruptions, does not plan work periods so that required amount of work is accomplished, avoids responsibility, does not complete assigned tasks in an acceptable manner, completes assigned tasks late.

7. *Take direction from work supervisor.* Acts in a hostile or aggressive manner when assigned work, does not follow directions given, is overly dependent on supervisor, provokes supervisor to the point of anger, unable to accept constructive criticism.

8. *Relationship to co-workers.* Is overly dependent, does not give assistance when requested, is unable to carry on a casual conversation with co-workers, responds to co-workers in a belligerent manner, makes derogatory remarks to co-workers, avoids co-workers during breaks and lunch hour, acts in such a way as to make co-workers feel uncomfortable.

9. *Response to norms of the work setting.* Does not dress appropriately, selects inappropriate topics of conversation, pace of work is markedly different from other workers, acts as if the work setting is designed to satisfy needs that are more appropriately satisfied in other settings, does not conform to the rules of the setting, cannot differentiate between the formal and informal structure.

Evaluative tools appropriate for assessment in the area of school and work are outlined in Chapter 16.

Play/Leisure/Recreation

1. *Age-appropriate play.* This continuum is particular to children and is concerned with the extent to which the child engages in play activities that are typical of his or her age. The evaluative procedures outlined in Chapter 16 can be used for assessment. Determining function or dysfunction in this area is based on the description of play activities for various age groups in Chapter 5.

2. *Leisure/recreation.* Minimal engagement in leisure/recreational activities, little variety in leisure/recreational activities, complains of boredom, states that leisure activities are not satisfying, leisure/recreational activities are not within the bounds considered acceptable by one's cultural group, activities are potentially self-destructive.

3. *Friendships.* States that he or she has no friends, does not know how to go about establishing friend relationships, spends little if any time with other people outside of the context of work or family interactions, states that there is no one he or she can talk to, most friendships seem to be casual in nature.

Evaluative tools for assessment in this area are outlined in Chapter 16.

Temporal Adaptation

1. *Temporal disorientation.* Disoriented relative to time, no discernible organization relative to time, needs direct guidance in knowing when to engage in basic activities of daily living.

2. *Organization.* Does not appear to have sufficient time and organizational ability to participate in all roles adequately, inadequate balance between roles, insufficient sleep, not able to organize tasks within a role so that a reasonable amount of tasks are accomplished, unable to establish priorities, does not have established routines, too much free time, use of time and routines is not satisfying to the self and acceptable to significant

others, when necessary cannot accommodate routines to other.

Evaluation of temporal adaptation is accomplished through a general interview and the Activity Configuration as outlined in Chapter 16.

POSTULATES REGARDING CHANGE

There are several general postulates regarding change in this frame of reference. Specific postulates are provided for each of the continuums. The following are *general postulates*.

- Long-term goals are set based on the client's expected environment.
- The sequence of the change process is generally task skills, interpersonal skills, social roles beginning with activities of daily living, and temporal adaptation.
- The sequence, however, need not be rigidly adhered to and is often best determined by the client.
- Task and interpersonal skills can be taught separately initially or they can be taught within the context of the learning of social roles.
- An adequate repertoire of behavior is acquired through (a) Activities that elicit, require, and permit the relevant behavior; (b) activities that are interesting to the client and allow for exploration and movement toward mastery; (c) activities that include socializing agents in particular role partners and role models; and finally, (d) through the selected application of the principles of learning.
- If intrapsychic content is shared by the client, it is accepted matter of factly by the therapist in conjunction with providing some reality testing (Remember that... "emphasis is on designing conditions [activities] which will change the behavior and thus alleviate the problem rather than delving into intrapsychic reasons for the problem.")
- The therapist must know very specifically what kind of behavior he wishes to promote or enhance. (This postulate, in conjunction with the other general and specific postulates, provides the basis for activity analysis and synthesis.)

Task Skills

As a general rule, if a client's task skills and interpersonal skills are both severly limited, it is best to teach beginning task skills in a one-to-one relationship with the therapist.

1. *Willingness to Engage in Doing Tasks.* Clients who have difficulty in doing simple tasks need support and encouragement. Frequently the therapist must spend considerable time establishing a relationship of trust between him- or herself and the client. The client may feel that other people do not understand how difficult it is for he or she to do anything that requires overt, self-initiated action. Learning is enhanced if the initial tasks are mutually shared by the client and therapist together. Later the therapist might introduce tasks in which the client does one part independently while the therapist does another part. Finally, the client is encouraged to do simple tasks alone. For clients who avoid participating in tasks because of fear of being judged, the change process is initiated with tasks where there are few measurable standards with graded movement to tasks that require self-judgment to tasks that can be judged by some measurable external standard.

2. *Adequate Posture for Task.* The therapist demonstrates and if necessary helps the client to take appropriate postures for various tasks. If the client is unable to take an adequate posture because of physical limitations, the therapist helps the client take the best possible position and/or makes adaptions in the activity. Considerable reinforcement for adequate posture is often necessary.

3. *Physical strength and endurance.* The therapist grades activities relative to strength required and length of time of involvement in activities. Initially, frequent rest periods are scheduled with these diminishing over time.

4. *Gross- and fine-motor coordination.* The therapist grades activities relative to the need for gross and fine-motor movements. If the client has difficulty in both areas, gross coordination is given attention first.

5. *Interest in tasks.* To help a client increase attention span, the therapist and client decide how long the client will work without interruption. This may be a very short period of time initially. Just being able to engage in a task for a limited period of time may be sufficiently reinforcing or the therapist may have to provide some additional reinforcement. The length of work periods is slowly increased at a rate that is comfortable for the client. Another method the therapist may use is to pay no attention to the client when the client is not engaging in an appropriate activity. The therapist gives the client attention and approval only when the client is engaging in appropriate task-oriented behavior.

The therapist can help clients who never seem to be able to finish a task by insisting they finish each task they start. Sometimes clients do not complete projects because they select ones that take a very long time to complete, or ones that are too complex or too repetitive for them. Thus, in the beginning of the change process, the client is helped to choose a task that is relatively short-term, fairly easy to do, and nonrepetitive. Once a task is chosen, the client is not permitted to select another task until the first task is finished. Initially, the client may need help in completing a task; if so, he or she is given assistance. However, it is made clear that such assistance is only temporary; the client will, at some point, be expected to finish tasks by him- or herself. As the change process progresses, the client is encouraged to select tasks that take an increasingly longer time to complete and are increasingly more complex.

6. *Rate of performance.* When a client works too slowly, a short time limit is set in the initial stages of the change process. This may be as little as 3 minutes. The client is asked to complete a part of the task that takes a specified period of time to do when it is done at a normal rate. If he or she finishes the assigned task in the specified time, some reward is given. If the client does not finish the task, a shorter time period is set. The client is allowed to rest for a few minutes and then is asked to work for the specified time again, and so on until the task is finished. The time periods are slowly increased in length. Activities should be short-term, allowing the client to complete an activity in one session. This helps the client to experience a sense of accomplishment. The client is never allowed to work on a task at her usual slow rate. Doing so may reinforce slowness. Simple tasks are usually best during the first stages of the change process, so that the client does not get delayed by having to figure out what to do.

7. *Ability to follow oral, demonstrated, pictorial, and written directions.* Clients who have difficulty following directions may not be able to follow one type of instruction. A type of direction which the client is able to follow is then paired with a type that causes difficulty. The type of direction that had been previously mastered is then slowly decreased. For example, a client may only understand how to do a task if shown how; verbal directions are not sufficient. The change process would begin with the therapist telling the client how to do the activity and demonstrating how to do it at the same time. Slowly the therapist decreases the demonstrated part of the instructions, eventually only giving verbal directions. On the other hand, some clients are only able to follow one-step instructions. When that is the case, the change process begins at that level. The therapist slowly increases the number of steps given with directions one at a time.

Some clients do not bother to read instructions. Or they read the instructions once and then go ahead with the project, never returning to the instructions to check if they are doing the project correctly. Such clients need to receive adequate reinforcement for reading instructions and periodically comparing what they are doing with the instructions.

Other clients repeatedly ask for verbal or demonstrated instructions to be given. This is often more of a way of getting attention than of actually forgetting what to do. If this is the case, it may be helpful for the therapist or another client to stay with the client after he or she has been given the directions. Time spent with the client is slowly decreased until the client is able to work alone for a reasonable period of time. It is also important that the client's need for attention be satisfied in many other kinds of ways; not just when, supposedly, unclear about the directions.

8. *Use of tools and materials.* When a client simply does not know how to use various tools and materials, he or she is given adequate instruction. Teaching should take place within the context of an activity rather than through repetition with no other purpose than learning to use a tool or material. Only one or two tools or materials that the client does not know how to use should be introduced in each new activity. The other aspects of the task should be familiar to the client.

In helping a client to use tools and materials in an appropriate manner, the therapist gives adequate instruction. After that the therapist stops the client each time he or she does something that is, for example, wasteful or unsafe. The therapist reminds the client of the "right" way and insists that he or she do it in that way. Positive reinforcement is given after the correction has been made. Positive reinforcement and feedback are also given while the client is using tools and materials in an appropriate manner. If the therapist gives attention to the client only when he or she is doing something wrong, the client may develop the habit of making mistakes just to receive attention.

9. *Acceptable level of neatness.* Clients who have difficulty creating a neat end product can be helped by initially involving them in tasks that require little neatness and by slowly introducing them to tasks that require increasing neatness. The client is encouraged to work in a tidy manner and is instructed in how to do so. When a sloppy end product can be changed to make it look neater, the client is urged to make these changes. When a client does not seem to have any idea what is or is not neatly done, the therapist sets standards, and then gives the client feedback about whether or not he or she has met the standards.

For a client who has difficulty cleaning up after a task, the therapist states the expectations clearly and may also find it useful to use shaping. The therapist initially helps the client to pick up and reinforces any attempts the client makes at cleaning up. Approximations of the desired behavior are reinforced. The therapist slowly decreases participation in cleaning up as the client is more able to take on responsibility. The therapist helps clients learn to do tasks in such a way that cleaning up is easier. Also, before the client starts a task, the therapist encourages the client to think about ways of doing the task that will make cleaning up less of a chore.

10. *Attention to detail.* Clients who give excessive attention to detail need to be encouraged to be a little less neat, to leave something undone or undone for the time being. The client is likely to need a considerable amount of reinforcement and reassurance that nothing horrible is going to happen if something is not done perfectly.

Clients who do not give sufficient attention to detail essentially need the opposite approach. Details they miss should be pointed out. Positive reinforcement is given when the client goes back and corrects an error and when the client does a task in which the majority of the details are taken into consideration.

11. *Ability to solve problems that arise in performing tasks.* For clients who have difficulty problem solving, the learning situation is designed so that they move slowly from tasks that usually present very few problems to tasks that require a fair amount of problem solving. In addition to grading tasks, the therapist encourages the client to reread the instruction or to go to some other source for possible solutions. When a client is afraid to try something he or she has never done before, the client is encouraged to engage in experimental efforts that are outside the context of the task. Clients are helped to study a problem, to look closely at what is involved, to identify specifically what the problem is, to think of various courses of action to take, and to determine the consequences of various ways of solving a problem. When the therapist must solve a problem for a client, the therapist explains how and why he or she arrived at a particular solution.

12. *Ability to organize task in a logical manner.* Clients who have difficulty in this area are helped to think about a task before it is begun. They are encouraged to consider the amount of time that will be needed, to locate all the items they will need for task completion, and to consider what should be done first, second, and so on. Activities are presented in a graded manner relative to the degree of organization required.

13. *Tolerates frustration.* It is important that the therapist be aware of what kinds of situations frustrate the client. With this knowledge, the therapist is able to grade activities so that initially the client is presented with minimal sources of frustration. Gradually the client is introduced to activities that are potentially more and more frustrating. The client is given suggestions about alternative and more adaptive ways of dealing with frustrating situations. Positive reinforcement is given when the client deals adequately with a potentially frustrating situation.

14. *Self-directed.* When a client has difficulty in this area, the therapist reinforces the client's ability to engage in new or different tasks. The therapist helps the client define the task and the necessary steps involved. A commitment to attempt the task is requested from the client. The client is encouraged to take one step at a time rather than rush into a complex project. Initial self-directed tasks should be well within the client's capacity to master. Considerable positive reinforcement is given for each part of a new task completed. Such reinforcement is diminished as the client receives positive reinforcement from a sense of being self-directed.

Interpersonal Skills

There are a few general postulates regarding change for the continuums in this category:

1. The teaching of interpersonal skills is facilitated by using thematic and topical groups which focus on the development of appropriate interpersonal behavior.

2. Learning is usually initiated in thematic groups with topical groups being used later in the change process. The need for practicing interpersonal skills within the context of the community cannot be over emphasized. Prescribed interactions with others outside the context of the group (within the treatment facility or in the community) are often very useful.

3. The activities used as a vehicle for learning should be such that they can reasonably be shared by the entire group or at least by several group members.

4. With some exceptions (which shall be mentioned later), it is best to use activities that are structured with a concrete end product. Such activities tend to elicit desired behavior and facilitate the organization of behavior into useful patterns. They also provide a gauge for measuring progress of group members.

5. Regardless of what particular interpersonal skill the therapist is attempting to develop, he or she designs the learning situation so that the client (a) is both aware of appropriate behavior and helped to engage in appropriate behavior and (b) receives reinforcement of or feedback about his or her behavior, or both. The therapist tells the client what behavior is expected before entering the group and periodically reminds group members what is and is not appropriate behavior in the group.

6. There are several things a therapist can do to elicit desired behavior so that it can be reinforced. Some of

the methods are the following: (a) Simply wait for the approximation of a desirable behavior and then reinforce that behavior selectively. This is the process of shaping. (b) Encourage the client to imitate another group member who is functioning fairly well in the group. (c) Suggest to the client that he or she try to act in a particular way, giving ideas about what the client might say and do. (d) Point out ways of acting that are ineffective or inappropriate and encourage the client to act in a different manner without any specific suggestion being given. (e) Encourage trial-and-error interactions, with the client receiving feedback about the appropriateness of experimental behavior. (f) Have the group pause periodically in their activity to examine what behavior has been useful to the group and to the individual and what behavior has been harmful or of minimal use to the group and the individual. This process both reinforces the learning of appropriate behavior and gives group members clues as to the kinds of behavior they might try. A discussion of this kind is kept as nonpersonal as possible. Group members are not singled out and told they did something right or wrong. Although using immediate examples of what is occurring in the group, the discussion is oriented to talking about what kind of behavior is useful and what is not. (g) Organize role-playing experiences. These may center around an incident that has recently occurred in the group or on a general problem area that several of the group members have in common.

7. The development of interpersonal skills is enhanced by group members providing reinforcement and feedback to each other. This can be facilitated by the therapist assisting group members not only to understand what behaviors are to be learned but also to learn to give and withhold reinforcement and to provide feedback.

Specific postulates regarding change for interpersonal skills are as follows:

1. *Ability to initiate, respond to, and sustain verbal interactions*. The therapist initially reinforces nonverbal responses but diminishes such reinforcement over time, with the major reinforcement being given to verbal behavior. At the beginning any kind of verbal response is reinforced even if it is not particularly appropriate; differential reinforcement is then given for more appropriate verbal behavior. Activities requiring little verbal interaction may be used at the beginning of the change process with gradation toward activities that require more verbal interaction. If at all possible, clients with difficulties in this area should be placed in groups where some group members have at least partially mastered this skill. This provides an opportunity for adequate role models.

2. *Express ideas and feelings*. For clients who are restricted in the expression of ideas and feelings, the therapist urges the client to say what he or she is thinking and to act out how he or she feels. The client usually needs considerable support to be able to do this. The process of shaping may be of assistance. Any expression of ideas and feelings is initially reinforced. Differential reinforcement is given later in the change process in regard to more adequate or appropriate expression. Clients are encouraged to find various ways of expressing their emotions in the protective circumstances of activity groups, in casual interactions in the treatment center, and in the community. Adequate feedback must be given to the client.

Staff members often serve as the primary models for imitation in this area. Thus it is important for staff members to be open in their expression of both positive and negative ideas and feelings. Affection for other staff members should be freely demonstrated and disagreements openly discussed.

Another approach to teaching this skill is to use activities that allow for and encourage the expression of ideas and feelings. Such activities are usually fairly unstructured and have no significant end product. It is sometimes easier for clients to recognize ideas and feelings when these are manifested in the doing process. The format for this type of group usually alternates between doing an activity and talking about the ideas and feelings that were aroused by the activity. It is important to remember that this process is not the exploration of ideas and feelings as was discussed in reconciliation of universal issues. Rather it is an opportunity for the client to learn to express ideas and feelings in an open and appropriate manner.

3. *Aware of others' needs and feelings*. Individuals with difficulty in this area frequently have little if any idea how their behavior affects other people. Such a deficit is primarily altered by massive amounts of feedback. The client is assisted in identifying what he or she is doing and the effect of that behavior on others. The client is helped to become "self-consious" about behavior—to know essentially, "What am I doing now?" The client is assisted in learning how to study the effects of actions. Another problem individuals have in this area is deficits in understanding rights and responsibilities relative to interpersonal relations. These should be made explicit by the therapist and, if possible, other group members. Respect for the rights of others is reinforced. The same is true for taking basic responsibilities such as sharing and providing assistance.

4. *Participation in cooperative and competitive situations.* Initially the therapist selects activities requiring minimal cooperation and competition. These may be fairly individualized activities in the context of a group. Activities are then graded so that increasingly more cooperative and/or competitive behavior is necessary. What is required for a cooperative venture is made very clear. After the first stages of the change process, it is recommended that the activity be designed so that success of the activity is dependent on adequate cooperation of those involved. Regarding competition, clients often need assistance in learning how to win and lose in a "graceful" manner. Appropriate behavior as a winner or loser and toward a winner or loser is emphasized and reinforced. This is done with full acceptance of the feelings of the involved individuals.

5. *Compromise and negotiation.* Group members selecting and planning activities together frequently provide the necessary stimuli for facilitating the development of this skill. Initially the therapist may need to provide assistance in helping clients understand the decision-making process. The client's interest in the decision to be made is all important. If the client has no interest, then he or she is not likely to participate in the learning of this skill. The reinforcement of appropriate compromise and negotiation behavior should be emphasized. Behaviors, for example, such as yielding one's position for the wrong reason or browbeating others into accepting one's ideas are not reinforced.

6. *Assertiveness.* Initially this skill can perhaps best be learned within the context of role playing situations. Such situations should be designed to allow the client to experiment with being assertive in a variety of interpersonal interactions which are similar to the interactions the client is likely to encounter in the expected environment. Role playing is graded so that the initial situations require less assertive behavior than those that follow. Planning assertive actions as a strategy for resolving a problem should be emphasized as well as a directly assertive confrontation. As a strategy for problem resolution, assertiveness is best learned within the context of a concurrent topical group.

7. *Takes appropriate group roles.* The teaching of this interpersonal skill is very similar to that described for the development of "mature group interaction skill" as outlined in recapitulation of ontogenesis. The only difference in teaching this skill as a part of an acquisitional frame of reference is in the grading of activities. Initial activities are designed so that only a few instrumental group membership roles are required, with the therapist taking the majority of the expressive roles. Gradation of the activity is along the dimensions of more instrumental roles being required and group members being assisted in taking on an increasing number of expressive roles.

Family Interaction

In dealing with problems in family interaction, the cultural background of the individual must be taken into consideration. This is, of course, true for all aspects of intervention, but it is particularly essential in this area. In addition, the dynamics of the family must be considered. When dealing with problems in family interaction, the capacities and limitations, interests and orientation of role partners must also be given considerable attention. Although, on occasion, one is only able to deal with disturbances in familial interaction by assisting the individual in isolation, it is far better to help all affected role partners.

There are three major approaches to dealing with deficits in family interaction. These approaches are not mutually exclusive but rather often are and should be used in conjunction one with the other. The first approach is individual centered and involves helping the individual develop the skill necessary for adequate family interaction within the context of nonfamilial situations. These situations are usually a one-to-one relationship with the therapist and/or involvement in a thematic group. Subsequent to the development of some basic skills necessary for family interaction, the individual, through the use of a concurrent topical group, begins to make use of these skills within the family constellation. The topical group provides the necessary support, opportunity for problem solving, and reinforcement that is needed for altering participation in the family constellation.

The second approach, role-partner centered, involves assisting role partners in altering their behavior in such a way that the "client" is able to engage more effectively in expected roles. It may involve helping the role partner give appropriate reinforcement for adequate role performance on the part of the client. On the other hand, it may involve helping the role partner alter behavior so that the client, given his or her present limitations, is able to carry out a role in a way that is satisfying to both partners. An example of the former would be assisting a parent to adequately discipline a child. An example of the latter would be helping children and husband take on more household tasks so that a woman who is working will have more time to fulfill her role as a mother and wife.

Third, the family-centered approach involves helping concerned family members engage in mutual problem solving relative to their difficulties in interaction. This is accomplished initially within a thematic group made up of the involved members of one family. Activities are selected to elicit interactional patterns that appear detrimental to comfortable participation in family roles. The family is assisted in identifying these patterns and the situations that provoke them. Alternative ways of dealing with these situations are identified by family members. Activities are then selected to help the family experiment with and practice new patterns of behavior. This type of a thematic group is often used in conjunction with or followed by participation in a concurrent topical group through which family members have an opportunity to try out their new skills in the reality of the home environment.

With these three approaches as background information, the following postulates regarding change relative to family interaction are suggested:

Child

A child whose family interaction role is deficient is probably best assisted through the use of an individual-centered and a role-partner centered approach. Regarding an individual-centered approach, the child is most likely to need assistance in controlling behavior and in accepting an appropriate degree of discipline. Second, the child is likely to need help in acquiring skill in sharing the attention of an adult with other family members. In dealing with the first problem area, the change process is often initiated in a dyadic relationship with the therapist. Play is used as the vehicle for change. In the first stages of the change process, the child, within broad limits, is allowed to engage in any kind of play that he or she wishes. In this atmosphere, the therapist begins to make graded demands on the child very slowly for more acceptable ways of interaction in the play environment. Some feedback may be given but differential positive reinforcement is really the key. The change process continues in this way until the child has demonstrated some capacity to respond to the external controls provided by the therapist.

The next phase of the change process involves the child's participation in a small thematic group consisting of not more than three or four children. Although other areas may be of concern in this group, such as interpersonal skills or task skills, emphasis is also given to assisting the child in sharing the attention of the therapist with other group members. Positive reinforcement is given for waiting one's turn for attention, assisting others, not making excessive demands, and so forth. The therapist continues to help the child to become somewhat independent in controlling his or her own behavior.

In the interim while the child is being assisted in developing more appropriate familial role behavior, the therapist assists the parents in fulfilling their role in a more effective manner. This is discussed shortly in the section on parenting.

Adolescents

Depending on the severity of the difficulty, the change process relative to adolescents is individually centered, family centered, or both. Inpatient or some kind of group home is frequently the best setting for change for the individual who has severe difficulty in managing the adolescent role. The focus of intervention is on helping the adolescent to develop self-discipline, the capacity to take responsibility, and the ability to share with others. This is best accomplished through the daily interactions of people working and playing together. Organizationally this frequently involves interaction in a variety of thematic groups throughout the day and perhaps evening. The groups, and the entire setting, are relatively highly structured with explicit expectations and the consequence of not meeting expectations known. Consistent and immediate feedback and reinforcement are essential. As the individual's repertoire of appropriate role behavior increases, anticipatory and concurrent topical groups are used to assist the adolescent in the transition back into the home. Focus is then on the specific problems the adolescent is having with family. The group serves as a source of support, assists in problem solving, and provides reinforcement.

For adolescents with less severe problems in role behavior, a family-oriented change process is often the most appropriate approach.

Parenting

A family-centered orientation may be used to assist individuals in their role of being a parent. This is particularly true in helping parents with the problems encountered in nurturing a handicapped child. In this case, several parents and children may participate in the group together. Play and recreational activities are used as the vehicle for intervention as well as for teaching some skills.

More typically, individuals are assisted in the role of being a parent through an individual centered approach in the context of a concurrent topical group. The group, made up of parents, is ideally led by a therapist who has had some experience in being a parent. In general, the group is designed to provide some information about the role of being a parent. This is usually done within the context of discussion and problem solving rather than lecture format. However, on occasion a guest speaker may be invited, such as a nutritionist or a parole officer, to discuss a particular topic. Group members are encouraged to share their feelings and anxieties about child rearing. Stereotypes of the "good parent" are avoided, for example, the myth that all mothers immediately love their child at birth or that a good parent is always consistent. It is emphasized that occasional feelings such as hostility, anger, disappointment, of being overwhelmed by the job, or resentment that a child is interfering with one's life, are normal reactions and not a sign of improper parenting. The use of community-based resources and support systems is encouraged. The major focus of the group is on problem solving relative to child rearing and development of a more adequate repertoire of role behavior. This is accomplished through discussion, prescribed activities, practice in altering less than satisfying parent-child interactions, and adequate feedback and reinforcement.

With these general remarks, postulates regarding change relative to each of continuums related to parenting are outlined below:

Care for child's physical needs. Difficulty in this area may be due to simple lack of knowledge—the client does not know how to physically care for the child. In this case, the therapist tells the client what needs to be done and explains or demonstrates how it should be done. At first the client may need direct assistance from the therapist or some other caretaker. On the other hand, the client may be able to manage alone through explicit instructions and considerable amount of positive reinforcement.

At other times difficulty in this area may be due to inadequate financial resources. The therapist, in this situation, helps the client in learning how to locate financial assistance. As above, initially forthright assistance may be necessary, or direction and reinforcement may be all that is needed. The therapist's knowledge of community resources is an important element in assisting a client in this area.

Care for a child's emotional needs. Difficulty in this area is sometimes due to a parent being overburdened by the demands of child rearing and other social roles. This is essentially a problem in temporal adaptation and should be dealt with as such. When temporal adaptation difficulties are under some degree of control, the client is assisted, initially, in identifying one need that the child might have at the moment and figuring out a behavioral interaction that might satisfy that need. The client is encouraged to initiate that interaction and is given positive feedback for doing so. This process is continued slowly, with the therapist encouraging increasingly greater amounts of emotional interaction with the child. Reinforcement for this continued behavior is most likely to come from the child's positive response to the parent and greater comfort on the part of the parent.

Play/recreational activities with child. Some parents have difficulty doing things with their children. They seem to have lost the ability to play. Often they themselves engage in few recreational activities. One way of assisting parents in this area is to encourage them to engage in play or recreational activities with their child for at least a few minutes every day or at least several times a week. What they do is unimportant and by no means should it be elaborate. The time spent in play is gradually increased until it is compatible with the child's age and the other responsibilities of the parent. For parents who have little idea of appropriate play or recreational activities, suggestions of activities are given. It is important that these activities are related to the interests of the parent. A parent is much more likely to engage in play or recreational activities if they are enjoyable to the parent. The child's interest is also, of course, taken into account. However, the enjoyment of the parent is often infectious and this will stimulate the child's interest. This is particularly true for children who have not yet reached middle adolescence.

The use of a role model also facilitates development of this parenting skill. For example, a member of a parent group who has minimal difficulty in this area may be paired with a member who has considerable difficulty and children of approximately the same age. These group members are encouraged to plan activities that they can do together with their children. Through participation in these activities, the parent is able to get some idea about what a parent-child play/recreation relationship is like. Hopefully, the parent will receive reinforcement from both the pleasure of play itself and the pleasurable response of the child.

Communication. There are two problems in this area—inaccurate communication and insufficient communication. To help the client make communication more accurate, the therapist first helps the parent identify what it is that the parent would like to communicate. With clarification of the message, the parent is helped to identify the way—time, place, tone of voice, etc.—the message is best communicated. At this point the client is encouraged to engage in delivering the message. Initially, communication is centered around relatively non-emotional and simple issues. Over the course of the change process, the parent is assisted in communicating in a more spontaneous manner and in communicating about more emotional and complex issues. In addition, the parent is encouraged to attend closely to the communication of the child; what is he or she trying to say? This can be facilitated by looking closely at various circumspect interactions between the parent and child. These interactions are explored to identify what message the child was trying to communicate. This process helps the parent become more sensitive to the child's communication.

The other problem is insufficient communication; parent and child simply do not spend enough time talking to each other. Change in this area is facilitated by the parent being encouraged to set aside time each day to discuss something with the child that is meaningful to both of them. What is discussed is not particularly important; what is important is that it not be a stereotyped interaction. For example, asking what a child did in school when one is neither particularly interested nor actually listening is not communication. The parent is encouraged to introduce topics of discussion which are interesting to the parent, without, of course, ignoring the child's interests. Increased communication is encouraged and reinforced until it is at a level that is satisfying to both parent and child.

Discipline. At the beginning of the change process, the parent is assisted in identifying expectations for the child. These are evaluated relative to their being realistic for both child and parent. Concerning the child, for example, are the expectations age-appropriate and within the capacity of the child? Concerning the parent, are the expectations those with which the parent can be comfortable? Parents at times feel that their expectations are too high, that they should not impose so many limits. It is important to help a parent understand that a parent has a right to expect behavior that is comfortable for the parent. The parent-child relationship is enhanced when the child is behaving in a way that is acceptable to the parent. As a general rule, if the parent is comfortable with the way the child is behaving, then the child will be comfortable.

After identification of at least some expectations, the parent is encouraged to select one expectation and to help the child act within this expectation. Initially, the expectation should be relatively simple and realistically possible to attain in a short period of time. The importance of using positive reinforcement rather than punishment is emphasized as well as the clear communication of the expectation to the child. It is often helpful if the parent devises a specific plan to assist the child in meeting the expectation. The parent's initiation of the plan is reinforced by the therapist and other group members. Success or failure is discussed, possible solutions to encountered problems are identified; again implementation is encouraged. It is important for both therapist and parent to remember that the child be given sufficient time to modify behavior. This will inhibit discouragement on the part of the parent. In the course of the change process, increasingly more complex issues relative to discipline are addressed.

Education. Parents do not get involved in their children's education for any number of reasons; they feel educationally inadequate, are intimidated by the school system, do not want to hassle over homework, are overburdened by other responsibilities, and so forth. Here again, a graded approach is used. The parent is encouraged initially, for example, to attend a meeting of some sort at the child's school, preferably one that does not entail discussion of any particular problem the child may be having. Or the parent may be encouraged to participate in some small way in the child's homework, e.g., checking simple math problems, quizzing the child on spelling words, reading over an assignment, and the like. Getting the child to do homework is essentially a matter of discipline. Involvement in the child's education is encouraged until the child shows evidence that he or she is aware of the parent's concern and is able to provide some assistance in this area of his life.

Responsibilities. In regard to not giving the child sufficent self-care and household responsibilities, a graded approach is used. The parent is helped in identifying appropriate responsibilities and, initially, in selecting one that will be required of the child. The parent is given support and guidance by the therapist and other group members as the parent requires increasing responsibilities on the part of the child. One problem often encountered is that the parent has difficulty in giving up responsibilities. Assistance in this area needs to be provided. Essentially, it involves giving reinforcement to the parent for not doing something, to leave something undone. This aspect of the change process must be given particular attention when the child is slow to take on responsibilities.

In some family situations, the child is given so much responsibility for household tasks and care of younger children that the child does not have sufficient time for participation in other roles. There are times when this cannot be altered because of the present situation of the family. If this is realistically the case, the parent should be encouraged to give the child considerable support and recognition. Taking the child's essentially excessive responsibilities for granted is a further detriment to the child's development. In most situations, however, something can be done to alleviate the child's excessive responsibilities. It may entail considerable problem solving on the part of the parent in terms of how responsibilities may be reallocated. Other family members, for example, may need to be assisted in taking on added responsibility. There are many community resources that can be called on to assist a family. The parent may well need considerable assistance in engaging in the necessary problem solving and in the process of implementation.

Relinquish the nurturing relationship. The major problem here is most often difficulty in giving up a role or some aspects of a role. The primary way of dealing with this problem is to assist the individual in developing other interests and/or to invest additional time and energy in other roles, be they familial, work, or leisure activities. The key to success is often identification of the particular needs that the nurturing role fulfilled for the individual. In this way the client is better able to make some informed decisions about how to meet these needs through other activities. The therapist offers guidance in this process but in no way imposes his or her own ideas. Once the client has made a decision about the best course of action, he or she is most likely to need considerable support in carrying it out. It is very likely that a degree of inertia will have to be overcome as well as some fear. The individual may also need assistance in establishing a nonnurturing parent-child relationship. A parent group is probably not appropriate for the learning of this altered role relationship. Change processes designed to deal with "general family interaction" are likely to be more suitable.

General Family Interaction

As mentioned previously, this continuum is concerned with all familial roles other than those specified above. Concurrent typical groups, previously described as individual centered and family centered, are recommended for facilitating learning in the area of family interaction. In the use of an individual-centered group, it is best if group members are concerned, at least in general, with the same kinds of problems. The difficulties experienced by each group member should be as clearly specified as possible. From this base, group members are able to engage in mutual and independent problem solving. Support is given, new behavior identified as a possible means of solving a particular problem is encouraged, the effectiveness of the new behavior is assessed, other solutions and thus behavior may be tried. Feedback, reinforcement, and prescribed activities are used to facilitate learning. During this process, information about various familial roles is provided. This is done in a manner similar to that described in the discussion of the parental role.

Role playing is also a useful means of enhancing learning. Group members are given an opportunity to practice new behavior in a protected environment. Also, in thinking about and playing the role of an absent role partner, the client frequently gains a better perspective of the partner's needs and feelings. This in turn helps the client to determine what behavior is likely to be the most effective.

Family-centered groups are perhaps the most effective way of dealing with general family interaction. The major problem in initiating such groups is to elicit the cooperation of key family members and to find a time that is suitable for all involved. The process within the group is similar to that outlined throughout this section. The major problem a therapist is likely to have in leading a family-centered group is maintaining a position of neutrality. This is particularly true if the therapist has had a more long-term relationship with one member of the family than with the others. As difficult as it may at times be, the therapist should not get involved in family arguments, take sides, or become caught up in cultural biases about how family members should behave toward each other. The therapist's role is to help the family identify their problems in functioning, to remedy these difficulties, and to acquire more effective patterns of interaction. This is accomplished through designing and prescribing appropriate learning experiences.

The occupational therapist's role in assisting clients in the area of sexuality is fairly new and thus not well defined in the profession. It is, however, generally agreed that the occupational therapist should be concerned about this aspect of family interaction. Therapists have been most active in assisting those clients who are physically disabled to deal with the physical problems that may be an impediment to satisfying sexual interactions. This has been done primarily through providing information about potential problems and outlining various possible solutions for the client and his or her partner to consider. Perhaps even more importantly, therapists have emphasized the necessity of open discussion within the clinical setting itself and between partners. Therapists have acted as role models by bringing up issues that need to be discussed and by acting in a comfortable, relaxed manner during discussion of sex-related issues.

Occupational therapists in the area of psychiatry have been less involved in dealing with sexuality as one aspect of family interaction. Why this is so is unclear. The ill-effects of stress, anxiety, and depression on sexual interests and activity are well documented. There is really no reason, then, why occupational therapists cannot take sexual matters into consideration in the process of assisting clients in the area of family interaction.

Good communication between partners has been identified as the key to the establishment or reestablishment and maintenance of compatible sexual relationships. Communication, however, should not and really cannot be considered by relating it to one area of a relationship only. Isolating communication so that it is related to sexual matters only is not wise. Thus, the intervention process relative to sexual difficulties or potential difficulties should be focused on facilitating general communication between partners across a broad number of areas. It is, in fact, often best to help partners to first learn to communicate about nonsexual issues. With some basic skills in communication as part of their shared repertoire, communication about sexual matters comes almost naturally, or at least more easily.

It should be noted that sex counseling, per se, is not an appropriate role for the occupational therapist. There are others specifically educated to assist people in this area. Clients who need such services should be referred by the occupational therapist. There are also experts in the area of sexuality and the physically handicapped. If such people are available, they should be consulted and/or the occupational therapist should establish a collaborative relationship with them.

Activities of Daily Living

Intervention relative to activities of daily living begins with an activity the client feels is of particular importance to him or her at the present time. It begins with something the client really wants to learn to do. However, when the client is unable to say what activity of daily living he or she would like to learn, the change process is initiated with a simple activity or with an activity that will make life easier for the client or those who are significant to the client.

Some activities of daily living are taught in a one-to-one situation. This is done either because the tasks to be learned are personal in nature such as dressing, or because the problem area is fairly unique. In other words, only one or two clients in the treatment center may be having difficulty with a particular activity of daily living. However, when several clients have common problem areas, a thematic and/or topical group is used. Some examples of groups concerned with daily living activities are grooming groups, cooking groups, homemaking groups, community survival groups (how to look for an apartment, open a checking account, and so forth). Although activities of daily living are learned in the context of a group, it is important that the client eventually be able to carry out the activities independently.

Ideally, the learning of most daily living activities takes place in the expected environment of the client. If at all possible, they are learned through actual doing in a real situation. Doing is preferred to talking about how to do an activity of daily living. Where appropriate, activities of daily living are demonstrated prior to the client practicing the activity. Role playing is also often useful. At times initial learning may take place in the treatment center and be followed by practice in the community. Concurrent topical groups are particularly appropriate for assisting the client in making the transition from the clinical center to the home and community.

In preparing to teach activities of daily living, the therapist analyzes the total activity breaking it down into its various parts and determines the sequential steps of the activity. This is done both to help the therapist identify what the client must learn and to figure out the best way to teach the activity. Some tasks, for example, may be best taught through chaining whereas others may be more easily learned through successive approximations. The therapist must also be aware of the client's assets and limitations as these are often a major factor in deciding the best way to approach the teaching of particular daily living activities to a given client.

Logical ordering and simplicity are emphasized in teaching activities of daily living. Logical ordering refers to thinking a task through before beginning it, i.e., deciding what should be done first, what second, and so forth. Simplicity refers to doing tasks in the easiest and least time-consuming manner.

The teaching of daily living activities should be as personal as possible. Learning is closely related to the individual's own community and home situation. For example, rather than learning how to prepare a budget by making one up for a hypothetical family, the client prepares a budget for her own family. In learning about meal preparation, the client uses the kinds of foods she and her family like and usually eat.

At times the problem is not that the client does not know how to perform various daily living activities. He or she knows how, but does not engage in the activity with any degree of frequency. It is then necessary for the client, the therapist, and the group to be concerned with identifying the reason or problem, discovering its immediate source, discussing ways of solving the problem, trying various solutions, and if that does not work, trying something else. Support, encouragement, and advice are offered as needed. All activities of daily living are looked at within the context of the client's life situation. This is done so that in some way the environment or the individual's actions can be structured so that the individual receives positive reinforcement. Few activities of daily living are maintained for any period of time if they are not at least occasionally reinforced.

Activities of daily living may seem fairly simple and routine to the therapist. But for the client who is unable to perform many of them, it is often a difficult area to master, and a source of considerable anxiety. Thus the therapist must take care to break down an activity into its various parts and to be sure that the client has learned all aspects of the activity. Also, the therapist must remember that many activities of daily living take considerable practice before they become an integrated part of the person's repertoire of behavior.

School

Ideally, when there are difficulties in the area of school, these are dealt with in an academic setting. A large treatment center usually has a school program with specially trained teachers to help the students. Or the client may be in a community school. Such schools are variable in terms of the amount of extra assistance which they are able to provide for students with school-related problems.

When the client is involved in a regular school, the therapist may serve as a consultant to the client's teachers. In such a role, the therapist assists the teacher in developing a plan designed to alter the student's behavior so that it is more appropriate to a school situation. Once this is done, the therapist is available for discussion and problem solving with the teachers, with changes being made in the plan as needed. The plan is essentially designed so that the child is able to experience mastery and recognition in some areas in conjunction with modifications of unacceptable behavior through differential reinforcement.

In addition to the school-oriented program, the client may be involved in a thematic group designed to develop interpersonal relations. Such a group is structured so that the therapist is in an authority position similar to that of a teacher; the relationship between group members then being like that of classmates. Both individual and group activities are used as the vehicle for intervention. Within the context of these activities, the therapist, through the grading of activities, feedback, and reinforcement, helps the client develop the task skills and interpersonal behavior that are appropriate for the role of a student.

For students older than apporximately 12 years, a concurrent topical group concerned with school-related problems is often appropriate. In this type of group, interpersonal and task difficulties are identified. Group members are encouraged to figure out ways of dealing with the various problems and of initiating a plan of action. If the plan is unsuccessful, another one is developed and implemented. Appropriate support and reinforcement are provided by the therapist and other group members. It is frequently helpful if a group concerned with school-related issues is co-led by a teacher. If this is not feasible, the therapist may want to make arrangements to consult regularly with a teacher. Finally, this type of activity group is also useful when a client is in the process of making a transition from a special to a regular school program.

More information related to working with clients within the school system is provided in Chapters 29 and 30.

Work

Learning the role of a worker is best accomplished in a situation that is a reasonable simulation of the realistic demands of a work environment. The opportunity must exist for the client to experience the full range of interpersonal relationships, time demands, and basic tasks that will be encountered on the job. Change is brought about primarily through interaction in a work-like situation where there is appropriate grading relative to required behavior, feedback, and reinforcement.

For clients who have little if any experience with work, the ideal situation for intervention offers the client an opportunity to participate sequentially in a work group, a sheltered workshop, a hospital job or a specially selected community job, a topical group concerned with work, and to receive the help of a vocational counselor. Of course, a given client may not need all of these services to develop work habits and find a suitable job, and the sequence may not be appropriate for every client. Clients, for example, who have some sense of what it is to be a worker, may not need to start in a work group. Intervention may begin in a sheltered workshop or even in a topical group concerned with work.

The following discussion will be divided into the various types of situations that may be used to help a client take on the role of a worker.

Work Groups

A work group is a thematic activity group designed primarily to help clients understand what kind of behavior is expected in a work situation and to begin to develop basic work habits. A client is usually ready for a work group when he or she has the ability to engage in an individual task in the presence of others and possesses simple task skills. The activities used as the vehicle for learning should be relatively simple but with sufficient variety to engage the interest of group members. Some appropriate activities might be making small wooden toys or candles using an assembly-line format, reproducing and collating hospital forms or other printed matter, making the noon meal for the other clients involved in the program, or taking care of the patient library. The usual atmosphere of the group is work-oriented and business-like. Group members are expected to come on time, stay for the whole period the group meets (usually about 2 hr), complete assigned tasks whether or not they enjoy the particular task, dress appropriately, not discuss personal problems unrelated to work, and to enter into casual conversation with fellow workers but in such a way that it does not interfere with the task the group is to accomplish. All work-related behavior is positively reinforced.

The therapist essentially acts in the role of a foreman, assigning tasks and making judgments about the quality of work. It is the therapist's responsibility to see that all the tools and materials needed to carry out the activity are available. Group members do not participate in selecting and planning the activity because that is not the usual situation in a work setting. While the group is working, the therapist gives individual assistance when it is needed. He or she may help someone who is having trouble with part of the task or talk with a group member who is experiencing a personal difficulty. The work of the group is not interrupted if at all possible. Although somewhat out of context here, the idea that the "show must go on" is emphasized. The therapist, in addition to maintaining an appropriate environment, gives support, feedback, and reinforcement to the clients—and encourages all group members to do likewise.

The therapist, however, may not always be in the role of the foreman. At times this role may be rotated among the group members who are able to take such a responsibility. Each client-foreman will vary somewhat in his or her way of organizing the task, assigning jobs, and evaluating work. Thus, group members learn something about the need to adjust to different styles of supervision. Rotating the job of foreman also allows clients to experience what it is like to be in a supervisory capacity. From that position, they are often better able to understand why they are expected to behave in a certain way in a work situation. The therapist helps the client-supervisor organize and plan for each work session and gives advice on ways of dealing with problems that arise. As much as possible, the therapist stays in the background, allowing the client-supervisor to manage whatever problems arise. It should be noted that a client-supervisor is not appropriate in all work groups. This is particularly true when the work habits of group members are just beginning to be developed.

After each group meeting, or perhaps once a week, group members may meet with the therapist to talk about problems that have been encountered. Different ways of behaving may be discussed or suggested to one of the group members. Feedback and encouragement are given as well as reinforcement for positive changes in behavior.

With some modifications, a work group may also be used to assist adolescents and young adults to become more familiar with the requirements of the worker role. The major difference is that more attention is given to exploring various types of jobs and the relationship between skills and interests and possible types of employment. This is frequently accomplished through visits to various work settings where the group members have an opportunity to observe people doing different types of jobs. These trips out into the community are usually followed by discussions about what was observed and related to each group member's interests and skills.

Sheltered Workshops

When a client has acquired some very basic work habits and is able to function in a work group with a minimal number of personal difficulties, he or she is likely to be ready for a sheltered workshop program. A sheltered workshop may be part of a large treatment facility or organizationally separated from any treatment facility. Regardless of where it may be located, a sheltered workshop is usually fairly large, offers several different kinds of job experience, and usually pays clients for the work that they do. Some sheltered workshops are oriented to providing employment for people who cannot hold a job in a competitive market. Others are concerned only with helping clients develop work habits. And still other workshops are concerned with teaching specific work skills such as preparation for office work or jobs in a particular industry. In the two latter situations, the client's participation in the program is seen as temporary and transitional. Occupational therapists are involved primarily with sheltered workshop programs that offer employment for people who are unable to work in a competitive job market and those that are designed to help clients develop work habits. Although both are important, only the latter is discussed in this section.

Participation in a sheltered workshop program is quite different from being in a work group. There are many more people, the atmosphere is more strongly work-oriented, one is required to punch a time clock, there is a definite foreman or work supervisor, and, perhaps for the first time, the client may be paid for work. In helping the client make the transition from a work group to a sheltered workshop, the therapist tells the client what it is going to be like and what the behavioral expectations are. It is often helpful if the client and therapist visit the workshop together before the client becomes involved in the program. Movement into a sheltered workshop may require another period of evaluation and the completion of forms. The therapist gives whatever support and direct assistances the client needs during this period.

The occupational therapist may be involved in a sheltered workshop program in a number of ways, e.g., in evaluation, work supervision, or as part of the support team. Evaluation in a sheltered workshop is in many ways similar to that outlined in the previous section of this chapter. However, it is likely to be more detailed, with particular focus on task skills and various aptitudes and interests. There are a number of standardized tests that are often used. As part of the evaluation process, the therapist is also likely to be involved in placing the client in a particular job in the workshop. This is done in conjunction with the client and is based on the client's interests, current assets, and limitations.

The therapist, in the role of a supervisor or foreman, assigns tasks and gives adequate instruction as to how they should be accomplished. The therapist makes certain the client knows how to do the assigned task before leaving him or her to work independently. Increased emphasis is placed on accuracy, neatness, and doing the job at the rate that would be expected in competitive employment. The therapist deals only with those problems a foreman working in the wider community would be expected to handle. Another person in the sheltered workshop is usually assigned to help the client with difficulties that might be encountered on the job or in other areas of life. (This is the supportive role, which is described shortly.) These two areas are separated in order to help the client experience a relatively realistic work setting. When the therapist is overly supportive and willing to talk extensively about nonwork-related matters, the client may think that this is the way that a typical foreman acts. This does not mean that the therapist takes a disinterested, authoritarian role. The therapist indicates interest in the client as a person and a desire and willingness to help the client learn the role of a worker. There is a middle position here between the traditional, warm, empathetic role of a therapist and the strict, impersonal role of a job foreman. The therapist identifies problems, manipulates those conditions of work that will help the client, provides appropriate feedback and reinforcement; and does all of this while "acting" like a real foreman.

As a member of the support team, the therapist meets with clients, usually in groups, to discuss the clients' progress in the sheltered workshop. The purpose of these concurrent topical groups is to provide support and reassurance. Clients talk about problems they have encountered on the job and are encouraged to think about other ways they might have dealt with the situation. Group members may offer suggestions or advice. Clients also report on the effects of new behavior they have tried on the job. A client is helped to overcome problems in interpersonal relations by assisting in identifying the expectations of a work setting and how the client's behavior is contrary to those expectations. More acceptable ways of interacting are suggested to the client and he or she is urged to try out these suggestions. Support and reinforcement are provided by the therapist and other group members. As the client begins to act in a more appropriate manner, the client receives reinforcement for the behavior within the actual work setting rather than from an outside source. The need for outside support gradually decreases.

If at all possible, it is suggested that the therapist who acts as part of the support team or discussion group leader not be the client's foreman in the work setting. These two roles are very different. Thus it may be confusing for some clients to need to relate to the therapist in such dissimilar ways. It may also be difficult for the therapist.

Hospital Jobs and Specially Selected Community Jobs

When a client seems to be functioning well in a sheltered workshop, he or she may be ready to go out and look for a job. However, some clients may be hesitant to take this large step or feel, for one reason or another, that they are not ready for the move into the wider community. When possible, these clients are assigned to a hospital job or a specially selected community job. Clients may also be assigned to these jobs without any experience in a work group or sheltered workshop or directly from a work group experience. A hospital job is a part- or full-time work assignment in the institution. These jobs may involve working in the mail room, library, grounds maintenance department, coffee shop, and so forth. It should be noted that most states have strict laws regarding clients working in an institution. The therapist should be familiar with these laws and, of course, adhere to them. A specially selected community job is a part- or full-time work assignment in a local business. The client may, for example, work as a cashier, carwash attendant, or waitress.

The therapist who coordinates the hospital/community job program is responsible for finding suitable jobs. This involves contacting work supervisors in the hospital and employers in the community, explaining the purpose of the program and convincing the supervisor or employer to participate in the program. The therapist may have to help the individuals in determining how they can best make use of the services of the clients. Occasionally, supervisors and employers are somewhat fearful of working with clients—these fears and anxieties must be allayed. The work supervisor is urged to interact with a client as he or she usually does with any employee. The client is given the same responsibilities and assignments that would be given to anyone in that position. Conversely, the client is allowed the usual coffee breaks and the opportunity to work without excess supervision. The therapist keeps in close contact with the supervisor or employer. The success of a hospital/community job placement program is determined to a great extent by the relationship between the responsible therapist and the supervisors and employers.

With the therapist's assistance, the client selects a job from the various positions available at the time. The therapist usually accompanies the client to work the first day and introduces the client to the supervisor. It is the supervisor's responsibility to orient the client to the work setting and the job he or she will be doing and to introduce the client to her co-workers. While a client is in a job placement, the therapist may occasionally visit him or her on the job. This is done in an unobtrusive way so as not to single the client out from among co-workers. Clients in hospital/community job programs usually participate in a work discussion group similar to the type mentioned in relation to a sheltered workshop.

Hospital or community jobs allow the client to experience a real work situation. He or she is able to observe other workers and compare behavior to their way of working and interacting. The therapist responsible for finding such jobs has assured him- or herself that work-related behavior is rewarded in that work situation. Thus the client receives direct reinforcement for appropriate behavior on the job. When a client is able to handle a hospital or community job comfortably, he or she is usually ready to begin to be involved in competitive employment.

Beginning employment

Looking for a job and beginning to work often poses problems with which clients may need help. Some clients have little idea about what types of jobs they would like, or what types of jobs would be suitable for them. A vocational rehabilitation counselor can be of considerable help in this case. A counselor may give various tests to determine what types of occupations the client is best suited for, describe various types of jobs, and inform the client about different training programs. The counselor may give direct assistance in getting a job or may help the client locate a suitable employment agency.

A client may not know very much about a job or training program that has been suggested for consideration. Ideally, rather than following the suggestion blindly, the client is encouraged to get further information before making a decision. In addition to talking to the vocational counselor about the suggested type of work, the client is advised to seek information in the community. The client might, for example, observe for a period of time in an appropriate work setting or talk to people who are employed in the suggested occupation. The more information the client has, the better able he or she is to make a wise decision about future employment.

Many treatment centers have an anticipatory concurrent topical group that focuses on the problems of seeking employment and on the beginning phase of employment. This may be led by a vocational counselor, an occupational therapist, or by both. Some typical topics discussed are: How do you go about looking for a job? How does one conduct oneself at an interview? What do you say about a period of unemployment? Problems encountered on the job. How one deals with various job-related situations. The group members share their various experiences and give encouragement, feedback, and advice as needed. A client usually continues to participate in the topical group until he or she feels able to make it on his or her own in the role of a worker.

Play

To facilitate the integration and mastery of play skills, a planned and guided experience is often required. Initially, it is often necessary to begin intervention in a one-to-one situation of therapist and child. This may be due to the child's age or the child's inability to engage in play when other children are around. The play activities provided—toys, games, equipment, and materials—should be compatible with the child's developmental age. Variety is important to enhance the possibility of engaging the child's attention and interest. The only time this would not be appropriate is when the child is highly distractable. In such a case the environment should be more limited even to the point of having only one activity available if necessary. The environment also should be such that it taps the child's desire to explore. This is usually accomplished by creating a relatively permissive environment but with sufficient external controls that the child is comfortable.

The therapist frequently plays with the child. As a companion in play, the therapist serves as a role model, demonstrating possibilities and, if appropriate, making suggestions. At other times the child may prefer to play alone. The therapist's role in this case is one of giving support and approval when requested. The therapist may also serve as a resource person. The therapist above all must be finely tuned to the child's needs, moving in and out of the play of the child in a flexible manner. It is, of course, also important that the therapist make each session with the child a fun and enjoyable experience.

When a child has acquired some play skills, he or she is usually involved in a thematic group focused on play. This is typically a group made up of children who are of approximately the same age. It is usually relatively small, consisting of from four to six children. A group of older children, however, may be somewhat larger. A play group is particularly useful because the children provide mutual stimulation to each other in exploring the environment and in practicing play skills. The description of an appropriate environment and of the role of the therapist is similar to that described above, with the added element of a group situation. Individual and cooperative kinds of activities are usually introduced in the initial stages of the group, with more competitive activities being offerred later.

Another way that play skills are enhanced is through the use of prescribed activities given to parents. The therapist, for example, might suggest certain toys and games that are compatible with the child's developmental age, interests, and capacities. Individual play activities and activities that can be shared with parents and/or siblings are usually suggested. The therapist may advise the parents of appropriate community play groups that the child might join. Follow-up, support, and reinforcement are of vital importance if the prescribed activities are to be effective in altering dysfunctional play patterns.

In the above discussion, it should be noted that the change process is directed toward the development of age-appropriate play. Play is not being described as a tool to facilitate the development of other skills. It is true that play involves task skills and, in a group, interpersonal skills. And it may well be necessary to facilitate the acquisition of these skills in the process of helping children learn how to play. There is a difference in emphasis, however, depending on whether the therapist is teaching play skills as opposed to task and/or interpersonal skills. Perhaps the best way to describe the difference is that in facilitating the acquisition of play skills, the therapist only teaches those task and interpersonal skills that will enhance the child's capacity to play, and no more.

Leisure/Recreation

Leisure/recreational skills are usually developed within the context of thematic and topical groups. The two types of groups, indeed, often blend together. In the initial phases of a recreational group, the focus is frequently on helping participants identify their leisure time interests. This is sometimes accomplished by group members engaging in a variety of recreational activities together. After participation in each of the activities, the group members are helped to identify what they liked and disliked about the activity. Some of the questions raised might be: Was it enjoyable and what made it so? What needs were satisfied? What made the activity disappointing? Is this something one would like to do with other people or might it be enjoyed alone? With these types of questions the activity is broken down into some of its component parts. Clients thus begin to look at the elements of recreational activities rather than just viewing them as global entities. In so doing, clients are helped to identify the parts of recreational activities that they find enjoyable. With this knowledge, clients are in a far better position to select future recreational activities having several elements that they enjoy.

A recreational group also emphasizes the use of leisure time independent from the protectiveness of the group. Members encourage each other to plan evening and weekend recreational activities which they will do alone and with others. Encouragement and support are given to those members who are hesitant in trying something new or venturing out on their own. The outcome of the recreational pursuit is discussed as well as possible reasons for success or failure. This information is used in planning recreational activities for the immediate future. The process continues until the client begins to experience pleasure in the use of leisure hours.

Some clients have little awareness of the recreational/leisure time activities available in their community. Thus, members of a recreational group often assign themselves the task of investigating leisure time activities in the community. This may involve going to such places as a "Y," settlement house, church or temple, museums, and academic institutions to find out what kind of programs they have for members or the general public. This information is shared with group members and often posted for the benefit of other persons in the treatment facility. Group members give each other encouragement and support in engaging in these newly identified recreational activities. Any problems encountered are brought back to the group for discussion. Reinforcement is provided until the engagement in these new activities provides their own reinforcement.

Some clients have no recreational skills. They may be able to identify possible interests but do not have the rudimentary skills that would enable them to begin to enjoy these activities. In this case the therapist is involved in the direct teaching of activities usually considered recreational in nature. This may involve, for example, teaching the basics of softball, tennis, chess, woodworking, appreciation of literature, using a knitting machine, and the like. To teach a recreational activity effectively, the therapist identifies its component parts. In this way both client and therapist are aware of what needs to be learned. For example, in playing softball a person has to know how to throw, catch and bat a ball, and the rules of the game. One must know how to cooperate with teammates and engage in friendly competition with the other team. Moreover, the person must be able to locate and join a softball team or get together a group of people who want to play softball. When the client has learned the basic elements of a recreational activity, the therapist encourages involvement with others in the community who are interested in the particular activity. Whether or not the recreational activity is one that is usually done individually, the therapist tries to help the client locate other people in the community with similar interests. This provides both a resource for help with the activity and an opportunity to make friends.

The potential of community service as a satisfying way of spending leisure time should not be neglected. Emphasis is often placed on this area, particularly when members of a recreational group live in the same community. People from the community may be invited to talk before a group meeting about the activities in which they are involved. They are able to outline the needs of the community and to help clients become aware of ways in which they can contribute to the community. A recreational group may help members to engage in community service or there may be another group concerned with this aspect of leisure activities. Such a group is usually a concurrent topical group. The group as a whole may participate in a community service, but more typically group members are encouraged to join in a community service of their choice. The purpose of this group is to acquaint clients with possible ways of serving the community and to help them acquire the skills necessary for such participation. A new member in a topical group with this orientation is told about community service activities and is helped to decide what he or she is able to do and the kinds of activities he or she would probably enjoy. Often a client will join in a community service with another client for a period of time. The other client is able to provide support and give the client direct assistance in the situation. Later the client is encouraged to engage in a community activity independently. This gives the client the opportunity to learn how to become part of a community group and to participate independent of the help of another client. Group members discuss problems they have encountered in their community activity. As in other concurrent topical groups, they help each other develop more useful patterns of interaction.

Loss of the worker role because of retirement, unemployment, physical limitations, or some other alteration in life circumstances can be a traumatic experience. There is usually a marked increase in free time, with leisure/recreational activities becoming far more significant in the individual's daily life. Such an individual may need assistance in exploring a variety of activities that may be both satisfying and feasible. This is often accomplished through the use of a concurrent topical group. The focus of this group is quite similar to that described above. Group members engage in a variety of activities to determine which ones are need-satisfying. Each client with the support of the group is then encouraged to begin engaging in these activities independent from the group. The client usually remains in the group until the activities he or she has selected are sufficiently reinforcing that the support of the group is no longer necessary. In helping clients select appropriate activities, consideration must be given to the individual's assets and limitations, financial circumstances, and available community resources. Many individuals who are unable to participate in the worker role experience the desire to do something "useful" or something for others. Various community service activities are helpful in satisfying this desire. Attention should also be given to exploring activities that are likely to satisfy the client's mastery and esteem needs. Temporal adaptation and finding a compatible circle of friends are two other areas frequently dealt with in a group concerned with adjustment to being a nonworker.

Chapter 30, Gerontology, provides additional information concerning retirement.

There is another group of people who often need assistance in the area of leisure/recreation. These are individuals who may have neglected this aspect of their life because of work or family responsibilities. Or the loss of an important role partner—e.g., children leaving home, divorce, or death of a spouse—may necessitate alteration in leisure/recreational activities. The focus of a concurrent topical group to assist people who want to modify their leisure/recreational patterns is quite similar to the various other groups discussed in this section. There are some special problems, however, that may be encountered in this population. Frequently individuals have little idea of what their leisure/recreational interests are; they really do not know what they do and do not enjoy. Having fun may not be something they have really thought very much about. Although group members may express an interest in altering leisure/recreational patterns, in actuality there may be considerable inertia that needs to be overcome. Considerable encouragement, direction, and positive reinforcement are often necessary to prompt action on the part of the client. Most individuals in this population have few friends or a narrow circle of friends who have constricted interests. Thus, attention must be given to the development of a new or broader circle of friends. This may be impeded by some deficit in social skills and/or excessive shyness. Difficulties in this area are discussed in the following section. Members in a group designed to modify leisure/recreational patterns may initially explore and engage in leisure/recreational activities together or in small subgroups. Indeed, lasting friendships may develop between some group members. However, independent participation in leisure/recreational activities alone and with people other than group members is encouraged, supported, and reinforced.

Friendships

Prior to engaging in the acquisition of the skills necessary to form and maintain friendships, the client must have at least some basic skills in interpersonal relationships. A person usually learns how to make friends by having friendly people with common interests available and by observing how friends interact.

Some clients have had no experience in making friends. They do not know how to talk to another person other than to deal with everyday interactions, how to ask someone to join them in an activity, how a friend usually behaves, and so forth. In helping such a client, the therapist often needs to talk with the client about what is involved in making and keeping friends. The client is urged to spend time with other people who have similar interests. This may be fellow clients in the same facility, acquaintances in the community, or people in some sort of community agency or center.

Initially, it is suggested that the client spend time with others in the context of an organized leisure/recreational activity. The therapist, for example, may suggest that the client participate in a specific task with another client who has similar interests, such as playing some game together or shopping. The task suggested should be well within the abilities of both clients, so that they do not become preoccupied with the task. This allows for more attention to personal interaction. The therapist may need to suggest shared tasks for some period of time before the individuals begin to do things together spontaneously.

Later the client is encouraged to interact with others outside the structure provided by an organized activity, e.g., eating lunch with another client or asking a person in the ceramic group he or she attends at the community center to go to the movies with him or her. The therapist offers support, advice, and reassurance and attempts to arrange the situation so that the client receives some sort of positive reinforcement for interactions designed to lead to the formation of friendship. This external reinforcement may be necessary until the client is able to get some degree of positive reinforcement from a friendship such as interactions with others.

People also learn about friendships by observing how friends interact. Thus, spontaneous friendships between clients in the treatment center are encouraged, giving other clients an opportunity to see friendship in action. Ideally, staff members allow their casual, friendly interactions to be evident to clients. They do not save the showing of affection, kidding around, and mild teasing just for the staff room or after-hours interactions. The clients should be allowed to see the staff as a group of people who have formed friend relationships with each other.

There are other individuals who have more advanced skills in friend relationships but who, for reasons previously mentioned, wish to broaden their circle of friends. Such individuals often need help in identifying places and situations in which they are likely to meet people with mutual interests. They may need practice in making overtures to others and engaging in small talk. A concurrent topical group may be used to assist people in this area. Group members may help each other in locating appropriate places and situations and involve themselves in these situations initially in pairs. This type of mutual support often facilitates interaction, and the members of the pair are able to give direct feedback to each other. Role playing may be used to gain beginning skills in making overtures to others and engaging in small talk. What does one do and what does one say are clearly spelled out, taking some of the mystery out of the whole process. Eventually, group members are encouraged to go out on their own to practice these skills. Knowing the group is "back there" often provides the needed impetus to demonstrate that one can do it and to provide the necessary reinforcement and feedback. As clients become more comfortable in forming friend relationships, the need for this type of concurrent topical group will gradually diminish.

Temporal Adaptation

For those individuals whose temporal adaptation is most severely impaired—the loss of all sense of time, doing almost nothing, or very disorganized manner of engaging in role responsibilities—it is frequently necessary to impose direct external controls. Gently, but firmly, the therapist provides a regular structure and routine for the client's daily life. This involves providing a schedule of daily activities that includes when one should engage in and appropriate amounts of time for daily living activities, work, play/recreation, and rest. Time for family interaction is also included if the client is living at home. Individuals this severely impaired, however, are usually in an institutional setting. As the individual begins to gain a sense of temporal organization, more flexibility in the scheduling of activities is introduced based on the client's preferences. The degree of control exercised by the therapist is gradually diminished as the client takes on more responsibility for managing his or her own time. Considerable positive reinforcement is necessary for this type of intervention to be successful.

The majority of clients are less severely impaired in the area of temporal adaptation. Their difficulties are primarily related to the use of time—i.e., not enough time to engage in fulfilling role responsibilities, or too much time. There are several steps involved in assisting clients in these areas. The steps, outlined below, may take place within the context of a client-therapist dyad or in a thematic or topical group. Whatever the setting, ultimately the client should be directly involved in organizing daily life in the community in a way that is both productive and need-satisfying for him or her and his or her various role partners.

The following sequence of events in the intervention process is suggested(578):

1. *Identification of the client's current state of temporal adaptation.* Although this may have been done in a preliminary way during the evaluation process, it is now done in considerably more detail. The "Activity Configuration" (see Chapter 16) is an ideal tool for determining how the client uses and manages time. Through this process, the client's particular problem can be identified.

2. *Planning.* Control over time involves bringing the future into the present so that one can do something about it. Planning, then, is the major way that one gains control over future time. Planning is initiated by making a list of all the things that the client must do—the normal daily routine kinds of things and the other things that one would like to do. Next, the client arranges the list in order of priorities. To do this properly, the client may need assistance in identifying the criteria being used to set priorities. The criteria used should, as much as possible, be what the client thinks is important rather than the expectations of others. In making this list, the client is also urged to identify those activities in which he or she does not really have to engage. Many activities are based on habit or past life situations rather than on current needs and circumstances. With the completion of the list or perhaps after several revisions, the client's priorities begin to become evident.

3. *Goal setting.* Through the identification of priorities, the client is in a position to set goals. These goals are first related to the establishment of some kind of a daily routine which allows the individual to satisfactorily engage in required roles. Second, these goals are related to something the individual wants to accomplish, such as looking for another job, making more friends, redecorating the living room, losing weight, and so forth. This type of goal is important because it helps the client realize that there is more to temporal adaptation than just organizing one's daily life. In addition, establishing and seeing the possibility of attaining this "future accomplishment" goal, helps motivate the individual maintain a daily routine. Future accomplishment goals are usually outlined in terms of short-term—what will the individual do next week, a month from now—and long-term goals—when will the goal be accomplished. If there are conflicts in goals, the individual needs to review priorities and perhaps revise them in a more realistic manner. Goal statements naturally lead to specifying activities that will lead to the goals.

4. *Establishing a schedule.* The schedule is usually made up for a week at a time. It includes blocks of time for familial roles, activities of daily living, work, leisure/recreation, and time for the future accomplishment goal(s). Effective scheduling has several characteristics. It is kept fairly loose to accommodate unavoidable interruptions, delays, and unforeseen problems. It takes into consideration the individual's own internal time, when he or she works most productively, and the best time to attend to other people (when they are available). Finally, it has build-in rewards above and beyond getting various tasks accomplished. This is usually done by scheduling an enjoyable activity subsequent to an activity that is not particularly pleasant.

5. *Implementation.* Setting priorities and making up a schedule are comparatively easy; staying within the schedule is often the difficult part. This is where support

and reinforcement from the therapist and/or fellow group members become particularly important. When there is serious difficulty in following the schedule, there are several things the individual may consider and do. First, the client should look at the priorities he or she has set. They may not be realistic; they may have changed; they may lead to a consequence one did not foresee; the "future accomplishment" goal may be too complex or time-consuming; or the future accomplishment goal may have some unpleasant associations and thus be emotionally difficult to accomplish. If any of these factors are operant, it is suggested that the client reestablish priorities and make up a new schedule. Other things that might be done to encourage maintaining some kind of schedule are to make tasks smaller, perhaps even 5 or 10 minutes; take advantage of a current mood rather than scheduled time; give oneself a peptalk; make a commitment to someone; do not allow oneself to become bored with the task; take more breaks; make a list and cross things off as they are accomplished; try not to let fear and anxiety get in the way; reward oneself.

It should be emphasized that staying with a schedule is only a tool in managing time; it is not an end in itself. The client should be encouraged to do his or her best and to consider that a success.

In addition to the method of time management outlined above, there are two other approaches to dealing with problems in the area of temporal adaptation. These approaches are primarily related to activities of daily living and consist of getting someone else to do the tasks, and finding an easier, less time-consuming way of doing tasks.

Getting someone else to do the tasks first involves consideration of whether other family members can, and perhaps should, take responsibility for more household and self-maintenance tasks. There are many people, particularly women, who believe they alone are responsible for most household tasks. This may be due to a traditional definition of roles based on age and gender, or it may simply be a matter of habit. Regardless of the reason, a woman, for example, may never indicate to household members that help would be appreciated. She may even indicate that she does not want any assistance. The woman may end up playing the role of a martyr or household drudge, or she may be completely exhausted and have no time for herself.

Clients with difficulties in this area need to learn how to ask for assistance and to provide appropriate and sufficient reinforcement to family members so that they consistently participate in designated household tasks. This is probably best accomplished in a concurrent topical group which focuses on both temporal adaptation and family interaction. Group members are assisted in identifying those tasks that can be done by other family members and which tasks would be appropriate for each family member. An appropriate task is one that is within the family member's capacity to perform, will not be too disruptive relative to the usual routine of the family member, and may possibly provide some intrinsic satisfaction. Next, group members are assisted in determining the best way to ask family members for help. A direct approach with the reason for the request being specified is probably the best. It is frequently useful to involve group members in role playing to learn this approach. Group members are reminded that they may need to teach family members how to do an assigned task. A plan is then devised as to how the client will provide the necessary reinforcement so that the family member performs the task in a consistent manner. Implementation may be somewhat of a lengthy matter. When one way of dealing with the problem does not work, the client is encouraged to try another solution. Group members provide support and reinforcement. One of the major possible pitfalls is the client giving up too soon and taking back responsibility for a task that has been assigned to another family member. The client must often be supported in persevering in tolerating complaints and a task poorly done and in leaving the task undone if it is not completed by the family member responsible.

Second, getting someone else to do the task entails using services that are available in the community. Although it may cost a little more money, the saving in time and energy may be worth the additional expense. It is, for example, not that expensive to have the groceries delivered and the dry cleaning picked up and delivered. There are services available that will thoroughly clean a house or an apartment once a month, or at least wash the windows. The client is helped to consider various services and to weigh them in terms of cost versus time and energy.

Adequate temporal adaptation can also be facilitated by finding an easier, less time-consuming way of doing a task. Sometimes referred to as work simplification or energy conservation, it essentially entails problem solving. Although originally developed in relationship to individuals who were physically disabled, this means of altering tasks is appropriate for any client who is experiencing problems in temporal adaptation. The following outline of principles of work simplification is taken from the description provided by Trombly and Scott (960). These principles are the following:

1. *Plan ahead.* A full day's activities to include appropriate periods of rest should be thought out ahead.

All supplies and equipment needed for the task should be gathered prior to doing the job.

2. *Organize storage.* Supplies and equipment should be located near where they are used and, if possible, within easy reach. Duplicate sets of equipment in different locations are often useful. If possible, things should not be stored behind or under other things because of the time and energy used in trying to get at them.

3. *Eliminate steps of a job or whole jobs.* There are many tasks that are not essential to one's life-style or if essential may not need to be done so frequently. Some examples of how to eliminate steps are: all family members wearing permanent-press clothes, making a bed by only going from side to side once, soaking dishes and letting them air dry, making double portions of various foods and freezing one portion, and so forth. The list is almost endless. Another very important way of eliminating steps is to shop by phone and/or through the use of catalogues.

When possible one should sit while working. The chair used should be comfortable and of the proper height.

Selecting the proper equipment and keeping it in good repair makes a job far easier. Electrically powered equipment such as a self-cleaning stove or garbage disposal can save considerable time and should be suggested if they are within the client's financial means.

The proper use of both hands can help make a task easier. Movements should be as symmetrical and smooth as possible. The muscle force of the proximal rather than the distal joint should be used as much as possible. This is particularly true in the case of lifting.

Whenever possible slide objects rather than lift them. This can be facilitated in the kitchen by arranging for contiguous counter space. Wheeled service carts and laundry baskets are also useful.

Avoid holding objects. Suction cup bases, nonskid mats, and wet towels are some examples of ways to stabilize pots and pans so that they do not have to be held. Heavy pots and pans can also be used but lifting them may be more energy consuming than necessary.

The location of switches and controls should be placed in a convenient place and in easy, safe reach. Be sure lighting is good.

Methods of work simplification can be taught in a client-therapist dyad, but they are probably best taught in the context of anticipatory or concurrent topical group. The group atmosphere stimulates thinking and the sharing of ideas and experiences. Regardless of the setting, the therapist describes some of the basic points outlined above. After that, the focus is on problem solving. There is no way the therapist can teach all the possible ways of work simplification. Thus, emphasis is on learning to think in terms of work simplification and to approach all tasks with that idea in mind. The basic principles outlined are important and provide an impetus for problem solving. However, they are only useful if they work for a particular client. The problem-solving approach that is an inherent part of work simplification is intriguing to many clients as well as a challenge. It is frequently viewed in a similar light by other family members. They often enjoy participating in the process, and this, of course, should be encouraged.

SUMMARY

Role Acquisition is an acquisitional frame of reference addressed to those behaviors considered important for adequate participation in the major social roles. The specific areas of concern can be viewed as hierarchical or pyramidal in nature, with task skills and interpersonal skills forming the base, family interactions, activities of daily living, school/work, and play/leisure/recreation forming the middle, and temporal adaptation making up the top portion of the pyramid. In the discussion of each area, behaviors indicative of dysfunction are outlined and evaluative tools suggested. In addition, general postulates regarding change are provided as well as specific postulates for each area.

Part 6

Areas of Specialization

The final part of this text is devoted to the discussion of the psychosocial components of occupational therapy within the context of the five areas of specialization recognized by the American Occupational Therapy Association (AOTA). These areas, in the order in which they are discussed, are mental health, physical disabilities, developmental disabilities, gerontology, and sensory integration. The general focus is on integration and application of all that has been described in the text up to this point. Although some new material will be introduced, the emphasis of Part 6 is on synthesis. Attention is given primarily to the special characteristics and problems of each population identified by AOTA's Special Interest Sections and to appropriate program planning.

Areas of specialization in occupational therapy cut across various diagnostic categories, age, and intervention needs. Thus, what is discussed in one chapter is often applicable to clients in addition to those to whom the chapter is addressed. Alternative living situations, for example, are discussed in Chapter 29, Developmental Disabilities. This is in no way to be taken to mean that this aspect of occupational therapy is not also applicable to other client populations.

27 Mental Health

The specialty area of mental health is primarily oriented to assist those individuals whose major problems are psychiatric in nature. This is, however, a somewhat narrow description. Occupational therapists who describe themselves as working in the area of mental health are also involved in working with such populations as refugees; abused women; individuals who are having difficulties in the area of role transitions, daily living activities, and leisure/recreation; juvenile offenders; and so forth.

This chapter is primarily devoted to a description of the various types of settings in and populations with which occupational therapists work. Typical programs will be outlined. These descriptions should be considered illustrative only. The variety of settings, populations, and programs is so great that a comprehensive survey is beyond the scope of this text. By way of introduction, the first section of this chapter briefly outlines some factors related to psychoactive drugs that should be taken into consideration by the occupational therapist. This is followed by a section each on general principles of program planning, settings for intervention, and types of programs.

PSYCHOACTIVE DRUGS

Psychoactive drugs have been a part of the medical treatment of psychiatric disorders since the mid-1950s. The four major groups of psychoactive drugs in current use are those that are effective in treating schizophrenic disorders, depression, manic disorders, and anxiety (77,461,470,546,568,911). Psychoactive drugs have become a powerful tool which has been both therapeutically used and abused. Although a part of medicine for 30 years, psychopharmacology remains more of an art than a science. There is such an individual reaction to various drugs and dosages that it is only the experienced, concerned, and wise physician who is able to effectively manage the prescription of psychoactive drugs.

It is questionable whether psychoactive drugs lead to a "cure" in the sense of permanently altering a pathological process. Nevertheless, they do markedly diminish the symptoms of specific disorders in the vast majority of cases. For example, antipsychotic drugs diminish blunted affect, withdrawal, hallucinations, delusions, hostility, and resistiveness. They contribute to the normalization of motor behavior and usually lead to a marked improvement in cognitive function. The judicious use of psychoactive drugs decreases the need for management and allows the client to participate in and benefit from the change process actively.

Despite the considerable therapeutic benefit of psychoactive drugs, there are many side effects, several of which are quite serious. Some of the major side effects are motor retardation, tremor, apathy, blunted affect, dry mouth and throat, weight gain, increased appetite, sedation and drowsiness, visual changes, sensitivity to the sun, orthostatic hypotension (a sudden drop in blood pressure causing dizziness or even fainting as a result of rapid postural changes), incoordination, changes in sexual functions, convulsions, and akasthesia (involuntary motor restlessness).

The most serious side effect is tardive dyskinesia. This is a condition characterized by repetitive involuntary movements affecting mainly the face and mouth. Symptoms include tongue protrusion, licking of the lips, smacking and sucking lip movements, chewing and jaw deviations, facial grimaces, grunting, and other peculiar sounds. The limbs and trunk may also be involved. It has been estimated that tardive dyskinesia occurs in 3% to 6% of a mixed population of psychiatric patients and in up to 40% of elderly, chronically institutionalized patients. Tardive dyskinesia may appear after a long uninterrupted course of treatment with antipsychotic medication or after the termination of chemotherapy. The medication itself may mask the symptoms of tardive dyskinesia, which is usually irreversible, although there have been some reports of recovery. The treatment of choice is to discontinue the use of antipsychotic medication. It should be noted that side effects vary from individual to individual in both type and intensity. Some antipsychotic drugs are more likely to produce specific side effects than other drugs.

In prescribing psychoactive medications, a responsible physician makes sure that the patient knows exactly what he or she is taking, what the dose is, and how the medication is administered. The physician ideally gives the patient a detailed and complete list of instructions and reviews it with the patient until satisfied that the patient understands the instructions and can follow them. Telling the patient about the probable and/or possible side effects is generally considered to be ethical responsible behavior. Such information appears to improve rather than diminish compliance.

It is important that the therapist know the side effects of psychoactive drugs. There are several current references for detailed information such as the *Physicians' Desk Reference*, the *Medical Letter*, and the *Adverse Drug Effect Bulletin*. Physicians who regularly prescribe psychoactive medication and the hospital should be aware of what specific drug(s) each client is receiving.

There are several reasons the therapist needs to know the side effects of psychoactive drugs. First, the side effects may be very uncomfortable, troublesome, and upsetting to the client. The patient is likely to need reassurance and encouragement to continue taking medication as prescribed. Second, as a member of the team the therapist is responsible for noting and reporting side effects and other changes in behavior. In this way the effects of medication can be monitored closely so that appropriate changes in medication can be made promptly. Third during evaluation the therapist should be aware that drug side effects must be taken into consideration in setting goals and designing activites for intervention. The purpose here is to capitalize on the therapeutic effects and, if possible, to diminish the negative side effects.

Following are some considerations and suggestions that may facilitate the intervention process:

- *Dry mouth and throat*. Water and low-calorie caffeine-free drinks should be readily available. Some clients also find it useful to chew gum or to suck on hard candy.
- *Sensitivity to the sun*. Time out in the sun should be limited. Some clients cannot tolerate being in the sun at all. When out in the sun clients should use a sun screen lotion and wear long sleeves and a hat.
- *Orthostatic hypotension*. Activities involving sudden postural changes such as bending and rapid movement from a sitting or squatting position to standing should be avoided.
- *Blurred vision*. Activities requiring minimal discrimination and the use of strongly contrasting colors are often helpful. As far-vision may also be affected, balls and other equipment used in active games should be brightly colored.
- *Akasthesia*. Simple, short-term, nonsedentary activities are the best for counteracting this side effect. The client may want to move from activity to activity as attention span is often short. This behavior need not be counterproductive if the client is doing something meaningful within the context of each activity.
- *Drowsiness*. Be aware that the client may be drowsy during some periods of the day. Arrange for rest periods but do not let the client stay in bed or on a couch the major portion of the day. Drowsiness is best combatted by keeping the client involved in activities that are meaningful.
- *Incoordination*. Select activities the client can accomplish despite incoordination, such as simple gross-motor activities. Observe the type of incoordination—for example, tremor, muscular rigidity, or spastic movements—before determining appropriate activities.
- *Convulsions*. Learn how to care for a person who is having a convulsion. A padded tongue depressor should be available at all times. Know which clients are prone to convulsions and watch them more carefully. Find out if a client can tell when a seizure is about to occur. If able to do so, encourage the client to share this information with you immediately.
- *Dizziness, faintness, and weakness*. Provide a place for the client to sit or lie down. Encourage the client to continue his or her usual activities when the episode passes.
- *Increased appetite and weight gain*. Have fruit and raw vegetables available for snacks. In groups that

use cooking as an activity, prepare foods that are low in calories. Give the client support relative to staying on a restricted diet. Encourage regular exercises.

It is important for the therapist to remember that side effects are real and uncomfortable. They are not a technique used by the client to get attention or to be excused from required activities. There are times when side effects become the predominant complaint of the client or cause the client to withdraw from activities and contact with others. The therapist should always be aware of the possibility that such effects may be significant contributors to the client's present thoughts, feelings, and actions.

GENERAL PRINCIPLES OF PROGRAM PLANNING

Program planning is the process of organizing and implementing the delivery of occupational therapy services in such a way as to meet the evaluation and intervention needs of a specified group of clients (235, 275,290,440,446,498,956). Program planning is concerned with a collectivity of clients such as a ward, unit, service, and the like. It is not directly concerned with evaluation and intervention relative to a particular client. Rather it provides the structure in which this may take place in the most optimal manner. Program planning is a continual process. It is not something that is done once and set for long periods of time. The occupational therapist is always concerned about the effectiveness of a given program and the ever changing needs of the population it is designed to serve. Thus, a program is always in the process of being evaluated and refined, with perhaps occasional major alterations.

The following principles of program planning are meant to be general in nature. That is, although outlined in this chapter, they apply to all areas of specialization. A good program in occupational therapy has the following characteristics:

A good program is based on the needs of the client population being served. It is designed to provide appropriate evaluation procedures and adequate intervention in all areas. Thus, it is not just concerned with the change process but also takes into consideration planning relative to prevention, meeting health needs, maintenance and management. The assessment of the needs of a particular client population involves identification of the major common problem areas experienced by the clients. This is often accomplished by assessing the health needs that are likely not to be met given the setting and the population, identifying typical maintenance and management problems, and delineating those performance components and occupational performances in which the majority of clients have deficits.

Demographic factors are taken into consideration when planning a program. This, in particular, includes the average age of the clients and the clients' typical sociocultural background. Activities designed to meet health needs, for example, will be different for young children than for a group of adolescents and young adults. The importance of the clients' sociocultural background in establishing rapport, evaluation, and intervention has been previously emphasized.

Good program planning makes provisions for assisting family members. All too often this aspect of the occupational therapy process is not taken into consideration in program planning. If attended to, it is frequently dealt with as an afterthought or something that will somehow be accomplished between more clearly specified parts of the program. This is not good program planning; the capacity of clients to adapt to their disability and living in the community is often dependent on the cooperation and knowledgable assistance of family members. Thus, good program planing takes into consideration the needs of family members. Specific aspects of the program are designed to meet these needs.

A good program is flexible. Although a program is developed for a given population, it must be sufficiently malleable to meet the unique needs of each client. A rigid, highly structured program, then, in most cases is not desirable. A planned program is probably best viewed as a framework on which an individualized program can be devised for each client.

A good program is realistic. It is fairly easy to plan a hypothetical program that offers more than optimal occupational therapy services. But no plan will be effective unless it is developed within the constraints that exist in a particular setting. For a program to have the potential of being effective it must be realistic in terms of personnel, time, facilities, and financial support. Concerning *personnel*, the planner must take into consideration the number of occupational therapists, assistants, and aids available and the capacity and limitations of these individuals. In addition, the planner should consider the number of other staff members who may effectively augment an occupational therapy program. For example, recreational therapists may be available to take responsibility for the play/leisure/recreational aspect of the program; the nursing staff may be able to take responsibility for those activities of daily living that are concerned with personal care; a social worker may be able to assist with problems that relate to family interaction.

In program planning, sufficient *time* must be scheduled for direct client care. In addition, time must be scheduled for meetings, documentation, and supervision. It goes without saying that no meetings should be scheduled for the lunch hour, nor should the therapist be expected to use that time for documentation. Insufficient time to accomplish all that is expected is one of the major sources of chronic stress for occupational therapists. This should be kept in mind in program planning.

A program must be realistic in terms of the *facilities* availalbe. It might, for example, be appropriate to client needs to have a small sheltered workshop program. However, if there is no available space for such a program, it is unrealistic to include this in one's plan. Similarly, if there is no gym facility, then activities requiring this type of facility are inappropriate.

The occupational therapy department is usually allocated a given sum of money that is to be used as financial support for departmental programs. Any program planned must take into consideration the cost of equipment and supplies. Developing a budget and taking responsibility for staying within that budget is an important part of program planning and implementation.

Being realistic in program planning does not mean that one should not try to manipulate the constraints of a particular setting. The therapist may, indeed, spend considerable time negotiating for more personnel and additional financial support. With some thought, space can be used quite creatively. Moreover, there may be facilities available in the community, such as a gymnasium or a swimming pool, that may be utilized in a program.

A means of assessing the effectiveness of the program is an integral part of the design. There are several ways this might be accomplished. One of the major ways is to determine the extent to which the goals set for each individual client are met by the time they leave the program. Client satisfaction with the program can be assessed by the general level of participation and by information provided by the client in the final interview before termination. Follow-up studies, although expensive, are also a useful device for program evaluation.

The program should be stated in such a way that it is understandable to others. An excellent program may be developed by the therapists, but if it is not able to be communicated to others—clients, families and, staff—then its possibility for success is limited. The objectives of the program need to be clearly stated, the means whereby those objectives are to be attained must be specifically outlined, and the rationale for the goals and means specified. When a plan includes intervention relative to a change process, the frames of reference being used should be stated. The extent to which the plan is able to be communicated is very likely to influence the amount of support the program will receive from others. In addition, the clarity of the plan is usually a good indication of how well it has been thought through by those responsible for its development.

The program must be acceptable to other members of the team. In order for an occupational therapy program to be seen as desirable, it must be compatible with the orientation of other members of the team. The orientation may be similar to that of others or it may be complementary. Lack of compatibility may lead to total rejection of the program or to the program becoming isolated from or peripheral to the other aspects of the facility's total program. An isolated or peripheral program is not likely to be effective. Active participation on the clients' part is likely to be low, and clients may be confused by the marked difference in orientation. Ideally, then, the occupational therapy program is an integral part of the clients' total program.

Implementation of a new or revised occupational therapy program should be fairly easy if the program has the characteristics outlined above. Ongoing communication with the other members of the team is essential. The therapist must also remember that the initial stages of implementation rarely go smoothly. There are likely to be problems encountered and refinements that need to be made. Above all, the therapist should not become discouraged. The process of implementation is similar to that outlined in Chapter 17 relative to putting into effect programs designed to meet health needs.

SETTINGS FOR INTERVENTION

The delivery of mental health services in the United States is extremely diverse. There is considerable variation in who is responsible and in the structure established for the delivery of such services. There are differences within and between particular geographical areas. The purpose of this section is to provide some orientation to the diversity of settings in which occupational therapists are involved (708,956). Various types of occupational therapy programs are described in the following section.

Large Public Institutions

Large public institutions include state hospitals and institutions operated by the Veterans Administration. These institutions, which have evolved over the past 125 years, are frequently found outside urban areas. They are often fairly self-sufficient communities which spread over many acres. Facilities, in addition to housing for clients, may include a farm, stores, post office, laundry, maintenance services, recreational center, a medical surgical hospital, chapels, housing for staff, and the like. The client population tends to be quite diverse and represents a wide range of problem areas. Many people in public institutions have multiple problems, with the common theme being severe difficulty in functioning in the community.

Traditionally, public institutions have been seriously understaffed, with a paucity of trained personnel. The structure tends to be centralized, with staff members' first loyalty to their own department (nursing, recreation, psychology, etc.) rather than to a unit of the institution. Staff members are often moved from unit to unit as the need arises. When clients first come to the institution, they are placed on an "admissions" unit. When a client improves fairly rapidly, he or she is sent home. If a client does not improve, he or she is sent to another ward; which specific ward depends on the client's level of functioning. Clients are moved from unit to unit as their condition improves or worsens. Various programs and services for clients, to the extent that they are available, usually take place off the unit in which the client lives.

The above description is of a traditional public institution. Although there are some institutions that remain as described above, many have undergone considerable change. The two major reasons for change have been the advent of relatively effective psychoactive drugs and the general belief that long-term care in large public institutions is not the best way to deal with mental health problems. The major changes that have occurred are decentralization and the development of satellite centers.

A decentralized institution is organized so that one unit is set aside for clients from a particular section of a city, town, or county. Clients are admitted directly to this unit and stay in the unit until they are discharged. The exceptions to this pattern might be clients who need special programs. There may, for example, be separate units for adolescents, individuals who have problems with substance abuse, court committed cases, and so forth.

The reason for unitization based on geographic location is the belief that treatment is more effective when clients are with people from their own community, people with whom they are likely to share common interests and experiences. Moreover, if a person needs to return to the institution at some later date, he will be returning to familiar surroundings.

Staff members are assigned to a specific unit, and it is expected that they will stay on that unit for an extended period of time. Their first loyalty is often to the unit, with day-to-day supervision being provided by the individual who is responsible for that unit. There continues to be departments of, for example, social work, but supervisors in the department structure serve more in an advisory, educational, and consulting capacity. They usually have little to do with the everyday work of staff members.

Many programs and services are unit-centered but special institutional-wide programs, such as a sheltered workshop, may also be utilized. These decentralized units are primarily concerned with short-term care during the acute phase of dysfunction, with much effort being made to prevent long-term institutionalization. Clients are transferred to other types of programs as soon as possible.

Satellite centers are located in and serve the same community as the decentralized units of a public institution. Staff members from the institution work in the satellite centers with a close relationship often being maintained between the institutionally located unit and its satellite center. These centers vary in the extent of the programs they offer, the majority being outpatient in nature. The major purpose of satellite centers is to offer sufficient services so that as many people as possible will be kept out of public institutions. Many satellite programs are essentially community mental health centers, a type of setting discussed shortly.

Many public institutions have a relatively stable population consisting of individuals who are severely, chronically disabled. The major diagnostic categories are organic mental disorders and schizophrenic disorders. These disorders may be complicated by other medical problems. A fairly large percentage of this population tends to be elderly. Programs for this group of clients may be directed toward preparation of the client for leaving the institution. The client's expected environment is usually residence in some relatively protected situation such as a group home or extended care facility. For those clients who are unlikely to leave the institution, programs ideally are designed to facilitate the highest level of functioning possible and to maintain that level as long as feasible. Essentially every effort is made to allow these individuals to live out their lives with dignity and comfort.

Private Psychiatric Services

Private psychiatric services may be located in an institution whose major purpose is the treatment of psychiatric disorders or in one unit of a general private hospital. The length of stay may be short term (less than two weeks), intermediate (up to 90 days), or long-term. Long-term care is more likely to take place in an institution whose major purpose is the treatment of psychiatric disorders rather than in a unit of a general hospital.

Regardless of where the service is located, there tend to be two types of staffing patterns: team-oriented and physician-oriented. In a team-oriented situation, psychiatrists and a group of other health professionals employed by the institution work together to provide all necessary services to the client. Programs are coordinated around clearly defined, shared goals for each client.

The other type of pattern is dominated by the physician, who is not employed by the institution but who has admitting privileges to the institution. The physician usually a psychiatrist, continues to see his or her client on a regular basis for individualized treatment. Occupational therapy programs in such settings tend to be less structured and primarily concerned with maintenance, management, and meeting health needs. It is possible to develop programs concerned with change if the physician is willing to cooperate in the venture. Such programs may be difficult to coordinate and require frequent and open communication between physician and therapist. The client must also be helped to recognize that participation in the occupational therapy program is as important as the individual treatment he or she is receiving from the physician. When this is not done, clients tend to view the occupational therapy program and other programs on the unit as inferior to verbal psychotherapy and/or medication or as only a good way to pass the time.

City and County General Hospitals

Most city and county hospitals have a psychiatric unit, the size varying from hospital to hospital. Clients are frequently admitted on an emergency basis or referred from some other unit of the hospital. The length of stay is usually short term. Care is primarily oriented to dealing with the client's acute phase of dysfunction and evaluation relative to the client's future needs for assistance. Depending on the nature of the client's dysfunction, he or she may be sent to a facility that offers intermediate or long-term care or discharged to the community with one plan or another for outpatient services.

Community Mental Health Centers

Community mental health centers are typically associated with, as mentioned, large public institutions or with private city or county institutions. There are, however, some which are free-standing, not associated with any type of hospital. These centers have evolved in order to take care of the mental health needs of people who live in a particular geographic area. The needs of the mentally retarded are also given attention. The development of community mental health centers has grown out of the belief, and some documented evidence, that clients will do better if they remain in their own community while receiving treatment. Continued contact with family and friends and familiar surroundings are believed to help the client maintain a sense of identity and desire to once again become a full participant in the community.

The types of services offered by a community mental health center vary. Some of the possible programs are day and evening programs oriented to change and/or maintenance; verbal psychotherapy and/or the prescription of therapeutic drugs; crisis intervention and a 24-hour telephone service; evaluation and referral to programs within the center or to other more appropriate community groups: emergency inpatient care: group homes as a permanent residence or as a temporary residence for individuals in the process of adjusting to the community; geriatric programs and programs for children and adolescents: programs oriented to dealing with problems in family interaction; and, programs designed to deal with substance abuse. Another type of service offered by the community mental health center is outreach programs, which may be concerned with such populations as residents of boarding homes for marginally adjusted former psychiatric patients; preschool children in city-run day care centers; political refugees and other recent immigrant groups; home programs for the elderly; and so forth.

The clients of a community mental health center may be former patients, but the vast majority are often members of the community who have never been hospitalized. The whole purpose of these centers is not only to attend to the mental health needs of the community, but to keep people in the community rather than in hospitals as much as possible.

Other Settings

This is a miscellaneous category that includes a variety of different types of centers or programs. One example is a day program for select clients supported by a psychotherapy or psychoanalytic training center. There are also facilities, not associated with any hospital, that have programs for discharged psychiatric patients. Some of these programs have one major focus such as the development of work habits. Others are more generalized, offering learning experiences in many areas and a social-recreational program. These nonhospital-related facilities also usually offer assistance and support relative to problems participants may face in the wider community. Other types of services that fall into this category are social-recreational programs for formally hospitalized psychiatric patients sponsored, for example by a church group or a "Y." The sponsoring organization may offer such programs as arts-and-craft instructions, planned trips, social coffee hours, and holiday parties.

The settings described above are not a complete listing of the programs concerned with helping individuals with problems in the area of mental health. The patterns suggested may also vary from community to community. What has been provided here is essentially a brief overview to give the beginning therapist some idea of the many settings in which the occupational therapy process takes place.

TYPES OF PROGRAMS

The purpose of this section is to orient the reader to various types of programs and, by extension, to working with different kinds of clients. What is presented is an overview rather than an in-depth discussion. These are simply examples of possible programs; each setting has its own particular program and special way of organizing itself.

Short-Term Care

This discussion focuses on short-term care in a setting that is designed for that purpose alone (206,306,440, 458,666,734,807). In this hypothetical setting, clients over the age of 18 years stay anywhere from 48 hr to 2 weeks. Thus there is rapid turnover, which limits the therapist's capacity to develop an in-depth understanding of each client. The majority of clients are in a severely disorganized state or profoundly depressed on admission. The major form of medical treatment is the use of psychoactive drugs and, in some settings, the use of electroconvulsive therapy (ECT) for those clients who are profoundly depressed. On discharge the client may return to the community without need for further treatment/intervention. More commonly, the client is referred to a community mental health center or for further inpatient treatment at another setting designed for intermediate or long-term care.

The three major overall goals of the occupational therapy program are:

1. To assist the client in reintegrating to the point that he has some sense of control over himself and the situation at hand. In general, the idea is to help the client return to somewhat near his state of functioning prior to his hospitalization.
2. To enhance the client's feelings of self-worth. Most clients who are hospitalized for short-term care feel that they have failed in their capacity to manage their own lives—a situation that can be seriously damaging to one's sense of worth.
3. To assess the client's need for further intervention and to assist in determining the type of intervention which would be most appropriate for the client.

The first two goals are accomplished through a program that includes maintenance, management, and meeting health needs. More specifically, they are accomplished through activities that are designed to do the following:

Provide an orientation to the hospital. Some clients experience hospitalization as a haven from the stresses of daily life. For other clients hospitalization is one more traumatic experience in addition to their basic difficulties in living in the community. It is this latter group that is of major concern to the therapist. However, even clients who view hospitalization in a relatively positive light need some orientation. There are several things that the therapist can do to assist a client in this area:

The therapist can recognize the client's fears relative to hospitalization and anxiety concerning other clients' hostility, bizarre behavior, and the like. The client is given support and an opportunity to discuss fears. Honest feedback regarding the reality of the client's fears is provided.

The client is helped to understand why he or she is in the hospital by being given honest and direct answers to questions.

The daily routine of the unit is discussed with the client and, if possible, a written schedule is provided. At the very least a schedule is posted in a central location. The physical layout of the unit is described; a simple map is useful for this purpose. The client is introduced to staff members and other clients. Socially appropriate introductions are made so that the client does not wonder about not knowing who people are.

The client is made aware of his or her privileges and responsibilities. Visiting hours and regulations regarding telephone calls, if any, are outlined. Regarding telephone calls, the client is assisted in making calls if necessary. There are times when the therapist must help the client determine who he or she should and should not call. The responsibilities of the client are outlined particularly relative to what is and is not considered acceptable behavior. The consequence of unacceptable behavior is described in a nonthreatening manner.

The client is given assistance in unpacking and putting away belongings. When the client's admission is an emergency, he or she is assisted in securing adequate clothing and toilet articles and in making any necessary arrangements such as paying bills and rent and seeing to the care of people who are depending on him.

The client should be made aware of any legal rights under the state's mental health laws by providing factual information about the law and how to contact a lawyer if that should be requested.

Orientation to the hospital may be the responsibility of the therapist, to an individual client who has been in the hospital for a few days, or it may take place in a group made up of relatively new clients as well as clients who have been hospitalized for a time. The latter is often the preferred means of general orientation, for "old" clients often present the necessary information and support in a way that is readily understandable to the client. They have had the experience of being new to the situation and often can present nuances that may be missed by the therapist. The opportunity to participate in a group orientation also gives the more experienced clients an idea of how far they have advanced since their first few days on the unit.

Help make adjustment to somatic treatment. This aspect of intervention was discussed in a previous section. The only point to be emphasized here is that clients in short-term care may be experiencing psychoactive drugs for the first time or may be experiencing a marked change in dosage or type of drug. The therapist, therefore, must be particularly alert to the client's response to the medication and to side effects.

Ensure satisfaction of current health needs. It is very likely that many health needs will not be satisfied in a facility concerned with short-term care if specific attention is not given to this area. Suggestions for meeting health needs were outlined in Chapter 17. The needs of primary importance for a client in a short-term care facility are likely to be psychophysical: safety, love, acceptance, and esteem. These, therefore, are given particular attention in program planning.

Provide an opportunity for meaningful communication. Most clients have a desire to communicate. The problem often is that they are hesitant in the strange environment of the hospital or that they communicate in such a way that it is difficult for others to comprehend.

At times the client may want to "just talk" outside the context of any other particular activity. Frequently the client's desire to communicate is motivated by some catastrophic event—surgery, loss of a job, the death of a family member—which has led to the client's hospitalization. Talking about such events is often helpful as it appears to be one way of integrating such events into one's totality of life experiences. In listening, the therapist must be patient. Attempting to bring the client to the point of problem solving relative to these events too soon is likely to lead to loss of rapport. Nevertheless, and with an appropriate sense of timing, the therapist needs to lead the client gently to the point of problem solving. Other clients may present a stereotyped repetition of their symptoms or a detailed demonstration of highly disordered thought processes. Although the therapist listens with empathy, such conversations should be turned as soon as possible to problem solving, reality testing, or at least to some other topic.

The client may wish to talk about less emotionally related issues. The client may, for example, wish to discuss current events, work, or a leisure time interest. Such a client may have little in common with other clients or, for whatever reason, have difficulty engaging them in conversation. The therapist initially spends time talking with the client but also helps the client engage in conversations with other clients.

When the client does not communicate easily in English and the therapist does not speak the client's language, attempts are made to find someone in the hospital who can talk with the client. This may be a staff member, another client, or someone in the maintenance or administration areas of the hospital. Ideally, regular meetings are arranged even if they are only a few minutes a day.

Initially, verbal communication may be difficult for the client. He or she may be more comfortable communicating through actions or through the use of the nonhuman environment. Participation in creative-expressive activities—art, dance, drama, or music—may be helpful. The client may or may not want to talk about the process or productions. This is the client's decision and it should be respected. It should be remembered that without validation from the client, it is risky to interpret what the client is communicating through creative-expressive processes and end products.

Maintain present functioning. Short-term care is designed to provide support and to give clients the opportunity and encouragement to function at the highest possible level. Particularly important is the maintenance of function in the areas of personal care, task skills, and interpersonal relations. The vast majority of clients are capable of doing something. Given the client's age, sex, assets and limitations, interests and cultural background, the therapist suggests appropriate activities. As the client is able to function on a higher level, more complex, demanding activities are suggested. Clients are encouraged to select activities themselves. If selection is a gross manifestation of a client's symptoms such as the manic client who decides to make a four-place setting of dishes using the slab method of ceramic construction, he or she is guided into selecting a more appropriate activity. A client who is extremely indecisive as to what he or she would like to do is told what to do. The depressed, withdrawn, regressed or catatonic client may at first refuse to engage in any activity. The therapist visits such a client several times a day. Verbal interaction with the client may be minimal at first, consisting of comments about the immediate surroundings. The level and type of verbal interaction is regulated by what the client is able to tolerate. Gently the client is guided into engaging in some activity: what is immaterial. To maintain function, a matter-of-fact, concrete, somewhat directive approach is usually appropriate. The therapist sets limits, provides structure, and offers an opportunity for reality testing as needed. Maintenance of function is significantly enhanced by adequate intervention relative to management. The reader is referred to Chapter 17 for a review of appropriate methods of management.

Help understanding of mental health and illness. It is important for the client to know the status of his or her physical health. If a good physical examination is not a routine part of short-term care, the therapist should make sure the client has such an examination. Clients frequently have inaccurate ideas about mental illness and how it is alleviated. Accurate information is given to the client either in a one-to-one discussion or in a group. Information about physical health and the relationship between mental health and good physical health—nutrition, sleep, exercise, weight control, care of chronic physical diseases—is shared with clients. The therapist emphasizes that mental illness may or may not be a disease in the usual sense and that it continues to be studied. Somatic treatment in conjunction with developing additional skills for living in the community is the best known form of care. In being honest with clients, the therapist discusses, in a matter-of-fact manner, that some types of psychosocial dysfunction are chronic in nature but that help is available if sought and used. Clients are also encouraged to learn how to identify signs of impending problems before becoming nonfunctional and/or in need of hospitalization.

Assist in problem solving for immediate stress-provoking life situations. This aspect of intervention is very similar to crises intervention outlined in Chapter 17. Clients are helped to understand the specific, concrete problems and events that led to their hospitalization. Assistance is given in identifying and trying different ways of solving current problems. This is best done in a group setting where support, feedback, and suggestions are freely given. Role playing and urging imitation of other clients who have solved similar problems are useful.

Facilitate adjustment to a return to the community and/or continued care. When the client is to return to the community, he or she is assisted in identifying people in the community who are able to provide situational support. These may be family members, friends, neighbors, and clergy. The client is urged to telephone these people and, if appropriate, invite them to visit in the hospital. With the client's permission, it is often helpful for the therapist to talk with these people, giving them information about how they may assist the client and giving them the necessary encouragement and support.

A client may express no interest in further assistance after discharge and assessment of his or her needs may be accurate. In most cases, however, the client will need further care. Helping the client to recognize this is best accomplished subsequent to evaluation. At that time, the therapist is often able to point out areas of difficulty that can be comfortably recognized by the client. The kinds of treatment/intervention programs available to the client are outlined, giving the client some idea of what participation in the program may be like. Some clients do not seek further assistance because they know little about it and do not know how to go about securing such assistance. Thus, it is important to provide as much information as possible as well as support and encouragement.

Help may also be needed in deciding what to tell friends and co-workers about one's hospitalization and with other practical problems relative to returning to the community. This is best accomplished in an anticipatory topical group.

Some clients will not be returning to the community immediately but rather will be going to an intermediate or long-term care facility. If possible the client should visit the new facility prior to discharge from the short-term treatment center. During such a visit the client is introduced to the staff and clients with whom he or she will be involved. When a visit is impossible, the therapist gives a detailed description of the new setting, the client's living arrangements, the program, and the behavior that will be expected. The client is likely to need concrete assistance and support as he or she moves from one facility to another.

The first two goals of intervention in a short-term care facility are accomplished, in part, through a general activity program. The organizing effect of purposeful activities, as discussed in Chapter 10, is used very deliberately. A regularly scheduled program of activities suitable for individuals with varying degrees of functional capacities is planned for the day, evening, and weekends. The schedule should include both active doing processes such as volleyball and calisthenics and more sedentary activities. These activities are interspersed with thematic and topical groups designed to meet some of the specific goals of the program outlined above.

Participation in the activity program is strongly encouraged for all clients. Sitting around doing nothing or ruminating about one's problems is not considered to be conducive to psychological reintegration or enhanced feelings of self-worth. When active participation is highly valued in the treatment center, there is usually very little difficulty in getting clients involved. There will, however, be some clients who initially refuse to participate in any kind of group activity. They may be so confused or preoccupied with their own problems that they have difficulty interacting with other clients and simply do not care about the concerns of others. This should not automatically be construed as a major deficit in the area of social interaction. Clients who initially refuse to participate are very likely to become involved after a few days. The probability of this occurring is higher if the client is given an adequate amount of personal attention by the staff. Once the client realizes that the staff is concerned about his or her welfare and that they are trustworthy, the client will begin to become involved in the organized program of activities.

Evaluation is the third major goal of short-term care. The purpose of the evaluation, as mentioned, is to assess the client's need for further intervention and the type of intervention which would be most appropriate. The suggested frame of reference to use as the basis for evaluation is role acquisition, because it is addressed to the majority of performance components and occupational performance. Because of the time factor, the evaluation procedures suggested in Chapter 26 may need to be abbreviated. Ideally, evaluation includes assessment of task skills and interpersonal relations using the procedures outlined in Chapter 16. When this is not possible given the constraints of time and the structure of the facility, the client's capacity relative to task skills and interpersonal relations can be assessed through observation of the client during participation in the usual activities of the center. An interview with the client is, however, essential. This should be a general interview but one that emphasizes the client's capacity to engage in the various occupational performances.

From these assessment procedures the therapist should have a general overview of the client's assets and limitations. This is shared with the client and other team members. The recommendations made to the client are based on this information. In general, if the client is so severely impaired that he or she is unable to function in the community, the client is referred to an intermediate or long-term care facility. If less impaired, the client is referred to a community-based program. The type of program will depend on the client's deficit in functioning and, pragmatically, on what is available in the community. It is very important that the therapist know what resources are available. With this knowledge the therapist is in a far better position to make appropriate recommendations. The support system of the client—family, friends, and so forth—is also important in deciding how best the client may be helped. The client should be an active participant both in the assessment process and in determining the type and extent of assistance needed after discharge. If at all possible, the client is given several options, with the pros and cons of each being spelled out. Finally,if the client is to be involved in some kind of treatment/intervention program the therapist's report of evaluation findings is sent to this facility.

It should be noted that the change process is not suggested as being part of short-term care. The rationale for this is that there is not sufficient time to implement a change program that has any real hope of being effective. Attempts to do so usually lead to a feeling of frustration on the part of therapist and client alike. It seems far more reasonable to focus attention on the three general goals and to feel confident that one can consistently meet these goals.

Intermediate-Term Care

For a description of a representative sample of intermediate-care programs see the following references: 68,78,216,227,241,257,290,296,411,431,451,482,489, 490,557,647,708,769,796,882,909. The discussion here will focus on intermediate care that takes place in an inpatient facility.

This hypothetical 30-bed-unit setting is designed for clients over 18 years of age who will stay anywhere from 1 to 3 months. Thus the therapist has a much better opportunity to develop an in-depth understanding of clients than is possible during short-term care. Intervention relative to the change process is possible in this setting. Any of the three types of frames of reference selected should, of course, be compatible with the overall orientation of the facility and with the functional level of the typical client population. In this hypothetical setting, reconciliation of universal issues is the frame of reference utilized.

The major overall goals of the occupational therapy program are (a) helping clients deal with unreconciled universal issues and (b) meeting health needs. Maintenance and management may be occasionally necessary, but on the whole, the client population in this setting does not require this type of intervention.

To give the reader some idea of what the program is like, it will be described in terms of a daily schedule. Prior to that, it should be mentioned that in addition to the medical staff, there are two occupational therapists on the unit and one recreational therapist. All staff members participate in the program, with the groups concerned with the change process often being co-led by an occupational therapist and perhaps a nurse, social worker, psychologist, or psychiatrist. Evaluation with the occupational therapist takes place 1 or 2 days after the client has been admitted to the unit. This short delay gives the client an opportunity to adjust to the unit, the staff, other clients, and the daily routine. Evaluation, which takes place over a 2-day period, consists of a general interview and participation in the Fidler Battery. The evaluative findings of the occupational therapist are pooled with those of other staff members. In conjunction with the client, the client's major problem areas are tentatively identified.

The daily schedule, with some flexibility, is as follows:

From 7:00 a.m. to 9:00 a.m. clients get up and dress, have breakfast, straighten up their rooms, and take care of other personal chores. The staff in the meantime have a meeting from 8:30 to 9:00 a.m.

The time from 9:00 a.m. to noon is divided into two periods. During one of these periods each client participates in a small (6 to 7 persons) task-oriented group. The group is designed primarily to facilitate that part of the change process which is concerned with communication. During the other period, clients participate in a variety of activities designed to meet health needs.

Lunch is served at noon with clients having free time until 1:00 p.m.

The time from 1:00 to 4:00 p.m. is again divided into two periods. During one of these periods each client is again involved in a task-oriented group. The group this time is primarily concerned with working through. It should be noted that communication and working through cannot be as easily separated as this division may indicate; rather it is a matter of emphasis. The groups concerned with communication are likely to make considerable use of unstructured activities with a high symbolic potential. The groups designed to enhance working through are likely to make use of activities that are more structured and have a specific end product or goal. The types of activities used and thus the group to which the clients are assigned are dependent on the kinds of universal issues that are being addressed. During the other period, clients, again, usually participate in activities designed to meet health needs. However, clients who are about to return to living in the community are involved in an anticipatory/concurrent topical group designed to facilitate transition to the community.

From 4:00 to 4:30 p.m., three times a week, there is a unit meeting which all clients and staff members attend. The purpose of this meeting is to attend to the business of the unit. There is discussion of current unit problems, interpersonal difficulties, and the like. The meeting has a problem-solving orientation designed to enhance the living and working together of the clients and staff. During this time on the other two days, smaller groups of clients and staff meet together to discuss and organize various evening and weekend activities.

After these meetings, the clients have free time, with dinner being served around 6:00 p.m.

Evening and weekend activities are less structured than those in the 9 to 5 schedule outlined above. Visiting family and friends and/or participation in various community-based activities are encouraged for clients who are able to engage comfortably in such activities. Visitors are also welcome on the unit either to join in the leisure/recreational activities taking place on the unit or to have a private chat with a client. Staff members are available to facilitate interaction between clients and their visitors, to help family members identify how they can be of assistance to the client, and to answer the questions of family members or friends.

Intermediate care on an inpatient unit may or may not be followed by some other type of treatment/intervention once the client has returned to the community. This is usually decided sometime near the end of the client's stay on the unit. If there is to be some further type of care, the client is assisted in moving into that program through participation in the transitional group as discussed above.

Long-Term Care

This discussion focuses on one aspect of long-term care—intervention with clients who have been hospitalized for some period of time and who are now considered able to return to the community (173,239,260, 364,613,639,757,767). Intervention with clients who will not be leaving the institution is discussed in Chapter 30. The population of concern in this section are those clients who have become institutionalized to such an extent that they have little idea of how to function in the community even on a marginal level. They are frequently quite deficient in both task and interpersonal skills. In terms of expected environment, most of these clients will be living in the community in some type of sheltered environment. Ideally, this would be a group home. In reality, it may well be a boarding house or a "single room occupancy" hotel.

The major goal of the program is to help clients become as independent as possible, recognizing the severe limitations that many of these individuals have. The program to be outlined below is based on role acquisition. Neither an analytical nor a developmental frame of reference would be appropriate for this client population.

This hypothetical program takes place in a large public institution on a unit specifically designed to facilitate movement into the community. It is a 20-bed unit. Clients come into the unit from other parts of the institution, with new clients entering as others leave to live in the community. Or, if intervention was not effective, clients return to other parts of the institution. Clients admitted to the unit are screened relative to the probability of being able to manage community living. The criteria used, in general, are, stabilized on medication; not actively psychotic; relatively good physical health; oriented relative to person, place, and time; the capacity to respond appropriately to direct questions; the ability to engage in personal care even if considerable prompting is necessary. The clients stay on the unit for approximately 6 months, although they may stay longer if there is evidence of continuing progress.

Evaluation on the unit is similar to the one outlined for the role acquisition frame of reference. However, much less attention is given to work because it is not anticipated that the majority of clients on the unit will be able to participate in the role of being a worker. Some clients, nevertheless, may be able eventually to participate in a very supportive sheltered workshop program. Less attention is also given to family interaction unless it is anticipated that the client will be returning to his or her family. This is, however, not the usual situation. Most of these clients have pretty much lost contact with their families. Evaluation also includes assessment relative to the need for maintenance and management and the extent to which the client requires assistance in meeting health needs.

It is important to remember that the clients on this unit are more than likely to be nonverbal, retarded in their movements, and functioning at a very low level. The program, therefore, must be highly structured and fairly directive. This is particularly true when clients first come onto the unit. As clients begin to gain some degree of autonomy and problem-solving skills, less structured, less directive approaches may be used. These clients tend to learn with considerable difficulty; thus progress is likely to be very slow. The best approach is direct experience, which includes considerable practice. Much encouragement and reinforcement are needed. In teaching skills, tasks need to be broken down into simple steps, with each step being patiently taught. Initially, tasks should be kept very simple. Finally, it should be noted that these clients often lack knowledge in a broad number of areas. For example, they may not have ever used even the most simple household appliance and have only a vague idea of the value of money. Their knowledge of the community is likely to be minimal.

The program designed for change essentially has four distinct parts: personal care, daily living groups, special skills, and recreation/temporal adaptation. Personal care is given considerable attention in the early morning when clients get up. They are taught how to bathe and groom themselves and how to select appropriate clothes. Such things as making a bed and putting their room in order may also be taught at this time. Personal care also involves assuming responsibility for taking one's own medication. This aspect of the program is graded from teaching the client to ask for medication at the appropriate times to the final step of giving the client a week's supply of medication with responsibility for taking it in the prescribed manner.

About 9:00 a.m., the staff and clients break up into four small groups. These groups, called daily living groups, are structured around the general needs of the unit. Each group, which lasts for the better part of the morning, has an assignment: preparing lunch, care of the unit, unit improvement, special projects, and the like. These assignments are generally rotated every week. The lunch group is responsible for planning the meal and ordering food from the institution's kitchen or purchasing supplies from a local grocery store. In addition to making and serving the meal, the group members are responsible for cleaning up the unit kitchen. (Breakfast and dinner and all weekend meals are served in the same way as they are throughout the institution.) Care of the unit involves daily cleaning of all public areas and the rooms of those clients who are not yet able to take responsibility for this task. Other tasks performed by the group concerned with unit care are such things as periodically waxing the floors or washing the windows. The group concerned with unit improvement takes responsibility for small repairs on the unit and other tasks such as making bookcases, painting the bathroom, and making curtains. They work within a budget provided by the institution. The group involved with special projects performs a variety of services for the unit. One responsibility is the unit laundry. (Each client is responsible for his or her own personal laundry, using facilities that are available on the unit.) Other responsibilities of this group are the care of the bulletin board, making holiday decorations, going on necessary errands, and so forth.

The above outlined tasks of the daily living groups may sound rather complex. However, if broken down appropriately and given adequate guidance, group members are able to carry out these tasks. In addition, the membership of the daily living groups is so structured that each of them include clients that are new to the unit as well as individuals who have been on the unit for some period of time. This variation in groups allows clients at a more advanced level to serve as role models. The more advanced clients often gain considerable satisfaction from being able to assist the newer clients; they also can, at times, be very understanding teachers.

Following lunch and some time for relaxation, clients are involved in learning special skills. This may include instruction in various daily living activities on the unit or out in the community, participation in groups focusing on task skills, or interpersonal skills. For those clients who are ready to leave the unit, there is a transitional group that deals with such topics as housing, financial matters, and use of community resources, planning what one is going to do each day, and the like. Attention is given to the individual situation of each client. This part of the program varies from day to day and from time to time in order to meet the learning needs of the clients on the unit in any given period.

The clients' evenings and weekends are primarily devoted to developing skills relative to recreation and temporal adaptation. Although specific recreational skills may be taught in the afternoon program, evening and weekends include participation in various recreational activities. These activities really have two purposes: developing an appreciation for and the capacity to engage in recreational activities and meeting health needs. The activities may take place on the unit, involve participation in the recreational activities that are part of the institution as a whole, or participation in community-based recreational activities. Temporal adaptation is of concern throughout the entire program, but particular attention is given to this area during evenings and weekends. Prior to admission to this unit clients were frequently used to a regimental schedule of meals and time for sleep. The rest of their day may have also been fairly regimented or a time of essentially nothing to do. On the unit, the clients' weekdays are fairly structured whereas evenings and weekends deliberately are not. Thus, clients are given the opportunity to experience the difference between structured and unstructured time and the opportunity to manage their own time. Adequate use of time in a way that is need-satisfying to the individual is emphasized.

The type of long-term care outlined above is most successful when the client is motivated to leave the institution and return to the community. However, the client usually has been out of the community for such a long time that there is frequently considerable hesitation about returning. The institution has come to be seen as a safe refuge. Thus, the therapist must make community living seem as attractive as possible but, nevertheless, present it in a realistic light. It is emphasized that successful participation in community living is, to a great extent, dependent on what the client does. It is also emphasized that there are support systems available to the client if only he or she is willing to seek them out and use them.

Community-Based Programs

Three programs are described in this section—one for adults, one for adolescents, and one for abusive parents and their children.

A day program for *adults* is one of the most common ways of helping individuals function more effectively in the community. Typically, these programs are conducted between 9:00 a.m. and 4:00 p.m. each weekday. Clients may be referred to the programs after discharge from a hospital, or they may be referred by an agency or individual in the community. The length of time clients participate in the program will depend on their particular needs. The usual length of stay, however, is about 3 months.

A combination of role acquisition and reconciliation of universal issues serves as the bases for most programs, with a greater emphasis on role acquisition. In other words, more attention is given to skills development as opposed to exploration of intrapsychic content. Various types of activity groups are a prominent parts of the program.

When clients enter the program they are assigned to a staff member who is responsible for evaluation with the client and for planning the client's course of intervention. This staff member, or "primary therapist," remains responsible for the client during his or her participation in the program and whatever follow-up is considered to be appropriate.

Although programs vary, typically a day's program is as follows: 9:00 to 10:00 a.m., morning coffee and community meeting; 10:00a.m. to noon, various thematic groups focusing on task skills, interpersonal skills, and daily living activities; noon to 1:00 p.m., lunch prepared by clients and free time just to relax; 1:00 to 4:00 p.m., various anticipatory and concurrent topical groups focusing on family roles; leisure/recreation, work and temporal adaptation. There may also be a task-oriented group for clients who have the capacity to engage in such a group; 4:00 to 5:00 p.m., a twice weekly staff meeting with the other 3 days being devoted to writing evaluation summaries, plans for intervention, and periodic notes. One evening a week, staff members meet with interested family members in a concurrent topical group.

Each client's program is tailored to meet his or her individual learning needs. Emphasis is also placed on providing support relative to dealing with events and situations which the client perceives as particularly stressful.

Most day programs make considerable use of community resources to enhance the development of skills. The gym at a local "Y," for example, may be used a few hours each week to help clients explore and learn various active recreational activities. The nearest supermarket is used to help clients learn how to shop for groceries.

Day programs that appear to be the most successful are those providing follow-up until the individual is able to live independently in the community. Continued follow-up may be necessary for some clients who will always need some guidance relative to dealing with daily life tasks. This is usually provided by a "case manager" who meets with the client on a weekly basis or less often if this is deemed to be appropriate.

The *adolescent* program described here is for individuals of both sexes between the ages of 13 and 18 years of age. It is designed for adolescents who have fairly serious psychosocial problems characterized by withdrawal and depression or acting out kinds of behavior. Individuals with serious substance abuse problems are not included in the program. The overall philosophy of the program is to keep the adolescent in the community and involved with family and school. The frame of reference used is role acquisition, with emphasis on the following areas: appropriate social behavior, in particular with authority and peers; the process of beginning separation from one's parents; adequate sex education; weight control and personal grooming; money management; proper study habits; occupational choice, in particular knowledge of one's skills and interests; and use of community recreational facilities.

This hypothetical program is situated in a large metropolitan area and physically located in a community center. One large room with a small kitchen is set aside for the program, with access to other facilities in the center and to small conference rooms. Participants are drawn from the large public school located near the center as well as from nearby private and parochial schools. Referral to the program is through the local community mental health center. There are approximately 15 participants at any one time. The program is staffed by an occupational therapist and a social worker, with other members of the community health center available for consultation and, when necessary, individual verbal therapy with clients.

The program takes place four afternoons a week and all day Saturday. The participants arrive at the center after their last class of the day. Subsequent to checking in they go to the gym for a program of gross physical activity. As participants arrive at different times, this part of the program is fairly loosely organized. Its purpose is to allow the adolescents to have an opportunity for physical activity after sitting in school all day and to get rid of excess energy. From 3:30 to 4:00 p.m., participants meet together with the two staff members to discuss any problems the group is having in their relationships with each other and in their working together. Plans are also made for the activities that will take place on Saturday.

After this meeting, from 4:00 to 5:30 p.m., activities vary from day to day. One day a week is devoted to activities of daily living. This is usually done in two small groups. The groups are divided by sex when personal grooming is being considered; otherwise they are mixed. Aspects of activities of daily living addressed depend on the needs of the group and may include such things as skin care, care of clothes, comparison shopping, banking transitions, meal preparation, nutritional needs, weight control, simple household repairs, and so forth. The focus of the group is on doing and, wherever possible and appropriate, this takes place in the community.

Two days a week, again between 4:00 and 5:30 p.m., there is a craft program. For clients who have difficulty in the area of task skills, individual arts or craft activities are selected by agreement between the client and therapist. Clients who have more difficulty in the area of social interaction are involved in a thematic group with a shared task. Group members are responsible for selecting, planning, and implementing projects. Emphasis is placed on realistic selection and planning, the decision-making process, and cooperative interaction. The therapist acts primarily as a resource person, moving into the group more actively only when the participants are unable to solve their own problems.

One day a week the 4:00 to 5:30 period is devoted to an anticipatory/concurrent topical group. On this day participants are divided into two groups. Discussion is focused on such problems as family interaction, studying, other school-related difficulties, friendships and recreation, dating and information regarding sexual matters. Temporal adaptation is also an area of concern, particularly in regard to setting aside a sufficient amount of time for study and using that time effectively. Organizing one's time relative to family interaction, activities of daily living and recreation are also discussed. The program ends at 5:30. The staff, however, is available for informal discussion until around 6:00 p.m.

Saturday morning is devoted to involvement in some sort of community project such as cleaning up a park, getting a petition signed, helping to take severely handicapped children on an outing, painting the basement of a local church, and so forth. The purpose of this aspect of the program is twofold: to encourage and to assist the participants in identifying their skills and interests. The latter is also dealt with in the twice weekly craft groups. The community project is selected by the group members. All members may work on one project or two or three projects may be selected. In making the decision, group members are encouraged to take into consideration relevant factors such as time commitment, interest and skills of group members, their values, and so forth. Emphasis is placed on how to negotiate and compromise.

Saturday afternoon is devoted to recreational activities in the community. The group, for example, may visit a museum or a flea market, go to a concert, play softball, or go swimming. The purpose of this activity is to introduce the adolescents to various recreational activities in the community and to assist them in identifying their recreational interests. The group as a whole may participate in one recreational activity together or two or three subgroups may be formed. Activities are selected by group members. The factors emphasized in making decisions regarding community projects are also stressed in decision-making relative to recreational activities. In addition, group members are urged to consider cost and making travel arrangements.

Candidates for the afterschool program are initially screened by the sponsoring community mental health center. On admission to the program, each client participates in an evaluation. Assessment is similar to that outlined for the role acquisition frame of reference. Emphasis is placed on those major areas of concern outlined at the beginning of the description of this program. Parents and the client's school advisor, with the client's permission, are also interviewed as part of the assessment procedure. Subsequent to evaluation the therapist and adolescent, through discussion, identify the adolescent's assets and limitations. The client is encouraged to select particular areas of concern to be worked on while in the program. Areas of concern may, of course, be altered during the client's participation in the program. Reevaluation takes place once a month.

The staff member who participates in evaluation with a given client becomes the client's "primary" therapist. A primary therapist coordinates the client's program, encourages involvement in appropriate learning experiences, and acts as the client's counselor and guide while he is in the program. The primary therapist also serves as the liaison between the program and the school and family.

The staff keeps in close touch with the adolescent's school and family. Telephone contact is encouraged, with an hour being set aside each day when the staff member can be reached. When the client first enters the program, the adolescent and staff members usually visit the client's school advisor. Together they identify problem areas, both academic and social, and seek to devise a plan whereby these problems can be effectively resolved. For example, arrangements for extra help might be made with instructors who teach subjects in which the client is doing poorly. A tutor is found if that is considered necessary. The therapist enlists the support of the school faculty and regularly follows up on all plans that were made.

The parents of the adolescents meet with one of the staff members one night a week for about an hour and a half. These meetings, which take the form of a concurrent topical group, are similar to the parent groups outlined in Chapter 26 to which the reader is referred. One night a month parents and adolescents meet together. These meetings may be structured as a concurrent topical group; a thematic group, in which the adolescent and parents are able to identify and practice more effective ways of relating to each other; or it may involve participating in a recreational activity together. The decision of what type of shared group meeting is preferred is left up to group members. On occasions parents and perhaps siblings join the adolescents in their Saturday afternoon recreational activity. The parents of the adolescents in the program are assisted in identifying ways in which they can help their child with his or her various problem areas. They are also assisted in developing appropriate expectations and more open channels of communication. Support, reinforcement, and encouragement are given at all times.

Adolescents usually participate in the above outlined program for one school semester, although they may, if deemed appropriate, stay for two semesters. There is also a summer program similar to the academic year program but structured somewhat differently. (For further discussion of intervention with adolescents see refs. 184,227,482,769,882,884,909,927).

A program for *abusive parents and their children* has been described by Colman (198). It will be briefly summarized here, with emphasis on the role of the occupational therapist. The project, referred to as the Extended Family Center, offered an alternative to separating children and parents, believing that intervention could best take place when families were allowed to remain intact. Supervision of the families was provided through the daily use of the Center, which was open 9 a.m. to 9 p.m., by the availability of a staff member by telephone 24 hours a day, and by making the Center available after hours as an emergency shelter. The program consisted of daily home visits, a day-care program for the children, verbal group therapy, occupational therapy, individual counseling, and services designed to help clients deal, for example, with community agencies, managing doctor appointments, and doing laundry and grocery shopping. The staff consisted of a director who was a social worker with experience in treating child-abuse families, two administrative assistants, three nonprofessional social workers, one head teacher, five nonprofessional teachers, one occupational therapist, and two "parent professionals." These parent professionals were individuals who had been designated as abusive parents 5 years before the opening of the program and had resolved their immediate problems relative to child abuse prior to their employment. Referrals to the Center were made by local hospitals, juvenile court, protective services, private physicians, and public health nurses. The frame of reference used for the entire program appears to be a combination of analytical and acquisitional.

The overall program was designed to give parents time away from their children, "in order to gain a perspective on their personal problems—separate from those problems exhibited in the relationship with that child" (ref. 198, p. 413). The day-care prgram for the children emphasized the development of age-appropriate skills.

The occupational therapy program, concerned with parents only, was designed to identify the characteristics common to abusive parents and as a nonverbal means of intervention. The description of the program does not outline the means used for evaluation. However, typical goals of the change process are identified as

> providing the parents with the means to develop a greater sense of their identity and self-worth, to learn ways of identifying and working with their process of problem solving, to develop skills to assess their abilities and limitations realistically, to learn to use support systems and to learn to work effectively within a structured situation (ref. 198, p. 415).

The occupational therapy program consisted of a social skills group, individual craft projects, individual informal sessions, a movement group, and a work group. Each of these is discussed briefly.

The social skills group took place in the homelike environment of the Center's living room. Craft projects (discussed shortly) were used to provide a focus around which social skills could be developed and practiced. Emphasis was placed on socially acceptable topics of conversation and on the mutual sharing of thoughts and feelings. Gossip and discussion of sex-related matters, which were inappropriate or caused discomfort to others, were discouraged. The therapist and parent professional acted as models as well as providing leadership.

While in the group each parent was required to work on an individual craft project. The purpose of this activity was to help the parents understand their behavior toward their children through experiencing how they dealt with the structure, problems encountered, and frustrations relative to the task. The projects were also used to assist the parents in making appropriate and well thought out decisions. This process was facilitated through the use of a contractual agreement. "A contract was made each time a parent was ready to choose a new project which stated that, as soon as the project was agreed upon, the parent was not to begin another until the one to which he was committed was completed" (ref. 198, p. 416). To aid in making a viable project decision and to offer a guide to follow when making other decisions, the process involved in doing each project was given in detail before the contract was made. This helped the parents to develop a sense of the investment of time and thought involved before making a decision. When enthusiasm waned or difficulties were encountered, parents were encouraged to "describe what was happening to their project and how they felt about themselves and their work. These discussions helped the parent to relate their behavior on the project to their behavior towards their children" (ref. 198, p. 416).

Individual informal sessions were held spontaneously during, for example, a car ride, over coffee, on a trip to get project supplies, or in the parents' home. The informality and spontaneity enhanced the parents' comfort and willingness to be receptive to learning about themselves. The purpose of these sessions was to deepen the relationship between parent and therapist and to assist the parent in developing an awareness of the therapeutic aspects of the project.

A movement group was begun to explore the discomfort with physical contact the parents seemed to exhibit in relationship to their children. This was a parent group only. Initially, individual exercises were designed to focus on the parents' own body space and how it related to the immediate environment. Later, group exercises were added to give the parents a sense of others in the immediate environment. When paired exercises were included, however, the parents became uncomfortable and group attendance quickly dropped. The group was discontinued. The author of the quoted article suggests that a parent-child movement group may have been more appropriate.

A work program was offered for unemployed parents. These parents, only a small percentage of those assisted through the project, were hired by the Center in various positions. This aspect of the program had two objectives. One was to help the parents develop work skills, take responsibility, and to follow a daily structure. The other objective was to help the parents understand something about their general problems in functioning through observation of their behavior within the context of a work situation. The occupational therapist supervised these parents in their daily work situation and met with them once a week as a group.

This demonstration project, which took place over a period of 2 years, provided services for 25 abusive families. Although not a typical program, it is outlined here to give the reader some idea of the variety of programs and settings in which the occupational therapist deals with problems in psychosocial dysfunction. (For other descriptions of community-based programs see refs. 53, 88, 133, 184, 226, 325, 431, 451, 503, 517, 564, 571, 757, 858,997.)

Outreach Programs

Although there are many types of outreach programs, in the interest of brevity only one will be described here. (For a description of other outreach and nontraditional programs see ref. 573,574,622,993,995.) The program to be outlined was developed by the Occupational Therapy Department at the University of Pennsylvania in conjunction with the Jewish Family Services (575). The program had a dual purpose in that it provided services as well as an educational experience for occupational therapy students. The major service objective of the program was to increase the level of independence in activities of daily living of recently arrived Indochinese refugees. Some of the problems of these refugees were lack of familiarity with the English language, limited financial resources, and dealing with extreme cultural and social differences. They were confronted with the need to make marked changes in established ways of accomplishing ordinary daily living activities, with many tasks having to be completely relearned.

The Jewish Family Service of Philadelphia, the official sponsoring agency for the refugees, took responsibility for providing resettlement services, arranging for adequate housing, necessary medical and dental care, appropriate educational and vocational programs, and obtaining public assistance. The staff, however, was often overwhelmed with simply providing basic social services and had little time to assist the refugees in learning how to adequately perform activities of daily living in their new environment. Thus, the program was developed to facilitate this aspect of the refugees' adjustment.

The frame of reference used as the basis for the program was acquisitional in nature and conceptualized around Maslow's hierarchy of human needs: physiological, safety, love and belonging, esteem and self-actualization. Four students each semester were assigned to the Agency. They worked with the refugees one-half day each week primarily in the client's home and community environment.

Initially, intervention focused on the development of rapport and on a viable means of communication. The latter was accomplished through the use of conversational dictionaries, "body" language (i.e., presenting and acting out the messages, written or drawn signs, and, when necessary, seeking out interpreters). The cultural differences often made it difficult to determine if nonverbal messages were correctly understood. Thus improvement of communication was an ongoing process.

Physiological needs were of primary importance to the refugees. Intervention focused on helping the clients learn to satisfy these needs in an unfamiliar environment.

> The major areas of concern for clients included *[sic]* 1) having enough money to meet rent, clothing and food costs; 2) knowing how to care for their apartments including making repairs, dealing with landlords and cleaning; 3) obtaining, preparing and preserving food; and 4) knowing how to dress and maintain their health in the unfamiliar cold Western climate (ref. 575, p. 12).

More specifically, the clients were assisted in developing housekeeping skills—which products to use for certain types of cleaning, how to prevent food spoilage, and maintaining the apartment free from insects and rodents. The clients were familiarized with American purchasing methods by visiting an open air market (a relatively familiar setting for these refugees), neighborhood supermarkets, and other stores. Some of the refugees had sewing skills which were capitalized on in encouraging them to make some of their own clothes.

The refugees' difficulty in meeting safety needs arose out of lack of familiarity with the neighborhood, the language, and the people. The surrounding environment was viewed as lacking in predictability; there were too many unknowns. Intervention involved orienting the refugees to the physical layout of the commuunty. This included trips into the neighborhood, showing the route to the nearest hospital and to various local shops, pointing out names and numbers of streets and local landmarks. A certain amount of safety initially was provided by the presence of the student-therapists. Clients were also assisted in learning how to read a city map, use the Yellow Pages, and to take public transportation. In order to further satisfy their safety needs, the refugees had to learn something about the social expectations of their new environment. This was accomplished through identifying for the clients modes of behavior that were clearly unacceptable by American standards and through providing feedback concerning the appropriateness of their behavior.

It was, in general, felt that the clients were able to satisfy their love and belonging needs independently. They seemed to do this though "identifying with each other as fellow refugees and redefining their 'family' in terms of their common association with Jewish Family Service" (ref. 575, p. 18). It was recommended, however, that space at the agency be found for the clients so that they would be able to meet together for informal social gatherings and planned group activities. Clients were also encouraged to become involved in social activities with refugees sponsored by agencies other than Jewish Family Service and in activities within the general community.

It was found that the refugees' esteem needs were not being met. This was felt to be due to lack of involvement in meaningful and productive activities. There was, thus, an attempt to identify former types of activities that satisfied esteem needs and, with the clients, decide whether these could be pursued satisfactorily in their new environment. One area where esteem needs could be met for some of the clients was through, once again, becoming adequate housekeepers and through improving the warmth, comfort, and appeal of their homes. The latter was accomplished, for example, through making wall posters, curtains, and pillow covers. For other clients esteem needs were met through taking English classes and through participation in programs designed to develop vocational skills. The student-therapists encouraged the clients to participate in these programs and were willing partners for clients who wished to practice their conversational English.

Self-actualization, the highest order need in Maslow's hierarchy, is believed to be addressed only after lower level needs are satisfied. On the whole, it was felt that the refugees were still in the process of satisfying these lower level needs. Thus, no real effort was made to assist the clients in satisfying their need for self-actualization at this time.

Although this program was limited in scope, it was felt to be very successful. The refugees and agency staff felt that there had been many personal gains for individual clients.

SUMMARY

This chapter has addressed psychosocial components of occupational therapy as they relate to intervention in the area of mental health. Several different types of settings and programs were outlined. As mentioned, these programs should be considered as illustrative only. There are other types of mental health settings and programs in which occupational therapists participate. Hopefully, this chapter has provided an overview of the occupational therapist's role in assisting those with problems in the area of mental health.

28 Physical Disabilities

The psychosocial aspects of physical disabilities are of paramount importance in assisting physically disabled individuals to function at the highest possible level (541,618,822,823,900,939,981). Some physical restoration and the development of compensatory skills alone are not sufficient. Although they are an extremely important part of the intervention process, they are only a part. Without attention to the psychosocial aspects of disabilities and to chronic illness, the individual is far less likely to create a life-style that is satisfying to him- or herself and compatible with the needs of others.

This chapter is primarily addressed to assisting individuals with acquired disabilities. For ease in presentation it is divided into five sections: meeting health needs, management, and maintenance; the change process; the family; intervention in the home; and program planning. Prior to reading this chapter it is suggested that the reader review the section on Chronic Illness/Disability in Chapter 5.

MEETING HEALTH NEEDS, MANAGEMENT, AND MAINTENANCE

The following discussion is fairly brief in that these areas of intervention have been described in Chapter 17 in greater detail. The purpose of this section is to highlight those points that are particularly pertinent to the care of hospitalized individuals who are physically disabled.

Meeting Health Needs

Attention should be given to meeting health needs immediately. In addition to humanitarian reasons, evaluation and intervention in the other aspects of practice are likely to be far easier and more effective through meeting health needs. Some suggestions in regard to meeting health needs are as follows:

Psychophysical needs. Some clients who are physically disabled are on a very strict diet. The therapist may assist them in adhering to that diet by listening to their complaints and agreeing with them that it may not be a pleasant experience. More positively, the therapist may assist the client by arranging for mealtime to be as satisfying as possible. Foods and trays can be made to look attractive, interesting herbs may be added to make food more palatable. Eating with others and good conversation make mealtime more enjoyable. These components should be given consideration whether the client is in the hospital or at home. Helping the client prepare satisfying meals within his or her dietary instructions should be given attention. There are many cookbooks that deal with special diets. These should be explored by the therapist and made readily available to clients. This is potentially a far better way to assist clients in staying on a particular diet than by giving them a list of foods that they should not eat.

Many people who are physically disabled are very concerned about their personal appearance. The physically disabled person, particularly in the initial period of disability, is often preoccupied with his or her body. Every effort should be made to assist the client in looking as attractive as possible. Clean, well-cut hair, a smooth shave or makeup, jewelry, and clothing that is both functional and stylish are all very helpful. The area of self-concept often needs to be dealt with in the change process. In the interim, however, looking as attractive as possible goes a long way in helping an individual to feel good about the self.

Clients who are bedridden for a period of time need a variety of stimuli and activities that will catch and hold their interest. There are many activities that can be done comfortably in bed. Some, however, require adaptations. Problem solving on the part of the therapist may be necessary. If at all possible, the client should also be involved in the problem solving. This in itself is a stimulating activity. The adaptations made should be reasonable. That is they should not be so extensive or bizarre that they destroy the nature of the activity or the pleasure in doing the activity.

The need for temporal balance and regularity. One of the major difficulties of clients in a rehabilitation center is that their day is likely to be filled with a tightly scheduled round of various therapies and other appointments. In addition, they are likely to have little to say in the matter of scheduling. There are many practical reasons for this. If at all possible, however, the scheduling of therapies and appointments should be sufficiently loose to allow for appropriate breaks or short rest periods. The client should also be consulted regarding alterations that may make the schedule more tolerable or even acceptable.

The busy weekday schedule of the client is often in sharp contrast to the long empty hours of the evening and weekend. This is particularly true for clients who have few visitors or who are unable to go out into the community. Although clients may need to relax during these times, a variety of recreational activities should also be available. The opportunity to select various activities and the time when one will participate in activities gives clients a sense of being in control of how they will use their time. Some clients may need assistance in selecting and actually getting to activities, particularly if they are depressed. The therapist, in this case, needs to provide both guidance and encouragement.

Difficulty in the area of temporal adaptation can present a serious problem for hospitalized clients who must stay in bed. This is particularly true for clients who are alert and feeling relatively well. Time tends to drag interminably, punctuated only by hospital routines and whatever suspense can be generated by daytime television. It is frequently helpful if the therapist assists the client in establishing his or her own routine, a time schedule for doing various different activities. This not only gives the client a sense of having control over time but it also gives the day and evening a predictable structure that is satisfying to the client's needs.

Problems relative to temporal adaptation for the client living in the community are discussed in the section on change process.

Safety. The lack of adequate and reliable information is one aspect of the need for safety that may not be met in a clinical setting. Information regarding the client's disability or illness, the various treatment and intervention methods being used, the expected course of events, and the probable degree of permanent impairment should be freely given. It is, however, important not to overload the client with information. Ideally the therapist and other staff members answer questions as they are raised. However, the majority of clients, if not most, are hesitant in raising questions. Thus, information should be given in the amount and detail that the client can understand and integrate.

Another aspect of safety that is often of concern to the physically disabled individual is the possibility of injury. They may be afraid that they will fall or that they will not be able to get help when it is needed. The client needs to be reassured and shown that every precaution is being taken to prevent injury. The use of various call bells should be demonstrated so that the client knows that it is quite easy to summon help at any time.

Love and acceptance. Many clients who are recently disabled do not see themselves as being lovable or acceptable. They have such negative feelings about their disability and perhaps their physical appearance that it spreads to their total concept of themselves as a person. This area frequently needs to be dealt with in the change process. But in the interim, clients need to experience a considerable amount of love and acceptance. Because of clients' negative feelings about themselves, it is often necessary to demonstrate love and acceptance in a somewhat exaggerated manner. There is a sense of having to get "through to" the client so that he or she is able to experience satisfaction of this need. Family members should also be assisted in demonstrating love and acceptance in a somewhat more pronounced way than may typically be their style.

Group association. Many people who are recently disabled have a tendency to isolate themselves from others. They feel badly about themselves, and being with other people who are disabled may remind them of their difficulties. Regardless of these actions and feelings, the individual does need the companionship of others. Gentle encouragement should be used to promote interactions with others. Helping the client to become involved with another client through a shared task mutually interesting to both is often the initial step. The task should be the focal point. This is not the time or situation where the discussion of problems is encouraged. Discussion of difficulties may occur spontaneously but that is not the purpose of the interaction in this situation. Although interaction with others is encouraged, the client may also need time to be alone to think or to engage in a solitary activity. This is particularly true in a setting where clients live in close quarters with each other and where it is difficult to avoid at least some level of interaction with others for a considerable portion of the day. It should be remembered that there is considerable variation in the degree to which an individual needs group association as opposed to time for being alone.

Clients confined to bed also are in need of group association. This may indeed be somewhat more difficult to arrange but it is often worth the effort. With, of course, the client's permission, ambulatory clients are encouraged to visit the client. Common interests, age, and cultural background of the client should be taken into consideration when selecting people as visitors. Bedridden clients should also be urged to call their friends and perhaps other bedridden clients.

Mastery. Many clients ultimately are able to gain a sense of mastery through their efforts to maximize function and perfect compensatory skills. Until this becomes a reality for clients, however, the therapist often needs to assist clients in finding activities through which they can experience a sense of mastery. Creative adaptations often allow clients to engage in preferred activities despite their physical limitation.

Esteem. Clients who have been recently disabled often have a very low level of self-esteem. This problem is frequently dealt with in the change process. Nevertheless, the therapist should attend to the client's self-esteem needs until the client is more independent in this area. Helping the client to receive recognition for something he or she has done or is doing may be somewhat difficult in an institutional setting. One way in which esteem needs can be satisfied is through the staff's explicit recognition of the work that the client is doing as he or she participates in the rehabilitation process. Clients' efforts should be acknowledged and commended. Each progressive step toward function should be cause for rejoicing. Another way that a client's esteem needs can be met is through helping the client be of assistance to others. Clients who have not been on the unit for some time, for example, can be given the responsibility of orienting new clients. Clients can be encouraged to help each other in any way possible and to visit others who may be confined to bed. One client helping another to deal with depression or anxiety can be of great benefit to both clients.

Sexual. Direct gratification of sexual needs within an institution may be somewhat difficult. However, one means of gratifying sexual needs is to interact with the client as a sexual being. Treating another individual as if he or she were asexual is often very destructive to the individual's sense of self. Home visits should be encouraged if that is at all possible. Sufficient privacy should be ensured when the client has visitors. If acceptable to the client, masturbation should be encouraged.

Pleasure. Although rehabilitation is demanding of time and energy and may, at times, be painful, it need not be dealt with as an entirely serious matter. The therapist's capacity to bring a light touch, a sense of humor, and a spirit of adventure to the rehabilitation process can make the process far more pleasurable than it might otherwise be. The therapist's mood, of course, should be differentially matched to that of the client. The therapist is also concerned with helping the client find activities, outside of the rehabilitation process, that are pleasurable.

Self-actualization. The vast majority of clients who are participating in a rehabilitation program are concerned with meeting the health needs described above. With this preoccupation, they frequently have little time or energy to attend to self-actualization needs. If this, however, is not the case, the therapist should provide every possible assistance to the client so that the need may be met.

Management

The various reactions to becoming physically disabled have been discussed in Chapter 5. These reactions are normal and, on the whole, a healthy part of the adjustment process. Nevertheless, there are times when these reactions are excessive either in terms of duration or intensity. In such an event the client may well need assistance in managing these reactions (900,979,981).

Of primary importance is indicating to clients that strong emotional reaction to disability is usual and to be expected; the client has a right to have these feelings. Clients should be encouraged to express fears, anxieties, and worries about their disability openly. The therapist needs to be accepting of these feelings and in no way minimize the seriousness or enormity of the client's problems. Cheerfulness and optimism are essential to being an effective therapist, but such attitudes should not be used to minimize clients' expressions of feelings or problems. Although cheerfulness and optimism are important, it is also helpful for the therapist to express irritation and anger when appropriate. This assists clients in realizing that expression will not lead to loss of the therapist's support. It may be useful to create situations where clients can safely express their strong feelings verbally, i.e., a situation where it is perfectly all right to blow off steam. Activities that allow and encourage the nonverbal expression of strong emotions should also be available.

Reality testing is an important part of helping clients manage their feelings. The therapist can be of assistance by outlining in a matter-of-fact way the problems facing the client. This allows the client to assess whether his or her fears are greater than warranted by the objective situation. Presentation of the actual facts surrounding the accident or medical incidents that have caused the client's disability often allows the client to view the past events in a more realistic way. This often diminishes the client's anger, that which is directed toward herself, other people, or fate.

Cultural groups and social classes have different beliefs about emotions and the appropriateness of their expression. As Verslays points out, some clients need help in identifying, labeling, accepting, and understanding reasons for their feelings and need support and guidance in dealing with them. Adequate management of reactions to disability greatly increases the amount of energy the client has available for participation in the change process and for making appropriate future plans.

Reactions to disability vary from individual to individual but the most common are depression, anger, denial, dependency, and anxiety. Some suggested means of managing these responses have been outlined in Chapter 17.

Maintenance

Concurrent maintenance of performance components and development tasks is of primary importance during the rehabilitation process (405,541,618,640,822,823, 981,982,1054). Inadequate concurrent maintenance may lead to serious deterioration of the client upon discharge or at least to a period of regression. In other words, the client may physically be able to perform at a fairly high level. However, if the other areas of human function have not been maintained, the client may be at a distinct disadvantage when she returns to the community.

Although attention may need to be given to specific performance components and developmental tasks, the overall orientation of the rehabilitation center is of primary importance. It is detrimental to the maintenance of function for the staff to be overprotective and authoritarian. Clients need as much as possible to have an opportunity to manage their own affairs. It is tempting to become dependent, especially when such behavior is encouraged by the attitudes of the staff. Clients should be encouraged to make decisions, engage in problem solving, and to take risks. Rather than being unduly protected from possible failure, most clients prefer to experiment, to test their abilities and limitations. Support should, of course, be provided when failure does occur.

Another important component of general maintenance of function is contact with family, friends, and co-workers. Through such interactions the client's relationships, repertoire of role behavior, and interests are much more likely to be maintained. If visiting is a problem because of distance, or other circumstances, liberal use of the telephone should be encouraged. Writing letters or short notes is also a way of maintaining contact. In addition, it helps to maintain cognitive function.

For more specific information regarding maintenance, the reader is referred to Chapter 17.

THE CHANGE PROCESS

Rehabilitation should be as much concerned with psychosocial components as with physical components. Adequate psychosocial adjustment, including the individual's acceptance of disability and the self as a worthy human being, is considered to be one of the most important factors in successful rehabilitation. Psychosocial components are a determining factor to the extent in which clients are able to become realistically independent and maintain independence after returning to the community. It is also, of course, a major factor in the degree to which the individual is able to live a satisfying life.

The change process involved in helping an individual adjust to a disability may be based on any of the three types of frames of reference that have been described. Most typically it is based on an analytical or acquisitional frame of reference or on a combination of these two. A combination is probably the best and the most often used. Regardless of the frame of reference being used as the bases for the change process, the following are a few general principles to be kept in mind (149,823).

It is essential that the client be involved in goal setting and planning intervention. The client and therapist need to see themselves as collaborators in a partnership. The client's goals initially may be somewhat unrealistic. As the client gains a greater understanding of her capacities and limitations, he or she is in a better position to establish more realistic goals.

Information about the client's medical condition, rehabilitation in general, and the occupational therapy process should be provided at a time and in a manner that make it meaningful for the client. The information needs to be repeated as often as necessary, and graciously.

The same staff members, if at all possible, should be responsible for the client's daily treatment/intervention. The staff members that a client sees regularly are likely to be the people with whom a client is most willing to discuss personal matters. It has also been suggested that each client select one staff member who will act as an advocate for the client. In this role the staff member would keep watch over the client's interests as defined by the client. Particularly in a large rehabilitation center, a client may feel that he or she has no one person to turn to for assistance. An advocate may fulfill this need.

The change process should be seen as preparation for living in the community, not oriented to adjustment to the clinical setting.

Only a small part of psychosocial adjustment is likely to take place in the clinical setting. This is a long-term process, which will continue for a matter of months if not years. Thus, realistic goals should be set in this area.

With these principles in mind the following discussion will briefly describe the use of reconciliation of universal issues and role acquisition respectively as the bases for the change process.

Reconciliation of Universal Issues

With the onset of a serious physical disability an individual's life situation is usually markedly altered. Because of this change the individual's current and typical way of reconciling the various universal issues is likely to no longer be effective (640,981,982). In addition, old fears and anxieties concerning universal issues may be reawakened. Thus the client may be:

- Uncertain about the nature of reality; the ideas others have about one's disability; how people feel about oneself; the best course of action to take relative to solving multiple problems;
- Mistrustful of others and the help they may offer;
- Fearful of any kind of intimacy. Having feelings of being unlovable, the client may reject the offer of love or affection from others;
- Overcome by feelings of inadequacy to the point where the individual cannot identify any positive personal characteristics;
- Concerned about being dependent on others or of having no one to be dependent on. Conversely, the individual may take the stance that the only acceptable course of action is to become totally dependent;
- Concerned about whether one will be seen by others as sexually desirable or whether one will be able to participate successfully in sexual activities;
- Unable to deal with aggression, directing it primarily toward the self or indiscriminately toward others;
- Unable to deal with the loss of physical function, cognitive capacity, usual appearance, or life plans.

The change process is designed to assist the client in being able to articulate the various ideas and feelings associated with the universal issues and to test them in a shared reality. It frequently becomes readily apparent that the client has a set of values and ideas that makes the reconciliation of universal issues, given one's current life situation, extremely difficult. Clients, as a product of their particular culture, frequently have negative feelings toward many types of disabilities, toward any alteration in physical appearance that deviates from the norm and from being dependent. Consequently, they often have negative feelings about themselves as a person and about their bodies in particular. In addition, clients are confronted with the very real prejudices of society against those who are disabled. A change process based on reconciliation of universal issues is designed to help clients become aware of their values and ideas and society's. Through communication, reality testing, and working through, clients are assisted in modifying their values and ideas in such a way that they are able to find more adaptive and satisfying ways to reconcile universal issues. All universal issues are important, but particular attention should be given to the issue of loss. This is discussed further in Chapter 30.

Role Acquisition

Emphasis in two particular areas has been found to be useful in helping an individual deal with the psychosocial components of disability (99,405,496,541,618, 640,643,748,822,823,878,900,979,981,982,1054). First there should be emphasis on the cognitive aspect of skill learning. Rather than demonstrating a particular skill and encouraging practice, the therapist should assist the individual in identifying the basic principles utilized in performing a particular task. This is particularly true for tasks that cannot be rehearsed during formal rehabilitation. An example of this idea is the teaching of energy conservation/work simplification. Although some methods of energy conservation may be taught for the purpose of illustration and reinforcement, considerable time should be spent on helping the client learn the basic principles behind these methods. These then may be applied in a variety of situations in the client's home.

Second, involvement with people who have successfully completed rehabilitation facilitates the learning process. Ideally, these should be individuals who have disabilities similar to those of the client. Successful rehabilitants can act as role models as well as providing very practical information. Some clients feel more comfortable talking with successful rehabilitants about various problems than with staff members. Contact or communication with disability-specific organizations or self-help groups while the client is still in a rehabilitation center is also useful. This provides an opportunity to interact with appropriate role models and gives clients an important source of support after return to the community.

The following, more specific discussion focuses on the various continuums of the role acquisition frame of reference as they apply to the physically disabled population.

Task skills. All of the various task skills are important, but two of them are likely to need particular attention—problem solving and frustration tolerance. With the onset of a disability, clients are confronted with a wide variety of problems; some very concrete as in how to perform a given task, others more complex or abstract as in how to deal with a son's or daughter's negative response to one's disability. Although a disabled person may have the usual amount of problem-solving skills, these skills often need to be refined. The major way that this is accomplished is through presenting all tasks and activities as problems to be solved. Solution giving should be avoided if at all possible. When a solution must be given, the therapist reviews the process of reaching the solution step by step. It is within this context that the articulation of basic principles is particularly important. These principles may be articulated by the therapist or, more fruitfully, by the client. All independent problem solving is reinforced, even when the client arrives at a solution that is not entirely compatible with the solution the therapist might have proposed.

Disabled individuals are frequently confronted with many tasks that are far more difficult to perform now than previously. They will, more than likely, find this a very frustrating experience. Typical ways of dealing with frustration may no longer be effective simply because the sense of frustration is so much greater. Initially, the therapist begins with activities that the client is able to accomplish, but frustrating tasks will also eventually need to be addressed. The client is cautioned to relax and proceed slowly, to take a break when a sense of frustration arises, and so forth. Approaching an activity as a problem to be solved also limits frustration. The client is encouraged to articulate feelings of frustration rather than keep them inside or act them out through excessively aggressive actions. The client should also be reassured that the performance of most tasks will become, with practice, less frustrating. Through the development of all task skills, the client is likely to once again have at least some sense of mastery over the environment.

Interpersonal skills. As with task skills, all of the interpersonal skills are important. In addition to those skills outlined in Chapter 26, most clients need to learn to (a) communicate effectively with medical personnel and others associated with the rehabilitation process; (b) make their needs known and to ask for help appropriately; to present their concerns and needs effectively to others; (c) cope with the nondisabled public; (d) deal wih staring, inappropriate questions, avoidance, and rejection; and (e) supervise those individuals who will provide various services in their home or relative to transportation.

These skills can be learned through role playing and through direct practice in the community. Sufficient practice is important here as it is in the development of any skill. A one- or two-time trial is not sufficient practice for the skill to be applied spontaneously and effectively. It also has been suggested that many of the above listed interpersonal skills can be acquired through the client attending and speaking for him- or herself at relevant conferences and meetings.

Family interaction. The most important concern here is to maintain the client's various roles within the family. Although there may be some cultural constraints that make this rather difficult, every effort should be made to support the client's familial roles. Because of deficits in physical function, the client may be unable to perform many of the task components usually associated with various familial roles. Strategies need to be developed to compensate for the loss of these components or to circumvent these tasks which the client can no longer perform. A problem-solving approach should be used to investigate alternative ways of fulfilling role requirements. This, of course, can only be accomplished with the cooperation of other family members. Enlisting the family's cooperation and dealing with the area of sexuality are discussed in a later section.

Activities of daily living. Developing skill in the performance of activities of daily living is tremendously important to an individual who is physically disabled. The more skill an individual has, the more likely he or she is to experience a sense of independence and competence. To facilitate adequate skill development, the teaching of activities of daily living should be individualized rather than presented in a routine manner. The skills to be practiced ought to be selected by the client, not those that have been stipulated by custom. Only adaptive equipment and assistive devices that are practical for use in the client's home should be introduced. Instruction in how to repair equipment and devices should be provided as well as information about how to secure replacements.

Two areas of activities of daily living that are frequently important to the disabled individual are transportation and dealing with financial matters. If necessary and appropriate, arrangements for driver training and car modifications should be made. For clients who are unable to drive, the means whereby the client can secure adequate transportation is carefully explained, including a listing of agencies through which such services can be obtained. Good transportation is often one of the major factors in allowing the individual to be employed and in being able to enjoy recreational activities in the community.

The onset of a disability frequently alters an individual's financial status. This is often true even if the individual is able to return to work. There are likely to be many ongoing medically related expenses as well as increased expenses for such things as household help and transportation, special diet, and so forth. The client may well need help in finding and applying for financial assistance. In addition, added expenses may require a substantial revision of the individual's or the family's budget. The therapist may be able to help directly in this area, or the client and/or family may be assisted in securing the help of a financial advisor. All possible aid should be given in this area since worry about financial matters can impede rehabilitation and adjustment to disability. When unresolved, it can also become a source of conflict in the family, something that a family with a disabled member does not need.

School/work. A rehabilitation center may have a formal school program. This is particularly true if the center is designed for long-term rehabilitation and has school-age clients. Other centers, often more short-term in nature, are likely to have a tutorial program provided by the local school district. Whatever the structure used for the continuation of clients' education, the therapist should be sure that clients' schedules are such that they are able to attend classes or tutorial sessions regularly. Time is also scheduled for study and a quiet place arranged for this activity. A good working relationship between therapist and teacher is important for the success of the total rehabilitation process. The teacher is often dealing with psychosocial problems similar to those of concern to the therapist, thus there needs to be coordination of approaches.

The continuing education of the college student is also important. Emphasis is placed on the client remaining in the student role during rehabilitation. Although a college education does not guarantee successful adaptation to a disability, it does help. The client is frequently better prepared for a job that does not require a good deal of physical activity, often a prerequisite if one is disabled. Remaining in the student role may be facilitated by assisting the client to arrange for taking extension courses. These may be courses that can be applied toward the client's degree or simply courses in areas that the client may like to explore. When extension courses are not feasible, the client should be encouraged to study further in the area of his or her college major. This may be a time when the student can read some of the books that were on the "suggested reading" lists given out in various courses. Whatever arrangements are made, specific time should be set aside in the client's daily schedule for study. This is not an activity that should be left for evenings, weekends, or whenever the client has some free time. Study is an important part of the rehabilitation process and should be dealt with as such. The therapist provides sufficient encouragement and reinforcement to keep the student at and enjoying the task of studying.

One of the major goals of intervention for a client who was in the worker role prior to the onset of a disability is to maintain the client in that role (262,425, 426,518,960). Early in the rehabilitation process, the client's capacity—physical, psychological, and cognitive—is assessed relative to his/her ability to return to former employment. When the possibility of returning to former employment is minimal or completely out of the question, vocational evaluation focuses on assessment of the client's assets and limitations for the purpose of determining the types of jobs which the client is likely to be able to perform successfully. This evaluation and subsequent steps necessary for a change in the type of employment is closely coordinated with the work of the vocational rehabilitation counselor.

With a young person who has never worked and who is able to work, the situation is somewhat more complex. Assessment is again addressed to what types of jobs the individual is capable of doing. There may be a need for the individual to develop basic work habits and assistance may be needed in helping the client to identify work interests. A vocational rehabilitation counselor should, of course, be involved in this process.

For some clients, work in the community is feasible if adequate transportation is available and if special adaptations can be made in the work setting. In this case the therapist must work closely with the client and employer for the special arrangements that need to be made. This may involve a change in work hours or providing an opportunity for periodic rest periods. On the other hand, it may involve extensive alteration in the work setting, including the installation of special equipment.

Whatever the special needs, it is often useful for the therapist to visit the work setting. On-site assessment enables the therapist to have a better understanding of the problems the client may encounter and ways of minimizing the problems.

In addition to adequate physical arrangement in the work setting, it may also be necessary for the therapist to help the employer and fellow workers adjust psychologically to the return or new employment of a disabled worker. One suggestion for accomplishing this is through exploring the ideas that people in the work setting have about what the worker will be like and what his or her needs may be. These ideas can then be discussed and subjected to reality testing. Ideally, misconceptions are eliminated so that people in the work setting are comfortable in interacting spontaneously and warmly with the client. If necessary, particular ways of interacting with the client may be suggested. The employer or the client's immediate supervisor is often the key person in the client's physical and psychological adjustment to the work setting. Thus, particular attention is given to helping this individual.

As mentioned, every effort should be made to enable the client to be employed in the community. When, however, this is not possible, employment in the home should be considered. The technical advances in communication make home-centered employment increasingly feasible (914). Knowledge of this area and the various opportunities for employment will help the therapist guide the client in exploring various possibilities. Home employment often requires some rearrangement of the home and the installation of equipment. This may necessitate alteration in the familiar use of space and in the scheduling of their daily activities. Thus, it is imperative that family members be involved in all phases of the planning for home employment.

There are times when even home employment is out of the question. When this is the situation and the individual has previously been a worker, attention must be given to the loss of a significant social role. Being faced with this loss is often exceptionally difficult as it is compounded by the loss of physical function. The client should be encouraged to identify and talk about this loss and to mourn for it in an appropriate manner.

Play/leisure/recreation. Play is discussed in Chapter 29, Developmental Disabilities. Thus, focus here is on leisure/recreational activities. This social role is sometimes considered secondary in the rehabilitation process, more attention being given to physical restoration, work, and general adjustment to disability. Attention should be given to this area, for leisure/recreation activities can be a profound source of pleasure. Important for all clients, this area needs to be given particular attention for those clients who are no longer able to work.

During evaluation, the client and therapist assess whether the client is likely to be able to participate in leisure/recreational activities that were enjoyed prior to the onset of disability. Those activities requiring considerable physical exertion, manual dexterity, and mobility outside the home, for example, may no longer be easily engaged in. The extent to which the individual will have to alter preferred leisure/recreational activities will, of course, be dependent on the nature and severity of the client's disability.

When intervention is required, the client is likely to need assistance in identifying interests. This is often best accomplished through trial participation in a variety of activities that take into consideration the client's assets and limitations. Many times these activities will be home centered, solitary, cognitive, and of a passive nature. Nevertheless, activities that encourage the client to go out into the community, require interaction with others, and allow for an optimal amount of physical exercise are also explored. Moreover, attention is given to participation in various community service activities. The availability of community recreational resources should also be investigated. When necessary, clients are assisted in developing specific recreational skills such as how to play chess or use a table loom.

Social isolation and insufficient friends may be a potential problem area. This is particularly true when interaction with friends was primarily in the context of activities in which the client is no longer able to participate. Thus, a new circle of friends may need to be developed. This may be particularly difficult when the individual is essentially homebound. However, there are organizations who match pen pals and other homebound people to whom the client can talk by telephone. The use of citizens band equipment and communication via ham radio are other ways to combat excessive solitude. There are also service organizations whose members visit homebound individuals. These organizations should be contacted and appropriate arrangements made by the client. Whether primarily homebound or fairly mobile, it is suggested that the disabled person cultivate friend relationships with both disabled and nondisabled people. A predominance of either type of friends is, on the one hand, likely to be excessively narrow in focus or, on the other hand, leave the client at times feeling like an outsider.

Participation in a variety of satisfying leisure/recreational activities and friend relationships is often dependent on the availability of adequate and relatively inexpensive transportation. It cannot be emphasized enough how important this factor is in the overall adjustment to a disability and to a satisfying life in the community.

Temporal adaptation. Temporal adaptation is likely to be a problem for many disabled persons. The organization of time and daily routines used prior to the onset of disability may no longer be effective. One of the reasons that clients need to alter their use of time is closely related to the necessity of revising life goals. It has, in fact, been suggested that the reshaping of life goals should constitute the primary focus of rehabilitation. This is particularly true when an individual has become severely disabled. In the process of setting priorities relative to temporal adaptation—as outlined in Chapter 26—the individual is given an opportunity to look at both immediate and long-term life goals. This process, sometimes referred to as value clarification, encourages the individual to formulate realistic life goals. The setting of life goals not only serves as a motivating force, but it also gives the individual a sense of personal control and responsibility.

The change process as outlined in this section has primarily focused on the client as an individual outside the context of any social matrix. However, rehabilitation is likely to be far more effective if family members are intimately involved in the process. It is to this aspect of intervention that the next section is addressed.

THE FAMILY

The family as a unit and as individual members are effected by the disability of a family member. They often need as much assistance in adjusting to the individual's disability as the individual (618,823,981,982,1054). The staff should never expect the family to demonstrate the ability to cope with a disabled family member immediately. Their adjustment process, as outlined in Chapter 5, is as complex and lengthy as that of the client.

The three major goals in working with a family are to enable them to (a) maintain the client's roles in the family; (b) give the client the kind of support that is needed at any particular time—being available, willing to listen, urging the client toward his goals, providing direct physical assistance, and so forth; and (c) allow the client to be as independent as possible.

As a major factor in facilitating the client's adjustment, the family should be intimately involved in making decisions with the individual and with health personnel and in planning for the future. Involvement should begin with the initial onset of the illness and be based on accurate and complete information about the illness and available options. Family members should be involved in clinics, conferences, and trips with the client into the community. This allows the family to gain a more accurate impression of the client's assets and limitations. Family members should be given adequate instruction in how to care physically for the client and, if appropriate, rehabilitation procedures. If the client's activities in the home must be restricted in some way, clear guidelines should be provided as to what is and is not permitted. This is particularly important for clients who have cardiac and pulmonary problems (99,748,878).

Education of the family in these matters may be done by the therapist or, preferably, by the client. Through assisting the client to educate family members, the therapist helps the client to be seen as a functional family member. If the therapist must take responsibility for educating the family, the client should be present at all therapist-family conferences. This diminishes any tendency toward suspiciousness on the part of the client. It also diminishes the possibility of client-family discord over conflicting messages.

In helping families adjust to a disabled family member and to the necessary adjustments in family life, the family as a whole, or particular members of the family, essentially become the client. Similar to working with the disabled individual, it is suggested that the change process be based on a combination of the reconciliation of universal issues and role acquisition frames of reference. Family members need an opportunity to articulate their ideas and feelings and to seek a different resolution of various universal issues. They also may need assistance in refining interpersonal skills, particularly in the area of being assertive. Components of all social roles may need to be altered or new roles taken on, as, for example, the wife who must return to work.

Not all families have the resources to care for a disabled family member. Attempting to keep the disabled member in the home may seriously undermine the stability of the family and impede family members in the continuing mastery of their developmental tasks. The decision of whether the disabled individual is to return to the family home should, ideally, be made by the client and family in consultation with the rehabilitation team. Prior to making any decision, the following questions should be addressed by all involved parties (1054):

1. Does the family sincerely want the individual to remain in the home and does the individual want to remain?
2. Is the family willing to accept the disability and the familial and social disruptions that may be caused by the individual's disability?
3. How readily is the family able to accept change in the individual's behavior, knowing the ramifications of such behavior?

4. Are there family members who are working against efforts toward habilitation/rehabilitation and why?
5. What resources can be utilized to maintain the individual in the home?
6. How much external support does the family have and need; how willing are they to accept assistance, and are the necessary resources available?
7. Are the alternative arrangements that might be made for the individual better than the living situation that can be provided by the family?

It is very important that family members are not made to feel guilty if they decide that it is best for them and the client that the client move to an alternative living situation. Rather, they should be given support and encouraged to remain involved with the client. Assistance should be given in selecting an appropriate sheltered environment with as much input as possible from the client. The family should be encouraged to visit the family member regularly and, if possible, arrange for him or her to return home for occasional weekends and holidays.

It has been found that even very severely disabled women, if they are married and have children, are able to return to the family home and maintain a part of their usual role function. The planning and organizing aspect of the homemaker role can be done by the disabled woman, with other family members carrying out the actual tasks. The therapist's role in this case would be to help the homemaker refine planning and organizational skills and develop skills in supervising family members. On the other hand, when a husband and father, who has been the primary wage-earner, is severely disabled and unable to engage in the worker role, the economic situation of the family is likely to deteriorate. In such a situation the stability of the family frequently becomes very precarious. This is a family at risk which may need special assistance and support (981).

Finally, as important as the family is, it should not be expected to compensate for the individual's deficits in occupational performances. The individual must be assisted in maintaining familial roles, but he or she must also be encouraged to develop an identity separate from that of being a family member. If this does not occur, family members, and ultimately the individual, will find their lives highly circumscribed and lacking in many areas of need satisfaction.

Sexuality

Sexual function or activity is a specific area of concern for many disabled individuals and their partners (201,729,837,895). Problems as a result of physical changes may require a great deal of adjustment for both partners. Partners must often learn new patterns of sexual behavior to compensate for deficits imposed by disability. Oral and manual manipulation and prosthetic devices may be used to satisfy a sexual partner. Different positions may be used to minimize spasticity or to compensate for weakness. Bowel and bladder disturbances often present embarrassing, logistical complications, which partners must manage within the context of sexual activity. The role of being a caretaker relative to one's partner's bowel, bladder, and menstruation needs and being an intimate sexual partner are sometimes difficult to integrate. Finding sufficient privacy when one or both partners need a nonpartner caretaker in close attendance may present problems.

The essentially mechanical problems and solutions mentioned above are important in the sexual adjustment of partners. However, the psychological component is far more significant. Perhaps the most important factor is the ability of the partners to communicate in an open and honest fashion with each other. Concerning alterations in sexual practices, for example, both partners need to be able to explore various possibilities and to be able to share whether a particular practice is acceptable and satisfying to them aside from the feelings of the other partner. Other important factors are the partner's acceptance of the disabled individual as an exciting, need-satisfying sexual being, the stability of the partnership, sexual compatibility prior to the onset of illness, the importance of sexual activity in the relationship, and the willingness of both partners to experiment. Although partners essentially have to work out their own sexual adjustment together, information about the sexual aspects of the particular disability and alternative means of sexual gratification is extremely helpful.

For some partners, brief counseling may also be useful. The types of counseling used will depend on the client's level of comfort. It may involve giving the client a book or pamphlet to read. This may be follwed by discussion between the therapist and client or discussion may take place without reference to the written material. The same methods may be used with the client's partner. In either case the therapist encourages the client and partner to discuss sexual issues together. It is often useful for the client to be involved in an anticipatory or concurrent topical group that is at least partly concerned with sex-related matters. Ideally, this group is made up of clients who have similar disabilities. The group may consist of clients only or clients and their partners. The latter is preferable if the group experience can be made comfortable for the partners.

The timing when sexual issues are raised is important. The client must be ready to consider this aspect of the rehabilitation process. The therapist, nevertheless, may need to take the initiative in bringing up sex-related matters. Many clients are hesitant to raise questions out of embarrassment or fear that the therapist thinks that such concerns are not appropriate for the client to entertain. As mentioned, it is very important that the therapist be comfortable in discussing sexual matters. The client may see the therapist's discomfort as rejection and thus not wish to engage in any further discussion. Lack of adequate sexual counseling is a criticism that some clients have raised about the rehabilitation process. Thus the therapist should give special attention to this area as part of the total intervention process.

It should be remembered, however, that not all partners are able to make a sexual adjustment that is acceptable to both. Termination of the relationship may ultimately be the best course of action in some cases.

INTERVENTION IN THE HOME

Home programs of intervention for individuals who are physically disabled are becoming increasingly available. One reason for this movement is economic. The increasing cost of hospitalization prompted those concerned with rehabilitation to seek alternative ways of delivering services. Second, occupational therapists have secured the right to third-party payment for their services outside an institutional setting (246,347,592,645).

Aside from economic issues, the prevalence of home programs has been influenced by recognizing the limitation of rehabilitation in an institutional setting. There is much that is artificial about a rehabilitation center: It is designed for the comfort and safety of disabled individuals, assistance is available when needed, meals are prepared and served by others, there is always someone around to talk to, recreational activities are available, and so forth. Returning to the community and one's home can be quite a shock. Although one may anticipate various problem areas, anticipation is quite different than being directly confronted with a vast array of difficulties. Thus, it has become increasingly evident that for many clients, some rehabilitation in an institution followed by intervention in the home is most effective.

Some of the general goals relative to physical restoration and maintenance are improvement in self-care and homemaking skills, altering architectural barriers if possible, assessing the need for and securing assistance/adaptive equipment, energy conservation, joint protection and the use of appropriate body mechanics, and assisting in the creation of a safe environment for the client. Attention to all of these areas will also assist the client in making a psychological adjustment to his or her disability.

More specifically, concerning psychosocial components, the client and therapist and, now more directly, the family need to be concerned about the following:

1. *The client's role in the family.* Beyond the necessity of perhaps rearranging tasks relative to familial roles, it is often helpful for the disabled person to take on one or more tasks that are of particular importance to the family as a whole. This allows the client to receive some satisfaction of esteem and indicates to the family that the individual is a valuable member.
2. *Leisure/recreation.* The leisure/recreational activities that family members have previously enjoyed together may have to be altered in some ways or markedly changed.
3. *Temporal adaptation.* Now is the time when the client will have to establish some kind of routine that is satisfying and compatible with the routine of other family members. At the same time, family members may need to alter their routines.
4. *Community resources.* The need for the use of community resources and some of the difficulties in using these resources now become more apparent to both the client and family members.

Intervention in the areas outlined above is in many ways similar to the methods described in "The Change Process" part of this chapter. Nevertheless, there are some real differences. When intervention takes place in the home, the therapist must be particularly concerned about:

1. *Support of the family.* The family that is given adequate encouragement and reinforcement is more likely to follow through and assist the client in a manner that was previously discussed with the family. Additional instruction and some alteration in the suggested regimen may be required to make it more appropriate to the situation of the family. At all times the therapists encourage the family to allow the client to be as independent as possible.
2. *Communication.* Adequate communication among family members is imperative to the adjustment of the disabled individual as well as the family as a whole. The therapist's job is essentially to keep everyone talking to everyone else. Ideas and feelings that are not shared can lead to considerable resentment and lack of need satisfaction. In facilitating communication, the therapist must be cautious that he or she does not become a barrier to direct communications. For example, a family member might tell the therapist something with the expectation that the therapist will tell the client. This is not the type

of communication which the therapist wishes to foster. Thus the therapist must take care not to become enmeshed in the family's channels of communication.

3. *Problem solving*. The therapist's approach in assisting the client and family should be one of problem solving. Emphasis is on developing problem-solving skills not on solving problems for the client and family. If possible, family members are helped to see difficulties as challenging and something to which they can apply their various knowledge and skills. With the development of a sense of competence in this area, the entire family feels more able to handle their affairs independently.

4. *Listening*. The therapist involved in home intervention needs to become a patient listener. Many times listening is the major form of intervention; suggestions, advice, and so forth are frequently not called for. With someone to act as a sounding board the client and family members are often able to effectively mobilize their resources and ultimately make the necessary personal and family adjustments.

The therapist's general approach and manner of interacting are somewhat different in the client's home than in a rehabilitation center. The therapist is a guest in the client's home. It is the client's space into which the therapist is invited and that space needs to be respected. The therapist, for example, does not rearrange furniture or use any object in the home without the expressed permission of the client. Everything in the home belongs to the client and must be treated with the utmost respect. The therapist acts as he or she would want any visitor in his or her home to act.

In going into the home, the therapist, in a very real sense, becomes the therapist for the whole family. The designated client is neither more nor less important than any other family member. This in itself may require some adjustment on the part of the client. As therapist to the whole family, the therapist must be highly sensitive to the situation of the family and to their cultural background. The privacy, integrity, structure, and idiosyncratic relationships of family members must be respected. Problems are assessed in terms of the family's definition of the situation and not solely on the basis of the client's assets and limitations. The goals set and plan for intervention must make sense not only in relation to the client's disability but also in relation to the family's attitudes and ideas about what should and should not be done. In other words, the therapist must attend to what the client and family members say is important to them and accept this as valid. The therapist must never enter the home with preconceived ideas of what is best or most appropriate. The therapist never imposes his or her point of view or tries to make any major changes in the lives of the people involved. The physical limitations of the home and the financial resources of the family must also be taken into consideration in setting goals and planing intervention.

To facilitate intervention in the home, a postdischarge referral for further intervention is important. When the original therapist does not follow the client into the community, a good working relationship between the clinically based therapist and the home therapist must be developed and maintained. This minimizes the need for redundant evaluation and provides for a smooth continuation of services. Home intervention should be terminated gradually in order to maintain the maximal functions of the client and the stable independence of the family. A plan for periodic follow-up should be specifically stated and carried out.

Home intervention can be highly successful. In some cases it is really preferable to a long course of care in a rehabilitation center. It is likely to become more prevalent in the future.

PROGRAM PLANNING

Program planning for the change process for a rehabilitation unit or center involves two major areas: the restoration of physical function and/or the development of compensating skills and psychosocial adjustment to being physically disabled. These goals may be dealt with separately or combined and worked toward simultaneously. The latter is usually preferable, although there are times when one goal may be emphasized more than another. When these goals are worked toward simultaneously, the therapist is using more than one frame of reference. Whenever this is the case, the therapist must be very clear what frames of reference are being used and that the frames of reference are compatible with each other. Confusion regarding goals, goal priorities, or the postulates regarding change that are being used is very likely to lead to muddled if not inadequate intervention.

The type of program developed to enhance psychosocial adjustment will vary with the nature of the client population and the typical length of stay in the rehabilitation center. Units that are fairly short term in nature tend to have a less elaborate program for psychosocial adjustment than units where the client's stay is considerably longer. The discussion below suggests a number of different ideas for dealing with psychosocial adjustment. Only some of these are likely to be appropriate for a particular setting (900,979,981,982).

Ideally, efforts toward psychosocial adjustment should be instituted as soon as the client's physical condition is stabilized. They certainly should be instituted by the time the client is actively involved in physical restoration. At the beginning the client may be in a state of psychological shock. When this is the case, it is usually most beneficial to encourage the client to talk and for the therapist to listen. This level of interaction may continue for some period of time and should not be rushed. Time is needed for the initial grief to subside and the mourning process to begin. When this has occurred, the client is usually ready to take a more active role in the adjustment process.

Regardless of specific activities or programs, there are certain environmental characteristics that promote psychosocial adjustment. The climate of the unit should be such that it

> acknowledges competency, arouses curiosity, feeds in universal knowledge, deepens appreciation and demands behavior across the full spectrum of a human's abilities. There should be a clear system of communication that is supportive and which provides realistic feedback in such a way that adaptation is encouraged and learning reinforced (ref. 981, p. 24).

The attitude of the staff is a crucial factor. Verslays has described this element as follows

> If the staff can accept the patient with deformity, show respect and recognize individuality there will be a positive effect on his self respect. Good social feedback from the non-disabled, empathy, and respect encourages maintenance of identity and self-respect. The patient who is accepted as he is by the staff can more easily accept himself (ref. 981, p. 22).

After the initial experience of grief has somewhat diminished, adjustment to disability is usually best facilitated by interaction in activity groups. Regardless of the type of group, the shared interaction provides a base of support and the opportunity to experiment with and practice coping skills.

If specialized groups—discussed shortly—cannot be implemented in the rehabilitation center, it is suggested that physical restoration and the development of compensatory skills take place in a group setting. There is usually very little reason, besides tradition, why this type of intervention cannot take place in a situation that facilitates group interaction. The therapist, in addition to focusing on goals relative to physical restoration, encourages the clients to share their ideas and feelings with each other and to give appropriate reinforcement and feedback.

The following are some of the many specialized activities groups that can be utilized more specifically to deal with psychosocial adjustment to disability. Some of these also include the development of physical skills while others are primarily concerned with psychosocial adjustment.

Homemaking group. This thematic group is designed to assist clients in becoming as independent as possible in such areas as food preparation, cleaning a home, doing laundry, shopping, and so forth. With these tasks as a focus, the group is also designed to help group members to gain skill in problem solving, test capacities and limitations, develop a sense of confidence, and provide support and encouragement to each other. It should be noted that this group is not just for women. It is for all clients—men and women, married and single, employed and unemployed.

A homemaking group is particularly important for men who will no longer be able to work. With their wives perhaps at or returning to work, these men, through taking some responsibility for household chores, are able to make a significant contribution to the maintenance of the home. There are two other advantages to the use of a homemaking group for men. The tasks involved in homemaking tend to be rather unfamiliar to many men. Thus they do not come to the group with a high level of expectation regarding the skills they think that they ought to have. Thus, they tend to be more relaxed and enter into the learning process at least with some spirit of adventure. The lack of a fear of failure and no previously set ideas about how specific tasks should be accomplished allow these men to experiment and be inventive in solving problems encountered. The other advantage of a homemaking group for men is that it encourages them to begin to look at the nature of social roles in a new light. The grumbling about "women's work" that is likely to occur is used as the basis for exploring their roles in the family and the possible changes that may need to be made regarding aspects of these roles.

In a homemaking group designed for women who have primary responsibility for taking care of a home, participants are given assistance in finding alternative ways of carrying out this responsibility. Attention is given to the practice of skills and work simplification. In addition, emphasis is placed on management techniques and on the supervision of other family members in doing household tasks. The participation of a disabled homemaker as a model and instructor in this type of group is particularly useful.

The above discussion may have implied separate homemaking groups for men and women. There need not, however, be such a separation. Although men and women may approach the task of learning or relearning homemaking skills somewhat differently, and some of the issues raised may be somewhat dissimilar, there is much that they can learn from each other. Besides, a mixed sex group may be a lot more fun.

Leisure/recreational group. The purpose of this group is to explore leisure/recreational interests and if necessary to develop new skills in this area. Solitary activities such as arts and crafts are explored as well as shared activities and activities requiring interaction outside the home. Emphasis is placed on consideration of a wide variety of activities that may be new to the individual. Consideration is also given to adaptations that might be made in order that the individual can participate in leisure/recreational activities that were enjoyed prior to the onset of disability. Again creative problem solving is emphasized. Within the context of enjoying shared interests and activities, group members are likely to develop new friendships, which may ultimately be a source of pleasure and support once the individuals return to the community.

Community-orientation group. This is a topical group, both anticipatory and concurrent, that is designed to sensitize group members to the difficulties they are likely to encounter in the community. Attention is given to identifying and expressing ideas and feelings about being disabled and coping with the feelings and ideas of the nondisabled. Ways of dealing with being stared at, rude questions, and rejection are discussed and practiced. This is best accomplished through group members going into the community—to a restaurant, a movie, shopping, and so forth. The reactions of oneself and others can then be dealt with concretely rather than through fantasizing various possibilities.

A community-orientation group is also concerned with helping clients identify community resources that they may need and/or want to use in the future. Again, this exploration should be experienced-based rather than simply being told about such resources. Visiting various agencies, going through the process of arranging for services, or participation in the programs of the agency is very useful. The more practice clients have in being out in the community, the more self assured they are likely to be about their capacity to function effectively as a member of the community. This is true both in a relationship to physically being able to manage themselves in the community as well as being able to deal with the psychosocial, interpersonal problems they are likely to encounter.

Creative-expressive groups. This type of thematic group is designed to assist group members to become aware of their ideas and feelings and better able to express them in a way that facilitates communication. Literature, music, painting, clay sculpting, and the like are used to stimulate group interaction, discussion, and learning. Although attention is given to feelings and ideas relative to being disabled, other areas of human concern are also explored. The purpose of the group is to help members become comfortable with internal experiences and their expression and thus should not be too narrowly focused. Through interaction in this type of group, members are encouraged to recognize their commonality with others regardless of whether they are or are not handicapped in some way. The realization that all people must continually reconcile universal issues, that others are anxious, fear rejection, and, at times, feel grossly incompetent helps disabled persons to see themselves as a member of the human family, unique but nonetheless quite similar to others.

Family groups. The major goal of a family group is to facilitate the mutual adjustment of the client and family members. Activities are used that are likely to enhance interaction, demonstrate the capacities and limitations of the client, and enable the entire family to enjoy being with each other. Structurally the group may be made up of one family but more typically it includes three or four families. The activities used may include preparing dinner together, attending concerts, visiting the zoo, craft activities, games of various sorts, and the like. Emphasis is on being with each other, sharing experiences, and having fun. These kinds of social activities give a structure to interactions that may initially be uncomfortable. They provide a context for learning to know each other on a different level and for the spontaneous expression of fears and concerns. They foster a sense of emotional closeness, which is essentially the key to mutual family adjustment. The therapist's role is to encourage interaction and to act as a role model for family members. There may be times when group members meet together for a serious discussion about various problem areas. However, this is only done when it occurs spontaneously and is not a regular part of the group format. Direct counseling of family members is accomplished outside the context of this type of group.

Transitional groups. This type of topical group has been previously discussed. Thus, only a few points will be made here. The focus of the group is on both the physical and the psychosocial problems of re-entry into the community. Attention is frequently given to architectural problems in the home and in the community, financial considerations, finding a new home, if it is necessary, arranging for adequate transportation, and so forth. When clients have not participated in a community group as outlined above, the transitional group also focuses on dealing with the nondisabled population. Prescribed activities are often used, especially for clients who are hesitant to experiment with various activities and interactions.

Participation in a transitional group should begin several weeks before discharge from the rehabilitation center. However, participation should not be instituted until the client is able to begin to contemplate return to the community. Timing is an important factor in the client being able to make effective use of a transitional group. Participation in a transitional group need not be terminated at the time of discharge. It is strongly suggested, in fact, that clients continue to participate in such a group until they feel that they have mastered the transitional process. Group members being at different stages in the transitional process can be an asset to the group. New members have models that they can emulate, and those more advanced in the process are able to provide guidance for those who are just beginning. There is often no better way of enhancing self-confidence than through realizing that one is able to help others.

The above description of various types of activity groups designed to facilitate the psychosocial adjustment of disabled clients is only illustrative. Other types of groups, such as ones concerned with vocational exploration or helping mothers who need to manage small children, may be appropriate for a particular rehabilitation center. In addition, the types of activity groups outlined above may be combined in a number of ways, depending on the client population and the availability of staff members.

CONCLUSION

The psychosocial adjustment of physically disabled individuals is an extremely important part of the rehabilitation process. It should never be assumed that it will take place automatically or that it is the responsibility of some other professional group. Facilitating psychosocial adjustment must be a conscious process, based on appropriate frames of reference and given considerable attention in program planning.

29 Developmental Disabilities

The developmentally disabled individual is often faced with serious problems in adaptation throughout the life cycle. What may seem ordinary and relatively easy to master for the nonhandicapped individual is often difficult for the individual who is developmentally disabled. The assistance by members of the health team is usually required not only during childhood but throughout the life-span.

Of paramount importance in the evaluation and intervention process is consideration of the individual's place in the life cycle (628). Both chronological and developmental age are taken into consideration—the areas of developmental delay and the developmental tasks that lie ahead. In addition, the developmentally disabled individual often has multiple areas of dysfunction which are interwoven and interactive. This compounds the evaluation and intervention process, making it a challenge to client, therapist, and those significant to the client. Finally, some developmentally disabling conditions are of such severity that the individual will, at best, only be able to function within a protected environment. For the benefit of all—client, therapist, and significant others—realistic goals must be set. Emphasis must be placed on maximizing the quality of the individual's life rather than on quantity or complexity of function. The setting of limited and realistic goals should not be construed as disregard for the client's welfare or rights as an individual. Rather, it is a humane effort directed toward making the individual's life as satisfying as possible given the individual's inherent limitations and the constraints of any given social system.

In assisting the developmentally disabled individual, all three types of frames of reference are used, either in combination or sequentially. Although there is much variation, in general, a developmental frame of reference is used as the basis for the change process during childhood and adolescence. When it is apparent that no further development is likely to take place in a particular area, an acquisitional frame of reference is used as the basis for the learning of compensatory skills. An acquisitional frame of reference is also usually used in assisting the adult who is developmentally disabled. The psychological problems related to the fact of being disabled are frequently dealt with through the use of an analytical frame of reference. The combination of an analytical and acquisitional frame of reference is utilized to help parents and significant others adjust to the disability of the client and to deal with the practical aspects of daily life as these are affected by living with a disabled individual.

This chapter focuses on the psychosocial related difficulties of the developmentally disabled with the exception of sensory integration deficit, which is discussed in the final chapter of this section. Many developmentally disabled individuals have deficits in the area of motor function. Thus, in the intervention process, the therapist usually combines physical restoration and the development of compensatory skills with remediation in the area of psychosocial dysfunction. There are times when these areas are dealt with separately, but it is usually more effective to deal with all areas of deficit in combination. There are times, however, when more emphasis is placed on one area as opposed to another.

There are many disorders that fall into the category of developmental disability. The most common diagnostic categories seen by occupational therapists are cerebral palsy, spina bifida, mental retardation, attention deficit disorders, conduct disorders, specific developmental disorders (learning disabilities), and pervasive developmental disorders, which include infantile autism.

For ease in presentation, this chapter is divided into three sections: the child, the school years, and the adult. This is, of course, somewhat of an artificial division as the life cycle is continuous. Various elements of evaluation and intervention which are discussed in one section may well be applicable across all age groups.

THE CHILD

Differential diagnosis of an infant or young child is often extremely difficult. The signs and symptoms of many conditions that are developmentally disabling are overlapping, and some are not readily apparent during the first few years of life. Thus, although it may be quite apparent that a child is not developing in a typical manner, a definitive diagnosis may not be able to be made for some period of time and, occasionally, never (33,182,569,913).

The lack of a differential diagnosis may be troubling to the therapist, but in the long run it is not a major impediment. The occupational therapist is primarily concerned with function and dysfunction—the performance components and occupational performances—rather than diagnoses. It is, of course, useful for the therapist to know the diagnosis, the course of the condition, prognosis, and likely future areas of difficulty. This can be used to facilitate evaluation, long-term goal setting, intervention, and identifying various precautions and counterindications.

Evaluation

The screening of a child who is suspected of developmental delay or at risk for such an eventuality should take place as soon as possible (74,339,384). Formal evaluation follows if it appears that the child has difficulties that fall within the occupational therapy domain of concern. Early evaluation and intervention is considered to be very important both as a means of alleviating blocks to development and of minimizing the possibility of secondary problems such as contractures and deviant behavior patterns.

The sequence and process of evaluation is as outlined in Chapter 15. In addition to the points made in that chapter, there are a few other factors to be taken into consideration in the evaluation of a child. The child and parent often come together to the evaluation situation (74,786). Thus, the therapist must establish rapport with two people simultaneously. Both are spoken to, with more direct attention usually being given to the parent at the onset of the interview. With a toddler or preschool child, it is often helpful to offer a toy. This helps to keep the child occupied and relaxed. It also gives the therapist an opportunity to observe the child's spontaneous behavior.

The child is usually gently separated from the parent and taken to another room for direct evaluation. When the child's anxiety level is high or the child is markedly hesitant to leave the parent, it is often useful to show the child the evaluation room with the parent present. Once the child has seen the room and investigated some of the available toys, the child usually shows little concern about the parent leaving. The child between 9 and 20 months, however, may not go along with this routine. A fear of strangers is fairly typical at this age, thus comfortable separation from the parent may not be possible. When this is the case, the parent is invited to stay in the room. When the child's anxiety is severe, it may be necessary for the parent to engage the child in various evaluation activities under the supervision of the therapist.

Information gained from the parent about the child's capacity to function in various areas is very important as is the data gathered from formal evaluative activities. Nevertheless, the question of what does the child actually do in situations where spontaneous activity is allowed or when the usual response may not be known is still in question. Thus, observation of the child in free play in a relaxed atmosphere with familiar, age-appropriate toys is often helpful (217). The therapist is able to observe how the child approaches and accomplishes a task and why further performance is difficult or impossible. Moreover, the various coexisting disturbances, how they interrelate and effect function, the child's compensatory behavior, and assets are able to be observed.

Data gathered in the evaluation of a child are usually not as reliable as that obtained from an adult. The child's current level of function is often more effected by interest, motivation, emotional state, fatigue, and so forth. This must be taken into consideration in the sharing and use of evaluative findings. Over a period of time there may be considerable fluctuation in the child's developmental level. This may be real fluctuation or an artifact of the evaluation situation and the child's desire and capacity to participate in evaluation at a given time. Thus, all evaluative findings must be considered tentative at best.

Intervention

As mentioned, intervention should begin as soon as possible. The earliest type of intervention, sometimes described as prevention, is directed toward infants who are identified as being at risk (74,225,384,558, 724,919,967,968). These infants may be of low birth weight (under 2,000 grams), have an identifiable condition at birth such as Down's syndrome, cerebral palsy, physical anomalies, etc., or they may be delayed in achieving typical developmental milestones. Such children are often involved in an "infant stimulation" program which is designed to facilitate motor, cognitive, and social development. The program consists of incorporating developmentally appropriate activities into the infant's daily routine which provide stimulation relative to the areas mentioned above. Visual, auditory, tactile, and postural stimulation are of primary importance. The goal is to facilitate normal development rather than teaching isolated skills.

Infant stimulation programs are considered to be particularly important for infants who are being treated in an acute-care nursery. The usual opportunity for interaction with the environment may be limited by confinement to an isolette or the use of physical restraint to prevent accidental dislodging of tubes. The occupational therapist may take direct responsibility for the infant stimulation program or act as a consultant to the nursery staff. Parents are often involved in this program, engaging in various activities with the child under the supervision of the therapist or the nursing staff.

Infant stimulation home programs for children at risk are also recommended by many therapists (967,968). In this situation the parents take primary responsibility for carrying out the program. The therapist suggests various appropriate activities, demonstrates them to the parents, and observes the parent participating with the child in the activities. Sequentially more advanced activities are suggested as the child achieves more advanced stages of development. Ways of helping parents to take the role of a home therapist will be discussed at the end of this section.

Two factors should be noted relative to infant stimulation programs. Overstimulation is probably as detrimental to the development of the child as understimulation. An immature nervous system is delicate. Thus, stimulation should be finely tuned to the response of the infant. Withdrawal and other signs of stress should be particularly noted and the program altered accordingly. Second, the effectiveness of early stimulation on later motor, cognitive, and social development is a controversial issue. Findings from animal studies support the importance of early stimulation. However, effectiveness has not been conclusively demonstrated relative to the human infant. In the absence of hard evidence, early stimulating programs are usually encouraged because of extrapolation from animal studies and for humanitarian reasons. This is an area that needs considerable further research.

Meeting health needs and the maintenance of function become particularly important areas of intervention for children who are hospitalized for a long period of time (196,384,389). In establishing appropriate programs, the chronological and developmental age of the children is given primary consideration. Activities are designed to be interesting and challenging. Independence is encouraged through giving the children an appropriate degree of freedom and responsibility. Participation in activities with both peers and adults is important. Many of the problems encountered by developmentally disabled individuals are the result of deficient life experiences. Impeded by their handicap(s) and/or environment, which by necessity must often be atypically protective, these children frequently do not have the opportunity to experience and learn about people, things, and events outside their circumscribed world. Thus, it is essential that the child participate in as many experiences as possible. Frequent trips outside the hospital should be arranged. When this is not possible, a variety of experiences should be brought to the hospital. A volunteer program to broaden the children's experiences and their general fund of knowledge is also very helpful.

Management may initially be the major focus of the intervention. This is particularly true in the case of severely disabled children, e.g., those who are profoundly retarded, deaf and blind, or autistic (205,428, 585,628,874). Excessive self-stimulation, abuse of self or others, destructiveness, and the like are fairly common. These undesirable behaviors need to be managed for the sake of the child's safety, the general welfare of the environment in which the child lives, and in order to allow the child to participate actively in the change process. Undesirable behaviors are frequently a reaction to the frustration that the child is experiencing and a response to an environment that does not meet the child's special needs. Once these undesirable behaviors are firmly entrenched, they are difficult to alter. The process is demanding of both time and energy. This is one of the major reasons why intervention should be begun as soon as possible. Early intervention tends to inhibit the acquisition of behaviors that interfere with satisfying environmental interaction and purposeful activity. It should be noted that management is an area in which parents often need assistance.

As mentioned, the change process is usually initially based on a developmental frame of reference. It is suggested that the reader review Chapter 24, which outlines recapitulation of ontogenesis. The change process with developmentally disabled children may proceed very slowly. This is particularly true with children who are severely disabled. Short-term goals that measure progress in small increments often provide the most rewards. Knowledge of the typical pace of the change process and the celebration of each small gain help to keep the child, parent, and therapist motivated to continue working toward the next goal and the long-term goals.

Within the limits inherent in the child's disability, all intervention should be directed toward assisting the child to be competent and to develop into a person who controls his or her own destiny (41,52,196,273,845). There are many ways in which this can be accomplished. The child should be allowed and encouraged to experience the excitement of discovery through involvement in appropriate activities. Self-confidence is fostered by permitting the child to act according to his or her own thoughts and feelings rather than according to imitation of set patterns of response. Every sign of originality in thought and action should be encouraged. Activities that maximize use of the senses and emphasize cause and effect encourage the child to view him- or herself as a participating, causal agent.

Esenther cautions against too much focus on the goal or task during intervention (273). Over-concern with goals or tasks may lead to the child becoming passive and responding with rote compliance to the demands of adults. Thus, spontaneity and the capacity to make decisions may be muted or lost. The child's ability to derive satisfaction from participating in a variety of activities may be impeded. Children who are helped or imposed on too much may not develop the capacity to manage their own transitions or acquire the ability to cope and adapt in new situations. The need on the part of therapist and parents to see "improvement" may inhibit the development of intrinsically motivated, competent children. Esenther emphasizes the importance of identifying and respecting the unique way each child functions. "Specific short-term goal attainment must be incorporated as much as possible by the child into the development of a healthy and flexible personality organization in order to produce personal and social competency" (273, p. 511).

The therapist's capacity to establish and maintain rapport with the child is a key element in the intervention process. Children seem to prefer staff members who are gentle but firm and consistent. The way in which the therapist moves and handles a child is also important. Children tend to respond to therapists who move with confidence, slowly, steadily, and precisely. The therapist should be sensitive to any discomfort the child may experience during intervention but nevertheless calmly proceed. In this way trust is developed through physical contact.

Children's suggestions about how the various activities which are a part of their intervention ought be organized should be elicited and, if at all possible, acted on. Many children prefer that activities be engaged in in a regular sequence and in a prescribed way; they make each session with the therapist into a ritual. This seems to provide a needed sense of security in a world over which the child may feel he or she has little control. Once the child feels secure, he or she is likely to become more spontaneous and delight in varying the ritual and adding new elements.

Although a realistic degree of physical and emotional independence is one of the long-term goals of intervention, movement toward this goal may not follow a straight trajectory. It may sometimes be wiser to accept dependence periodically until the child has accumulated sufficient resources to continue on his or her own. For example, independence in appropriate self-care activities may be deliberately delayed until the child is physically more capable of handling these tasks or until he or she has a better sense of autonomy. As the child's desire for independence will vary over time, so must the expectations.

Developmentally disabled children are, above all, children. They must, like all children, deal with the developmental tasks that are particular to their place in the life cycle. And like all children, they will manage them in their own way, in their own style, and according to their own timetable. And like all children, development will be uneven, episodic, and marked by periods of regression.

Play

The major vehicle used in the intervention process with developmentally disabled children is play (74,78, 205,232,305, 363, 377,384,431,462,463,552,610,625, 680,681,801,883,910,946,977,1002,1019). This is usually an effective tool because, given an optimal environment, most children play spontaneously. The pleasure derived from play motivates the child to participate in intervention and to meet the challenges inherent in that process. Well-designed intervention often looks to the casual observer like supervised play, with all involved, child or children and the therapist, having a good time. And that is as it should be. Intervention is a serious endeavor but it need not and usually should not be perceived as such by the young child.

Play is an effective vehicle for intervention when the child knows how to play. However, there are some children, particularly those who are severely retarded or neurologically impaired or autistic, who do not play spontaneously. Left to their own devices such children usually engage in stereotyped or other nonpurposeful activities. If this is the case, the therapist needs to assist the child in learning how to play. Some suggestions regarding how this may be accomplished are outlined in Chapter 26.

Wheman and Marchant describe a program to improve the play skills of severely retarded children (1002). They suggest the use of reactive toys, toys that respond or "act back" in some way when played with. The program takes place with children and staff members together in a play area. Each child or children in pairs are given verbal instructions about how to play with a specific toy. If this proves to be ineffective, the child is shown how to use the toy through modeling and demonstration. When necessary, manual guidance is used to show the child how the toy works. Verbal praise and physical affection is given for any appropriate response. Once the child has begun to play, even at a fairly primitive level, the play situation can be structured to facilitate the attainment of more specific goals of intervention.

Although play is the major vehicle used for intervention with the developmentally disabled child, activities of daily living can also serve as a medium for intervention. Most of the initial stages of the adaptive skills described in recapitulation of ontogenesis can also be developed within the context of feeding, bathing, dressing, and so forth. In order for this aspect of human experience to be used in intervention, the child must be an active participant in the process, not acted on. It will, more than likely, take a somewhat longer time to accomplish activities of daily living when they are used as a vehicle for intervention. Nevertheless, the extra time is often well worth the effort. The child's exploration and experimentation during participation in daily living activities also enhance the likelihood of eventual independence in these areas.

Parent Participation

Some of the problems encountered by the parents of developmentally disabled children were outlined in Chapter 5. Some suggestions of how to assist parents in dealing with these difficulties are outlined in this section (74, 153,695,814,966,968,1053).

The area in which the parents may initially need assistance is coping with the shock of having a disabled child and the grief and mourning that follow. The therapist encourages the parents to talk about their disappointment, anger, fears, and guilt. Comfort and support are given as well as reality testing. The therapist also provides information about the child's condition. It should be remembered that adjustment to a child's disability is a long-term process that may take a matter of several years.

The therapist's assistance in this area will ultimately be of great importance to the child. A child's adjustment to disability and active participation in the habilitation process is strongly influenced by the parents' response to the disability.

The parents should be involved as soon as possible in planning for the child's habilitation. Sufficient information is given to the parents so that they can make informed decisions. Planning should be so structured that the parents realize they are in control of the situation, that their wishes and decisions will be respected. The parents' cultural background may well influence their plans and aspirations for the child. The degree to which they want to pursue habilitation vigorously and their acceptance of adaptive equipment, for example, will often be dependent on cultural beliefs and taboos. The therapist's own ideas about appropriate habilitation are secondary to what the parents believe is the best course of action.

Parents will often need assistance in learning how to care physically for their disabled child. Very specific instructions should be given. The therapist should also demonstrate what needs to be done as well as give the parents an opportunity to practice the necessary skills. Instructions should also be written so that the parents have these at home for easy reference. Many disabled infants are hospitalized for a period before they are able to go home. If at all possible, the parents should be given an opportunity to assist with the care of the infant during this time. This helps the parents feel a sense of involvement with the child, increases their degree of comfort in handling the child, and facilitates the transition from hospital to home.

As mentioned in Chapter 5, parents' attachment to their disabled child, the bonding process, is often delayed and occasionally may not occur at all. This appears to happen because the disabled child is often less responsive than the nondisabled child, or may respond in a way that is not expected. The therapist may assist the parents in forming an adequate attachment by providing information about how the child is likely to respond and some idea about when the child may reach various developmental milestones. In addition, the therapist helps the parents learn how to play with the child. This not only facilitates the child's responsiveness, but it allows the parents to experience pleasurable interactions with the child. The therapist suggests appropriate play activities and demonstrates these activities with the child. In suggesting play activities, the therapist is careful not to make these prescriptive in nature. These should be activities that are fun, not a specified program of intervention. The parents are encouraged to experiment with a variety of play activities in order to identify those that are pleasurable to them and the child. The bonding process is most likely to occur when there is a considerable amount of interesting, enjoyable interaction between the child and parents. Everything possible should be done to facilitate this type of activity.

The long-term adjustment of the parents to raising a developmentally disabled child needs to be an ongoing concern of the therapist. Many of the problems the parents are likely to encounter are outlined in Chapter 5. By way of review, some of these are alteration of life-style and temporal adaptation, dealing with the reality of the child's disability, disciplining the child, finding sufficient leisure time, satisfying the needs of other family members, and so forth. In assisting parents, the therapist listens, encourages the expression of feelings, emphasizes the importance of a problem-solving approach, gives information concerning the child and resources available to help the child, and provides support. It may seem at times that the therapist is spending more time in assisting the parents than in dealing directly with the child. And this often is as it should be. Through helping the parents, the therapist is indirectly helping the child and allowing the parents to take appropriate responsibility for the habilitation of their child.

Parent support groups have also been found to be effective in helping the parents of developmentally disabled children. These groups, which usually meet regularly over a long period of time, provide a forum for the sharing of information and mutual problem solving. The group may also engage in advocacy activities to ensure that their children receive optimal services and have access to community facilities. Parent support groups may be available in the community, in which case the therapist should encourage the parents to join one of them. If no such group is available, it is suggested that the therapist start such a group. The therapist is usually fairly active in the initial phase of the group. As the group begins to function effectively, the therapist acts as a resource person, only occasionally attending group meetings.

As briefly discussed in Chapter 5, there are some inherent conflicts in parents taking on the additional role of being a therapist. Being a therapist takes time and energy, it requires making demands that parents usually do not have to make on a child, and it is a role that requires a self-conscious studied approach to the child. Nevertheless, parent and child involvement in a home program may well be the only means by which adequate habilitation can occur.

The way in which the home program is introduced and guided by the therapist appears to have an impact on the effectiveness of the program and the quality of the parent-child interaction (967). Without adequate support and follow-up, it has been found that parents: (a) engage in a high frequency of demanding, commanding, requesting, and asking behavior relative to the child; (b) progressively reduce their amount of warm and positive behavior (smiling, positive verbal statements, physical closeness) both during play and while engaged in intervention; (c) become preoccupied with positioning at the expense of the child's satisfaction and comfort; (d) often fail to support the child's less-than-successful efforts to comply; (e) repeatedly call the child's errors to the child's attention; (f) seem determined to continue with a frustrating activity long after the child becomes irritable and uncooperative; and (g) view the child's inability to perform as a demonstration of their own inadequacies in working with the child.

It appears that initiation of a home program should only occur subsequent to the parents having accepted the child's disability, at least to some degree; the formation of the parent-child bond; and the development of play interaction between parent and child. To make the parents' adaptation to their new role as smooth as possible, a home program should be introduced slowly with graded steps so that change can be worked gradually into the established parent-child relationship.

With the prerequisites described above, Tyler and Kogan have outlined a method for facilitating parent-child participation in a home program (967). Instruction and demonstration were used to orient the parent to the program, but the unique aspect was personalized instruction through the use of videotaped interaction between child and parent. Each of eight sessions was taped and reviewed with the parent. Areas of behavior the parent saw as problems at home were discussed, with an effort made to relate the videotaped observations to the problem areas. The information gained through the discussion was jointly translated into specific behavioral suggestions for the parent to follow in the playroom during the weekly interaction sessions. The therapist also observed the parent and child through a one-way mirror and, via a microphone in the parent's ear, made suggestions to the parent and gave positive reinforcement for appropriate interactions with the child. In the weekly discussions between parent and therapist, videotaped segments were identified as examples of interactions that were helpful to the child's habilitation and those that were not helpful.

After the series of eight-week sessions, the parent and child continued participation in a home program under the guidance of a therapist. However, the videotaping and personalized instruction were not used. A nine-month follow-up study indicated that the interaction between parent and child remained positive. There was no evidence of the negative behavior outlined above.

In conclusion, the quality of parents' involvement with the disabled child is a crucial factor in the habilitation process. It is the responsibility of the therapist to ensure that the needs of the parent are given sufficient attention and that a positive parent-child relationship is fostered and supported.

THE SCHOOL YEARS

The occupational therapist traditionally has worked with school-age disabled children and adolescents within a clinical setting or within the context of special schools. The passage of Public Law 94-142, Education for All Handicapped Children, in 1975 has led to a marked change in the delivery of health services for developmentally disabled individuals (423,424,662,970,971,989). This law, other previous legislation and court decisions are based on the "belief that handicapped children are best served by providing more opportunities for integration into regular education settings, greater individualization of instruction and increased opportunity to participate in community life" (38, p. 640). Further, it is based on the belief that handicapped individuals have a legal and moral right to the opportunities enjoyed by all. In essence Public Law 94-142 mandates that all handicapped children be educated in the least restricted environment (e.g., an environment that is as close as possible to the mainstream of the educational system) and that relevant health services be offered to support these students within the educational system. Occupational therapy was identified as one of the services that should be available to assist handicapped students in meeting their educational needs. As a consequence of this mandate, both disabled students and members of the health team have moved into the school system in rather large numbers.

To work effectively in the school system, the occupational therapist needs considerable knowledge regarding the educational process and the school system. The information needed is beyond the scope of this text. Thus, this section is only an introduction to provide the reader with a brief orientation to this area of practice (31,38,209,338,340,507,535,688,752,797,964,965).

In its definition of related services, Public Law 94-142 states that occupational therapy is and should be concerned with:

1. Improving, developing, or restoring functions impaired or lost through illness, injury, or deprivation;
2. Improving the ability to perform tasks for independent functioning when functions are impaired or lost;
3. Preventing, through early intervention, initial or further impairment or loss of function.

Within the school system, occupational therapy services must have a direct bearing on the student's ability to learn and benefit from educational programs. Thus, the therapist must assess the student's areas of function and dysfunction relative to learning and to optimal interaction within the school environment. Goals must be set and intervention take place in a way that is compatible with educational programming. The occupational therapy program must be designed so that it is integrated with the student's total experience and not a separate entity, for example, that takes place a few times a week.

The role and function of the occupational therapist within the school system has been defined as follows:

1. Screening of those students with suspected educational handicaps; referring these students to appropriate services, including occupational therapy; and formal evaluation of students referred to occupational therapy;
2. Setting goals for the individual student and designing a plan for intervention;
3. Participating in educational program planning for the individual student to coordinate occupational therapy goals and program plans with the child's total educational program;
4. Implementing an occupational therapy program to facilitate the student's optimal functioning and to enhance the student's ability to learn and develop;
5. Consulting with school personnel and parents regarding services provided by occupational therapy;
6. Promoting ongoing evaluation, making appropriate alteration in goals and program, and determining the time when occupational therapy services should be terminated;
7. Developing, managing, and supervising school-based occupational therapy programs;
8. Engaging in appropriate communication and documentation of activities;
9. Providing direct and indirect services in accordance with legal regulations and ethical standards.

To carry out these roles and functions the occupational therapist must have an understanding of the educational delivery system, i.e., its structure, philosophies, traditions, conflicts, priorities, vocabulary, and theories. To work effectively, one must know the role and functions of administrators, regular classroom teachers, teachers in special education, resource teachers (in reading, mathematics, etc.), teacher aides, and the school maintenance staff. In addition, it is important to know the role of the parent in the educational system and the aspirations of parents relative to their children's education.

A therapist who has been educated or worked within the context of clinical medicine often finds the culture of the school system very different, if not somewhat alien. Not only must the therapist learn about the new culture but he or she must be accepted by the members of the culture. This may well be a somewhat long-term endeavor that includes a socialization process. The therapist must learn to think like an educator while maintaining the capacity to conceptualize and reason like an occupational therapist.

Ottenbacker emphasizes the importance of therapists and educators working together and states that,

> All professions involved must develop an understanding of their historical and philosophical differences and similarities and a realization that all conceptual and treatment models are limited in their capacity to deal effectively with the many and varied problems existing within the developmentally disabled population (ref. 752, p. 84).

The problems encountered by developmentally disabled students are multiple and varied. Many students have difficulties in mobility, which may limit their ability to fully participate in a school program. Some common difficulties encountered are transportation to and from school, toileting and other personal care activities, lunch, gym, recess, and transition time between activities and classes. These difficulties are usually dealt with in several ways: direct remediation, development of compensatory skills, use of adaptive equipment, a buddy system with a nondisabled student, assistance from an adult, and modification of the environment.

Dealing with difficulties in mobility are essentially outside the parameters of this text. However, a few points are worth mentioning. Surmounting difficulties in mobility frequently require a good deal of problem solving. This should by no means be the sole responsibility of the therapist. If at all possible, the student and teacher(s) should be involved in the process. Where appropriate, suggestions from parents, administrators, other students, teacher aides, and maintenance staff should also be elicited. This allows all involved parties to feel that they are a part of the problem-solving process. They are also much more likely to willingly participate in the solution of the problem. Successfully dealing with difficulties in mobility enables the disabled student to be a more active participant in the affairs of the school. This, in turn, allows students to be involved in a wide variety of different kinds of experiences and thus increase their general fund of knowledge. Finally, the capacity to participate actively in the affairs of the school is likely to increase self-esteem, a factor that may well enhance academic performance.

Many developmentally disabled students have difficulties in the area of learning (401,679,965,1023). These children may be mentally retarded, they may have serious psychological and/or social interaction problems that inhibit their capacity to engage in age-appropriate learning experiences, or they may have specific learning disabilities. The nature of the students' problem relative to diagnoses may not be at all clear. The occupational therapist's task and that of other members of the health/educational team is to assess the child's functional capacities and to devise an individualized educational program. A developmental approach is usually used to assist these students.

Many students with difficulty in learning are so severely impaired that they are placed in special classes for all or the majority of the school day. Every effort is usually made to include them in some activities with nondisabled students, but this is sometimes not possible. Special classes for the younger severely learning-impaired students are usually designed to develop preacademic skills. Particular attention is frequently given to the development of cognitive and group interaction skills. Play and activities of daily living are used as the means for learning. Older severely learning-impaired students are usually introduced to academic skills with emphasis on simple reading, writing, and mathematics. Activities of daily living relative to interaction in the community and basic work habits are also taught. The overall goal of the educational program is to help the students become as independent as possible in regard to managing environmental interactions. The gestalt of activities taught are sometimes referred to as community survival skills. There are, of course, some students who are not able to master these skills.

Not so severely learning-impaired students may spend most of the school day in regular classes. Their educational program is usually supplemented by participation in the activities of various "resource rooms." The activities in a resource room may include such things as occupational therapy, speech therapy, the use of learning aids for the visual- or hearing-impaired student, and tutoring. Although the use of resource rooms is a valuable addition to students' education, they should not be overused. The student should spend as much time as possible in the regular classroom; that is the whole point of not being in a special class. Through problem solving and being somewhat inventive, ways of assisting the child to learn while in the regular classroom can often be found.

Further discussion of the learning-disabled individual and sensory integration is presented in Chapter 31.

Many developmentally disabled students, regardless of the nature or severity of their disability, have difficulty in the areas of dyadic interaction, group interaction, self-identity, and sexual identity. It is in these areas that the occupation therapist can be of great assistance, using recapitulation of ontogenesis as a guide for the change process. Programs may be designed to focus directly on these areas, or intervention may occur in the context of the usual school program. In the latter case, the occupational therapist usually acts as a consultant to the regular classroom teachers and special educators. Conversely, these teachers may act as a consultant to the occupational therapist in that academic learning can be incorporated into programs designed primarily to focus on adaptive skills.

As discussed in Chapter 5, the developmentally disabled child and adolescent pass through various stages in the process of adjusting to being disabled and accepting it as part of the self. The process of giving up the fantasy of someday being nondisabled and of accepting one's limitations frequently comes to the forefront during adolescence. It occurs at a time that has its own complex developmental tasks, and the disabled adolescent often needs assistance in dealing with universal issues. The use of reconciliation of universal issues to facilitate this process is recommended. The opportunity to identify and communicate ideas and feelings in a shared reality and to work through various issues is often welcomed by disabled students. This process not only assists students in ultimately being able to take full advantage of the educational experience, it assists them in making realistic plans for the future.

The therapist and other members of the education/health team also have a responsibility for helping the nondisabled students adjust to their disabled classmates. Nondisabled students often bring to the school setting many fears and prejudices relative to disabled people. A well-designed education program that provides for multiple positive interactions between nondisabled and disabled students goes a long way in eliminating fears and prejudices. In addition, nondisabled students should be provided with appropriate information about various disabilities and the problems that disabled individuals face. The need to respect and support each other should be fostered among all the students. This provides a growth-facilitating environment for disabled students as well as nondisabled students.

In their role of consultant to teachers, occupational therapists are often confronted with a variety of requests for assistance (538). Some of the common concerns of teachers are how to (a) interpret therapeutic goals relative to such areas as adaptive equipment, proper positioning, specific exercises, psychosocial adjustment, and the like; (b) incorporate the goals into educational plans and implement them daily; (c) fill in gaps in learning that are characteristic of developmentally disabled students because of their lack of typical life experiences; (d) cope with physical, cognitive, psychological, and social limitations that involve daily functioning; (e) plan for the future based on prognostic information; (f) use multisensory teaching techniques; (g) manage a variety of school situations for the disabled child; and (h) deal with hospitalization and frustrations of handicapped children.

It should be remembered that some teachers have negative ideas and feelings about disabled individuals, culturally based ideas and feelings that may be essentially unconscious. When this is the case, the occupational therapist may need to help the teacher in this area before any meaningful consultation can take place.

The parents of developmentally disabled children have the right, by law, to participate in the educational planning for their children. This right must be respected and, indeed, their participation should be encouraged. Parents should be consulted regularly and invited to planning or problem-solving meetings that concern their child. Their concerns and suggestions should be elicited and given careful consideration, and they should be helped to realize that they have a great deal of control relative to their child's educational experience. A support group, as outlined in the previous section, continues to be helpful for many parents. However, such a support group should not replace the parents' involvement in the various parent groups and activities associated with their child's school. Participation in such groups should be encouraged.

An adequate educational program in the mainstream of the school system is felt to be the best preparation for taking on the roles, responsibilities, and privileges of being an adult. Although hard evidence to support this belief is not yet available, it is supported by a good deal of logic and reason.

THE ADULT

Many developmentally disabled individuals are able to take on adult roles with little if any assistance from members of the health team. Others, however, will need continued or periodic assistance in managing developmental tasks, three of which are of major concern to the occupational therapist—alternative living situations, selected occupational performances, and special problems of the mentally retarded.

Alternative Living Situations

Typically, after completion of high school, young adults begin to prepare to leave the home of their parents. For some developmentally disabled individuals, particularly those who are severely impaired, this major life event involves decisions that are difficult to make—for them and for their family. The occupational therapist can help in this process by assessing the individual's potential for managing various living situations and by outlining the pros and cons of various possible living situations. Although the individual and the family must make decisions, the therapist is often in a position to provide reality testing and support while decisions are being made. Ultimately, it may be decided that the individual will live alone, continue to live with her parents, that institutionalization is the wisest course of action, or that a living situation that is an alternative to one of these first three choices would be most suitable for the individual.

This section deals with the last decision and the occupational therapist's role in this area (32,38,523,574, 814,874). It should be noted that an alternative living situation is also a possible option for disabled individuals who are currently residing in an institution and for individuals with an acquired disability who have completed a course of rehabilitation. The following discussion reflects this broader application of alternative living situations.

The two major types of alternative living situations are boarding homes and group homes. A boarding home, usually run for profit, basically provides each resident with a room and meals. Other services such as attendants to assist residents with activities of daily living and interactions with the community, a leisure time/recreational program, programs designed to increase and/or maintain function, social services, and the like may or may not be available.

A group home usually consists of three to eight disabled individuals living together in a family-like environment. There may be a home manager who lives full time in the home or who is only there during the day. Or, there may be no one who regularly assists in the management of the home. The individuals who live in a group home share as much as possible in meal preparation, cleaning, and other household chores. When feasible, establishing and enforcing basic rules for living together are the responsibility of the residents as well as making other kinds of decisions about the living situation that will affect all group members. Members of a health team may or may not visit regularly to provide services, help with tasks that the residents are unable to manage on their own, or act as consultants and resource persons for the residents.

The overall orientation of alternative living situations is to give the individual an opportunity "to have primary responsibility for his/her life choices and to rely minimally on others for the decision-making process and performance of personal care and home-community activities within the limits of the individual's physical, emotional, social, mental and economic abilities" (32 p. 812). The goal is to help the individual to achieve as full participation in the life of the alternative living situation and the community as possible and to achieve a satisfying and meaningful quality of life. "Full participation in the life of the alternative living situation" by no means should be taken to indicate that the individual's continued relationship with family members is not fostered. The individual and family members are encouraged to visit regularly and to engage in shared recreational activities. The same is true for old friends.

Preparation for moving to an alternative living situation should begin wherever the client is currently living, e.g., a parents' home, a rehabilitation facility, or institutional setting. However, the process should be completed in the individual's new home and community environment. Adequate preparation is often the key to successful transition from the old to the new living situation. Adequate time and attention, thus, should be devoted to this process (399).

The occupational therapist may be involved in the transition process and/or in the provision of services within the context of alternative living situations. The role may entail direct service or be consultive in nature. In either case, the occupational therapy program needs to be integrated with other community health and rehabilitation services.

An adequate transitional program can be divided into the following four parts:

1. *Evaluation and program planning*. The client's current and potential capacity for independent living is assessed and compared with the functional requirements of various alternative living situations. Through comparing the client's assets and limitations with the demands of the selected alternative living situation, the therapist is in a position to design a program for intervention.

2. *Program implementation*. The program, usually based on an acquisitional frame of reference, is oriented toward the development of the highest possible level of independence. Focus may be on performance components or occupational performances or both. Periodically during the transition program, the client is encouraged to visit his or her home so as to become familiar with the setting and its demands and to begin to become acquainted with the other residents.

3. *Movement into the alternative living situation*. Any necessary physical modification of the new home should be complete. In addition, the client, or the therapist if the client is severely impaired, should have made contact with and know how to use appropriate community resources and services. It is the therapist's responsibility to be sure that the client has a support system that provides for adequate safety and that maintains the client's optimal level of function.

4. *Follow-up*. The therapist continues the intervention process until the client has made the initial adjustment to the new home. Some additional skills that will foster adaptation to group living may be taught at this time. After the initial adjustment phase has been completed, the transition program is brought to a close. The therapist may periodically follow-up on the client's adjustment to the new home. This is only done, however, if it is acceptable to the client.

In the role of providing services to residents of alternative living situations, the occupational therapist may be involved in a variety of endeavors. Of major concern to the therapist is the maintenance of function. A separate program may not be needed for this. Rather, the therapist helps residents to organize their daily life in such a way that they are making optimal use of all of their capacities. After participation in an alternative living situation, it may become apparent that a residence's potential level of function is considerably higher than was previously suspected. The types of stimulation available and demands made in an alternative living situation may encourage the unfolding of heretofore unsuspected capacities. When this occurs, the therapist supports such growth and/or builds on this potential through involving the resident in a change process. In addition to activities of daily living and interpersonal skills, other areas of concern to the therapist are leisure/recreation and, if appropriate, work. Community resources are used to enhance and maintain function in these areas. Temporal adaptation may also be an issue needing attention.

In addition to providing services for residents, the occupational therapist may act as a consultant to the managers of alternative living situations (574). This may involve a program of education to help managers identify the needs of their residents and to develop skills in meeting these needs. The task of being the manager of an alternative living situation is not easy. Thus, the therapist often needs to provide considerable support. It is also very useful for the therapist to help managers develop their own support system through regular meetings of managers from various settings. As a consultant, the therapist's usual approach is to assist managers by guiding them in problem solving. Given encouragement and support, managers are usually quite able to identify appropriate ways to deal with the various situations that they encounter in their daily work.

Selected Occupational Performances

Many developmentally disabled individuals want to expand their family interaction roles. They wish to marry or form long-term intimate partnerships and to have children. The areas in which these individuals may need assistance are sex education, including an understanding of the particular problems they may encounter in engaging in satisfying sexual relationships, the development of social skills necessary for dating and courtship, and acquisition of the skills necessary for the care of a child and home (814).

Adequate sex education should be provided for all developmentally disabled individuals regardless of their ultimate decision to marry or form a partnership. Some of this can and should be gained through school-based sex education programs. The adequacy of these programs vary, however, from one school district to another. Even if the program is adequate for the nondisabled student, it is unlikely to be totally adequate for developmentally disabled students. A supplementary program often needs to be arranged to deal with such issues as appropriate contraceptive measures; appropriate positioning to facilitate comfortable and satisfying sexual intercourse; the variables to be taken into consideration in deciding whether to have a child, including hereditary factors, the health of the mother, and the physical and emotional capacities to take care of a child.

Some developmentally disabled individuals, because of the lack of appropriate life experiences, do not have the necessary social skills to engage in dating and courtship. An anticipatory/concurrent topical group is usually an effective way of dealing with this area of deficit. Learning occurs most easily if group participants are involved in social situations where there are suitable persons to date. Finding and participating in these situations may, indeed, be the initial focus of the group.

The physical care of a child and home may present some problems for developmentally disabled individuals, particularly those with impaired motor function (636,960). Prior to the birth of the child, parents should be given an opportunity to practice child care skills with a realistic life-size doll. Through guidance, problem solving, and practice, the parents are able to develop skill and to determine the most appropriate way for them to deal with the child's needs. They are also able to determine the type of equipment they will require to facilitate care.

In addition to physical care, the disabled parent may need assistance in the nurturing aspects of child rearing. The parent is likely to be very busy, thus it is important that sufficient time in the daily routine be allowed for playing with the child. The parent must learn to be an effective and consistent disciplinarian because the child's safety will often be dependent on coming when called and stopping an activity when told. A disabled parent must teach the child to accommodate to the parent's disability. The parent can learn to direct a child's activities verbally for the benefit of all and in such a manner that the child's self-esteem is maintained and the child is not made to feel imposed on. The child cannot only be very helpful to the parent, but is also able to learn important personal skills and values in the process of helping a parent.

A severely disabled parent may not be able to participate fully in the care of a child. In deciding what the parent can and cannot do, it is suggested that the parent reserve those things that he or she finds most enjoyable and delegate the other, perhaps more mechanical tasks to a child-care helper. It is important for many disabled parents to have emergency help easily, quickly, and consistently available. This is particularly true when caring for an infant and toddler. Such help not only ensures the safety of the parent and child, but also provides the parent with the sense of security that is such a necessary part of adequate parenting.

Severely disabled adults may have some difficulty in adequately using their leisure/recreational time (935). This is true particularly for individuals who are not able to work. Whether an individual lives with parents, other family members, or in an alternative living situation, it is important that he or she engages in activities outside the home. This not only increases the possibility that an optimal degree of independent functioning will be maintained, but also increases the quality of his or her life experience.

There are many community-based leisure/recreational programs for severely disabled adults. The types of programs vary, depending to a great extent on the level of functioning of the participants (691). Typically, the program takes place for 4 or 5 hours in the middle of the day, 3 to 5 days a week. Some of the programs also have weekend activities. The major emphasis of the program is leisure/recreational activities, which take place both in the center and out in the immediate community. The program is also concerned with maintenance of function in all areas. At times specific skills may be taught, such as greater independence in self-care and skills that allow the individual to be more comfortable in participating in community-based activities.

Staff members from these programs sometimes also take responsibility for bringing leisure/recreational activities to disabled individuals who are unable to regularly leave an alternative living situation or the family home. The focus of these satellite programs is often to facilitate the entry of the individual into the community-based program.

An occupational therapist may be responsible for these leisure/recreation programs or may be a consultant to the staff. Regardless of the nature of involvement, however, the therapist working with severely developmentally disabled adults should encourage their participation in such programs. It is one more way in which the therapist assists the individual in making use of community resources.

Some developmentally disabled individuals need assistance in learning to work (230,352,727,999). Ideally, this process begins at the usual time in the life cycle, being fostered by the young person's family and school. This, however, sometimes does not occur and the individual, as an adult, lacks the basic skills and habits needed for adjustment to the worker role. Participation in a sheltered workshop is one of the major ways utilized to assist developmentally disabled individuals to acquire the necessary role behaviors.

In addition to what was outlined in Chapter 26 regarding sheltered workshops, there are two other areas that need to be given attention. Some developmentally disabled individuals are unaware of their skills and interests and therefore have little idea of what jobs might be appropriate for them. The factors contributing to this delay in development are multiple. Some of the major factors, however, appear to be the following (999):

1. Difficulty in following the process of making a vocational choice because of cognitive deficits;
2. Family or cultural beliefs that adversely affect passage through the choice process;
3. Difficulty in understanding feedback from the environment and/or altering behavior on the basis of feedback;
4. Fewer occupations to choose from;
5. An occupational choice being forced on the individual or making a premature choice.

The sheltered workshop program, then, must also include a component that allows individuals to explore skills and interests and to learn more about the types of jobs that are appropriate, given their capacities and limitations. Ways of doing this were also discussed in Chapter 26.

The other area of concern relative to helping a developmentally disabled individual prepare for the role of a worker is activities of daily living. More specifically, they may need assistance in dressing and grooming. There is a stigma attached to looking different in our society in general and particularly in the world of work. Thus the therapist may need to provide assistance in helping program participants learn more about and attend to these aspects of personal care. Clients may also need guidance in learning how to use public transportation. The capacity to move more freely about the community may enhance the possibility of their finding a suitable and satisfying job.

The transition from a sheltered workshop to a community job may not be an easy one (230). The rapport that clients may have established with the workshop staff is not likely to be available, at least not immediately in a community job. They may also miss the social contact with those who are like themselves. It is important, therefore, that the clients be given adequate support during this transition period. Continued involvement with the sheltered workshop in some way may be a necessary component of the transition.

Some developmentally disabled individuals will never be able to participate in a competitive employment situation. Nevertheless, they are quite able to work in a protected, properly supervised environment. Every effort should be made to assist such individuals in finding an appropriate work environment. Participation in some type of work situation goes a long way in helping the individual to gain and maintain an adequate identity and sense of self-worth.

Special Problems of the Mentally Retarded

Keilhofner and associates have written a series of papers about the world view of some mentally retarded adults and suggest ways of facilitating evaluation and intervention (520,526,527). The population of concern are individuals, most previously institutionalized, who are now living in boarding homes. Mentally retarded adults are described as:

- Not taking expected social roles at the usual time in the life cycle. They are in a sense "frozen in time," acting as if they were children and often being treated that way.
- Perceiving nonretarded people as being very powerful.
- Establishing a dependency relationship with staff; dependency becomes a way of life. This state of helplessness, however, may be considered to be adaptive in that it can be used to manipulate others.
- Being concerned with the here and now—not long-term planning.
- Engaging in considerable ritualism—actions that have the form and appearance but not the purpose of true social interaction. There is planning without anticipation, recreation without enjoyment, waiting is something to do.
- Being, nevertheless, knowledgeable about the circumscribed world in which they live. They have a set of common-sense interpretations about the nature of that world and how to deal with the required interactions of daily life.

Much of the behavior of retarded adults is a consequence of the environment in which they live. The physical and social environment of boarding homes is designed to facilitate eating, sleeping, sitting, wandering around, and watching. There is little interaction between residents because there is no place arranged for congregation and visiting. There is little privacy and no safe place to store belongings. Leaving the premises is not encouraged, and therefore there is little contact with people outside the boarding home. Inactivity and passivity are rewarded because such behavior is considered the least troublesome by the staff.

Within this context, the goals of intervention are seen as the development of skill in (a) basic self-care; (b) self-management in home, neighborhood, and peripheral community; (c) social interaction behavior; (d) discovery and use of community resources and public transportation; (e) productive use of leisure time; and (f) recreation. The last is seen as particularly important, since mentally retarded adults have a decreased response to those stimuli which ordinarily arouse people to engage in play or recreational activities.

In order to reach these goals, Keilhofner and associates suggest several factors that they believe will facilitate the evaluation and intervention process.

Assessment should take into consideration the unique historical and environmental conditions that have shaped the lives of retarded persons. An individual's repertoire of behavior comes into being through the meaning the person has given to his or her own actions, the environment, and the totality of life experiences. Evaluation, therefore, must focus on determining under what conditions and in what personal sense of the world observed behavior may be described as functional and adaptive.

When historical and environmental circumstances are not taken into consideration, competence may be underestimated and more negative than positive characteristics identified.

Intervention must be designed to take into consideration the way that retarded clients experience and make sense of the world, given their past and current life situation. This includes being sensitive to the temporal differences between retarded and nonretarded persons, which may alter the meaning of activities.

Skills are best learned through repeated interactions in an environment that demands an adequate response to variation and flexibility, capacities that are necessary for interaction in the community. Skills cannot be learned outside a context that is meaningful to the client.

Activities used as the basis for intervention should be stimulating but nevertheless graded in complexity. Required skills should be demonstrated directly and indirectly by the therapist acting as a model. Thus, the therapist should join in activities with clients so that his or her behavior can be observed and imitated.

The therapist's relationship with mentally retarded clients should be as equals rather than that of helper/helpee. In this horizontal relationship the therapist is able to make demands for competence that cannot reasonably be made within a superordinate-subordinate relationship. Clients, for example, should be equally responsible for deciding what will be done in the program. A horizontal relationship contributes to a marked decrease in client's dependent behavior.

CONCLUSION

Developmentally disabled individuals may need assistance in adapting throughout the life cycle. This assistance should be provided in such a way that independence is fostered. Nevertheless, expectations must be set at a realistic level, with emphasis placed on the quality of the individual's life.

30 Gerontology

Occupational therapists have been involved with the elderly population probably since the formal beginning of the profession. This involvement, however, has not been extensive. It has increased over the years, but has not kept pace with the real and proportional increase of individuals over the age of 65 years. During the past 15 years, the occupational therapy literature has repeatedly called for greater involvement of therapists with this age group (397,399,471,597,598,637,670,819,880,897,1031). This appeal has emphasized our expertise in the area of purposeful activities, adapting the environment to meet the needs of disabled individuals and considering the individual as a holistic entity existing in a social matrix.

The current lack of involvement of occupational therapists with the elderly population appears to be influenced by three major factors: deficient knowledge, the average age of occupational therapists, and lack of financial support. There is little attention given to gerontology in basic professional education, major emphasis being placed on the previous phases of the life cycle. There are few advanced professional programs with specialization in gerontology and only occasional continuing education courses. The average age of registered occupational therapists and certified occupational therapy assistants is 31 years and 28 years, respectively (*personal communication*, Francis A. Acquaviva). Younger people tend not to elect to work with the elderly. Some of the reasons for this phenomenon were outlined in Chapter 8. There is comparatively little financial support available for dealing with the problems encountered by the elderly. Although positions for occupational therapists are available, many of these are in institutions. These are frequently undesirable places of employment because of a serious lack of adequate funding. Whether our society will decide to spend more money to enhance the quality of life of the elderly is unknown. The elderly population, given its ever-increasing number, may well become a political force that is able to demand appropriate services. On the other hand, the state of the economy may mitigate against any increase in the expenditure of additional public funds for the elderly.

The above remarks were by no means meant to imply that occupational therapy's involvement in gerontology is a wasteland. Much work has and is being done in this area. This chapter focuses on programs designed to enhance the psychosocial function of the elderly population. The chapter is divided into four sections: the healthy elderly population, the disabled elderly population in the community, the elderly population in institutional settings and in the process of dying. These sections are, of course, arbitrary. The various programs and issues discussed are often applicable relative to the entire aged population regardless of where they may be living or whether or not they are disabled. Prior to proceeding, it is suggested that the reader review "Sixty-Five Years of Age to Death," "Chronic Illness/Disability," and "Death and Loss," all in Chapter 5.

THE HEALTHY ELDERLY POPULATION

The term "healthy" as used here refers to those individuals over 65 years of age who have no major disability. Their state of physical and emotional health is good with only minor deficits due to the aging process. This section is divided into three parts: pre- and postretirement programs, senior citizen organizations, and adjustment to the aging process. There is, of course, some overlapping here.

Pre- and Postretirement Programs

One of the first developmental tasks of individuals over the age of 65 years is to successfully master the process of retirement. The role of worker must be given up and its loss mourned, leisure time interests developed and expanded, and new adjustments made relative to temporal adaptation. The occupational therapist can provide assistance with this life task through involvement in pre- and postretirement planning programs. Such programs may be sponsored by management, labor unions, fraternal organizations, and the like. They usually deal with many aspects of retirement, e.g., financial, legal, and personal. It is the latter aspect of the program to which occupational therapists may lend their expertise.

The hypothetical program to be described here is based on the role acquisition frame of reference and is very similar to the program outlined by Cantor (164). Although it may be conducted on an individual basis, intervention is probably more effective if it takes place within the context of an anticipatory/concurrent topical group.

The purpose of the pre- and postretirement program is to plan for a purposeful and healthful use of time during the individual's retirement years. Although planning is for the near future or present, emphasis is also placed on using a similar method of planning in the future when life circumstances may require a change in one's usual routines and activities. The focus of the program is the exploration of interests, needs, values, use of time, and the reciprocal relationship between these elements. The program has five sequential steps, although progress through these steps may not be linear. The five steps are:

1. *Fact finding*. This step involves participant's identifying the current activities in which they engage and their use of time. This is best accomplished through making out a schedule of activities for a typical week. A form similar to the one used for assessment of temporal adaptation, the activity configuration, is a useful tool to assist in this process.
2. *Assessment*. Each activity is then looked at separately, relative to several dimensions: its source of motivation, the needs that it satisfies, how well one does it, the extent to which the activity will be engaged in during retirement, and so forth. In addition, participants look at their pattern of activities and use of time over the period of the week. This is assessed in the same way as individual activities. Ultimately, participants are encouraged to make some decisions about what activities they would like to maintain, what activities they would like to change, and how they would like to structure the use of their time.
3. *Option Search*. This step involves exploration of various activities, alterations in activities, and ways of structuring time. A brainstorming method whereby many options are identified with due consideration being given to all is suggested. This method allows participants to entertain a variety of ideas, even those that may seem somewhat outlandish at first glance.
4. *Selection of options and planning strategies*. Ultimately participants are encouraged to decide what options they would like to implement. Priorities are set and participants assisted in determining a step-by-step procedure for implementing the desired changes.
5. *Implementation*. At this point participants begin to implement the changes in their life which they have decided they would like to make. Support and feedback are provided by group members. At times it may be necessary for a participant to go back to earlier steps if choices or plans are not found to be satisfactory.

The choices made by the participants are their own. Although the therapist and other group members may make suggestions and give feedback, each participant selects the gestalt of activities he or she wishes to engage in and the way in which these activities will be patterned relative to time. The only guidelines that the therapist might suggest is that participants consider some activities that will satisfy their need for association with others, recognition, the use of their knowledge and skills, expression of feeling, and activities that reduce anxiety and provide an outlet for anger and frustration. Above all, emphasis should be placed on selecting activities that are interesting and pleasurable to the individual.

Participation in pre- and postretirement programs are not, of course, appropriate for all individuals. Some people are quite able to manage this role transition with relative ease and without any outside assistance. Other individuals do, however, need help. Perhaps the best indicators of the need for participation in a pre- and postretirement program is the expression of considerable anxiety regarding retirement and/or evidence of considerable nonpurposeful behavior after retirement. It should be noted that initial adjustment to retirement may appear to be very good. It is only somewhat later, after the individual has completed a variety of tasks or activities that had been postponed until retirement, that the individual may begin to experience difficulty.

Senior Citizen Organizations

Many communities have centers or clubs specifically designed to meet the educational and recreational needs of the healthy, elderly population (471,540,745,880,992). These clubs or centers may be freestanding or affiliated with some larger organization such as a church, temple, or a fraternal group. They are usually managed by the members and supported, at least in part, by members' dues. Physical facilities vary, but ideally they include an area for visiting and conversation; exercise room and showers; a game room; a craft room; a kitchen; a large multipurpose room for the presentation of educational programs and large group activities such as dancing, dining, and the like; and office space.

Occupational therapists sometime act as a consultant to these groups. In this capacity, the occupational therapist may help the board of managers identify the needs and interests of the members, facilitate the problem solving and decision making, and act as a resource person regarding services and facilities in the community. Occasionally the therapist may provide direct services. The occupational therapist's overall purpose is to assist members with the various developmental tasks of this part of the life cycle and to enhance their general sense of security and well-being.

The therapist's role in the educational aspect of the center's program may be to suggest areas of interest, to identify appropriate speakers, and to present information that is within his or her area of expertise. As to the last, the therapist, for example, may prepare presentations regarding work simplification and energy conservation, or the adaptation of one's home to accommodate for diminished vision and physical agility (399). Examples of other topics that may be presented in educational programs are social security and medicare benefits, income taxes, security in the home and street, first aid, nutrition, living on a reduced income, organizing for political action, how to use the library effectively, and special discounts and services for the elderly.

The therapist's role in the recreational aspect of the program may be to help the board of managers or groups of members to identify activities that are likely to be of interest. This is often best accomplished through brainstorming. A variety of activities are important, e.g., active, sedentary, individual, group, sports, cultural, and arts and crafts. These activities may be located in the center, in the community, may be service-orientation, and so forth. The cultural, ethnic background of members should be capitalized on relative to the preparation of special food and the celebration of holidays.

Some elderly people are not particularly interested in formal activities, primarily using the center as a place for dropping in, meeting friends, and gossiping. The area set aside for conversation, therefore, should be made as comfortable as possible, with appropriate grouping of chairs and simple refreshments available.

Regarding direct service, the occupational therapist may facilitate adjustment to the latter phase of the life cycle by assisting members of the center in reconciling various universal issues. Many elderly people are pleased to have an opportunity to express their thoughts and feelings about the aging process and the adjustments and adaptations that they need to make now or will need to make in the future. This is probably best accomplished in a task-oriented group. The universal issues of major concern are adequacy, dependence/independence, and loss.

Regarding adequacy, the individual may experience a diminished degree of self-esteem owing to the aging process, retirement, or to the necessity of living on a fixed income. On the other hand, the individual may see this phase of the life cycle as a second chance, a time to make a new start. There may be a desire to undo old patterns, to develop new interests. With this awakening desire, the individual may initially question his or her adequacy to bring about these changes. Ideally, the issue is reconciled in the direction of taking on the challenge of exploring new possibilities.

The issue of dependence/independence frequently focuses on the individual's concern about being able to manage his affairs independently. There is often a fear of becoming a burden to others. The need for autonomy and connectedness with others is sometimes viewed as a dichotomous position rather than as a dimension along which one may move comfortably according to the current needs and inclination (155,453). Adequate reconciliation is characterized by less extreme values being placed on dependence and independence and flexibility in accepting an appropriate dependent/independent position.

The elderly individual is faced with managing and anticipating many losses. Ultimately, the individual is confronted with the reality of his or her own death. Reconciliation of this universal issue occurs through reaching some degree of accommodation with the inevitable and making appropriate plans.

A task-oriented group that allows elderly individuals to express and explore their thoughts and feelings in a safe, supportive environment is often viewed as an invaluable experience. It provides a shared reality that allows the individual to deal more effectively with the self and the external environment.

THE DISABLED ELDERLY POPULATION IN THE COMMUNITY

It is somewhat difficult to identify the disabled elderly population through the use of any specific criteria (399,540,645,670,880,954,955,992,1031). The objective presence and degree of a disability is a poor indicator of functional ability. The individual's personal interpretation of his or her state of health and current life circumstances most often determines how the individual views the quality of life. The value the individual places on health and his or her particular limitations will influence the ability to cope and the way in which he or she identifies need priorities. In general, all that can be safely said is that an individual's health status is determined by the mutual interdependence of physical health, capacity to adapt, and emotional health.

Except in the case of rather severe illness, it is generally felt that it is better for disabled elderly persons to stay within the community. It is economically more advantageous, and, furthermore, research indicates that those who stay in the community have a greater sense of need satisfaction and a better self-concept than individuals who reside in an institution. It is unknown, however, if the poor self-perception of the institutionalized elderly is a factor in their being institutionalized or if it has arisen because of institutionalization. Recognition of the benefits of keeping the disabled elderly in the community has led to a growing movement to develop adequate support systems for this population. It has been found that such support systems are most effective when (a) an effort is made to seek out and respect the input of potential consumers; (b) there is recognition that clients are usually able to identify their major problems and to decide which services would be most effective in helping them to solve these problems; and (c) there is continuous communication between the various agencies involved which results in the coordination of services.

It has been found that adequate community supports increase disabled persons' sense of security. This, in turn, allows the individual to cope with environmental problems more successfully.

The difficulties encountered by disabled elderly persons are many and varied. Briefly, the major problems are difficulties in dealing with the mental and physical changes of aging: failing health, loss of family members and peers, a sense of social isolation and loneliness, lack of income security, inadequate health care, poor transportation, and inadequate services to facilitate home maintenance and continued residence in one's own home. Concerning the last area, it has been found that the most important tasks for independence in the home are the ability to use the telephone, shop, cook, clean, take care of the laundry, being able to take responsibility for one's own medication, and handling personal finances.

It is to all of the above problem areas that support systems must be addressed. The remaining portion of this section describes some programs in which occupational therapists have been involved that have been designed to provide services for the disabled elderly in the community.

One approach to providing at least the beginning of a support system is the formation of an activity group. Menks, et al. describe such a group that was designed to meet the mental health and maintenance needs of the elderly in a rural community (675). Participants are described as individuals at high risk: they had previously been hospitalized or had experienced emotional problems, they were living in social isolation, taking psychoactive drugs, had extrapyramidal symptoms, or they had rather serious hearing and/or vision loss. Activities used included participating in crafts, team games, the sharing of stories, eating together, and trading recipies. The last reflected the culinary heritage of the region.

Auerbach describes a community group in San Francisco named the Bernal Heights Ladies Club (53). It existed previous to the occupational therapist's involvement, meeting once a week in the basement of the local library. Members were lonely older women from the community who were gathered together by a natural group leader—a strong, motherly woman. Meetings included eating a bag lunch and working on craft and needlework projects. Informal discussion involved the sharing of local gossip, discussion of problems, exchange of information, and general support. The occupational therapist heard about the group and joined it with one of her clients who was about to return to the community after a psychiatric hospitalization. The therapist continued to participate in the group, bringing suitable clients with her as prospective members. The therapist did not take a leadership position in the group. She participated as a member, acting as a role model for the clients that she periodically brought to the group. The group, able to tolerate some deviant behavior, provided a means of transition for elderly clients and a base for reintegration into the community.

A more comprehensive support system for the disabled elderly is outlined by Hasselkus and Kumat (399). The project had three major parts: education, home consultation, and transportation. Relative to education, several mini-courses (three class sessions) were designed to provide information about coping with various disabilities. Some examples of the focus of courses offered were caring for the self when confined to a wheel chair, remaining independent when one-handed, solving daily living problems associated with being arthritic, how best to regulate daily activities for individuals with cardiac problems, and daily adjustment to the loss of vision. Much of this information was later made available at the local library.

Home consultation involved an occupational therapist visiting a client's home (at the client's invitation) for the purpose of assessment. The home was evaluated relative to its safety and the extent to which it facilitated the functioning of the client. Recommendations were made to the client about alterations that could be easily made. The therapist also assessed the client's need for services such as mobile meals, visisting nurse, homemaker help, and so forth. Referrals were made when appropriate, but, again, only with the consent of the client.

Lack of adequate transportation in the geographic area covered by the project interfered with the elderly making adequate use of community resources. A minibus was bought to provide regular transportation for going to a shopping center, appointments with health personnel, and other essential visits.

The report of this project ends with some brief comments on the occupational therapist working in the community. The therapist must find a way through a maze of community organizations, by no means an easy task. The therapist is required to define his or her role not only within various community organizations but also to the elderly. The use of technical terms and jargon should be avoided in written reports as well as in face-to-face communication. Finally, working in the community can be a lonely experience. There may be no one with whom to exchange ideas and share decision-making; feedback, both positive and negative, may be lacking.

Hasselkus has also reported on another type of support system, a small group home for the elderly (397). The home was in a residential neighborhood and specially renovated for the residents. This was a relatively independent alternative living situation with minimal support services. The occupational therapist acted as a consultant to the residents, with the general goal of promoting an environment conducive to meaningful social relationships. It was found that the group dynamics of the residents represented the most difficult and vulnerable component of the program. Problem areas centered around the use of the kitchen and bathroom, daily household chores, and the upkeep of common living space. Other sources of tension were differences in mobility, the amount of attention paid by family, and a resident leaving or a new resident coming into the home. The therapist's role was to help the group express feelings and ideas, communicate effectively with each other, make compromises, and engage in joint decision-making. It was also necessary to assist the residents in learning how to give support and positive feedback to each other.

A very different approach to developing an adequate support system for the disabled elderly is day-hospital programs (50,528,540,1025). The general goal of such programs is to provide comprehensive services so as to prevent or delay institutionalization. Specific goals include rehabilitation (if that is realistic for the individual client), maintenance, and meeting health needs. Some day-hospital programs also define one of their goals as providing relief for the family. Clients come to the program for a full day two to four times a week, depending on their needs and those of the family.

The usual role of the occupational therapist is to engage in regular evaluations with each client, provide rehabilitation programs, supervise the activity program, make home visits, and work with the team to maintain an appropriate milieu. Evaluation, rehabilitation, and home visits have been previously discussed. Brief attention is given here to the activity program and to creating an appropriate milieu.

The activity program is designed to maintain function or to impede deterioration and to meet health needs. Activities are used to revive or discover skills and interests, to establish social contacts, to encourage mobility, and to help each individual find a personal role in the day-hospital setting. Games, arts and crafts, kitchen activities, and discussion groups (current events, controversial issues, etc.), and trips to engage in community-based activities are some of the activities utilized.

The general milieu created by the staff is considered one of the most important factors in the program. It is designed to emphasize respect for each individual and to foster active participation. Participants are, as fully as possible, involved in making decisions and planning daily activities. The expression of ideas and feelings are encouraged. When complaints are voiced, participants are urged to consider ways to deal with the offending situation. The staff gives considerable support and consistently attempts to demonstrate an attitude of caring.

Finally, the use of volunteers should not be overlooked in planning programs for the disabled elderly. They not only provide valuable services but are also an effective way of educating the community about the needs of the elderly population. Some tasks that volunteers may perform are regular visits to the elderly, particularly those who are essentially homebound; assistance with transportation; home maintenance and meal preparation; and staying with an elderly individual so that family members are able to engage in leisure activities outside the home. It has been found that the effectiveness of a volunteer program is dependent on appropriate education and supervision of the participants by an occupational therapist or some other individual with skill in this area.

THE ELDERLY POPULATION IN INSTITUTIONS

As used here, the term institution refers to a nursing home, extended care facility, and the like that is concerned with providing adequate care for an elderly individual who is no longer able to live in the community. An elderly person may enter an institution with the expectation of remaining there for the rest of his or her life or the individual's stay may be temporary. The major emphasis in an institution for the elderly is on meeting health needs, maintenance, and management. Residents occasionally may be involved in a change process but, on the whole, this is not the major focus.

In the interest of clarity, this section is divided into three parts: relocation stress, factors to consider in program planning, and special types of programs (8,211, 398,471,597,637,682,897,953,991).

Relocation Stress

Relocation stress refers to the physiological, mental, and emotional disequilibrium that occurs when an individual moves his or her place of residence from one location to another (398,453). It may occur during preparation for the move, during the move itself, or during the necessary adjustments that follow a move. Factors that appear to give rise to a stress reaction are deprivation of familiar cues and environmental supports and the need to cope with a new set of stimuli in an unfamiliar environment. Although the focus here is on the relocation stress that may arise in moving from the community to an institution, it may also occur with any change in permanent or temporary residence. Some elderly individuals tend to move rather frequently: temporary housing with relatives, moves to apartments and retirement villages, limited stays in nursing homes, to a hospital for acute care. The possibility of relocation stress should always be kept in mind whenever there is a change in residence.

Men appear to be more vulnerable than women to the strain of relocation. Other personal factors that increase vulnerability are psychosis, senility, feelings of helplessness and/or despair, and close and long-term association with a particular neighborhood. Environmental factors also influence the likelihood of relocation stress. Some of these factors are (a) the degree of similarity between the old and new environment and the degree of continuity between these environments; (b) the extent of disruption in social relationships with family and friends either due to geographic distance or to lack of apparent interest; (c) the amount of curtailment of personal choice, independence, and privacy; and (d) the predictability of the new environment.

The elderly, particularly those who are disabled, are dependent on the surrounding environment. At the same time, they often feel, at times rightly so, that control over their life space is diminishing.

Relocation stress relative to movement into an institution can be minimized by adequate preparation and appropriate policies on the part of the institution. Preparation for relocation begins with an assessment of the individual's capacity to remain in the community. This involves evaluation of the individual's ability to engage in self-care and other daily living tasks and the adequacy of community, family, and personal support systems. The individual should be intimately involved in the evaluation, for the data gathered will be at least somewhat influential in the individual's ultimate decision. Family members are also closely involved in this assessment, for they are very often participants in this decision. If at all possible, ample time should be allowed for decision-making and for determining the most suitable institution for the individual. The emotional issues involved—for the individual and the family—are as important, if not more so, than the practical issues. Sufficient time should be given for the expression of feelings, exploration, and reality testing. If at all possible, the ultimate decision should be left to the elderly individual. When this is not feasible, the individual should be as involved in the process as possible.

Movement into the institution, ideally, proceeds gradually. The individual, for example, may visit the institution and join the residents for lunch or dinner. Arrangements might be made for the individual to stay overnight. When the individual is unable to visit the institution, it is often possible for a staff member and perhaps a resident to visit the individual. A family member may take photographs inside and outside the institution, thus providing the individual with a sense of at least the physical facilities.

Some of the policies of an institution that tend to minimize relocation stress are as follows:

1. A bedroom that can be personalized by each resident and that is respected as a place of privacy;
2. Integration of the institution into the surrounding community so that there is a flow of community

members through the institution and regular use of community resources by residents;
3. The provision of adequate transportation so that residents are able to participate in social, religious, and cultural programs;
4. The encouragement of visitors and regular telephone contact with family and friends;
5. The opportunity to engage in light household tasks and simple meal preparation;
6. A varied program of regular activities;
7. An orientation program that provides a detailed overview of the institution—its physical layout, roles of the various staff members, schedule of regular activities, methods for dealing with grievances—and a description of the privileges, responsibilities, and rights of the residents.

Transition from the community to an institution is never an easy process. The reality of the emotional and practical issues involved should not be denied. Nevertheless, with proper planning and enlightened policies, the transition can be designed to minimize the amount of stress involved.

Factors to Consider in Program Planning

To engage in effective program planning, the therapist must be aware of the many components of a long-term care facility—the resident population, staff, the concerns of family members, sensitivity of volunteers, involvement of the attending physicians, the clergy (682). This is the matrix within which program planning must take place.

The residents in a nursing home or extended care facility vary in the type and degree of their disability. Miller has identified six groups that need to be considered (682):

1. Those who are substantially physically and cognitively intact;
2. Those who are physically disabled and cognitively intact;
3. Those who are ambulatory with advanced organic mental disorders;
4. Those who are severely physically handicapped with advanced organic mental disorders;
5. Those who are cognitively intact, ambulatory, and terminally ill;
6. Those who are cognitively intact, debilitated, and terminally ill.

Because all groups may not be able to be provided with adequate services, difficult decisions often need to be made regarding the allocation of services. Programs tend to be provided for those who are able to speak up and demand services. These are also the residents that are likely to be the most independent and capable of being creative and puposeful in their use of time. The most disadvantaged groups are those who are severely cognitively impaired—they have the least number of visitors and are least likely to leave the institution for visits and trips. These are also the residents who need the most guidance in engaging in purposeful activities.

In program planning the therapist is often overly concerned with group activities. This may be due to a shortage of staff, but it also may be a reflection of a value system that places a high premium on group interaction. Not all residents share that value. Some subscribe to the tenet of rugged individualism, others simply are not all that fond of involvement in group activities. Thus, individually oriented activities as well as group activities should be planned and encouraged.

Long-term care institutions tend to breed loneliness (or more correctly, a sense of aloneness), helplessness, a sense of despair, and inertia. Program planning should be designed to combat this endemic condition. The occupational therapist alone is not responsible for maintaining the human spirit but certainly is obligated to participate actively in the process.

The therapist's role in the institution includes evaluation and intervention. The purpose of evaluation is both to determine the resident's general functional capacity and to determine if there are aspects of dysfunction that can be remedied. Focus is usually on the resident's potential for greater independence in activities of daily living. If increase in function appears to be feasible, the resident is involved in a change process. Data from the assessment of the resident's functional capacity are also used to determine the types of tasks the client is able to engage in and the adaptations that may need to be made to allow the individual to participate more fully in the activities of the institution.

As in the discussion of day-hospitals, the activity program in an institution is usually separated from that aspect of the total program which is concerned with the change process. The goal of the activity program is to meet health needs and to maintain function. The program emphasizes the client's strengths. Expectations are individualized so that they are neither too high nor too low. Demand, then, is closely calibrated to the capacity of each resident. Recognizing the importance of activities for the maintenance of physical and emotional health, the staff should strongly urge residents to participate in the activity program. Nevertheless, the residents' right to not participate should be recognized and respected. Finally, the activity program should be challenging and ever changing. New activities should be regularly introduced. This not only facilitates the satisfaction of different needs and interests but it also helps to combat the inflexible and constant part of the institution.

Some of the activities usually included in the general activity program are quiet and active games, exercise, sports, arts and crafts, hobbies, social activities, educational programs, music and dance, community service, and religious activities. Various specialized groups are also a part of many activity programs. Examples of such groups are:

- *New residence group*. Such a group is concerned with learning about living in an institution and how to deal with some of the problems inherent in group living;
- *Men's group*. Men, a minority in most institutions, often need a time to be together to discuss their particular concerns and/or to pursue special interests;
- *A couples group*. This type of group is made up of couples who have come to the institution together or who have met in the institution;
- *Out-reach group*. Through this group, members keep in contact with residents who have been hospitalized and write letters of condolence to relatives of residents who have died;
- *Current events group*. Such a group is concerned not only with the discussion of current events but also with the active participation in influencing these events through letter writing, attending rallies, and telephone campaigns.
- *Various committees*. Some of the activities in which these groups may be involved are self-government of a unit of the facility, negotiating complaints lodged by residents, an advisory group to the administration, and other services such as dietary, organization of special events, preparation for holiday celebrations, and so forth.

Participation in the events and activities of the surrounding community should be an integral part of the activity program. Adult education courses, cultural events, visiting theme parks, going to movies and plays, eating in restaurants, walks in the city or countryside, visiting the local library, going to the lake or ocean are just some examples of the activities that may be enjoyed by residents.

The activity program should also be addressed to the needs and concerns of family members. A group that provides an orientation to the institution and an opportunity to express the feelings and ideas associated with the institutionalization of a family member is often beneficial for the relatives of new residents. Evening and weekend, as well as some weekday activities should be designed to include family members and friends. Participating in activities together is often a welcome diversion and an opportunity to share mutual interests. Family and friends should also be invited to special events and holiday celebrations. Visits outside the institution with family and friends should, of course, be encouraged.

Volunteers can make a valuable contribution to an activity program. They may well bring a variety of experience and expertise that can add new dimensions to the program. They allow residents who are unable to leave the institution regularly to have contact with members of the community. Volunteers are sometimes able to offer home hospitality to residents who have no family with whom to visit. Participation of grade school, high school, and college students should not be overlooked. Besides their usual natural exuberance and energy, they bring a sense of the life cycle, the continuation of life, the promise of the younger generation.

Another area in which the occupational therapist can make a contribution to a long-term care institution is the enhancement of the physical environment. The occupational therapist should be concerned not only about the safety of the environment but also about the organization of the environment so that it facilitates function. Some examples of the adaptations that might be made are environmental modifications that take into consideration resident's limitations in mobility, vision, and hearing. The therapist's knowledge of the significance of the nonhuman environment is a further resource for assisting in the design of a living space that is conducive to optimal function.

The occupational therapist may be involved in a nursing home or extended care facility as a full-time employee or as a consultant. The latter role was briefly discussed in Chapter 8. Miller makes some interesting additional comments on the role of a consultant in a nursing home (682). She describes the consultant as being at somewhat of a disadvantage because of the part-time nature of his or her services and of the lack of responsibility for implementation. Nevertheless, the therapist is responsible for informing and guiding the administration in the successful accomplishment of a quality program. The therapist/consultant is most likely to be effective when he or she thoroughly documents needs and provides explicit plans for improving the quality and life of the residents. Miller describes the competent consultant as an individual who is independent, objective and informed, able to stimulate creative approaches, make valid judgments and appropriate decisions—and above all, who is involved.

Special Types of Programs

This section includes a brief description of three programs frequently used to assist the elderly. The first two—reality orientation (sometimes referred to as remotivation) and sensory stimulation—are designed to assist the cognitively impaired elderly individual become more aware of and involved in the environment (374,598). The third program—life review—is designed to assist individuals in assessing their past life, resolving old conflicts, and, in general, giving meaning to their life.

A program of reality orientation is designed to ameliorate disorientation and confusion and to increase clients interest in the surrounding environment. Emphasis is placed on orientation to person, place, and time and on other basic facets of the environment. This is accomplished by repeatedly giving basic information to the client such as his or her name, where the client is, the time of day and the date, the name of common objects, what the client is doing or should be doing at the present time, and so forth. The client is requested to repeat this information or act on the basis of the information and is given reinforcement for doing so. This aspect of reality orientation is most effective if it is a 24-hour a day process. Staff, family members, and volunteers, whenever they are in contact with the client, should identify and reinforce the client's awareness of person, place, time, and the surrounding events that are occuring. The prominent display of clocks, calenders with the day and date indicated, and the daily schedule of events are useful. The individual's room, bed, clothes, and other personal belongings should be marked with his or her name or initials. It is often useful if the staff and residents wear large name tags to assist the individual in sorting out the people in the immediate environment. (It should be remembered, however, that some people find name tags offensive and dehumanizing.)

Reality orientation, as described above, is informal. It sometimes, however, is formalized into a specific program. As described in the literature, the program takes place within the context of a thematic group which meets at least twice a week. Each group meeting is described as having four phases:

1. *Opening*. Each participant is greeted by name and some positive remark is made about his or her appearance. Group members are encouraged to greet each other by name. The leader identifies the day and date and comments on some immediate event such as the weather, what was on the lunch menu, and the like. Every effort is made to create an atmosphere of warmth and acceptance.

2. *Introduction of a topic*. A topic for discussion is introduced by the leader. This may be a poem, news story, controversial issue, a coming holiday, seasonal change, and so forth. The leader presents the topic in some detail to provide immediate stimuli for discussion. Audiovisual aids are particularly useful.

3. *Discussion*. The discussion portion of the meeting is focused through the leader asking a series of direct, objective questions. This allows group members to respond and participate at a fairly low level. Each group member is asked at least one question. If he or she does not know the answer, the therapist provides it and asks the client to repeat it. The therapist also encourages group members to ask questions. A general free-flowing group discussion may not be possible in this type of group. But if such a discussion should occur spontaneously, it is encouraged.

4. *Closing*. The high points of the discussion are reviewed and each member is personally thanked (by name) for his or her participation. Members are encouraged to bid farewell to each other. The time and date of the next meeting is announced, and the topic for discussion identified.

The topics selected and the level of presentation and discussion questions will vary, depending on the general cognitive capacity of group members. An individual may participate in a reality-oriented group for an indeterminate amount of time, or the group may be used as a transition to participating in other, more demanding aspects of the activity program.

A program of sensory stimulation is also used to orient the elderly, cognitively impaired individual to the environment. It has been found to be particularly useful for individuals who demonstrate severe psychomotor retardation and deficits in discriminating between and responding appropriately to environmental stimuli. It is hypothesized that such individuals are experiencing sensory deprivation resulting from disuse or malfunction of sensory receptors, or generalized retreat from the environment.

A sensory stimulation program usually takes place in a thematic group and involves the stimulation of the major sensory receptors individually, then simultaneously in a multisensory approach. The group itself offers general social and cognitive stimulation and feedback and consensual validation of the individual's reactions. Activities are designed to provide stimulation and require an adaptive response. The response might be to identify an object, to describe one's reactions to a particular stimuli, or to share the associations brought to mind by a given stimuli.

Each group meeting begins in a manner similar to that outlined for a reality orientation group. Some of the activities used are:

- *Kinesthetic*. The use of exercises that emphasize movement of body parts in space and proprioceptive input. The leader may ask each individual to move and identify a body part following demonstration by the leader on some group member.
- *Tactile*. Group members are asked to identify and describe objects placed in their hand without looking at them. Objects of various size and texture are used. Tactile stimulation is also provided through touching, hugging, handshaking, and clapping.
- *Auditory*. Group members are asked to identify different sounds such as a ball bouncing, various types of whistles, traditional songs, the crackle of a fire, paper being shaken, and so forth. A group member may be placed out of sight, with the remaining members being asked to imitate the sounds (clapping, humming, tapping) made by the individual.
- *Olfactory*. Group members are presented with a variety of odors which they are asked to identify and, if possible, to share associations to particular odors. Differentiation between odors is another activity that may be used.
- *Gustatory*. Group members are given a variety of foods to taste while vision is occluded. It is best to present well-liked very familiar foods initially. Along with the taste, the individual may be asked to also focus on the texture.

At the end of each session, group members participate in an activity involving multiple stimuli such as square dancing or a rhythm band.

There are many ways to provide sensory stimuli which require an adaptive response. The therapist must be somewhat creative in order to present a variety of activities. This type of group is most effective when there is considerable novelty.

Life review has been identified by some authorities as being a natural-occuring, universal, and necessary part of the last phase of the life cycle (155,272,453.) It is so described because it appears to be engaged in spontaneously by many individuals cross-culturally. Evidence for this phenomenon is the tendency of the elderly to reminisce, tell stories about their past life, and indulge in mild nostalgia. The elderly may make pilgrimages back to places that were significant to them in the past; it is the elderly who tend to write autobiographies.

It is believed that life review is prompted by the realization of approaching death. It appears to be initiated by the progressive return to consciousness of past experiences, particularly those that entail unresolved conflicts. The function of life review seems to be twofold: First, the recognition of what one has achieved and the adversities and losses that one has overcome; the realization that one's life has mattered and that it was worth living. And second, the review of revived experiences and conflicts, the correction of old judgments, the reintegration of negative and positive experiences so that the individual is able to come to terms with old wounds, sadness, and disappointments.

Ultimately, life review frequently leads to a reconciliation of estranged family relationships and the desire to transmit knowledge and values to those who follow. Moreover, the individual becomes comfortable in taking responsibility for creating a meaningful life for the time that remains.

Life review then should not be seen as a sign of self-preoccupation, meaningless, or morbid. As a natural and necessary process, the therapist should do whatever possbile to encourage involvement in this activity (487,529,597). Some of the methods used to facilitate this process are compiling family photo albums and scrapbooks of other memorabilia, searching out and preparing a family geneology, and making an oral history of one's life experiences. Life review is often structured as a group activity where memories and experiences can be shared. Audiovisual material and music may act as memory aids that trigger reminiscing. The celebration of religious and ethnic holidays also tends to trigger memories.

Above all, it is important that the therapist and other staff members be available as interested and caring listeners. One need say very little, just being there to listen to the sad parts as well as to the good times is usually all that is needed. This is the client's task—to remember, to resolve, and, eventually, to gain a sense of pride, serenity, and an acceptance of mortal life.

THE PROCESS OF DYING

Many of the issues and problems associated with loss, dying, grief, and mourning were discussed in "Death and Loss," Chapter 5. Some ways of assisting individuals with these problems and issues were outlined in Chapter 22. It is suggested that the reader review these sections. This section briefly describes some ways in which the occupational therapist may assist the dying individual and the family. The discussion is general in nature and not specifically applicable to any particular age group or to a long-term care facility (151,328,487,597,746, 747,775,1018). It is primarily based on a modification of role acquisition.

There are three major areas of concern in assisting an individual in the dying process: (a) helping the client to relinquish current social roles and accept the role of a dying person, (b) meeting the client's various needs, and (c) helping those close to the client in their adjustment.

Although it may sound somewhat cruel, it is usually considered important for the dying individual to realize that he or she can no longer fulfill former social roles and that these roles are now inappropriate. It is only through relinquishing these roles that the individual is able to engage in what is now the most important role—that of a dying person. One way to assist a client in giving up former roles is to help the dying person instruct others in the assumption of various roles. A husband, for example, may be helped to teach his wife how to manage family finances; a mother to teach her oldest son some homemaking skills. In helping the client assume the role of a dying person more directly, the therapist may need to instruct the individual how to play that role effectively. The client, for example, may be helped to be more assertive in making requests or urged to minimize behavior, such as excessive complaining, that causes others to withdraw. In teaching appropriate role behaviors, the therapist should emphasize that these behaviors are in the best interest of the client and that certain types of behavior will lead to positive responses from staff members and family. The dying role is essentially selfish in nature, as it should be. The client needs support at this time and has the right to learn how to get that support.

A dying individual has several needs that he or she may require help in satisfying. First, the client has the need to clarify and understand his or her own feelings and those of others. There are concerns about the past; dealing with these may be facilitated by a life review process. There are concerns about the present; the trajectory of the dying process, the welfare of loved ones. Some reality testing is useful here, but the therapist's participation as an active listener is probably the best way of helping the individual. For a child, the use of activities such as drawing, painting, or making objects out of clay facilitates the expression of feelings and ideas.

Second, the individual needs to have a sense of control over self and the environment. One of the major ways that self-control can be experienced in a concrete way is independence in activities of daily living. Independence in this area should be encouraged as long as feasible. Emphasis should be placed on self-care, and, in particular, on grooming. For many people, being well-groomed and nicely dressed minimizes the feeling of vulnerability, of not being master of the immediate situation. Control over the environment can be enhanced by such things as the client making a living will (as outlined in Chapter 5), determining the length of visits of family and friends, deciding the daily menu, and the like.

The third major need of the dying individual is related to temporal adaptation. With the recognition of approaching death, the individual's perspective regarding time is frequently altered. Time is now limited, circumspect, a newly precious commodity. Ideally, the therapist helps the individual develop an orientation to present and future time that is both wise and expedient. Regarding present time, the individual is assisted in learning to live one day at a time, each to its fullest. Regarding future time, the client is helped to appreciate and become aware of the need to structure the time that is left. The individual is encouraged to plan feasible strategies and alternatives to make the remaining life and time as comfortable and productive as possible.

Taking the above needs into consideration and the client's life-style and personal interests, the client and therapist together develop a plan for intervention. Emphasis is placed on what the individual is still able to do. Initially, activities may be quite creative and challenging. As the client's condition deteriorates, structured and familiar activities may be more appropriate. The pleasure that can be derived from being of service to others should not be overlooked. Many individuals have a desire to leave something of themselves for others to enjoy after their death. Thus, some of the activities selected may involve the making of final presents for family members and friends. In addition to leaving of a small legacy, making and presenting these gifts is one way of marking and giving reality to the separation that is soon to come.

The third area of concern for the therapist is to help the family adapt to the dying of one of its members. Again, it is important for the therapist to be an active listener. The family may need particular assistance in expressing their feelings of anger and guilt and may also need reassurance that these feelings are natural. At times family members will neglect their other social roles, feeling that they must spend all their time with the dying individual. The therapist should help family members to realize that continued participation in other roles is important and that the dying individual does, indeed, need time to be alone.

Open communication between the family and the dying individual is important. This can be facilitated by the therapist providing support and by assuring that there is adequate privacy. The therapist may enhance the degree of comfort between the family and client by encouraging them to engage in a variety of activities together. Specific activities are suggested, based on the interests and abilities of both client and family members. The process of "doing together" tends to diminish anxiety and increase communication, both verbal and nonverbal. A shared activity often provides a sense of companionship that cannot be experienced in any other way.

Engaging family members in activities when the client's condition has progressed to the point of profound incapacity is also helpful. These activities can be done while sitting with the client or in an appropriate room away from the client. Activities at this time can be used to combat anxiety and, literally, to occupy time.

Although the task of dying and of watching someone die is a serious and emotionally draining experience, it need not take place in a somber atmosphere. The creation and enjoyment of pleasurable experiences, no matter how small, should be emphasized. One way of maintaining a more joyous atmosphere is through the use of humor. Humor tends to diminish social distance, relieves tension, and brings people closer together. Pain and anxiety may be momentarily forgotten. Thus, it is often helpful to expose the humorous side of everyday events, occasionally to tell a funny story, to watch comedies on television, and to develop private jokes with the client and family. The human experience in all of its manifestations is often tragic. On the other hand, it is also humorous—a factor that assists us in mastering all phases of the life cycle.

CONCLUSION

This chapter has described some of the ways in which occupational therapists assist elderly individuals adapt to the many changes that take place in this phase of the life cycle. As mentioned, this is an area in which occupational therapists are just beginning to become involved. It is also an area that is just beginning to receive the attention of the medical sciences and technology. The development of knowledge in both areas is likely to enhance the quality of life for the elderly. The role of occupational therapists in assisting the elderly will probably be somewhat different in the future than it is today.

31 Sensory Integration

Sensory integration has been previously defined both as an area of human function and as a frame of reference. As an area of human function, sensory integration is a subcortical process that involves receiving, selecting, sorting, and organizing vestibular, proprioceptive, and tactile information (somatosensory input) for functional use. As a frame of reference, sensory integration is a type of intervention using direct, primary somatosensory input to normalize neural functions affecting posture, lateralization, space orientation, and motor planning. It usually includes the elicitation of an adaptive motor response as a means of facilitating feedback and integration.

The following discussion of sensory integration is organized around the primary client groups described as being deficit in this area—learning disabilities and schizophrenic disorders—and is followed by some brief additional comments.

LEARNING DISABILITIES

Occupational therapy's involvement in the remediation of sensory integrative deficits arose out of Ayres' concern with children who are now referred to as learning disabled (55,58,60,64,65,231). Some of the confusion and controversy surrounding sensory integration can best be understood within the context of the field of learning disabilities. Thus, an overview of the field is outlined in this section. Moreover, an overview is presented because the occupational therapist may assist learning-disabled individuals in ways other than through remediation of sensory integration deficits.

This section is divided into nine parts: definitions and prevalence, historical perspective, evaluation and remediation, social-emotional issues, adolescents, parents, preschool children, adults, and role of the occupational therapist.

Definitions and Prevalence

There are currently two ways of defining learning disabilities—the federal definition and the medical definition.

The federal definition itself has two parts. The first part appears in the major body of the rules and regulations of PL 94-142 (971). It reads as follows:

> 'Specific learning disability' means a disorder in one or more of the psychological processes involved in understanding and in using language, spoken or written, which may manifest itself in an imperfect ability to listen, think, speak, read, write, spell or do mathematical calculations. The term includes such conditions as perceptual handicaps, brain injury, minimal brain dysfunction, dyslexia, developmental aphasia. The term does not include children who have learning problems which are primarily the result of visual, hearing or motor handicaps, of mental retardation, of emotional disturbance or of environmental, cultural, or economic disadvantages.

The second part of the definition appeared in a second set of regulations applying to PL 94-142 and is designed to provide guidelines for determining whether a child has a specific learning disability. A child is considered to be learning disabled if (972):

1. The child does not achieve commensurate with his or her age and ability level in one or more of seven specific

areas when provided with learning experiences appropriate for the child's age and ability levels.

2. The team finds that a child has severe discrepancy between achievement and intellectual ability in one or more of the following areas:
   a. Oral expression
   b. Listening comprehension
   c. Written expression
   d. Basic reading skills
   e. Reading comprehension
   f. Mathematical calculations
   g. Mathematical reasoning.

Some of the elements of this definition may need to be clarified (143,587,808,835):

This definition is behavioral in orientation rather than neurological. This causes difficulty for some people who view the individual with a learning disability as having some type of central nervous impairment. A neurological condition related to a learning problem is often difficult, if not impossible, to determine by medical examination. Medical diagnoses, when made, are usually primarily based on observation of the individual's behavior. Despite the shift to a behavioral and educational emphasis, many people believe that more refined research will substantiate the relationship between central nervous system pathology and learning disability. On the whole, occupational therapists who ascribe to the concept of sensory integrative dysfunction belong to this group.

This definition assumes that cognitive ability related to academic performance is not a single capacity but rather a collection of many underlying abilities. For the individual with learning disabilities, some of these abilities mature at an anticipated rate while others lag in their development, thus causing or appearing as symptoms of a learning problem. It is the concept of uneven growth patterns that has become the primary basis for evaluation and remediation in education and occupational therapy.

The definition lists specific learning problems that are evidence of a learning disability. Such specificity does not deal with the issue of whether these areas of deficit are discrete entities or an indication of some underlying, more comprehensive problem. Further, the listing of specific academic areas has created some conflicts within education. If, for example, the child's problem is described as a deficit in reading skill, the reading specialist in the school may consider the child's problem within his or her area of expertise. If the deficit is described as being a language disorder, the speech and language teacher or the speech therapist may view the problem as their responsibility. This specificity has, at times, led to fragmentation of services. The learning disability teacher in the school, if there is one, is responsible for coordinating the remedial programs for each child. Good practice as well as federal regulation emphasize the importance of a team effort.

Learning disability is described as a descrepancy between achievement and potential. Assessment involves identification of a gap between what the child is potentially capable of doing and what, in fact, the child has learned or achieved. The problem with this method of defining a learning disability is in determining (a) what the individual's potential for learning is; (b) what the individual's achievement level is; and (c) what degree of discrepancy between potential and achievement is considered "severe."

Finally, the above definition of learning disability states that in order to be considered learning disabled, the problem must not be primarily the result of other causes, such as mental retardation, emotional disturbance, visually handicapped, and so forth. Such a distinction is often difficult to make in practice. On the other hand, some exceptional children may have two handicaps—their primary impairment plus learning disabilities. It is, in addition, often difficult to determine which problems are primary and which are secondary. The exclusion clause was included in the definition to establish learning disabilities as a separate and discrete category. This was done to facilitate appropriate legislation, funding, and research, and to focus remediation.

Medicine does not use the term learning disabilities to identify the phenomena described above. Rather, they use the label "attention deficit disorder" and/or "specific developmental disorders." Attention deficit disorders are divided into two types: with and without hyperactivity.

Attention deficit disorders are described as (ref 35, pp. 43–44):

> . . . developmentally inappropriate inattention, impulsivity, and hyperactivity. In the classroom, attentional difficulties and impulsivity are evidenced by the child's not staying with tasks and having difficulty organizing and completing work. The children often give the impression that they are not listening or that they have not heard what they have been told. Their work is sloppy and is performed in an impulsive fashion. On individually administered tests, careless, impulsive errors are often present. Performance may be characterized by oversights, such as omissions or insertions, or misinterpretations of easy items even when the child is well motivated, not just in situations that hold little intrinsic interest. Group situations are particularly difficult for the child, and attentional difficulties are exaggerated when the child is in the classroom where sustained attention is expected.
>
> At home, attentional problems are shown by a failure to follow through on parental requests and instructions and by the inability to stick to activities, including play for periods of time appropriate for the child's age.

Hyperactivity in young children is manifested by gross motor activity, such as excessive running or climbing. The child is often described as being on the go, "running like a motor," and having difficulty sitting still. Older children and adolescents may be extremely restless and fidgety. Often, it is the quality of the motor behavior that distinguishes this disorder from ordinary overactivity in that hyperactivity tends to be haphazard, poorly organized and not goal directed.

In order for a diagnosis of attention deficit disorder to be made, the onset of the condition must occur before the age of 7 and the duration must be of at least 6 months. Additional points made about attention deficit disorders are as follows:

The symptoms of this disorder are likely to vary in any given child with situation and time. An individual rarely displays signs of the disorders in all settings or even in the same setting all the time.

Specific developmental disorders (to be discussed momentarily) are often associated with attention deficit disorders as are obstinacy, stubbornness, negativism, bossiness, bullying, increased mood liability, low frustration tolerance, temper outbursts, low self-esteem, and lack of response to discipline.

EEG abnormalities and nonlocalized "soft" neurological signs may be present. The latter refers to neurological abnormalities that are mild or slight and difficult to detect, as contrasted with the gross or obvious neurological abnormalities. The soft signs include mild coordination difficulties, minimal tremors, motor awkwardness, visual-motor disturbances, finger agnosia, delay in speech, and the like. However, in only about 5% of the cases is attention deficit disorders associated with a diagnosable neurological disorder.

The disorder is apparently more common in family members than in the general population.

The course of the disorder varies: (a) all of the symptoms persist into adolescent and adult life, (b) the disorder is self-limited and all of the symptoms disappear at puberty, (c) the hyperactivity disappears, but the attentional difficulties and impulsivity persist into adolescence or adult life (residual type).

The relative frequency of these three courses is unknown as is any method of determining the course for a specific individual.

Attention deficit disorders without hyperactivity is similar to that described above except for the absence of hyperactivity. The associated features and impairment are generally milder.

Specific developmental disorders refer to impairment in the areas of reading, arithmetic, and language (expressive type, receptive type, articulation). These disorders may be associated with attention deficit disorders or they may occur without any evidence of attention deficit disorder.

Regarding course, the various specific developmental disorders are stable through childhood and adolescence, and many individuals continue to show some signs of the disorder in adult life. In some milder cases there is marked improvement in (or even disappearance of) all symptoms in time.

The difference between the legal and the medical definition of the phenomena of concern here is the identification of inattention as being of primary importance in the medical definition. This is not meant to imply, however, that the American Psychiatric Association believes that poor attention skills alone are sufficient to account for the learning deficits these individuals often exhibit. The legal definition does not mention either inattention or hyperactivity. This does not mean that legislators, educators, and parents are unaware of these behavior patterns in many learning-disabled children. Definition of a phenomena often reflects the concerns of the definers. Physicians are able to prescribe medication which, in many cases, can minimize inattention and hyperactivity; the major focus of legislators, educators, and parents is primarily the development of academic skills.

Estimates of the prevalence of children who are learning disabled range from 1% to 30% of the school population (587). The number arrived at depends on the criteria used to determine the disability and the identification procedures used. According to the U.S. Office of Education, for the school year 1977 to 1978, children defined as learning disabled constituted 1.89% of the total school-aged population and 25.7% of the identified handicapped population (973). Actual prevalence is believed to be higher, being estimated at 3%. Thus 1.11% either remain unidentified, unserved, or both. It is unknown whether these figures are comparable in the adult population (587).

Regarding sex ratio, the American Psychiatric Association states that attention deficit disorders are 10 times more common in boys than in girls. There is no information available for developmental arithmetic disorders. It is reported that the other specific developmental disorders are all about twice as common in males as in females (35).

Historical Perspective

Wiederholt and Lunner (587,1022) have divided the history of learning disabilities into the following four distinct periods:

The Foundation Phase (1800–1930)

This period was marked by basic scientific investigation of brain function and its disorders. Scientists gathered information by studying the behavior of those who had lost some function, such as the ability to speak or read, through acquired brain damage. They then examined these individuals' brains after death in an attempt to correlate loss of function with specific damaged areas of the brain. It was hypothesized that specific localized areas of the brain governed particular activities. This localized theory was criticized by many, with the contention that the human brain was more than a collection of independent centers. Rather, it was hypothesized that the parts of the brain were intimately linked and that damage to one part would reduce overall general function.

James Hinshelwood, Sir Henry Head, and Kurt Goldstein were three important figures in this stage. Hinshelwood (1917), reporting on the case of an intelligent boy who was unable to learn to read, speculated that the problem was due to a deficit in the angular gyrus (435). Head (1926), through clinical observations, devised a system for data collection and developed a test for aphasia (404). He emphasized that individuals who were aphasic did not suffer from generalized impairment of intellectual ability, even though they had sustained brain damage. Goldstein (1939) studied brain injured soldiers after World War I (356). He hypothesized that brain damage affected an individual's behavior in a generalized kind of way. Among the characteristics he identified were figure-ground difficulties, distractability to external stimuli, perservation, and a low tolerance for stress and frustration.

The Transition Phase (1930–1960)

This period was characterized by studies of the brain that focused on children, the development of instruments for assessment and remediation, and the examination of specific kinds of learning disorders found in children.

One of the pioneers in the field at this time was Alfred Strauss, a physician who built on the work of Goldstein after emigrating to the United States from Germany in 1937 (934). The subjects of his study were children with severe behavioral disturbances who frequently had medical histories indicating that brain injury had occurred at some time. Strauss felt that the behavior and learning patterns of these children were a manifestation of brain damage. Some of the characteristics Strauss noted in the children he categorized as brain injured were (a) perceptual disorders—seeing the parts of an object instead of a whole and seeing a shifting background and foreground; (b) perseveration—the continuation of an activity once it has started and difficulty in changing to another activity; (c) conceptual disorders—the inability to organize materials and thoughts in the usual manner and the confusion of one concept with another, such as radio and radiator; (d) behavioral disorders—hyperactive, explosive, erratic, or otherwise uninhibited behavior; low frustration tolerance; and easy distraction from the task at hand.

Because children known to be brain injured exhibited the above characteristics, Strauss concluded that children who exhibited the same characteristics could be presumed to have suffered brain damage at some time.

Strauss introduced the term "brain injured" to identify this group of children in his classic work *Psychopathology and Education of the Brain Injured Child*, written with Laura Lehtinen in 1947 (934). There were many questions raised about the assumptions and implications of the work. Nevertheless, Strauss and his coworkers laid the foundation for the field of learning disabilities by:

1. Alerting physicians to many pre- and postpartum events that could be related to injury to the brain;
2. Perceiving a homogeneity in a diverse group of children who had been (a) misdiagnosed by specialists as mentally retarded, emotionally disturbed, lazy, or careless; (b) a source of much confusion for parents who had often been blamed for causing psychological problems that created learning difficulties for their children, and who could rarely find anyone who could guide them in the management of their children; (c) discarded by society as uneducatable;
3. Devising diagnostic tests to specify and evaluate the characteristics of these children;
4. Planning and implementing educational procedures to teach such children successfully; and
5. Alerting many professions to the existence of a new category of exceptional children (587).

Nevertheless, the term "brain-injured" proved to be confusing and emotionally laden (436,760). Not all children with obvious brain injury—many children with cerebral palsy, for example—have learning disorders. The diagnosis was based on behavior, with frequently no evidence of brain injury. Educators were reluctant to use the term because it was essentially medical. They also questioned the usefulness of " brain-injured child" as a guide for evaluating and teaching such children. Parents understandably reacted negatively when told their child had a brain injury and felt that it was excessively condemning on the child's school record.

Because of the generally adverse reaction to "brain-injured child" other labels were developed and frequently used interchangeably. One label, perhaps most commonly used at this time, was "minimal brain dysfunction." This term was devised to differentiate the mildly involved child from the child with a major brain disorder. Critics of the term note that the so-called major brain injuries on the conceptualized scale may or may not be accompanied by difficulties in learning; and they ask, how much is minimal?

One of the first writers to suggest the term "learning disabilities" was Samuel Kirk (542). Rather than emphasizing presumed cause, it focuses on the problem the individual faces. Although it does not specify the area in which the individual has learning difficulties, nor the learning process in which the individual is deficit, it seems to be the most acceptable term currently available.

The other major concern during this period was the development of teaching strategies that would facilitate education of learning-disabled children. With some variation, it was recommended that the learning environment be characterized by (a) reducing unessential visual and auditory environmental stimuli, (b) reducing to a minimum the space in which the child works, (c) providing a highly structured, daily school schedule, and (d) increasing the stimulus value of the teaching material (934).

The Integration Phase (1960–1980)

This period was characterized by a rapid growth of school programs for the learning-disabled child and by the development of a number of theories to serve as the basis for evaluation and remediation. Many teachers were trained, programs initiated, and teaching methods and materials developed. A concerted effort was made to identify learning-disabled children and to provide them with appropriate services. All of this activity was, in many ways, encouraged by the formation of a well-organized and vocal parents group, the Association for Children and Youth with Learning Disabilities; federal legislation; and the involvement of many professional groups with the learning-disabled population. The last included, to name just a few, psychology, speech, and language pathology; linguistics and psycholinguistics; ophthalmology and optometry; audiology; and occupational therapy.

Various theories regarding learning disabilities were articulated. Although there is some overlapping, these theories seem to fall into two categories: "psychological processing," which focuses on the underlying abilities and disabilities within the child, and "academic skill mastery," which concentrates on the tasks to be learned. These two orientations are discussed in the following section.

The Contemporary Phase (1980 to the Present)

The 1980s are a time of emerging directions for the field of leaning disabilities. Three of the major trends are briefly outlined here. One direction is the extension of the age group of concern (12,14,208,214,514,589,638). Up until this time, the focus had been primarily on the elementary school age child. Interest now includes individuals younger and older than that initial age group. There is particular concern for the child aged 3 to 5 years and in many cases even younger. The hope is that if children with learning disabilities, or at high risk relative to the development of such a disability, can be identified early and receive appropriate intervention, that learning failure may be prevented or mitigated. At the other end of the continuum are adolescents and adults. Their special needs are just beginning to be recognized both in the school setting and in the wider community.

Within education the entire field of special education is undergoing change. Until recently the field was categorized largely by the physical or medical characteristics of a particular group of exceptional children—mentally retarded, emotionally disturbed, and so forth. It is now being recognized that the categories of exceptionality are not discrete and separate entities but have much in common with each other (178,543,587,677). Thus, many states are moving toward the "generic" certification of special education teachers with training that allows them to work in several areas. This is likely to prepare teachers who are better able to work with multiply handicapped children and to provide a more integrated educational experience for disabled children regardless of the nature of their disability.

The final major trend in learning disabilities is in the direction of expanded and more refined research. This is reflected in the areas of increasing reliability and validity of tools used for assessment, testing, and refining theory and in evaluation of the effectiveness of remedial techniques.

Evaluation and Remediation

The most common medical treatment for children with attention deficit disorders is medication (16,539,568). The current drugs of choice are methylphenidate (Ritalin®) and dextroamphetamine (Dexedrine®), which are central nervous system stimulants. Their mode of action is unclear. Until recently it was widely held that the drugs provoked a "paradoxical reaction" in that they have a sedative effect on the child with an attention deficit disorder. They produce a decrease in motor activity and an increase in attentiveness and task persistence. Recent research, however, suggests that the "paradoxical reaction" model of stimulant reaction is unlikely. On the basis of research findings, some authors, in particular Wender, suggest that children with attention deficit disorders are characteristically underaroused and that this state is ameliorated by the administration of a stimulant. Data derived from research to substantiate this view have, however, been inconclusive.

Studies of outcome in the use of stimulant drug treatment for attention deficit disorders indicate that about two-thirds of the children improve in behavior, while 5% to 10% worsen. Both drugs are active for 4 to 5 hours and are usually given as a single dose in the morning or as a divided dose at morning and mid-day. The most common side effects of both drugs are anorexia, insomnia, headache, stomachache, nausea, tearfulness, and pallor. Stimulants are not considered to produce euphoria in children, and children on such medication rarely become drug abusers. For unknown reasons, hyperactive behavior is often substantially reduced at the onset of puberty, and medication is typically stopped at that time. Careful follow-up during the course of treatment is essential to regulate dosage and to evaluate the side effects and behavioral effects of treatment. It is important to note that drug treatment by itself is rarely considered to be a sufficient remedy for the child's total set of difficulties. Other methods of intervention and remediation continue to be required. The adequate prescription of drugs simply facilitates the intervention process.

Nonmedical evaluation and intervention, as previously mentioned, has been described as having two general approaches: psychological processing and academic skill mastery (143,323,324,326,383,515,543,587,679,808, 834,980,1038,1039). These will be discussed separately, initially followed by an integrated perspective. Although presented separately, these two theoretical orientations need not be viewed as diametrically opposed nor as mutually exclusive alternatives.

Psychological processes refers to the analysis, storage, synthesis, and symbolic (relative to language) use of information. The various theories in this category hypothesize a deficit in one or more of these areas as a causal factor in learning disabilities. Some of the underlying processing abilities identified are auditory processing, visual processing, kinesthetic and tactile processing, memory abilities, language abilities, and so forth. Conceptualized another way, the basic premise of these theories is that certain children fail to learn effectively in school because of deficits in perceptual development, motor development, and memory.

Ayres' theory of sensory integration belongs to this category of theories because it hypothesizes deficits in underlying processes (58). It is different from these theories in that it is concerned with processing at the subcortical as opposed to the cortical level. Ayres' theory, as currently stated, places vestibular-proprioceptive-tactile processing as being more basic or ontogenetically more fundamental than perceptual-motor-memory processing. On the whole, she considers the latter to be functions that take place at the cortical level. Proponents of the sensory integrative approach would recommend that individuals with somatosensory deficits receive adequate intervention in these areas prior to remediation relative to perceptual-motor-memory processing. Although considered more fundamental than the other theories included in this category, the criticism of this entire approach applies equally to sensory integration.

To return to a more general discussion of this orientation, students' strengths and weaknesses are assessed through tests and observations. This information leads to a plan for remediation. Three different approaches are used:

1. *Addressing the deficit process.* Using this approach, the student is helped to develop those processing functions that are weak in order to eliminate the disability and prepare the child for further learning. (This is the approach that is usually used in dealing with deficits in sensory integration.)
2. *Teaching through the preferred process.* This approach uses the child's processing strengths as the basis of teaching in the hopes of circumventing processing weaknesses.
3. *The combined approach.* The child is helped to learn through methods that emphasize processing strengths in conjunction with strategies designed to strengthen the processing weaknesses.

Theories of psychological processing dysfunctions as a way of understanding children with learning disabilities became predominant during the early years of the fields development. In more recent times, however, questions are being raised about the orientation (587). Some of these questions are examined briefly:

Do psychological processing deficits cause learning failures? The theories in this category appear to *assume* that psychological processing deficits are the cause of learning disabilities. The evidence supporting this relationship is correlational, and correlation does not indicate causation. A causative relationship has not been established. Further, since the evidence for underlying psychological processes is indirect—they are not observable phenomena—they may not, in fact, exist.

Can psychological processes be measured through existing tests? A review of the research literature on such tests indicates that reliability and validity are quite low, particularly in application to the younger age group. It is thus questionable whether these tests alone should be used to make serious decisions about a child's educational needs. It should be noted that tests used to measure academic achievement are subject to the same criticism of inadequate reliability and validity.

Does teaching based on psychological processing of information help the child to learn? Each of the approaches has been criticized separately. Addressing the deficit process has been the focus of most of the critical research. The research itself has raised considerable controversy regarding methodology and appropriate statistical treatment of the data. In general, although the findings are by no means conclusive, it appears that addressing psychological processes in isolation will not improve academic skills. It is still necessary to teach these skills. Research also indicates that the age of the child and the severity of the problem also have an impact on the success of the method.

Specific evaluative research regarding the effect of sensory integration intervention relative to learning-disabled children without any other identified handicap is sparse and has not been directly related to academic achievement. Primarily it has been directed toward assessing degree of improvement relative to the process being addressed or some other related process. Similar to all research in this area, findings are inconclusive (590).

Teaching through the preferred process has not received as much research attention as focus on deficit processes. What studies have been conducted are primarily in the area of reading. Results, in general, show no significant relationship between tailoring the method of reading instruction to the child's processing strength and successful learning. The combined approach to remediation has received little research attention.

What is being altered in remediation of deficit psychological processes? This question has not been subjected to empirical research but some of the subquestions it raises are: To what extent are psychological processing deficiencies the result of maturational delay as opposed to a potentially identifiable pathological situation? Does remediation make use of already existing but underdeveloped neuronal connections or are new anatomical pathways being developed? Does remediation lead to a way of processing information that is similar to the way in which information is processed by the nonlearning-disabled individuals or does it lead to the development of compensatory skills?

Academic skill mastery has been proposed as an alternative to the psychological processing orientation. Several terms have been used to refer to this collection of theories: task analysis, specific skills training, directed teaching, sequential skills teaching, and mastery learning. Proponents of this school of thought recommend that educators concentrate on the academic skills a child needs to learn rather than on the proposed disabilities within the child. The essence of this approach is the analysis of the academic tasks in terms of the collection of skills needed to accomplish that task. The skills are then placed in an ordered and logical sequence. Evaluation involves testing to determine which of these skills the child does and does not possess. Teaching is directed toward helping the student acquire the subskills that are not yet mastered. The academic skills mastery approach does not recognize any special learning problems or ability deficits other than the child's lack of experience and practice with the task.

The use of the academic skills mastery orientation as the sole basis for thinking about learning disabilities also raises many questions (587).

1. Is learning comprised of a set of separate and distinct skills? It is doubtful if many types of learning can be conceptualized as a set of separate skills. There is, for example, disagreement about what skills constitute reading, how many there are, and what order they are acquired. Exactly what is involved in the act of reading and learning to read remains a mystery. The same can be said for most of the other academic areas.
2. Can skills be ordered in a hierarchy? Specific skills may be ordered logically from an adult point of view. The problem is that there is little evidence that children learn in a logical and orderly fashion.
3. Is the establishment of a set of skills a method of teaching? Identifying skills to be learned is not a method of instruction; it says nothing about how the skills should be taught.
4. Are individuals with learning disabilities different from other kinds of underachievers? This orientation has become the recommended approach for teaching underachievers as well as learning-disabled children. But there is something very different about these two groups of students. Lerner has stated the dilemma here by likening learning disabilities to pornography: each is "impossible to define but you always know it when you see it" (587, p.178).

It appears that an integrated perspective is necessary. Neither the psychological processing orientation nor the academic skills mastery orientation alone seem to provide the basis for effective remediation of learning disabilities. The debate persists, often with more passion than logic. The problems being considered in this "processing versus skills" debate are complex; much more needs to be known about learning, and probably the central nervous system, to resolve the issues. What is likely to emerge is a theory that integrates the two perspectives in a manner that cannot be identified at the present time. In the interim, one cannot wait for the development of a verified theory to act. Learning-disabled individuals are in need of assistance regardless of how less than perfect that assistance may be. At present it is perhaps wisest to use both a psychological processing approach and an academic skills mastery approach in designing an individualized educational program for a given child (543,588,677).

Social-Emotional Issues

Psychosocial difficulties are common in learning-disabled children. Two factors, which are not necessarily mutually exclusive, appear to account for these problems (35,143,383,543,587,835). Some authorities describe children who are unable to engage in social activities that are consistent with their chronological age and intelligence as being deficient in social perception. This is viewed as evidence of a learning disability that may or may not be associated with deficits in academic learning. Children with social perception problems do not seem to be able to anticipate social expectations, i.e., confirm whether their actions match what is expected, or to adjust their behavior in light of the results. As a consequence, such children have been described as performing poorly in independent activities expected of children of the same chronological age; poor in judging moods and attitudes of other people; insensitive to the general atmosphere of social situations; continually doing or saying the inappropriate thing; unable to establish a close relationship with those with whom they wish to be friends; and having difficulty in interacting with family members and acquiring appropriate status as a family member.

It is important to note that not all learning-disabled children are deficient in social perception. Some have developed a high degree of social awareness and interaction skill. This ability is often used fairly effectively in negotiating their way through the perils of being an exceptional child. Such children may use their social skills as a means of taking a leadership position in the classroom and among their friends. This, in some ways, may serve as a means of compensating for deficits in academic skills.

The other factor related to the psychosocial problems of learning-disabled children is the consequence of being learning disabled. Attempts at mastering various tasks frequently lead to failure and feelings of frustration rather than to a sense of accomplishment. Instead of increasing self-esteem, the child's activities produce an attitude of self-derision. Observing the child's failures, parents experience anxiety and frustration, which may finally lead to overprotection or rejection. The insult to the child's developing personality continues and increases in school. The expectations for competency in academic skills cannot be met. The child invariably compares him- or herself with nonlearning-disabled children and finds him- or herself wanting. The characteristic unevenness in academic ability and occasional moments of achievement in areas of difficulty may make matters worse for the child. Parents and teachers may be convinced that the child could do better if he or she just tried harder. Failure may be viewed in terms of laziness and poor attitude.

Learning-disabled children, then, often do not receive the normal satisfaction of their needs for recognition, achievement, and affection. The feelings within themselves plus feedback from the environment lead them to view the world as a threatening place and themselves as inept and undesirable. The child is very likely to experience frustration and confusion and to have a generally poor self-concept. The child may react to all these very negative experiences in any number of ways: conscious refusal to learn, overt hostility, displacement of hostility, resistance to pressure, dependency, quick discouragement, withdrawal, or absorption in a private world.

The psychosocial difficulties of the child—whether they are due to faulty social perception, the consequence of being learning disabled, or both—must be taken into consideration. The emotional status of the child has an impact not only on academic progress but also on the capacity to interact effectively in other social roles.

Adolescents

Learning-disabled adolescents are confronted with two major problems: accomplishing the developmental tasks of this phase of the life cycle and dealing with the limitations of being learning disabled (14,214,233,587,638). Many gradeschool students who received assistance relative to this disability are still in need of help when they reach secondary school. Other adolescents are not identified as being learning disabled until they reach the secondary level. This may be because of the more subtle nature of their problems, because the demands of the secondary curriculum are more stringent, or because they attended an elementary school where programs for learning-disabled students were not available.

The secondary school differs in many respects from the elementary school. It tends to be larger, more complex to negotiate, and somewhat less concerned with the individual learning needs of students. There are increased demands for independent study, reading, written work, and abstract thinking. On the whole, teacher training programs have not prepared special education to work with secondary school students. High school content-area teachers are usually less sensitive to the special problems of the learning-disabled student. Since content-area teachers are primarily interested in their specialization, they are often not prepared to make the necessary adjustments in curriculum or mode of teaching that may facilitate learning for special students.

The matter of course credit is another issue. Should credit be given for work accomplished in the learning-disabilities program, or should it be considered supplementary to the regular program? The establishment of credit, of course, requires decisions by school administrators at the local and, most likely, the state level. The decisions made may also affect the types of diploma the individual receives.

Finally, it is generally believed that simply transplanting methods and teaching approaches from the elementary to the secondary school is not effective. However, because the establishment of secondary level programs for learning-disabled students is so new, there has not been sufficient time to conduct research and to develop adequate assessment tools and methods of remediation.

The turmoil, increased demands, and developmental tasks that accompany puberty create additional problems for the learning-disabled adolescent. They enter this phase of the life cycle with less than an even start. They not only have specific problems in learning, self-management, and dealing with the external environment, they come to this phase with years of failure, low self-esteem, poor motivation, and often inadequate peer acceptance. The typical learning-disabled adolescent can best be characterized as engaging in such behavior as task avoidance, impulsivity, emotional swings, overreaction, disorganized study habits, poor use of time, procrastination, and lack of attention. These patterns of behavior not only interfere with academic learning, they also interfere with mastery of other developmental tasks.

Some of the areas in which the adolescent is likely to have difficulty is in establishing an appropriate degree of autonomy, recreation/friendship, heterosexual interactions, and vocational choice. Regarding autonomy, the learning-disabled youth often has difficulty making decisions, finding his or her way around town, reading menus, filling out forms, managing money; everywhere there are words and more words, and numbers. In illustration, one of the rites of passage of the adolescent stage is getting a driver's license. Some learning-disabled youths have visual processing and motor problems that make it very difficult and at times impossible to learn how to drive. Some cannot read the signs in order to respond appropriately on the road and to find their way about. Getting a license usually entails passing a written test with special permission needed to take it verbally. The struggle for autonomy is hampered by the learning-disabled adolescent's deficits and by the need for real and continued assistance in many areas.

In the area of recreation/friendships, adolescence is a time when groups splinter off around particular interests, e.g., athletics, academics, special pursuits. For many learning-disabled youths, their lack of motor coordination precludes participation in many sports. Interest in any particular academic area such as history or science may be difficult to cultivate because of deficits in reading skills. Special interests such as computer games, board or card games, listening to music and dancing may not be areas in which the learning-disabled adolescent is able to participate comfortably. Finding satisfying recreational pursuits and friends with whom to share these pursuits may be difficult. The adolescent may retreat to stereotyped, not really satisfying recreational activities, or to primarily solitary endeavors.

Regarding heterosexual interactions, the learning-disabled adolescent often comes to the beginning of the dating and courtship period with low self-esteem, poor social skills, and mistrust of others. The increasingly subtle cues one has to decipher for properly testing out and learning how to relate to members of the opposite sex are often missed by learning-disabled adolescents. They are also prone to expect failure and to be particularly sensitive to rejection.

Vocational choice and more direct preparation for the work role is an important developmental task of adolescence. The learning-disabled youth may avoid after-school and summer jobs because of fear that the disability will be discovered, the necessity to fill out job applications, concern about being able to meet expectations, and so forth. Thus, there is little opportunity to explore and test one's interests and skills. Parental aspirations for a learning-disabled youth may be unrealistic in either direction, i.e., too high or too low. Accepting parental aspirations as realistic may lead the youth into contemplating jobs that are totally unsuited to his or her interests and skills. Finally, the learning-disabled adolescent, through unsatisfying relationships with teachers, may have developed a negative attitude toward authority. This, in combination with difficulty in peer interactions, may interfere with engaging satisfactorily in the interpersonal aspect of the work role.

Adolescence, probably more than any other period in the life cycle, is a time when frustration is acted out rather than being dealt with in a more intrapsychic manner. Learning-disabled youths are considered to be at risk relative to asocial behavior—delinquency, dropping out of school, teenage pregnancy—for two reasons. First, failure and frustration at school lead to attempts to satisfy needs in another manner. Second, some learning-disabled youths are impulsive and lack sound judgment. They do not anticipate the consequences of their acts, they do not control behavior, or learn from their experiences. It should, of course, be noted that all learning-disabled youths do not deal with frustration and lack of need satisfaction through engaging in asocial behavior (214,233,510,1052).

Programs for learning-disabled students at the secondary school level are neither as prevalent nor as innovative as those found at the primary level. This is still a very new area. Some of the types of learning-disability programs available in the secondary schools are as follows (214,233,510,1052):

Skills remediation. This approach focuses on improving the student's basic academic skills by providing remedial instruction primarily in reading, spelling, writing, and math. Programs are based on the academic skills mastery orientation. The psychological processing orientation does not appear to be used at the secondary school level.

Functional curriculum. This approach is designed to equip students to function in society. Students are taught what is often referred to as "survival skills," i.e., specific skills that will allow them to manage outside of the world of home and school. Content is presented at a practical level and is concerned with everyday life, e.g., consumer information, completion of applications and other types of forms, reading street maps, deciphering road signs, money management, self-care, sex education, and the like. The importance of sex education is emphasized both because learning-disabled students are less likely to get adequate information on their own by reading or from their peers and because of the impulsivity of some learning-disabled youths.

Tutorial. This approach is designed to provide additional instruction in academic content areas (i.e., literature, biology) that the student is currently studying.

Learning strategies. Learning strategies are techniques, principles, or rules that will facilitate the acquisition, manipulation, integration, storage, and retrieval of information across situations and settings. It is concerned with teaching adolescents how to learn rather than the teaching of specific content.

Career and vocational education. It is generally believed that without prior preparation, the prospects for success in the work role for the learning-disabled individual is poor. PL 94-142 provides for educational services up to the age of 21, a provision that enhances the possibility that learning-disabled youths will receive adequate help in career planning and training.

Some learning-disabled students have the desire and capacity to attend college. They may, however, need special guidance in preparing for college and help in realizing that accomplishing this goal will not be an easy task. Fortunately, there are now some colleges that have programs designed to meet the particular needs of learning-disabled students (294).

Other students will move directly into the job market. One fairly innovative approach for these students is a work-study program. Students typically spend half the day on the job and the remainder of the day in school. Academic work may involve the study of material directly related to the job experience, or the student may take regular courses in the high school. Other programs, which may take place in the secondary school or in a sheltered workshop, emphasize general work skills. Rather than preparing students for one specific job—that may soon be outmoded—it is recommended that students be instructed in marketable skills that apply to many occupations. A positive attitude toward work and the importance of work as a source of need satisfaction should be fostered. Skilled career counseling with someone knowledgeable in the special problems of the learning-disabled individual is important. Because of limited possible choices, learning-disabled individuals often need assistance in matching their occupational strengths with specific job requirements.

The above programs are by no means mutually exclusive. Many individuals can benefit from a variety of programs provided concurrently or sequentially. One of the difficulties with most of the current programs is that they take place within the context of resource rooms or self-contained classrooms. Thus, one of the current challenges is to find effective ways to integrate the learning-disabled adolescent into the regular classroom.

In conclusion, the learning-disabled adolescent is faced with both the need to master academic material and to deal with the tasks inherent in being an adolescent. The youth's specific difficulties in learning can not be considered outside the context of his or her place in the life cycle.

Parents

Much has previously been mentioned about the parents of disabled children: their relationship to their child, the role they may play in facilitating their child's growth, and programs designed to help these parents. This section, therefore, only briefly outlines a few additional guidelines that have been found useful to the parents of learning-disabled children and adolescents (81,213,320, 683,835):

1. Match tasks to the child's level of functioning. This includes helping the child to figure out ways to deal with the practical tasks of daily life and giving the child tasks that are appropriate to his or her level of functioning. It also is important for the child to have tasks for which he or she alone is responsible.
2. Do not push the child into activities for which he or she is not ready. By forcing the child to meet standards that are inappropriate, learning becomes painful and associated with failure.
3. Be alert to what the child is good at doing. Through emphasizing such activities, the child is given an opportunity for success. Encourage nonacademic activities such as sports, hobbies, work, travel—anything that bypasses his or her most difficult area of learning.
4. Structure and organize the home environment to facilitate the child's capacity to cope. This may include keeping the child's room simple and a quiet place for relaxation and retreat, keeping all household objects in specified places, and establishing simple and regular daily routines. Consistent discipline is also important.
5. Parents should not take the role of a teacher in the home. They can, however, be of great help in the area of homework. This may, for example, be done by identifying a place and creating an atmosphere conducive to study, assisting the child in organizing the necessary materials, reviewing directions, being available to answer specific questions, and structuring the time so that each assignment is completed.
6. Help the child to realize that he or she must learn to live with other people in a world that does not revolve around him or her. Parents may have to go out of their way to plan and guide social experiences.
7. Help the child to learn to be a responsible and contributing member of the family. This may be more important than acquiring the academic skills demanded by the school.

Preschool Children

There is growing concern about early identification of preschool children (3–5 years) who are likely to encounter difficulties in academic learning and the provision of appropriate services for these children (12,328,436,514,589). This is based on the hope that appropriate remediation will prevent potential learning failures from occurring.

Programs for early identification and remediation include evaluation, placement of some children in early childhood classes, and making recommendations for future educational placement. Evaluation involves two phases: screening to identify high-risk children and formal, in-depth assessment of selected children to determine the nature of the problem and to make further referrals if appropriate. There are a number of methods and instruments used for screening. In general, the areas examined are sensory, motor, affective (anxiety, emotional stability, etc.) social, conceptual sorting, demonstrating spacial concepts, following verbal directions, and language. It has also been suggested that evaluation includes assessment of neurophysiological maturity.

Programs for children with potential learning disabilities are still in the process of evolving. In general, however, they include four areas:

1. *Cognitive development*. Focus is on improvement of concept formation, acquisition of general knowledge, problem-solving ability, memory, and discriminate learning;
2. *Psychological processing*. This includes sensory integration, visual discrimination, visual-motor integration, and gross and fine motor skills;
3. *Language*. The areas stressed are oral language development, listening skills, vocabulary and sentence development;
4. *Social development*. Focus is on age-appropriate group interaction skills and cooperation with the professional and other staff members.

Critics of evaluation and remediation programs for preschool children have raised a number of issues (587). First, children do not mature at the same rate. Some children have developmental lags, which may disappear by the time they are ready for formal schooling. Second, early identification and labeling of a child may serve to impose limits on teachers' expectations and create an environment that reinforces the child's learning problems (436). This process is sometimes referred to as "self-fulfilling prophecy"; if an individual is expected to have problems, he or she will have problems. Another issue is that evaluative instruments for this age group are fairly unreliable and have low predictive validity (36). An inappropriate label may stigmatize the child. Further, evaluative instruments for this age group are imprecise, making it difficult to discern the exact nature of the child's problem: learning disability, mental retardation, emotional disturbances, language disorder, and so forth. However, many people believe that a differential diagnosis is not as important as it is to find and help the child.

Concerning remediation, effectiveness of a program is difficult to determine (1047). At the time the child is identified, the learning disability has not yet occurred. If not involved in a program, the child may or may not develop a problem. When a child who has been in a remediation program is successful in a regular school situation, one cannot be certain if that success was due to early identification and remediation.

Nevertheless, most specialists in the area of learning disabilities feel that these programs accomplish much in preventing or reducing learning disorders. Further, it is felt that programs are most effective when they (a) provide intervention at an early age, (b) include parents as active participants, and (c) involve a number of professions in assessment and planning for the child (12,589).

Adults

At the other end of the life cycle are learning-disabled adults. The problems encountered by these individuals in childhood and adolescence may continue to plague them in the adult years (208,214). There is actually very little known about learning-disabled adults, for minimal research has been done in this area. However, sketchy reports in the literature indicate various possible patterns.

Some adults never identified themselves or were identified as learning-disabled during childhood or adolescence. They may only recently have developed awareness of past or current difficulties in this area through television programs and magazine articles designed to increase public knowledge of learning disabilities. Others may come to recognize problems through the history-taking that accompanied the evaluation of their own child who is suspected of being learning disabled.

There are many well-known people—Nelson Rockefeller, Thomas Edison, Auguste Rodin, Woodrow Wilson, and Albert Einstein to name just a few—who had problems in learning (587,952). These eminent people, and the less than eminent, were somehow able to find ways of learning. Whether the disability or some aspect of it disappeared or they were able to develop compensatory skills is unknown. An understanding of how they were able to do this is more than a matter of curiosity. Knowledge in this area may well help those concerned with the learning disabled to develop more effective methods of prognosis and remediation.

The types of problems experienced by learning-disabled adults is to a great extent dependent on the severity of their disability. Many report that they have difficulty in finding their place in the world. They have trouble securing and keeping a job and may have had to compromise their personal occupational goals because of their disability. They may also have difficulty in developing an adequate social life and in coping with many activities of daily living. For those who cannot read, this deficit may be seen as a continual threat, and much energy may be spent on hiding it from public notice. It appears that many learning-disabled adults continue to be dependent on their parents for a longer than usual time. Dependency later is often transferred to a spouse.

Some of the other characteristics of learning-disabled adults are a poor sense of direction, with a tendency to get lost or an avoidance of unknown areas; motor incoordination, especially in balance and in sports involving the use of a ball; discomfort in places where there is a high degree of auditory and visual stimuli; a sense of disorientation in new surroundings; difficulty in reading the social responses of others or a hypersensitivity to responses; fear of failure; difficulty in following verbal or written directions; problems in writing letters and reports; little if any time spent in reading for enjoyment; dependency on others in dealing with financial matters; and dependency on a pocket calculator for simple daily mathematical problems. It should, of course, be noted that all adults with residual or pronounced learning problems do not exhibit all the characteristics outlined above. Nor are these problems necessarily indicative of problems in learning.

The Role of the Occupational Therapist

After this somewhat lengthy discussion of learning disabilities, it is somewhat easier to put intervention relative to sensory integration into some perspective. The issue of psychological processing versus academic skills mastery prevalent in education can be rephrased using the vocabulary of occupational therapy. The issue then becomes should the occupational therapist (a) focus on intervention in the area of sensory integration deficit; (b) focus on intervention relative to motor and psychological function, social interaction, and occupational performances; or (c) focus on both?

Proponents of the first point of view identify adequate sensory integration processing as fundamental to all other aspects of function (58,64,433,434,537). Intervention in this area is seen as being of utmost importance. Some attention may be given to the individual's emotional responses, but the other performance components and occupational performances would not be considered a priority. Proponents of this point of view believe that attention to these other areas would result in the development of "splinter skills," an orientation to which they are strongly opposed.

Proponents of the second point of view would point to the lack of strong research findings to support a sensory integration orientation (590). They feel that occupational therapists provide a more meaningful service through assisting individuals relative to psychological function, social interaction, and occupational performances. They do not believe that they are engaged in the development of splinter skills.

Proponents of the third approach believe all areas of dysfunction should be taken into consideration, with priority being based on the current needs of the client.

Until there is more empirical data available, the third approach is probably the soundest, on both theoretical and ethical grounds.

The age of the client may, however, be a factor in the therapist's decision about what approach is appropriate. Although the theoretical base supporting the sensory integration approach is still in the process of being formulated, in part it is based on the plasticity of the brain (58). Plasticity refers to the degree to which neural structures and functions can be modified through interaction with the environment. It is generally felt that neurological organization is virtually completed within the first decade of life. However, there is some recent research to support lesser but continued brain plasticity subsequent to preadolescence. The therapist who ascribes to termination of plasticity prior to preadolescence would only use a sensory integrative approach with preschool and elementary school children, the assumption being that nothing positive can be accomplished relative to sensory integrative deficit of adolescents and adults. With these age groups, then, the therapist would direct intervention to other identified areas of dysfunction. The therapist who ascribes to continued brain plasticity would, of course, give attention to sensory integration deficit when working with adolescents and adults.

A note regarding the evaluation of sensory integration relative to adolescents and adults. The assessment instruments used for elementary school children are not suitable for this population. Evaluation is perhaps best dealt with through observation of the individual performing tasks that are purported to require a high degree of sensory integration. This should be done with full recognition of the lack of normative data. Data gained from the evaluative interview may also be useful.

Leaving the issue of sensory integration aside, the remaining portion of this section briefly outlines some ways in which the therapist deals with the nonsensory integrative deficits of learning-disabled individuals.

Prevention. Focus here would be on the preschool child who is at risk relative to the development of a learning disability (358).

Meeting health needs. The learning-disabled individual may experience most difficulty in the area of satisfying mastery and esteem needs. These needs often must be met fairly directly until the individual develops sufficient capacity to meet these needs independently.

Maintenance. Maintenance is usually only a problem in the case of elementary school children. Intervention may not occur during the summer months while the child is out of school. A simple home program planned in conjunction with the child and parents may minimize any regression that could possibly occur.

Management. Grossly inappropriate behavior is likely to be most prevalent in the elementary school age group. It may also, however, occur in the preschool age group and in adolescence. In addition to the various techniques mentioned in Chapter 17, some strategies for managing disruptive behavior in the classroom are (589): *Contracting:* The student and teacher or therapist agree to simple contracts for improving behavior, with the responsibilities of each outlined. *Peer-mediated strategies:* Students with inappropriate behavior are paired with students who are judged to be socially mature, reliable, and sensible. This method relies on peer modeling. *Time-out:* A student is isolated from the group for a short period of time immediately after engaging in a previously defined inappropriate behavior. *Self-directed exclusion:* The child is encouraged to go to a specified quiet place (e.g., the library, the bench at the end of the hall, an unused classroom) for a period of time when he or she is experiencing the classroom situation as overwhelming.

One additional problem in management may be seen in learning-disabled adolescents. Some youths are initially resistant to any kind of assistance because they see such help as indicative of being different. Adolescents tend to want to be very much like their peers. Resistance is best dealt with through slowly establishing a trust relationship and letting the adolescent take the lead in identifying problem areas.

Another aspect of intervention somewhat related to management is helping the learning-disabled individual, particularly elementary and secondary school students, understand the nature of his or her problems. Emphasis, of course, should be placed on what the child is able to do, without denying the areas of specific difficulty. Repeated emphasis should be placed on the fact that the student's difficulty in learning is not the student's fault.

The change process. In dealing with faulty social perception, the psychosocial consequence of being learning disabled, or both in conjunction, any of the three frames of reference as described in Part 5 or combination of these is appropriate. Recapitulation of ontogenesis may be used, with particular emphasis on group interaction and self-identity skills. Deficits in social perception are perhaps best dealt with through the use of role acquisition, with considerable attention given to developing sensitivity to other people, how to handle various social situations, and establishing friend relationships. This frame of reference is also useful as the basis for dealing with deficits in occupational performances. All areas are of equal importance. However, difficulties in activities of daily living and in temporal adaptation may be experienced as most troublesome by the client. The use of reconciliation of universal issues may be useful in helping adolescents manage the emotional components of being learning disabled. It is particularly helpful if this type of intervention takes place in a task-oriented group.

In conclusion, learning-disabled individuals may or may not have a deficit in sensory integration. When there is a deficit, the factor of age is important in determining whether the deficit should be addressed directly or the individual assisted in developing compensatory skills. Regardless of the presence or absence of problems in sensory integration, the majority of learning-disabled individuals need some help in mastering the other performance components and occupational performances.

SCHIZOPHRENIC DISORDERS

The other major client population identified as having a deficit in sensory integration are some individuals described as having a schizophrenic disorder. As in considering learning disabilities, this section begins with a survey of schizophrenic disorders (48,387,600,719,726, 1042). This is done with the hope that it will facilitate an understanding of some of the issues and controversies surrounding the use of a sensory integration orientation in intervention with this population. More specifically, the parts of this section are diagnoses and classification, factors in research design, factors associated with schizophrenic disorders, research regarding treatment outcomes, sensory integration, and the role of the occupational therapist.

Diagnoses and Classification

The diagnostic category of schizophrenia was first identified by Kraepelin and elaborated upon by Bleuler (110,563). Since their time, schizophrenia has been redefined in any number of ways (33–35,513,788,810). The major redefinitions have focused on what should or should not be included in the broad category of schizophrenia and on identification of the subtypes of schizophrenia. Of particular concern has been differentiation between schizophrenia and the affect disorders (depressive and/or manic), and schizophrenia and paranoid disorders.

In addition, there has been considerable controversy regarding "reactive" versus "process" schizophrenia (726). Reactive schizophrenia is characterized by onset in early adulthood, abrupt development of symptoms often following an identifiable stressful life event, a good premorbid history, emotional components such as anxiety and depression, and a good prognosis for recovery. In contrast, process schizophrenia is characterized by gradual development of the disorder beginning in early childhood, poor premorbid social and psychological development distinguished by a constriction of interests and avoidance of social interaction, the absence of any specific precipitating life crisis, blunt affect, a relative absence of emotionality, and a poor prognosis with a tendency toward continued deterioration. The controversy has essentially centered around whether reactive and process schizophrenia are one entity differing only in severity or separate distinct entities.

The most current, widely disseminated description of schizophrenic disorders is that recommended by the American Psychiatric Association in *The Diagnostic and Statistical Manual of Mental Disorders (DSM-III)* (35). Schizophrenic disorders are described as a group of conditions characterized by certain psychotic features during the active phase of the illness, deterioration from a previous level of functioning, onset before age 45, and a duration of at least 6 months. The last characteristic esentially precludes reactive schizophrenia from the major category of schizophrenic disorders. Also excluded are depressive and manic syndromes having certain psychotic features and paranoid disorders that are not accompanied by hallucinations, incoherence, loosening of associations, or bizarre delusions.

The behavioral symptoms of schizophrenic disorders are problems in the area of:

- *Content of thought.* The major disturbances in this area are delusions that are often multiple, fragmented, and bizarre. Common types of delusions are persecutory, delusions of reference, belief that one is being controlled by external forces, and the belief that one's thoughts are known by others.

- *Form of thought*. The client demonstrates illogical thinking, loosening of associations, poverty of content, and speech that is overly abstract, concrete, repetitive, or stereotyped.
- *Perception*. Various froms of hallucinations may occur in all sensory systems, with auditory being far the most common. Other perceptual abnormalities that may occur are sensations of bodily changes and hypersensitivity to sound, sight, and smell.
- *Affect*. The disturbances often include blunting, flattening, or inappropriateness of affect.
- *Sense of self*. Difficulties in this area are manifested by extreme perplexity about one's own identity, exaggerated concern about the meaning of existence, or by some specific delusions regarding the self.
- *Volition*. A disturbance in self-initiated, goal-directed activity that may take the form of inadequate interest, inability to follow a course of action to its logical conclusion, or pronounced ambivalence regarding alternative courses of action.
- *Relationship to external world*. There is a tendency to withdraw from the external world, to become involved with egocentric and illogical ideas and fantasies, and to appear emotionally detached from others.

It should be noted that no single feature mentioned above is invariably present in an individual diagnosed as having a schizophrenic disorder or that any of these features are seen only in schizophrenia.

The course of the illness is typically characterized by a prodromal stage in which there is a clear deterioration from a previous level of functioning. During the active phase psychotic symptoms are prominent. The residual phase is similar to the prodromal phase, with affective blunting or flattening and impairment in role function being common. Some of the psychotic symptoms such as delusions of hallucinations may persist but are no longer accompanied by strong affect. A complete return to premorbid functioning is unusual. The most common course is one of acute exacerbations, with increasing residual impairment between episodes.

The types of schizophrenia disorders are defined by a major presenting symptom or stage in the course of the illness, e.g. acute or chronic. These types are disorganized, catatonic, paranoid, undifferentiated, and residual.

Issues Related to Research Design

Considerable research has been conducted regarding the nature of schizophrenia. Investigations have been concerned with the identification of behavioral and biological characteristics of the disorder, the elucidation of etiological variables, and the effectiveness of various therapeutic procedures. A wide range of factors has been considered by various disciplines, including epidemiology, genetics, biochemistry, neurology, psychophysiology, pharmacology, sociology, and psychology. This diversity in orientation and marked differences in research procedures has led to a complex body of literature but one marked by some inconsistencies and contradictions. In reviewing research findings, there are a number of methodological and conceptual issues, common to most areas of schizophrenic research, that need to be taken into consideration (43,159,392,642,655,725, 726,804,833).

General Design

In true experimental design, which hypothesizes cause and effect relationships, subjects are randomly assigned to conditions that have been created or manipulated by the experimenter. In any comparison of those diagnosed as schizophrenic with other individuals, subjects are not randomly assigned to groups by the investigator. Investigators must rely on the identification of a group of individuals who have already developed the disorder. Therefore, investigation using schizophrenic patients can never be truly experimental. The exception to this is in the case of studies designed to determine effectiveness of treatment.

To overcome the problems outlined above, investigators have often made use of experimental analogous research. This type of design involves an attempt to reproduce schizophrenia (or something like it) in a group of animal or human subjects. The independent variables are therefore under experimental control. There are three problems that make this type of research questionable:

1. The usefulness of the findings is dependent on the degree to which experimentally created behavior resembles the disorder it is intended to mimic. The degree to which experimentally induced behavior truly resembles schizophrenia is a matter of much debate.
2. There are a large number of experimental conditions—hallucinogenic drugs, sensory deprivation, hypnosis, to name just a few—that produce schizophrenic-like symptoms. Because there are so many conditions, the validity of the argument for any one of them is questionable.
3. A relationship demonstrated by analog research can not be assumed to occur in the natural environment. Extreme caution must be used in drawing inferences.

Given the limitations imposed by experimental and analog research, most investigators use a correlational design. There are, however, two problems with such a design. First, no distinction between cause and effect can be made. To infer cause and effect is a misinterpretation of research findings. Second, the relationship between the diagnostic category and the dependent variable could be produced by the operation of some *third* variable.

Selection of Subjects

Three major problems are apparent in the selection of a sample of individuals diagnosed as schizophrenic. Psychiatric diagnosis is highly unreliable. First, there is considerable variation between physicians, clinical settings, and geographical areas. Second, there are many different sets of diagnostic criteria for schizophrenia. The diagnostic criteria specified in *DSM-II*, for example, are far different than those outlined in *DSM-III*.

Third, schizophrenia is a highly heterogenous category characterized by considerable variation in performance. Traditional subtypes have usually not been helpful in accounting for this variation. Samples of patients used in research projects, then, are not likely to be very similar, and by some criteria participants may not even be considered to be schizophrenic. All of the above limit comparison of research findings and generalization to the schizophrenic population as a whole.

Contrast groups typically consist of normal individuals or a heterogenous group of nonschizophrenic patients. A simple demonstration of schizophrenic/normal difference is usually quite trivial. Cognitive, perceptual, and motor differences are quite easy to find. Physiological and biochemical distinctions, although less common, are also able to be identified.

A heterogeneous group of nonschizophrenic patients has often been used in an attempt to control for the effects of hospitalization. Regardless of the criteria used to calculate length of hospitalization, it is frequently difficult to find a heterogeneous group of patients who have been hospitalized as long as schizophrenic patients.

Matching has sometimes been used to control for the effects of nuisance variables. In this case an attempt is made to match schizophrenics and the contrast group on variables that have been found or are believed to be significantly related to the diagnosis and dependent measures. The first problem is that the variable being controlled for may be an important factor in accounting for the real difference that exists between the groups. Also, matching groups on one variable may result in a systematic mismatching on another. It would be methodologically impossible to simultaneously control for all of the plausible variables.

It should be noted that matching does not in any way rule out the possibility of a third, unknown variable, which may account for the correlation observed. Third-variable explanations are particularly troublesome in schizophrenic research. Complex statistical procedures are often required to solve this problem.

Antipsychotic Medication

Phenothiazines, used almost universally in the United States for treatment of patients diagnosed as schizophrenic, may well represent another explanation of the behavioral and biological differences observed between schizophrenics and other groups of individuals who are not receiving these same drugs. Drugs may represent a nuisance variable whose effect must be controlled. However, medication effects are probably more than a methodological annoyance. They may represent an important link in the network of relationships defining schizophrenia. If this is so, then research should be designed to consider the relationship between antipsychotic medication and other variables that are potentially relevant to an understanding of schizophrenia.

Longitudinal Designs

Many of the relationships currently of interest in understanding schizophrenia are developmental in nature and can only be studied appropriately through longitudinal research designs. Another reason for the support of longitudinal studies is that most other designs study individuals who are already schizophrenic. Thus, it is unknown whether the traits observed are truly antecedent to the disorder or the results of factors associated with the life experiences that arise as a consequence of the condition and/or factors associated with identification and treatment.

The most promising longitudinal studies are likely to be those focusing on individuals who are at high risk for becoming schizophrenic in the future but who have not yet manifested clinical signs of disturbance. Individuals in this category are children who have a parent who is schizophrenic. Problems related to this type of study are great expense, a high rate of attrition, and any number of events—known and unknown to the investigator—that may occur with the passage of time.

Demand Characteristics and Impression Management

Demand characteristics refer to those factors within the research project which are interpreted by the subjects and which serve as a basis for their response. In other words, subjects may formulate ideas about the nature of the study and make judgments about what is expected of them in response to various aspects of the experimental situation. Some examples of demand characteristics are the research setting, rumors about the investigation, explicit as well as implicit instructions, various characteristics of the experimenter and his or her behavior, the degree of attention paid to the subjects, and so forth. Response to demand characteristics may produce artifactual results and thus may lead to erroneous conclusions.

Impression management is the subject's manipulation of his or her responses in a way that he or she feels is in his or her own best interests. For example, a schizophrenic patient may respond in one way as opposed to another, depending on the desire or lack of desire to be discharged from the hospital. The extent or which schizophrenics are able to manipulate voluntarily the quality of their responses is likely to depend on the nature of the performance required.

Response to demand characteristics and impression management should be taken into consideration in the interpretation of any research finding.

As the above discussion indicates, research designed to study schizophrenic disorders is permeated with conceptual and methodological problems. Some of these difficulties can be alleviated to some degree by more sophisticated research design and statistical manipulation. Other difficulties are inherent in the nature of the phenomena being studied and cannot be controlled for at this time. Although the discussion was focused on research relative to the schizophrenic disorders, the problems identified are similar to those that are likely to be encountered in research projects involving many of the populations with which occupational therapists are concerned.

Factors Associated with Schizophrenic Disorders

In general, research findings have led to the following conclusions (ref. 726, p.464):

> Schizophrenia is not, in all likelihood, a distinct disease entity that will ultimately be explained by the discovery of a single necessary and sufficient cause. The etiological models that seem the most applicable in the light of current knowledge emphasize a complex interactional sequence of unspecified organismic and environmental events. Preschizophrenics apparently inherit a trait or set of traits, that make them vulnerable to further events, which, in turn, may precipitate the overt clinical manifestations of the disorder and lead to intervention and possible hospitalization. Once the clinical disorder has appeared, it is often relieved by the administration of psychopharmacological agents. With or without drugs, most patients recover sufficiently to leave the hospital, although many return within several months following an exacerbation of symptoms.

The remaining portion of this section will focus on some of the areas of research that may facilitate the occupational therapist's understanding of the schizophrenic disorders.

Language and Information Processing

Many schizophrenics appear to have difficulty at the level of controlled information processing (109,158,180, 829,870). It is in the area of active, conscious mental operations involving short-term memory that problems are encountered. Complex, higher-level cognitive functions appeared to be impaired. Linguistic performance, which depends on the interaction of grammatical knowledge and of complex cognitive skills, is often disturbed. The unusually long hesitation before emitting sentences, which is typical of many schizophrenics, seems to indicate that schizophrenics' processing is impaired at the point where decisions regarding the direction of speech are presumably made. One possible explanation for this phenomenon is that the selective attention mechanism, which protects the speaker from intrusion of irrelevant material, is malfunctioning in schizophrenics. Thus, the individual's train of thought or plan for verbal response becomes disorganized.

There also appears to be difficulty in subjectively organizing stimulus units into manageable sets of information. This is particularly evident in tasks requiring short-term recall. There does not seem to be any difficulty in perceiving attributes of the environment around which organization might occur nor in normal patterns of storage. The problem seems to be a failure in selective attention. Research findings indicate that not all schizophrenics have difficulty in language and information processing and that the difficulty is not a uniquely schizophrenic characteristic.

Biochemical Factors

There are several biochemical theories regarding the etiology of schizophrenia (218,430,511,642,729,824). Owing to the complexity of the research area, there are many methodological problems that make it difficult to either confirm or refute many of the theories. Interpretation is also plagued by the question of an unknown third variable that may account for biochemical abnormalities and the behavioral symptoms of schizophrenia. In addition, the distinct possibility of multiple etiological factors is suggested by a biochemical abnormality that has not been found in all patients diagnosed as schizophrenic or in any one subtype of schizophrenia.

The dopamine hypothesis is considered to be the most promising of the current biochemical theories of schizophrenia (204,674,726,918,978.) The theory essentially states that there is an excess of dopamine in the brain caused either by increased synthesis or faulty feedback regulation of the amount of dopamine. Support for this hypothesis is (a) drugs that are clinically effective in treating schizophrenia are known to block dopamine receptors, and (b) drugs, such as the amphetamines, that stimulate dopamine release can exacerbate schizophrenic symptoms. The correlation between clinical effectiveness of the phenothiazines and their ability to block dopamine receptors is impressive, although not perfect. Such evidence does not substantiate the conclusion that schizophrenia is due to dopamine excess or receptor overactivity. Among the many questions unanswered are what causes the dopamine excess and why does such an excess lead to the behavioral manifestation of schizophrenia?

Psychophysiological Factors

In psychophysiological studies the electrical activity of various biological systems is studied. Some of the findings that appear to be consistent and statistically significant are (146,308,387,719,726,1042): First, skin conductance and the frequency of spontaneous fluctuations in conductance levels have both been found to be higher in some schizophrenics—particularly in those who are chronic or high in severity—than in controls. Second, electrochemical-orienting response differentiates schizophrenics from controls. Approximately 50% of schizophrenics do not have any orienting response at all. Those who do tend to have a higher resting level of skin conductance, more frequent spontaneous fluctuations, and a slower than normal habituation of the orienting response. Some patients also show higher amplitude-orienting responses from their right to their left hand.

Early theoretical approaches to this body of data focused on the concept of arousal—that schizophrenics were high in arousal. But low correlation among different measures of arousal made this theoretical stance difficult to defend. Another interpretation of these findings is that they indicate a left-hemisphere dysfunction in the temporal lobe. Considerably more evidence is needed to substantiate this hypothesis.

There have been many studies of the central nervous system psychophysiological responses, with the majority of the studies focusing on electroencephalogram (EEG) responses. Some of the findings are:

1. Schizophrenics have less alpha rhythm than controls; a possible indication that they are higher in arousal. They also show less variability over time in the amplitude of the EEG.
2. During sleep, some schizophrenics show less REM time and less stage-4 sleep.
3. Studies of responses to discrete stimuli indicate that schizophrenics' responses are more variable and show smaller amplitudes of the early components of the evoked response than controls.

All the data, which are fairly consistent, cannot be fit together into any one theoretical system. This is essentially information in need of a theory.

Finally, studies indicate that schizophrenics and their first-degree relatives appear to have problems in following a moving target. There is a deficit in smooth-pursuit eye movements. The significance of these data are also unclear.

Genetics

The data from twin, family, and adoption studies strongly indicate an inherited predisposition to schizophrenia (295,361,500,832,834). The specific nature of the heredity factor remains unknown. Most of the data, for example, are compatible with either a polygenetic model or a single-locus model. Further studies may support the hypothesis that schizophrenia is a heterogenous disorder that can be transmitted in more than one fashion. Although a predisposition is evident, the exact nature of that predisposition in biological terms is not known.

Environmental Factors

Research dealing with environmental factors has not contributed a great deal to the understanding of schizophrenia. Nevertheless, it is quite evident that environmental factors are important. The problem is that the nature of significant environmental factors and the manner in which they interact with equally ill-defined genetic factors remain unknown.

Family interaction has received considerable attention as a potentially significant environmental factor (42,294, 331,795,832). Various kinds of disturbances have been noted in the interaction of families with a schizophrenic daughter or son. The direction of the relationship, however, is unclear. Earlier theorists argued that the parents' interactional problems contributed to the poor adjustment of the offspring. Recent studies suggest that the parents' difficulties may be a response to the problems of living with a seriously disturbed individual.

Another environmental factor—stress—has also received considerable attention (43,138,240,476,869). In the past, the etiology of schizophrenia was sought in radical, traumatic environmental events. More recent research does not support this hypothesis. Neale and Oltmanns suggest, on the basis of current research, that (ref. 726, p. 341):

> Given a genetically determined vulnerability, *routine* experience may be sufficient to precipitate the disorder. It may not be necessary for preschizophrenics to experience a greater number of stressful events. These people may simply be less able to handle the same events to which others are able to adjust (e.g., social dating during adolescence, academic pressure, child birth, and so on). Thus the environmental events in schizophrenia may not be abnormal in themselves; the problem may be in the response of the preschizophrenic to routine life events.

Developmental Studies

The purpose of developmental research is to identify the characteristics of individuals prior to the onset of the schizophrenia (314,330,407,502,579,700,804,812, 816,1044). The major research strategies used have been follow-up of child guidance populations, the follow-back of adult schizophrenics, and longitudinal studies of high-risk populations.

Follow-up studies of guidance clinic populations indicate that those children who later become schizophrenic were aggressive and antisocial as children (withdrawn children were not more likely than controls to become schizophrenic), demonstrated the presence of neurological soft signs, and lived in a generally disordered family environment. Conclusions drawn from the data should be tempered by the fact that most schizophrenics are not seen at guidance clinics as children and most children seen at guidance clinics used in these studies were referred for aggressive behavior disorders.

Follow-back studies have been primarily based on school records. Findings indicate a low childhood IQ; abrasive, disagreeable social behavior for boys; and introverted, passive social behavior on the part of girls. Although these findings are consistent, it is questionable whether they are specific indicators of schizophrenia.

Most of the high-risk longitudinal studies are still in progress. The majority of the data now available have been derived from high-risk versus low-risk cross-sectional studies. The data show that in many ways the high-risk children perform similarly to an adult schizophrenic on tasks reflecting attentional and cognitive performance. High-risk children also show low social competence and increased levels of neurological soft signs. Results from these studies are difficult to interpret because the studies do not compare children of schizophrenics with children of parents in other specific groups (e.g., children of manics or of depressives).

Research Concerning Treatment Outcomes

The literature regarding treatment emphasizes the long-term nature of schizophrenic disorders. The most effective treatment provides for both the resolution of acute episodes and the remediation of chronic social impairment (89,156,162,350,353,354,420,612,655,713,768, 851,924,1030). Antipsychotic drugs are able to improve the conditions of many but not all patients. However, they are by no means a cure for schizophrenia, having little impact on the patient's capacity to engage effectively in various social roles. Individual and group verbal psychotherapy has not been found to be an effective form of treatment. Most patients can be maintained in the community if they are involved in programs designed to help them develop interpersonal skills, resolve routine problems, and to minimize the effects of stressful life events.

A study of the effectiveness of 10 aftercare programs for schizophrenic clients provides some information regarding the type of program that facilitates maintenance in the community (612). The most effective programs—using the criteria of social function, symptoms, attitudes, and relapse rate—had the following characteristics: Formal methods to evaluate the client's progress; the assignment of each client to one staff member during his or her tenure in the program and for follow-up; a sustained nonthreatening environment; significantly less group psychotherapy and family counseling; and greater participation in occupational therapy.

In conclusion, knowledge regarding the etiology of schizophrenic disorders is limited, although there is considerable information regarding behavioral and biological characteristics associated with the disorders. Regarding the effectiveness of treatment, many schizophrenic clients are able to achieve at least a moderately successful adjustment to the community through a combination of psychopharmacology and psychosocial intervention.

Sensory Integration

King has hypothesized a relationship between sensory integrative deficit and schizophrenia. She states that (ref. 533, p. 529):

> Some individuals have defective proprioceptive feedback mechanisms, the vestibular component in particular being first underactive, and secondly underactive in its role in the sensorimotor integration process. This defect, whether genetic, developmental or the result of trauma, constitutes an important etiological or prodromal factor in process and reactive schizophrenia.

Schizophrenia paranoid type is seen by King as a related but different syndrome than reactive-process schizophrenia. Deficit in sensory integration is not considered to be a factor in paranoid schizophrenia. When King formulated her theory, "reactive" schizophrenia was identified as one type of schizophrenia. It no longer is identified as such in *DSM-III*. Here again is evidence of the ever-changing classification of schizophrenia and schizophrenia-like disorders.

Putting the problems and classification aside, King provides considerable evidence to support her theory. She states that deficits in the processing of vestibular, proprioceptive, and tactile information at the subcortical level leads to the following:

1. Severe anxiety arising from the feeling of being, literally and figuratively, unsteady on one's feet. This is accompanied by a fear of falling, which accounts for a typical posture of flexion, adduction, and internal rotation.
2. The need to use cortical processing of information to compensate for the subcortical deficit. Thus, the individual must consciously think about common movements that would otherwise be initiated automatically. A much slower way of processing information, this leads to disruptions in the motor patterns of speech and general retardation in movement.
3. Inadequate integration of auditory and visual stimuli, which in turn results in inadequate visual size and form consistency and unreliable localization of auditory stimuli. The lack of perpetual consistency is considered to be the mechanism that produces hallucinations.
4. Inadequate processing of information at the cortical level leading to concrete associations, inability to think in abstract terms, and bizarre associations.
5. Anxiety, which in turn leads to tension in the facial musculature. A decrease in the mobility of the facial muscles is said to inhibit the extent to which emotions are experienced. This accounts for the flattening affect so often seen in schizophrenics.

King's theory regarding the relationship between sensory integrative deficit and schizophrenia may be questioned on many points. Some of the major issues that need to be addressed are:

Sensory integrative deficit as an etiological or prodromal factor. The cause, or more accurately, the probably multiple causes of the schizophrenic's disorders—is unknown. To hypothesize that sensory integrative deficit accounts for the majority of the symptoms associated with schizophrenic disorders seems to be somewhat of an overstatement. A more conservative theoretical position is that sensory integrative deficit is a prodromal factor. The term "prodromal" as used in medicine refers to a biological or behavioral manifestation of a disorder prior to development of the clinical signs and symptoms traditionally associated with the disorder. Prodromal factors are not in any way considered to be causal. Sensory integrative deficit, as a prodromal factor, would then be considered one of the presymptoms of schizophrenic disorders.

To postulate that a factor is etiological *or* prodromal relative to a particular disorder is at best risky. Etiological theories are concerned with the identification of cause. Prodromal theories are concerned with linking a biological or behavioral factor to a known or unknown cause and to the clinical signs and symptoms of a disorder. The starting point in the reasoning process is somewhat different, and using the medical model, what one does with the information is also different. Although King states that sensory integrative deficit may be either an eitological factor or a prodromal factor, taken as a whole her writings seem to favor an etiological position.

If sensory integrative deficit is a causal factor relative to some schizophrenic disorders, then why do the vast majority of individuals with hypothesized defects in this area not develop schizophrenic disorders? Severity may be a factor here but that does not really answer the question. Another more conservative position that may be taken is that sensory integrative deficit is only a contributing factor to the etiology of some schizophrenic disorders when there is a genetic predisposition.

A hypothesized sensory integrative deficit has been suggested as a causal factor in schizophrenia and learning disabilities. There are two elements that might be indicative of some similarity. Neurological soft signs have been identified in some children with learning disabilities and in some children of schizophrenic parents. Learning disabilities are associated with a medical diagnosis of attention deficit disorders. It has been suggested that depletion of norepinephrine and excessive dopamine lead to general arousal as opposed to focused alertness, an indication of some type of attention deficit (559,726,744,846,950). However, taken collectively, the difficulties associated with learning disabilities and those associated with reactive-process schizophrenia are very different. There is no empirical evidence to support a close link between these two disorders. It would seem that two disorders with a common etiological factor are likely to be somewhat more similar in their clinical manifestation.

King uses a particular postural stance as being typical of reactive and process schizophrenia as one element to support a sensory integrative deficit. This postural stance has been identified as the consequence of long-term institutionalization as differentiated from a behavior associated with schizophrenia (86,936,1030). The posture in question—flexion, adduction, and internal rotation—is felt to be a response to the elements inherent in institutionalization. Some of these elements include being treated as somewhat less than human, leading to a marked deficit in self-esteem, beds that provide inadequate postural support, improperly fitting clothes and shoes, poor nutrition. Anxiety, fatigue, illness, and insufficient exercise may also be contributing factors.

Institutionalization probably does result in diminished sensory stimulation. However, lack of a typical or normal amount of sensory stimuli in the external environment does not lead to sensory integrative deficit. Sensory depreciation and sensory integrative deficit are not the same thing.

Study of the relationship between sensory integration and schizophrenia has focused on exploring the hypothesized theory and the effectiveness of sensory integration intervention. Theoretical research has primarily focused on vestibular reactivity as measured by postrotary nystagmus in the schizophrenic population (456,537). The evidence seems to indicate some problem with vestibular system function in schizophrenia. The nature of that problem, however, is not clear.

Most of the studies regarding vestibular reactivity have rather serious methodological flaws in that there were insufficient controls relative to medication, length of illness and hospitalization, age, sex, and subtypes of schizophrenia. More importantly, vestibular responsiveness was measured with techniques that are not reliable and/or valid or techniques that never have been standardized with adults. Aside from methodological flaws, the major problem with these studies is the assumption that abnormal vestibular reactivity is indicative of sensory integrative deficit. Although there may be some circumstantial evidence for this relationship, adequate empirical data are not available.

Research relative to the effectiveness of sensory integration intervention with schizophrenic clients does not offer a great deal of support for this orientation (70, 210,264,591,609,806). Some positive changes were evident in the areas of activities of daily living, relevance of verbalization, person drawing scores, gait, and "general behavior." These findings have not been replicated, and there are many reports of no significant change relative to target behavior.

Some of the methodological problems of these studies are less than rigorous criteria for placing subjects in diagnostic categories, small sample size, and poorly matched experimental and control groups. Cross-study comparison is difficult because of sketchy reports regarding the activities used for intervention and differences in the outcome measures used. The efficacy of sensory integration intervention cannot be compared with other types of treatment/intervention because, with one exception, the studies did not use generally accepted psychiatric status tests (537). It should be noted that research relative to the effectiveness of sensory integration intervention is relatively recent and not extensive.

The research findings regarding the effectiveness of intervention can be interpreted from two different perspectives: success and lack of success. Positive research findings may be explained by the following:

1. Individuals diagnosed as reactive/process schizophrenics do have a sensory integrative deficit which can be altered by direct intervention in that area. Selection of clients, the intervention process, and research methodology, however, need to be refined.
2. Individuals diagnosed as reactive/process schizophrenics do not have a sensory integrative deficit. Successful intervention is due to the special attention given to clients and/or the general physiological benefits of gross motor exercise. In the latter case, clients physically feel better and therefore are able to respond in a more normal manner.

Reasoning from the other perspective, the lack of documented successful intervention may be due to:

1. Methodological flaws,
2. Individuals diagnosed as reactive/process schizophrenics who do not have a sensory integrative deficit,
3. Individuals diagnosed as reactive/process schizophrenics who do have a sensory integrative deficit, but in whom diminished brain plasticity makes intervention in this area ineffective.

There is much unknown about sensory integration and about schizophrenic disorders. The future, hopefully, will erase some of these unknowns.

The Role of the Occupational Therapist

Given the above information regarding schizophrenic disorders and sensory integration, what is the best course of action for the occupational therapist to take? This question cannot be answered categorically, for it depends on how one interprets the research findings and how one fills in the blanks relative to all of the unknowns.

In reading King's work, there appears to be a distinct impression that once an individual can adequately process vestibular, proprioceptive, and tactile information at the subcortical level, no other type of intervention is necessary. If King actually means this, then it is likely that this orientation is promising more than it can deliver. Individuals diagnosed as having a reactive or process schizophrenic disorder are severely disabled in many areas of human function. It seems unlikely that intervention directed only to the enhancement of sensory integration will enable an individual to master spontaneously the various skills necessary for successful interaction in the environment. What King probably means is that facilitating the development of more adequate sensory integrative processing should be the therapist's first priority. Concurrently or subsequently, other areas of dysfunction would be addressed in the intervention process.

It is the author's opinion that given our present level of knowledge, intervention directed toward altering sensory integration dysfunction should be initiated only if there is strong evidence of deficit in this area. It should be initiated only after thorough evaluation and not solely on the basis of the client's diagnosis. It should not be initiated at the expense of attention to the client's other areas of dysfunction.

Setting sensory integrative dysfunction aside, the body of literature concerning schizophrenic disorders provides some guidelines for occupational therapists. Typically, individuals with schizophrenic disorders are initially hospitalized for a period of time and discharged to some type of care in the community. For many individuals the disorder is chronic in nature, being characterized by periods of exacerbation and some degree of remission. During the acute phases (initial and periodic), the short-term care as outlined in Chapter 27 is probably the best approach. Clients who are to some degree in remission are usually involved, at least periodically, in community-based programs. The literature certainly emphasizes the importance of these types of programs. There are some individuals with relatively severe chronic schizophrenic disorders who are in long-term care institutions. Some of these individuals, provided with proper forms of intervention, are able to return to the community, although their adjustment is likely to be marginal at best. A program designed to facilitate deinstitutionalization and movement into the community is also outlined in Chapter 27. Finally, some individuals diagnosed as chronic schizophrenics will never be able to return to the community, indeed, should not be returned to the community. Programs designed for such individuals are focused on meeting health needs, maintenance, and, if necessary, management.

Individuals with schizophrenic disorders have deficits in many areas of human function. The areas in which occupational therapists can probably contribute most are cognitive function, social interaction, and the various occupational performances.

Guidelines for selecting an appropriate frame of reference are as follows: In general, reconciliation of universal issues is not an appropriate frame of reference for the change process. The vast majority of individuals with schizophrenic disorders do not have sufficient cognitive function to participate successfully in a change process with this orientation. Recapitulation of ontogenesis is an appropriate frame of reference, particularly for the younger population of individuals with schizophrenic disorders. This frame of reference is most appropriate when the change process is to be concerned with the enhancement of sensory integration and cognitive function. The role acquisition frame of reference is also very appropriate and suitable for all age groups. The application of recapitulation of ontogenesis and role acquisition has been discussed previously and will not be elaborated on further here.

SOME ADDITIONAL COMMENTS

The study of sensory integration has received a good deal of attention by occupational therapists. In addition to the research cited in previous sections, attention has been given to:

- Refinement of the sensory integration syndromes as described by Ayres (55,57,60,61).
- Theoretical research concerning variation in sensory integrative function between and within various populations (63,177,188,301,615,662,730,751,754,755, 756,805,898,930,931,1001).
- Study of the reliability and validity of the Southern California Sensory Integration Tests and the California Postratory Nystagmus Test (56,228,393,454,509, 530,693,763,789,836,1055).
- The effectiveness of intervention relative to many different populations (40,62,65,66,71,118,130,187, 256,417,499,508,668,724,742,803,976).

Theoretical and evaluative research, on the whole, has been inconclusive. In addition, findings, whether they be negative or positive, are limited in their general applicability because of methodological flaws. This is an area that is just beginning to be studied. Nevertheless, it is important to note that it has been studied more than any other area of occupational therapy, a point that should not be forgotten in criticism. (For further critical study of sensory integration see refs. 279,590,753,1046.)

The two major concerns of the profession regarding sensory integration are that some therapists have arrived at some conclusions that are unfounded given the current data available and have focused on sensory integrative deficit to such an extent that other areas in which the client needs assistance have been neglected.

Finally, the validation of any area of practice is difficult. King has described the situation well (ref. 537, p. 20). She has said that any area of practice is justified only

> . . . if current scientific knowledge can be used to rationalize or explain the therapeutic benefit. . . . The first question to ask about any treatment for any condition is "Does it work?" If the answer to that is negative, we need go no further. If the answer is positive, we then need to narrow the question to: "For which patient is it most successful?" The answer to that question, by helping to define the characteristics of a certain group, will assist with answering the third question, "Why does it work?"

King has defined the situation and identified the essential steps. Read another way, she has presented the challenge for all of us.

Part 7

Conclusion

This text has presented an overview of the psychosocial components of occupational therapy. It has outlined a number of taxonomies, theories, and frames of reference. It has described evaluation and intervention with a variety of client populations.

The text, however, can only serve as a foundation. Out of this matrix the neophyte therapist must, with guidance, fashion and refine a repertoire of clinical skills.

And yet clinical skills are not sufficient alone. They must be applied with wisdom in an atmosphere of respect and caring. They must be applied in association with the art of practice.

The content of this text represents only a moment in time; the theoretical base and practice of occupational therapy is ever evolving. It will be transformed and improved over time through research, theory development, and resourceful responses to the continually changing needs of society.

The reader, I hope, is concerned with taking the profession beyond what it is today and with building on the foundation that has been laid by generations of occupational therapists. May you engage in that process critically, creatively, and with the exercise of judicious restraint and defined direction.

References

1. Abels, P. (1977): *The New Practice of Supervision and Staff Development*. Association Press, New York.
2. Abreu, B. C. (1981): Interdisciplinary approach to the adult visual perception function-dysfunction continuum. In: *Physical Disabilities Manual*, edited by B. C. Abreu, Raven Press, New York.
3. Abreu, B. C. (1981): Evaluation. In: *Physical Disabilities Manual*, edited by B. C. Abreu. Raven Press, New York.
4. Abt, L., and Bellak, L. (1950): *Projective Psychology*. Charles C Thomas Publisher, Chicago.
5. Ackerknicht, E. H. (1959): *A Short History of Psychiatry*. Hafner, New York.
6. Adams, J. E., and Lindeman, E. (1974): Coping with long term disability. In: *Coping and Adaptation*, edited by G. Grelko, D. Hamburg and J. Adams. Basic Books, New York.
7. Adler, A. (1964): *Problems of Neurosis*. Harper & Row Publishers, New York.
8. Aitken, M. J. (1982): Self-concept and functional independence in the hospitalized elderly. *Am. J. Occup. Ther.*, 36:243–250.
9. Alexander, F. (1956): *Psychoanalyis and Psychotherapy*. W. W. Norton & Co., New York.
10. Alexander, F. G., and Selesnick, S. T. (1966): *The History of Psychiatry*. Mentor, New York.
11. Alexander, T. (1969): A Biological *Approach to Psychological Development*. Aldine Publishing Company, Chicago.
12. Allen, K., Holm, V., and Schiafebusch, R., editors (1978): *Early Intervention: A Team Approach*. University Park Press, Baltimore.
13. Allen, M. J., and Yen, W. M. (1979): *Introduction to Measurement Theory*. Brooks/Coles, Monterey.
14. Alley, G., and Deshler, D. (1979): *Teaching the Learning Disabled Adolescent: Strategies and Methods*. Love Publishing, Denver.
15. Allport, G. (1965): *Becoming*. Yale University Press, New Haven.
16. Aman, M. (1980): Psychotropic drugs and learning problems—a selective review. *J. Learning Disabilities*, 13:87–97.
17. American Journal of Occupational Therapy (1967): 50th anniversary issue. *Am. J. Occup. Ther.*, 21:259–342.
18. American Journal of Occupational Therapy (1968): Special section: theories of psychiatric occupational therapy. *Am. J. Occup. Ther.*, 22:397–546.
19. American Journal of Occupational Therapy (1971): Occupational therapy: an historical perspective. *Am. J. Occup. Ther.*, 25:226–246.
20. American Journal of Occupational Therapy (1971): (Occupational behavior). *Am. J. Occup. Ther.*, 25:271–307.
21. American Journal of Occupational Therapy (1977): AOTA 60th anniversary 1917–1977: commemorative issue. *Am. J. Occup. Ther.*, 31:625–712.
22. American Journal of Occupational Therapy (1979): Specialization. *Am. J. Occup. Ther.*, 33:14–49.
23. American Occupational Therapy Association (1967): *Then—and Now: 1917–1967.* AOTA, Rockville, Md.
24. American Occupational Therapy Association (1972): Report of the task force on social issues. *Am. J. Occup. Ther.*, 26:332–359.
25. American Occupational Therapy Association (1973): *Essentials of an Accredited Program for Occupational Therapists*. AOTA, Rockville, Md.
26. American Occupational Therapy Association (1975): Model occupational therapy practice act. *Am. J. Occup. Ther.*, 29:48–52.
27. American Occupational Therapy Association (1978): *Manual on Administration*. AOTA, Rockville, Md.
28. American Occupational Therapy Association (1979): The philosophical base of occupational therapy. *Am. J. Occup. Ther.*, 33:785.
29. American Occupational Therapy Association (1979): *Uniform Terminology System for Reporting Occupational Therapy Services*. AOTA, Rockville, Md.
30. American Occupational Therapy Association (1980):

Principles of occupational therapy ethics. *Am. J. Occup. Ther.*, 34:896–899.
31. American Occupational Therapy Association (1980): Standards of practice for occupational therapists in schools. *Am. J. Occup. Ther.*, 34:900–905.
32. American Occupational Therapy Association (1981): Official position paper: occupational therapy's role in independent or alternative living situations. *Am. J. Occup. Ther.*, 35:812–814.
33. American Psychiatric Association (1952): *Diagnostic and Statistical Manual of Mental Disorders I.* American Psychiatric Association, Washington, D.C.
34. American Psychiatric Association (1968): *Diagnostic and Statistical Manual II.* American Psychiatric Association, Washington, D.C.
35. American Psychiatric Association (1980): *Diagnostic and Statistical Manual of Mental Disorders III.* American Psychiatric Association, Washington, D.C.
36. Anastasi, A. (1976): *Psychological Testing.* Macmillan, New York.
37. Anderson, N. (1974): *Man's Work and Leisure.* E. J. Bull, Leiden.
38. Anderson, R. N., Greer, J. G., and McFadden, S. M. (1976): Providing for the severely handicapped: a case for competency based preparation of occupational therapists. *Am. J. Occup. Ther.*, 30:640–645.
39. Andre, R. (1981): *Homemakers: The Forgotten Workers.* University of Chicago Press, Chicago.
40. Angels, J. K. B. (1980): Effects of sensory integration treatment on the low achieving college student. *Am. J. Occup. Ther.*, 34:671–675.
41. Angliss, V. E. (1974): Habilitation of upper-limb-deficient children. *Am. J. Occup. Ther.*, 28:407–414.
42. Anthony, E. J., and Koupernik, C., editors (1974): *The Child in His Family--Children at a Psychiatric Risk.* John Wiley and Sons, New York.
43. Appley, M. H., and Turnbull, R., editors (1967): *Psychological Stress: Issues in Research.* Appleton-Century-Crofts, New York.
44. Ardrey, R. (1966): *The Territorial Imperative.* Atheneum, New York.
45. Argyris, C., and Schon, D. A. (1974): *Theory in Practice.* Jossey-Boss Publishers, San Francisco.
46. Arieti, S. (1959): *American Handbook of Psychiatry.* Basic Books, New York.
47. Arieti, S. (1967): *The Intrapsychic Self.* Basic Books, New York.
48. Arieti, S. (1974): *Interpretation of Schizophrenia.* Basic Books, New York.
49. Arnheim, R. (1967): *Towards a Psychology of Art.* University of California Press, Berkeley.
50. Aronson, R. (1976): Programs I. The role of an occupational therapist in a geriatric day hospital setting—Maimonides Day Hospital. *Am. J. Occup. Ther.*, 30:290–292.
51. Aschenbrenner, J. (1955): *Lifelines: Black Families in Chicago.* Holt, Rinehart & Winston, New York.
52. Atkins, J. A., and Chapman, R. L. (1975): Occupational therapy in a myelomeningocele clinic. *Am. J. Occup. Ther.*, 29:403–406.
53. Auerbach, E. (1974): Community involvement: the Bernal Heights Ladies' Club. *Am. J. Occup. Ther.*, 28:272–273.
54. Ayd, F. J., and Blackwell, B., editors (1970): *Discoveries in Biological Psychiatry.* J. B. Lippincott, Philadelphia.
55. Ayres, A. J. (1963): The development of perceptual-motor abilities: a theoretical basis for the treatment of dysfunction. *Am. J. Occup. Ther.*, 17:221–225.
56. Ayres, A. J. (1969): Relationship between Gesell developmental quotients and later perceptual motor performance. *Am. J. Occup. Ther.*, 23:11–17.
57. Ayres, A. J. (1971): Characteristics of types of sensory integrative dysfunction. *Am. J. Occup. Ther.*, 25:329–334.
58. Ayres, A. J. (1972): *Sensory Integration of Learning Disorders.* Western Psychological Services, Los Angeles.
59. Ayres, A. J. (1972): *Southern California Sensory Integration Tests Battery.* Western Psychological Services, Los Angeles.
60. Ayres, A. J. (1972): Types of sensory integrative dysfunction among disabled learners. *Am. J. Occup. Ther.*, 26:13–18.
61. Ayres, A. J. (1977): Cluster analysis of measurements of sensory integration. *Am. J. Occup. Ther.*, 31:362–366.
62. Ayres, A. J. (1977): Effects of sensory integrative therapy on the coordination of children with choreoathetoid movements. *Am. J. Occup. Ther.*, 31:291–293.
63. Ayres, A. J. (1977): Listening performance in learning disabled children. *Am. J. Occup. Ther.*, 31:441–446.
64. Ayres, A. J. (1979): *Sensory Integration and the Child.* Western Psychological Services, Los Angeles.
65. Ayres, A. J., and Mailloux, Z. (1981): Influence of sensory integrative procedures on language development. *Am. J. Occup. Ther.*, 35:383–391.
66. Ayres, A. M., and Tickle, L. S. (1980): Hyper-responsivity to touch and vestibular stimulation as a predictor of positive response to sensory interaction procedures by autistic children. *Am. J. Occup. Ther.*, 34:375–381.
67. Azima, H., and Azima, F. J. (1959): Outline of a dynamic theory of occuptional therapy. *Am. J. Occup. Ther.*, 13:215–219.
68. Bailey, D. M. (1968): Suitability of work program placements at Massachusetts Mental Health Center. *Am. J. Occup. Ther.*, 22:311–318.
69. Bailey, D. M. (1971): Vocational theories and work habits related to childhood development. *Am. J. Occup. Ther.*, 25:298–302.
70. Bailey, D. M. (1978): Effect of vestibular stimulation on verbalization of chronic schizophrenics. *Am. J. Occup. Ther.*, 32:445–450.
71. Baker-Nobles, L., and Bink, M. P. (1979): Sensory integration in the rehabilitation of blind adults. *Am. J. Occup. Ther.*, 33:559–564.
72. Baldwin, A. L. (1967): *Theories of Child Development.* John Wiley and Sons, New York.
73. Baltes, P. B., and Schaie, K. W. (1973): *Life Span Developmental Psychology: Personality and Socialization.* Academic Press, New York.
74. Banus, B. S., editor (1979): *The Developmental Therapist.* Charles B. Slack, Thorofare, N.J.
75. Barber, B., and Wirsch, W., editors (1962): *The Sociology of Science.* Free Press, Glencoe, N.Y.

76. Barber, R. C., Wright, B. A., and Gonick, H. R. (1973): *Adjustment to Physical Handicap and Illness*. Social Science Research Council, Bulletin 55, New York.
77. Barchas, J. D., Berger, P. A., Ciaranello, R. D., and Elliot, G. R. (1977): *Psychopharmacology from Theory to Practice*. Oxford University Press, New York.
78. Barker, P., and Muir, A. M. (1969): The role of occupational therapy in a children's inpatient psychiatric unit. *Am. J. Occup. Ther.*, 23:431–436.
79. Barnett, R. C. (1975): Sex differences and age trends in occupational preferences and occupational prestige. *J. Psychol.*, 22:35–38.
80. Barris, R. (1982): Environmental interactions: an extension of the model of occupations. *Am. J. Occup. Ther.*, 36:637–644.
81. Barsch, R. (1967): Counseling the parent of the brain-damaged child. In: *Educating Children with Learning Disabilities*, edited by E. Frieson and W. Barke. Appleton-Century-Crofts, New York.
82. Barton, J. G. (1968): Consolation house: fifty years ago. *Am. J. Occup. Ther.*, 22:340–345.
83. Baum, C. M. (1980): Independent living: a critical role for occupational therapists. *Am. J. Occup. Ther.*, 34:773–774.
84. Baum, M. C. (1978): Management and documentation of services. In: *Willard and Spackman's Occupational Therapy*, edited by H. Hopkins and H. Smith. J. B. Lippincott, Philadelphia.
85. Bazeldon, D. L. (1974): The perils of wizardry. *Am. J. Psychiatry*, 13:1317–1322.
86. Beck, M. A., and Callahan, D. K. (1980): Impact of institutionalization on the posture of chronic schizophrenic patients. *Am. J. Occup. Ther.*, 34:332–335.
87. Becker, E. (1974): *Revolution in Psychiatry.* Free Press, Glencoe, N.Y.
88. Becker, R. E., and Page, M. S. (1973): Psychotherapeutically oriented rehabilitation in chronic mental illness. *Am. J. Occup. Ther.*, 27:34–38.
89. Bellack, A. S., Hersen, M., and Turner, S. M. (1976): Generalization effects of social skills training in chronic schizophrenics: an experimental analysis. *Behav. Res. Ther.*, 14:391–398.
90. Bendroth, S., and Southam, M. (1973): Objective evaluation of projective material. *Am. J. Occup. Ther.*, 27:78–80.
91. Benjamin, A. (1969): *The Helping Interview.* Houghton Mifflin Company, Boston.
92. Bentham, J. (1962): *The Works of Jeremy Bentham* (1748–1832). Russell and Russell, New York.
93. Berenson, B. G., and Corkhuff, R. R. (1967): *Sources of Gain in Counseling and Psychotherapy.* Holt, Rhinehart & Winston, New York.
94. Berger, M. M. (1977): *Working with People Called Patients.* Brunner Mazel, New York.
95. Berger, P. L., and Luckman, T. (1966): *The Social Construction of Reality.* Doubleday, New York.
96. Bernard, J. (1975): *Women, Wives, Mothers: Values and Options.* Aldine Press, Chicago.
97. Berni, R., and Readey, H. (1974): *Problem-Oriented Medical Record Implication: Applied Health Peer Review.* C. V. Mosby, St. Louis.
98. Bernstein, L., and Bernstein, R. S. (1980): *Interviewing: a Guide for the Health Professions.* Appleton-Century-Crofts, New York.
99. Berzins, G. F. (1970): An occupational therapy program for the chronic obstructive pulmonary disease patient. *Am. J. Occup. Ther.*, 24:181–186.
100. Bidgood, F. E. (1974): Sexuality and the handicapped. *SIECUS Report*, Vol. II, No. 3.
101. Bing, R. K. (1981): Eleanor Clarke Slagle Lectureship—1981—occupational therapy revisited: a paraphrastic journey. *Am. J. Occup. Ther.*, 35:499–518.
102. Bion, W. R. (1959): *Experiences in Groups.* Basic Books, New York.
103. Bird, C. (1979): *The Two-Paycheck Marriage.* Rawson, Wade Publishers, New York.
104. Birdwhistell, R. L. (1970): *Kinesics and Context: Essays on Body Motion and Communication.* Ballantine, New York.
105. Birren, J. E., and Schaie, K. W., editors (1977): *Handbook of the Psychology of Aging.* Van Nostrand Reinhold, New York.
106. Black, M. M. (1976): Adolescent role assessment. *Am. J. Occup. Ther.*, 30:73–79.
107. Black, M. M. (1976): The occupational career. *Am. J. Occup. Ther., 30:225–228.*
108. Blackwell, W. S., and Blackwell, M. F. (1979): *Working Partners, Working Parents.* Broadman Press, Nashville.
109. Blaney, P. H. (1974): Two studies on the language behavior of schizophrenics. *J. Abnorm. Psychol.*, 83:23–31.
110. Bleuler, E. (1950): *Dementia Praecox or the Group of Schizophrenics.* International Universities Press, New York.
111. Bloomer, J. (1978): The consumer of therapy in mental health. *Am. J. Occup. Ther.*, 32:621–627.
112. Bloomer, J., and Williams, S. (1979): *The Bay Area Functional Performance Evaluation.* Task Oriented Assessment and Social Interaction Scale (Limited), San Francisco.
113. Blos, P. (1962): *On Adolescence: A Psychoanalytic Interpretation.* Free Press, Glencoe, N.Y.
114. Blungart, H. L. (1973): The art and the science. In: *Hippocratic Revisited*, edited by R. J. Bulger. Medcom Press, New York.
115. Bockhoven, J. S. (1963): *Moral Treatment in American Psychiatry.* Springer Publishing Company, New York.
116. Bockhoven, J. S. (1971): Legacy of moral treatment—1890's to 1910. *Am. J. Occup. Ther.*, 25:223–225.
117. Bolotin, S. (1982): Voices from the past—feminist generation. *The New York Times Magazine*, Oct. 17, p. 28.
118. Bonadonna, P. (1981): Effects of vestibular stimulation program on stereotypic rocking behavior. *Am. J. Occup. Ther.*, 35:775–781.
119. Borg, W. R., and Gall, M. D. (1971): *Educational Research.* David McCay Company, New York.
120. Boss, B. M., and Barrett, G. V. (1972): *Man, Work and Organizations.* Allyn and Bacon, Boston.
121. Bouchard, V. C. (1972): Hemiplegic exercise and discussion group. *Am. J. Occup. Ther.*, 26:330–331.
122. Boulding, K. G. (1968): General systems theory: skeleton of science. In: *Modern Systems Research for the Behavioral Scientist*, edited by W. Buckly. Aldine Publishing Company, Chicago.

123. Bowers, J. Z., and Purcell, S., editors (1976): *Advances in American Medicine: Essays at the Bicentennial*. Joseph Macy, Jr. Foundation, New York.
124. Bowlby, J. (1969): *Attachment and Loss*. Basic Books, New York.
125. Bowlby, J. (1973): *Separation*. Basic Books, New York.
126. Braginsky, B. M., Braginsky, D. D., and Ring, K. L. (1969): *Methods of Madness: The Mental Hospital as Last Resort*. Holt, Rinehart & Winston, New York.
127. Brantl, V. M., and Brown, M. R. (1973): *Readings in Gerontology*, C. V. Mosby, St. Louis.
128. Brawn, D., Wyne, M. D., Blackburn, J. E., and Powell, W. C. (1979): *Consultation: Strategy for Improving Education*. Allyn and Bacon, Boston.
129. Briggs, A. K., Duncombe, L. W., Howe, M. C., and Schwartzberg, S. L. (1979): *Case Simulations in Psychosocial Occupational Therapy.* F. A. Davis, Philadelphia.
130. Bright, T., Bittick, K., and Brandt, K. D. (1981): Reduction of self-injurious behavior using sensory integrative techniques. *Am. J. Occup. Ther.*, 35:167–172.
131. Brightbill, C. K. (1961): *Man and Leisure*. Prentice-Hall, Englewood Cliffs.
132. Brightbill, C. K., and Mobley, T. A. (1977): *Education for Leisure-Centered Living*. John Wiley and Sons, New York.
133. Brockema, M. C., Danz, K. H., and Schloemer, C. V. (1975): Occupational therapy in a community after care program. *Am. J. Occup. Ther.*, 29:22–27.
134. Bronfenbrenner, V. (1972): *Two Worlds of Childhood: U.S. and U.S.S.R.* Simon and Schuster, New York.
135. Bronfenbrenner, V. (1974): *Is Early Intervention Effective?* United States Department of Health, Education and Welfare, Government Printing Office (Publication Number OHD 74-25), Washington, D.C.
136. Bronfenbrenner, V. (1979): *The Ecology of Human Development*. Harvard University Press, Cambridge.
137. Brown, E. L. (1963): Meeting patients' psychosocial needs in the general hospital. *Ann. Am. Acad. Polit. Soc. Sci.*, 346:117–125.
138. Brown, G. W., and Birley, J. L. T. (1968): Crises and life changes and the onset of schizophrenia. *J. Health Soc. Behav.*, 9:203–214.
139. Brown, J. (1963): *Understanding Other Cultures*. Prentice-Hall, Englewood Cliffs.
140. Bruner, J. S. (1966): *Towards a Theory of Instruction*. The Belknap Press, Cambridge.
141. Bruner, J. S., et al. (1967): *Studies in Cognitive Growth*. John Wiley and Sons, New York.
142. Bryant, C. D. (1972): *The Social Dimensions of Work*. Prentice-Hall, Englewood Cliffs.
143. Bryant, T., and Bryant, J. (1978): *Understanding Learning Disabilities*. Alfred Publishing, Sherman Oaks, CA.
144. Buber, M. (1965): *Between Man and Man*. Macmillan, New York.
145. Buch, R. C. (1956): On the logic of general behavior systems theory. In: *Minnesota Studies in the Philosophy of Science*. Vol. I, edited by H. Feigl and M. Scriven. University of Minnesota Press, Minneapolis.
146. Buchsbaum, M. S. (1977): Psychophysiology and schizophrenia. *Schizophr. Bull.*, 3:7–14.
147. Bulger, R. J., editor (1973): *Hippocratic Revisited*. Medcom Press, New York.
148. Bullock, T. H. (1977): *Introduction to Nervous Systems*. W. H. Freeman, San Francisco.
149. Burnett, S. E., and Yerxa, E. J. (1980): Community-based and college-based needs assessment of physically disabled persons. *Am. J. Occup. Ther.*, 34:201–207.
150. Burnett-Beaulieu, S. (1982): Occupational therapy profession dropouts: escape from the grief process. *Occup. Ther. Ment. Health* 2(2):45–56.
151. Burton, L. (1974): *Care of the Child Facing Death*. Routledge and Kegan Paul, Boston.
152. Burton, L. E., and Smith, H. H. (1975): *Public Health and Community Medicine for the Allied Medical Professions*. Williams and Wilkins, Baltimore.
153. Buscaglia, L. (1975): *The Disabled and Their Parents*. Charles B. Slack, Thorofare, N.J.
154. Busse, E. W., and Pfeiffer, E., editors (1969): *Behavior and Adaptation in Late Life*. Little Brown & Co., Boston.
155. Butler, R. N., and Lewis, M. J. (1977): *Aging and Mental Health: Positive Psychological Approaches*. C. V. Mosby, St. Louis.
156. Caffey, E. M., Galbrecht, C. R., and Klett, C. J. (1971): Brief hospitalization and aftercare in the treatment of schizophrenia. *Arch. Abnorm. Psychol.*, 24:81–86.
157. Caillois, R. (1961): *Man, Play and Games*. Free Press, Glencoe, N.Y.
158. Cairns, H. S., and Cairns, C. E. (1976): *Psycholinguistics: A Cognitive View of Language*. Holt, Rinehart and Winston, New York.
159. Cambell, D. T., and Stanley, J. C. (1966): *Experimental and Quasi-Experimental Designs for Research*. Rand McNally, Chicago.
160. Campbell, J. (1959): *The Mask of God: Primitive Mythology*. Viking Press, New York.
161. Campbell, J., editor (1971): *The Portable Jung*. Viking Press, New York.
162. Cancro, R., Fox, N., and Shapiro, L. E., editors (1974): *Strategic Intervention in Schizophrenia: Current Developments in Treatment*. Behavioral Publications, New York.
163. Candland, D. K., and Moyer, R. S. (1978): *Psychology: The Experimental Approach*. McGraw-Hill, New York.
164. Cantor, S. G. (1981): Occupational therapists as members of pre-retirement resource teams. *Am. J. Occup. Ther.*, 35:638–643.
165. Caplan, G. (1961): *An Approach to Community Mental Health*. Grune and Stratton, New York.
166. Caplan, G. (1964): *Principles of Preventive Psychiatry.* Basic Books, New York.
167. Caplin, F. (1973): *The First Twelve Months of Life*. Grosset and Dunlap, New York.
168. Caplow, T. (1954): *The Sociology of Work*. McGraw-Hill, New York.
169. Caplow, T., and Bohr, M. (1982): *Middletown Families: Fifty Years of Change and Continuity.* University of Minnesota Press, Minneapolis.
170. Carr, S. H. (1969): Documentation of services. *Am. J. Occup. Ther.*, 23:335–338.
171. Carter, E. A., and McGoldrich, M., editors (1980): *The Family Life Cycle: A Framework for Family Therapy.* Gardner Press, New York.

172. Cartwright, D., and Zander, A. (1968): *Group Dynamics: Research and Theory*. Harper & Row Publishers, New York.
173. Casanoria, J. S., and Ferber, J. (1976): Comprehensive evaluation of basic living skills. *Am. J. Occup. Ther.*, 30:101–105.
174. Cassidy, H. G. (1962): *The Sciences and the Arts: A New Alliance*. Harper & Bros., New York.
175. Caudill, W. (1958): *The Psychiatric Hospital as a Small Society*. Harvard University Press, Cambridge.
176. Cermak, S. A. (1976): Community Based learning in Occupational Therapy. *Am. J. Occup. Ther.*, 30:157–161.
177. Cermak, S. A., Cermak, L. S., and Henny, R. (1978): The effect of concurrent manual activity in dichotic listening performance of boys with learning disabilities. *Am. J. Occup. Ther.*, 32:493–499.
178. Chalfant, J., Pysh, M., and Poultrie, R. (1979): Teacher assistance teams: a model for within-building problem solving. *Learn. Disabil. Q.*, 2:85–96.
179. Chapin, F. S. (1974): *Human Activity Patterns in the City*. John Wiley and Sons, New York.
180. Chapman, L. J., and Chapman, J. P. (1973): *Disordered Thought in Schizophrenia*. Appleton-Century-Crofts, New York.
181. Cheek, N. H., and Burch, W. R. (1967): *The Social Organization of Leisure in Human Society*. Harper & Row Publishers, New York.
182. Chess, S., and Hassibi (1978): *Principles and Practices of Child Psychiatry*. Plenum Press, New York.
183. Child, D. (1977): *Psychology of the Teacher*. Holt Rinehart & Winston, London.
184. Christiansen, C. H., and Davidson, D. A. (1974): A community health program with low achieving adolescents. *Am. J. Occup. Ther.*, 28:346–350.
185. Clark, D. D. (1974): Nationally speaking—accountability. *Am. J. Occup. Ther.*, 28:389–390.
186. Clark, D. W., and Mahon, B. (1967): *Preventive Medicine*. Little Brown & Co., Boston.
187. Clark, F. A., Miller, L. R., Thomas, J. A., Kuscherawy, D. A., and Azen, S. P. (1978): A comparison of operant and sensory integrative methods on developmental parameters of profoundly retarded adults. *Am. J. Occup. Ther.*, 32:86–92.
188. Clark, F. A., and Steingold, L. (1982): A potential relationship between occupational therapy and language development. *Am. J. Occup. Ther.*, 36:42–44.
189. Clark, P. N. (1979): Human development through occupation: theoretical frameworks in contemporary occupational therapy practice, part 1. *Am. J. Occup. Ther.*, 33:505–514.
190. Clark, P. N. (1979): Human development through occupation: a philosophy and conceptual model for practice, part 2. *Am. J. Occup. Ther.*, 33:577–585.
191. Clausen, J. A. (1968): *Socialization and Society*. Little, Brown, Boston.
192. Clayre, A. (1975): *Work and Play*. Harper & Row Publishers, New York.
193. Clayton, T. E. (1965): *Teaching and Learning: A Psychological Perspective*. Prentice-Hall, Englewood Cliffs.
194. Clendening, L., editor (1942): *Source Book of Medical History*. Davis Publications, New York.
195. Coles, R. (1970): *Erik H. Erikson: The Growth of His Work*. Little Brown & Co., Boston.
196. Coley, J. L. (1972): The child with juvenile rheumatoid arthritis. *Am. J. Occup. Ther.*, 26:325–329.
197. Collins, A., and Pancoast, E. (1976): *Natural Helping Networks: A Strategy for Prevention*. National Association of Social Workers, Washington, D.C.
198. Colman, W. (1975): Occupational therapy and child abuse. *Am. J. Occup. Ther.*, 29:412–417.
199. Combs, A. W. (1965): *The Professional Education of Teachers*. Allyn and Bacon, Boston.
200. Conger, J. J. (1973): *Adolescence and Youth: Psychological Development in a Changing World*. Harper & Row Publishers, New York.
201. Conine, T. A., Christie, G. M., Hammond, G. K., and Smith, M. F. (1979): An assessment of occupational therapist's role and attitudes towards sexual rehabilitation of the disabled. *Am. J. Occup. Ther.*, 33:515–519.
202. Connaughton, J. P. (1979): Psychiatry. In: *Preventing Physical and Mental Disability: Multidisciplinary Approaches*, edited by P. J. Valletutti and F. Christopher. University Park Press, Baltimore.
203. Cooley, C. H. (1956): *Human Nature and the Social Order*. Free Press, Glencoe, N.Y.
204. Cooper, J. E., Bloom, F. E., and Roth, R. H. (1974): *The Biochemical Base of Neuropharmacology*. Oxford University Press, New York.
205. Copeland, M., Ford, L., and Solon, G. (1976): *Occupational Therapy for Mentally Retarded Children*. University Park Press, Baltimore.
206. Corry, S., Sebastian, V., and Mosey, A. C. (1974): Acute short term treatment in psychiatry. *Am. J. Occup. Ther.*, 28:401–406.
207. Coser, L., and Rosenberg, B. (1957): *Sociological Theory*. Macmillan, New York.
208. Cox, S. (1977): The learning disabled adult. *Acad. Ther.*, 13:79–86.
209. Creighton, C. (1979): The school therapist and vocational education. *Am. J. Occup. Ther.*, 33:373–375.
210. Crist, P. (1979): Body image changes in chronic nonparanoid schizophrenics. *Can. J. Occup. Ther.*, 46:61–65.
211. Cristarella, M. C. (1977): Visual functions of the elderly. *Am. J. Occup. Ther.*, 31:432–440.
212. Cross, K. P. (1981): *Adults as Learners*. Jossey-Boss Publishers, San Francisco.
213. Cruichshank, W. (1967): *The Brain-Injured Child in Home, School and Community*. Syracuse University Press, Syracuse.
214. Cruichshank, W. M., Morse, W. C., and Johns, J. S. (1980): *Learning Disabilities: The Struggle from Adolescence Towards Adulthood*. Syracuse University Press, Syracuse.
215. Cull, J. G., and Hardy, R. E., editors (1974): *Administrative Techniques of Rehabilitation Facility Operations*. Charles C. Thomas Publisher, Springfield.
216. Cumming, J., and Comming, E. (1966): *Ego and Milieu*. Atherton Press, New York.
217. Currie, C. (1969): Evaluating function of mentally retarded children through the use of toys and play activities. *Am. J. Occup. Ther.*, 23:35–42.
218. Curtis, B. A. (1972): *An Introduction to Neurosciences*. W. B. Saunders, Philadelphia.

219. Curtis, J. E. (1979): *Recreation: Theory and Practice*. C. V. Mosby, St. Louis.
220. Cynkin, S. (1979): *Occupational Therapy: Toward Health Through Activities*. Little Brown & Co., Boston.
221. Danto, A., and Morgenbesser, S. (1960): *Philosophy of Science*. The World Publishing Company, Cleveland.
222. Daub, M. M. (1978): The human development process. In: *Willard and Spackman's Occupational Therapy*, edited by H. L. Hopkins and H. D. Smith, J. P. Lippincott, Philadelphia.
223. Davidson, S. V. S. (1976): *PSRO Utilization and Audit in Patient Care*. C. V. Mosby, St. Louis.
224. Davy, J. D., and Peters, M. (1982): State licensure for occupational therapists. *Am. J. Occup. Ther.*, 36:429–432.
225. Day, S. (1982): Mother-infant activities as providers of sensory stimulation. *Am. J. Occup. Ther.*, 36:579–585.
226. Deacon, S., Dunning, E., and Dease, R. (1974): A job clinic for psychotic patients in remission. *Am. J. Occup. Ther.*, 28:144–147.
227. De Angeles, G. G. (1976): Theoretical and clinical approaches to the treatment of adolescent drug addiction. *Am. J. Occup. Ther.*, 30:87–93.
228. Deitz, J. C., Siegner, C. B., and Crowe, T. K. (1981): The Southern California Postrotory Nystagmus Test: test-retest reliability for preschool children. *Occup. Ther. J. Res.*, 1:165–178.
229. Delougherty, G. W., Gebbie, K. M., and Neuman, B. M. (1971): *Consultation and Community Organization in Community Mental Health Nursing*. Williams and Wilkins, Baltimore.
230. De Mars, P. S. (1975): Training adult retardates for private enterprise. *Am. J. Occup. Ther.*, 29:39–42.
231. de Quiros, J. B. (1976): Diagnoses of vestibular disorders in the learning disabled. *J. Learn. Disabil.*, 9:50–58.
232. de Renne-Stephan, C. (1980): Imitation: a mechanism of play behavior. *Am. J. Occup. Ther.*, 34:95–102.
233. Deshler, D., Lourey, N., and Alley, G. (1979): Programming alternatives for learning disabled adolescents: a nation wide survey. *Acad. Ther.*, 14:389–398.
234. Deutsch, H. (1973): *The Psychology of Women*. Bantam Edition, New York.
235. Devereaux, E. B. (1978): Community home health care in the rural setting. In: *Willard and Spackman's Occupational Therapy*, edited by H. L. Hopkins, and H. D. Smith. L. J. Lippincott, Philadelphia.
236. Diasio, K. (1968): Psychiatric occupational therapy: search for a conceptual framework in the light of psychoanalytic ego psychology and learning theory. *Am. J. Occup. Ther.*, 22:400–414.
237. Diasio, K. (1971): The Modern era—1960 to 1970. *Am. J. Occup. Ther.*, 25:237–242.
238. Dicmonas, E. (1981): A Psychoneurophysiologically based activity analysis. In: *Physical Disabilities Manual*, edited by B. Abreu. Raven Press, New York.
239. Distefano, M. K., and Pryer, M. W. (1970): Vocational evaluation and successful placement of psychiatric clients in a vocational rehabilitation program. *Am. J. Occup. Ther.*, 24:205–207.
240. Dohrenwend, B. S., and Dohrenwend, B. P., editors (1974): *Stressful Life Events: Their Nature and Effects*. John Wiley and Sons, New York.
241. Donohue, M. V. (1982): Designing activities to develop a women's identification group. *Occup. Ther. Ment. Health*, 2(1):1–20.
242. Dragastin, S. E., and Elder, G. H., editors (1975): *Adolescence in the Life Cycle: Psychological Changes and the Social Context*. Halsted Press, New York.
243. Dubin, S. S. (1972): Obsolescence or life long education: a choice for the professional. *American Psychologist*, 27:486–498.
244. Dundes, A., editor (1968): *Every Man His Way*. Prentice-Hall, Englewood Cliffs.
245. Dunham, H., and Weinberg, K. (1960): *The Culture of the State Mental Hospital*. Wayne State University Press, Detroit.
246. Dunleavey, E. (1974): Utilizing the occupational therapist in home health. *Am. J. Occup. Ther.*, 28:484–487.
247. Dunning, H. (1970): The territorial instinct and its relevance to the occupational therapy process. *Am. J. Occup. Ther.*, 24:569–571.
248. Dunning, R. E. (1973): Philosophy and occupational therapy. *Am. J. Occup. Ther.*, 27:18–23.
249. Dunning, R. E. (1975): An accountability model for occupational therapists. *Am. J. Occup. Ther.*, 29:35–38.
250. Dunphy, D. C. (1972): *The Primary Group: A Handbook of Analyses and Field Research*. Appleton-Century-Crofts, New York.
251. Dunton, W. R. (1928): *Prescribing Occupational Therapy*. Charles C Thomas, Springfield.
252. Durbin, R. L., and Springall, W. H. (1974): *Organization and Administration of Health Care: Theory, Practice, Environment*. C. V. Mosby, St. Louis.
253. Duvall, E. M., editor (1971): *Family Development*. J. B. Lippincott, Philadelphia.
254. Dyer, E. D. (1979): *The American Family: Variety and Change*. McGraw-Hill, New York.
255. Eccles, J. C. (1977): *The Understanding of the Brain*. McGraw-Hill, New York.
256. Ecker, D. M. (1973): The effects of tactile stimulation on EEG recordings and seizures. *Am. J. Occup. Ther.*, 27:392–395.
257. Edelson, M. (1964): *Ego Psychology, Group Dynamics and the Therapeutic Community*. Grune and Stratton, New York.
258. Ekstein, R., and Wallerstein, R. (1972): *The Teaching and Learning of Psychotherapy*. Basic Books, New York.
259. Ellsworth, P. D. (1979): Role of the occupational therapist in the promotion of health and prevention of disability. *Am. J. Occup. Ther.*, 33:50–51.
260. Ellsworth, P. D., and Colman, A. D. (1969): Application of operant conditioning principles to work group experience. *Am. J. Occup. Ther.*, 23:495–501.
261. Ellsworth, P. D., and Rumbaugh, J. H. (1980): Community organization and planning consultation: strategies for community-wide assessment and preventative program design. *Occup. Ther. Ment. Health*, 1(1):33–56.
262. Ellsworth, P., et al. (1980): Position paper—the role of occupational therapy in the vocational rehabilitation process. *Am. J. Occup. Ther.*, 34:881–883.

263. Enby, H. (1975): *Let There Be Love—Sex and the Handicapped*. Taplinger Publishing, New York.
264. Endler, P. B., and Eimon, M. C. (1978): Postural reflex integration in schizophrenic patients. *Am. J. Occup. Ther.*, 32:456–459.
265. Engel, G. (1962): *Psychological Development in Health and Disease*. W. B. Saunders, Philadelphia.
266. Engel, G. L., and Morgan, W. L. (1973): *Interviewing the Patient*. W. B. Saunders, London.
267. Engelhardt, H. T. (1977): The meaning of therapy and the value of occupation. *Am. J. Occup. Ther.*, 31:666–672.
268. English, H. B., and English, A. C. (1958): *A Comprehensive Dictionary of Psychological and Psychoanalytical Terms*. David McKay Company, New York.
269. Epstein, J. (1974): *Divorced in America*. E. P. Dutton, New York.
270. Epstein, J. (1975): *Divorce: The American Experience*. Jonathan Cape, London.
271. Erikson, E. (1950): *Childhood and Society.* Norton, New York.
272. Erikson, E. (1967): *Adulthood*. W. W. Norton & Co., New York.
273. Esenthy, S. (1978): Use of goal attainment scales in the treatment and ongoing evaluation of neurologically handicapped children. *Am. J. Occup. Ther.*, 32:511–516.
274. Eshleman, J. R. (1974): *The Family*. Allyn and Bacon, Boston.
275. Ethridge, D. A. (1976): The management view of the future of occupational therapy in mental health. *Am. J. Occup. Ther.*, 30:623–628.
276. Etzioni, A., editor (1962): *Complex Organizations*. Holt Rinehart & Winston, New York.
277. Etzioni, A., editor (1969): *The Semi-Professions and Their Organization: Teachers, Nurses, Social Workers*. Free Press, Glencoe, N.Y.
278. Evans, H. S. (1977): Mental status. In: *Physical Diagnoses: The History and Examination of the Patient*, edited by J. A. Prior and J. S. Silberstein. C. V. Mosby, St. Louis.
279. Evans, P., and Peham, M. (1981): *Testing and Measurement in Occupational Therapy: A Review of Current Practice with Special Emphasis on the Southern California Sensory Integration Tests*. University of Minnesota Institute for Research on Learning Disabilities, Monograph No. 15.
280. Fahl, M. (1970): Emotionally disturbed children: effects of cooperative and competitive activity on peer interaction. *Am. J. Occup. Ther.*, 24:31–33.
281. Fairbairn, W. R. (1954): *An Object-Relations Theory of Personality*. Basic Books, New York.
282. Farber, S. (1966): *The Ways of the Will*. Basic Books, New York.
283. Fearing, V. G. (1978): An authors group for extended care patients. *Am. J. Occup. Ther.*, 32:526–527.
284. Feldman, S. D., and Ghielbar, G. W., editors (1972): *Life Styles: Diversity in American Society.* Little Brown & Co., Boston.
285. Felstein, J. (1970): *Sex in Later Life*. Penguin Books, Baltimore.
286. Fidler, G. S. (1966): Learning as a growth process: a conceptual framework for professional education. *Am. J. Occup. Ther.*, 20:1–8.
287. Fidler, G. S. (1969): The task oriented group as a context for treatment. *Am. J. Occup. Ther.*, 23:43–48.
288. Fidler, G. S. (1981): From crafts to competence. *Am. J. Occup. Ther.*, 35:567–573.
289. Fidler, G. S., and Fidler, J. W. (1954): *Introduction to Psychiatric Occupational Therapy*. Harper & Row Publishers, New York.
290. Fidler, G. S., and Fidler, J. W. (1963): *Occupational Therapy: A Communication Process in Psychiatry*. Macmillan, New York.
291. Fidler, G. S., and Fidler, J. W. (1978): Doing and becoming: purposeful action and self-actualization. *Am. J. Occup. Ther.*, 32:305–310.
292. Field, J. (1970): Medical education in the United States: late nineteenth and twentieth centuries. In: *History of Medical Education*, edited by V. E. Hald. University of California Press, Los Angeles.
293. Fielder, F. E. (1967): *A Theory of Leadership Effectiveness*. McGraw-Hill, New York.
294. Fielding, P., editor (1975): *A National Directory of Four-Year Colleges, Two-Year Colleges and Post High School Training Programs for Young People with Learning Disabilities*. Partners in Publishing,Tulsa.
295. Fiene, R. R., Rosenthal, D., and Brill, H., editors (1975): *Genetic Research in Psychiatry.* Johns Hopkins University Press, Baltimore.
296. Fine, S. B. (1980): Psychiatric treatment and rehabilitation: what's in a name? *J. Natl. Assoc. Private Psychiatr. Hosp.*, 2(5):8–13.
297. Fink, M., Katz, S. S., and McGant, J. (1974): *Psychobiology of Convulsive Therapy.* Winston and Sons, Washington, D.C.
298. Finn, G. L. (1972): The occupational therapist in prevention programs. *Am. J. Occup. Ther.*, 26:59–66.
299. Finn, G. L. (1977): Update of Eleanor Clark Slagle lecture: the occupational therapist in prevention programs. *Am. J. Occup. Ther.*, 31:658–659.
300. Fishbein, M. (1967): The changing scene in medicine. *Am. J. Occup. Ther.*, 21:376–381.
301. Fisher, A. G., and Bundy, A. C. (1982): Equilibrium reactions in normal children and boys with sensory integrative dysfunction. *Occup. Ther. J. Res.*, 2:171–183.
302. Flavell, J. (1963): *The Developmental Psychology of Jean Piaget*. Van Nostrand, New York.
303. Flexner, A. (1910): Medical Education in the United States and Canada. Bulletin No. 4, Carnegie Foundation for the Advancement of Teaching, New York.
304. Florey, L. (1971): An approach to play and play development. *Am. J. Occup. Ther.*, 25:275–280.
305. Florey, L. L. (1981): Studies of play: implications for growth, development and clinical practice. *Am. J. Occup. Ther.*, 35:519–524.
306. Florey, L. L., and Michelman, S. M. (1982): Occupational history: a screening tool for psychiatric occupational therapy. *Am. J. Occup. Ther.*, 36:301–308.
307. Ford, D., and Urban, H. (1963): *Systems of Psychotherapy.* John Wiley and Sons, New york.
308. Fowles, D., editor (1975): *Clinical Applications of Psychophysiology.* Columbia University Press, New York.

309. Fox, J. V. D., and Jirgal, D. (1967): Therapeutic properties of activities as examined by the clinical council of the Wisconsin schools of occupational therapy. *Am. J. Occup. Ther.*, 21:29–33.
310. Fraiberg, S. (1959): *The Magic Years: Understanding and Handling the Problems of Early Childhood.* Charles Scribner's Sons. New York.
311. Frank, I., Hoehn-Savic, R., Imher, S., Leberman, B., and Stone, A. (1978): *Effective Ingredients of Successful Psychotherapy.* Bruner Mazel, New York.
312. Frank, J. (1958): The therapeutic use of self. *Am. J. Occup. Ther.*, 12:215–225.
313. Frank, J. (1974): *Persuasion and Healing: A Comparative Study of Psychotherapy.* Schocken Books, New York.
314. Frazee, H. E. (1953): Children who later become schizophrenics. *Smith College Studies in Social Work*, 23:125–149.
315. Freedman, A. M., Kaplin, H. I., and Sadock, B. S., editors (1975): *Comprehensive Textbook of Psychiatry.* Williams and Wilkins, Baltimore.
316. Freud, A. (1965): *Normality and Pathology in Childhood.* International Universities Press, New York.
317. Freud, S. (1966): *Standard Edition of the Complete Psychological Works of Sigmund Freud.* Hogarth Press, London.
318. Freudenberger, H., and Richelson, G. (1980): *Burnout: The High Cost of Achievement.* Anchor Press, Garden City, N.Y.
319. Friday, N. (1977): *My Mother, My Self.* Dell Publishing, New York.
320. Friedman, B. (1982): A program for parents of children with sensory integrative dysfunction. *Am. J. Occup. Ther.*, 36:586–589.
321. Friedson, E. (1970): *Profession of Medicine.* Dodd, Mead & Co., New York.
322. Fromm, E. (1941): *Escape from Freedom.* Holt, Rinehart & Winston, New York.
323. Frostig, M. (1964): *Frostig Program for Development of Visual Perception.* Follett Publishing, Chicago.
324. Frostig, M. (1964): *Teachers Guide: The Frostig Program for Development of Visual Perception.* Follett Educational Corp., Chicago.
325. Gabriel, J. (1981): Day treatment. *Mental Health Special Interest Section Newsletter*, AOTA. Vol. 4, 4:1.
326. Gagne, R. (1970): *The Conditions of Learning.* Holt Rinehart & Winston, New York.
327. Gaines, B. (1978): Goal-oriented treatment plans and behavioral analysis. *Am. J. Occup. Ther.*, 32:512–516.
328. Gammage, P. S., McMahon, P., and Shanahan, P. (1976): The occupational therapist and terminal illness: learning to cope with death. *Am. J. Occup. Ther.*, 30:294–399.
329. Gans, H. (1962): *The Urban Villager.* Free Press, New York.
330. Gardner, G. G. (1967): The relationship between childhood neurotic symptomatology and later schizophrenics. *J. Nerv. Ment. Dis.*, 144:97–100.
331. Garmezy, N. (1974): Children at risk: the search for the antecedents of schizophrenia: II. Ongoing research programs, issues and intervention. *Schiz. Bull.*, 9:55–125.
332. Garrison, K. C., and Garrison, K. C., Jr. (1975): *Psychology of Adolescence.* Prentice-Hall, Englewood Cliffs.
333. George, N. M., Braun, B. A., and Walker, J. M. (1982): A prevention and early intervention mental health program for disadvantaged pre-school children. *Am. J. Occup. Ther.*, 36:99–106.
334. Gesell, A. (1940): *The First Five Years of Life.* Harper & Row Publishers, New York.
335. Gesell, A., and Ilg, F. S. (1946): *The Child from Five to Ten.* Harper & Row Publishers, New York.
336. Gilbard, G. S., Hartman, J. J., and Mann, R. D., editors (1976): *Analysis of Groups.* Jossey-Bass Publishers, San Francisco.
337. Gilfoyle, E. M. (1980): Caring: a philosophy for practice. *Am. J. Occup. Ther.*, 34:517–521.
338. Gilfoyle, E., and Farace, J. (1981): The role of occupational therapy in an education-related service (Official position paper, The American Occupational Therapy Association). *Am. J. Occup. Ther.*, 35:811.
339. Gilfoyle, E. M., Grady, A. P., and Moore, J. C. (1981): *Children Adapt.* Charles B. Slack, Thorofare, N.J.
340. Gilfoyle, E. M., and Hays, C. (1979): Occupational therapy roles and functions in the education of school-based handicapped children. *Am. J. Occup. Ther.*, 33:565–576.
341. Gillespie, C. C. (1960): *The Edge of Objectivity.* Princeton University Press, Princeton.
342. Gillette, N., and Kielhofner, G. (1979): The impact of specialization on the professionalization and survival of occupational therapy. *Am. J. Occup. Ther.*, 33:20–28.
343. Ginott, H. (1965): *Between Parent and Child.* Macmillan, New York.
344. Ginott, H. (1969): *Between Parent and Teenager.* Macmillan, New York.
345. Ginzberg, E. (1972): Towards a theory of occupational choice: a restatement. *Educ. Guid.* 2.20:169–176.
346. Glaser, R. (1976): Cognitive psychology and instructional design. In: *Cognition and Instruction*, edited by D. Klahr, pp. 303–315. John Wiley and Sons, New York.
347. Goble, R. E. A. (1969): The role of the occupational therapist in a home setting. *Am. J. Occup. Ther.*, 23:141–145.
348. Goffman, E. (1961): *Asylums: Essays on the Social Situation of Mental Patients and Other Inmates.* Doubleday, New York.
349. Goffman, E. (1963): *Stigma.* Prentice-Hall, Englewood Cliffs.
350. Goldberg, S. C., Schooler, N. R., Hogarty, G. E., and Roper, M. (1977): Prediction of relapse in schizophrenic outpatients treated by drug and sociotherapy. *Arch. Gen. Psychiatry*, 34:171–184.
351. Goldhammer, R., Anderson, R. H., and Krajewski, R. J. (1980): *Clinical Supervision: Special Methods for the Supervision of Teachers.* Holt, Rinehart & Winston, New York.
352. Goldman, L. E. (1975): Behavioral skills for the employment of the intellectually handicapped. *Am. J. Occup. Ther.*, 24:539–546.
353. Goldsmith, J. B., and McFall, R. M. (1975): Development and evaluation of an interpersonal skill training program for psychiatric inpatients. *J. Abnor. Psych.*, 85:51–58.
354. Goldstein, A. P., Gershaw, N. J., and Sprafkin, R. P. (1975):

Structural learning therapy—skill training for schizophrenics. *Schizophr. Bull.*, 14:83–86.

355. Goldstein, A. P., Gershaw, N. J., and Sprafkin, R. P. (1979): Structured learning therapy: development and evaluation. *Am. J. Occup. Ther.*, 33:636–639.
356. Goldstein, K. (1939): *The Organism*. American Book, New York.
357. Goldstein, P. K. (1979): Occupational therapy. In: *Preventing Physical and Mental Disability: Multidisciplinary Approaches*, edited by P. J. Valletritti and F. Christoplos. University Park Press, Baltimore.
358. Goldstein, P. K., O'Brien, J. D., and Katz, G. M. (1981): A learning disability screening program in a public school. *Am. J. Occup. Ther.*, 35:451–455.
359. Good, T. L., and Brophy, J. E. (1977): *Educational Psychology.* Holt Rinehart & Winston, New York.
360. Goslin, D. A., editor (1969): *Handbook of Socialization: Theory and Research*. Rand McNally, Chicago.
361. Gottesman, S. S. (1972): *Schizophrenia and Genetics: A Twin Study Vantage Point*. Academic Press, New York.
362. Graig, G. J. (1974): *Human Development*. Prentice-Hall, Englewood Cliffs.
363. Gralewicz, A. (1973): Play deviation in multi-handicapped children. *Am. J. Occup. Ther.*, 27:70–72.
364. Gralewicz, A., Hill, B., and Mackinson, M. (1968): Restoration therapy: an approach to group therapy for the chronically ill. *Am. J. Occup. Ther.*, 22:294–299.
365. Gray, M. (1972): Effects of hospitalization on work-play behavior. *Am. J. Occup. Ther.*, 26:180–185.
366. Gray, M. (1977): Competence assurance: applying the concept. *Am. J. Occup. Ther.*, 31:580–581.
367. Greenblatt, M., Levenson, D., and Williams, R. (1957): *The Patient and the Mental Hospital*. Free Press, Glencoe, N.Y.
368. Greenson, R. (1965): The problem of working through. In: *Drives, Affect and Behavior*, edited by M. Schur. International Universities Press, New York.
369. Greenstein, L. R. (1977): Bioethics: occupational therapy attitudes towards the prolongation of life. *Am. J. Occup. Ther.*, 31:77–80.
370. Griffith, E. R., Trieschman, R., Hohman, G., Cole, T., Tobis, J., and Cummings, V. (1975): Sexual dysfunctions associated with physical disabilities. *Arch. Phys. Med. Rehab.*, 56:8–21.
371. Grossman, J. (1974): Community experiences for students. *Am. J. Occup. Ther.*, 28:589–591.
372. Grossman, J. (1977): Preventive health care and community programming. *Am. J. Occup. Ther.*, 31:351–354.
373. Group for the Advancement of Psychiatry (1960): *Administration of the Public Psychiatric Hospital*. Group for the Advancement of Psychiatry, New York.
374. Gubrium, J. F., and Ksander, M. (1975): On multiple realities and reality orientation. *Gerontology*, 15:142–145.
375. Guerin, P., editor (1976): *Family Therapy: Theory and Practice*. Gardner Press, New York.
376. Guilford, J. P. (1967): *The Nature of Human Intelligence*. McGraw-Hill, New York.
377. Gunn, S. L. (1975): Play as occupation: implications for the handicapped. *Am. J. Occup. Ther.*, 29:222–225.
378. Guttmacher, A. F. (1973): *Pregnancy, Birth and Family Planning*. The New American Library, New York.
379. Haas, L. J. (1925): *Occupational Therapy for the Mentally and Nervously Ill*. Bruce Publishing, Milwaukee.
380. Haberman, M., and Stinnett, T. M. (1973): *Teacher Education and the New Profession of Teaching*. McCutcheon Publishing Corporation, Berkeley.
381. Haimann, T. (1973): *Supervisory Management for Health Care Institutions*. Catholic Hospital Association, St. Louis.
382. Hall, E. (1961): *The Silent Language*. Premier Book, Fawcett, Greenwich.
383. Hallahan, D., and Cruickshank, W. (1973): *Psychoeducational Foundations of Learning Disabilities*. Prentice-Hall, Englewood Cliffs.
384. Hamant, C. (1978): Pediatrics. In: *Willard and Spackman's Occupational Therapy*, edited by H. L. Hopkins and H. D. Smith. J. B. Lippincott, Philadelphia.
385. Hammeke, P. L., and Ganti, A. R. (1974): A method of quality control in occupational therapy. *Am. J. Occup. Ther.*, 28:154–157.
386. Hammer, E. (1967): *The Clinical Application of Projective Drawings*. Charles C Thomas, Springfield.
387. Hammer, M., Salzinger, K., and Sutton, S., editors (1973): *Psychopathology: Contributions from the Social, Behavioral and Biological Sciences*. John Wiley and Sons, New York.
388. Hampton, D. R., Summer, C. E., and Webber, R. A. (1973): *Organizational Behavior and the Practice of Management*. Scott, Foreman and Company, Glenview, Il.
389. Hardgrove, C. B. (1972): *Parents and Children in the Hospital*. Little Brown & Co., Boston.
390. Hare, A., Borgatta, E., and Bales, R. (1960): *Group Dynamics: Research and Theory.* Harper & Row Publishers, New York.
391. Hare, A., Borgatta, E., and Bales, R. (1965): *Small Groups: Studies in Interaction*. Alfred A. Knopf, New York.
392. Hare, R. D. (1970): *Psychopathology: Theory and Research*. John Wiley and Sons, New York.
393. Harris, P. H. (1981): Duration and quality of the prone extension position in four-, six-, and eight-year-old normal children. *Am. J. Occup. Ther.*, 35:26–30.
394. Hartley, R. E., and Goldenson, R. M. (1963): *The Complete Book of Children's Play.* Apollo Editions, New York.
395. Harwood, A., editor (1981): *Ethnicity and Medical Care*. Harvard University Press, Cambridge.
396. Haspel, A. A., and Musaph, H., editors (1979): *Psychosomatics in Peri-Menopause*. University Park Press, Baltimore.
397. Hasselkus, B. R. (1977): A small group home for the elderly. *Am. J. Occup. Ther.*, 31:525–529.
398. Hasselkus, B. R. (1978): Relocation stress and the elderly. *Am. J. Occup. Ther.*, 32:631–636.
399. Hasselkus, B. R., and Kiemat, J. M. (1973): Independent living for the elderly. *Am. J. Occup. Ther.*, 27:181–188.
400. Havighurst, R. J. (1972): *Developmental Tasks and Education*. David McKay Company, New York.
401. Hawisher, M., and Calhoun, M. (1978): *The Resource Room*. Charles E. Merrill, Columbus.
402. Haynes, S. N., and Wilson, C. C. (1979): *Behavioral Assessment*. Jossey-Bass, San Francisco.

403. Hays, C. (1978): General medicine and surgery. In: *Willard and Spackman's Occupational Therapy*, edited by H. L. Hopkins and H. D. Smith. J. B. Lippincott, Philadelphia.
404. Head, H. (1926): *Aphasia and Kindred Disorders of Speech*. Vols. I and II. Cambridge University Press, London.
405. Heard, C. (1977): Occupational role acquisition: a perspective on the chronically disabled. *Am. J. Occup. Ther.*, 31:243–247.
406. Hease, J. B., Trother, A. B., and Flynn, R. T. (1970): Attitudes of stroke patients towards rehabilitation and recovery. *Am. J. Occup. Ther.*, 24:285–289.
407. Heath, E. B., Albee, G. W., and Lane, E. A. (1965). Predisorder intelligence of process and reactive schizophrenics and their siblings. *Proceedings of the 73rd Annual Convention of the American Psychological Association*. pp. 221–222.
408. Hebb, D. O. (1964): *The Organization of Behavior: A Neurophysiological Theory*, Wiley, New York.
409. Hebb, D. O. (1972): *Textbook of Psychology.* W. B. Saunders, Philadelphia.
410. Hein, E. C. (1973): *Communications in Nursing Practice*. Little Brown & Co., Boston.
411. Heine, D. B. (1975): Daily living group: focus on transition from hospital to community. *Am. J. Occup. Ther.*, 29:628–630.
412. Hemphill, B. J. (1980): Mental health evaluations used in occupational therapy. *Am. J. Occup. Ther.*, 34:721–726.
413. Hemphill, B. J., editor (1982): *The Evaluation Process in Psychiatric Occupational Therapy.* Charles B. Slack, Thorofare, N.J.
414. Hendin, D. (1976): *The Life Givers*. William Morrow, New York.
415. Henton, B. L., and Reitz, N. J., editors (1971): *Groups and Organizations: Integrated Reading in the Analysis of Social Behavior.* Wadsworth Publishing, Belmont, CA.
416. Hergenkahn, B. R. (1976): *An Introduction to Theories of Learning*. Prentice-Hall, Englewood Cliffs.
417. Herman, B. E. A sensory integrative approach to psychotic children. *Occup. Ther. Ment. Health*, 1(1):57–68.
418. Herron, R. C., and Sutton-Smith, B. (1971): *Child's Play.* John Wiley and Sons, New York.
419. Herskovitz, M. J. (1972): *Cultural Relativism*. Random House, New York.
420. Herz, M. J., Endicott, J., and Spitzer, R. L. (1979): Brief hospitalization: a two-year follow-up. *Arch. Gen. Psychiatry*, 36:701–705.
421. Hess, A. K. (1980): *Psychotherapy Supervisors: Theory Research and Practice*. John Wiley and Sons, New York.
422. Heyel, C., editor (1973): *The Encyclopedia of Management*. Van Nostrand, New York.
423. Hightower-Vandamm, M. D. (1979): Nationally speaking—developmental disabilities acts: an historic perspective. Part 1. *Am. J. Occup. Ther.*, 33:355–359.
424. Hightower-Vandamm, M. D. (1979): Nationally speaking—developmental disabilities acts: an historic perspective. Part 2. *Am. J. Occup. Ther.*, 33:421–423.
425. Hightower-Vandamm, M. D. (1981): The role of occupational therapy in vocational evaluation, part 1. *Am. J. Occup. Ther.*, 35:563–565.
426. Hightower-Vandamm, M. D. (1981): The role of vocational evaluation, part 2. *Am. J. Occup. Ther.*, 35:631–634.
427. Hilgard, E., and Bower, G. (1975): *Theories of Learning*. Appleton-Century-Crofts, New York.
428. Hill, L. (1977): Working with the blind pre-schooler. *Am. J. Occup. Ther.*, 31:417–419.
429. Hill, W. F. (1977): *Learning: A Survey of Psychological Interpretations*. Thomas Y. Crowell, New York.
430. Himwich, H. E., editor (1971): *Biochemistry, Schizophrenia and Affective Illnesses*. Williams and Wilkins, Baltimore.
431. Hindmarsh, W. A. (1979): Play diagnoses and play therapy. *Am. J. Occup. Ther.*, 33:770–774.
432. Hinkle, L. E. (1980): The effect of exposure to cultural change, social change and changes in inter-personal relations in health. In: *Readings in Medical Sociology*, edited by D. Mechanic. Free Press, Glencoe, N.Y.
433. Hinojosa, J., et al. (1982): Occupational therapy for sensory integrative dysfunction (draft). *Occupational Therapy Newspaper*, April, p. 6.
434. Hinojosa, J., Anderson, J., Goldstein, P. K., and Becker-Lewin, M. (1982): Roles and function of the occupational therapist in the treatment of sensory integrative dysfunction (draft). *Occupational Therapy Newspaper*, April, p. 6.
435. Hinshelwood, J. (1917): *Congenital Word Blindness.* Lewis, London.
436. Hobbs, N. (1975): *The Future of Children: Categories, Labels and Their Consequence*. Jossey-Bass, San Francisco.
437. Hollingshead, A., and Redlick, F. (1958): *Social Class and Mental Illness*. John Wiley and Sons, New York.
438. Hollis, L. I. (1974): Skinnerian occupational therapy. *Am. J. Occup. Ther.*, 28:208–212.
439. Hollis, L. I. (1979): Remember?, *Am. J. Occup. Ther.*, 33:493–499.
440. Holmes, C., and Bauer, W. (1970): Establishing an occupational therapy department in a community hospital. *Am. J. Occup. Ther.*, 24:219–226.
441. Holmes, L. D. (1965): *Anthropology: An Introduction*. Ronald Press, New York.
442. Homans, G. (1950): *The Human Group*. Harcourt, Brace and World, New York.
443. Hopkins, H. L. (1978): An historical perspective of occupational therapy. In: *Willard and Spackman's Occupational Therapy*, edited by H. Hopkins and H. Smith. J. B. Lippincott, Philadelphia.
444. Hopkins, H. L. (1978): Methods of instruction. In: *Willard and Spackman's Occupational Therapy*, edited by H. L. Hopkins and H. D. Smith. J. B. Lippincott, Philadelphia.
445. Hopkins, H. L., and Smith, H. D., editors (1978): *Willard and Spackman's Occupational Therapy.* J. B. Lippincott Company, Philadelphia.
446. Hopkins, H. L., Smith, H. D., and Tiffany, E. G. (1978): The activity process. In: *Willard and Spackman's Occupational Therapy*, edited by H. L. Hopkins and H. D. Smith. J. B. Lippincott, Philadelphia.
447. Horney, K. (1937): *The Neurotic Personality of Our Time.* W. W. Norton & Co., New York.

448. Houle, C. D. (1980): *Continued Learning in the Professions*. Jossey-Bass, San Francisco.
449. Howard, J. (1978): *Families*. Simon and Schuster, New York.
450. Howe, M. C., and Briggs, A. K. (1982): Ecological systems model for occupational therapy. *Am. J. Occup. Ther.*, 36:322–327.
451. Howe, M. C., Weaver, C. T., and Dulay, J. (1981): The development of a work-oriented day center program. *Am. J. Occup. Ther.*, 35:711–718.
452. Howe, M. J. A. (1980): *The Psychology of Human Learning*. Harper & Row Publishers, New York.
453. Howells, J. G., editor (1975): *Modern Perspectives in the Psychiatry of Old Age*. Brunner Mazel, New York.
454. Hsu, Y. T., and Nelson, D. L. (1981): Adult performance on the Southern California Kinesthesia and Tactile Perception Tests. *Am. J. Occup. Ther.*, 35:788–791.
455. Huber, J., editor (1973): *Changing Women in a Changing Society*. University of Chicago Press, Chicago.
456. Huddleston, C. I. (1978): Differentiation between process and reactive schizophrenia based on vestibular reactivity, grasp strength and posture. *Am. J. Occup. Ther.*, 32:438–444.
457. Hughes, E. C., editor (1973): *Education for the Professions of Medicine, Law, Theology and Social Work*. McGraw-Hill, New York.
458. Hughes, P., and Mullins, L. (1981). *Acute Psychiatric Care: An Occupational Therapy Guide to Exercises in Daily Living Skills*. Charles B. Slack, Thorofare, N.J.
459. Huizinga, J. (1955). *Homo Luden: A Study of Play Elements in Culture*. Beacon Press, New York.
460. Hunt, M., and Hunt, B. (1977): *The Divorce Experience*. McGraw-Hill, Boston.
461. Hunter, R. H. (1973): Psychiatry and neurology. Psychosyndrome or brain disease. *Proc. Soc. Med.*, 66:355–364.
462. Hurff, J. (1974): A play skill's inventory. In: *Play as Exploratory Learning*, edited by M. Reilly, Sage Publications, Beverly Hills.
463. Hurff, J. M. (1980): A play skill inventory: a competency monitoring tool for 10 year olds. *Am. J. Occup. Ther.*, 34:651–656.
464. Huss, A. J. (1977): Touching with care or a caring touch. *Am. J. Occup. Ther.*, 31:11–18.
465. Huss, A. J. (1981): From kinesiology to adaptation. *Am. J. Occup. Ther.*, 35:574–580.
466. Hyman, M., and Melzher, J. P. (1970): Occupational therapy in an emergency setting. *Am. J. Occup. Ther.*, 24:280–283.
467. Hymens, D., editor (1964): *Language in Culture and Society. A Reader in Linguistics and Anthropology.* Harper & Row Publishers, New York.
468. Ingelman-Sundberg, A., and Wersen, C. (1966): *A Child Is Born: The Drama of Life, Before Birth*. Dell Publishing, New York.
469. Isaacs, S. (1933): *Social Development in Young Children: A Study of Beginnings*. G. Routledge and Sons, London.
470. Iversen, S. D., and Iversen, L. L. (1975): *Behavioral Pharmacology*. Oxford University Press, New York.
471. Jackson, B. N. (1970): The occupational therapist as consultant to the aged. *Am. J. Occup. Ther.*, 24:572–575.
472. Jaco, E. G., editors (1972): *Patients, Physicians and Illness: A Sourcebook on Behavioral Sciences and Health*. Free Press, Glencoe, N.Y.
473. Jacobi, J. (1959): *Complex/Archetype/Symbol*. Pantheon Books, New York.
474. Jacobs, A., and Spradlen, W. W., editors (1974): *The Group as an Agent of Change*. Behavioral Publications, New York.
475. Jacobs, M. (1964): *Patterns in Cultural Anthropology.* Dorsey Press, Homewood, Il.
476. Jacobs, S., and Myers, J. (1976): Recent life events and acute schizophrenic psychosis: a controlled study. *J. Nerv. and Mental Diseases*, 162:75–87.
477. Jaffe, E. (1980): The role of the occupational therapist as a community consultant: primary prevention in mental health programs. *Occup. Ther. Ment. Health*, 1(2):47–62.
478. Janeway, E. (1971): *Man's World, Woman's Place*. Delta, New York.
479. Jaques, E. (1970): *Work, Creativity and Social Justice*. International Universities Press, New York.
480. Jeffers, C. (1967): *Living Poor*. Ann Arbor Publishers, Ann Arbor.
481. Jersild, A. T., Telford, C. W., and Sawrey, J. M. (1975): *Child Psychology.* Prentice-Hall, Englewood Cliffs.
482. Jodrell, R. D., and Sanson-Fisher, R. (1975): An experiment involving adolescent girls. *Am. J. Occup. Ther.*, 29:620–624.
483. Johnson, J. et al. (1972): Report on the task force on social issues. *Am. J. Occup. Ther.*, 26:332–359.
484. Johnson, J. A. (1973): Occupational therapy: a model for the future. *Am. J. Occup. Ther.*, 27:1–7.
485. Johnson, J. A. (1977): Humanitarianism and accountability: a challenge for occupational therapy on its 60th aniversary. *Am. J. Occup. Ther.*, 31:631–637.
486. Johnson, J. A. (1978): Sixty years of progress: questions for the future. *Am. J. Occup. Ther.*, 32:209–213.
487. Johnson, L. A. (1978): Gernontology. In: *Willard and Spackman's Occupational Therapy.* Edited by H. L. Hopkins and H. D. Smith. J. B. Lippincott, Philadelphia.
488. Johnson, T. P., Vinnicombe, B. J., and Merrill, G. W. (1981): The independent living skills evaluation. *Occup. Ther. Ment. Health*, 1:5–18.
489. Jones, M. (1953): *The Therapeutic Community.* Basic Books, New York.
490. Jones, M. (1968): *Beyond the Therapeutic Community.* Yale University Press, New Haven.
491. Jones, W. M., and Jones, R. A. (1980): *Two Careers—One Marriage*. AMACOM, New York.
492. Jung, C. G. (1922): *Collected Papers on Analytic Psychology.* Bailliere, Tindall and Cox, London.
493. Jung, C. (1933): *Modern Man in Search of a Soul*. Harcourt, Brace and World, New York.
494. Jung, C. (1964): *Man and His Symbols*. Doubleday, New York.
495. Kadushin, A. (1977): *Consultations in Social Work*. Columbia University Press, New York.
496. Kales-Rogoff, L. (1979): Community skills for rheumatic disease patients. *Am. J. Occup. Ther.*, 33:394–395.
497. Kalish, R. A. (1975): *Late Adulthood: Perspectives on Human Development*. Brooks Cole Publishing, Monterey.

498. Kannegieter, R. B. (1980): Environmental interactions in psychiatric occupational therapy—some inferences. *Am. J. Occup. Ther.*, 34:715–720.
499. Kantner, R. M., Kantner, B., and Clark, D. L. (1982): Vestibular stimulation effect on language development in mentally retarded children. *Am. J. Occup. Ther.*, 36:36–40.
500. Kaplan, A., editor (1972): *Genetic Factors in Schizophrenia*. Charles C Thomas Publisher, Springfield.
501. Kaplin, M. (1978): *Leisure: Perspectives on Education and Policy.* National Education Association, Washington, D.C.
502. Kasanin, J., and Veo, J. (1932): A study of the school adjustment of children who later in life became psychotic. *Am. J. Orthopsychiatry*, 2:212–230.
503. Kaseman, B. M. (1980): Teaching money management skills to psychiatric outpatients. *Occup. Ther. Ment. Health*, 1(3):59–72.
504. Kastenbaum, R. J. (1977): *Death, Society and Human Experience*. C. V. Mosby, St. Louis.
505. Katchadourian, H. A. (1976): Medical perspectives on adulthood. In: *Adulthood*, edited by E. Erikson. W. W. Norton & Co., New York.
506. Kaufman, L. (1974): *Sight and Mind: An Introduction to Visual Perception*. Oxford University Press, London.
507. Kaufman, N. A. (1978): Occupational therapy assessment and treatment in educational settings. In: *Willard and Spackman's Occupational Therapy*, edited by H. L. Hopkins and H. D. Smith. J. B. Lippincott, Philadelphia.
508. Kawar, M. (1973): The effects of sensorimotor therapy on the dichotic listening in children with learning disabilities. *Am. J. Occup. Ther.*, 27:226–231.
509. Keating, N. R. (1979): A comparison of duration of nystagmus as measured by the Southern California Postrotary Nastagmus Test and electronystagmography. *Am. J. Occup. Ther.*, 33:92–97.
510. Keilitz, S., Zremba, B., and Broder, P. (1979): The link between learning disabilities and juvenile delinquency: some issues and answers. *Learn. Disabil. Q.*, 2 (Spring):2–11.
511. Keith, S. J., Gunderson, J. G., Reifman, A., Buchsbaum, S., and Mosher, L. R. (1974): Special report: schizophrenia. *Schizophr. Bull.* 2:509–565.
512. Kellerman, H. (1979): *Group Psychotherapy and Personality: Intersecting Structures*. Grune and Stratton, New York.
513. Kendell, R. E. (1975): *The Role of Diagnosis in Psychiatry.* Blackwell, London.
514. Keogh, B., and Becker, L. (1973): Early detections of learning problems: questions, cautions and guidelines. *Except. Child.*, September:5–13.
515. Kephart, N. (1960): *The Slow Learner in the Classroom*. Charles E. Merrill, Columbus.
516. Kerlinger, F. N. (1973): *Foundations of Behavioral Research*. Holt, Rinehart & Winston, New York.
517. Kessler, J. F. (1978): The soap opera: a dynamic group approach for psychiatric patients. *Am. J. Occup. Ther.*, 32:317–319.
518. Kester, D. L. (1978): Prevocational and vocational assessment. In: *Willard and Spackman's Occupational Therapy.* edited by H. L. Hopkins and H. D. Smith. J. B. Lippincott, Philadelphia.
519. Kielhofner, G. (1977): Temporal adaptation: a conceptual framework for occupational therapy. *Am. J. Occup. Ther.*, 31:235–242.
520. Kielhofner, G. (1979): The temporal dimensions in the lives of retarded adults. *Am. J. Occup. Ther.*, 33:161–168.
521. Kielhofner, G. (1980): A model of human occupations, part 2. Ontogenesis from the perspective of temporal adaptation. *Am. J. Occup. Ther.*, 34:657 663.
522. Kielhofner, G. (1980): A model of human occupations, part 3. Benign and vicious cycles. *Am. J. Occup. Ther.*, 34:731–737.
523. Kielhofner, G. (1981): An ethnographic study of deinstitutionalized adults: their community settings and early life experiences. *Occup. Ther. J. Res.*, 1:125–142.
524. Kielhofner, G., and Burke, J. P. (1980): A model of human occupations, part 1. Structure and content. *Am. J. Occup. Ther.*, 34:572–581.
525. Kielhofner, G., Burke, J. P., and Igi, C. H. (1980): A model of human occupations, part 4. Assessment and intervention. *Am. J. Occup. Ther.*, 34:777–788.
526. Kielhofner, G., and Meyake, S. (1981): The therapeutic use of games with mentally retarded adults. *Am. J. Occup. Ther.*, 35:375–382.
527. Kielhofner, G., and Takata, M. (1980): A study of mentally retarded persons: applied research in occupational therapy. *Am. J. Occup. Ther.*, 34:252–258.
528. Kiernat, J. M. (1976): Geriatric day hospitals: a golden opportunity for therapists. *Am. J. Occup. Ther.*, 30:285–289.
529. Kiernat, J. M. (1979): The use of life review activities with confused nursing home residence. *Am. J. Occup. Ther.*, 33:306–310.
530. Kimball, J. G. (1981): Normative comparison of the Southern California Postrotary Nystagmus Test: Los Angeles vs. Syracuse data. *Am. J. Occup. Ther.*, 35:21–25.
531. Kimmel, D. C. (1974): *Adulthood and Aging*. John Wiley and Sons, New York.
532. King, I. M. (1971): *Towards a Theory for Nursing*. John Wiley and Sons, New York.
533. King, L. J. (1974): A sensory integrative approach to schizophrenia. *Am. J. Occup. Ther.*, 28:259–536.
534. King, L. J. (1978): Occupational therapy research in psychiatry: a perspective. *Am. J. Occup. Ther.*, 32:15–18.
535. King, L. J. (1978): Towards a science of adaptive responses. *Am. J. Occup. Ther.*, 32:429–437.
536. King, L. J. (1980): Creative caring. *Am. J. Occup. Ther.*, 34:522–528.
537. King, L. J. (1981): Occupational therapy and neuropsychiatry. Paper presented at Rusk University Symposium, "A Multi-Faceted Look" at Sensory Integration, Chicago.
538. Kinnealey, M., and Morse, A. B. (1979): Educational mainstreaming of physically handicapped children. *Am. J. Occup. Ther.*, 33:365–372.
539. Kinsbourne, M., and Caplan, P. (1979): *Children's Learning and Attention Problems*. Little Brown & Co., Boston.
540. Kirchman, M. K., Reichenback, V., and Gambalvo, B.

(1982): Preventitive activities and services for the well elderly. *Am. J. Occup. Ther.*, 36:236–242.
541. Kirchman, M. M., and Loomis, B. (1980): A longitudinal study assessing the quality of occupational therapy. *Am. J. Occup. Ther.*, 24:285–289.
542. Kirk, S. (1963): Behavioral diagnosis and remediation of learning disabilities. *Conference on Exploration into the Problems of the Perceptually Handicapped Child.* Fund for Perceptually Handicapped Children, Evanston.
543. Kirk, S., and Gallagher, J. (1979): *Educating Exceptional Children.* Houghton Mifflin, Boston.
544. Klaus, M. H., and Kennell, N. J. (1976): *Maternal-Infant Bonding*, C. V. Mosby, St. Louis.
545. Klein, C. (1973): *The Single Parent Experience.* Walker and Company, New York.
546. Klein, D., and Glittleman-Klein, R. (1975): *Progress in Psychiatric Drug Treatment*, Bruner Mazel, New York.
547. Kleinman, B. L., and Bulkley, B. L. (1982): Some implications of a science of adaptive responses. *Am. J. Occup. Ther.*, 36:15–19.
548. Klucholn, C., and Murray, H. A. (1961): *Personality in Nature, Society and Culture.* Alfred A. Knopf, New York.
549. Knapp, P. (1963): *Expressions of the Emotions in Man.* International Universities Press, New York.
550. Kneller, G., editor (1963): *Foundations of Education.* John Wiley and Sons, New York.
551. Knox, A. B. (1977). *Adult Development and Learning: A Handbook on Individual Growth and Competence in the Adult Years for Education and the Helping Professions.* Jossey-Bass Publishers, San Francisco.
552. Knox, S. H. (1974): A play scale. In: *Play as Exploratory Learning*, edited by M. Reilly, Sage Publications, Beverly Hills.
553. Koch, R., and Dobson, J., editors (1971): *The Mentally Retarded Child and His Family.* Brunner Mazel, New York.
554. Koch, S. (1959): *A Study of Science, Volume II.* McGraw-Hill Company, New York.
555. Kohen-Roz, R. (1974): *The Child from Nine to Thirteen*, Jason Aronson, New York.
556. Kohler, E. S. (1980): The effect of activity/environment on emotionally disturbed children. *Am. J. Occup. Ther.*, 34:446–451.
557. Kolodner, E. (1973): Neighborhood extension of activity therapy. *Am. J. Occup. Ther.*, 27:381–383.
558. Komich, M. P., Lansford, A., Lord, L. B., and Tearney, A. (1973): The sequential development of infants with low birth weight. *Am. J. Occup. Ther.*, 27:396–342.
559. Kopfstein, J. H., and Neale, J. M. (1972): A multivariate study of attention dysfunction in schizophrenia. *J. Abnorm. Psychol.*, 80:294–298.
560. Kornhaber, A., and Woodward, K. L. (1981): *Grandparents/Grandchildren.* Anchor Press, Garden City, N.Y.
561. Kottak, C. P. (1975): *Cultural Anthropology.* Random House, New York.
562. Kraeplin, E. (1921): *Clinical Psychiatry: A Textbook for Students and Physicians.* (translated from German). Macmillan, New York.
563. Kraeplin, E. (1971): *Dementia Praecox and Paraphrenia.* Krieger, Huntinton, N.Y. (originally published 1919).
564. Kramer, L. P., and Beidel, C. C. (1978): Job seeking skills groups: a review and application to a chronic psychiatric population. *Occup. Ther. J. Ment. Health* 2(2):37–43.
565. Kris, E. (1952): *Psychoanalytic Exploration in Art.* International University Press, New York.
566. Kroeber, A. L. (1963): *Anthropology: Cultural Patterns and Processes.* Harcourt, Brace and World, New York.
567. Kruger, R., and Lieb, J. (1981): The craft of clinical interviewing. In: *Clinical Psychiatric Medicine*, edited by A. E. Staby, L. R. Tancredi and J. Lick. Harper & Row Publishers, Philadelphia.
568. Kruger, R., and Lieb, J. (1981): Psychopharmacology. In: *Clinical Psychiatric Medicine.* Edited by A. E. Slaby, L. R. Tancredi, and J. Lieb. Harper & Row Publishers, Philadelphia.
569. Kruger, R., and Lieb, J. (1981): Psychological and behavioral disorders in children. In: *Clinical Psychiatric Medicine.* edited by A. E. Slaby, L. R. Tancredi and J. Lieb. Harper & Row Publishers, Philadelphia.
570. Kubler-Ross, E. (1971): *On Death and Dying.* Macmillan, New York.
571. Kuenstler, G. (1976): A planning group for psychiatric outpatients. *Am. J. Occup. Ther.*, 30:634–639.
572. Kuhn, T. (1974): *The Structure of Scientific Revolutions.* University Press, Chicago.
573. Labovitz, D. R., and Domke, L. (1981): Shelter for abused women: occupational therapy intervention strategies. Paper presented at 1981 Annual Conference, American Occupational Therapy Association, San Antonio.
574. Labovitz, D. R., and Imbody, S. (1980): Activity program: living skills for boarding house residence. Paper presented at 1980 Annual Conference, American Occupational Therapy Association, Denver.
575. Labovitz, D. R., Williams, M., Zernick, D. and Katz, S. (1981): ADL Skills for Indochinese refugees: prototype of nontraditional fieldwork. Paper presented at the 1981 Annual Conference, American Occupational Therapy Association, San Antonio.
576. Lacoursiere, R. B. (1980): *The Life Cycle of Groups: Group Development and Stage Theory.* Human Science Press, New York.
577. La Duca, A., Madigan, M. J., Grofman, H., Sajid, A., Risley, M. S., and Giannini, G. (1975): *Professional Performance Situational Model for Health Professions Education: Occupational Therapy.* Area Health Education System, Chicago.
578. Lakein, A. (1973): *How to Get Control of Your Time and Life.* Peter H. Wyden, New York.
579. Lane, E. A., and Albee, G. W. (1968): On childhood intellectual decline and adult schizophrenics: a reassessment of an earlier study. *J. Abnorm. Psychol.*, 73:174–177.
580. Langer, S. K. (1956): *Philosophy in a New Key: A Study in Symbolism of Reason, Rite and Art.* Mentor, New York.
581. Langner, T. S., and Michael, S. T. (1963): *Life Stress and Mental Health: The Midtown Manhattan Study.* Free Press, Glencoe, N.Y.
582. Laszlo, E. (1972): *The Systems View of the World.* Doubleday, New York.
583. Laukaran, V. H. (1977): Nationally speaking: towards a

model of occupational therapy for community health. *Am. J. Occup. Ther.*, 31:71–79.

584. Lawn, E. C., and O'Kane, C. P. (1973): Psychosocial symbols as communications media. *Am. J. Occup. Ther.*, 27:30–33.
585. Lenke, H. (1974): Self-abusive behavior in the mentally retarded. *Am. J. Occup. Ther.*, 28:94–98.
586. Leopold, R. L. (1968): Consultant and consultee: an extraordinary human relationship. *Am. J. Occup. Ther.*, 22:72–81.
587. Lerner, J. W. (1981): *Learning Disabilities: Theories, Diagnosis and Teaching Strategies*. Houghton Mifflin, Boston.
588. Lerner, J. W., Dawson, D., and Horvath, L. (1980): *Cases in Learning and Behavioral Problems: A Guide to Individualized Education Programs*. Houghton Mifflin, Boston.
589. Lerner, J., Mandell-Czudnowski, G., and Goldenberg, D. (1981): *Special Education for the Early Childhood Years*. Prentice-Hall, Englewood Cliffs.
590. Lerner, R. J. (1981): An open letter to an occupational therapist. *J. Learn. Disabil.*, 14:3–4.
591. Levine, J., O'Connor, H., and Stacey, B. (1977): Sensory integration with chronic schizophrenics. *Can. J. Occup. Ther.*, 44:17–21.
592. Levine, R. E. (1978): Community home health care: in the urban setting. In: *Willard and Spackman's Occupational Therapy* edited by H. L. Hopkins and H. D. Smith. J. P. Lippincott, Philadelphia.
593. Levinson, D. J. (1978): *The Seasons of a Man's Life*. Alfred A. Knopf, New York.
594. Lewin, K. (1935): *A Dynamic Theory of Personality*. McGraw-Hill, New York.
595. Lewin, K. (1951): *Field Theory in Social Science*. Harper & Bros., New York.
596. Lewis, C. E. (1973): The quandary of quality: incompetence among the excellence. *Am. J. Occup. Ther.*, 27:59–63.
597. Lewis, S. (1975): Occupational therapy and geriatrics: assuming a leadership position. *Am. J. Occup. Ther.*, 29:459–460.
598. Lewis, S. C. (1979): *The Mature Years: A Geriatric Occupational Therapy Text*. Charles B. Slack, Thorofare, N.J.
599. Licht, S. (1948): *Occupational Therapy Source Book*. Williams and Wilkins, Baltimore.
600. Lidz, T. (1973): *The Origin and Treatment of Schizophrenic Disorders*. Basic Books, New York.
601. Lieb, J., Lipstick, S. S., and Slaby, A. E. (1973): *The Crisis Team: A Handbook for the Mental Health Professional*. Harper & Row Publishers, New York.
602. Lieberman, J. N. (1977): *Playfulness: Its Relationship to Imagination and Creativity*. Academic Press, New York.
603. Liebow, E. (1967): *Talby's Corner: A Study of Negro Streetcorner Men*. Little Brown & Co., New York.
604. Lifton, W. M. (1972): *Groups: Facilitating Individual Growth and Societal Change*. John Wiley and Sons, New York.
605. Lilley, M. L. (1967): *Friedrich Troebel: A Selection From His Writings*. Cambridge University Press, Cambridge.
606. Lillie, M. D., and Armstrong, H. E. (1972): Contributions to the development of psychoeducational approaches to mental health service. *Am. J. Occup. Ther.*, 36:438–443.
607. Lindemann, E. (1979): *Beyond Grief: Studies in Crisis Intervention*. Jason Aronson, New York.
608. Linder, S. B. (1970): *The Harried Leisure Class*. Columbia University Press, New York.
609. Lindquist, J. E. (1981): Activity and vestibular function in chronic schizophrenics. *Occup. Ther. J. Res.*, 1:56–78.
610. Lindquist, J. E., Mack, W. M., and Parham, L. D. (1982): A synthesis of occupational behavior and sensory integration concepts in theory and practice, part 2. Clinical application. *Am. J. Occup. Ther.*, 36:433–437.
611. Lindzey, G. (1954): *Handbook of Social Psychology*. Addison-Wesley Publishing Company, Cambridge.
612. Linn, M. W. et al. (1979): Day treatment and psychotropic change in the aftercare of schizophrenic patients. *Arch. Gen. Psychiatry*, 36:1055–1066.
613. Linnell, K. G., Sleckman, A. M., and Watson, C. G. (1975): Resocialization of schizophrenic patients. *Am. J. Occup. Ther.*, 29:288–290.
614. Llorens, L. (1967): Projective techniques in occupational therapy. *Am. J. Occup. Ther.*, 21:4–8.
615. Llorens, L. A. (1968): Identification of Ayres' syndrome in emotionally disturbed children: an exploratory study. *Am. J. Occup. Ther.*, 22:286–288.
616. Llorens, L. A. (1970): Facilitating growth and development: the promises of occupational therapy. *Am. J. Occup. Ther.*, 24:93–101.
617. Llorens, L. A. (1971): Occupational therapy in community child health. *Am. J. Occup. Ther.*, 25:335–339.
618. Llorens, L. A. (1976): *Application of a Developmental Theory for Health and Rehabilitation*. AOTA, Rockville, Md.
619. Llorens, S., and Shuster, J. (1977): Occupational therapy sequential client care recording system: a comparative study. *Am. J. Occup. Ther.*, 31:367–371.
620. Lofland, L. H. editor, (1976): *Towards a Sociology of Death and Dying*. Sage Publications, Beverly Hills.
621. Lorenz, C. (1963): *On Aggression*. Harcourt, Brace and World, New York.
622. Loveland, C. A., and Little, V. L. (1974): The occupational therapist in the juvenile correction system. *Am. J. Occup. Ther.*, 28:537–539.
623. Lucci, J. A. (1977): *Occupational Therapy Case Studies*. Medical Examination Publishing Company, New York.
624. Lusted, L. B. (1968): *Introduction to Medical Decision Making*. Charles C Thomas Publisher, Springfield.
625. Mack, W. M., Parham, L. D., and Lindquist, J. E. (1982): The use of play in pediatric occupational therapy, part 1. An organizing framework for a model of play development. *Am. J. Occup. Ther.*, 36:365–373.
626. Mackenzie, R. A. (1972): *The Time Trap*. AMACON, New York.
627. Madge, J. (1962): *The Origins of Scientific Sociology*. Free Press, Glencoe, N.Y.
628. See ref. 691a.
629. Mager, R. (1963): *Preparing Instructional Objectives*. Fearon Publishers, Palo Alto.
630. Magraw, R. M. (1973): Science and humanism. In: *Hy-*

pocratic Revisited, edited by R. J. Bulger. Medcom Press, New York.
631. Mahoney, E. A., Verdisco, L., and Shortridge, L. (1976): *How to Collect and Record a Health History.* J. B. Lippincott, New York.
632. Maier, H. W. (1969): *Three Theories of Child Development.* Harper & Row Publishers, New York.
633. Maier, N. R. T. (1970): *Problem Solving and Creativity in Individuals and Groups.* Brooks Cole, Belmont, CA.
634. Malick, M. H. (1978): Upper extremity orthotics. In: *Willard and Spachman's Occupational Therapy*, edited by H. L. Hopkins and H. D. Smith. J. P. Lippincott, Philadelphia.
635. Malick, M. H., and Sherry, B. (1978): Evaluation and assessment: Life work tasks. In: *Willard and Spackman's Occupational Therapy*, edited by H. L. Hopkins and H. D. Smith. J. B. Lippincott, Philadelphia.
636. Malick, M. H., and Sherry B. (1978): Activities of daily living and homemaking. In: *Willard and Spackman's Occupational Therapy*, edited by H. L. Hopkins and H. D. Smith, L. B. Lippincott, Philadelphia.
637. Maloney, C. C. (1976): The occupational therapist on a geriatric rehabilitation team. *Am. J. Occup. Ther.*, 30:300–304.
638. Mann, L., Goodman, L. and Wiederholt, J., editors (1978): *Teaching the Learning Disabled Adolescent.* Houghton Mifflin, Boston.
639. Mann, W. C. (1976): A quarterway house for adult psychiatric patients. *Am. J. Occup. Ther.*, 30:646–647.
640. Mann, W., Godfrey, M. E., and Dowd, E. T. (1973): The use of group counseling procedures in the rehabilitation of spinal cord injured patients. *Am. J. Occup. Ther.*, 27:73–77.
641. Mann, W. C., and Sobsey, R. (1975): Feeding programs for the institutionalized mentally retarded. *Am. J. Occup. Ther.*, 29:471–474.
642. Marholin, D., and Phillips, D. (1976): Methodological issues in psychopharmacological research—a case in point. *Am. J. Orthopsychiatry*, 46:477–495.
643. Marmo, N. A. (1975): Discovering the lifestyle of the physically disabled. *Am. J. Occup. Ther.*, 29:475–478.
644. Marram, G. D. (1973): *The Group Approach in Nursing Practice.* C. V. Mosby, St. Louis.
645. Marshall, E., Kerr, J., Foto, M., and Farace, J. (1981): The role of occupational therapy in home health care (official position paper, the American Occupational Therapy Association) *Am. J. Occup. Ther.*, 35:809–810.
646. Marx, M., and Hillix, W. (1963): *Systems and Theories in Psychology.* McGraw-Hill Company, New York.
647. Muslin, D. (1982): Rehabilitation training for community living skills. *Occup. Ther. Ment. Health* 2(1):35–40.
648. Maslow, A. (1962): *Towards a Psychology of Being.* D. Van Nostrand, Princeton.
649. Masserman, J. H. (1971): *A Psychiatric Odyssey.* Science House, New York.
650. Martin, W. H., and Johnson, V. E. (1969): *Human Sexual Response.* Little Brown & Co., Boston.
651. Matsutsuyu, J. S. (1969): The interest check list. *Amer. J. Occup. Ther.*, 23:323–328.
652. Matsutsuyu, J. (1971): Occupational behavior: a perspective on work and play. *Am. J. Occup. Ther.*, 25:291–294.
653. Maurer, P. (1971): Antecedents of work behavior. *Am. J. Occup. Ther.*, 25:295–297.
654. Maxey, M. et. al. (1979): The issue—professional prescription. *Am. J. Occup. Ther.*, 33:397–398.
655. May, P. R. A., Tuma, A. H., and Dixon, W. J. (1974): Schizophrenia—a follow-up study of results of treatment: I. design and other problems. *Arch. Gen. Psychiatry*, 33:474–478.
656. Mazer, J. (1968): *Final Report: Rehabilitation Services Administration Grant #123-T-68 for Field Consultant in Psychiatric Rehabilitation.* American Occupational Therapy Association, Rockville, MD.
657. Mazer, J. (1968): Towards an integrated theory of occupational therapy. *Am. J. Occup. Ther.*, 22:451–456.
658. Mazer, J., and Mosey, A. C. (1968): Introduction to special section: theories of psychiatric occupational therapy. *Am. J. Occup. Ther.*, 22:398–399.
659. Mazer, J. L. (1969): The occupational therapist as a consultant. *Am. J. Occup. Ther.*, 23:417–421.
660. Mazer, J. L., Fidler, G. S., Kovalenko, L. J. and Overly, K. (1970): *Exploring How a Think Feels.* AOTA, Rockville, MD.
661. McAshan, H. H. (1970): *Writing Behavioral Objectives.* Harper & Row Publishers, New York.
662. McCormick, L. and Lee, C. (1979): Public Law 94–142: mandated partnership. *Am. J. Occup. Ther.*, 33:586–589.
663. McCrocken, A. (1975): A tactile function in educatable retarded children. *Am. J. Occup. Ther.*, 29:397–402.
664. McDaniel, J. W. (1969): *Physical Disability and Human Behavior.* Pergamon Press, New York.
665. McFadden, M. (1974): *Bachelor Fatherhood: How to Raise and Enjoy Your Children as a Single Parent.* Walker and Company, New York.
666. McGlothlin, W. (1964): *The Professional Schools.* The Center for Applied Research in Education, New York.
667. McGraw, M. B. (1969): *The Neuromuscular Maturation of the Human Infant.* Harper & Row Publishers, New York.
668. McKibbin, E. H. (1973): The effect of additional tactile stimulation in a perceptual motor treatment program. *Am. J. Occup. Ther.*, 27:191–197.
669. McLellan, J. (1970): *The Question of Play.* Pergamon Press, London.
670. Mcquire, G. A. (1979): Volunteer program to assist the elderly to remain in home settings. *Am. J. Occup. Ther.*, 33:98–101.
671. Mead, G. (1934): *Mind, Self and Society.* University of Chicago Press, Chicago.
672. Mechanic, D., editor (1980): *Readings in Medical Sociology.* Free Press, Glencoe, N.Y.
673. Meltzer, H. and Wickert, F. editors (1976): *Humanizing Organizational Behavior.* Charles C Thomas Publisher, Springfield.
674. Meltzer, H. Y., and Stahl, S. M. (1976): The dopamine hypothesis of schizophrenia: a review. *Schizophr. Bull.*, 2:19–76.
675. Menks, F., Sittler, S., Weaver, D., and Yanow, B. (1977): A psychogeriatric activity group in a rural community. *Am. J. Occup. Ther.*, 31:376–384.
676. Menzel, F. S., and Teegarden, K. (1982): Quality assur-

ance: a tri-level model. *Am. J. Occup. Ther.*, 36:163–169.
677. Merton, R. K. (1968): *Social Therory and Social Structure*. Free Press, Glencoe, N.Y.
678. Meyer, A. (1977): The philosophy of occupational therapy. *Am. J. Occup. Ther.*, 31:639–642.
679. Meyer, G., Vergason, G., and Whelan, R. editors (1979): *Instructional Planning for Exceptional Children*. Lone Publishing, Denver.
680. Michelman, S. (1971): The importance of creative play. *Am. J. Occup. Ther.*, 25:285–290.
681. Michelman, S. S. (1974): Play and the deficient child. In: *Play as Exploratory Learning*, edited by M. Reilly. Sage Publications, Beverly Hills.
682. Miller, D. B. (1978): Reflections concerning an activity consultant by a nursing home administrator. *Am. J. Occup. Ther.*, 32:375–384.
683. Miller, J. (1973): *Helping Your Young Child at Home*. Academic Therapy Publications, San Rafael, CA.
684. Miller, S. (1968): *The Psychology of Play*. Penguin Books, Middlesex.
685. Mills, C. M. (1967): *The Sociological Imagination*. Oxford University Press, New York.
686. Mills, T. M. (1967): *The Sociology of Small Groups*. Prentice-Hall, Englewood Cliffs.
687. Minuchin, S. (1974): *Families and Family Therapy.* Harvard University Press, Cambridge.
688. Mitchell, M. M., and Lindsay, D. A. (1979): A model for establishing occupational therapy and physical therapy services in public schools. *Am. J. Occup. Ther.*, 33:361–364.
689. Mitford, J. (1963): *The American Way of Death*. Hutchinson, London.
690. Moersch, M. S. (1977): Training the deaf-blind child. *Am. J. Occup. Ther.*, 31:425–431.
691. Moersch, M. S. (1978): Developmental disabilities. *Am. J. Occup. Ther.*, 32:93–99.
691a. Moersch, M. S. (1982): Developmental disabilities—an ambiguous term. *Am. J. Occup. Ther.*, 36:111–115.
692. Monnier, M. (1975): *Functions of the Nervous System, Vol. 3: Sensory Functions and Perception*. Elsevier, Amsterdam.
693. Montgomery, P. C., and Rodel, D. A. (1982): Effect of state on myctagmosis duration on the Southern California Postrotary Nystagmus Test. *Am. J. Occup. Ther.*, 36:177–182.
694. Mooney, T., Cole, T. M., and Chilgren, R. (1975): *Sexual Options for Paraplegics and Quadraplegics*. Little Brown & Co., Boston.
695. Moore, C. B., and Morton, K. G. (1976): *A Readers Guide for Parents of Children with Mental, Physical or Emotional Disabilities*. U.S. Department of Health, Education and Welfare, Rockville, Md.
696. Moore, J. C. (1977): Individual differences and the art of therapy. *Am. J. Occup. Ther.*, 31:663–665.
697. Moore, W. E. (1970): *The Professions: Roles and Rules*. Russell Sage Foundation, New York.
698. Moorehead, L. (1969): The occupational history. *Am. J. Occup. Ther.*, 23:329–334.
699. Morris, D. (1967): *The Naked Ape*. McGraw-Hill, New York.
700. Morris, D. P., Soroker, E., and Burruss, G. (1954): Follow-up studies of shy, withdrawn children. *Am. J. Orthopsychiatry*, 24:743–754.
701. Morris, V. C., and Pai, Y. (1976): *Philosophy and the American School*. Houghton Mifflin Company, Boston.
702. Mosey, A. C. (1968): *Occupational Therapy: Theory and Practice*. Pothier Brothers, Medford, Ma.
703. Mosey, A. C. (1968): Recapitulation of ontogenesis. *Am. J. Occup. Ther.*, 22:426–438.
704. Mosey, A. C. (1969): The treatment of pathological distorting of body image. *Am. J. Occup. Ther.*, 23:413–416.
705. Mosey, A. C. (1970): *Three Frames of Reference for Mental Health*. Charles B. Slack, Thorofare, N.J.
706. Mosey, A. C. (1970): The concept and use of developmental groups. *Am. J. Occup. Ther.*, 24:272–275.
707. Mosey, A. C. (1971): Involvement in the rehabilitation movement—1942 to 1960. *Am. J. Occup. Ther.*, 25:234–236.
708. Mosey, A. C. (1973): *Activities Therapy.* Raven Press, New York.
709. Mosey, A. C. (1973): Meeting health needs. *Am. J. Occup. Ther.*, 27:14–17.
710. Mosey, A. C. (1974): An alternative: the biopsychosocial model. *Am. J. Occup. Ther.*, 28:137–140.
711. Mosey, A. C. (1981): *Occupational Therapy: Configuration of a Profession*. Raven Press, New York.
712. Mosey, A. C. (1981): Introduction: the art of practice. In: *Physical Disabilities Manual*, edited by B. Abreu, Raven Press, New York.
713. Marker, L. R., and Menn, A. Z. (1978): Community residential treatment for schizophrenia: two-year follow-up. *Hosp. Community Psychiatry*, 29:715–723.
714. Muller, P. (1970): *The Tasks of Childhood*. McGraw-Hill, New York.
715. Murphy, E. A. (1976): *The Logic of Medicine*. The Johns Hopkins University Press, Baltimore.
716. Mussen, P. H., and Conger, J. J. (1974): *Child Development and Personality.* Harper & Row Publishers, New York.
717. Musto, D. (1977): What happened to community mental health centers? *Psychiatr. Ann.*, 7:30–55.
718. Muuss, R., editor (1975): *Theories of Adolescence*. Peter Smith Publishers, Gloucester, Ma.
719. Nader, M. H., editor (1975): *Studies of Schizophrenia*. Headley, Ashford, England.
720. Nagel, E. (1961): *The Structure of Science*. Harcourt, Brace and World, New York.
721. National Conference of Social Work (1954): *Administration, Supervision and Consultation*. Family Services of America, New York.
722. Naumburg, M. (1950): *Schizophrenic Art: Its Meaning in Psychotherapy.* Grune and Stratton, New York.
723. Naumburg, M. (1953): *Psychoneurotic Art: Its Function in Psychotherapy.* Grune and Stratton, New York.
724. Neal, M. V. (1968): Vestibular stimulation and developmental behavior of premature infants. *Nurs. Res. Report*, 3:3–5.
725. Neale, J. M., and Liebert, R. M. (1980): *Science and Behavior: An Introduction to Methods of Research*. Prentice-Hall, Englewood Cliffs.

726. Neale, J. M., and Oltmanns, T. F. (1980): *Schizophrenia*. John Wiley and Sons, New York.
727. Neff, W. S. (1968): *Work and Human Behavior*. Atherton Press, New York.
728. Neff, W., editor (1971): *Rehabilitation Psychology*. American Psychiatric Association, Washington, D.C.
729. Neistadt, M., and Baker, M. F. (1978): A program for sex counseling the physically disabled. *Am. J. Occup. Ther.*, 32:646–647.
730. Nelson, D., Nitzberg, L., and Hollander, T. (1980): Visually monitored postrotory nystagmus in seven autistic children. *Am. J. Occup. Ther.*, 34:382–386.
731. Nelson, D. L., Thompson, G., and Moore, J. A. (1982): Identification of factors of affective meaning in four selected activities. *Am. J. Occup. Ther.*, 36:381–387.
732. Neufeld, P. S. (1981): Neurobehavioral evaluation and management. In: *Physical Disabilities Manual*, edited by B. C. Abreu. Raven Press, New York.
733. Neugarten, B. L., editor (1968): *Middle Age and Aging*. University of Chicago Press, Chicago.
734. Neville, A. (1980): Temporal adaptation: application with short-term psychiatric patients. *Am. J. Occup. Ther.*, 34:328–331.
735. Newcomb, T. M., Koenig, K. E., Flacks, R., and Warwick, D. P. (1967): *Persistence and Change: Bennington College and Its Students After Twenty-five Years*. John Wiley and Sons, New York.
736. New York Times (1982): Poll says most women perceive job bias. August 15, section 1, p. 28.
737. New York Times (1982): Lack of beds seen in nursing homes. October 17, section 1, p. 1.
738. Nidditch, P. H., editor (1968): *The Philosophy of Science*. Oxford University Press, London.
739. Noback, C. R. (1967): *The Human Nervous System*. McGraw-Hill, New York.
740. Norman, C. W. (1976): Behavior modification: a perspective. *Am. J. Occup. Ther.*, 30:491–494.
741. Norman, D. A. (1976): *Memory and Attention*. John Wiley and Sons, New York.
742. Norton, Y. (1975): Neurodevelopment and sensory integration for the profoundly retarded multiply handicapped child. *Am. J. Occup. Ther.*, 29:93–100.
743. Nasow, S., and Form, W., editors (1962): *Men, Work and Society*. Basic Books, New York.
744. Neuchterlein, K. H. (1977): Reaction time and attention in schizophrenia: a critical evaluation of the data and theories. *Schizophr. Bull.*, 3:373–428.
745. Nystrom, E. P. (1974): Activity patterns and leisure concepts among the elderly. *Am. J. Occup. Ther.*, 28:337–345.
746. Occupational Therapy Newspaper (1981): Terminally ill people need activity. American Occupational Therapy Association, July, p.7.
747. Oelrich, M. (1974): The patient with a fatal illness. *Am. J. Occup. Ther.*, 28:429–432.
748. Ogden, L. D. (1979): Activity guidelines for early subacute and high-risk cardiac patients. *Am. J. Occup. Ther.*, 33:291–298.
749. O'Kane, C. (1968): *The Development of a Projective Technique for Use in Psychiatric Occupational Therapy*. Monograph. State University of New York, Buffalo.
750. Ostrow, P. C. (1980): The care and feeding of theories. *Am. J. Occup. Ther.*, 34:272–273.
751. Ottenbacher, K. (1978): Identifying vestibular processing dysfunction in learning disabled children. *Am. J. Occup. Ther.*, 32:217–221.
752. Ottenbacher, K. (1982): Occupational therapy and special education: some issues and concerns related to public law 94-142. *Am. J. Occup. Ther.*, 36:81–84.
753. Ottenbacher, K. (1982): Sensory integration therapy: affect or effect. *Am. J. Occup. Ther.*, 36:571–578.
754. Ottenbacher, K. (1982): Patterns of postrotory nystagmus in three learning disabled children. *Am. J. Occup. Ther.*, 36:657–663.
755. Ottenbacher, K., Watson, J. P., and Short, M. A. (1979): Association between nystagmus hyporesponsivity and behavioral problems in learning disabled children. *Am. J. Occup. Ther.*, 33:317–322.
756. Ottenbacher, K., Watson, P. J., Short, M. A., and Biderman, M. D. (1979): Nystagmus and occular fixation difficulties in learning disabled children. *Am. J. Occup. Ther.*, 33:717–721.
757. Palmer, F., and Gatti, D. (1982): Transitional employment project. *Occup. Ther. Ment. Health*, 2(2):23–36.
758. Papalia, D., and Olds, S. (1975): *A Child's World: Infancy Through Adolescence*. McGraw-Hill, New York.
759. Parad, H., editor (1965): *Crisis Intervention: Selected Readings*. Family Service Association of Social Workers, Washington, D.C.
760. Park, G. (1968): The etiology of learning disabilities: an historical perspective. *J. Learn. Disabil.*, 1:313–330.
761. Parke, R. D. (1981): *Fathers*. Harvard University Press, Cambridge.
762. Parker, S. (1972): *The Future of Work and Leisure*. Praeger Publishers, New York.
763. Parmenter, C. L. (1975): The asymmetrical tonic neck reflex in normal first and third grade children. *Am. J. Occup. Ther.*, 29:463–468.
764. Parsons, T. (1951): *The Social System*. Free Press, Glencoe, N.Y.
765. Parsons, T. (1965): *Social Structure and Personality*. Free Press, Glencoe, N.Y.
766. Parsons, T., and Bales, R. F. (1955): *Family, Socialization and Interaction Process*. Free Press, Glencoe, N.Y.
767. Pasework, R., Hall, J., and Fitzgerald, B. (1969): Attitudes towards industrial therapy of mental hospital patients and staff. *Am. J. Occup. Ther.*, 23:244–248.
768. Paul, G. L., and Levitz, R. J. (1977): *Psychosocial Treatment of Chronic Mental Patients: Milieu versus Social Learning Programs*. Harvard University Press, Cambridge.
769. Paulson, C. P. (1980): Juvenile delinquency and occupational choice. *Am. J. Occup. Ther.*, 34:565–571.
770. Pearce, J., and Newton, S. (1963): *The Conditions of Human Growth*. Citadel Press, New York.
771. Petrie, A. (1967): *Individuality in Pain and Suffering*. University of Chicago Press, Chicago.
772. Pezzuti, L. (1979): An exploration of adolescent feminine and occupational behavior development. *Am. J. Occup. Ther.*, 33:84–91.
773. Piaget, J. (1952): *Play, Dreams and Imitation in Childhood*. Norton, New York.

774. Piaget, J. (1966): *The Origins of Intelligence in Children*. International Universities Press, New York.
775. Picard, H. B., and Magno, J. B. (1982): The role of occupational therapy in hospice care. *Am. J. Occup. Ther.*, 36:597–598.
776. Pi Lambda Theta (1966): *The Body of Knowledge Unique to the Profession of Education*. Pi Lambda Theta, Washington, D.C.
777. Pittinger, O. E., and Gooding, C. T. (1971): *Learning Theories in Educational Practice*. John Wiley and Sons, New York.
778. Plokker, J. H. (1964): *Art from the Mentally Disturbed*. Little Brown & Co., Boston.
779. Pochert, L. (1970): Our new role challenge: the occupational therapy consultant. *Am. J. Occup. Ther.*, 24:106–110.
780. Popper, K. P. (1972): *Objective Knowledge: An Evolutionary Approach*. Oxford University Press, London.
781. Posthuma, B. W., and Posthuma, A. B. (1972): The effect of small-group experience on occupational therapy students. *Am. J. Occup. Ther.*, 26:415–418.
782. Pratt, C. (1948): *The Logic of Modern Psychology.* Macmillan, New York.
783. Price, A. (1967): An early statement about occupational therapy. *Am. J. Occup. Ther.*, 21:281–282.
784. Price, A. (1977): Sensory integration in occupational therapy. *Am. J. Occup. Ther.*, 31:287–289.
785. Price, A. (1980): The issue—neurotherapy and specialization. *Am. J. Occup. Ther.*, 34:809–815.
786. Prior, J. A., and Silberstein, J. S. (1977): *Physical Diagnosis: The History and Examination of the Patient*. C. V. Mosby, St. Louis.
787. Professional Examination Service (1975): *Development of Occupational Therapy Proficiency.* PES, New York.
788. Professional Staff of the U.S.-U.K. Cross-National Project (1974): The diagnoses and psychopathology of schizophrenia in New York and London. *Schizophr. Bull.*, 2:80–102.
789. Punwar, A. (1982): Expanded normative data: Southern California Postrotory Nystagmus Test. *Am. J. Occup. Ther.*, 36:183–187.
790. Purteta, R. (1973): *The Allied Health Professional and the Patient*. W. B. Saunders, Philadelphia.
791. Rance, C., and Price, A. (1973): Poetry as a group project. *Am. J. Occup. Ther.*, 27:252–255.
792. Random House Dictionary of the English Language (1966): edited by J. Stein. Random House, New York.
793. Read, H. (1965): *Icon and Idea*. Schocker Books, New York.
794. Reed, K., and Sanderson, S. R. (1980): *Concepts of Occupational Therapy.* Williams and Wilkins, Baltimore.
795. Reed, S. C., Hartley, C., Anderson, V. E., Phillips, V. P., and Johnson, N. A. (1973): *The Psychoses: Family Studies*. W. B. Saunders, Philadelphia.
796. Reese, C. C. (1974): Forced treatment of the adolescent drug abuser. *Am. J. Occup. Ther.*, 28:540–544.
797. Regan, N. N. (1982): The implementation of occupational therapy services in the rural school system. *Am. J. Occup. Ther.*, 36:85–89.
798. Reilly, M. (1962): Occupational therapy can be one of the greatest ideas of 20th century medicine. *Am. J. Occup. Ther.*, 16:1–9.
799. Reilly, M. (1969): The educational process. *Am. J. Occup. Ther.*, 23:299–307.
800. Reilly, M. (1971): The modernization of occupational therapy. *Am. J. Occup. Ther.*, 25:243–246.
801. Reilly, M., editor (1974): *Play as Exploratory Learning*. Sage Publications, Beverly Hills.
802. Rerek, M. D. (1971): The depression years—1929 to 1941. *Am. J. Occup. Ther.*, 25:231–233.
803. Resman, M. H. (1981): Effect of sensory stimulation on eye contact in a profoundly retarded adult. *Am. J. Occup. Ther.*, 35:31–35.
804. Ricks, D., Thomas, A., and Roff, M. (1974): *Life History Research in Psychopathology* (Vol. 3). University of Minnesota, Minneapolis.
805. Rider, B. A. (1974): Abnormal postural reflexes in dysphasic children. *Am. J. Occup. Ther.*, 28:351–353.
806. Rider, B. A. (1978): Sensory motor treatment of chronic schizophrenics. *Am. J. Occup. Ther.*, 32:451–455.
807. Rider, B. B., and Gramblin, J. T. (1980): An activities approach to occupational therapy in a short-term acute mental health unit. *Mental Health Specialty Newsletter, AOTA*. Vol. 3, 4:1.
808. Rie, H., and Rie, E. (1980): *Handbook of Minimal Brain Dysfunction: A Critical View.* John Wiley and Sons, New York.
809. Riessman, F., Cohen, J., and Pearl, A. (1964): *Mental Health and the Poor*. Free Press, Glencoe, N.Y.
810. Ritzler, B. A., and Smith, M. (1976): The problem of diagnostic criteria in the study of paranoid subclassification of schizophrenia. *Schizophr. Bull.*, 2:209–217.
811. Roberts, K. (1978): *Contemporary Society and the Growth of Leisure*. Longman, London.
812. Robins, L. (1966): *Deviant Children Grow Up*. Williams and Wilkins, Baltimore.
813. Robinson, A. L. (1977): Play: the arena for acquisition of rules for competent behavior. *Am. J. Occup. Ther.*, 31:248–253.
814. Robmault, J. P. (1978): *Sex, Society and the Disabled*. Harper & Row Publishers, New York.
815. Rock, I. (1975): *An Introduction to Perception*. Macmillan, New York.
816. Roff, J. D., Knight, R., and Westheim, E. A. (1976): A factor analysis study of childhood symptoms antecedent to schizophrenia. *J. Abnorm. Psychol.*, 85:543–549.
817. Rogers, C. R. (1951): *Client-Centered Therapy.* Houghton Mifflin Company, Boston.
818. Rogers, C. R. (1961): *On Becoming a Person*. Houghton Mifflin Company, Boston.
819. Rogers, J. C. (1981): Gerontic occupational therapy. *Am. J. Occup. Ther.*, 35:663–666.
820. Rogers, J. C. (1982): Order and disorder in medicine and occupational therapy. *Am. J. Occup. Ther.*, 36:29–35.
821. Rogers, J. C. (1982): Sponsorship: developing leaders for occupational therapy. *Am. J. Occup. Ther.*, 36:309–313.
822. Rogers, J. C., and Figone, J. J. (1978): The avocational pursuits of rehabilitants and traumatic quadriplegia. *Am. J. Occup. Ther.*, 32:571–576.
823. Rogers, J. C., and Figone, J. J. (1979): Psychosocial pa-

rameters in treating the person with quadriplegia. *Am. J. Occup. Ther.*, 33:432–439.

824. Romano, J., editor (1967): *The Origins of Schizophrenia*. Excerpta Medica Foundation, New York.
825. Rood, M. S. (1958): Everyone counts. *Am. J. Occup. Ther.*, 12:326–329.
826. Rose, A. M., editor (1962): *Human Behavior and Social Processes*. Houghton Mifflin Company, Boston.
827. Rosen, G. (1975): *Preventive Medicine in the United States—1900–1975*. Science History Publications, New York.
828. Rosenberg, C. E., editor (1979): *Healing and History*. Dawson, Science History Publications, New York.
829. Rosenberg, S., editor (1977): *Sentence Production: Developments in Theory and Research*. Erlbaum, New York.
830. Rosenfeld, M. S. (1982): A model of activity intervention in disaster-stricken communities. *Am. J. Occup. Ther.*, 36:229–236.
831. Rosenfeld, M. S. (1982): Nuclear task approach: a unified system for teaching crisis intervention methods to occupational therapy students. Paper presented to the Commission on Education, American Occupational Therapy Association Conference, Philadelphia.
832. Rosenthal, D., and Kety, S. S., editors (1968): *The Transmission of Schizophrenia*. Pergamon Press, New York.
833. Rosenthal, R., and Rosnow, R. L., editors (1969): *Artifacts in Behavioral Research*. Academic Press, New York.
834. Rosenthal, S. (1977): Searchers for the mode of genetic transmission in schizophrenia: reflections and loose ends. *Schizophr. Bull.*, 3:268–276.
835. Ross, H. (1976): *Psychological Aspects of Learning Disabilities*. McGraw-Hill, New York.
836. Royeen, C. B. (1980): Factors affecting test-retest reliability of the Southern California Postrotory Nystagmus Test. *Am. J. Occup. Ther.*, 34:37–39.
837. Rozycha, M. (1978): Human sexuality. In: *Willard and Spackman's Occupational Therapy*, edited by H. L. Hopkins and H. D. Smith. J. Lippincott, Philadelphia.
838. Rubenstein, R., and Lasswell, H. (1966): *The Sharing of Power in a Psychiatric Hospital*. Yale University Press, New Haven.
839. Rubins, J. L. (1967): Self-awareness and body image, self-concept and identity. In: *The Ego*, edited by J. M. Mosserman. Grune and Stratton, New York.
840. Ruch, F. (1963): *Psychology and Life*. Scott, Foresman and Company, Chicago.
841. Ruesch, J. (1963): *Disturbed Communication*. W. W. Norton & Co., New York.
842. Ruesch, J. (1973): *Therapeutic Communication*. W. W. Norton & Co., New York.
843. Rugh, R., et al. (1971): *From Conception to Birth: The Drama of Life's Beginnings*. Harper & Row Publishers, New York.
844. Runes, D. D. (1962): *Living Schools of Philosophy*. Littlefield, Adams and Company, Paterson.
845. Rutter, M. (1975): *Helping Troubled Children*. Penguin Books, New York.
846. Saffir, J. S. (1978): The theoretical implications of chlorpromazine as a sensory integrative theory. *Am. J. Occup. Ther.*, 32:460–466.
847. Safifios-Rothschild, C. (1970): *The Sociology and Social Psychology of Disability and Rehabilitation*. Random House, New York.
848. Sahakian, W. S. (1968): *Outline: History of Philosophy*. Barnes & Noble, New York.
849. Salpino, A. O. (1979): Thanatology. In: *Preventing Physical and Mental Disabilities*, edited by P. J. Valletutti and F. Christopher. University Park Press, Baltimore.
850. Samson, E. E., and Marthas, M. S. (1977): *Group Process for the Health Professions*. John Wiley and Sons, New York.
851. Sanders, D. H. (1972): Innovative environments in the community: a life for the chronic patient. *Schizophr. Bull.*, 1:49–59.
852. Sargent, W., and Slater, E. (1972): *An Introduction to Physical Methods of Treatment in Psychiatry*. Science House, New York.
853. Saunders, C. (1959): *Care of the Dying*. Macmillan, New York.
854. Saxton, L. (1980): *The Individual, Marriage, and the Family*. Wadsworth Publishing, Belmont, Ca.
855. Scanzoni, J. (1978): *Sex Roles, Woman's Work, and Marital Conflict*. Lexington Books, Lexington, Ma.
856. Scardina, V. (1981): From pegboards to integration. *Am. J. Occup. Ther.*, 35:581–589.
857. Scarry, R. (1968): *What People Do All Day*. Random House, New York.
858. Schechter, L. (1974): Occupational therapy in a psychiatric day hospital. *Am. J. Occup. Ther.*, 28:151–153.
859. Scheff, T. J. (1966): *Being Mentally Ill: A Sociological Theory*. Aldine Publishing Company, Chicago.
860. Scheflin, A. (1973): *Body Language and Social Order: Communication as Behavioral Control*. Prentice-Hall, Englewood Cliffs.
861. Schein, E. H. (1972): *Professional Education*. McGraw-Hill, New York.
862. Schilder, P. (1950): *The Image and Appearance of the Human Body*. John Wiley and Sons, New York.
863. Schlesinger, B. (1975): *The One Parent Family: Perspectives and Annotated Bibliography*. University of Toronto Press, Buffalo.
864. Schneck, J. M. (1960): *A History of Psychiatry*. Charles C Thomas Publishing, Springfield.
865. Schontz, F. (1975): *The Psychological Aspects of Physical Illness and Disability*. Macmillan, New York.
866. Schulman, E. D. (1974): *Intervention in Human Services*. C. V. Mosby, St. Louis.
867. Schulman, J. (1964): *The Structure and Fate of Innovations in an Elite Psychiatric Hospital*. (Unpublished Dissertation) Columbia University.
868. Schulz, D. A. (1976): *The Changing Family: Its Function and Future*. Prentice-Hall, Englewood Cliffs.
869. Schwartz, C. C., and Myers, J. K. (1977): Life events and schizophrenia: I. comparison of schizophrenics with a community sample. *Arch. Gen. Psychiatry*, 31:557–560.
870. Schwartz, S., editor (1978): *Language and Cognition in Schizophrenia*. Erlbaum, Hillsdale, N.J.
871. Scott, A. H., and Neuhaus, B. E. (1981): Documentation and clinical research. In: *Physical Disabilities Manual*, edited by B. C. Abreu. Raven Press, New York.

872. Scott, D. (1970): *The Psychology of Work*. Gerald Duckworth and Company, London.
873. Searles, H. F. (1960): *The Nonhuman Environment*. International Universitites Press, New York.
874. Sebelist, R. M. (1978): Mental retardation. In: *Willard and Spackman's Occupational Therapy*, edited by H. L. Hopkins and H. D. Smith. J. B. Lippincott, Philadelphia.
875. Sechehaye, M. (1951): *Symbolic Realization*. International Universities Press, New York.
876. Sechehaye, M. (1956): *A New Psychotherapy in Schizophrenia*. Grunc and Stratton, New York.
877. Selltiz, C., Wrightsman, L. S., and Cook, S. W. (1976): *Research Methods in Social Relations*. Holt, Rinehart & Winston, New York.
878. Semmler, C., and Semmler, M. (1974): Counseling the coronary patient. *Am. J. Occup. Ther.*, 28:609–614.
879. Shaevitz, M. H., and Shaevitz, M. H. (1980): *Making It Together as a Two-Career Couple*. Houghton Mifflin Company, Boston.
880. Shafer, A. L. (1971): Providing support systems for the elderly. *Am. J. Occup. Ther.*, 25:423–427.
881. Shaffer, J. B., and Galinsky, M. D., editors (1974): *Models of Group Therapy and Sensitivity Training*. Prentice-Hall, Englewood Cliffs.
882. Shannon, P. D. (1970): Work adjustment and the adolescent soldier. *Am. J. Occup. Ther.*, 24:111–115.
883. Shannon, P. D. (1972): Work-play theory and the occupational therapy process. *Am. J. Occup. Ther.*, 26:169–172.
884. Shannon, P. D. (1974): Occupational choice: decision-making play. In: *Play as Exploratory Learning*, edited by M. Reilly. Sage Publications, Beverly Hills.
885. Shannon, P. D. (1977): The derailment of occupational therapy. *Am. J. Occup. Ther.*, 31:229–234.
886. Shapiro, D. (1981): Laws, motivation and activity. In: *Bereavement of Physical Disability: Recommitment to Life, Health and Function*, edited by J. Downey, G. Reidel, and A. Kutscher. Arno Press, New York.
887. Shaw, C. (1982): The interview process. In: *The Evaluation Process in Psychiatric Occupational Therapy*, edited by B. J. Hemphill. Charles B. Slack, Thorofare, NJ.
888. Sheehy, G. (1976): *Passages: Predictable Crises of Adult Life*. E. P. Dutton and Company, New York.
889. Sheridan, C. L. (1971): *Fundamentals of Experimental Psychology*. Holt, Rinehart & Winston, New York.
890. Shorres, E. (1981): *Politics of Middle Management*. Anchor Press, Garden City, NY.
891. Shorter, E. (1975): *The Making of the Modern Family*. Basic Books, New York.
892. Shryock, R. H. (1947): *The Development of Modern Medicine*. Alfred A. Knopf, New York.
893. Shuff, F. L., and Kramer, J. (1971): Organizational concepts, part I: components of administration. *Am. J. Occup. Ther.*, 25:360–363.
894. Shuff, F. L., and Kramer, J. (1971): Organizational concepts, part II: communication. *Am. J. Occup. Ther.*, 25:428–431.
895. Sidman, J. M. (1977): Sexual function of the physically disabled adult. *Am. J. Occup. Ther.*, 31:81–85.
896. Sieg, K. (1974): Applying the behavioral model to the O.T. model. *Am. J. Occup. Ther.*, 28:421–428.
897. Sieg, K. W. (1977): The nursing home: occupational therapy services in an institution. *Am. J. Occup. Ther.*, 31:516–524.
898. Silberzahn, M. (1975): Sensory integrative dysfunction in a child guidance clinic population. *Am. J. Occup. Ther.*, 29:28–34.
899. Siller, J. (1968): *Studies in Reaction to Disabilities*. New York University Press, New York.
900. Simon, J. I. (1971): Emotional aspects of physical disabilities. *Am. J. Occup. Ther.*, 25:408–410.
901. Simon, J. L. (1978): *Basic Research in Social Sciences*. Random House, New York.
902. Singer, D. G., and Singer, J. L. (1977): *Partners in Play*. Harper & Row Publishers, New York.
903. Skinner, B. F. (1953): *Science and Human Behavior*. Macmillan, New York.
904. Slagle, E. C. (1922): *Training Aides for Mental Patients: Paper on Occupational Therapy*. State Hospital Press, Utica.
905. Slagle, E. C. (1924): A year's development of occupational therapy in New York State hospitals. *Mod. Hosp.*, 22:1.
906. Slagle, E. C. (1934): Occupational therapy: recent methods and advances in the United States. *Occup. Ther. Rehab.*, 13:5.
907. Slagle, E. C., and Robeson, H. A. (1933): *Syllabus for Training of Nurses in Occupational Therapy*. State Hospital Press, Utica.
908. Slavson, S. R. (1952): *Introduction to Group Psychotherapy*. International Universities Press, New York.
909. Slobitz, F. W. (1970): The role of occupational therapy in heroin detoxification. *Am. J. Occup. Ther.*, 24:340–346.
910. Smiley, C. W. (1975): Playgrounds for the mentally retarded. *Am. J. Occup. Ther.*, 28:474–477.
911. Smith, D. A. (1981): Effects of psychotropic drugs on the occupational therapy process. *Mental Health Specialty Section Newsletter, AOTA*. Vol. 4, 1:1.
912. Smith, D. W., and Bierman, E. L. (1973): *The Biological Ages of Man: From Conception Through Old Age*. W. B. Saunders, Philadelphia.
913. Smith D. W., and Marshall, R. E., editors (1972): *Introduction to Clinical Pediatrics*. W. B. Saunders, Philadelphia.
914. Smith, E. J. (1973): The employment and functioning of the homebound disabled in information technology. *Am. J. Occup. Ther.*, 27:232–238.
915. Smith, H. D. (1978): Specific evaluation procedures. In: *Willard and Spackman's Occupational Therapy*, edited by H. S. Hopkins and H. D. Smith. J. B. Lippincott, Philadelphia.
916. Smith, H. D., and Tiffany, E. C. (1978): Assessment and evaluation: evaluation overview. In: *Willard and Spackman's Occupational Therapy*, edited by H. S. Hopkins and H. D. Smith. J. B. Lippincott, Philadelphia.
917. Snelbecher, G. E. (1974): *Learning Theory, Instructional Theory and Psycho-educational Design*. McGraw-Hill, New York.
918. Snyder, S. H., Banerjec, S. P., Yamamura, H. T., and Greenberg, D. (1974): Drugs, neurotransmitters and schizophrenia. *Science*, 184:1243–1253.
919. Solkoff, N., and Maturzak, D. (1975): Tactile stimulation

and behavioral development among low birthweight infants. *Child Psychiatry Hum. Dev.*, 6:33–37.

920. Spackman, C. S. (1968): A history of the practice of occupational therapy for restoration of physical dysfunction: 1917–1967. *Am. J. Occup. Ther.*, 22:67–71.
921. Spelbring, L. M. (1976): Nationally speaking: outcome measures in occupational therapy . . . the quality assurance method of choice? *Am. J. Occup. Ther.*, 30:539–540.
922. Sperry, R. W. (1964): The great cerebral commissure. *Sci. Am.*, 1:42–52.
923. Spitz, R. (1965): *The First Year of Life*. International Universities Press, New York.
924. Spitzer, R. L., and Klein, D. F., editors (1976): *Evaluation of Psychological Therapies*. Johns Hopkins University Press, Baltimore.
925. Srole, L., Langner, T. S., Michael, S. T., Opler, M. K., and Rennie, T. A. C. (1962): *Mental Health in the Metropolis: The Midtown Manhattan Study*. McGraw-Hill, New York.
926. Stanton, A. H., and Schwartz, M. S. (1954): *The Mental Hospital*. Basic Books, New York.
927. Stein, F. (1972): Community rehabilitation of disadvantaged youth. *Am. J. Occup. Ther.*, 26:277–283.
928. Stein, M. R., Vidick, A. J., and White, D. M., editors (1960): *Identity and Anxiety*. Free Press, Glencoe, N.Y.
929. Stephens, L. C. (1973): Introducing a stroke service in a general hospital setting. *Am. J. Occup. Ther.*, 29:418–422.
930. Stilwell, J. M. (1981): Relationship between development of body righting reaction and normal midline crossing behavior in the learning disabled. *Am. J. Occup. Ther.*, 35:391–398.
931. Stilwell, J. M., Crowe, T. K., and McCallum, L. W. (1978): Postrotory nystagmus duration as a function of communication disorders. *Am. J. Occup. Ther.*, 32:222–228.
932. Stogdell, R. J. (1974): *Handbook of Leadership: A Survey of Theory and Research*. Free Press, Glencoe, N.Y.
933. Stonequist, E. V. (1937): *The Marginal Man*. Charles Scribner's Sons, New York.
934. Strauss, A., and Lehtinen, L. (1947): *Pathology and Education of the Brain-Injured Child*. Grune and Stratton, New York.
935. Strauss, A. L. (1975): *Chronic Illness and the Quality of Life*. C. V. Mosby, St. Louis.
936. Strauss, M. E. (1973): Behavioral difference between acute and chronic schizophrenics: course of psychoses, effects of institutionalization or sampling bias. *Psychol. Bull.*, 79:468–473.
937. Strub, R. L., and Black, W. F. (1977): *The Mental Status Examination in Neurology*. F. A. Davis, Philadelphia.
938. Sullivan, H. S. (1953): *The Interpersonal Theory of Psychiatry*. W. W. Norton & Co., New York.
939. Super, D. E. (1957): *The Psychology of Careers*. Harper & Row Publishers, New York.
940. Susser, M. W. (1971): *Sociology in Medicine*. Oxford University Press, London.
941. Sutherland, J. W. (1973): *A General Systems Philosophy for the Social and Behavioral Sciences*. George Braziller, New York.
942. Swartz, M. J., and Jordan, D. K. (1980): *The New Anthropological Perspective*. John Wiley and Sons, New York.
943. Szalai, A., editor (1972): *The Use of Time: Daily Activities of Urban and Suburban Populations in Twelve Countries*. Mouton, The Hague.
944. Takata, N. (1969): The play history. *Am. J. Occup. Ther.*, 23:314–318.
945. Takata, N. (1971): The play milieu: a preliminary appraisal. *Am. J. Occup. Ther.*, 25:281–284.
946. Takata, N. (1974): Play as a prescription. In: *Play as Exploratory Learning*, edited by M. Reilly. Sage Publications, Beverly Hills.
947. Talbot, N. R. (1979): *Raising Children in Modern America*. Little, Brown & Co., Boston.
948. Tempon, V., and Smith, A. (1968): Psychiatric occupational therapy within a learning theory context. *Am. J. Occup. Ther.*, 22:415–425.
949. Terkel, S. (1972): *Working: People Talk About What They Do All Day and How They Feel About What They Do*. Pantheon Books, New York.
950. Thayer, J., and Silber, D. E. (1971): Relationship between levels of arousal and responsiveness among schizophrenics and normal subjects. *J. Abnorm. Psychol.*, 77:162–173.
951. Thibaut, J. W., and Kelley, H. H. (1959): *The Social Psychology of Groups*. John Wiley and Sons, New York.
952. Thompson, L. (1971): Language disabilities in men of eminence. *J. Learn. Disabil.*, 4:34–45.
953. Thralow, J. V., and Watson, C. G. (1974): Remotivating geriatric patients using elementary school children. *Am. J. Occup. Ther.*, 28:469–473.
954. Tickle, L. S., and Yerxa, E. J. (1981): Need satisfaction of older persons living in the community and in institutions, part 1. The environment. *Am. J. Occup. Ther.*, 35:644–649.
955. Tickle, L. S., and Yerxa, E. J. (1981): Need satisfaction of elderly persons living in the community and in institutions, part 2. Role of activity. *Am. J. Occup. Ther.*, 35:650–655.
956. Tiffany, E. G. (1978): Psychiatry and mental health. In: *Willard and Spackman's Occupational Therapy*, edited by H. Hopkins and H. Smith. J. B. Lippincott, Philadelphia.
957. Torjesen, H. (1979): *The House-Husband's World*. The Garden, Eden Prairie, MN.
958. Torrey, E. F. (1974): *The Death of Psychiatry*. Chilton, Radnor, Pa.
959. Towle, C. (1954): *The Learner in Education for the Professions*. University of Chicago Press, Chicago.
960. Trombly, C. A., and Scott, A. D. (1977): *Occupational Therapy for Physical Dysfunction*. Williams and Wilkins, Baltimore.
961. Truex, C. R., and Carpenter, M. B. (1969): *Human Neuroanatomy*. Williams and Wilkins, Baltimore.
962. Tuke, D. H. (1892): *Reform in the Treatment of the Insane: An Early History of the Retreat, York; It's Objectives and Influences*. J. and A. Churchill, London.
963. Tumin, M. M. (1967): *Social Stratification*. Prentice-Hall, Englewood-Cliffs.
964. Turgang, N. T., and Yerxa, E. J. (1979): Expectations of teachers for physically handicapped and normal first grade students. *Am. J. Occup. Ther.*, 33:697–703.

965. Turnbull, A., and Schulz, J. (1979): *Mainstreaming Handicapped Children: A Guide for the Classroom Teacher*. Allyn and Bacon, Boston.
966. Turnbull, A. P., and Turnbull, H. R., III (1979): *Parents Speak Out: Growing with a Handicapped Child*. Charles E. Merrill, Columbus.
967. Tyler, N. B., and Kogan, K. L. (1977): The reduction of stress between mothers and their handicapped children. *Am. J. Occup. Ther.*, 31:151–155.
968. Tyler, N. B., Kogan, K. L., and Turner, P. (1974): Interpersonal components of therapy with young cerebral palsied. *Am. J. Occup. Ther.*, 28:395–400.
969. Ullmann, L. P., and Krasner, L., editors (1965): *Case Studies in Behavioral Modification*. Holt, Rinehart & Winston, New York.
970. U.S. Office of Education (1976): Education of handicapped children: assistance to states; proposed rule-making. *Federal Register* 41, Washington, D.C.
971. U.S. Office of Education (1977): Education of handicapped children. Implementation of part B of the education of the handicapped act. *Federal Register*, Part II. U.S. Department of Health, Education and Welfare, Washington, D.C.
972. U.S. Office of Education (1977): Education of handicapped children. assistance to states; procedures for evaluating specific learning disabilities. *Federal Register*, Part III. Department of Health, Education and Welfare. Washington, D.C.
973. U.S. Office of Education (1979): *Progress Towards a Free, Appropriate Education: A Report to Congress on the Implementation of PL94-142, The Education for All Handicapped Children Act*. Department of Health, Education and Welfare, Washington, D.C.
974. Vacher, C. D., and Stratas, N. E. (1976): *Consultation—Education: Development and Validation*. Human Services Press, New York.
975. Valletutti, P. J., and Christopher, F., editors (1979): *Preventing Physical and Mental Disabilities: Multidisciplinary Approaches*. University Park Press, Baltimore.
976. Van Benschoten, R. (1975): A sensory integration program for blind campers. *Am. J. Occup. Ther.*, 29:620–624.
977. Vandenberg, B., and Kielhofner, G. (1982): Play in evolution, culture and individual application: implications for therapy. *Am. J. Occup. Ther.*, 36:20–28.
978. Van Praag, H. M. (1977): The significance of dopamine for the mode of action of neuroleptics and the pathogenesis of schizophrenia. *Br. J. Psychiatry*, 130:463–474.
979. Vargo, J. W. (1978): Some psychological effects of physical disabilities. *Am. J. Occup. Ther.*, 32:31–34.
980. Vellutino, F. R., Stiger, B. M., Moyer, S. C., Harding, C. J., and Niles, J. A. (1977): Has the perceptual deficit hypothesis led us astray? *J. Learn. Disabil.*, 10:375–384.
981. Versluys, H. (1977): Psychological adjustment to physical disabilities. In: *Occupational Therapy for Physical Dysfunction*, edited by C. A. Trombly and A. D. Scott. Williams and Wilkins, Baltimore.
982. Versluys, H. P. (1980): The remediation of role disorders through focused group work. *Am. J. Occup. Ther.*, 34:609–614.
983. von Bartalonfly, L. (1968): *General Systems Theory: Foundations, Development, Application*. George Braziller, New York.
984. von Bartalonfly, L. (1968): General systems theory: a critical review. In: *Modern Systems Research for the Behavioral Scientist*, edited by W. Buckly. Aldine Publishing Company, Chicago.
985. Vygotsky, L. S. (1962): *Thought and Language*. M.I.T. Press, Cambridge.
986. Wade, B. (1947): Occupational therapy for patients with mental diseases. In: *Principles of Occupational Therapy*, edited by H. S. Willard and C. S. Spackman. J. B. Lippincott Co., Philadelphia.
987. Wain, H. (1970): *A History of Preventive Medicine*. Charles C Thomas Publishing, Springfield.
988. Walizer, M. H., and Wienir, P. L. (1978): *Research Methods and Analysis: Searching for Relationships*. Harper & Row Publishers, New York.
989. Walker, L. (1971): Occupational therapy in the well community. *Am. J. Occup. Ther.*, 25:345–347.
990. Wanderer, Z. W. (1974): Therapy as learning: behavior therapy. *Am. J. Occup. Ther.*, 28:207–208.
991. Ward, R. (1971): Review of research related to work activities for aged residents of long-term care facilities. *Am. J. Occup. Ther.*, 25:348–351.
992. Warren, H. H. (1974): Self-perception of independence among urban elderly. *Am. J. Occup. Ther.*, 28:329–336.
993. Wataonabe, S. A. (1967): The developing role of occupational therapy in psychiatric home service. *Am. J. Occup. Ther.*, 21:353–356.
994. Wataonabe, S. (1968): The activities configuration. In: *Materials from the 1968 Regional Institutes Sponsored by the American Occupational Therapy Association*, edited by J. Mazer. AOTA, Rockville, Md.
995. Wataonabe, S. (1968): Four concepts basic to the occupational therapy process. *Am. J. Occup. Ther.*, 22:439–450.
996. Watzlawick, P., Beaven, J., and Jackson, D. (1967): *Pragmatics of Human Communications: A Study of Interactional Patterns, Pathologies, and Paradoxes*. W. W. Norton & Co., New York.
997. Webb, L. (1973): The therapeutic social club. *Am. J. Occup. Ther.*, 27:81–84.
998. Weber, J. W. (1978): Chaining strategies for teaching sequential motor tasks to mentally retarded adults. *Am. J. Occup. Ther.*, 32:385–389.
999. Webster, P. S. (1980): Occupational role development in the young adult with mild mental retardation. *Am. J. Occup. Ther.*, 34:13–18.
1000. Weed, L. L. (1970): *Medical Research, Medical Education and Patient Care*. Year Book Medical Publications, Chicago.
1001. Weeks, Z. R. (1979): Effects of the vestibular system on human development, part 2: effects of vestibular stimulation on mentally retarded, emotionally disturbed and learning disabled individuals. *Am. J. Occup. Ther.*, 33:450–457.
1002. Wehman, P., and Abramson, M. (1976): Three theoretical approaches to play: application for exceptional children. *Am. J. Occup. Ther.*, 30:551–559.

1003. Weidiger, P. (1976): *Menstruation and Menopause*. Alfred A. Knopf, New York.
1004. Weller, J. (1966): *Yesterday's People*. University of Kentucky Press, Lexington.
1005. Welles, C. A. (1976): Ethics in conflict: yesterday's standards—outdated guide for tomorrow. *Am. J. Occup. Ther.*, 30:44–47.
1006. Werner, V., Maddigan, R. F., and Watson, C. G. (1969): A study of two treatment programs for chronically mentally ill patients in occupational therapy. *Am. J. Occup. Ther.*, 23:132–136.
1007. West, W. L., editor (1959): *Changing Concepts and Practices in Psychiatric Occupational Therapy.* American Occupational Therapy Association, New York.
1008. West, W. L. (1968): Professional responsibilities in times of change. *Am. J. Occup. Ther.*, 22:9–15.
1009. West, W. L. (1969): The growing importance of prevention. *Am. J. Occup. Ther.*, 23:226–231.
1010. West, W. L. (1976): Problems and policies in the licensure of occupational therapists. *Am. J. Occup. Ther.*, 30:40–43.
1011. West, W. L. (1979): Historical perspectives. In: *Occupational Therapy: 2001 A.D.*, edited by American Occupational Therapy Association, Rockville, Md.
1012. West, W. L. (1982): In memoriam—Winifred Conrick Kahmann. *Am. J. Occup. Ther.*, 36:472–475.
1013. Whitaker, D. S., and Lieberman, M. A. (1964): *Psychotherapy through the Group Process*. Atherton Press, New York.
1014. White, R. (1967): Motivation reconsidered: the concept of competence. In: *Sourcebook in Abnormal Psychology*, edited by L. Rabkin and J. Carr. Houghton Mifflin Company, Boston.
1015. White, R. (1967): Competence and the growth of personality. In: *The Ego*, edited by J. M. Massiman. Grune and Stratton, New York.
1016. White, R. (1971): The urge towards competence. *Am. J. Occup. Ther.*, 25:271–274.
1017. Whitely, J. S., and Gordon, J. (1979): *Group Approaches in Psychiatry.* Routledge and Kegan Paul, London.
1018. Whitley, S. B., Brancomb, B. V., and Moreno, H. (1979): Identification and management of environmental problems of children with cancer. *Am. J. Occup. Ther.*, 33:711–716.
1019. Whyman, P., and Marchant, J. A. (1978): Improving free play skills of severely retarded children. *Am. J. Occup. Ther.*, 32:100–104.
1020. Whyte, W. F. (1943): *Street Corner Society: The Social Structure of an Italian Slum*. University of Chicago Press, Chicago.
1021. Wickelgren, W. (1977): *Learning and Memory.* Prentice-Hall, Englewood Cliffs.
1022. Wiederholt, J. L. (1974): Historical perspectives in the education of the learning disabled. In: *The Second Review of Special Education*, edited by L. Mann and D. Sabatino. Journal of Special Education Press, Philadelphia.
1023. Weiderholt, J., Hammill, D., and Brown, V. (1978): *The Resource Teacher.* Allyn and Bacon, Boston.
1024. Wiemer, R. B. (1972): Some concepts of prevention as an aspect of community health. *Am. J. Occup. Ther.*, 26:1–9.
1025. Williams, R., and Benes, N. (1976): Program II. The day hospital at the Burke rehabilitation center. *Am. J. Occup. Ther.*, 30:293.
1026. Williamson, G. G. (1981): Pediatric overview. In: *Physical Disabilities Manual*, edited by B. C. Abreu. Raven Press, New York.
1027. Williamson, M. (1961): *Supervision: New Patterns and Processes.* Association Press, New York.
1028. Wilson, M. A. (1977): A competency assurance program. *Am. J. Occup. Ther.*, 31:573–579.
1029. Winch, R. F., and Spanier, G. B., editors (1974): *Selected Studies in Marriage and the Family.* Holt, Rinehart & Winston, New York.
1030. Wing, J. K., and Brown, G. W. (1970): *Institutionalism and Schizophrenia*. Cambridge University Press, London.
1031. Winston, E. B. (1981): An older population: meeting major needs through occupational therapy. *Am. J. Occup. Ther.*, 35:635–637.
1032. Winston, E. I. (1976): Motivation for licensure. *Am. J. Occup. Ther.*, 30:27–31.
1033. Winters, E. E., editor (1957): *Collected Papers of Adolf Meyer.* Johns Hopkins Press, Baltimore.
1034. Wisconsin Occupational Therapy Association (1963): *Proceedings of the Wisconsin Council Workshops on Student Supervision and Counseling*. Wisconsin Occupational Therapy Association, Milwaukee.
1035. Wold-Tortelli, N., Chioteli, S., and Miron-Bernstein, S. (1981): Adult perceptual motor evaluation and management. In: *Physical Disabilities Manual*, edited by B. C. Abreu. Raven Press, New York.
1036. Wollmer, H., and Mills, D., editors (1966): *Professionalism*. Prentice-Hall, Englewood Cliffs.
1037. Wolpe, J., and Lazarus, A. A. (1966): *Behavior Therapy.* Pergamon Press, New York.
1038. Wong, B. (1979): The role of theory in learning disabilities, part I: analysis of problems. *J. Learn. Disabil.*, 12:585–595.
1039. Wong, B. (1979): The role of theory in learning disabilities, part II: a selective review of current conceptual frameworks in learning disabilities and/or reading disability. *J. Learn. Disabil.*, 12:649–658.
1040. Woodside, H. H. (1971): The development of occupational therapy—1910 to 1929. *Am. J. Occup. Ther.*, 25:226–230.
1041. Wright, B. A. (1960): *Physical Disabilities—A Psychological Approach*. Harper & Row Publishers, New York.
1042. Wynne, L. C., Cromwell, R. L., and Matthysse, S., editors (1978): *The Nature of Schizophrenia*. John Wiley and Sons, New York.
1043. Yalom, I. D. (1975): *Theory and Practice of Group Psychotherapy.* Basic Books, New York.
1044. Yarrow, M. R., Campbell, J. D., and Barton, R. V. (1970): Recollections of childhood: a study of the retrospective method. *Monographs of the Society for Research in Child Development* 35.
1045. Yerxa, E. J. (1979): The philosophical base of occupational therapy. In: *Occupational Therapy: 2001 A.D.*,

edited by American Occupational Therapy Association, Rockville, MD.

1046. Yerxa, E. J. (1982): A response to testing and measurement in occupational therapy: a review of current practice with special emphasis on the Southern California Sensory Integration Tests. *Am. J. Occup. Ther.*, 36:399–404.

1047. Ysseldyke, J. (1977): *Assessing the Learning Disabled Youngster: The State of the Art.* Research Report No. 1. Institute for Research on Learning Disabilities, University of Minnesota.

1048. Zaltman, G., Duncan, R., and Holbek, J. (1973): *Innovations and Organizations.* John Wiley and Sons, New York.

1049. Zander, A. (1971): *Motives and Goals in Groups.* Academic Press, New York.

1050. Zborowski, M. (1969): *People in Pain.* Jossey-Bass Publishers, San Francisco.

1051. Zilboorg, G. (1941): *A History of Medical Psychology.* W. W. Norton & Co., New York.

1052. Zinkus, P. W., Gottlieb, M. S., and Zinkus, C. B. (1979): The learning disabled juvenile delinquent: a case for early intervention of perceptually handicapped children. *Am. J. Occup. Ther.*, 33:180–184.

1053. Zisserman, L. (1978): Sex of a parent and knowledge about cerebral palsy. *Am. J. Occup. Ther.*, 32:500–504.

1054. Zisserman, L. (1981): The modern family and rehabilitation of the handicapped: a macrosociological view. *Am. J. Occup. Ther.*, 35:13–20.

1055. Ziviani, J., Paulsen, A., and O'Brien, A. (1982): Correlation of the Bruininks-Oseretsky Test of Motor Proficiency with the Southern California Sensory Integration Tests. *Am. J. Occup. Ther.*, 36:519–524.

1056. Zubin, J., and Freyhen, F. A., editors (1968): *Social Psychiatry.* Grune and Stratton, New York.

Index

Page numbers in italic indicate tables.